Muller & Kirk's

SMALL ANIMAL
DERMATOLOGY

DANNY W. SCOTT, D.V.M.

Professor of Medicine
College of Veterinary Medicine
Cornell University
Ithaca, New York

WILLIAM H. MILLER, JR., V.M.D.

Associate Professor of Medicine
College of Veterinary Medicine
Cornell University
Ithaca, New York

CRAIG E. GRIFFIN, D.V.M.

Animal Dermatology Clinic
San Diego, California

Muller & Kirk's
SMALL ANIMAL
DERMATOLOGY

5 TH
EDITION

W.B. SAUNDERS COMPANY
A Division of Harcourt Brace & Company

Philadelphia   London   Toronto   Montreal   Sydney   Tokyo

W.B. SAUNDERS COMPANY
A Division of
Harcourt Brace & Company

The Curtis Center
Independence Square West
Philadelphia, Pennsylvania 19106

Library of Congress Cataloging-in-Publication Data

Muller, George H.

[Small animal dermatology]

Muller and Kirk's small animal dermatology. — 5th ed. / Danny W. Scott, William H. Miller, Jr., Craig E. Griffin.

p.   cm.

Includes bibliographical references and index.

ISBN 0–7216–4850–9

1. Dogs—Diseases.   2. Cats—Diseases.   3. Veterinary dermatology.   4. Pets—Diseases.   I. Kirk, Robert Warren. II. Scott, Danny W.   III. Miller, William H. (William Howard). IV. Griffin, Craig E.   V. Title.   VI. Title: Small animal dermatology.

SF992.S55M85 1995 636.089′65—dc20

DNLM/DLC   94-4949

Muller and Kirk's Small Animal Dermatology, 5th Edition   ISBN 0–7216–4850–9

Last digit is the print number: 9   8   7   6   5   4   3

In the preface to the first edition of *Small Animal Dermatology* in 1969, Drs. Muller and Kirk wrote

This textbook of small animal dermatology is designed for students and clinicians. The authors have attempted to present a complete discussion of the entire subject in one volume. The book covers basic science, clinical aspects, and therapeutic methods in a manner designed primarily for those who struggle daily with clinical dermatologic problems.

These words launched the career of one of the most enduring and successful textbooks in the history of veterinary medicine. *Small Animal Dermatology* was the brain child, the blood, sweat, and tears, the labor of love, of Drs. George H. Muller and Robert W. Kirk. As their dermatologic legacy enters its fifth edition in 1995, we dedicate the finished product to George and Bob.

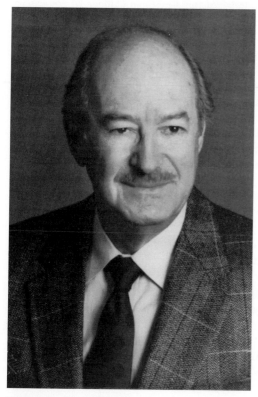

GEORGE H. MULLER

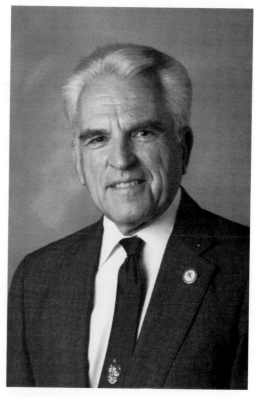

ROBERT W. KIRK

GEORGE H. MULLER

Dr. George Muller attended Washington State University and Texas A & M University (D.V.M. in 1943). During World War II he served as Captain in the United States Army in the China, Burma, and India theater (1943 to 1946) and received the China War Memorial Medal.

While in small animal practice, Dr. Muller realized how little was known about skin diseases of dogs and cats, even though dermatologic disorders constituted over 25 per cent of small animal practice. So in 1958, he decided to learn more about dermatology and, under the tutelage of Eugene M. Farber, M.D., Professor and Head of the Dermatology Department at Stanford University, Dr. Muller monitored the Department's courses and clinics to apply that knowledge to comparative and veterinary dermatology. In 1959, Dr. Muller joined the clinical faculty of the Dermatology Department of the Stanford University Medical School. He eventually became a clinical professor and had an office there for over 30 years. At Stanford, he conducted research; taught courses; wrote articles, chapters, and books; and prepared seminars.

Dr. Muller owned and operated a small animal hospital in Walnut Creek, California. During the past 25 years, before his retirement, he restricted his practice to dermatology, thereby establishing the first full-time small animal dermatology practice in the world. Working part-time in his dermatology practice and part-time in the academic environment of Stanford was a good combination. Dr. Muller's increasing understanding of dermatology and his more than 6000 clinical photographs led to the writing of the first edition of *Small Animal Dermatology* in 1969.

Dr. Muller also published other books (*Canine Skin Lesions,* 1968; *Feline Skin Lesions,* 1974) as well as numerous articles and chapters on small animal dermatology. He presented over 150 seminars around the world, including dermatology seminars at the annual American Animal Hospital Association meeting for 18 years in a row!

Dr. Muller was co-founder of the American Academy of Veterinary Dermatology in 1964, and was its president in 1968. He was the co-founder of the American College of Veterinary Dermatology and its president in 1980. Dr. Muller was also co-founder and honorary charter member of the European Society of Veterinary Dermatology in 1983. Awards received for his work in veterinary dermatology include the McCoy Memorial Award (Washington State University in 1968), the American Animal Hospital Association Merit Award in 1970, the American Academy of Veterinary Dermatology Service Award in 1978, the American Veterinary Medical Association Gaines FIDO Award in 1980, and the American College of Veterinary Dermatology Award of Excellence in 1991.

Dr. Muller is currently Clinical Professor of Dermatology Emeritus at Stanford University School of Medicine, and Program Co-Chairman and speaker at the 1-week annual George H. Muller Stanford Veterinary Dermatology Seminar.

ROBERT W. KIRK

Dr. Robert Kirk attended the University of Connecticut and Cornell University (D.V.M. in 1946). He served as Captain in the United States Air Force from 1950 to 1952. Although acknowledged around the world as an authority in all areas of small animal medicine, Dr. Kirk had a special interest in and love for dermatology. He spent a 1-year sabbatical leave with Dr. Muller in Stanford and became co-author of the first edition of *Small Animal Dermatology* in 1969.

Dr. Kirk was in private practice in Vermont and Connecticut from 1946 to 1950, and then joined the faculty of Cornell University in 1952. Before his retirement in 1985, Dr. Kirk held several positions in the College of Veterinary Medicine: Head of the Department of Small Animal Medicine and Surgery, Director of the Small Animal Clinic, and Director of the Veterinary Medical Teaching Hospital.

Dr. Kirk published numerous articles and chapters and five editions of the *Handbook of Veterinary Procedures and Emergency Treatment* with co-author Dr. S. I. Bistner. However, his most stunning contribution to veterinary medicine, and certainly that for which he is world renowned, is his editorship of 11 editions of *Current Veterinary Therapy.* He also presented over 400 continuing education seminars!

Bob was the president of the American College of Veterinary Internal Medicine in 1974, and president of the American College of Veterinary Dermatology from 1985 to 1987. He was a member of the organizing committee of the American Board of Veterinary Practitioners and was its president from 1982 to 1983. Awards he received for work in veterinary dermatology and medicine include the World Small Animal Veterinary Association International Prize for Scientific Achievement in 1984, the British Small Animal Veterinary Association Bourgelat Award in 1987, the American College of Veterinary Internal Medicine Distinguished Service Award in 1988, the New York State Veterinary Medical Society Centennial Commendation for Outstanding Professional Contributions to the Practice of Veterinary Medicine in 1990, and the American College of Veterinary Practitioners' Award for Excellence in 1991, and the American College of Veterinary Dermatology Award of Excellence in 1991.

Dr. Kirk is currently Professor of Medicine Emeritus at Cornell University and enjoying retirement in Ithaca.

As "dermoids," we remember George and Bob as individuals who brought standardization in nomenclature and diagnostic approach, science, integrity, credibility, and enthusiasm to veterinary dermatology. As just plain "folks," we remember George and Bob for their warmth, friendship, and encouragement. Guys, you are very special to us. And George, you still have the best photographs!

Although some aspects of this fifth edition of *Small Animal Dermatology* have changed— and change we must—we have attempted to carry on the science, integrity, and enthusiasm, the *tradition,* of George Muller and Bob Kirk. May our efforts be pleasing to you and something we can all be proud of.

Small Animal Dermatology V must now speak for itself. Again, words taken from that first edition in 1969 seem appropriate in 1995

The authors dedicate this book to clinicians who deal daily with small animal dermatoses, and to those who for years have requested that it be written. We hope they will find encouragement in it, and answers to many of their questions.

DANNY W. SCOTT
WILLIAM H. MILLER, JR.
CRAIG E. GRIFFIN

Preface and Acknowledgments ■

In veterinary medicine, very little information is available concerning the demographics of canine and feline skin disorders. It has been estimated that between 20 per cent and 75 per cent of the small animals seen in the average practice have skin problems as a chief or concurrent owner complaint.[1–5] A 1978 Ralston Purina Company survey indicated that 25 per cent of all small animal practice activity was involved with the diagnosis and treatment of problems with skin and haircoat.[6] A nationwide survey by the Alpo Company in 1985 of 2540 small animal practitioners in the United States revealed that skin disorders were the most common reason for patient visits to the veterinarian's office.[7] Dermatologic disorders accounted for 18.8 per cent of the dogs and 15.2 per cent of the cats examined at a university teaching hospital.[8]

Using data gathered from 17 North American veterinary teaching hospitals for the year 1983, Sischo and associates reported that the 10 most commonly diagnosed canine skin disorders were, in decreasing order of frequency, flea bite hypersensitivity, skin cancer, bacterial pyoderma, seborrhea, allergy, demodicosis, scabies, immune-mediated dermatoses, endocrine dermatoses, and acral lick dermatitis.[9] Significant differences were noted in the frequency of those skin diseases in the various geographic regions studied. A survey conducted in 1981 by the American Academy of Veterinary Dermatology revealed the most common feline dermatologic disorders to be, in decreasing order of frequency, parasitic dermatoses, miliary dermatitis, eosinophilic granuloma complex, endocrinologic disorders, fungal diseases, hypersensitivity reactions, bacterial diseases, psychogenic dermatoses, seborrheic conditions, neoplastic tumors, and autoimmune dermatoses.[10]

During a 1-year period at a university teaching hospital,[8] the most common dermatoses in dogs and cats were as follows:

Dogs—bacterial folliculitis and furunculosis (25.3 per cent of the cases), atopy (12.7 per cent), food hypersensitivity (4.7 per cent), flea bite hypersensitivity (3.4 per cent), hyperadrenocorticism (3.4 per cent), and hypothyroidism (2.7 per cent).

Cats—abscesses (18.5 per cent), otodectic mange (12.9 per cent), cheyletiellosis (8.1 per cent), flea bite hypersensitivity (6.5 per cent), atopy (5.6 per cent), flea infestation (4.9 per cent), neoplasia (4.9 per cent), and food hypersensitivity (4 per cent).

Clearly, dermatology is a ''big ticket item'' in small animal practice; bacterial infections, ectoparasitisms, allergies, fungal infections, and neoplasia are common problems.

It is probably safe to say that no other specialty area in veterinary medicine has witnessed the information explosion that has occurred in veterinary dermatology in the past decade. As one clear indication of this explosion and of both the importance of veterinary dermatology and the practitioner's hunger for information, one has only to note the number of veterinary dermatology textbooks published in the past 10 years (see Chap. 21).

This fifth edition of *Small Animal Dermatology* has undergone many changes: extensive revision of subject matter, style, and organization. With the departure of George Muller and Bob Kirk, the book welcomes two new co-authors: William Miller and Craig Griffin. Discussions of over 40 diseases have been added. Diagnostic methods and therapeutic protocols have, in many instances, undergone radical rethinking since the fourth edition was published in 1989. In order to gain precious space, many diagrams and pearls of knowledge have been eliminated. An attempt has been made, where practical, to separate the canine and feline aspects of the various dermatoses. Many new clinical and pathologic illustrations have been added. In addition, because of the increasing popularity of small mammals (''pocket pets''), it was believed that the time had come to include a chapter on the dermatoses of these pets as well.

We also sought to make this edition an international treatise on veterinary dermatology. Our colleagues in the field throughout the world responded mightily with their photographs and thoughts. To list every name would greatly weary the reader, yet to omit any seems akin to gross ingratitude. You know who you are, and we are forever grateful. Still, special thanks must go to, in alphabetical order, Zeineb Alhaidari, Didier Carlotti, David Chester, Robert Dunstan, Carol Foil, Tracy French, Jay Gould, Thelma Lee Gross, Eric Guaguère, Jay Harvey, Richard Harvey, Peter Ihrke, John King, George Kollias, Ken Mason, Manon Paradis, Karen Helton Rhodes, Keith Thoday, and Emily Walder.

We cannot emphasize enough our appreciation for the love and support of those so close to us: Kris, Travis, and Tracy (DWS); Kathy, Steven, Julia, and Andrew (WHM); and Bud, Mary, Wayne, and Vicki (CEG).

Finally, we gratefully acknowledge the dedication, enthusiasm, patience, and support of the W. B. Saunders Company, and especially our ''partner-in-crime'' Ray Kersey. Well . . . as they say . . . ''Let's rock and roll!''

REFERENCES

1. Schwartzman, R.M., Orkin, M.: A Comparative Study of Skin Diseases of Dog and Man. Charles C Thomas, Springfield, 1962.
2. Ihrke, P.J., Franti, C.E.: Breed as a risk factor associated with skin diseases in dogs seen in northern California. Calif. Vet. 39:13, 1985.
3. Nesbitt, G.H.: Canine and Feline Dermatology: A Systematic Approach. Lea & Febiger, Philadelphia, 1983.
4. Wilkinson, G.T.: Color Atlas of Small Animal Dermatology. Williams & Wilkins, Baltimore, 1985.
5. Grant, D.I.: Skin Diseases in the Dog and Cat. Blackwell Scientific Publications, Oxford, 1986.
6. Ralston Purina Company. An Introduction to the Nutrition of Dogs and Cats. Veterinary Learning Systems, Trenton, 1989.
7. Alpo Veterinary Panel. Dermatological problems head problem list. DVM Magazine, August, 1985.
8. Scott, D.W., Paradis, M.: A survey of canine and feline skin disorders seen in a university practice: Small Animal Clinic, University of Montréal, Saint-Hyacinthe, Québec (1987–1988). Can. Vet. J. 31:830, 1990.
9. Sischo, W.M., et al.: Regional distribution of 10 common skin diseases in dogs. J. Am. Vet. Med. Assoc. 195:752, 1989.
10. Nesbitt, G.H.: Incidence of feline skin disease: A survey. Proc. Am. Acad. Vet. Dermatol., Las Vegas, 1982.

D. W. Scott
W. H. Miller, Jr.
C. E. Griffin

Notice

■

Companion animal practice is an ever-changing field. Standard safety precautions must be followed, but as new research and clinical experience grow, changes in treatment and drug therapy become necessary or appropriate. The authors of this work have carefully checked the generic and trade drug names and verified drug dosages to assure that dosage information is precise and in accord with standards accepted at the time of publication. Readers are advised, however, to check the product information currently provided by the manufacturer of each drug to be administered to be certain that changes have not been made in the recommended dose or in the contraindications for administration. This is of particular importance in regard to new or infrequently used drugs. Recommended dosages for animals are sometimes based on adjustments in the dosage that would be suitable for humans. Some of the drugs mentioned here have been given experimentally by the authors. Others have been used in dosages greater than those recommended by the manufacturer. In these kinds of cases, the authors have reported on their own considerable experience. It is the responsibility of those administering a drug, relying on their professional skill and experience, to determine the dosages, the best treatment for the patient, and whether the benefits of giving a drug justify the attendant risk. The authors cannot be responsible for misuse or misapplication of the material in this work.

THE PUBLISHER

Contents

For a more detailed listing of the subjects covered in this book, see the outlines at the beginning of each chapter.

Structure and Function of the Skin

■

Chapter Outline

What a glorious organ it is! The skin is the largest organ of the body and the anatomic and physiologic barrier between animal and environment. It provides protection from physical, chemical, and microbiologic injury, and its sensory components perceive heat, cold, pain, pruritus, touch, and pressure. In addition, the skin is synergistic with internal organ systems and thus reflects pathologic processes that are either primary elsewhere or shared with other tissues. Not only is the skin an organ with its own reaction patterns; it is also a mirror reflecting the *milieu interieur* and, at the same time, the capricious world to which it is exposed. The skin, hair, and subcutis of a newborn puppy represent 24 per cent of its body weight.[39, 103] By the time of maturity, these structures constitute only 12 per cent of body weight.

■ GENERAL FUNCTIONS OF THE SKIN

The general functions of animal skin are as follows:*

1. *Enclosing barrier.* The most important function of skin is to make possible an internal environment for all other organs by maintaining an effective barrier to the loss of water, electrolytes, and macromolecules.

2. *Environmental protection.* A corollary function is the exclusion of external injurious agents—chemical, physical, and microbiologic—from entrance into the internal environment.

3. *Motion and shape.* The flexibility, elasticity, and toughness of the skin allow motion and provide shape and form.

4. *Adnexa production.* Skin produces keratinized structures such as hair, claws, and the horny layer of the epidermis.

5. *Temperature regulation.* Skin plays a role in the regulation of body temperature through its support of the hair coat, regulation of cutaneous blood supply, and sweat gland function.

6. *Storage.* The skin is a reservoir of electrolytes, water, vitamins, fat, carbohydrates, proteins, and other materials.

7. *Indicator.* The skin may be an important indicator of general health, internal disease, and the effects of substances applied topically or taken internally.

8. *Immunoregulation.* Keratinocytes, Langerhans' cells, and lymphocytes together provide the skin with an immunosurveillance capability that effectively protects against the development of cutaneous neoplasms and persistent infections.

9. *Pigmentation.* Processes in the skin (melanin formation, vascularity, and keratinization) help determine the color of the coat and skin. Pigmentation of the skin helps prevent damage from solar radiation.

10. *Antimicrobial action.* The skin surface has antibacterial and antifungal properties.

11. *Sensory perception.* Skin is a primary sense organ for touch, pressure, pain, itch, heat, and cold.

12. *Secretion.* Skin is a secretory organ by virtue of its apocrine (epitrichial), eccrine (atrichial), and sebaceous glands.

13. *Excretion.* The skin functions in a limited way as an excretory organ.

14. *Vitamin D production.* Vitamin D is produced in the skin through stimulation by solar radiation. In the epidermis, vitamin D_3 (cholecalciferol) is formed from provitamin D_3 (7-dehydrocholesterol), via previtamin D_3, on exposure to sunlight.[35, 49] The vitamin D–binding protein in plasma translocates vitamin D_3 from the skin to the circulation. Vitamin D_3 is then hydroxylated in the liver to 25-hydroxyvitamin D_3 and again hydroxylated in the kidney to form 12,25-dihydroxyvitamin D_3, which is important in the regulation of epidermal proliferation and differentiation.

---

*See references 38, 39, 43, 49, 82, 119, 124, 133, and 140.

■ ONTOGENY

Initially, the embryonic skin consists of a single layer of ectodermal cells and a dermis containing loosely arranged mesenchymal cells embedded in an interstitial ground substance. The ectodermal covering progressively develops into two layers (the basal cell layer, or *stratum germinativum,* and the outer *periderm*), three layers (the *stratum intermedium* forms between the other two layers), and then into an adult-like structure.[39, 43, 49, 89, 119] Melanocytes (neural crest origin) and Langerhans' cells (bone marrow origin) become identifiable during this period of ectodermal maturation.

Dermal development is characterized by an increase in the thickness and number of fibers, a decrease in ground substance, and the transition of mesenchymal cells to fibroblasts. This process of building a fiber-rich matrix has been referred to as a *ripening* of the dermis. Elastin fibers appear later than do collagen fibers. Histiocytes, Schwann cells, and dermal melanocytes also become recognizable. Fetal skin contains a large percentage of Type III collagen compared with the skin of an adult, which contains a large proportion of Type I collagen.[49] Lipocytes (adipocytes, fat cells) begin to develop into the subcutis from spindle-shaped mesenchymal precursor cells *(prelipoblasts)* in the second half of gestation.

The embryonal stratum germinativum differentiates into hair germs (primary epithelial germs), which give rise to hair follicles, sebaceous glands, and apocrine (epitrichial) sweat glands.[9, 129] Hair germs initially consist of an area of crowding of deeply basophilic cells in the basal layer of the epidermis. Subsequently, the areas of crowding become buds that protrude into the dermis. Beneath each bud lies a group of mesenchymal cells, from which the dermal hair papilla is later formed.

As the hair peg lengthens and develops into a hair follicle and hair, three bulges appear. The lowest (deepest) of the bulges develops into the attachment for the arrector pili muscle; the middle bulge differentiates into the sebaceous gland; and the uppermost bulge evolves into the apocrine sweat gland. These appendages develop on the ental side of primary hair follicles; secondary hair follicles develop on the extal side. In general, the first hairs to appear on the fetus are vibrissae and tactile or sinus hairs that develop on the chin, eyebrows, and upper lip as white, slightly raised dots on otherwise smooth, bare skin.[119, 129] The general body hair appears first on the head and gradually progresses caudally.

Eccrine (atrichial) sweat gland germs also begin as areas of crowding of deeply basophilic cells in the basal layer of the epidermis. They initially differ from hair germs only slightly, by being narrower and by showing fewer mesenchymal cells at their base.

Cell interaction plays a central role in the formation of skin appendages. Several new adhesion molecule families that mediate cell-to-cell and cell-to-substrate adhesion have been identified: (1) neural cell adhesion molecules (N-CAM), which belong to the immunoglobulin (IgG) gene superfamily; (2) cadherins, which mediate adhesion in the presence of calcium; (3) tenascin, which is a unique matrix molecule similar to the epidermal cell growth factor (EGF); (4) fibronectin and fibrinogen; (5) and integrins, which serve as cellular receptors for fibronectin, collagen, and other extracellular matrix molecules.[27, 49] Thus, in each step of the morphogenesis of skin appendages, different adhesion molecules are expressed and are involved in different functions: induction, mesenchymal condensation, epithelial folding, and cell death.

All vessels in fetal skin develop first as capillaries.[8, 49] They have been suggested to organize in situ from dermal mesenchymal cells into single-layered endothelial tubes. Branches from large subcutaneous nerve trunks extend into the dermis and organize into deep and superficial plexuses related to the vascular plexus.

■ GROSS ANATOMY AND PHYSIOLOGY

At each body orifice, the skin is continuous with the mucous membrane located there (digestive, respiratory, ocular, urogenital). The skin and haircoat vary in quantity and quality among species, among breeds within a species, and among individuals within a breed; they also vary from one area to another on the body, and in accordance with age and sex.

In general, skin thickness decreases dorsally to ventrally on the trunk and proximally to distally on the limbs.[39, 94, 119, 124, 134, 142] The skin is thickest on the forehead, dorsal neck, dorsal thorax, rump, and base of the tail. It is thinnest on the pinnae and on the axillary, inguinal, and perianal areas. The reported average thickness of the general body skin of cats is 0.4 to 2.0 mm[124, 134]; of dogs, it is 0.5 to 5.0 mm.[39, 82] The haircoat is usually thickest over the dorsolateral aspects of the body and thinnest ventrally, on the lateral surface of the pinnae, and on the undersurface of the tail.

The skin surfaces of haired mammals are, in general, acidic. The pH of normal feline and canine skin has been reported to range from about 5.5 to 7.5.[37, 82, 116, 124]

The metabolism of the skin is not well understood. All the enzymes of the glycolytic pathway and those of the tricarboxylic acid cycle have been demonstrated in skin, but actual glucose metabolism seems to be anomalous.[17, 49, 56, 80] Glucose is preferentially metabolized to lactate, rather than fully oxidized to CO_2.

Studies of the surface markings of the muzzle and nose have shown that there are individual, genetically determined differences similar to those of human fingertips.[119] It has been suggested that imprints (''fingerprints''!) of these special skin areas (termed *labiograms* or *nasolabiograms*) could be used for the identification of animals.

Hair

Hair, which is characteristic of mammals, is important in thermal insulation and sensory perception and as a barrier against chemical, physical, and microbial injury to the skin.[49, 95, 129, 133] The ability of a haircoat to regulate body temperature correlates closely with its length, thickness, and density per unit area, and with the medullation of individual hair fibers. In general, haircoats composed of long, fine, poorly medullated fibers, with the coat depth increased by piloerection, are the most efficient for thermal insulation at low environmental temperatures. Coat color is also of some importance in thermal regulation; light-colored coats are more efficient in hot, sunny weather. The glossiness of the haircoat is important in reflecting sunlight. Transglutaminase is a marker of early anagen hair follicles, and it is important in the protein cross-linking that contributes to the shape and remarkable physical strength of hair.[49, 90]

Both primary (outercoat, guard) and secondary (undercoat) hairs are medullated in dogs and cats; thus, the term *lanugo,* meaning nonmedullated, is incorrect when applied to nonfetal dogs and cats. In cats, secondary hairs are far more numerous than primary hairs (10:1 dorsally, 24:1 ventrally).[124] The hairs of the cat have been divided into three types based on gross appearance: (1) guard hairs (thickest, straight, evenly tapered to a fine tip), (2) awn hairs (thinner, possessing subapical swelling below the hair tip), and (3) down hairs (thinnest, evenly crimped or undulating).[115, 129] In general, the shape of the hair fiber is determined by the shape of the hair follicle, with straight follicles producing straight hairs and curly follicles producing curly hairs.[119, 129]

In general, no new hair follicles are formed after birth. All hair follicles grow obliquely (30 to 60 degrees) in relation to the epidermis. The direction of the slope of the hairs, which varies from one region of the body to another, gives rise to the *hair tracts.*[129] The study of hair tract patterns is called *trichoglyphics.* The true significance and the origin of hair tracts are unknown. With the hair slope generally running caudally and ventrally, benefits include minimal impediment to forward motion and the ability of water to flow off the body to the ground without soaking the haircoat, which would reduce its thermal-insulating properties.

Hair Cycle

Analysis of the factors controlling or influencing hair growth is complicated by evolutionary history.[49] The pelage changes as a mammal grows, and that of the adult often differs markedly from that of the juvenile, reflecting different requirements for heat regulation, camouflage, and sexual and social communication. In addition, the cyclic activity of the hair follicles and the periodic molting of hairs have provided a mechanism by which the pelage can be adapted to seasonal changes in ambient temperature or environmental background. This mechanism is influenced by changes in the photoperiod, which acts through the hypothalamus, hypophysis, and pineal gland, altering levels of various hormones (including those of gonadal, thyroidal, and adrenocortical origin) and modifying the inherent rhythms of the hair follicle.

Hair growth cycles involve the repeated induction of hair follicle anlagen and their concurrent downward growth and invasion through the dermis.[143] Signals controlling hair follicle induction, development, regression, and reactivation have not been identified; however, multiple growth factors or their receptors (e.g., EGF, transforming growth factor [TGF-β_1, TGF-β_2]) have been localized to hair follicles and the surrounding mesenchyme. These control cellular proliferation and collagenase release from cultured hair follicles. In addition, an interplay between class I major histocompatibility complex (MHC) expression, chondroitin proteoglycans, and activated macrophages is involved in the regulation of hair growth, especially during the catagen phase.[48]

Hairs do not grow continuously but rather in cycles (Fig. 1:1). Each cycle consists of a growing period *(anagen)*, during which the follicle is actively producing hair, and a resting period *(telogen)*, during which the hair is retained in the follicle as a dead (or *club*) hair that is subsequently lost. There is also a transitional period *(catagen)* between these two stages. It is often stated that certain breeds of dogs, such as poodles, Old English sheepdogs, and Schnauzers, have continuously growing hair coats,[34] but there has been no scientific investigation that would substantiate such a statement. The relative duration of the phases of the cycle varies with the age of the individual, the region of the body, the breed, and the sex, and it can be modified by a variety of physiologic and pathologic factors.

The hair cycle, and thus the haircoat, are controlled by photoperiod, ambient temperature, nutrition, hormones, general state of health, genetics, and poorly understood intrinsic factors.*

---

*See references 1, 2, 16, 24, 49, 53, 55, 95, 118, 120, 129, and 140.

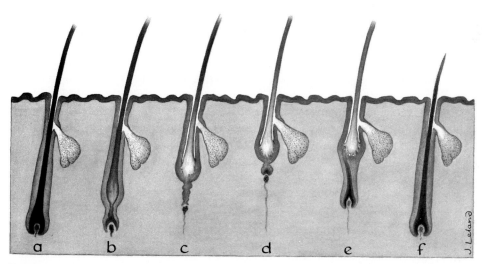

Figure 1:1. The hair cycle. *a*, Anagen: During this growing stage, hair is produced by mitosis in cells of the dermal papilla. *b*, Early catagen: In this transitional stage, a constriction occurs at the hair bulb. The hair above this will become a "club." *c*, Catagen: The distal follicle becomes thick and corrugated and pushes the hair outward. *d*, Telogen: This is the resting stage. The dermal papilla separates and an epithelial strand shortens to form a secondary germ. *e*, Early anagen: The secondary germ grows down to enclose the dermal papilla and a new hair bulb forms. The old "club" is lost. *f*, Anagen: The hair elongates as growth continues.

Hair replacement in dogs and cats is mosaic in pattern because neighboring hair follicles are in different stages of the hair cycle at any one time. Replacement is unaffected by castration; it responds predominantly to photoperiod and, to a lesser extent, to ambient temperature. Dogs and cats in temperate latitudes such as the northern United States and Canada may shed noticeably in the spring and fall. Hair follicle activity, and thus hair growth rate, are maximal in summer and minimal in winter. For example, up to 50 per cent of hair follicles may be in telogen in the summer, but this proportion may increase to 90 per cent in the winter. Catagen hairs always constitute a small proportion of the total number of hairs, usually accounting for 4 to 7 per cent of the total.[3, 103] Many dogs and cats exposed to several hours of artificial light (e.g., animals housed indoors) shed, sometimes profusely, throughout the year.[103, 124]

Hair grows until it attains its preordained length, which varies according to body region and is genetically determined; it then enters the resting phase, which may last for a considerable amount of time. Each region of the body has its own ultimate length of hair beyond which no further growth occurs. This phenomenon is responsible for the distinctive coat lengths of various breeds and is genetically determined. In mongrel dogs, it was shown that hair growth rates varied at different sites and that the speed of growth was related to the ultimate length of the hair in each particular site.[53] For example, in the shoulder region, where ultimate hair length was about 30 mm, the average rate of hair growth was 6.7 mm/wk, whereas in the forehead region, which had ultimate hair length of about 16 mm, the growth rate was 2.8 mm/wk. Other investigators have reported daily hair growth rates in dogs of 0.04 to 0.18 mm (Greyhound)[24, 28] and 0.34 to 0.40 mm (beagle).[1] In the cat, daily hair growth rate has been reported to be 0.25 to 0.30 mm.[16]

Because hair is predominantly protein, nutrition has a profound effect on its quantity and quality (see Chap. 16). Poor nutrition may produce a dull, dry, brittle, or thin haircoat with or without pigmentary disturbances.

Under conditions of ill health or generalized disease, anagen may be considerably shortened; accordingly, a large percentage of body hairs may be in telogen at one time. Because telogen hairs tend to be more easily lost, the animal may shed excessively. Disease states may also lead to faulty formation of hair cuticle, which results in a dull, lusterless hair coat. Severe illness or systemic stress may cause many hair follicles to enter synchronously and precipitously into telogen. Shedding of these hairs (telogen defluxion; see Chap. 10) thus occurs simultaneously, often resulting in visible thinning of the coat or actual alopecia.

The hair cycle and haircoat are also affected by hormonal changes.[24, 49, 55, 95] In general, anagen is initiated and advanced, and hair growth rate is accelerated, by thyroid hormones. Conversely, excessive amounts of glucocorticoids or estrogens inhibit anagen and suppress hair growth rate. Dermal papilla cells, which are a mesenchymal component of the hair bulb, are considered to play a fundamental role in the induction of epithelial differentiation. These cells are morphologically and functionally differentiated from dermal fibroblasts and are thought to be the primary target cells that respond to hormones and mediate growth-stimulating signals to the follicular epithelial cells.[69]

Hair growth is a confusing subject that needs much research. It should be remembered that the haircoat of pet animals is a cosmetic or ornamental feature. Every effort should be made to minimize procedures (clipping and shaving) that may affect the animal's appearance for many weeks. Although generalizations can be misleading, normal or short coats usually take about 3 to 4 months to regrow after shaving and long coats may take as long as 18 months.[103] Occasionally, an unexplained and extremely frustrating failure to regrow hair in an area of skin occurs, usually following clipping and surgical scrubbing.[103] The skin in affected areas appears grossly normal, but biopsy reveals catagenization, or occasionally telogenization, of the hair follicles. This frustrating *follicular arrest* disappears spontaneously in 6 months to 2 years after clipping (see Chap. 10).

Attention has been focused on the usefulness of *hair analysis* as a diagnostic tool.[132, 158] It is well recognized by most dermatologists and nutritionists in human medicine that mineral and trace element analysis of hair samples is not a clinically useful tool in the assessment of nutritional status. The reasons for variability and unreliability include environmental effects (topical agents, geographic location, occupational exposures), differing hair growth rates (health, drugs, age, sex), and lack of standardization in analysis techniques. Until and unless adequate scientific documentation of the validity of such multi-element analysis is performed, it is necessary for both health professionals and the public to be aware of the very limited value of hair analysis and of the potential to be confused and misled by it. Scientifically oriented nutritionists do not use hair analysis as a primary method of detecting nutritional problems. Cautious consumers and health professionals should regard practitioners who rely solely on this test with suspicion.[158]

Small (0.16 to 0.42 mm in diameter), hairless, knoblike structures are present in the haired skin of cats and dogs.[39, 122, 124] These *tylotrich pads* serve as slow-adapting mechanoreceptors.

Cell proliferation kinetic values have been established for the hair follicle epithelium of normal beagles and Cocker spaniels.[86a] These values were established by intradermal pulse-labeling injections of tritiated thymidine, examination of skin biopsies, and autoradiographs. The basal cell labeling index was 1.46 ± 0.78 per cent in beagles and 1.07 ± 0.42 per cent in Cocker spaniels.

Hair Colors and Types

DOG

Although hair types in dogs are extremely diverse, various authors have attempted to classify them on the basis of color, length, type of bristle, and characteristics of the medulla and cortex.[39, 103] Hair types among dogs can be divided into normal (intermediate length), short, and long coats.

■ *Normal Coat.* The normal coat is typified by that seen in the German shepherd, the Welsh corgi, and wild dogs such as wolves and coyotes. It is composed of primary hairs (coarse guard hairs or bristles) and secondary hairs (fine hairs or undercoat). A high proportion of the hairs, by number but not by weight, are secondary hairs.

The next two classes of hair coats are also made up of primary and secondary hairs, but the relative sizes of the hairs and their numbers vary markedly from those of the normal coat.

■ *Short Coat.* The short coat can be classified as coarse or fine. The coarse short coat is typified by the Rottweiler and many of the terriers. This type of coat has a strong growth of primary hairs and a much lesser growth of secondary hairs. The total weight of hair is lower, and the secondary hairs, especially, weigh less and are fewer in number than those in the normal coat. The fine short coat is exemplified by boxers, dachshunds, and miniature pinschers. This type of coat has the largest number of hairs per unit area. The secondary hairs are numerous and well developed, and the primary hairs are reduced in size as compared with those of the normal coat.

■ *Long Coat.* The long coat can also be arranged into two subdivisions: the fine long coat and the woolly or coarse long coat. The fine long coat is found in the Cocker spaniel, the Pomeranian, and the Chow Chow. This coat has a greater weight of hair per unit area than does the normal coat, except in the toy breeds (in which the weight of the hair may be less because it is finer). The woolly or coarse long coat is found in the Poodle and in the Bedlington terrier and the Kerry blue terrier. Secondary hairs make up 70 per cent of the total weight of these coats and 80 per cent of the number of hairs; compared with other secondary-type hairs, these are relatively coarse. The three breeds mentioned have less tendency to shed hair than do many breeds.

The genetic aspects of coat color in dogs constitute a complex subject.[92, 103] Pigmentation in individual hairs may be uniform throughout the length of the shaft, or it may vary. In the agouti-type hair (German shepherd, Norwegian elkhound), the tip is white or light, the heavy body is pigmented brown or black, and the base is a light yellow or red-brown. Pigment cells in the bulb of the hair deposit pigment in or between the cortical and medullary hair cells. The amount of pigment deposited in the hair and its location there produce different optical effects; however, there are only two types of pigment. The black-brown pigment is called *eumelanin,* and the yellow-red pigment is called *pheomelanin.* In addition, the melanocytes of the follicle may or may not produce pigment throughout the period of growth. In black hair, pigment production obviously remains active throughout the period.

CAT

The colors and types of hair coat in cats have been studied in some detail.[113, 115, 154] A self (solid) cat is a single color throughout. No patterning, shading, ticking, or other variation of color is observed, although it is common for kittens to have slightly tabby markings and scattered white hairs that disappear with maturity. Whatever their coloring, all cats are genetically tabbies, possessing the Abyssinian, mackerel, or blotched tabby genes or a combination of two of these types. Solid white is dominant over all colors but may be associated with various abnormalities; for example, white cats with blue eyes often have cochlear degeneration and deafness.

The tabby is the basic type of cat, the wild type from which all others evolved. The complex tabby coloration arises from two component patterns governed by two separate sets of genes. The underlying pattern is agouti, which is characterized by hairs with a bluish base and black tip separated by yellow banding. The tabby genes determine whether a cat has narrow, vertical, gently curving stripes (mackerel), larger patches (blotch), or an Abyssinian pattern.

Tipped hair coats are characterized by hairs that have colored tips (e.g., blue, red, black) overlying a paler color. Differences in the degree of tipping are great, with the greatest in the smokes and least in the chinchillas (silver). Pointed hair coats are characterized by pale-colored hair on the body with darker hairs on the extremities or points (nose, ears, feet, tail). Points arise through a temperature-dependent mechanism present in breeds such as Siamese, Himalayan, Balinese, and Birman. In these breeds, the dark hair color *(acromelanism)* is due to a temperature-dependent enzyme that converts melanin precursors into melanin by a process of oxidation.[124] With higher temperatures, the hair is light colored; with low temperatures, it is darker. Thus, kittens are light at birth, and cats kept indoors or in tropical climates are lighter than those kept outdoors or in cold climates. Inflammation and hyperemia result in more lightly colored new hair. The poor peripheral circulation that accompanies senility and shaving to remove hair often result in more darkly colored new hair.

Multicolored coats include the tortoiseshell and piebald spotting patterns. The archetypal tortoiseshell is a patchwork of black and orange, but there is range of color variation among torties. The hair may be chocolate (chestnut), cinnamon, blue, or lilac (lavender) in the nonorange areas. The tortoiseshell pattern occurs in females or in males with two X chromosomes. White spotting in piebald cats varies in degree from white gloves on the feet, a nose smudge, or a white bib, to extensive white over most of the body.

The *Maltese dilution,* which dilutes black to blue, orange to cream, and seal-point (Siamese) to blue, is inherited as an autosomal recessive trait.[112] In normal black-haired cats, numerous small, round melanin granules are scattered uniformly throughout the cortex and medulla of the hair and skin. In the skin from Maltese dilution cats, a nonuniform distribution of very large, irregularly sized melanin granules results from the clumping of small granules.

In a typical short-haired cat, the longest primary hairs average about 4.5 cm in length. By contrast, the silky coat of a good show cat has primary hairs that may exceed 12.5 cm in length. The short-hair is the fundamental wild type and is dominant to the others. Various mutant hair coat types have occurred that have been perpetuated as a breed characteristic. The rex mutant is characterized by curly hairs and occurs in two major breeds, the Devon rex and the Cornish (German) rex. The Cornish rex lacks primary hairs, and the Devon rex has primary hairs that resemble secondary hairs. Cornish rex whiskers are often short and curly, but Devon rex whiskers are often absent or stubbled. In some Devon rexes, the coat is completely absent on the chest, belly, and shoulders, a fault many breeders try to eliminate. Cornish and Devon rexes may partially or completely molt, especially during estrus or pregnancy, resulting in a symmetric alopecia that may be mistaken for an endocrine dermatosis.[40] These breeds are occasionally recommended as hypoallergenic cats to humans with animal dander hypersensitivities, but there appears to be no scientific documentation for this claim.

The wire-hair mutation, seen in the American wirehair, is characterized by a coat that looks and feels wiry because it is coarse, crimped, and springy. All hairs are curled in an irregular fashion, and the awn hairs resemble a shepherd's crook.

One survey attempted to relate feline coat color to personality.[114] Results suggested that cats with solid black, black and white, or gray tabby coats tended to have good personalities, to handle stress well, and to make excellent pets. By contrast, calicos were most likely to be aggressive and to have litter pan problems.

There are a number of cutaneous patterns or *lines* that are evoked to explain certain distributions of skin lesions encountered clinically.[73] *Voight's lines* are the boundaries of the areas of distribution of the main cutaneous nerve stems. *Langer's lines* reflect the course of blood vessels or lymphatics. *Blashko's lines* form the pattern assumed by many different nevoid and acquired skin diseases on human skin; their embryologic and structural causes are unknown. *Tension lines* are determined by muscle action, connective tissue fiber orientation and traction, and gravity.[68]

Footpads

The canine and feline footpad is a specialized area of integument.[101, 119] The thick epidermis protects against mechanical trauma, and the large fat deposits provide shock-absorbing elasticity. A copious nerve supply provides an important sensory function. Numerous eccrine sweat glands produce a secretion that may improve traction during running and climbing and may also be important in scent marking.

■ MICROSCOPIC ANATOMY AND PHYSIOLOGY

The microscopic anatomy and physiology of the skin of dogs and cats have been the subjects of numerous studies.*

Epidermis

The outer layer of the skin, or epidermis, is composed of multiple layers of cells ranging from columnar to flat in shape (Figs. 1:2 and 1:3 *A*). These are of four distinct types: keratinocytes (about 85 per cent of the epidermal cells), melanocytes (about 5 per cent), Langerhans' cells (3 to 8 per cent), and Merkel's cells, which are associated with tylotrich pads. For purposes of identification, certain areas of the epidermis are classified as layers and are named, from inner to outer, as follows: basal layer (stratum basale), spinous layer (stratum spinosum), granular layer (stratum granulosum), clear layer (stratum lucidum), and horny layer (stratum corneum).

---

*See references 38, 39, 82, 94, 95, 102, 103, 115a, 119, 121, 123, 124, 134, 136, and 156.

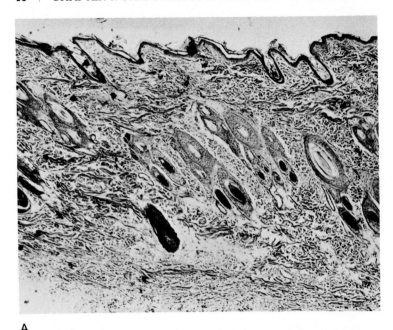

A

Figure 1:2. *A*, Normal canine skin. *B*, Normal feline skin.

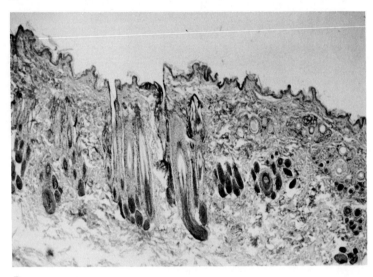

B

Figure 1:3. *A*, Normal canine skin (H & E stain). *B*, Elastin (black) and collagen (pink) fibers (AOG stain). *C*, Mucin (blue) separating dermal collagen bundles (pink) (H & E stain). *D*, Melanin (black) in keratinocytes and epidermal and dermal melanocytes (H & E stain). *E*, Keratohyalin granules (dark blue) below stratum corneum (H & E stain). *F*, Trichohyalin granules (red) in the inner root sheath of a hair follicle (H & E stain). Note vacuolated (glycogen) appearance of outer root sheath keratinocytes. *G*, Trichilemmal keratinization (red) of central hair follicle (H & E stain). *H*, Basement membrane zone (violet) (PAS stain).

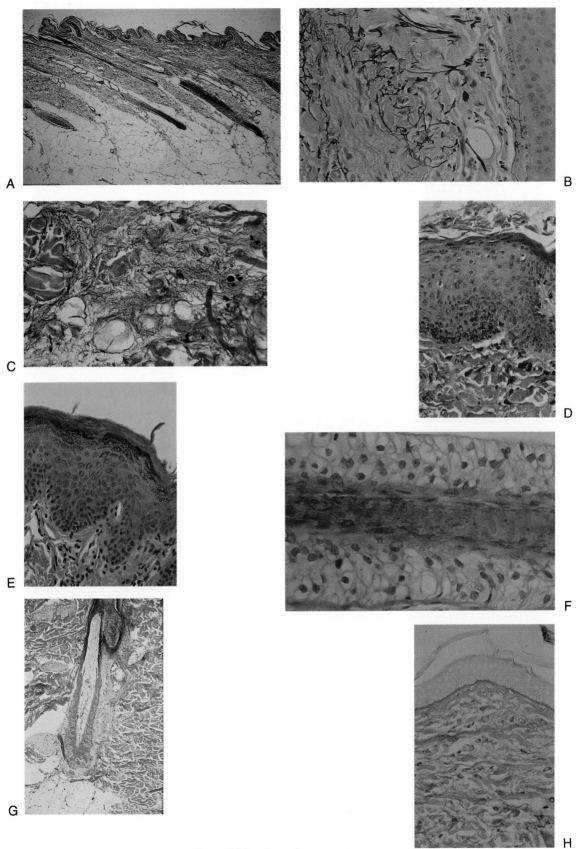

Figure 1:3 *See legend on opposite page*

In general, the epidermis of cats and dogs is thin (two to three nucleated cell layers, not counting the horny layer) in haired skin, ranging from 0.1 to 0.5 mm in thickness or in depth.[39, 93, 124, 134, 142] The thickest epidermis is found on the footpads (Fig. 1:4) and nasal planum (Fig. 1:5), where it may measure 1.5 mm. The surface of the footpad epidermis is smooth in cats but papillated and irregular in dogs. Rete ridges (projections of the epidermis into the underlying dermis) are not found in the normal hair-bearing skin of cats and dogs. Rete ridges, however, may be found in normal footpad and nasal planum epidermis and in the lightly haired scrotum (Fig. 1:6).

BASAL LAYER

The stratum basale is a single row of columnar to cuboidal cells resting on the basement membrane zone that separates the epidermis from the dermis (Fig. 1:7).[49, 119] Most of these cells are keratinocytes, which are constantly reproducing and pushing upward to replenish the epidermal cells above. The daughter cells move into the outer layers of the epidermis and are ultimately shed as dead horny cells. Mitotic figures and apoptotic keratinocytes are occasionally seen, especially in areas of skin with thicker epidermis (e.g., nasal planum, footpad, mucocutaneous junction). There is morphologic and functional heterogenicity in basal keratinocytes;[49] some populations serve primarily to anchor the epidermis and others serve a proliferative and reparative (stem cell) function. The tips of the deep epidermal rete ridges (in glabrous skin) and the bulge (Wulst) region of the hair follicle (site of attachment of the arrector pili muscle) are the presumed sites of the epidermal and hair follicle stem cells.[87, 88]

MELANOCYTES AND MELANOGENESIS

Melanocytes, the second type of cell found in the basal layer of the epidermis, are also found in the outer root sheath and hair matrix of hair follicles and in the ducts of sebaceous and sweat glands.[49, 89, 103, 124, 155] Traditionally, melanocytes are divided structurally and functionally into two compartments: epidermal and follicular.[49, 52] Because melanocytes do not stain readily with hematoxylin and eosin (H&E) and because they undergo artifactual cytoplasmic shrinkage during tissue processing, they appear as clear cells (Fig. 1:7). In general, there is one melanocyte per 10 to 20 keratinocytes in the basal cell layer. They are derived from the neural crest and migrate into the epidermis in early fetal life. Although melanocytes are of nondescript appearance, with special stains (dopa reaction, Fontana's ammoniacal silver nitrate) they can be shown to have long cytoplasmic extensions (dendrites) that weave among the keratinocytes. There is an intimate relationship between melanocytes and keratinocytes in which both cells interact and exist as epidermal symbionts—a functional and structural unit called the *epidermal melanin unit*.[49, 140] Ultrastructurally, melanocytes are characterized by typical intracytoplasmic melanosomes and premelanosomes and a cell membrane–associated basal layer lamina (Fig. 1:8). Most of the melanin pigment in skin is located in the basal layer of the epidermis, but in dark-skinned animals melanin may be found throughout the entire epidermis as well as within superficial dermal melanocytes (see Fig. 1:3 *D*).

Melanin pigments are chiefly responsible for the coloration of skin and hair. Melanins embrace a wide range of pigments, including the brown-black eumelanins, yellow or red-brown pheomelanins, and other pigments whose physicochemical natures are intermediate between the two. Despite the different properties of the various melanins, they all arise from a common metabolic pathway in which dopaquinone is the key intermediate.[43, 49, 52] Tyrosine is converted to dopa, which is then oxidized to dopaquinone. Both reactions are catalyzed by the same copper-containing enzyme, tyrosinase. Dopaquinone then undergoes a series of oxidative reactions to form either eumelanin or pheomelanin. Synthesis of these two pigment classes is under genetic control.[22]

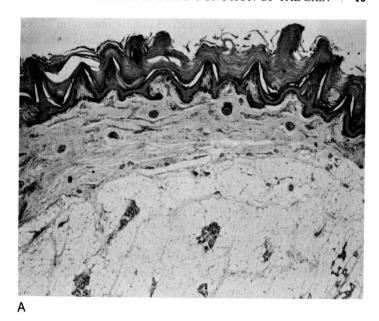

A

Figure 1:4. *A*, Histologic section of canine footpad. Note papillated surface. *B*, Histologic section of feline footpad. Note smooth surface.

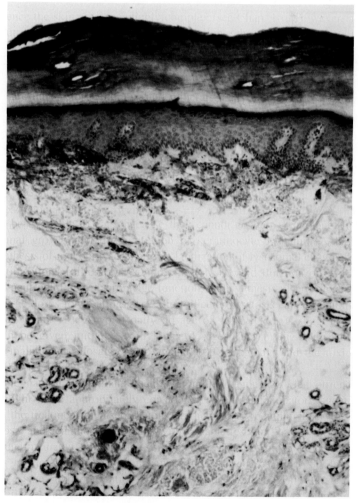

B

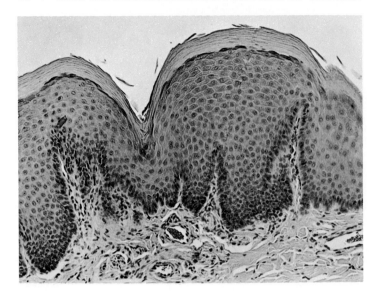

Figure 1:5. Histologic section of the nasal planum.

Figure 1:6. Histologic section of canine scrotal skin. Note muscle bundles *(arrow)*.

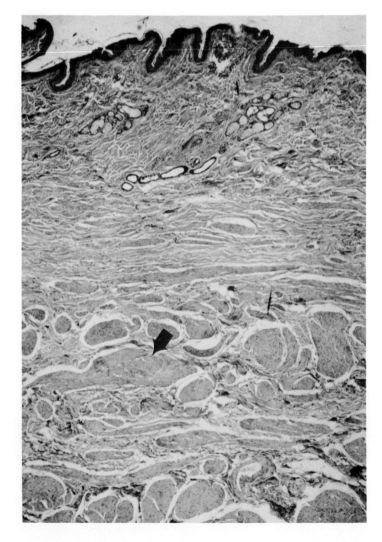

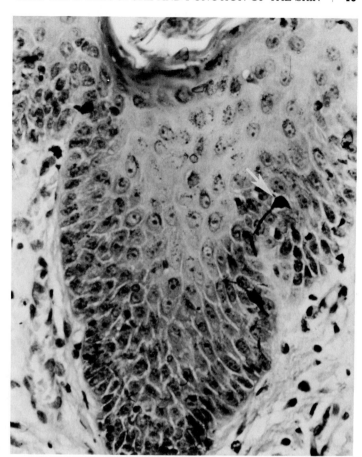

Figure 1:7. Melanocytes *(arrow)* in the basal layer of the epidermis.

Classically, melanin production has been thought to be under the control of genetics and melanocyte-stimulating hormone (MSH) from the pituitary gland.[43, 49, 52, 140] However, data are accumulating to indicate that β-MSH is not a physiologic hormone, has no role in the regulation of pigmentation, and is probably an artifact produced during isolation of β-lipotropin (β-lipotropin is derived from the primordial peptide, pro-opiomelanocortin, produced in the pars intermedia of the pituitary gland).[49] α-MSH is also a fragment of β-lipotropin, and is two to four times **less** potent a pigmenting agent than β-lipotropin. β-Lipotropin may be the physiologic hormone. Recent interest has focused on the theory that melanogenesis and melanocyte proliferation are, in fact, regulated locally by the keratinocyte and Langerhans' cell more than by distant factors in the pituitary gland.[49, 155] Basic fibroblast growth factor (bFGF) is an important growth factor for melanocytes; it is produced by dermal fibroblasts and by keratinocytes.[155] Arachidonic acid and its metabolites (leukotrienes, prostaglandins) are known to affect melanogenesis and melanocyte proliferation. In addition, ultraviolet light and inflammation increase the production of melanin locally in affected skin.[49, 52] Hormones—especially androgens, estrogens, glucocorticoids, and thyroid hormones—are also able to modulate melanogenesis through mechanisms that are poorly understood at present.[49, 52]

Melanogenesis takes place in membrane-bound organelles called melanosomes,[49, 89, 140] designated Types I through IV according to maturation. Melanosomes originate from the Golgi apparatus, where the tyrosinase enzyme is formed. Type I melanosomes contain no melanin and are electron-lucent. As melanin is progressively laid down on protein matrices, melanosomes become increasingly electron-dense. At the same time, they migrate to the periphery of the dendrites, where transfer of melanin to adjacent epidermal cells takes place. Transfer involves the endocytosis of the dendrite tips of the incorporated Type IV melanosomes by the

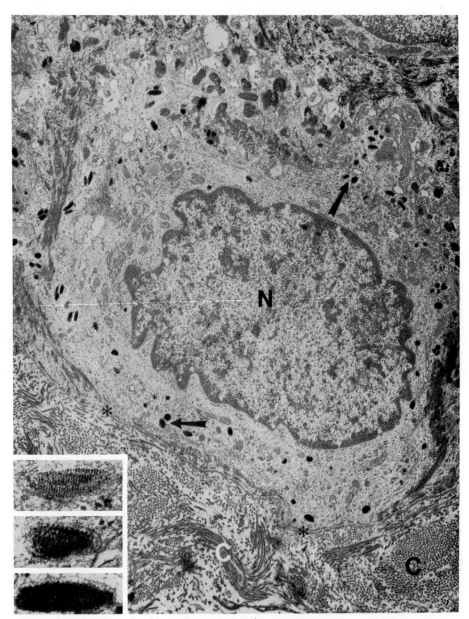

Figure 1:8. Melanocyte. N, nucleus of melanocyte; arrows, melanosomes; C, collagen in the dermis; asterisk, basal lamina (×10,000). Insets: Melanosomes in different stages of development: upper inset, Stage II; middle inset, Stage III; lower inset, Stage IV (×75,000). (From Lever, W. F., Schaumburg-Lever, G.: Histopathology of the Skin, 7th ed. J. B. Lippincott Co., Philadelphia, 1990, p. 861.)

adjacent keratinocytes. Melanocytes eject melanosomes into keratinocytes by a unique biological transfer process called cytocrinia.[49] Dermal melanocytes are often referred to as *continent* melanocytes, because they do not transfer melanosomes as do the epidermal or *secretory* melanocytes. Skin color is determined mainly by the number, size, type, and distribution of melanosomes. Melanins not only are responsible for coloration but also play important roles in photoprotection and free radical scavenging.[43, 49, 52]

MERKEL'S CELLS

Merkel's cells are epidermal clear cells confined to the basal cell layer, or just below, and occur only in tylotrich pads.[49, 54, 89, 122–125] These specialized cells (slow-adapting mechanoreceptors) contain a large cytoplasmic vacuole that displaces the cell nucleus dorsally (Fig. 1:9). They possess desmosomes and characteristic dense-core cytoplasmic granules and paranuclear whorls on electron microscopic examination (see Chap. 19). Merkel's cells also contain cytokeratin, neurofilaments, and neuron-specific enolase, suggesting a dual epithelial and neural differentiation. Current evidence suggests that Merkel's cells are derived from a primitive epidermal stem cell.[49, 116a]

SPINOUS LAYER

The stratum spinosum (prickle cell layer) is composed of the daughter cells of the stratum basale.[49, 123, 124, 134, 142] In haired skin, this layer is one or two cells thick. The stratum spinosum

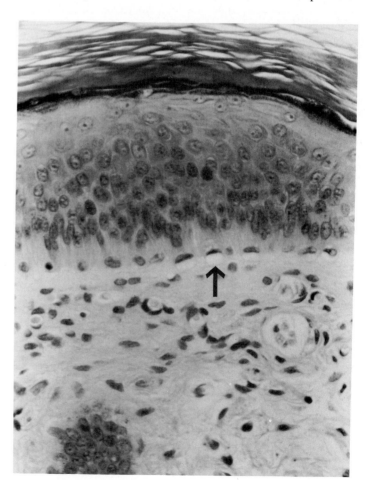

Figure 1:9. Merkel's cells *(arrow)* in a tylotrich pad.

becomes much thicker at the footpads, nasal planum, and mucocutaneous junctions, where it may occasionally approach 20 cell layers. The cells are lightly basophilic to eosinophilic, nucleated, and polyhedral to flattened cuboidal in shape. The keratinocytes of the stratum spinosum appear to be connected by intercellular bridges (prickles), which are more prominent in nonhaired skin (Fig. 1:10). Ultrastructurally, keratinocytes are characterized by tonofilaments and desmosomes (Fig. 1:11).[49] Calcium and calmodulin are crucial for desmosome and hemidesmosome formation. At least three keratinocyte-derived calmodulin-binding proteins participate in a flip-flop regulation (calcium concentration–dependent) of calcium-calmodulin interactions: caldesmon, desmocalmin, and spectrin.[49] Immunohistochemically, keratinocytes are characterized by the presence of cytokeratins.[49] All epithelia express a *keratin pair:* one keratin chain from the acidic subfamily (Type I keratins) and one chain from the neutral-basic subfamily (Type II keratins).[46, 49, 69a,110a, 132a, 136–138] The keratin pairs change with different epithelia, and in the same epithelia at various stages of differentiation or proliferation. A number of workers have published electrophoretic patterns of proteins isolated from the keratins of a variety of animals and, on the basis of observed differences in banding patterns, have suggested that the technique might be useful as an aid to taxonomy, animal classification, and identification.[49] The keratinocytes of the stratum spinosum synthesize lamellar granules (keratinosomes, membrane-coating granules, Odland bodies), which are important in the barrier function of the epidermis (see Epidermopoiesis and Keratogenesis in this chapter).[49]

Because of the research efforts directed at defining the pathomechanism of pemphigus, much has been learned concerning the structure and chemical composition of epidermal desmosomes.[49] Desmosomes are presently known to consist of keratinocyte tonofilaments and their attachment plaques, the keratinocyte plasma membrane, and the desmosomal core (desmoglea), which is interposed between two adjacent keratinocyte plasma membranes. Numerous desmosomal plaque proteins (tentatively grouped as desmoplakins) and desmosomal core glycoproteins (tentatively grouped as desmogleins) have been characterized. The immunohistochemical staining pattern seen with human pemphigus foliaceus antibody is identical to that seen with an antibody directed at desmoglein I (desmosomal core glycoprotein).

LANGERHANS' CELLS

Langerhans' cells are mononuclear dendritic cells located suprabasally.[49, 89, 98a] They are epidermal clear cells that do not stain for melanin with dopa. Langerhans' cells in many species have characteristic intracytoplasmic organelles (Birbeck's or Langerhans' granules), which are observed by means of electron microscopy.[49, 89] However, the Langerhans'-like cell studied in

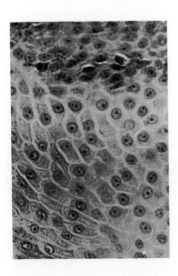

Figure 1:10. Prickle cells from footpad showing intercellular bridges (high power).

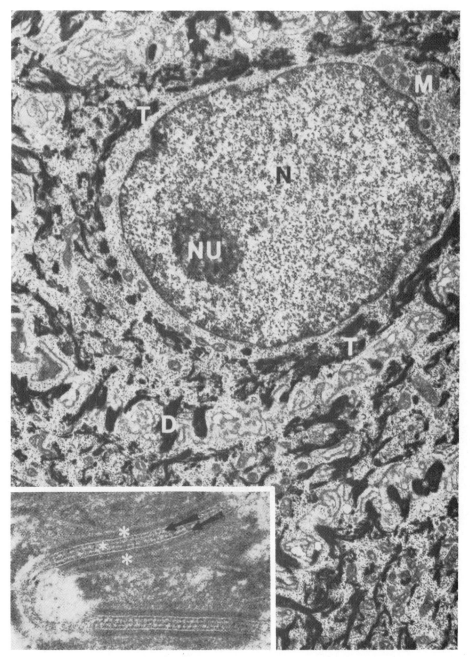

Figure 1:11. Squamous cell. N, nucleus; NU, nucleolus; T, tonofilaments; D, desmosome; M, mitochondria (×12,500). Inset: Desmosomes at higher magnification (×100,000). A desmosome connecting two adjoining keratinocytes consists of nine lines: five electron-dense lines and four electron-lucid lines. The two peripheral dense, thick lines *(large asterisks)* are the attachment plaques. The single electron-dense line in the center of the desmosome *(small asterisk)* is the intercellular contact layer. The two electron-dense lines between the intercellular contact layer and the two attachment plaques represent the cell surface coat together with the outer leaflet of the trilaminar plasma membrane of each keratinocyte *(arrows)*. The two inner electron-lucid lines adjacent to the intercellular contact layer represent intercellular cement. The two outer electron-lucid lines are the central lamina of the trilaminar plasma membrane. (From Lever, W. F., Schaumberg-Lever, G.: Histopathology of the Skin, 7th ed. J. B. Lippincott Co., Philadelphia, 1990, p. 858.)

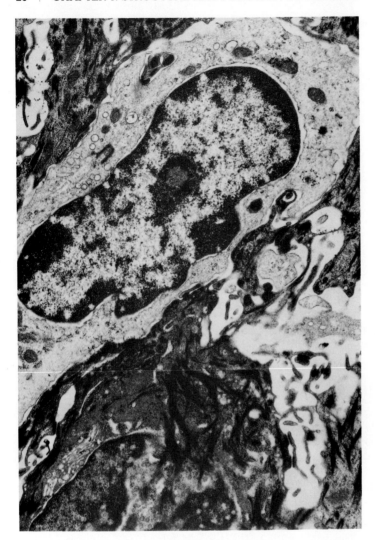

Figure 1:12. Electron micrograph of an epidermal Langerhans' cell.

dogs does not contain these granules (Fig. 1:12).[50, 98a, 156] Langerhans' cells are aureophilic (i.e., they stain with gold chloride), and they contain membrane-associated adenosine triphosphatase as well as vimentin and S-100 protein (immunohistochemical markers). They also have Fc fragment (Fc)-IgG and complement 3 (C3) receptors, and they synthesize and express antigens associated with the immune response gene. These cells are of bone marrow origin, of mono-cyte-histiocyte lineage, and serve antigen-processing and alloantigen-stimulating functions. Studies in humans have shown that the number of Langerhans' cells per unit of skin varies from one area of skin to another in the same individual, emphasizing the need to use adjacent normal skin as a control when counting Langerhans' cells in skin lesions.[49, 89, 98a]

THE SKIN AS AN IMMUNOLOGIC ORGAN

Advances in the past decade have demonstrated that normal mammalian epidermis functions as the most peripheral outpost of the immune system. Langerhans' cells, keratinocytes, epider-motropic T lymphocytes, and draining peripheral lymph nodes are thought to form collectively an integrated system of *skin-associated lymphoid tissue* (SALT) that mediates cutaneous immunosurveillance.[49, 140] *Langerhans' cells* (see previous discussion) stimulate the proliferation of relevant helper T lymphocytes by the presentation of antigen; they also induce cytotoxic

T lymphocytes directed to allogeneic and modified self-determinants, produce interleukin (IL) 1 and other cytokines, contain numerous enzymes, and are phagocytic.[49, 140]

The *keratinocyte* also plays an active role in epidermal immunity.[49, 140] Keratinocytes (1) produce IL 1, (2) produce various cytokines (e.g., IL 3, prostaglandins, leukotrienes, interferon), (3) are phagocytic, and (4) can express antigens associated with the immune response gene in a variety of lymphocyte-mediated skin diseases (presumably as a result of gamma interferon secretion by activated lymphocytes).[49, 140]

Ultraviolet light and topical or systemic glucocorticoids are known to depress Langerhans' cell numbers and function as well as other cutaneous and systemic immune responses.[49] The areas of photoimmunology and photocarcinogenesis are receiving much attention, especially because they are relevant to the pathogenesis of skin cancer.[49]

GRANULAR LAYER

The stratum granulosum is variably present in haired skin; it ranges from one to two cells thick in areas where it occurs.[123, 124, 134, 142] In nonhaired skin or at the infundibulum of hair follicles, the stratum granulosum may be four to eight cells thick (Fig. 1:13). Cells in this layer are flattened and basophilic, and they contain shrunken nuclei and large, deeply basophilic keratohyalin granules in their cytoplasm (Fig. 1:3 *E*). Keratohyalin granules are not true granules; they lack a membrane and are more accurately described as insoluble aggregates. Keratohyalin granules are the morphologic equivalents of the structural protein profilaggrin, which is the precursor of filaggrin[49] and is synthesized in the stratum granulosum. The function of keratohyalin granules is incompletely understood, but it is thought to be concerned with keratinization and barrier function. The sulfur-rich component of keratohyalin granules has been implicated as a precursor to the cornified cell envelope. Filaggrin has at least two functions. First, it aggregates, packs, and aligns keratin filaments and produces the matrix between the keratin filaments in the corneocytes. Second, it is a source of free amino acids, which are important for the normal hydration of the stratum corneum.

CLEAR LAYER

The stratum lucidum is a fully keratinized, compact, thin layer of dead cells.[123, 124, 134, 142] This layer is anuclear, homogeneous, and hyaline-like, and it contains refractile droplets (eleidin)

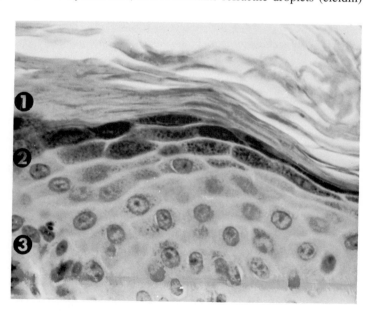

Figure 1:13. Horny layer (1), granular layer (2), and prickle cell layer (3) from the nasal planum (high power).

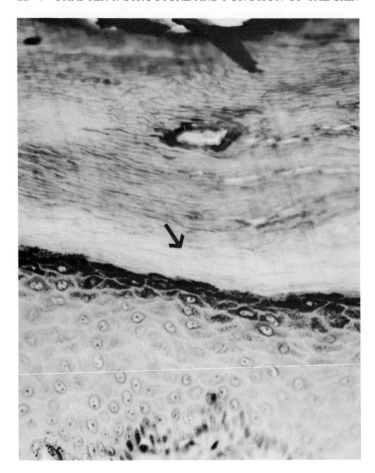

Figure 1:14. Stratum lucidum *(arrow)* in footpad epithelium.

(Fig. 1:14). The stratum lucidum is best developed in the footpads; it is less developed in the nasal planum and is absent from all other areas of normal skin.

HORNY LAYER

The stratum corneum is the outer layer of completely keratinized tissue that is constantly being shed.[123, 124, 134, 142] This layer, which consists of flattened, anuclear eosinophilic cells (corneocytes), is thicker in lightly haired or glabrous skin (Fig. 1:13). Its gradual desquamation is normally balanced by proliferation of the basal cells, which maintains a constant epidermal thickness.

The terminally differentiated corneocyte has a highly specialized structure in the cell periphery, the *cell envelope,* which assumes protective functions.[49] It develops beneath the plasma membrane of stratified epidermal cells, cells of the inner root sheath and medulla of the hair follicle, and the cuticle of the claw. Cell envelope formation is associated with the increased activity of calcium-dependent epidermal or hair follicle transglutaminases that catalyze the cross-linking of soluble and particulate protein precursors into large, insoluble polymers. Major cytoplasmic protein precursors synthesized in the stratum spinosum of the cell envelope include involucrin, keratolinin, cornifin, and loricrin.[49, 83, 132a] The cornified envelope provides structural support to the cell and resists invasion by microorganisms and deleterious environmental agents; however, it does not appear to have a significant role in regulating permeability.

In routinely processed sections, the stratum corneum varies in thickness from 3 to 35 μm in cats and from 5 to 1500 μm in dogs. However, clipping and histologic preparation involving

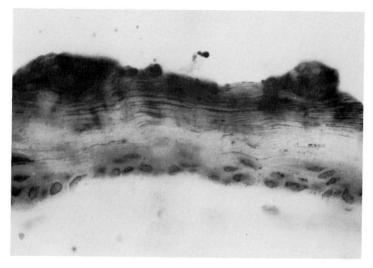

Figure 1:15. Frozen section of skin treated with an alkaline buffer to swell the cornified cells. Sudanophilic material (dark layers) is present in intercellular spaces of the distal stratum corneum (× 900). (From Lloyd, D. H., Garthwaite, G.: Epidermal structure and surface topography of canine skin. Res. Vet. Sci. 33:99, 1982.)

fixation, dehydration, and paraffin embedding result in the loss of about one half of the stratum corneum. The stratum corneum of canine truncal skin, when measured in cryostat sections, was found to have a mean thickness of 47 cell layers that measured 13.3 μm.[93] The loose, basket-weave appearance of the stratum corneum is an artifact of fixation and processing.[89, 93]

Topographic studies have shown that the epidermal surface varies from gently undulating on the densely haired skin of the back to heavily folded on the skin of the abdomen (Fig. 1:15).[93, 123] The hairs arise from the follicle infundibula, which are seen as pits in the skin (Figs. 1:16 and 1:17). At their bases the hairs tend to be joined by amorphous material that can also be seen around the squames adhering to hairs. The surface of the stratum corneum is uneven, especially in the hairy areas (Fig. 1:16). It is covered with a homogeneous film that tends to conceal the structure of the squames and their intercellular junctions. Globular masses that are partially concealed by this film can be seen (Fig. 1:18). On closer examination, the surface can be seen to be composed of hexagonal cells and an amorphous substance that appears to be oozing to the surface of the margins of the cells (Fig. 1:19). The bases of the hair follicle infundibula are sealed by an amorphous substance (sebaceous and cutaneous lipids) and squames. There is no evidence that sebum flows from the hair pore to the interfollicular region,

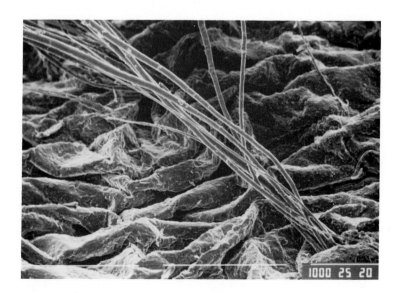

Figure 1:16. Scanning electron micrograph of freeze-dried skin from the posterior abdomen. The skin is heavily folded. White bar marker indicates 1000 μm. (From Lloyd, D. H., Garthwaite, G.: Epidermal structure and surface topography of canine skin. Res. Vet. Sci. 33:99, 1982.)

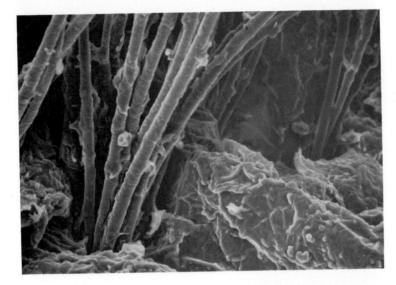

Figure 1:17. Scanning electron micrograph of freeze-dried skin from the anterior abdomen. (From Lloyd, D. H., Garthwaite, G.: Epidermal structure and surface topography of canine skin. Res. Vet. Sci. 33:99, 1982.)

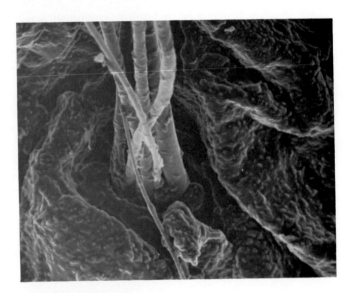

Figure 1:18. High-power view of hair follicle shown in Figure 1:16 ($\times$170). Note globular masses on surface. (From Lloyd, D. H., Garthwaite, G.: Epidermal structure and surface topography of canine skin. Res. Vet. Sci. 33:99, 1982.)

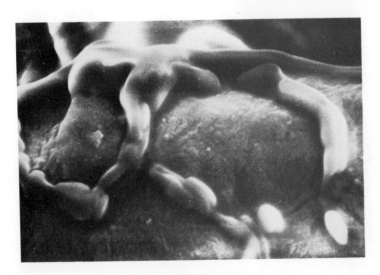

Figure 1:19. Surface of the stratum corneum in the interfollicular region. Amorphous material appears to be oozing onto the surface at the margins of the squames ($\times$2300). (From Lloyd, D. H., Garthwaite, G.: Epidermal structure and surface topography of canine skin. Res. Vet. Sci. 33:99, 1982.)

which suggests that rubbing and grooming are important in spreading this emulsion over the skin.

Lipids are considered to play an important role in the differentiation, structure, and function of the epidermis. Epidermal lipid composition changes dramatically during keratinization, beginning with large amounts of phospholipids and ending with predominantly ceramides, cholesterol, and fatty acids. Skin surface lipids of cats and dogs were studied by thin-layer chromatography and found to contain more sterol esters, free cholesterol, cholesterol esters, and diester waxes, but fewer triglycerides, monoglycerides, free fatty acids, monester waxes, and squalene, than those of humans.* It was suggested that the surface lipids of cats and dogs are mainly of epidermal origin, whereas those of humans are mainly of sebaceous gland origin.

EPIDERMOPOIESIS AND KERATOGENESIS

Normal epidermal homeostasis requires a finely tuned balance between growth and differentiation of keratinocytes. This balance must be greatly shifted in the direction of proliferation in response to injury and then must return to a state of homeostasis with healing. In addition, epidermal keratinocytes have important functions as regulators of cutaneous immunity and inflammation.

The most important product of the epidermis is keratin, a highly stable, disulfide bond–containing fibrous protein. This substance is the major barrier between animal and environment, the so-called miracle wrap of the body. Prekeratin, the fibrous protein synthesized in the keratinocytes of the stratum basale and stratum spinosum, appears to be the precursor of the fully differentiated stratum corneum proteins.[49, 140]

The epidermis is ectodermal in origin and normally undergoes an orderly pattern of proliferation, differentiation, and keratinization.[49] The factors controlling this orderly epidermal pattern are incompletely understood, but the protein kinase C/phospholipase C second messenger system, the calcium/calmodulin second messenger system, the receptor-linked tyrosine kinases, and the adenylate cyclase/cAMP-dependent protein kinases are important in coupling extracellular signals to essential biological processes such as the immune response, inflammation, differentiation, and proliferation.[49] Among the intrinsic factors known to play a modulating role in these processes are the dermis, EGF, FGFs, insulin-like growth factors, colony-stimulating factors, platelet-derived growth factor, TGFs, neuropeptides, interleukins, tumor necrosis factor, epidermal chalone, epibolin, interferons, acid hydrolases, arachidonic acid metabolites, proteolytic enzymes (endopeptidases and exopeptidases or peptidases) and various hormones (particularly epinephrine, vitamin D_3, and cortisol).[35, 49, 108, 111, 157] In addition, there appears to be a host of hormones and enzymes that can induce, increase, or both induce and increase the activity of the enzyme ornithine decarboxylase.[49] This enzyme is essential for the biosynthesis of polyamines (putrescine, spermidine, and spermine), which encourage epidermal proliferation. Numerous nutritional factors are also known to be important for normal keratinization, including protein, fatty acids, zinc, copper, vitamin A, and the B vitamins.[49]

Modern research in epidermal cellular and molecular biology recognizes four distinct cellular events in the process of cornification:[49] (1) keratinization (synthesis of the principal fibrous proteins of the keratinocyte), (2) keratohyalin synthesis (including the histidine-rich protein filaggrin), (3) the formation of the highly cross-linked, insoluble stratum corneum peripheral envelope (including the structural protein involucrin), and (4) the generation of neutral, lipid-enriched intercellular domains, resulting from the secretion of distinctive lamellar granules. The lamellar granules are synthesized primarily within the keratinocytes of the stratum spinosum and are then displaced to the apex and periphery of the cell as it reaches the stratum granulosum. They fuse with the plasma membrane and secrete their contents (neutral sugars linked to lipids, proteins, or both; hydrolytic enzymes; and sterols). Intercellular lipids then undergo

*See references 49, 91, 104, 105, 107, 131, 145, and 146.

substantial alterations and assume an integral role in the regulation of stratum corneum barrier function and desquamation.

Tritiated thymidine labeling techniques have shown that the turnover (cell renewal) time for the viable epidermis (stratum basale to stratum granulosum) of dogs is approximately 22 days.[12] Clipping the hair shortened the epidermal turnover time to approximately 15 days.[13] Surgically induced wounds in the skin of normal dogs greatly increased epidermal mitotic activity.[153] Epidermal turnover time in seborrheic Cocker spaniels and Irish setters was approximately 7 days.[14]

The growth characteristics, differentiation, cell surface markers, and morphology of canine keratinocytes grown in vitro have been reported.[135–138, 149–151] Cultured canine keratinocytes express pemphigus vulgaris, pemphigus foliaceus, and bullous pemphigoid antigens, and deposit laminin and Type IV collagen.[151] The use of cultured canine keratinocytes should provide a useful model for in vitro studies of epidermal kinetics, the pathogenesis of various dermatologic diseases, and the cutaneous effects of various pharmacologic agents.

CUTANEOUS ECOLOGY

The skin forms a protective barrier without which life would be impossible. This defense has three components: physical, chemical, and microbial.[49] Hair forms the first physical line of defense to prevent contact of pathogens with the skin and to minimize external physical or chemical insult to the skin. Hair may also harbor microorganisms.

The stratum corneum forms the basic physical defense barrier. Its thick, tightly packed keratinized cells are permeated by an emulsion of sebum and sweat that is concentrated in the outer layers of keratin, where it also functions as a physical barrier. In addition to its physical properties, the emulsion provides a chemical barrier to potential pathogens. Water-soluble substances in the emulsion include inorganic salts and proteins that inhibit microorganisms. Sodium chloride and the antiviral glycoprotein interferon, albumin, transferrin, complement, glucocorticoid, and immunoglobulins are in the emulsion.[49, 93] In the normal skin of dogs, (1) IgG and IgM are found in the interstitial spaces in the dermis, in dermal blood vessels, and in hair papillae; (2) IgM is found at the basement membrane zone of the epidermis, hair follicles, and sebaceous glands; (3) IgA is found in the apocrine sweat glands (suggesting that it functions as a cutaneous secretory immunoglobulin); and (4) C3 is found in the stratum corneum and in the dermal interstitial spaces.[46a, 47, 127, 128] In the cat, IgM has been detected at the basement membrane zone of the nasal planum.[78] The polymeric immunoglobulin receptor, secretory component, is expressed and synthesized by keratinocytes and the secretory and ductal epithelium of sweat glands.[63] This receptor can interact with IgA and IgM; this interaction may be a mechanism for protecting the skin from microbial agents and foreign antigens.

The single factor with the greatest influence on the flora is the degree of hydration of the stratum corneum.[26, 49] Increasing the quantity of water at the skin surface (increased ambient temperature, increased relative humidity, or occlusion) enormously increases the number of microorganisms. In general, the moist or greasy areas of the skin support the greatest populations of microorganisms. In addition to effects on microflora, epidermal water content appears to be important in the regulation of epidermal growth, keratinization, and permeability.[26]

The normal skin microflora also contributes to skin defense. Bacteria and, occasionally, yeasts and filamentous fungi are located in the superficial epidermis (especially in the intercellular spaces) and in the infundibulum of hair follicles. The normal flora is a mixture of bacteria that live in symbiosis. The flora may change with different cutaneous environments, which include such factors as pH, salinity, moisture, albumin level, and fatty acid level. The close relationship between the host and the microorganisms enables bacteria to occupy microbial niches and inhibit colonization by invading organisms.

Some organisms are believed to live and multiply on the skin, forming a permanent population; these are known as *residents,* and they may be reduced in number but not eliminated by degerming methods.[49, 107a] The resident skin flora is not spread out evenly over the surface but is aggregated in microcolonies of various sizes. Other microorganisms, called *transients,* are merely contaminants acquired from the environment and can be removed by simple hygienic measures. Recently, a third class of organisms, whose behavior falls between that of residents and transients, has been called the *nomads.*[107a] These are organisms that are readily able to take advantage of changes in the microenvironment of the skin surface and, thus, frequently become established and proliferate on the skin surface and deeper.

Most studies of the normal microbial flora of the skin of cats and dogs have been strictly qualitative. The skin is an exceedingly effective environmental sampler, providing a temporary haven and way station for all sorts of organisms. Thus, only repeated quantitative studies allow the researcher to make a reliable distinction between resident and transient bacteria.

In cats, most studies indicate that *Micrococcus* spp., coagulase-negative staphylococci, α-hemolytic streptococci, and *Acinetobacter* spp. are normal residents of the skin (see Chap. 4).[86, 103, 124] Coagulase-negative and coagulase-positive staphylococci are often isolated from the skin of normal cats.[33, 36] Of the coagulase-negative staphylococci, *Staphylococcus simulans* was isolated most frequently and is probably a normal resident. *S. capitis, S. epidermidis, S. haemolyticus, S. hominis, S. sciuri,* and *S. warneri* were isolated primarily from household cats as opposed to cattery cats, suggesting that cats acquire these species of staphylococci through human contact. Of the coagulase-positive staphylococci, *S. aureus* and *S. intermedius* were isolated more commonly from household cats than from cattery cats. Cats may be asymptomatic carriers of the dermatophyte *Microsporum canis* as well (see Chap. 5).[124]

In dogs, most studies indicate that *Micrococcus* spp., coagulase-negative staphylococci, α-hemolytic streptococci, and *Acinetobacter* spp. are normal residents of the skin (see Chap. 4).[33a, 103] Coagulase-negative and coagulase-positive staphylococci (especially *S. epidermidis, S. xylosus,* and *S. intermedius*) are regularly isolated from the skin and haircoat of normal dogs, and there are no significant quantitative or qualitative differences in the staphylococci of skin and hair or between species of staphylococci and body site.[2b, 2c, 33a, 85, 93a, 147] The anal, nasal, and oral mucocutaneous regions are also important sites of *S. intermedius* carriage.[2a, 36a] Recent findings[56a] indicate that *Propionibacterium acnes* can be found on the skin surface and in the hair follicles of dogs in sufficient numbers to be considered part of the normal canine flora. In addition, it is well known that many saprophytic fungi—including *Malassezia pachydermatis, Alternaria* spp., *Aspergillus* spp., and *Penicillium* spp.—can be cultured from the skin and hair of normal dogs and cats (see Chap. 5).[103, 124–126]

EPIDERMAL HISTOCHEMISTRY

Histochemical studies of normal cat and dog epidermis have demonstrated distinct oxidative enzyme activity in all layers except the stratum corneum.[59, 75, 99, 100] In addition, strong reactions to nonspecific esterases were demonstrated, especially in the stratum granulosum. Oxidative enzymes that were demonstrated included cytochrome oxidase, succinate dehydrogenase, malate dehydrogenase, isocitrate dehydrogenase, lactate dehydrogenase, glucose-6-phosphate dehydrogenase, nicotinamide-adenine dinucleotide phosphate, nicotinamide-adenine dinucleotide, and monoamine oxidase. Hydrolytic enzymes that were demonstrated included acid phosphatase, arylsulfatase, β-glucuronidase, and leucine aminopeptidase. Positive reactions for cholinesterases were not observed. Thus, the enzyme pattern of normal cat and dog epidermis shows only limited similarities to that of humans, especially regarding esterase distribution.

BASEMENT MEMBRANE ZONE

Basement membrane zones are the physicochemical interface between the epidermis and other skin structures (appendages, neural, vascular, smooth muscle) and the underlying or adjacent connective tissue (dermis).[42, 49, 140] This zone is important in (1) anchoring the epidermis to the dermis, (2) maintaining a functional and proliferative epidermis, (3) maintaining tissue architecture, (4) wound healing, and (5) functioning as a barrier. It is now believed that basement membranes may influence many aspects of cell and tissue behavior, including adhesion, cytoskeletal organization, migration, and differentiation.[31] The basement membrane zone is often poorly differentiated in H&E preparations, but it stains nicely with periodic acid–Schiff (PAS) stain (see Fig. 1:3 *H*).[123, 124, 134, 142] It is most prominent in nonhaired areas of the skin and at mucocutaneous junctions. As observed by light microscopy, the basement membrane zone comprises only the fibrous zone of the sublamina densa area and is about 20 times thicker than the actual basal lamina.

Ultrastructurally, the basement membrane zone can be divided into the following four components, proceeding from epidermis to dermis (Fig. 1:20): (1) the basal cell plasma membrane, (2) the lamina lucida (lamina rara), (3) the lamina densa (basal lamina), and (4) the sublamina densa area (lamina fibroreticularis), which includes the anchoring fibrils and the dermal microfibril bundles. The first three components appear to be primarily of epidermal origin. The precise biochemical and functional aspects of the basement membrane zone and its various components are still being unraveled. Presently recognized basement membrane zone components, their localization, and their presumed functions are listed in Table 1:1.[42, 49] The involvement of the basement membrane zone in many important dermatologic disorders has prompted most of the current research interest.

Dermis

The dermis (corium) is an integral part of the body's connective tissue system and is of mesodermal origin.[49] In areas of thick-haired skin, the dermis accounts for most of the depth, whereas the epidermis is thin. In very thin skin, the decreased thickness results from the thinness of the dermis. The dermis is composed of fibers, ground substance, and cells. It also

Table 1:1. Characteristics of Basement Membrane Zone Components

Component	Localization	Function
Bullous pemphigoid antigen	Basal cell hemidesmosome and lamina lucida	Adherence
19-DEJ-1	Basal cell hemidesmosome and lamina lucida	?
Kalinin	Basal cell hemidesmosome and lamina lucida	?
Cicatricial pemphigoid antigen	Lamina lucida	Adherence
Laminin	Lamina lucida (partly lamina densa)	Adherence
Nidogen/entactin	Lamina lucida (partly lamina densa)	Adherence
AA3	Lamina lucida	?
GB3	Lamina lucida and lamina densa	?
Type IV collagen	Lamina densa	Adherence, networking
Type V collagen	Lamina densa (partly lamina lucida)	?
LDA-1	Lamina densa	?
KF-1	Lamina densa	Adherence
Heparan sulfate	Lamina densa	Networking, electrical charge barrier
Chondroitin-6-sulfate	Lamina densa	Networking, electrical charge barrier
Fibronectin	Lamina densa and lamina lucida	Networking
Epidermolysis bullosa acquisita antigen	Sublamina densa area (partly lamina densa)	Adherence
Type VII collagen	Anchoring fibrils	Anchorage
AF1	Anchoring fibrils	Anchorage
AF2	Anchoring fibrils	Anchorage

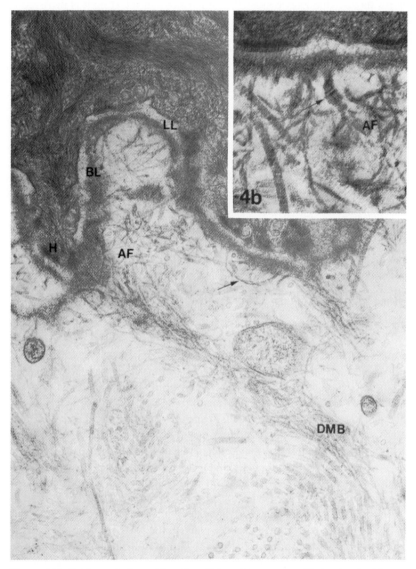

Figure 1:20. Epidermal–dermal junction. H, hemidesmosome; LL, lamina lucida. Anchoring fibrils (AF) form a meshwork beneath the lamina densa. A dermal macrofibril bundle (DMB) extends from the basal lamina (BL) into the dermis (×49,700). Inset: Sub–basal lamina fibrous components of the epidermal–dermal junction. Anchoring fibrils *(arrow)* with a central, asymmetric, cross-banded section. AF, interlocking meshwork of anchoring fibrils (×86,000). (From Briggaman, R., Wheeler, C. E., Jr.: The epidermal–dermal junction. J. Invest. Dermatol. 65:71–84, 1975.)

contains the epidermal appendages, arrector pili muscles, blood and lymph vessels, and nerves. Because the normal haired skin of cats and dogs does not have epidermal rete ridges, dermal papillae are not usually seen. Thus, a true papillary and reticular dermis, as described for humans, is not present in cats and dogs. The terms *superficial* and *deep* dermis are preferred. The dermis accounts for most of the tensile strength and elasticity of the skin; it is involved in the remodeling, maintenance, and repair of the skin; and it modulates the structure and function of the epidermis. The dermis of scrotal skin is unique in that it contains numerous large smooth muscle bundles (see Fig. 1:6).

DERMAL FIBERS

The dermal fibers are formed by fibroblasts and are collagenous, reticular, and elastic. *Collagenous fibers* (collagen) have great tensile strength and are the largest and most numerous fibers (accounting for approximately 90 per cent of all dermal fibers and 80 per cent of the dermal extracellular matrix) (see Fig. 1:3 *B*). They are thick bands composed of multiple protein fibrils and are differentially stained by Masson's trichrome. Collagen is a family of related molecules whose diverse biological roles include morphogenesis, tissue repair, cellular adhesion, cellular migration, chemotaxis, and platelet aggregation.[49] Collagen contains two unusual amino acids—hydroxylysine and 4-hydroxyproline—whose levels in urine have been used as indices of collagen turnover. *Reticular fibers* (reticulin) are fine, branching structures that closely approximate collagen with age. They can be detected best with special silver stains. *Elastin fibers* are composed of single fine branches that possess great elasticity and account for about 4 per cent of the dermal extracellular matrix. They are well visualized by Verhoeff's and van Gieson's elastin stains (see Fig. 1:3 *B*). The major component of elastic fibers is elastin, which contains two unique cross-linked amino acids (desmosine and isodesmosine) that are not found in other mammalian proteins.[49]

There are numerous (at least 13) genetically and structurally different types of collagen molecules.[49] Types I, III, and V collagen predominate in the dermis and account for approximately 87 per cent, 10 per cent, and 3 per cent, respectively, of the dermal collagen. Types I, III, V, and VI collagen appear to be distributed uniformly throughout the dermis. Types III and V collagen are also concentrated around blood vessels. Types IV (lamina densa) and V (lamina lucida) collagen are found in the basement membrane zone, and Type VII collagen is found in the anchoring fibrils of the basement membrane zone. The biosynthesis of collagen is a complex process of gene transposition and translation, intracellular modifications, packaging and secretion, extracellular modifications, and fibril assembly and cross-linking. Collagen abnormalities may result from genetic defects; from deficiencies of vitamin C, iron, and copper; and from β-aminopropionitrile poisoning (lathyrism). Collagen synthesis is stimulated by ascorbic acid (vitamin C), TGF-β, IL-1, insulin-like growth factor 1 (somatomedin C), insulin-like growth factor 2, superoxide generating systems, and bleomycin.[49] Collagen synthesis is inhibited by glucocorticoids, retinoids, vitamin D_3, parathormone, prostaglandin (PG) E_2, interferon-γ, D-penicillamine, and minoxidil.

Collagenases occupy a crucial position in both the normal and pathologic remodeling of collagen.[49] In the skin, a number of cell types contribute to connective tissue destruction by their capacity to synthesize and release collagenase. Dermal fibroblasts are the major source of skin collagenase under normal conditions of remodeling as well as in many pathologic conditions. However, under certain conditions keratinocytes, neutrophils, eosinophils, and macrophages can release a variety of proteolytic enzymes, including collagenase, and contribute to local connective tissue destruction in disease.

In general, the superficial dermis contains fine, loosely arranged collagen fibers that are irregularly distributed and a network of fine elastin fibers. The deep dermis contains thick, densely arranged collagen fibers that tend to parallel the skin surface and elastin fibers that are thicker and less numerous than those in the superficial dermis. In the superficial dermis, elastic fibers, known as *elaunin* fibers, are organized in an arcade-like arrangement.[49] From these, still thinner elastic fibers, called *oxytalan* fibers, ascend almost vertically to terminate at the dermoepidermal junction. Although elaunin and oxytalan fibers are part of the elastic fiber network, their exact biochemical composition and relation to mature elastic fibers are unknown. Elastases are proteolytic enzymes capable of degrading elastic fibers, and a variety of tissues and cells are capable of producing elastolytic enzymes. The elastases that are present in neutrophils and eosinophils are the most potent, and they readily degrade elastic fibers in disease states.

The indigenous interstitial cell of the dermis has been generically called a *fibroblast* and described as spindle-shaped (based on its appearance in paraffin- or plastic-embedded fixed tissue sections).[57] However, if tissues are studied by oxidative enzyme preparations on frozen sections or by electron microscopy, these cells are highly dendritic. It has been proposed that the so-called fibroblast would be more appropriately called the dermal dendrocyte.[57] These cells have been shown to be phagocytic (e.g., tatoo ink, melanin, hemosiderin) and positive for clotting enzyme factor XIIIa.

DERMAL GROUND SUBSTANCE

The ground (interstitial) substance is a viscoelastic gel-sol of fibroblast origin composed of glycosaminoglycans (formerly called mucopolysaccharides) usually linked in vivo to proteins (proteoglycans) and consisting principally of hyaluronic acid, dermatan sulfate (chondroitin sulfate B, decorin), chondroitin-4-sulfate (chondroitin sulfate A), and chondroitin-6-sulfate (chondroitin sulfate C).[49, 140] It fills the spaces and surrounds other structures of the dermis but allows electrolytes, nutrients, and cells to traverse it in passing from the dermal vessels to the avascular epidermis. The proteoglycans are extracellular and membrane-associated macromolecules that function in water storage and homeostasis; in the selective screening of substances; in the support of dermal structure; in lubrication; and in collagen fibrillogenesis, orientation, growth, and differentiation.

Fibronectins are widespread extracellular matrix and body fluid glycoproteins capable of multiple interactions with cell surfaces and other matrix components.[31, 32] They are produced by many cells, including keratinocytes, fibroblasts, endothelial cells, and histiocytes. The fibronectins moderate cell-to-cell interaction and cell adhesion to the substrate, and they modulate microvascular integrity, vascular permeability, basement membrane assembly, and wound healing. Fibronectin has been implicated in a variety of cell functions, including cell adhesion and morphology, opsonization, cytoskeletal organization, oncogenic transformation, cell migration, phagocytosis, hemostasis, and embryonic differentiation. Fibronectins are present in the dermis, especially perivascularly and perineurally, and within the lamina lucida and lamina densa of the basement membrane.

Small amounts of *mucin* (a blue-staining, granular- to stringy-appearing substance with H&E stain) are often seen in normal feline and canine skin, especially around appendages and blood vessels (see Fig. 1:3 *C*). In the Chinese Shar Pei, however, large amounts of mucin are normally found throughout the dermis, which could be confused with pathologic mucinosis (myxedema) in other breeds and species.

DERMAL CELLULAR ELEMENTS

The dermis is usually sparsely populated with cells.[49, 123, 124, 142] *Fibroblasts* are present throughout. *Melanocytes* may be seen near superficial dermal blood vessels, especially in dark-skinned dogs. They may also be seen around the hair bulbs in darkly colored dogs, especially Doberman pinschers and black Labrador retrievers.

Mast cells are most abundant around superficial dermal blood vessels and appendages. In dogs, as in cats, many mast cells are easily recognized with routine H & E stain. In cats, the cells have a ''fried-egg'' appearance, with the lightly stained intracytoplasmic granules giving the cytoplasm a stippled appearance. In both species, the mast cells are more easily recognized with special stains such as toluidine blue and acid orcein-Giemsa. In general, normal cat skin contains 4 to 20 mast cells per high-power microscopic field around superficial dermal blood vessels; normal dog skin contains 4 to 12 cells per high-power microscopic field.[103, 124, 148a]

Other cells that are occasionally seen in very small numbers in normal feline and canine skin include *neutrophils, eosinophils, lymphocytes, histiocytes,* and *plasma cells.*

Hair Follicles

Hair follicle morphogenesis is a complex process that occurs during the development of the skin, as part of the hair cycle, when skin repairs superficial wounds, and in response to certain pharmacologic agents.[49, 62] It is a complex, multistage process in which the epithelial cells of the hair follicle and the associated mesenchymal cells undergo a number of collaborative interactions. At each stage, the participating cells have different phenotypic properties and produce different products.

The hair shaft is divided into medulla, cortex, and cuticle.[49, 89, 120, 123, 124, 129] The *medulla,* the innermost region of the hair, is composed of longitudinal rows of cuboidal cells, or cells flattened from top to bottom. The cells are solid near the hair root, but the rest of the hair shaft contains air and glycogen vacuoles. The *cortex,* the middle layer, consists of completely cornified, spindle-shaped cells, whose long axis is parallel to the hair shaft. These cells contain the pigment that gives the hair its color. Pigment may also be present in the medulla, but there it has little influence on the color of the hair shaft. In general, the cortex accounts for one-sixth to one-third of the width of the hair shaft, and it contributes the most to the mechanical properties of hair fibers. The *cuticle,* the outermost layer of the hair, is formed by flat, cornified, anuclear cells arranged like slate on a roof, with the free edge of each cell facing the tip of the hair (Fig. 1:21). Secondary hairs have a narrower medulla and a more prominent cuticle than do primary hairs, and lanugo hairs have no medulla. In the cat, the profile of the hair shaft is distinctly serrated. The epicuticle is an amorphous external layer derived from cuticular cells, as an exocellular secretion, or from the outer portion of cuticular cell membranes.[129]

Hair follicles are usually positioned at a 30- to 60-degree angle to the skin surface. Cats and

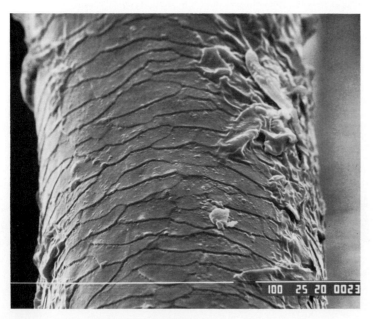

Figure 1:21. Scanning electron micrograph of canine hair showing shingle-like hair cuticle with globs of amorphous material on its surface.

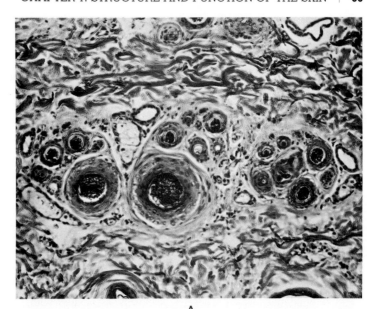

A

Figure 1:22. *A*, Three multiple hair follicle units (high power). *B*, Three apopilosebaceous complexes, each showing primary and secondary hairs, sebaceous and apocrine glands, and arrector pili muscles (high power).

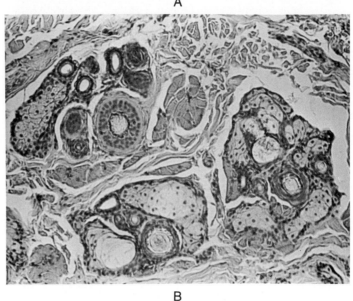

B

dogs have a compound hair follicle arrangement (Fig. 1:22). In general, a cluster consists of two to five large primary hairs surrounded by groups of smaller, secondary hairs. One of the primary hairs is the largest (central primary hair), and the remaining primary hairs are smaller (lateral primary hairs). Each primary hair has sebaceous and sweat glands and an arrector pili muscle. Secondary hairs may be accompanied only by sebaceous glands. The primary hairs generally emerge independently through separate pores; the secondary hairs emerge through a common pore. From five to 20 secondary hairs may accompany each primary hair. Hairs are present in groups of 100 to 600/cm² in the dog, with two to 15 hairs per group. In cats, there are 800 to 1600 groups/cm², with 10 to 20 hairs per group.[103, 124]

The hair follicle has five major components: the dermal hair papilla, the hair matrix, the hair itself, the inner root sheath, and other outer root sheath. The pluripotential cells of the hair matrix give rise to the hair and the inner root sheath. The outer root sheath represents a downward extension of the epidermis. Large hair follicles produce large hairs. For descriptive purposes, the hair follicle is divided into these three anatomic segments: (1) the *infundibulum,* or pilosebaceous region (the upper portion, which consists of the segment from the entrance of the sebaceous duct to the skin surface), (2) the *isthmus* (the middle portion, which consists of the segment between the entrance of the sebaceous duct and the attachment of the arrector pili muscle), and (3) the *inferior segment* (the lowest portion, which extends from the attachment of the arrector pili muscle to the dermal hair papilla).

The inner root sheath is composed of three concentric layers; from inside to outside these include (1) the *inner root sheath cuticle* (a flattened, single layer of overlapping cells that point toward the hair bulb and interlock with the cells of the hair cuticle), (2) the *Huxley layer* (one to three nucleated cells thick), and (3) the *Henle layer* (a single layer of non-nucleated cells). These layers contain eosinophilic cytoplasmic granules called *trichohyalin granules* (see Fig. 1:1 *F*). Trichohyalin is a major protein component of these granules, which are morphologic hallmarks of the inner root sheath and medullary cells of the hair follicle. Trichohyalin functions as a keratin-associated protein that promotes the lateral alignment and aggregation of parallel bundles of intermediate filaments in inner root sheath cells.[49, 109] The expression of trichohyalin is not unique to the hair follicle; it is found to occur normally in a number of other epithelial tissues, where it is closely associated with the expression of filaggrin, the major keratohyalin granule protein. The inner root sheath keratinizes and disintegrates when it reaches the level of the isthmus of the hair follicle. The prime function of the inner root sheath is to mold the hair within it, which it accomplishes by hardening in advance of the hair. The amino acid citrulline occurs in high concentrations in hair and trichohyalin granules; it has been used as a marker for hair follicle differentiation.

The outer root sheath is thickest near the epidermis and gradually decreases in thickness toward the hair bulb. In its lower portion (from the isthmus of the hair follicle downward), the outer root sheath is covered by the inner root sheath. It does not undergo keratinization, and its cells have a clear, vacuolated cytoplasm (glycogen). In the middle portion of the hair follicle (isthmus), the outer root sheath is no longer covered by the inner root sheath, and it does undergo trichilemmal keratinization (keratohyalin granules are not formed) (see Fig. 1:1*G*). In the upper portion of the hair follicle (infundibulum), the outer root sheath undergoes keratinization in the same fashion as occurs in the surface epidermis.

The outer root sheath is surrounded by two other prominent structures: a basement membrane zone, or glassy membrane (a downward reflection of the epidermal basement membrane zone), and a fibrous root sheath (a layer of dense connective tissue). Perifollicular mineralization of the basement membrane zone has been described in healthy Toy Poodles and Bedlington terriers.[51a, 130] This may also occur as a senile change in other breeds of dogs and must be differentiated from the perifollicular mineralization seen in dogs with naturally occurring or iatrogenic Cushing's syndrome.

The dermal hair papilla is continuous with the dermal connective tissue and is covered by a thin continuation of the basement membrane. The inner root sheath and hair grow from a layer of plump, nucleated epithelial cells that cover the papilla. These cells regularly show mitosis and are called the *hair matrix.* The importance of the papilla in the embryogenesis and subsequent cycling of hair follicles is well known.[31, 49] Additionally, the morphology of the dermal papilla changes throughout the hair growth cycle, being maximal in volume in mature anagen and minimal at telogen. This is mostly a result of changes in the amount of extracellular matrix within the papilla. In the anagen hair follicle, dermal papilla volume is proportional to the volume of the hair.

The hair follicles of animals with straight hair are straight, and those of animals with curly hair tend to be spiral in configuration. Follicular folds have been described in the hair follicles of animals. These structures represent multiple (1 to 23) corrugations of the inner root sheath, which project into the pilar canal immediately below the sebaceous duct opening. These folds are believed to be artifacts of fixation and processing because they are not seen in unprocessed sections cut by hand.[124, 129]

Two specialized types of tactile hairs are found in mammalian skin: sinus hairs and tylotrich hairs.[49, 103, 124, 129] *Sinus hairs* (vibrissae, whiskers) are found on the muzzle, lip, eyelid, face, and throat and on the palmar aspect of the carpus of cats (pili carpalis, carpal gland). These hairs are thick, stiff, and tapered distally. Sinus hairs are characterized by an endothelium-lined blood sinus interposed between the external root sheath of the follicle and an outer connective tissue capsule (Fig. 1:23). The sinus is divided into a superior, nontrabecular ring (or annular) sinus and an inferior, cavernous (or trabecular) sinus. A cushion-like thickening of mesenchyme *(sinus pad)* projects into the annular sinus. The cavernous sinuses are traversed by trabeculae containing many nerve fibers. Skeletal muscle fibers attach to the outer layer of the follicle. Pacinian corpuscles are situated close to the sinus hair follicles. Sinus hairs are thought to function as slow-adapting mechanoreceptors.

Tylotrich hairs are scattered among ordinary body hairs. The hair follicles are larger than surrounding follicles and contain a single stout hair and an annular complex of neurovascular tissue that surrounds the follicle at the level of the sebaceous glands. Tylotrich hairs are thought to function as rapid-adapting mechanoreceptors. Each tylotrich follicle is associated with a tylotrich pad (haarscheiben, touch corpuscle, touch dome, or Pinkus corpuscle) (see Fig. 1:9). Tylotrich pads are composed of a thickened and distinctive epidermis underlaid by a convex area of fine connective tissue that is highly vascularized and well innervated. Unmyelinated nerve fibers end as flat plaques in association with Merkel's cells, which serve as slow-adapting touch receptors.

The histologic appearance of hair follicles varies with the stage of the hair follicle cycle.[2, 49, 89] The *anagen* hair follicle is characterized by a well-developed, spindle-shaped dermal papilla, which is capped by the hair matrix (the ball-and-claw appearance) to form the hair follicle bulb (Fig. 1:24). Hair matrix cells are often heavily melanized and show mitotic activity.

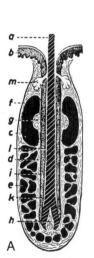
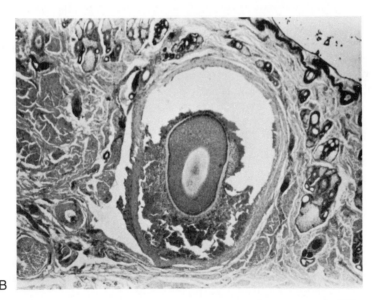

Figure 1:23. *A,* Hair follicle of sinus hair of cat in longitudinal section, semidiagrammatic (× 150): *a,* hair; *b,* epidermis; *c,* outer, *d,* inner layer of the dermal follicle; *e,* the blood sinus (this sinus has been differentiated into a nontrabecular annular sinus *f,* into which projects the sinus pad *g*); *h,* hair papilla; *i,* glassy membrane of the follicle; *k,* outer root sheath; *l,* inner root sheath; *m,* sebaceous glands. *B,* Tactile hair from upper lip of dog showing blood sinus (high power). (*A* from Trautmann, A., Fiebiger, J.: Fundamentals of the Histology of Domestic Animals. Cornell University Press, 1952, p. 342.)

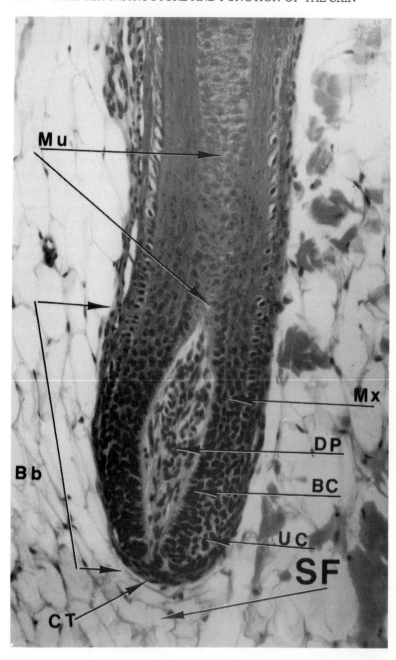

Figure 1:24. Anagen hair follicle. Longitudinal section of a secondary hair follicle at anagen stage, from the saddle region of a 28-month-old beagle. The bulb (Bb) extends into the subcutaneous fat (SF). The spindle-shaped dermal papilla (DP) extends toward the medulla of the hair (Mu); the base of the dermal papilla is continuous with the connective tissue (CT) of the hair follicle. The dermal papilla is surrounded by the matrix cells (Mx) of the bulb (Bb). The basal cells of the matrix are columnar (BC). The lower part of the bulb contains undifferentiated matrix cells (UC). (×350, H & E.) (From Al-Bagdadi, F. K., Titkemeyer, C. W., Lovell, J. E.: Histology of the hair cycle in male beagle dogs. Am. J. Vet. Res. 40:1734, 1979.)

The anagen hair follicle extends into the deep dermis and often into the subcutis. Anagen has been divided into six stages: Stages I through IV, referred to as *proanagen* (differentiation); Stage V, referred to as *mesanagen* (transition to rapid growth); and Stage VI, referred to as *metanagen* (posteruptive hair elongation).[129]

The *catagen* hair follicle is characterized by a thickened, irregular, undulating basement membrane zone, a thickened basement membrane zone between the hair matrix and the dermal papilla, a smaller bulb, and an ovoid or round dermal papilla (Fig. 1:25). The *telogen* hair follicle is characterized by the small dermal papilla that is separated from the bulb, by the lack of melanin and mitotic activity, and by the absence of the inner root sheath and the presence of club (brushlike) hair (Figs. 1:26 and 1:27).

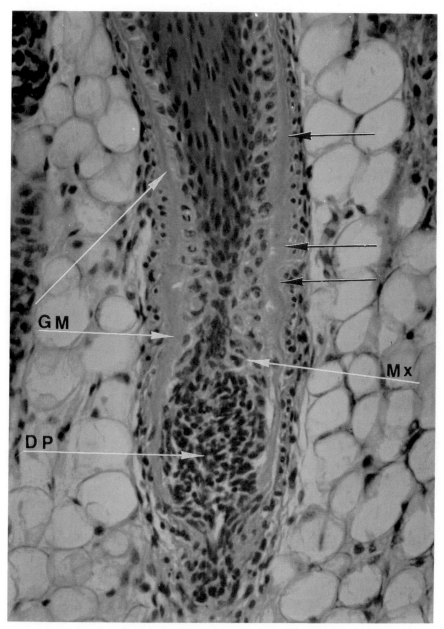

Figure 1:25. Catagen. Longitudinal section of a hair follicle at catagen stage from the saddle region of a 2-week-old beagle. The dermal papilla (DP) is oval in shape. The nuclei are crowded and the matrix cells (Mx) that border the dermal papilla have lost their orientation. The glassy membrane (GM) is thick and straight at the upper part of the hair follicle (single black unlabeled *arrow* in the upper part of the picture) while above the bulb, the glassy membrane is undulating (two black unlabeled *arrows* in the lower part of the picture) (×395, H & E). (From Al-Bagdadi, F. K., Titkemeyer, C. W., Lovell, J. E.: Histology of the hair cycle in male beagle dogs. Am. J. Vet. Res. 40:1734, 1979.)

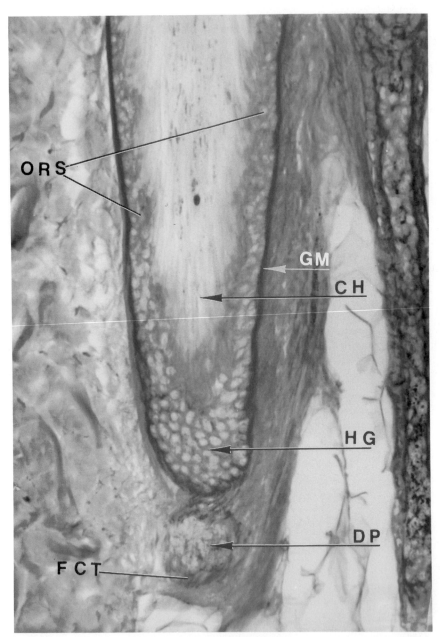

Figure 1:26. Telogen. Longitudinal section of a main hair follicle at telogen stage from the saddle region of a 3-month-old beagle. The dermal papilla (DP) is separated from the matrix cells of the hair follicle. It is surrounded by fibrous connective tissue (FCT) and appears to contact the base of the follicle at one point. The hair germ cells (HG) are located at the base of the club hair (CH). The cells of the outer root sheath (ORS) lack glycogen granules. The glassy membrane (GM) is thick and PAS positive. The hair follicle at this stage is surrounded by connective tissue that separates the follicle from the adipose tissue (×400). (From Al-Bagdadi, F. K., Titkemeyer, C. W., Lovell, J. E.: Histology of the hair cycle in male beagle dogs. Am. J. Vet. Res. 40:1734, 1979.)

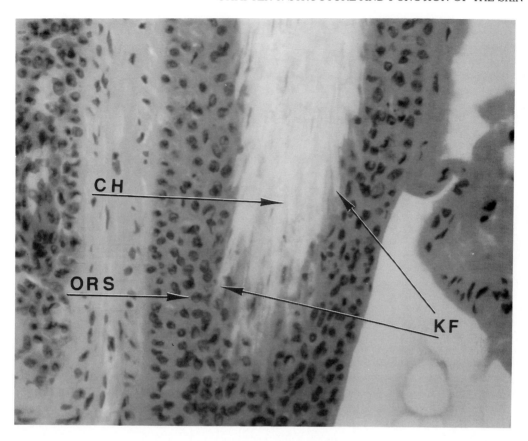

Figure 1:27. Club hair of telogen. Longitudinal section of a main hair follicle at telogen stage from the saddle region of a 24-month-old beagle. The club hair (CH) has many keratinized fibers (KF) that extend between the cells of the outer root sheath (ORS). These keratinized fibers give the club hair a brushlike appearance. (×465, H & E.) (From Al-Bagdadi, F. K., Titkemeyer, C. W., and Lovell, J. E.: Histology of the hair cycle in male beagle dogs. Am. J. Vet. Res. 40:1734, 1979.)

A hair plucked in anagen shows a larger expanded root that is moist and glistening, often pigmented and square at the end, and surrounded by a root sheath (see Chap. 2). A hair plucked in telogen shows both a club root, with no root sheath or pigment, and a keratinized sac.

Sebaceous Glands

Sebaceous (holocrine) glands are simple or branched alveolar glands distributed throughout all haired skin.[49, 77, 106, 123, 124] The glands usually open through a duct into the pilary canal in the infundibulum (pilosebaceous follicle). Sebaceous glands tend to be largest in areas where hair follicle density is lowest. They are largest and most numerous near mucocutaneous junctions, in the interdigital spaces, on the dorsal neck and rump, on the chin (submental organ), and on the dorsal tail (tail gland, supracaudal organ, preen gland). The submental organ (chin gland) also contains large nerve fibers, so it may serve tactile and scent-marking functions.[119] Sebaceous glands are not found in the footpads and nasal planum.

Sebaceous lobules are bordered by a basement membrane zone, on which there sits a single layer of deeply basophilic basal cells (called *reserve* cells) (Fig. 1:28). These cells become progressively more lipidized and eventually disintegrate to form sebum toward the center of the lobule. Sebaceous ducts are lined with squamous epithelium.

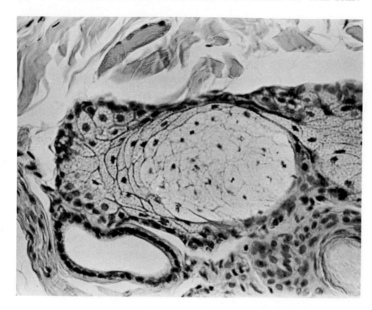

Figure 1:28. Canine sebaceous gland (apocrine duct in lower left corner, hair follicle and hair in lower right corner) (high power).

The oily secretion (sebum) produced by the sebaceous glands tends to keep the skin soft and pliable by forming a surface emulsion that spreads over the surface of the stratum corneum to retain moisture and thus maintain proper hydration. The oil film also spreads over the hair shafts and gives them a glossy sheen. During periods of illness or malnutrition, the haircoat may become dull and dry as a result of inadequate sebaceous gland function. In addition to its action as a physical barrier, the sebum-sweat emulsion forms a chemical barrier against potential pathogens (see Cutaneous Ecology in this chapter). Many of sebum's fatty acid constituents (linoleic, myristic, oleic, and palmitic acids) are known to have antimicrobial actions. Sebum may also have pheromonal properties.[77]

Sebaceous glands have an abundant blood supply and appear to be innervated. Their secretion is thought to be under hormonal control, with androgens causing hypertrophy and hyperplasia, and estrogens and glucocorticoids causing involution. The skin surface lipids of cats and dogs have been studied in some detail and are different from those of humans (see Horny Layer in this chapter). Enzyme histochemical studies have indicated that all mammalian sebaceous glands contain succinate acid dehydrogenase, cytochrome oxidase, and a few esterases.[102]

Sweat Glands

Because of investigations into the physiology and ultrastructural aspects of sweat production by sweat glands, it has been suggested that the *apocrine* and *eccrine* sweat glands would be more accurately called the *epitrichial* and *atrichial* sweat glands, respectively.[77] However, the terms *apocrine* and *eccrine* are still in common use and are therefore retained in this book.[38, 39, 43, 89, 119]

APOCRINE (EPITRICHIAL) SWEAT GLANDS

Apocrine sweat glands are generally coiled and saccular or tubular and are distributed throughout all haired skin.* They are not present in footpads or nasal planum. These glands are located below the sebaceous glands, and they usually open through a duct into the pilary canal in the infundibulum, above the sebaceous duct opening. Apocrine sweat glands tend to be larger in areas where hair follicle density is lower. They are largest and most numerous near mucocutaneous junctions, in interdigital spaces, and over the dorsal neck and rump.

---

*See references 39, 49, 76, 77, 106, 123, 124, and 134.

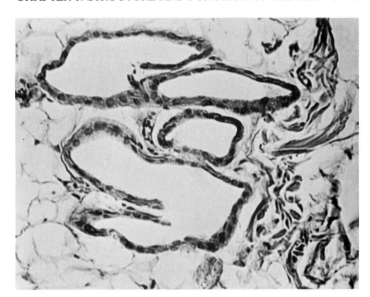

Figure 1:29. Section through coiled portion of apocrine sweat gland (high power).

The secretory portions of apocrine sweat glands consist of a single row of flattened to columnar epithelial (secretory) cells and a single layer of fusiform myoepithelial cells (Figs. 1:29 and 1:30). The apocrine sweat gland excretory duct is lined by two cuboidal to flattened epithelial cell layers and a luminal cuticle, but no myoepithelial cells.[72] In general, apocrine sweat glands do not appear to be innervated. Apocrine sweat probably has pheromonal and antimicrobial properties (IgA content).[77]

Enzyme histochemical studies have demonstrated alkaline phosphatase and acid phosphatase in apocrine sweat gland secretory epithelium.[71, 97, 102] Immunohistochemical studies show that the acini and ducts of canine apocrine sweat glands are positive for cytokeratin; associated myoepithelial cells are positive for both cytokeratin and S-100 protein.[41]

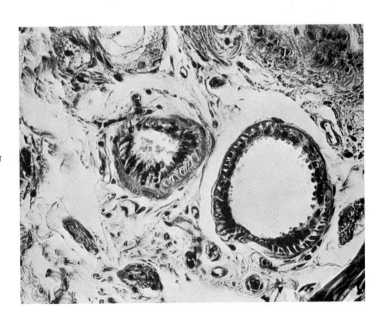

Figure 1:30. Apocrine gland showing secretory epithelium (high power).

ECCRINE (ATRICHIAL) SWEAT GLANDS

Eccrine (merocrine) sweat glands are found only in the footpads.[39, 124, 134, 142] These glands are small and tightly coiled, and they are located in the deep dermis and subcutis of the footpads. Secretory coils consist of a single layer of cuboidal to columnar epithelial cells and a single layer of fusiform myoepithelial cells (Fig. 1:31). The intradermal portion of the excretory duct consists of a double row of cuboidal epithelial cells. The excretory duct opens directly to the footpad surface.

Enzyme histochemical studies have demonstrated cytochrome oxidase, succinate and other dehydrogenases, phosphorylases, and alkaline phosphatase in eccrine sweat glands.[102] They are richly supplied with cholinesterase-positive nerves.[5, 7, 59, 102, 124, 152]

SWEATING AND THERMOREGULATION

The skin of cats and dogs does not possess the extensive superficial arteriovenous shunts of humans and swine that are designed to disseminate heat in hot weather. Carnivores also lack eccrine sweat glands in the hairy skin.

The frequency of sweating and the circumstances under which sweating occurs in cats and dogs are unclear. Some authors have stated that the dog shows great variation in the degree of apocrine sweating that takes place and that some breeds (especially German shepherds, Labrador retrievers, and other large breeds) may show visible sweating in the axillae, groin, and ventral abdomen.[103] Other authors have noted that apocrine sweating is occasionally seen in certain febrile and excited dogs.[106] Still others have reported the absence of apocrine sweating in dogs subjected to severe generalized temperature stress and in dogs that were struggling violently.[30] Eccrine sweating may be seen on the footpads of excited or agitated cats and dogs.[103]

In dogs, localized apocrine sweating can be produced by local heat applications and by the intradermal injection of various sympathomimetic (epinephrine, norepinephrine) and parasympathomimetic (acetylcholine, pilocarpine) drugs.[3, 4, 29, 70, 106] Because responses to all of these can be blocked by atropine, the final physiologic stimulus appears to be cholinergic. It has also been reported that asphyxiation or the intravenous injection of epinephrine or norepinephrine has produced generalized apocrine sweating in dogs.[70] Because these responses could not be blocked by adrenal medullectomy but were blocked by sympathetic denervation of skin, it was

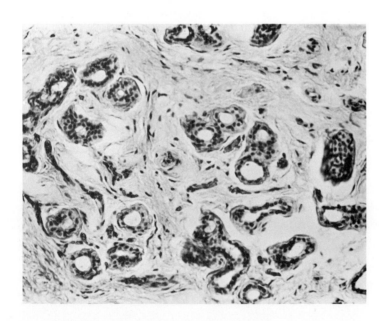

Figure 1:31. Eccrine sweat glands from canine footpad (high power).

concluded that canine apocrine sweating is primarily regulated by neural mechanisms and that humoral mechanisms play a subsidiary role. One group of researchers concluded—on the basis of available local and systemic pharmacologic data, local and generalized thermal responses, hypothalamic stimulation, and electron microscopic examinations—that canine apocrine sweat glands were not directly innervated and had little, if any, thermoregulatory importance.[18, 30] It was also suggested that because the only physiologic stimulus noted to produce apocrine sweating consistently in dogs was copulation, apocrine sweating in dogs served a predominantly pheromonal function.[30]

Eccrine sweating from the footpads of cats and dogs can be provoked by cholinergic stimuli and, less so, by adrenergic stimuli.[5–7, 124, 139] Atropine blocks glandular responses to these agents. Feline eccrine sweat contains lactate, glucose, sodium, potassium, chloride, and bicarbonate, and it differs from that of humans in that it is hypertonic and alkaline and contains much higher concentrations of sodium, potassium, and chloride.[21, 45, 134]

■ *Mechanisms to Conserve Heat.* When the environmental temperature falls, the body attempts to reduce heat loss by vasoconstriction in the skin and erection of the hairs to improve the insulating qualities of the skin and coat. The external temperature at which the heat-retaining mechanisms are no longer able to maintain a constant body temperature and at which heat production has to be increased is known as the *critical temperature*. Normal dogs with intact pelage had a critical temperature of 14°C (57°F); when their coats were shaved off, however, they had a critical temperature of 25°C (77°F).[103] Thick subcutaneous fat also acts as efficient insulating material. Nonfasting animals have a lower critical temperature than fasting individuals; therefore, the former are better able to tolerate a low environmental temperature. When the aforementioned mechanisms of heat conservation are no longer effective in preventing a fall in body temperature, an increase in heat production begins. A rapid increase in heat production is accomplished mainly by shivering. In normal dogs, shivering begins when the rectal temperature falls 1°C.

■ *Mechanisms to Dissipate Heat.* Heat is regularly lost from the body by radiation, conduction, and convection; vaporization of water from the skin and respiratory passages; and excretion of urine and feces. The excretory losses are relatively unimportant in heat dissipation. Ordinarily, 75 per cent of the heat loss is attributable to radiation, conduction, and convection. The efficiency of these mechanisms varies with the external temperature and humidity, and it is modified further by the animal's vasomotor and pilomotor responses. These become ineffective at higher temperatures, when heat loss by vaporization of water from the skin and lungs becomes more influential. Because they do not produce an abundance of eccrine sweat, dogs and cats have developed the ability to vaporize large volumes of water from their respiratory passages. In dogs, as the environmental temperature rises above 27 to 29°C (81 to 84°F), the rate of breathing also rises, but the depth of breathing (tidal volume) is markedly reduced. This helps prevent excess carbon dioxide blowoff and severe blood gas changes. At a rectal temperature of 40.5°C (105°F), the dog is in danger of thermal imbalance; at 43°C, collapse is imminent.

The rectal temperature of the cat begins to rise at an environmental temperature of 32°C (90°F), but as the respiratory rate increases, the tidal volume is only slightly reduced. As a result, the cat is more susceptible to a lowering of its blood CO_2 level (i.e., to respiratory alkalosis). The cat possesses an additional compensatory mechanism; a hot environment, or sympathetic stimulation, produces a copious flow of watery saliva from the submaxillary gland. The cat spreads this on its coat for additional water vaporization, and cooling results. Similar stimulation in dogs produces only a scanty secretion of thick saliva that cannot help the cooling process.[103]

The problem of temperature regulation in dogs and cats is often complicated by the physical condition of the coat and by the environmental temperature. Breeds with heavy coats intended for cold climates sometimes suffer when they are moved to regions of high temperatures. The problem is greatly accentuated by a matted, unkempt coat that stifles air circulation through the hair. Proper grooming greatly increases the comfort of these animals (see Chap. 3, Care of the Skin and Haircoat).

Specialized Glands

Specialized glands include the perianal (circumanal) glands, the glands of the external auditory canal, and the anal sacs (see Chap. 18), as well as the tail gland.

The *tail gland* (supracaudal gland, preen gland) of the dog is an oval-shaped area located on the dorsal surface of the tail over the fifth to seventh coccygeal vertebrae, about 5 cm distal to the anus.[39, 103] This gland is consistently present in wild Canidae; it is regarded as an atavism in dogs, however, because it is somewhat different in structure, is lacking in function, and is clearly visible in only about 5 per cent of all normal male dogs. The gland is present histologically in most dogs. The haircoat of the region is characterized by stiff, coarse hairs, each of which emerges singly from its follicle. The surface of the skin may be yellow and waxy from the abundant secretion of the numerous large glands in the area. This secretion may aid in olfactory species recognition. This area of the tail may be severely affected in seborrheic skin diseases and may also develop hyperplasia, cystic degeneration, infection, adenoma, and adenocarcinoma.

Histologically, the canine tail gland is composed predominantly of *hepatoid* cells, which are identical to those in the hepatoid (perianal, circumanal) glands. The glandular ducts empty into hair follicles. The tail gland and the circumanal glands are dependent on testosterone and form a topographic-ethnologic unit.

The tail gland (supracaudal organ) of the cat consists of numerous large sebaceous glands that run the entire length of the dorsal surface of the tail.[124, 134] Excess accumulation of glandular secretion in this area is called *stud tail.*

Arrector Pili Muscles

Arrector pili muscles are of mesenchymal origin and consist of smooth muscle with intracellular and extracellular vacuoles.[39, 49, 124, 134, 142] They are present in all haired skin and are largest in the dorsal neck and rump. Arrector pili muscles originate in the superficial dermis and insert approximately perpendicularly on a bulge of the primary hair follicles (see Fig. 1:34). Branching of these muscles is often seen in the superficial dermis. Arrector pili muscles are about one fourth to one half the diameter of central primary hair follicles in most haired skin areas but of equal diameter in the dorsal lumbar, dorsal sacral, and dorsal tail areas.

These muscles receive cholinergic innervation and contract in response to epinephrine and norepinephrine, producing piloerection. Arrector pili muscles probably function in thermoregulation and in the emptying of sebaceous glands.

Blood Vessels

Cutaneous blood vessels are generally arranged in three intercommunicating plexuses of arteries and veins (Fig. 1:32).[39, 49, 103, 119, 124] The deep plexus is found at the interface of the dermis and subcutis. Branches from this plexus descend into the subcutis and ascend to supply the lower portions of the hair follicles and the apocrine sweat glands. These ascending vessels continue upward to feed the middle plexus, which lies at the level of the sebaceous glands. The middle plexus gives off branches to the arrector pili muscles, ascending and descending branches that supply the middle portions of the hair follicles and the sebaceous glands, and ascending branches to feed the superficial plexus. Capillary loops that are immediately below the epidermis emanate from the superficial plexus and supply the epidermis and upper portion of the hair

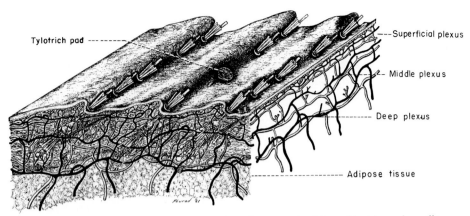

Tylotrich pad

Superficial plexus

Middle plexus

Deep plexus

Adipose tissue

Figure 1:32. Schematic section of skin of the dog, showing tylotrich pad (epidermal papilla, haarscheiben) and blood vessels (veins in black). (Modified from Evans, H. E.: Miller's Anatomy of the Dog, 3rd ed. W. B. Saunders Company, Philadelphia, 1993.)

follicles. Blood vessel endothelial cells are characterized (1) ultrastructurally by a peripheral basement membrane and intracytoplasmic Weibel-Palade bodies (rod-shaped tubular structures enveloped in a continuous single membrane), (2) by their possession of factor VIII antigen, plasminogen activators, and prostaglandins, and (3) by being phagocytic.[49, 89] Angiogenesis (new vessel formation) is controlled, at least in part, by mast cells (histamine), macrophages (tumor necrosis factor-α [TNF-α]), and TGF-β.[79]

Arteriovenous anastomoses are normal connections between arteries and veins that allow arterial blood to enter the venous circulation without passing through capillary beds.[49, 89, 103] Because of the size and position of these anastomoses, they can alter circulation dynamics and the blood supply to tissues. They occur in all areas of the skin but are most common over the extremities (especially the legs and ears). These anastomoses occur in all levels of the dermis but especially in the deep dermis.

Arteriovenous anastomoses show considerable variation in structure, ranging from simple, slightly coiled vessels to such complex structures as the *glomus,* a special arteriovenous shunt located within the deep dermis. Each glomus consists of an arterial segment and a venous segment. The arterial segment (Sucquet-Hoyer canal) branches from an arteriole. The wall shows a single layer of endothelium surrounded by a basement membrane zone and a tunica media that is densely packed with four to six layers of glomus cells. These cells are large and plump, have a clear cytoplasm, and resemble epithelioid cells. Glomus cells are generally regarded as modified smooth muscle cells. The venous segment is thinly walled and has a wide lumen.

Arteriovenous anastomoses are associated with thermoregulation. Constriction of the shunt restricts and dilatation enhances the blood flow to an area. Acetylcholine and histamine cause dilatation; epinephrine and norepinephrine cause constriction.

Pericytes, which vary from fusiform to clublike in appearance, are aligned parallel to blood vessels on their dermal side.[49, 89] They are contractile cells, containing actin-like and myosin-like filaments, and they are important in regulating capillary flow. The origin of pericytes is uncertain.

Veil cells are flat, fibroblast-like cells that surround all dermal microvessels.[49] Unlike pericytes, which are an integral component of the vascular wall and are enmeshed in the mural basement membrane material, veil cells are entirely external to the wall. The veil cell demarcates the vessel from the surrounding dermis and can be considered to be adventitial.

Lymph Vessels

Lymphatics arise from capillary networks that lie in the superficial dermis and surround the adnexa.[49, 89] The vessels arising from these networks drain into a subcutaneous lymphatic plexus. Lymph vessels are not usually seen above the middle dermis in routine histologic preparations of normal skin.

The lymphatics are essential for nutrition because they control the true microcirculation of the skin, the movement of interstitial tissue fluid. The supply, permeation, and removal of tissue fluid are important for proper function. The lymphatics are the drains that take away the debris and excess matter that result from daily wear and tear in the skin. They are essential channels for the return of protein and cells from the tissues to the blood stream and for linking the skin and regional lymph nodes in an immunoregulatory capacity.

In general, lymph vessels are distinguished from blood capillaries by (1) possessing wider and more angular lumina, (2) having flatter and more attenuated endothelial cells, (3) having no pericytes, and (4) containing no blood (Fig. 1:33). However, even the slightest injury disrupts the wall of a lymphatic or blood vessel or the intervening connective tissue. Consequently, traumatic fistulae are commonplace. These account for the common observation of blood flow in the lymphatics in inflamed skin.

Nerves

In general, cutaneous nerve fibers are associated with blood vessels (dual autonomic innervation of arteries), various cutaneous endorgans (tylotrich pad [see Fig. 1:9], Pacini's corpuscle, Meissner's corpuscle), sebaceous glands, hair follicles, and arrector pili muscles. The fibers occur as a subepidermal plexus (Fig. 1:34).[49] Some free nerve endings even penetrate the epidermis. The motor innervation of skin is attributable to sympathetic fibers of the autonomic nervous system. Although ordinarily considered somatic sensory nerves, the cutaneous nerve trunks carry myelinated postganglionic sympathetic fibers. Under the light microscope, small cutaneous nerves and free nerve endings can be demonstrated satisfactorily only by methylene blue staining, metallic impregnation, or histochemical techniques.

In addition to the important function of sensory perception (touch, heat, cold, pressure, pain, and itch), the dermal nerves promote the survival and proper functioning of the epidermis (i.e., the so-called trophic influences).

The area of skin supplied by the branches of one spinal nerve is known as its dermatome. Dermatomes have been mapped out for the cat[58, 84] and dog.[10, 11, 81, 144]

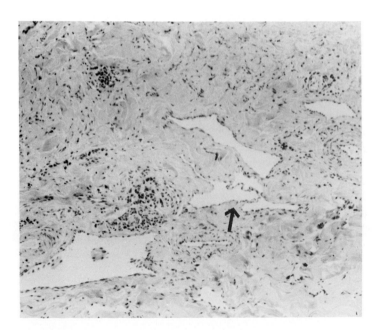

Figure 1:33. Lymphatic vessels *(arrow).* Note angular outline and absence of intravascular blood cells.

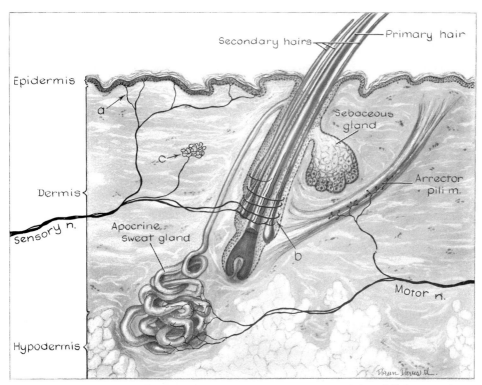

Figure 1:34. Nerve supply of the canine skin. *a*, dermal nerve network; *b*, hair follicle network; *c*, specialized end organs.

OVERVIEW OF CUTANEOUS SENSATION

The skin is a major sensory surface. Signals about external events and about the internal state of the skin are sent to the central nervous system by an array of receptor endings. *Thermoreceptors* fall into two categories: cold units, which are excited by falling skin temperatures, and warm units, which are excited by rising skin temperatures.[49] Cold units have C axons and A δ axons. Cold unit nerve terminals are branches of a small myelinated axon, ending in a small invagination in the basal cells of the epidermis.[49, 60, 61] Warm units also have C axons and A δ axons, but no morphologic nerve terminal has been identified.

Four types of sensitive *mechanoreceptor* units with A β axons are present in most skin regions.[49] Pacinian corpuscle units are extremely sensitive to small high-frequency vibrations and to very rapid transients.[49, 64, 96] Rapidly adapting units, which arise from Meissner or other encapsulated corpuscles, are primarily sensitive to the velocity of skin movement.[49, 74] In hairy skin, there are many afferent units that are excited by hair movement and have both A β and A δ axons. These provide the major tactile input from such regions. Guard and down hairs receive many nerve terminations of the lanceolate type. Such units can be subdivided into two major classes: (1) those excited only by movement of large guard or tylotrich hairs (G and T hair units), and (2) those excited by movement of all hairs, but especially by the fine down hairs (D hair units).[20, 23, 49, 66, 98, 148] The units driven from large hairs nearly always have A β axons; those driven from down hairs have A δ axons. G and T hair units are activated by rapid hair movements, and D hair units respond to slow movements. An additional class of units activated by static deflection of hairs is associated with large sinus hairs such as vibrissae.[49, 51] Finally, a characteristic class of unit with an unmyelinated axon, the C mechanoreceptor, is frequently encountered in cat haired skin.[49, 65] Slowly adapting Type I endings from Merkel's cell complexes signal about steady pressure.[49, 66, 67, 74] Slowly adapting Type II units, which are associated with Ruffini endings,[25, 49] show directional sensitivity in response to skin stretch and may play a proprioceptive role.

Most *nociceptor* units fall into two categories: A δ high-threshold mechanoreceptor units with A δ axons, and polymodal nociceptor units with C axons.[49] The latter afferents are classic pain receptors, responding to intense mechanical and thermal stimuli and to irritant chemicals. C-polymodal nociceptor units are involved with hyperalgesia and itch. They are responsible, through the local release of vasoactive agents, for the flare around skin injuries.[19, 49, 141]

PRURITUS

Pruritus, or itching, is an unpleasant sensation that provokes the desire to scratch.[49, 103, 140] It is the most common symptom in dermatology and may be due to specific dermatologic diseases or may be generalized without clinically evident skin disease. Pruritus may be sharp and well localized (epicritic), or it may be poorly localized and have a burning quality (protopathic).

The skin is richly endowed by a network of sensory nerves and receptors (see Fig. 1:33). The sensory nerves subserve hair follicles as well as encapsulated structures such as Pacini's, Meissner's, and Ruffini's corpuscles.[49] In addition, sensory nerves may end as free nerve endings, referred to as *penicillate* nerve endings. The penicillate endings arise from the terminal Schwann cell in the dermis as tuftlike structures and give rise to an arborizing network of fine nerves, and they terminate either subepidermally or intraepidermally. These unmyelinated penicillate nerve endings are limited to the skin, mucous membranes, and cornea.

Although several morphologically distinct end organs have been described, a specific end organ for pruritus has not been found. There is a clear association between C-polymodal nociceptor activation and itch that appears to involve a subpopulation of specific itch afferent fibers.[49, 141]

On the basis of the properties of afferent units, somatosensory activity can be subdivided into mechanoreceptors, thermoreceptors, and nociceptors. The nociceptors are involved in itch and pain. Nociceptors are supplied by A δ and C fibers. The A δ fibers (myelinated) conduct at about 10 to 20 m/sec and carry signals for spontaneous (physiologic), well-localized, pricking itch (epicritic itch). The C fibers (nonmyelinated) conduct more slowly (2 m/sec) and subserve unpleasant, diffuse burning (pathologic) itch (protopathic itch). Both fibers enter the dorsal root of the spinal cord, ascend in the dorsal column, and cross to the lateral spinothalamic tract. From there, they ascend to the thalamus and, via the internal capsule, to the sensory cortex. There, the itch sensation may be modified by emotional factors and competing cutaneous sensations.

At present, it has not been possible to isolate a universal mediator to explain pruritus, but a host of chemical mediators have been implicated (Table 1:2).[49, 129a, 129b] However, the pathophysiology of pruritus is complicated and poorly understood for most diseases in most species. The relative importance of these putative mediators and modulators of pruritus in any given species, disease, or individual is rarely known.

Table 1:2. Mediators and Modulators of Pruritus

Histamine	Proteases	Peptides
Eicosanoids	Kallikrein	Bradykinin
Leukotrienes	Cathepsins	Neuropeptides (opioids)
Prostaglandins	Trypsin	Substance P
Serotonin	Chymotrypsin	Vasoactive intestinal peptide
Platelet-activating factor	Fibrinolysin	
	Leukopeptidases	
	Plasmin	
	Microbial proteases	

For years it has been stated, on the basis of studies performed in humans, that proteolytic enzymes are the most important mediators of pruritus in dogs and cats and that histamine is relatively unimportant. Although there is no evidence to support the importance of proteolytic enzymes in dogs and cats, clinical studies have suggested that histamine and leukotrienes are important, and more so in cats than in dogs (see Chap. 8).[129a, 129b]

Central factors such as anxiety, boredom, or competing cutaneous sensations (e.g., pain, touch, heat, cold) can magnify or reduce the sensation of pruritus by selectively acting on the gate-control system.[49] For instance, pruritus is often worse at night because other sensory input is low. Although the mechanisms involved here are not clear, it has been suggested that stressful conditions may potentiate pruritus through the release of various opioid peptides (central opinergic pruritus).[49] Various neuropeptides, such as enkephalins, endorphins, and substance P, have been demonstrated to participate in the regulation of such cutaneous reactions as pruritus, pain, flushing, pigmentary changes, and inflammation.[49]

Subcutis

The subcutis (hypodermis) is of mesenchymal origin and is the deepest and usually thickest layer of the skin.* However, there is no subcutis in some areas for functional reasons (e.g., lip, cheek, eyelid, external ear, anus); in these areas, the dermis is in direct contact with musculature and fascia. Fibrous bands that are continuous with the fibrous structures of the dermis penetrate and lobulate the subcutaneous fat into lobules of lipocytes (adipocytes, fat cells) and form attachments of the skin to underlying fibrous skeletal components such as fascial sheets and periosteum. The superficial portion of the subcutis projects into the overlying dermis as *papillae adiposae*; these surround hair follicles, sweat glands, and vasculature to assist in protecting these structures from pressure and shearing forces. The subcutis is about 90 per cent triglyceride by weight, and it functions (1) as an energy reserve, (2) in thermogenesis and insulation, (3) as a protective padding and support, and (4) in maintaining surface contours. It is also important as a steroid reservoir, and as the site of steroid metabolism and estrogen production. The mature lipocyte is dominated by a large lipid droplet that leaves only a thin cytoplasmic rim and pushes the nucleus to one side.

Senility

Senile changes have been reported in the skin of aged dogs[15] and cats.[124] The hair of some dogs was dull and lusterless, with areas of alopecia and callus formation over pressure points. An increase in the number of white hairs on the muzzle and body was often seen. The footpads and noses of some dogs were hyperkeratotic, and claws tended to become malformed and brittle.

Histologically, one may see orthokeratotic hyperkeratosis of the epidermis and hair follicles, the latter often being atrophic and containing no hairs. Atrophy of the epidermis may be manifested as a single layer of flattened keratinocytes with pyknotic nuclei. Dermal changes may include decreased cellularity, fragmentation and granular degeneration of collagen bundles, and occasional diminution and fragmentation of elastic fibers. The solar elastosis (basophilic degeneration of elastic fibers) that characterizes aging human skin is not usually seen in aged dogs and cats. It is probable that the dense hair coat of dogs and cats protects them from the damaging effects of ultraviolet light.

Variable changes may be seen in the glands of the skin, including cystic dilatation of apocrine sweat glands and large, yellow, refractile granules in the secretory cells of the apocrine sweat glands. Arrector pili muscles become more eosinophilic, fragmented, and vacuolated.

Extensive studies in humans have demonstrated the following changes in senile skin: (1)

See references 38, 39, 117, 119, 123, 124, 134, and 142.

epidermal atrophy, decreased adherence of corneocytes, and flattening of the dermoepidermal junction; (2) decreased numbers of melanocytes and Langerhans' cells; (3) dermal atrophy (relatively acellular and avascular) and altered dermal collagen, elastin, and glycosaminoglycans; (4) atrophy of the subcutis; (5) attenuation of the eccrine and apocrine glands and decreased sebaceous gland secretion; (6) reduction of hair follicle density; (7) thinning, ridging, and lusterless nail plates; (8) decreased growth rate of the epidermis, hair, and nails; (9) delayed wound healing; (10) reduced dermal clearance of fluids and foreign materials; (11) compromised vascular responsiveness; (12) diminished eccrine and apocrine secretions; (13) reduced sensory perception; (14) reduced vitamin D production; (15) and impairment of the cutaneous immune and inflammatory responses.[49] Clinical correlates in humans of these intrinsic aging changes of the skin include alopecia, pallor, xerosis (dry skin), increased incidence of benign and malignant neoplasms, increased susceptibility to blister formation, predisposition to injury of the dermis and underlying tissues, increased risk of wound infections, and thermoregulatory disturbances.[49] Wounds in aged beagles and boxers healed less rapidly than in young dogs.[110]

REFERENCES

1. Al-Bagdadi, F. A., et al.: Hair follicle cycle and shedding in male beagle dogs. Am. J. Vet. Res. 38:611, 1977.
2. Al-Bagdadi, F. A., et al.: Histology of the hair cycle in male beagle dogs. Am. J. Vet. Res. 40:1734, 1979.
2a. Allaker, R. P., et al.: Population sites and frequency of staphylococci at mucocutaneous sites on healthy dogs. Vet. Rec. 103:303, 1992.
2b. Allaker, R. P., et al.: Occurrence of *Staphylococcus intermedius* on the hair and skin of normal dogs. Res. Vet. Sci. 52:174, 1992.
2c. Allaker, R. P., et al.: Colonization of neonatal puppies by staphylococci. Br. Vet. J.. 148:523, 1992.
3. Aoki, T. Wada, M.: Functional activity of the sweat glands in the hairy skin of the dog. Science 114:123, 1951.
4. Aoki, T.: Stimulation of the sweat glands in the hairy skin of dogs by adrenaline, noradrenaline, acetylcholine, mecholyl and pilocarpine. J. Invest. Dermatol. 24:545, 1955.
5. Aoki, T.: Cholinesterase activities associated with the sweat glands in the toe pads of the dog. Nature 202:1124, 1964.
6. Aoki, T.: Evidence for the discharge of cholinesterase into canine eccrine sweat. Nature 211:886, 1966.
7. Aoki, T.: Postnatal development of secretory function of sweat glands in the dog foot pads and cholinesterase activities associated with these glands. Tohoku J. Exp. Med. 110:173, 1973.
8. Badawi, H., et al.: Morphogenesis of the cutaneous vasculature in fetal dogs. Assiut. Vet. Med. J. 18:30, 1987.
9. Badawi, H., et al.: Histogenesis of the pilosebaceous apparatus in dogs. Assiut. Vet. Med. J. 18:38, 1987.
10. Bailey, C. S., et al.: Cutaneous innervation of the thorax and abdomen of the dog. Am. J. Vet. Res. 45:1689, 1984.
11. Bailey, C. S., et al.: Spinal nerve root origins of the cutaneous nerves of the canine pelvic limb. Am. J. Vet. Res. 49:115, 1988.
12. Baker, B. B., et al.: Epidermal cell renewal in the dog. Am. J. Vet. Res. 34:93, 1973.
13. Baker, B. B., et al.: Epidermal cell renewal in dogs after clipping of the hair. Am. J. Vet. Res. 35:445, 1974.
14. Baker, B. B., Maibach, H. I.: Epidermal cell renewal in seborrheic skin of dogs. Am. J. Vet. Res. 48:726, 1987.
15. Baker, K. P.: Senile changes of dog skin. J. Small Anim. Pract. 8:49, 1967.
16. Baker, K. P.: Hair growth and replacement in the cat. Br. Vet. J. 130:327, 1974.
17. Bell, R. L., et al.: Oxidative metabolism in perfused surviving dog skin. J. Invest. Dermatol. 31:13, 1958.
18. Bell, M., Montagna, W.: Innervation of sweat glands in horses and dogs. Br. J. Dermatol. 86:160, 1972.
19. Bessou, P., Perl, E. R.: Response of cutaneous sensory units with unmyelinated fibers to noxious stimuli. J. Neurophysiol. 32:1025, 1969.
20. Brown, A. G., Iggo, A.: A quantitative study of cutaneous receptors and afferent fibers in the cat and rabbit. J. Physiol. 193:707, 1967.
21. Brusilow, S. W., Munger, B.: Comparative physiology of sweat. Proc. Soc. Exp. Biol. Med. 110:317, 1962.
22. Burchill, S. A.: Regulation of tyrosinase in hair follicular melanocytes of the mouse during the synthesis of eumelanin and phaeomelanin. Ann. N.Y. Acad. Sci. 642:396, 1991.
23. Burgess, P. R., et al.: Receptor types in cat hairy skin supplied by myelinated fibers. J. Neurophysiol. 31:833, 1968.
24. Butler, W. F., Wright, A. I.: Hair growth in the greyhound. J. Small Anim. Pract. 22:655, 1981.
25. Chambers, M. R., et al.: The structure and function of the slowly adapting type II mechanoreceptor in hairy skin. Q. J. Exp. Physiol. 57:417, 1972.
26. Chesney, C. J.: Water and the skin—the forgotten molecule. Vet. Dermatol. News. 24:44, 1992.
27. Chuong, C. M., et al.: Adhesion molecules in skin development: Morphogenesis of feather and hair. Ann. N.Y. Acad. Sci. 642:263, 1991.
28. Comben, N.: Observations on the mode of growth of the hair of the dog. Br. Vet. J. 107:231, 1951.
29. Cotton, D. W. K., van Hasselt, P.: Sweating on the hairy surface of the beagle. J. Invest. Dermatol. 59:313, 1972.
30. Cotton, D. W. K., et al.: Nature of the sweat glands in the hairy skin of the Beagle. Dermatologica 150:75, 1975.

31. Couchman, J. R., et al.: Proteoglycans and glycoproteins in hair follicle development and cycling. Ann. N.Y. Acad. Sci. 642:243, 1991.
32. Couchman, J. R., et al.: Fibronectin-cell interactions. J. Invest. Dermatol. 94:7S, 1990.
33. Cox, H. U., et al.: Distribution of staphylococcal species on clinically healthy cats. Am. J. Vet. Res. 46:1824, 1985.
33a. Cox, H. U., et al.: Temporal study of staphylococcal species on healthy dogs. Am. J. Vet. Res. 49:747, 1988.
34. Craig, J. A., et al.: A practical guide to clinical oncology—4: Chemotherapy and immunotherapy. Vet. Med. 81:226, 1986.
35. DeLuca, H. F.: New concepts of vitamin D functions. Ann. N.Y. Acad. Sci. 669:59, 1992.
36. Devriese, L. A., et al.: Identification and characterization of staphylocci isolated from cats. Vet. Microbiol. 9:279, 1984.
36a. Devriese, L. A., DePelsmaecker, K.: The anal region as a main carrier site of *Staphylococcus intermedius* and *Streptococcus canis* in dogs. Vet. Rec. 121:302, 1987.
37. Draize, H. H.: The determination of the pH of the skin of man and common laboratory animals. J. Invest. Dermatol. 5:77, 1942.
38. Dyce, K. M., et al.: Textbook of Veterinary Anatomy. W.B. Saunders Co., Philadelphia, 1987.
39. Evans, H. E., Christensen, G. C.: Miller's Anatomy of the Dog, 2nd ed. W.B. Saunders Co., Philadelphia, 1979.
40. Feinman, J. M.: The Rex cat: A mutation for the masses. Vet. Med. (S.A.C.) 78:1717, 1983.
41. Ferrer, L., et al.: Immunocytochemical demonstration of intermediate filament proteins, S-100 protein and CEA in apocrine sweat glands and apocrine gland derived lesions of the dog. J. Vet. Med. A 37:569, 1990.
42. Fine, J. D.: Structure and antigenicity of the skin basement membrane zone. J. Cutan. Pathol. 18:401, 1991.
43. Fitzpatrick, T. B., et al.: Dermatology in General Medicine, 3rd ed. McGraw-Hill Book Co., New York, 1993.
44. Fjellner, B., et al.: Pruritus during standardized mental stress. Acta Derm. Venereol. (Stockh) 65:199, 1985.
45. Foster, K. A.: Composition of the secretion from the eccrine sweat glands of the cat's foot pad. J. Physiol. 184:66, 1966.
46. Galvin, S., et al.: The major pathways of keratinocyte differentiation as defined by keratin expression: An overview. Adv. Dermatol. 4:277, 1989.
46a. Garrot, C.: Les techniques peroxydase-antiperoxydase et immunofluorescence directe appliquée à la détection d'immunoglobulines et de complément C3 dans la peau saine du chien. Proc. GEDAC 7:14, 1991.
47. Garthwaite, G., et al.: Location of immunoglobulins and complement (C3) at the surface and within the skin of dogs. J. Comp. Pathol. 93:185, 1983.
48. Gibson, W. T., et al.: Immunology of the hair follicle. Ann. N.Y. Acad. Sci. 642:291, 1991.
49. Goldsmith, L. A. (ed.): Physiology, Biochemistry, and Molecular Biology of the Skin, 2nd ed. Oxford University Press, New York, 1991.
50. Goodell, E. M., et al.: Canine dendritic cells from peripheral blood and lymph nodes. Vet. Immunol. Immunopathol. 8:301, 1985.
51. Gottschaldt, K. M., et al.: Functional characteristics of mechanoreceptors in sinus hair follicles of the cat. J. Physiol. 235:287, 1973.
51a. Gross, T. L., et al.: Veterinary Dermatopathology. Mosby–Year Book, St. Louis, 1992.
52. Guaguère, E., et al.: Troubles de la pigmentation mélanique en dermatologie des carnivores Ire partie: Éléments de physiopathologie. Point Vét. 17:549, 1985.
53. Gunaratnam, P., Wilkinson, G. T.: A study of normal hair growth in the dog. J. Small Anim. Pract. 24:445, 1983.
54. Halata, Z.: Postnatale Entwicklung sensibler Nervenendigungen in der Unbehaarten Nasenhaut der Katze. Bib. Anat. 19:210, 1981.
55. Hale, P. A. Periodic hair shedding by a normal bitch. J. Small Anim. Pract. 23:345, 1982.
56. Halprin, K. M., Chow, D. C.: Metabolic pathways in perfused dog skin. J. Invest. Dermatol. 36:431, 1961.
56a. Harvey, R. G., et al.: Distribution of *propionibacteria* on dogs: A preliminary report of the findings on 11 dogs. J. Small Anim. Pract. 34:80, 1993.
57. Headington, J. T., Cerio R.: Dendritic cells and the dermis: 1990. Am. J. Dermatopathol. 12:217, 1990.
58. Hekmatpanah, J.: Organization of tactile dermatomes, C_1 through L_4 in cat. J. Neurophysiol. 24:129, 1961.
59. Hellman, K.: Cholinesterase and amine oxidase in the skin: A histochemical investigation. J. Physiol. 129:454, 1955.
60. Hensel, H., et al.: Structure and function of cold receptors. Pflug. Arch. 352:1, 1974.
61. Hensel, H.: Thermoreception and Temperature Regulation. Academic Press, New York, 1981.
62. Holbrook, K. A., Minami, S. I.: Hair follicle embryogenesis in the human. Characterization of events in vivo and in vitro. Ann. N.Y. Acad. Sci. 642:167, 1991.
63. Huff, J. C.: Epithelial polymeric immunoglobulin receptors. J. Invest. Dermatol. 94:74S, 1990.
64. Hunt, C. C.: On the nature of vibration receptors in the hindlimb of the cat. J. Physiol. 155:175, 1961.
65. Iggo, A.: Cutaneous mechanoreceptors with afferent C fibers. J. Physiol. 152:337, 1960.
66. Iggo, A.: Specific sensory structures in hairy skin. Acta Neuroreg. 24:175, 1962.
67. Iggo, A., Muir, A. R.: The structure and function of a slowly adapting touch corpuscle in hairy skin. J. Physiol. 200:763, 1969.
68. Irwin, D. H. G.: Tension lines in the skin of the dog. J. Small Anim. Pract. 7:593, 1966.
69. Itum, S., et al.: Mechanism of action of androgen in dermal papilla cells. Ann. N.Y. Acad. Sci. 642:385, 1991.
69a. Ivanyi, D., et al.: Patterns of expression of feline cytokeratins in healthy epithelia and mammary carcinoma cells. Am. J. Vet. Res. 53:304, 1992.
70. Iwabuchi, T.: General sweating on the hairy skin of the dog and its mechanism. J. Invest. Dermatol. 49:61, 1967.
71. Iwasaki, T.: An electron microscopic study on secretory process in canine apocrine sweat gland. Jpn. J. Vet. Sci. 43:733, 1981.

72. Iwasaki, T.: Electron microscopy of the canine apocrine sweat duct. Jpn. J. Vet. Sci. 45:739, 1983.
73. Jackson, R.: The lines of Blashko: A review and reconsideration. Br. J. Dermatol. 95:349, 1976.
74. Janig, W.: Morphology of rapidly and slowly adapting mechanoreceptors in the hairless skin of the cat's hind foot. Brain Res. 28:217, 1971.
75. Jenkinson, D. M., Blackburn, P. A.: The distribution of nerves, monoamine oxidase and cholinesterase in the skin of the dog and cat. Res. Vet. Sci. 9:521, 1968.
76. Jenkinson, D. M.: Myoepithelial cells of the sweat glands of domestic animals. Res. Vet. Sci. 12:152, 1971.
77. Jenkinson, D. M.: Sweat and sebaceous glands and their function in domestic animals. In: von Tscharner, C., Halliwell, R. E. W. (eds.). Advances in Veterinary Dermatology 1. Baillière Tindall, Philadelphia, 1990, p. 229.
78. Kalaher, K. M., et al.: Direct immunofluorescence testing of normal feline nasal planum and footpad. Cornell Vet. 80:105, 1990.
79. Karasek, M. A.: Mechanisms of angiogenesis in normal and diseased skin. Int. J. Dermatol. 30:831, 1991.
80. Kealey, T., et al.: Intermediary metabolism of the human hair follicle. Ann. N.Y. Acad. Sci. 642:301, 1991.
81. Kitchell, R. L., et al.: Electrophysiologic studies of the cutaneous nerves of the thoracic limb of the dog. Am. J. Vet. Res. 41:61, 1980.
82. Kral, F., Schwartzman, R. M.: Veterinary and Comparative Dermatology. J. B. Lippincott Co., Philadelphia, 1964.
83. Kubilus, J., et al.: Involucrin-like proteins in non-primates. J. Invest. Dermatol. 94:210, 1990.
84. Kuhn, R. A.: Organization of tactile dermatomes in cat and monkey. J. Neurophysiol 16:169, 1953.
85. Kwochka, K. W.: Qualitative and quantitative incidence of staphylococci on normal canine skin and haircoat: An investigation into the possibility of two different microbial populations. Proc. Annu. Meet. Am. Acad. Vet. Dermatol. and Am. Coll. Vet. Dermatol., 1986.
86. Kwochka, K. W.: Differential diagnosis of feline miliary dermatitis. In Kirk, R. W. (ed.). Current Veterinary Therapy, 9th ed. W.B. Saunders Co., Philadelphia, 1986, p. 538.
86a. Kwochka, K. W., Rademakers, A. M.: Cell proliferation of epidermis, hair follicles, and sebaceous glands of beagles and Cocker Spaniels with healthy skin. Am. J. Vet. Res. 50:587, 1989.
87. Lane, E. B., et al.: Stem cells in hair follicles. Cytoskeletal studies. Ann. N.Y. Acad. Sci. 642:197, 1991.
88. Lavker, R. M., et al.: Stem cells of pelage, vibrissae, and eyelash follicles: The hair cycle and tumor formation. Ann. N.Y. Acad. Sci. 642:214, 1991.
89. Lever, W. F., Schaumburg-Lever, G.: Histopathology of the Skin, 7th ed. J.B. Lippincott Co., Philadelphia, 1990.
90. Lichti, U.: Hair follicle transglutaminases. Ann. N.Y. Acad. Sci. 642:82, 1991.
91. Lindholm, J. S., et al.: Variation of skin surface lipid composition among mammals. Comp. Biochem. Physiol. [B]. 69:75, 1981.
92. Little, C. C.: The Inheritance of Coat Color in Dogs. Comstock Publishing Associates, Ithaca, NY, 1957.
93. Lloyd, D. H., Garthwaite, G.: Epidermal structure and surface topography of canine skin. Res. Vet. Sci. 33:99, 1982.
93a. Lloyd, D. H., et al.: Carriage of *Staphylococcus intermedius* on the ventral abdomen of clinically normal dogs and those with pyoderma. Vet. Dermatol. 2:161, 1991.
94. Lovell, J. E., Getty, R.: The hair follicle, epidermis, dermis, and skin glands of the dog. Am. J. Vet. Res. 18:873, 1957.
95. Lyne, A. G., Short, B. F.: Biology of the Skin and Hair Growth. American Elsevier Publishing Co., New York, 1965.
96. Lynn, B.: The nature and location of certain phasic mechanoreceptors in the cat's foot. J. Physiol. 201:765, 1969.
97. Machida, H., et al.: Histochemical and pharmacological properties of the sweat glands of the dog. Am. J. Vet. Res. 117:566, 1966.
98. Mann, S. J., Straile, W. E.: Tylotrich (hair) follicle: Association with a slowly adapting tactile receptor in the cat. Science 147:1043, 1965.
98a. Marchal, T.: Characterisation antigenique et distribution de la cellule de Langerhans du chien. Proc. GEDAC 7:3, 1991.
99. Meyer, W., Neurand, K.: The distribution of enzymes in the epidermis of the domestic cat. Arch. Dermatol. Res. 260:29, 1977.
100. Meyer, W., Neurand, K.: Zur Leuzinaminopeptidase-aktivitat in normaler und geschadigter Katzenhaut. Zbl. Vet. Med. 24:601, 1977.
101. Meyer, W., et al.: Zur Struktur und Funkten der Fussballen der Katze. Kleintierpraxis 35:67, 1990.
102. Montagna, W.: Comparative anatomy and physiology of the skin. Arch. Dermatol. 96:357, 1967.
103. Muller, G. H., et al.: Small Animal Dermatology, 4th ed. W.B. Saunders Co., Philadelphia, 1989.
104. Nicolaides, N., et al.: The skin surface lipids of man compared with those of eighteen species of animals. J. Invest. Dermatol. 51:83, 1968.
105. Nicolaides, N., et al.: Diesterwaxes in surface lipids of animal skin. Lipids 5:299, 1970.
106. Neilsen, S. W.: Glands of the canine skin—morphology and distribution. Am. J. Vet. Res. 14:448, 1953.
107. Nikkari, T.: Comparative chemistry of sebum. J. Invest. Dermatol. 62:257, 1974.
107a. Noble, W. C.: The Skin Microflora in Health and Disease. Cambridge University Press, Cambridge, 1993.
108. Nozaki, S., et al.: Keratinocyte cytokines. Adv. Dermatol. 7:83, 1992.
109. O'Guin, W. M., Manabe, M.: The role of trichohyalin in hair follicle differentiation and its expression in nonfollicular epithelia. Ann. N.Y. Acad. Sci. 642:51, 1991.
110. Orentreich, N., Selmanowitz, V. J.: Levels of biological functions with aging. Trans. N.Y. Acad. Sci. 31:992, 1969.
110a. Peaston, A. E., et al.: Evaluation of commercially available antibodies to cytokeratin. Intermediate filaments and laminin in normal cat pinna. J. Vet. Diagn. Invest. 4:306, 1992.

111. Pittelkow, M. R.: Growth factors in cutaneous biology and disease. Adv. Dermatol. 7:55, 1992.
112. Prieur, D. J., Collier, L. L.: The Maltese dilution of cats. Feline Pract. 14:23, 1984.
113. Queinnec, B.: Nomenclatures des robes du chat. Rev. Méd. Vét. 134:349, 1983.
114. Rach, J.: Coat color and personality. Cat Fancy, July 1988, p. 58.
115. Robinson, R.: Genetics for Cat Breeders. Pergamon Press, Oxford, 1977.
115a. Rook, A. J., Walton, G. S. Comparative Physiology and Pathology of the Skin. Blackwell Scientific Publications, Oxford, 1965.
116. Roy, W. E.: Role of the sweat gland in eczema in dogs. J. Am. Vet. Med. Assoc. 124:51, 1954.
116a. Rutner, D., et al.: Merkel cell carcinoma. J. Am. Acad. Dermatol. 29:143, 1993.
117. Ryan, T. J., Curri, S. B.: The structure of fat. Clin. Dermatol. 7:37, 1989.
118. Ryder, M. L.: Seasonal changes in the coat of the cat. Res. Vet. Sci. 21:280, 1976.
119. Schummer, A., et al.: The Circulatory System, the Skin, and the Cutaneous Organs of the Domestic Mammals. Verlag Paul Parey, Berlin, 1981.
120. Schwarz, R.: Haarwachstum und Haarwechsel—eine Zusätzliche funktonelle Beanspruchung der Haut—am Beispiel markhaltiger Primärhaarfollikel. Kleintierpraxis 37:67, 1992.
121. Schwarz, R., et al.: Die gesunde Haut von Hund und Katze. Kleintierpraxis 37:67, 1992.
122. Schwarz, R., et al.: Die gesunde Haut von Hund und Katze. Kleintierpraxis 26:395, 1981.
123. Schwarz R., et al.: Micromorphology of the skin (epidermis, dermis, subcutis) of the dog. Onderstepoort J. Vet. Res. 46:105, 1979.
124. Scott, D. W.: Feline dermatology 1900–1978: A monograph. J. Am. Anim. Hosp. Assoc. 16:331, 1980.
125. Scott, S. W.: Feline dermatology 1979–1982: Introspective retrospections. J. Am. Anim. Hosp. Assoc. 20:537, 1984.
126. Scott, D. W.: Feline dermatology 1983–1985: "The secret sits." J. Am. Anim. Hosp. Assoc. 20:537, 1984.
127. Scott, D. W., et al.: Pitfalls in immunofluorescence testing in canine dermatology. Cornell Vet. 73:131, 1983.
128. Scott, D. W., et al.: Pitfalls in immunofluorescence testing in dermatology. II. Pemphigus-like antibodies in the cat, and direct immunofluorescence testing of normal dog nose and lip. Cornell Vet. 73:275, 1983.
129. Scott, D. W.: The biology of hair growth and its disturbances. In: von Tscharner, C., Halliwell, R. E. W. (eds.). Advances in Veterinary Dermatology 1. Baillière Tindall, Philadelphia, 1990, p. 3.
129a. Scott, D. W., Miller, W. H., Jr.: Nonsteroidal anti-inflammatory agents in the management of canine allergic pruritus: J. S. Afr. Vet. Assoc. 64:52, 1993.
129b. Scott, D. W., Miller, W. H., Jr.: Medical management of allergic pruritus in the cat, with emphasis on feline atopy. J. S. Afr. Vet. Assoc. 64:103, 1993.
130. Seaman, W. J., Chang, S. H.: Dermal perifollicular mineralization of toy poodle bitches. Vet. Pathol. 21:122, 1984.
131. Sharaf, D. M., et al.: Skin surface lipids of the dog. Lipids 12:786, 1977.
132. Sheretz, E. C.: Misuse of hair analysis as a diagnostic tool. Arch. Dermatol. 121:1504, 1985.
132a. Smack, D. P., et al.: Keratin and keratinization. J. Am. Acad. Dermatol. 30:85, 1994.
133. Spearman, R. I. C.: The Integument. Cambridge University Press, London, 1973.
134. Strickland, J. H., Calhoun, M. L.: The integumentary system of the cat. Am. J. Vet. Res. 24:1018, 1963.
135. Suter, M. M., et al.: Extracellular ATP and some of its analogs induce transient rises in cytosolic free calcium in individual canine keratinocytes. J. Invest. Dermatol. 97:223, 1991.
136. Suter, M. M., et al.: Monoclonal antibodies: Cell surface markers for canine keratinocytes. Am. J. Vet. Res. 40:1367, 1987.
137. Suter, M. M., et al.: Keratinocyte differentiation in the dog. In: von Tscharner, C., Halliwell, R. E. W. (eds.). Advances in Veterinary Dermatology 1. Baillière Tindall, Philadelphia, 1990, p. 252.
138. Suter, M. M., et al.: Comparison of growth and differentiation of normal and neoplastic canine keratinocyte cultures. Vet. Pathol. 28:131, 1991.
139. Takahashi, Y.: Functional activity of the eccrine sweat glands in the toe-pads of the dog. Tohoku J. Exp. Med. 83:205, 1964.
140. Thoday, A. J., Friedmann, P.S.: Scientific Basis of Dermatology. A Physiological Approach. Churchill Livingstone, New York, 1986.
141. Tuckett, R. P., Wei, J. Y.: Response to an itch-producing substance in the cat. II. Cutaneous receptor populations with unmyelinated axons. Brain Res. 413:95, 1987.
142. Webb, A. J., Calhoun, M. L.: The microscopic anatomy of the skin of mongrel dogs. Am. J. Vet. Res. 15:274, 1954.
143. Weinberg, W. C., et al.: Modulation of hair follicle cell proliferation and collagenolytic activity by specific growth factors. Ann. N.Y. Acad. Sci. 642:281, 1991.
144. Whalen, L. R., Kitchell, R. L.: Electrophysiologic studies of the cutaneous nerves of the head of the dog. Am. J. Vet. Res. 44:615, 1983.
145. Wheatley, V. R., Sher, D. W.: Studies of the lipids of dog skin. I. The chemical composition of dog skin lipids. J. Invest. Dermatol. 36:169, 1961.
146. Wheatley, V. R., et al.: Studies of the lipids of dog skin. II. Observations of the lipid metabolism of perfused surviving dog skin. J. Invest. Dermatol. 36:237, 1961.
147. White, S. D., et al.: Occurrence of *Staphylococcus aureus* on the clinically normal canine haircoat. Am. J. Vet. Res. 44:332, 1983.
148. Whitehorn, D., et al.: Cutaneous receptors supplied by myelinated fibers in the cat. I. Number of receptors innervated by a single nerve. J. Neurophysiol. 37:1361, 1974.
148a. Wilkie, J. S. N., et al.: Morphometric analyses of the skin of dogs with atopic dermatitis and correlations with cutaneous and plasma histamine and total serum IgE. Vet. Pathol. 27:179, 1990.

149. Wilkinson, J. E., et al.: Long-term cultivation of canine keratinocytes. J. Invest. Dermatol. 88:202, 1987.
150. Wilkinson, J. E., et al.: Ultrastructure of cultured canine oral keratinocytes. Am. J. Vet. Res. 50:1161, 1989.
151. Wilkinson, J. E., et al.: Antigen expression in cultured oral keratinocytes from dogs. Am. J. Vet. Res. 52:445, 1991.
152. Winkelmann, R. K., Schmit, R. W.: Cholinesterase in the skin of the rat, dog, cat, guinea pig and rabbit. J. Invest. Dermatol. 33:185, 1959.
153. Winstanley, E. W.: The rate of mitotic division in regenerating epithelium in the dog. Res. Vet. Sci. 18:144, 1975.
154. Wright, M., Walter, S.: The Book of the Cat. Summit Books, New York, 1980.
155. Yaar, M., Gilchrest, B. A.: Human melanocyte growth and differentiation: A decade of new data. J. Invest. Dermatol. 97:611, 1991.
156. Yager, J. A., Scott, D. W. The skin and appendages. In: Jubb, K. V. F., et al. (eds.). Pathology of Domestic Animals, 4th ed. Vol. 1. Academic Press, New York, 1993, p. 531.
157. Yates, R. A., et al.: Epidermal growth factor and related growth factors. Int. J. Dermatol. 30:687, 1991.
158. Zlotkin, S. H.: Hair analysis. A useful tool or a waste of money? Int. J. Dermatol. 24:161, 1985.

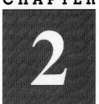

Diagnostic Methods

■

Chapter Outline

■ THE SYSTEMATIC APPROACH

Dermatologic diseases offer several unique opportunities for the practitioner. The progression of skin lesions and diseases can often be determined with a good history. Incomplete histories may eventually be amended because the chronic, recurrent nature of many diseases allows the practitioner to instruct clients in what observations they should try to make. The educated client may then add relevant information about the course of the disease. The physical examination reveals the gross pathologic lesions that are present for direct examination. With no other organ system is this great amount of information so readily available.

To benefit optimally from these opportunities, the clinician uses a systematic approach; this greatly increases the probability of determining the correct diagnosis in the most cost-effective manner. Ideally, a thorough examination and appropriate diagnostic procedures are accomplished the first time that the patient is seen and before any masking treatment has been initiated. However, in practice, many clients are reluctant to spend money on diagnostic tests, particularly for the initial occurrence of a problem. This makes a thorough history and physical examination even more important, as they often are the only tools available for arriving at a differential diagnosis.

At the first visit, it is important to establish the client's reliability as a historian and observer. The least expensive tool available to the practitioner is the education of the client about signs and symptoms to look for. The clinician can develop a better relationship with clients and gain valuable information by training clients in what they should observe and watch for, especially if there is a poor response to treatment or a recurrence. Spending some time educating the client in the value of this information often leads to better acceptance of the costs associated with future treatment.

A rational approach to the accurate diagnosis of dermatologic diseases is presented in Table 2:1.

Table 2:1. Steps to a Dermatologic Diagnosis

Major Step	Key Points to Determine or Questions to Answer
Chief complaint	Why is the client seeking veterinary care?
Signalment	Record the animal's age, breed, sex, and weight
Dermatologic history	Obtain data about the original lesion's location, appearance, onset, and rate of progression. Also determine the degree of pruritus, contagion to other animals or people, and possible seasonal incidence. Relationship to diet and environmental factors and the response to previous medications are also important
Previous medical history	Medical history that does not directly seem to relate should also be reviewed
Client credibility	Determine what the clients initially noticed that indicated a problem. Repeat questions and ask in a different way to determine how certain the clients are and whether they understand the questions
Physical examination	Determine the distribution pattern and the regional location of lesions. Certain patterns are diagnostically significant
	Closely examine the skin to identify primary and secondary lesions
	Determine skin and hair quality (e.g., thin, thick, turgid, elastic, dull, oily, or dry)
	Observe the configurations of specific skin lesions and their relationship to each other
Differential diagnosis	Differential diagnosis is developed on the basis of the preceding data. The most likely diagnoses are recorded in order of probability
Diagnostic or therapeutic plan	A plan is presented to the client. The client and the clinician together then agree on a plan
Diagnostic and laboratory aids	Simple and inexpensive office diagnostic procedures that confirm or rule out any of the most likely (first three or four) differential diagnostic possibilities should be done
	More complex or expensive diagnostic tests or procedures are then recommended
	Clients may elect to forgo these tests and pursue less likely differential diagnostic possibilities in attempts to save money. Often, this approach is not cost effective when the expense of inefficient medications and repeated examination is considered
Trial therapy	Clients may elect to pursue a therapeutic trial instead of diagnostic procedures. Trial therapies should be selected so that further diagnostic information is obtained. Generally, glucocorticoids and progestational drugs are not acceptable because little diagnostic information is obtained
Narrowing the differential diagnosis	Plan additional tests, observations of therapeutic trials, and re-evaluations of signs and symptoms to narrow the list and provide a definitive diagnosis

■ RECORDS

Recording historical facts, physical examination findings, and laboratory data in a systematic way is particularly important for patients with skin disease. Many dermatoses are chronic, and skin lesions may be slow to change. For this reason, many practitioners use outline sketches of the patient, which enable the clinician to draw the location and the extent of lesions.

Figure 2:1 is a record form for noting physical examination and laboratory findings for dermatology cases. Most importantly, the form leads the clinician to consider the case in a systematic manner. It also enables one to apply pertinent descriptive terms, saves time, and ensures that no important information is omitted. This form details only dermatologic data and should be used as a supplement to the general history and physical examination record. A

NEW YORK STATE COLLEGE OF VETERINARY MEDICINE—VETERINARY TEACHING HOSPITAL

DERMATOLOGY

DATE: _____

REF. DVM _____

CLINICIAN _____

SECONDARY # _____

PRIMARY LESIONS (Circle)

Macule	Patch	Papule	Plaque
Vesicle	Bulla	Pustule	Wheal
Nodule	Tumor		

SECONDARY LESIONS (Circle)

Scale   Epidermal collarette   Scar
Ulcer   Erosion   Crust   Excoriation
Fissure   Comedone   Cyst   Abscess
Hypopigmentation   Hyperpigmentation   Erythema
Hyperkeratosis   Callus   Alopecia

Pruritus:

Parasites:

SKIN CHANGES

Elasticity + −   Extensibility + −
Thickness + −

QUALITY OF HAIR COAT   OTHER FACTORS

Epilation: + −   Footpads
Pelage is: Dry,   Nails
  Brittle, Dull, Oily   Hyperhidrosis

CONFIGURATION OF LESIONS

Linear   Annular (Target)   Grouped

DIFFERENTIAL DIAGNOSIS

DISTRIBUTION OF LESIONS

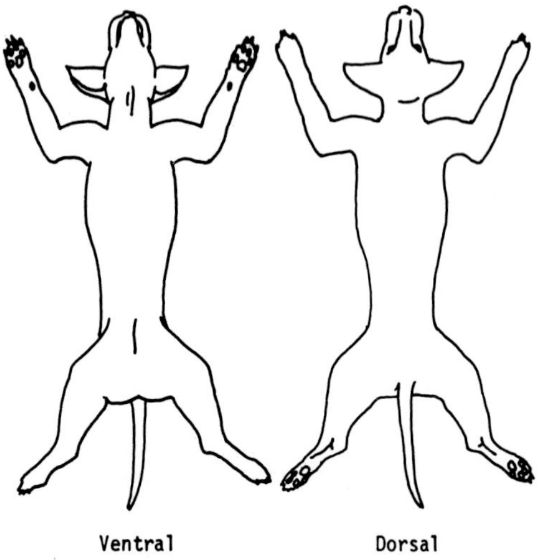

Ventral   Dorsal

LABORATORY TESTS

Scotch Tape: _____Wood's Light + −
Skin Scraping: _____
KOH Digestion: _____
Direct Smear: _____
Fungal Culture: _____
Bacterial Culture: _____
Sensitivity: _____
Allergy: _____
_____
Endocrine: _____
Immune:
  D.I.T.: _____
  I.I.T.: _____
  ANA: _____
  Other: _____
Biopsy:

Figure 2:1. Dermatology examination sheet.

special dermatologic history form is also useful, especially for patients with allergies and chronic diseases (Fig. 2:2).

The disadvantage of the forms is that many chronic cases have tremendous variations in the type of lesions and their distribution, making a map confusing. For example, how would one draw the following alopecia lesion? A 10-cm plaque in the flank fold has a central (8-cm) zone of lichenification, hyperpigmentation, alopecia, and crusts. The outer (2-cm) margin is alopecic and has a papular dermatitis with mild hyperpigmentation of lattice configuration. Peripheral to the plaque are occasional papules and pustules. Representing several different lesions on a small diagram is difficult or, if done, is often unreadable. This can make a diagram unsatisfactory to use. Therefore, the authors have found that brief written descriptions of lesions in various body regions are preferable to diagrams in complicated cases.

■ HISTORY

General Concepts

The pet's disease is like an unsolved mystery in which the client is the witness to what has occurred and the veterinarian is the detective who must ascertain what the client observed. As this information is extracted, the veterinarian becomes the lawyer to determine whether the client is a credible or qualified witness. Obtaining a thorough history and being attentive to clues from the client are skills that must be practiced and developed by the clinician in order to develop a tentative diagnosis. A comprehensive history in conjunction with a thorough dermatologic examination is helpful for another practical reason: this is often when the veterinarian initially establishes her or his credibility as a professional with the client. In veterinary dermatology, the client-veterinarian relationship is often important for a successful outcome. Because many chronic diseases necessitate lifelong control and can be frustrating for client and veterinarian alike, it is critical for the client-veterinarian relationship to start well. If the veterinarian is thorough and obtains the most information possible from the history and the dermatologic examination, the client is more likely to recognize the effort and expertise of the veterinarian. These clients are often more agreeable to pursuing diagnostic tests or trial therapies if the information from the initial exhaustive examination is not sufficient for a diagnosis. Cursory examinations leave a sense of insecurity in some clients, making them reluctant to follow recommendations based on such examinations.

Owner's Chief Complaint

The owner's chief complaint, or chief cause of concern, is often one of the major signs initially used in establishing a differential diagnosis. Addressing the client's chief complaint is an important step in achieving satisfaction of clients and obtaining their confidence and often initiates a favorable client-veterinarian relationship. Other findings not directly related to the chief complaint may be uncovered. Although these additional findings are important to discuss, the client's chief complaint must always be addressed.

Age

Some dermatologic disorders are age related, so age is important in the dermatologic history.[5–8] For example, demodicosis usually begins in young dogs before sexual maturity. Allergies tend to appear in more mature animals, probably because repeated exposure to the antigen must occur and the immune response has to occur before clinical signs develop. Reactivity to intradermal testing in cats has also been correlated with age.[40] Hormonal disorders tend to occur more frequently in animals between 6 and 10 years of age, and most neoplasms develop in mature to older patients. Most of the ages listed in Table 2:2 refer to the usual age at the beginning of the disease, not necessarily the age at which the animal presents.

NEW YORK STATE COLLEGE OF VETERINARY MEDICINE—VETERINARY TEACHING HOSPITAL

DATE: _____

DERMATOLOGY HISTORY SHEET

CHIEF COMPLAINT(S) _____

_____

_____

_____

_____

AGE PURCHASED _____

KENNEL ____PET SHOP ____PRIVATE ____WHERE ____

REF. DVM _____

CLINICIAN _____

SECONDARY #_____

HAS ANIMAL BEEN OUT OF AREA? YES ____NO _____

IF YES—WHERE _____

Date Problem First Noticed _____ Age _____Is It Year Round? Yes _____No _____

If Seasonal, Is It Worse: Spring _____Summer _____Fall _____Winter _____

Where Did Problem Begin? _____

What Did It Look Like Then? _____

How Has It Changed or Spread? _____

Are Other Animals or People Affected? Yes _____No _____If So Describe _____

When Did You Last See Fleas? _____

Describe Animal's Indoor Environment _____

Time Indoors _____% _____

Describe Animal's Outdoor Environment _____

Time Outdoors _____%_____

Does Animal Itch? Yes _____ No _____ When? Constantly _____Sporadically _____Night _____

Animal's Diet _____

What Medications Have Been Used? List Effects and Dates Used _____

_____

_____

Other Illnesses of Animal _____

What Other Facts Do You Think Would Be Helpful? _____

_____

_____

_____

(Use Reverse Side If Needed)

Figure 2:2. Dermatology history sheet.

Table 2:2. Skin Disease With Frequent Age-Related Onset (Strong Clinical Impression)

Age	Disease
Younger than 6 months	Alopecia universalis
	Black hair follicle dysplasia
	Canine muzzle furunculosis
	Cutaneous asthenia
	Demodicosis
	Dermatomyositis
	Dermatophytosis
	Ectodermal defect
	Epidermolysis bullosa
	Hypotrichosis
	Ichthyosis
	Impetigo
	Juvenile cellulitis
	Lymphedema
	Other congenital hereditary defects
	Pituitary dwarfism
	Tyrosinemia
	Viral papillomatosis (oral)
1 to 3 years	Allergic diseases, especially atopy
	Color dilution alopecia
	Hyposomatotropism in the mature dog
	Primary idiopathic seborrhea
Older than 6 years	Cushing's disease
	Feminization with testicular tumor
	Neoplasms
Senile dogs	Alopecia
	Decubital ulcer
	Necrolytic migratory erythema
	Thin, fragile skin

Breed

Breed predilection determines the incidence of some skin disorders (Table 2:3).[9, 10] For example, primary seborrhea is common in Cocker spaniels; acanthosis nigricans usually occurs in dachshunds; adult-onset hyposomatotropism occurs in Keeshonds; hypogonadism in intact males is found in Chow Chows; adrenal sex hormone imbalances occur in Pomeranians; dermatomyositis is found in Shetland sheepdogs (shelties) and collies; zinc-responsive dermatosis occurs in Siberian huskies and Alaskan Malamutes; and many of the wire-coated terrier breeds (Scottish, Cairn, Sealyham, West Highland white, Irish, and Welsh) seem to be particularly predisposed to allergic skin disease. See Chapter 19 for a review of breed predilections for cutaneous neoplasms.

In a study of dogs in northern California conducted at the University of California at Davis, 31 breeds were found to be at elevated risk for skin diseases, including Doberman pinscher, Irish setter, Dalmatian, dachshund, Golden retriever, various terrier breeds, Shar Pei, Chow Chow, and Akita.[9] In the same study, decreased risk of skin disease was found for dogs of mixed breeding and for 12 purebred breeds, including St. Bernard, Standard Poodle, beagle, Basset hound, German shorthaired pointer, Afghan hound, and Australian shepherd.

Sex

The sex of the patient affects the incidence of certain problems. Obviously, male feminization with testicular tumors occurs only in male animals. Other sex-related problems occur (e.g.,

Text continued on page 67

Table 2:3. Breed Predilection for Non-Neoplastic Skin Diseases (Strong Clinical Impression)

Breed	Disease
Abyssinian cat	Follicular dysplasia
	Idiopathic ceruminous otitis externa
	Psychogenic dermatitis or alopecia
Afghan hound	Hypothyroidism
Airedale	Adult-onset demodicosis
	Atopy
	Follicular dysplasia, flank
Akita	Pemphigus foliaceus
	Sebaceous adenitis
	Uveodermatologic syndrome
Basenji	Immunoproliferative enteropathy
Basset hound	Atopy
	Malassezia dermatitis
	Seborrhea, primary
	Skin fold intertrigo
Beagle	Atopy
	Demodicosis
	Immunoglobulin A (IgA) deficiency
Belgian sheepdog (Belgian Tervuren)	Vitiligo
Berger de Beauce	Epidermolysis bullosa
Borzoi	Hypothyroidism
Boston terrier	Atopy
	Demodicosis
	Facial fold intertrigo
	Hyperadrenocorticism
	Patterned alopecia
	Tail fold intertrigo
Boxer	Atopy
	Demodicosis
	Food hypersensitivity
	Follicular dysplasia (flank)
	Hyperadrenocorticism
	Hypothyroidism
	Muzzle furunculosis, bacterial
	Pedal furunculosis, bacterial
	Solar dermatitis (white dogs)
	Sterile pyogranuloma syndrome
	Sternal callus
Bullmastiff and Mastiff	Follicultis and furunculosis, bacterial
Bull terrier	Atopy
	Furunculosis, scarring, and bacterial
	Lethal acrodermatitis
	Solar dermatitis
	Zinc-responsive dermatosis
Chesapeake Bay retriever	Atopy
	Folliculitis and furunculosis, bacterial
Chihuahua	Demodicosis
	Pinnal thrombovascular necrosis
Chow Chow	Adrenal sex hormone abnormalities
	Pemphigus foliaceus
	Color dilution alopecia
	Demodicosis
	Hyposomatotropism
	Hypothyroidism
Collie	Bullous pemphigoid
	Dermatomyositis
	Discoid lupus erythematosus
	Idiopathic ulcerative dermatosis
	Nasal furunculosis, bacterial

Table 2:3. Breed Predilection for Non-Neoplastic Skin Diseases (Strong Clinical Impression) *Continued*

Breed	Disease
Collie *(Continued)*	Pemphigus erythematosus
	Pyotraumatic dermatitis
	Systemic lupus erythematosus
Curly-coated retrievers	Follicular dysplasia
Dachshund	Acanthosis nigricans
	Color dilution alopecia
	Demodicosis
	Folliculitis and pedal furunculosis, bacterial
	Hyperadrenocorticism
	Hypothyroidism
	Idiopathic onychodystrophy
	Juvenile cellulitis
	Linear IgA dermatosis
	Malassezia dermatitis
	Nodular panniculitis (sterile)
	Pattern alopecia (ears)
	Pattern alopecia (ventral)
	Pemphigus foliaceus
	Sterile pyogranuloma syndrome
	Sternal callus
	Vasculitis (idiopathic)
Dalmatian	Atopy
	Demodicosis
	Folliculitis and furunculosis, bacterial
	Solar dermatitis
Doberman pinscher	Acral furunculosis, bacterial
	Acral lick dermatitis
	Color dilution alopecia
	Demodicosis
	Drug reaction (sulfas)
	Flank sucking
	Follicular dysplasia
	Folliculitis and pedal furunculosis, bacterial
	Hypothyroidism
	Muzzle furunculosis, bacterial
	Vitiligo
Dogue de Bordeaux	Hereditary footpad hyperkeratosis
	Sterile pyogranuloma syndrome
English bulldog	Atopy
	Demodicosis
	Facial fold intertrigo
	Folliculitis and pedal furunculosis, bacterial
	Follicular dysplasia (flank)
	Hypothyroidism
	Malassezia dermatitis
	Muzzle furunculosis, bacterial
	Sterile pyogranuloma syndrome
	Tail fold intertrigo
German shepherd	Atopy
	Cellulitis (folliculitis and furunculosis), bacterial
	Collagen disorder of footpads
	Contact hypersensitivity
	Discoid lupus erythematosus
	Flea bite hypersensitivity
	Fly dermatitis of ear tips
	Food hypersensitivity
	Lupoid onychodystrophy

Table continued on following page

Table 2:3. Breed Predilection for Non-Neoplastic Skin Diseases (Strong Clinical Impression) *Continued*

Breed	Disease
German shepherd *(Continued)*	Insect- or arachnid-related eosinophilic furunculosis (face)
	Mucocutaneous bacterial pyoderma
	Nasal furunculosis, bacterial
	Otitis externa
	Pemphigus erythematosus
	Pituitary dwarfism
	Pyotraumatic dermatitis
	Seborrhea, primary
	Systemic lupus erythematosus
	Tarsal fistulae
	Vitiligo
Golden retriever	Acral furunculosis, bacterial
	Acral lick dermatitis
	Atopy
	Folliculitis and furunculosis, bacterial
	Hypothyroidism
	Juvenile cellulitis
	Nasal hypopigmentation
	Pyotraumatic dermatitis
	Pyotraumatic folliculitis and furunculosis, bacterial
	Sterile pyogranuloma syndrome
Gordon setter	Atopy
	Hypothyroidism
	Juvenile cellulitis
Great Dane	Acral furunculosis, bacterial
	Acral lick dermatitis
	Callus formation, hygroma
	Demodicosis
	Hypothyroidism
	Muzzle furunculosis, bacterial
	Pedal furunculosis, bacterial
	Solar dermatosis in Harlequin
Great Pyrenees	Demodicosis
	Pyotraumatic dermatitis
Greyhound	Vasculopathy
Himalayan cat	Cheyletiellosis
	Dermatophytosis (*Microsporum canis*)
Irish setter	Acral furunculosis, bacterial
	Atopy
	Acral lick dermatitis
	Color dilution alopecia
	Folliculitis and furunculosis, bacterial
	Granulocytopathy
	Hypothyroidism
	Seborrhea, primary
Irish water spaniel	Follicular dysplasia
	Idiopathic onychodystrophy
Irish wolfhound	Elbow hygroma
	Hypothyroidism
Keeshond	Hypogonadism of intact male
	Hyposomatotropism
	Hypothyroidism
Labrador retriever	Acral furunculosis, bacterial
	Acral lick dermatitis
	Atopy
	Folliculitis and furunculosis, bacterial
	Food hypersensitivity
	Pyotraumatic dermatitis

Table 2:3. Breed Predilection for Non-Neoplastic Skin Diseases (Strong Clinical Impression) *Continued*

Breed	Disease
Labrador retriever *(Continued)*	Seborrhea, primary
	Waterline disease
Lhasa apso	Atopy
	Injection reaction
	Malassezia dermatitis
Malamute	Zinc-responsive dermatosis
Newfoundland	Folliculitis and furunculosis, bacterial
	Pemphigus foliaceus
	Pyotraumatic dermatitis
Old English sheepdog	Atopy
	Demodicosis
	Pedal furunculosis, bacterial
Pekingese	Facial fold intertrigo
Persian cat	Cheyletiellosis
	Dermatophytosis
	Facial fold intertrigo
	Hair mats
	Seborrhea, primary
Pointers	Acral mutilation
	Demodicosis
	Follicular dysplasia (flank)
	Hereditary lupoid dermatosis
Pomeranians	Adrenal sex hormone abnormalities
	Hyposomatotropism
Poodle	Ectodermal defect
	Epiphora
	Hyperadrenocorticism
	Hyposomatotropism
	Hypothyroidism
	Injection reactions
	Otitis externa
	Sebaceous adenitis (standard)
Portuguese water dog	Follicular dysplasia
Pug	Atopy
	Facial fold and tail fold intertrigo
Rex cat	Hypotrichosis
Rhodesian Ridgeback	Dermoid sinus in midline of back
Rottweiler	Folliculitis and furunculosis, bacterial
	Idiopathic vasculitis
	Vitiligo
Schipperke	Pemphigus foliaceus
Shar Pei	Atopy
	Demodicosis
	Fold intertrigo
	Folliculitis, bacterial
	Food hypersensitivity
	Hypothyroidism
	Idiopathic mucinosis
	IgA deficiency
Schnauzer, miniature	Atopy
	Aurotrichia
	Hypothyroidism
	Schnauzer comedo syndrome
	Subcorneal pustular dematosis
	Superficial suppurative necrolytic dermatitis
Shetland sheepdog	Dermatomyositis
	Discoid lupus erythematosus

Table continued on following page

Table 2:3. Breed Predilection for Non-Neoplastic Skin Diseases (Strong Clinical Impression) *Continued*

Breed	Disease
Shetland sheepdog *(Continued)*	Folliculitis, bacterial
	Idiopathic ulcerative dermatosis
	Systemic lupus erythematosus
Shih tzu	Atopy
Siamese cat	Food hypersensitivity
	Hypotrichosis
	Periocular leukotrichia
	Psychogenic dermatitis or alopecia
	Vitiligo
Siberian husky	Discoid lupus erythematosus
	Eosinophilic granuloma
	Follicular dysplasia
	Hypogonadism in intact male
	Idiopathic onychodystrophy
	Zinc-responsive dermatosis
Spaniels (Cocker and Springer)	Atopy (American Cocker)
	Cutaneous asthenia (English Springer)
	Food hypersensitivity
	Hypothyroidism
	Idiopathic onychodystrophy (Springer)
	Lip fold intertrigo
	Malassezia dermatitis
	Otitis externa (especially proliferative)
	Psoriasiform-lichenoid dermatosis (English Springer)
	Seborrhea, primary
St. Bernard	Acral lick dermatitis
	Follicultis and furunculosis, bacterial
	Pyotraumatic dermatitis
Terriers	
Cairn	Atopy
Irish	Hereditary footpad hyperkeratosis
Jack Russell	Atopy
	Demodicosis
	Dermatophytosis (*Trichophyton mentagrophytes*, var. *erinacei*)
Kerry blue	Footpad keratoses (corns)
	Otitis externa
	Spiculosis
Scottish	Atopy
	Folliculitis and furunculosis, bacterial
	Hereditary nasal pyogranuloma and vasculitis
West Highland white	Atopy
	Epidermal dysplasia
	Ichthyosis
	Malassezia dermatitis
	Seborrhea, primary
Wire-haired fox	Atopy
Yorkshire	Color dilution alopecia
	Dermatophytosis (*M. canis*)
	Injection reactions
	Traction alopecia
Vizsla	Sebaceous adenitis
Weimaraner	Sterile pyogranuloma syndrome
Whippet	Idiopathic onychodystrophy

perianal adenomas are seen almost exclusively in male dogs). In addition, sex-related behaviors may affect the incidence of certain diseases, such as abscesses in fighting tomcats. One should determine whether the patient is sexually intact; in intact females, it should be determined whether the skin problem bears any relationship to the estrus cycle.

Color

The color of an animal may also be related to certain problems—most notable is the association of solar dermatitis and squamous cell carcinoma of the pinna in white-eared cats. In addition, solar dermatitis, actinic keratoses, solar-related hemangioma, hemangiosarcoma, and squamous cell carcinoma occur in white-skinned, thinly haired regions of dogs, particularly in white bull terriers, Staffordshire bull terriers (pit bull terriers), boxers, Dalmatians, beagles, whippets, and Great Danes.

Coat color may also relate to disease, as in color dilution alopecia. Although most commonly described in Doberman pinschers, this hair disorder occurs in any breed that has diluted coat colors and may occur in piebald breeds as well.[41] The color of the eyes and coat may be helpful in diagnosis, as in yellow-eyed, ''smoky'' Persian cats with the Chédiak-Higashi syndrome. Also, an association between positive intradermal skin test results and coat colors was observed in normal cats.[40]

Medical History

The clinician should obtain a complete medical history in all cases.[3] This should initially include questions about previous illnesses and problems. Some dermatologists prefer to examine the skin quickly first, so that pertinent questions may be emphasized in taking the history, while inappropriate items can be omitted. However, it is vital to use a systematic, detailed method of examination and history taking so that important information is not overlooked.

The clinician who can draw out a complete history in an unbiased form has a valuable skill. It is important that the questions presented to the client do not suggest answers or tend to shut off discussion. Some owners purposely or unconsciously withhold pertinent facts, especially about neglect, diet, previous medication, or other procedures they think may not be well received by the examining veterinarian. Other pertinent information may be left out because some owners are not aware of what is normal. They may not know how much licking or chewing it takes to consider a dog's behavior abnormal. Therefore, they may not supply valuable information because they do not perceive the information to be significant or abnormal. In other cases, they may recognize something as abnormal but attribute the observation to some other, unrelated cause (e.g., paw licking that the client interprets as behavior to obtain attention and does not list as a problem in the history).

The clinician must become skillful at extracting all the relevant history and observations, regardless of the client's perception of their importance. The skillful clinician is ever tuned to listen for side comments by the client or by the children. These may be veritable ''pearls'' of information in a mass of trivia. They also help to establish the client's accuracy and credibility.

Next, the following information about the skin lesions should be obtained from the owner: the date and age at onset, the original locations, the initial appearance, the tendency to progression or regression, factors affecting the course, and previous treatment (home, proprietary, or pet shop remedies used, as well as veterinary treatment). In addition, treatments of other problems should be determined and recorded. The relationships between all treatments and the onset of or changes in the disease should be recorded and a possible drug reaction considered. Drug reactions are diagnosed only when they are suspected, and because they may mimic any disease, the history is what raises the question.

Almost all animals with skin disorders have been bathed, dipped, sprayed, or treated with one or more medications, and the owner may be reluctant or unable to disclose a complete list of previous treatments. It is important that the types of medication and the dates of application are completely divulged, because a modification of pertinent signs may have resulted.

Although the patient cannot relate subjective findings (symptoms such as itching, burning sensation, and pain), it is possible to determine the degree of pruritus reasonably well. The presence and severity of pain may also be evaluated in some cases by the patient's response to stimuli: exhibiting shyness, pulling away, exhibiting skin twitching, and responding with aggressiveness may be manifested when pain is provoked.

Pruritus is one of the most common presenting complaints and, in many cases, is a hallmark of allergy. The presence, location, and degree of itching are important criteria in the differential diagnosis of many skin diseases. The owner's idea of the intensity of itching, however, may vary considerably from that of the veterinarian. Consequently, it is helpful to ask questions, "How many times daily do you see your dog scratch?" "Does it itch in many sites, or just a few?" "Does it shake its head?" "Does it lick its paws?" "Does it lick the front legs or other areas?" "Does it roll on its back or rub its chin, ears, or body against things?" It is also very helpful to determine, when possible, whether the pruritus involves initially normal-appearing skin (an itch that rashes, typical of allergy), or whether skin lesions precede or appear at the same time as the pruritus (a rash that itches).

Many times, owners disassociate other problems that their pet is having. For example, a dog is presented for paw licking and groin pruritus. The dog has also had multiple ear infections during the past few years but has only recently had pruritus of the paws and groin. The owners may not mention, unless specifically asked about, the ear problems, the itching, or treatments for the ears, because they assume it is not important or it is an unrelated problem.

The same types of specific questions are helpful when discussing diets, as the owner often states the typical feedings and leaves out treats and supplements. A more representative answer is often secured if one asks, "What did your pet eat yesterday, or during the past 48 hours?" Also: "What treats does your pet receive and what supplements do you add to its diet?" Specifically, the clinician asks whether any vitamins or flavored chewable medications are given. The clinician also asks about rawhide chew toys or other edible toys.

Because contact irritants or allergens are important contributors to or causes of skin disease, it is necessary to inquire about the animal's environment. Does it live in an apartment or is it outdoors in the fields and forests? Does it sleep in a doghouse or in the owner's house? If it sleeps in the house, in what room is it and is there carpeting? If it sleeps in a person's bedroom, is it on the floor or on the bed? Are there feather pillows or comforters or wool blankets? If the pet sleeps in a doghouse, in a garage, or outside, does the bedding consist of straw, wool blankets, or some other material? Are symptoms worse when the pet first awakens, sometimes suggesting exposure throughout the night?

If the pet is boarded or hospitalized, do the symptoms improve? If the pet travels, does it improve while traveling or while in other homes? Symptoms that resolve in a different environment are highly suggestive of a reaction to an environmental allergen or irritant. Questions regarding sexual behavior may also reveal important information, particularly when endocrine disorders are suspected. Other more organ-specific questions may also be asked, depending on the clinical suspicions of possible diseases. Questions regarding changes in water consumption, appetite, weight, and urination or defecation habits should be included in history taking.

In determining contagion, one should inquire about the skin health of other animals on the premises. The presence of skin disease in the people living with the patient may also be highly significant in some disorders (scabies, cheyletiellosis, and dermatophytosis).

At this point, the clinician usually has a general idea of the problem and is ready to proceed with a careful physical examination. In some cases, the clinician may want to come back to the medical history if further examinations indicate a more serious or underlying systemic disease.

■ PHYSICAL EXAMINATION

General Observations

A good examination necessitates adequate lighting. Normal daylight without glare is best, but any artificial light of adequate candlepower is sufficient if it produces bright, non–color-changing, uniform lighting. The lamp should be adjustable to illuminate all body areas. A combination loupe and light provides magnification of the field as well as good illumination.

Before the clinician concentrates on the individual lesions, the entire animal should always be observed from a distance of a couple of meters to obtain a general impression of abnormalities and to observe distribution patterns.

Does the pet appear to be in good health? Is it fat or thin, unkempt or well-groomed? Is the problem generalized or localized? What is the distribution and configuration of the lesions? Are they bilaterally symmetric or unilaterally irregular (Fig. 2:3)? Is the haircoat shiny or dull, and if dull, what is the pattern of those changes? Is it an appropriate color and pattern of colors for its breed? Are coat changes in quality or color lifelong, or did they develop before or after the symptoms for which the pet is presented?

To answer some of these questions, the clinician must examine the patient more closely. The dorsal aspect of the body should be inspected by viewing it from the rear, as elevated hairs and patchy alopecia may be more obvious from that angle. Then, the head, the lateral trunk, and the extremities should be observed. Next, the clinician should complete a thorough dermatologic examination.

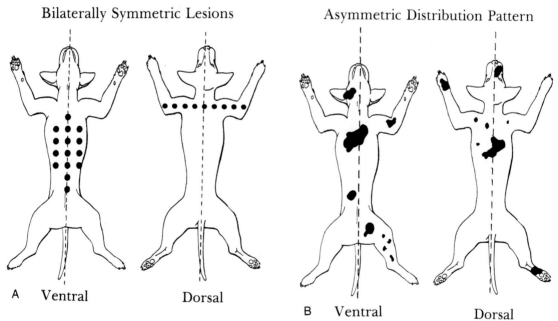

Bilaterally Symmetric Lesions   Asymmetric Distribution Pattern

A   Ventral   Dorsal   B   Ventral   Dorsal

Figure 2:3. *A,* When a line is drawn from the tip of the nose to the end of the tail and the distribution of the lesions is relatively the same on the right and left sides, the pattern is called bilaterally symmetric. Most such skin disorders have an internal cause, and the skin reflects internal disease. Examples are hypothyroidism, hyperadrenocorticism, Sertoli's cell tumor, and autoimmune diseases such as pemphigus foliaceus. Allergies may also present symmetric lesions. *B,* When a line is drawn from the tip of the nose to the end of the tail and the lesions on one side are not identical to those on the other side, the distribution pattern is asymmetric. External environmental causes, such as ectoparasites, fungi, or contact allergens, are examples of disorders that cause asymmetric lesions.

Dermatologic Examination

After an impression is obtained from a distance, the skin should be examined more closely and palpated.[3] It is important to examine every centimeter of skin and visible mucous membranes. Many subtle clues are located where the client is unaware of problems. The authors have seen many cases in which ventrally located lesions and interdigital, paronychial, and oral lesions went unobserved by a veterinarian. These lesions may add valuable diagnostic information. It is difficult to complete a dermatologic examination without rolling animals on their sides or back. All the paws must be picked up or handled so that the ventral interdigital skin is also examined.

Many observations need to be made. What is the texture of the hair? Is it coarse or fine, dry or oily? Does it epilate easily? A change in the amount of hair is often a dramatic finding, although subtle thinning of the haircoat should also be noted. *Alopecia* is a partial or complete lack of hair in areas where it is normally present. *Hypotrichosis* implies partial hair loss and is a form of alopecia. Is the thinning diffuse, or are there numerous small focal areas of alopecia (the latter being often seen with folliculitis)? *Hypertrichosis* is excessive hair and, although rare in animals, usually has hormonal or developmental causes.

The texture, elasticity, and thickness of the skin should be determined and impressions of heat or coolness recorded. It is easier to find skin lesions in some breeds than in others, depending on the thickness of the coat. Additionally, there is variation in an animal's coat density in different body areas, with skin lesions often being discerned more readily in sparsely haired regions. Therefore, the clinician must part or clip the hair in heavily haired areas to observe and palpate lesions that are present but obscured.

When abnormalities are discovered, it is important to establish their morphologic features, configuration, and general distribution. The clinician should try to appreciate the different lesions and their patterns. Together they often represent the natural history of the skin disease.

Morphology of Skin Lesions

The morphologic characteristics of skin lesions, together with their history, are an essential feature of dermatologic diagnosis.[1, 3] Morphologic features and the medical and dermatologic history are often the only guides if laboratory procedures cannot be performed or do not yield useful information. The clinician must learn to recognize primary and secondary lesions. A primary lesion is the initial eruption that develops spontaneously as a direct reflection of underlying disease. Secondary lesions evolve from primary lesions or are artifacts induced by the patients or by external factors such as trauma and medications. Primary lesions (pustules, vesicles, papules) may appear quickly and then disappear rapidly. However, they may leave behind secondary lesions (such as focal alopecia, epidermal collarettes, scaling, hyperpigmentation, and crusts), which may be more chronic and give clues about the presence of previous primary lesions. Therefore, the identification and the characterization of both primary and secondary lesions are important.

Careful inspection of the diseased skin frequently reveals a primary lesion, which may suggest a limited differential diagnosis. For example, pustules most commonly represent a bacterial pyoderma, whereas sterile pustular diseases occur infrequently. Close inspection of primary lesions may also reveal elusive differences. In assessing the subtle morphologic features of lesions, the clinician may find it helpful to focus on individual lesions and examine them minutely with good light and a hand-held lens or a head loupe with 4- to 6-power magnification. This may allow better identification (e.g., whether pustules are follicular or nonfollicular).

A primary lesion may vary slightly from its initial appearance to its full development. Later, through regression, degeneration, or traumatization, it may change in form and become a secondary lesion. Although classic descriptions and textbooks refer to lesions as primary or secondary, some lesions can be either (e.g., alopecia can be primary [from endocrine disorders] or secondary [from chewing because of pruritus]). Follicular casts, scales, pigment changes, crusts, and comedones may also be primary or secondary. In some cases, such as primary seborrhea and zinc-responsive dermatosis with secondary bacterial pyoderma, crusts may appear in the same animal as both primary and secondary lesions.

Secondary lesions may also be informative. A ring of orthokeratotic scaling usually follows a point source of inflammation, either a papule or a pustule. This is also true of small focal circular areas of alopecia. Hyperpigmentation that has a lattice- or lacelike configuration generally reflects an area of previous inflammation such as erythematous macules, papules, and pustules. Yellow- to honey-colored crusts usually follow the rupture and drying of pustules. In many cases, however, the significant lesion must be differentiated from the mass of secondary debris. Variations of lesions and their configurations are common, because early and advanced stages coexist in most skin diseases. The ability to discover a characteristic lesion and understand its significance is an important aspect of mastering dermatologic diagnoses.

The following illustrations can help the clinician to identify primary and secondary lesions. Also, the character of the lesions can vary, implying a different pathogenesis or cause. The definitions and examples in Figures 2:4 to 2:24 explain the relationship of skin lesions to canine and feline dermatoses.

PRIMARY LESIONS

Macule or patch (Fig. 2:4)
Papule or plaque (Fig. 2:5)
Pustule (Fig. 2:6)
Vesicle or bulla (Fig. 2:7)

Wheal (Fig. 2:8)
Nodule (Fig. 2:9)
Tumor or cyst (Fig. 2:10)

LESIONS THAT MAY BE PRIMARY OR SECONDARY

Alopecia (Fig. 2:11)
Scale (Fig. 2:12)
Crust (Fig. 2:13)

Follicular casts (Fig. 2:14)
Comedo (Fig. 2:15)
Pigmentary abnormalities (Figs. 2:16 and 2:17)

SECONDARY LESIONS

Epidermal collarette (Fig. 2:18)
Scar (Fig. 2:19)
Excoriation (Fig. 2:20)
Erosion or ulcer (Fig. 2:21)

Fissure (Fig. 2:22)
Lichenification (Fig. 2:23)
Callus (Fig. 2:24)

Two special techniques of close examination of the skin, although infrequently used, are noteworthy:

1. Diascopy is performed by pressing a clear piece of plastic or glass over an erythematous lesion. If the lesion blanches on pressure, the reddish color is due to vascular engorgement. If it does not, there is hemorrhage into the skin (petechia or ecchymosis).
2. Nikolsky's sign is elicited by applying pressure on a vesicle or at the edge of an ulcer or erosion or even on normal skin.[42] It is positive when the outer layer of the skin is easily rubbed off or pushed away. It indicates poor cellular cohesion, as found in the pemphigus complex, toxic epidermal necrolysis (Fig. 2:25), and erythema multiforme major.

Configuration of Lesions

The configuration of skin lesions may be helpful in establishing a differential diagnosis (Fig. 2:26).[3] Some diseases often have lesions present in certain configurations, and although excep-

Text continued on page 89

PRIMARY LESION—MACULE

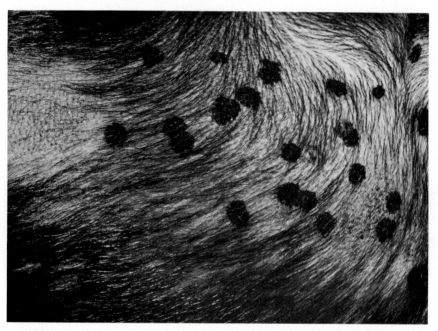

Figure 2:4. *Macule*—a circumscribed, nonpalpable spot up to 1 cm in diameter and characterized by a change in the color of the skin. *Patch*—a macule over 1 cm in size. The discoloration can result from several processes: an increase in melanin pigmentation, depigmentation, and erythema or local hemorrhage. Examples are the hyperpigmentation patches in endocrine or postinflammatory hyperpigmentation, hypopigmentation, and vitiligo. Discoloration also occurs after inflammation of the erythematous macules in many types of acute dermatitis, lentigo, and pigmented nevi. (The photograph illustrates lentigo.) Types of macules are as follows: *purpura*— bleeding into the skin (these are usually dark red but change to purple as absorption proceeds); *petechiae*—pinpoint macules that are much less than 1 cm in diameter and are caused by hemorrhage; and *ecchymoses*—patches greater than 1 cm in diameter that are caused by hemorrhage.

PRIMARY LESION—PAPULE

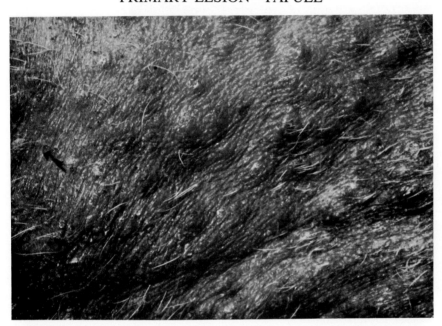

Figure 2:5. *Papule*—a small, solid elevation of the skin up to 1 cm in diameter that can always be palpated as a solid mass. Many papules are pink or red swellings produced by tissue infiltration of inflammatory cells in the dermis, by intraepidermal and subepidermal edema, or by epidermal hypertrophy. They may or may not involve hair follicles. Examples are the erythematous papules seen in scabies and flea bite hypersensitivity. In the dog, another common cause of papules is superficial bacterial folliculitis. (Photograph illustrates allergic contact dermatitis.) *Plaque*—a larger, flat-topped elevation formed by the extension or coalition of papules. A plaque that is made up of closely packed, projecting elevations often covered by crusts is called a *vegetation*.

PRIMARY LESION—PUSTULE

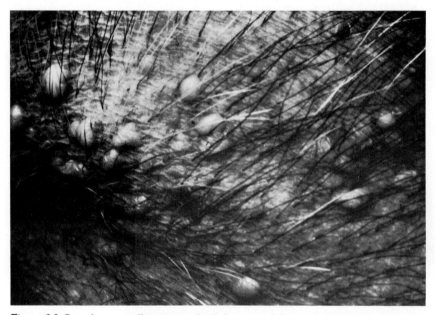

Figure 2:6. *Pustule*—a small, circumscribed elevation of the epidermis that is filled with pus. Pustules may be intraepidermal, subepidermal, or follicular in location. Their color is usually yellow but may be green or red. Most commonly, pustules primarily contain neutrophils and are infectious in origin; however, eosinophils may predominate (especially in parasitic or allergic disorders) and may be sterile (subcorneal pustular dermatosis, pemphigus foliaceus, sterile eosinophilic pustulosis). Size and color may be clues to the cause of the condition. Larger flaccid pustules (bullous impetigo) are more often associated with Cushing's disease, iatrogenic Cushing's disease, immune-suppressed cases, or pemphigus foliaceus. Larger green pustules imply gram-negative infections or marked toxic changes. Examples are acne, folliculitis, and the pustules found on the abdomen of puppies with impetigo. (Photograph illustrates nonfollicular pustules from subcorneal pustular dermatosis.) *Abscess*—a demarcated fluctuant lesion resulting from a dermal or subcutaneous accumulation of pus. The pus is not visible on the surface of the skin until it drains to the surface. Abscesses are larger and deeper than pustules.

PRIMARY LESION—VESICLE

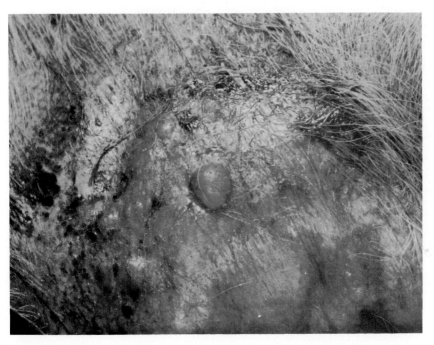

Figure 2:7. *Vesicle*—a sharply circumscribed elevation of the epidermis filled with clear fluid. It can be intraepidermal or subepidermal. Vesicles are rarely seen in dogs and cats because they are fragile and transient. They occur in viral or autoimmune dermatoses, or in dermatitis caused by irritants. Vesicles are lesions up to 1 cm in diameter; those with a diameter greater than 1 cm are called *bullae*. (Photograph illustrates several vesicles caused by a chemical irritant.)

PRIMARY LESION—WHEAL

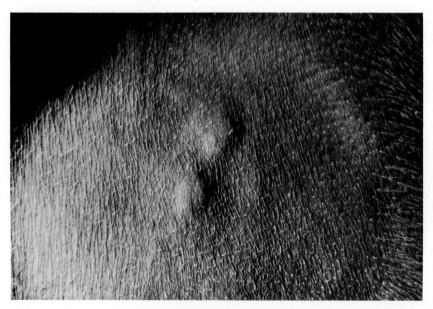

Figure 2:8. *Wheal*—a sharply circumscribed, raised lesion consisting of edema that usually appears and disappears within minutes or hours. Wheals usually produce no changes in the appearance of the overlying skin and haircoat. Wheals are characteristically white to pink, elevated ridges or round edematous swellings that only rarely have pseudopods at their periphery. They blanch on diascopy (viewing the skin through glass slide that is pressed firmly against the lesion). A huge hive of a distensible region such as the lips or eyelids is called *angioedema*. Examples of wheals are urticaria, insect bites, and positive reactions to allergy skin tests. (Photograph illustrates hives.)

PRIMARY LESION—NODULE

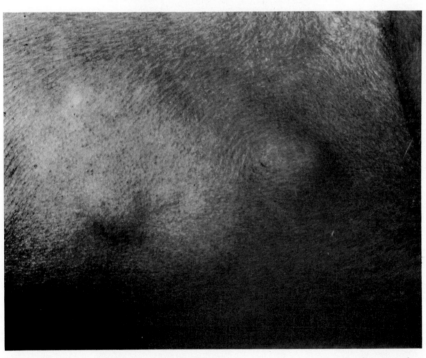

Figure 2:9. *Nodule*—a circumscribed, solid elevation greater than 1 cm in diameter that usually extends into the deeper layers of the skin. Nodules usually result from massive infiltration of inflammatory or neoplastic cells into the dermis or subcutis. Deposition of fibrin or crystalline material also produces nodules. (Photograph illustrates panniculitis.)

PRIMARY LESION—TUMOR

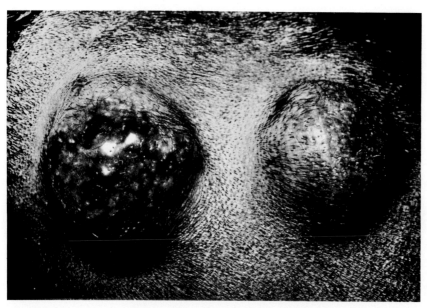

Figure 2:10. *Tumor*—a large mass that may involve any structure of the skin or subcutaneous tissue. Most tumors are neoplastic or granulomatous in origin. (Photograph illustrates pilomatrixoma.) *Cyst*—an epithelium-lined cavity containing fluid or a solid material. It is a smooth, well-circumscribed, fluctuant to solid mass. Skin cysts are usually lined by adnexal epithelium (hair follicle, sebaceous, or apocrine) and filled with cornified cellular debris or sebaceous or apocrine secretions.

PRIMARY OR SECONDARY LESION—ALOPECIA

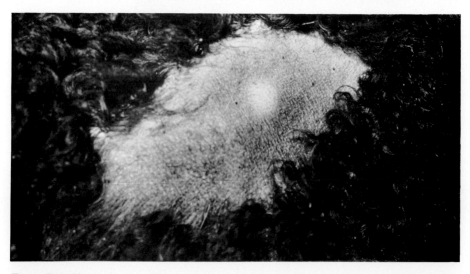

Figure 2:11. *Alopecia* is loss of hair and may vary from partial to complete. It may be primary, such as alopecia with endocrine disorders and follicular dysplasias, or it can occur secondary to trauma or inflammation. (Photograph illustrates alopecia from an injection reaction.)

PRIMARY OR SECONDARY LESION—SCALE

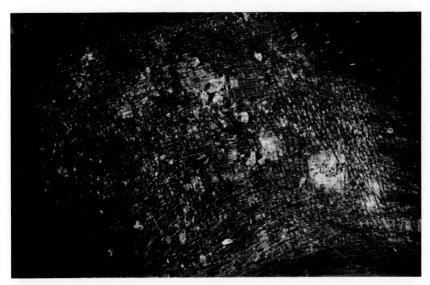

Figure 2:12. *Scale*—an accumulation of loose fragments of the horny layer of the skin (cornified cells). The corneocyte is the final product of epidermal keratinization. Normal loss occurs as individual cells or small clusters not visible to the naked eye. Abnormal scaling is the loss in larger flakes. Flakes vary greatly in consistency; they can appear branny, fine, powdery, flaky, platelike, greasy, dry, loose, adhering, or "nitlike." The color varies from white, silver, yellow, or brown to gray. (Photograph illustrates seborrhea.) Scales may be the primary lesions in some cases of color dilution alopecia, follicular dysplasia, primary idiopathic seborrhea, and ichthyosis. They are common secondary lesions in chronic inflammation.

PRIMARY OR SECONDARY LESION—CRUST

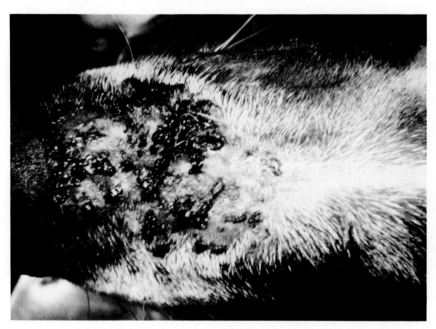

Figure 2:13. *Crust*—is formed when dried exudate, serum, pus, blood, cells, scales, or medications adhere to the surface. Unusually thick crusts are found in hairy areas because the dried material tends to adhere more tightly than in glabrous skin. Crust may be primary as in idiopathic seborrhea and zinc-responsive dermatosis, or secondary as in pyoderma, fly strike, or pruritus. Hemorrhagic crusts in pyoderma are brown or dark red; yellowish green crusts appear in some cases of pyoderma; tan, lightly adhering crusts are found in impetigo. *Vegetations*—heaped-up crusts seen in pemphigus vegetans. (Photograph illustrates nasal furunculosis.) Dark crusts imply deeper tissue damage or hemorrhage and may be seen more with traumatic wounds, furunculosis, fly strike dermatitis, and vasculitis. Honey-colored crusts are more commonly infectious in nature; thicker dry yellow crusts are more typical of scabies and zinc-responsive dermatosis. Tightly adherent crusts are typical in zinc-responsive dermatosis and necrolytic migratory erythema, and they also occur in some cases of seborrhea.

PRIMARY OR SECONDARY LESION—FOLLICULAR CAST

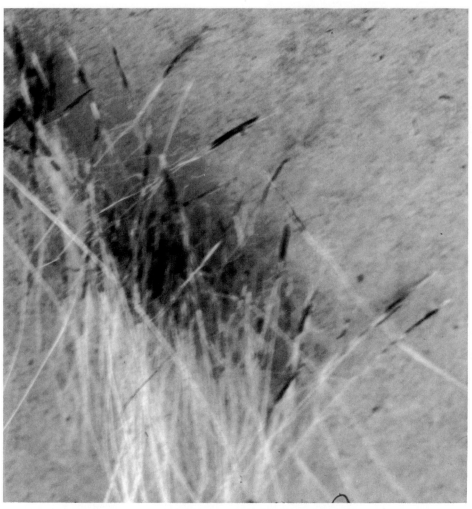

Figure 2:14. *Follicular cast*—an accumulation of keratin and follicular material that adheres to the hair shaft extending above the surface of the follicular ostia. It is a primary lesion in vitamin A–responsive dermatoses, primary idiopathic seborrhea, and sebaceous adenitis. (Photograph illustrates hair epilated from a dog with sebaceous adenitis; the clumps of material at the base of multiple hairs are the casts.) Follicular casts may be secondary lesions in demodectic mange and dermatophytosis.

PRIMARY OR SECONDARY LESION—COMEDO

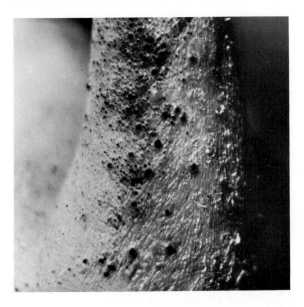

Figure 2:15. *Comedo*—a dilated hair follicle filled with cornified cells and sebaceous material. It is the initial lesion of feline acne and may predispose the skin to bacterial folliculitis. A comedo may be produced secondary to seborrheic skin disease, to occlusion with greasy medications, or to the administration of systemic or topical corticosteroids. (Photograph illustrates comedones of the skin on the tail of a dog.) When comedones are present diseases of the hair follicle should be considered such as infection with *Demodex* and dermatophytosis. Comedones may be primary lesions in feline acne, vitamin A–responsive dermatosis, Schnauzer comedo syndrome, Cushing's disease, sex hormone dermatoses, and some idiopathic seborrhea disorders.

PRIMARY OR SECONDARY LESION—PIGMENTARY ABNORMALITIES

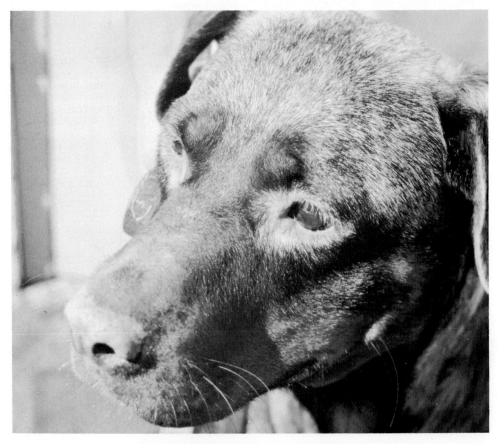

Figure 2:16 *See legend on opposite page.*

PRIMARY OR SECONDARY LESION—PIGMENTARY ABNORMALITIES

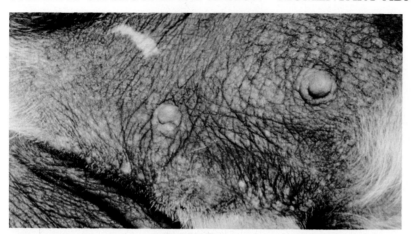

Figure 2:17. *Hyperpigmentation* (hypermelanosis, melanoderma)—increased epidermal and, occasionally, dermal melanin. Melanophages may be found in the superficial dermis. (Postinflammatory, chronic, traumatic, and endocrine skin lesions.) Excess pigment in hair is called *melanotrichia*. (Photograph illustrates postinflammatory hyperpigmentation.) The pattern of hyperpigmentation is helpful in determining the etiology. Endocrine hyperpigmentation tends to be diffuse increase, whereas postinflammatory hyperpigmentation has a latticework appearance.

Figure 2:16. *Abnormal pigmentation*—skin coloration caused by a variety of pigments but most commonly melanin, which is responsible for many skin colors: black—melanin present throughout the epidermis (lentigo); blue—melanin within melanocytes and melanophages in the middle and deep dermis (dermal melanocytoma); gray—diffuse dermal melanosis or superficial dermal melanosis from pigment incontinence; tan, brown, black—various shades of normal skin color in breeds are due to melanin; brown—hemochromatosis is due primarily to melanin, not hemosiderin. Other pigments are as follows: red, purple—hemorrhage in the skin is red at first, becoming dark purple with time (bruises); yellow, green—accumulations of bile pigments (icterus). In *hypopigmentation* (hypomelanosis), loss of epidermal melanin may be primary, as with vitiligo-like disease, or secondary, as in postinflammatory change. (Photograph demonstrates Rottweiler with leukoderma and leukotrichia.) *Leukoderma* is a general term for white skin, whereas vitiligo refers to a specific disease. Lack of pigment in hair is called *leukotrichia* or *achromotrichia*.

SECONDARY LESION—EPIDERMAL COLLARETTE

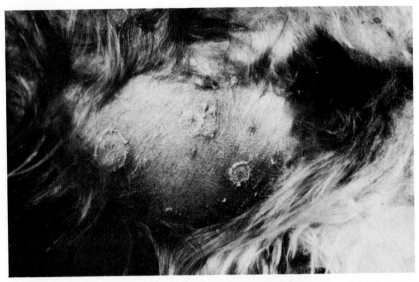

Figure 2:18. *Epidermal collarette*—a special type of scale arranged in a circular rim of loose keratin flakes or "peeling" keratin. It represents the remnants of the "roof" of a vesicle, bulla, pustule, or papule, or the hyperkeratosis caused by a point source of inflammation as seen with papules and pustules. (Photograph illustrates a healing pustule of staphylococcal folliculitis.)

SECONDARY LESION—SCAR

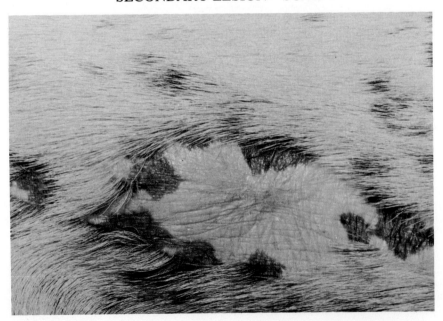

Figure 2:19. *Scar*—an area of fibrous tissue that has replaced the damaged dermis or subcutaneous tissue. Scars are the remnants of trauma or dermatologic lesions. Most scars in dogs and cats are alopecic, atrophic, and depigmented. Proliferative scars do occur, and in dark-skinned dogs scars can be alopecic and hyperpigmented. Scars are observed following severe burns and in deep pyoderma. (Photograph illustrates burn scarring.)

SECONDARY LESION—EXCORIATION

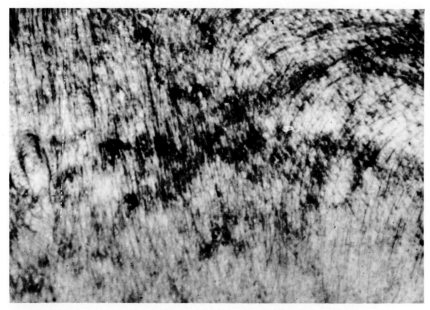

Figure 2:20. *Excoriation*—erosions or ulcers caused by scratching, biting, or rubbing. Excoriations are self-produced and usually result from pruritus; they invite secondary bacterial infection. They are often partly recognized by their linear pattern. (Photograph illustrates linear excoriations on the side of a dog with scabies.)

SECONDARY LESION—EROSION, ULCER

Figure 2:21. *Erosion*—a shallow epidermal defect that does not penetrate the basal laminar zone and consequently heals without scarring; it generally results from epidermal diseases and self-inflicted trauma. *Ulcer*—there is a break in the continuity of the epidermis, with exposure of the underlying dermis. A deep pathologic process is required for an ulcer to form. It is important to note the structure of the edge: Is it undermined, fibrotic and thickened, or necrotic (vasculitis, neoplastic, fibrosing, vascular)? The firmness of the ulcer depth and the type of exudate in the crater should also be noted. A scar is often left after an ulcer heals. Examples are feline indolent ulcer, severe deep pyoderma, and vasculitis. (Photograph illustrates bullous pemphigoid-like disease in a shelty.)

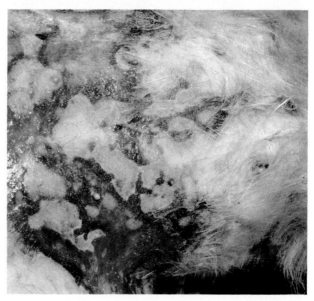

SECONDARY LESION—FISSURE

Figure 2:22. *Fissure*—a linear cleavage into the epidermis, or through the epidermis into the dermis, caused by disease or injury. Fissures may be single or multiple tiny cracks or large clefts several centimeters long. They have sharply defined margins and may be dry or moist and straight, curved, or branching. They occur when the skin is thick and inelastic and then subjected to sudden swelling from inflammation or trauma, especially in regions of frequent movement. Examples are found at ear margins, and at ocular, nasal, oral, and anal mucocutaneous borders. (Photograph illustrates two fissures in a footpad.)

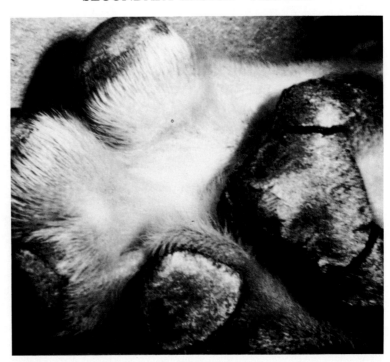

SECONDARY LESION—LICHENIFICATION

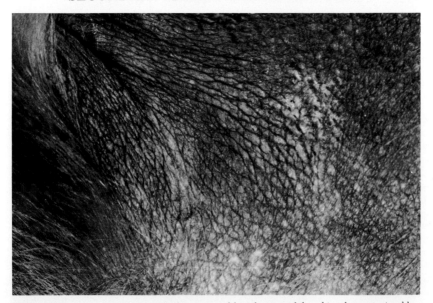

Figure 2:23. *Lichenification*—a thickening and hardening of the skin characterized by an exaggeration of the superficial skin markings. Lichenification areas often result from friction. They may be normally colored but are more often hyperpigmented. Crusted lichenified plaques usually have a bacterial component and improve with antibiotic therapy. Occasionally, *Malassezia* is found with these lesions. Examples are the axillae in acanthosis nigricans. (Photograph illustrates the axilla of a dog with chronic atopic dermatitis. The lichenification here is a result of rubbing.)

SECONDARY LESION—CALLUS

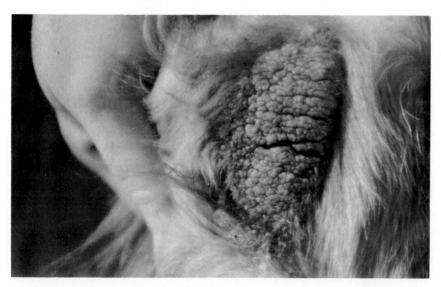

Figure 2:24. *Callus*—a thickened, rough, hyperkeratotic, alopecic, often lichenified plaque that develops on the skin. Most commonly, calluses occur over bony prominences and result from pressure and chronic low-grade friction. (Photograph illustrates an elbow callus.)

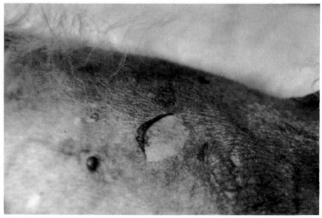

Figure 2:25. Photograph illustrates a case of toxic epidermal necrolysis (drug-induced) with a positive Nikolsky sign.

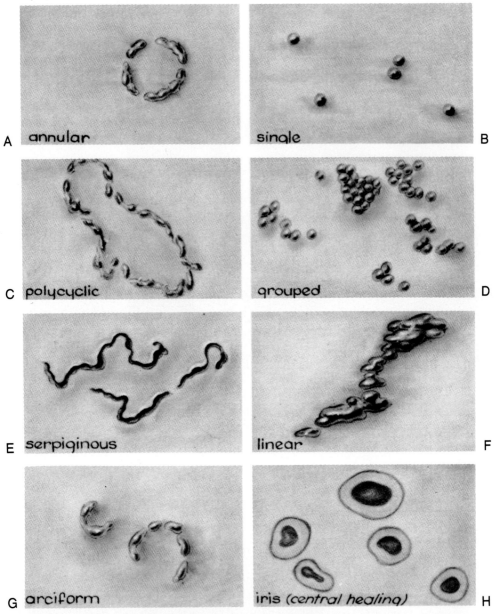

Figure 2:26. Configuration of skin lesions. *A,* The annular configuration has a clear or less involved center and is found in superficial spreading bacterial folliculitis, local seborrhea, demodicosis, and dermatophytosis. *B,* Single lesions are typified by feline acne, acral lick dermatitis, cysts, and many tumors. *C,* Polycyclic configurations often result from the confluence of lesions or a spreading process. Examples are superficial spreading bacterial folliculitis, demodicosis, or pyotraumatic dermatitis. *D,* Grouped lesions are clusters, often the result of new foci developing around an old lesion. They are seen in folliculitis, insect bites, contact dermatitis, and calcinosis cutis. *E,* Serpiginous lesions develop as a result of spreading, such as in canine scabies or demodicosis. They may also occur as a result of the confluence and partial resolution of polycyclic lesions. *F,* Linear configurations are best typified by the linear form of eosinophilic granuloma of cats or by contact with irritant materials streaked along the skin. *G,* Arciform lesions usually result from the partial resolution of polycyclic lesions such as spreading folliculitis, but they may result from spreading, as in canine scabies and demodicosis. *H,* Central-healing (target) configurations are produced when the skin heals behind an advancing front of a disease process. It is typical of certain dermatophytoses, demodicosis, and bacterial folliculitis.

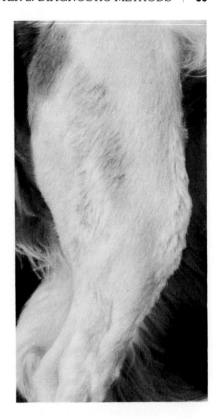

Figure 2:27. A linear epidermal nevus in a spaniel was a congenital malformation.

tions exist, recognizing the pattern of lesions adds information for decision making. Lesions may be single, such as the solitary dermatophytosis lesion and a foreign-body reaction. Multiple lesions are most commonly seen in skin diseases of dogs and cats.

When lesions are linear, external forces such as scratching, being scratched by something, and having something applied to the skin are often responsible. In other cases, linear lesions may reflect the involvement of a blood or lymphatic vessel, a dermatome, or a congenital malformation (Fig. 2:27). Diffuse areas of involvement tend to suggest a metabolic or systemic reaction, such as endocrine disorders, keratinization, and immunologic or hypersensitivity disorders. Annular lesions are often associated with peripheral spreading of a disease. Common examples of annular lesions are superficial spreading bacterial folliculitis (Fig. 2:28) and

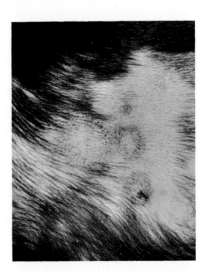

Figure 2:28. Annular lesions in a case of superficial spreading bacterial folliculitis.

dermatophytosis. Coalescing lesions occur when multiple lesions are present and spread so that they overlap.

Different Stages

A skin disease and its individual lesions progress from an earliest appearance to a fully developed state and, in many cases, to a chronic or resolved stage. The distribution, the configuration, and the histologic appearance of lesions change. The evolution of lesions should be determined either by obtaining the history or by finding different stages of lesions on the patient. Papules often develop into vesicles and pustules, which may rupture to leave erosions or ulcers and finally crusts. An understanding of these progressions helps in the diagnostic process.

As lesions develop in specific patterns, they also involute in characteristic ways. The lesions themselves, as well as their histologic appearance, change. For example, a macule may develop into a pustule and then a crust or crusted erosion. It may then spread peripherally, occurring as a ring of lesions; the lesion then appears as a circular patch with multiple pustules or crusts on the margins and central alopecia. The fully developed lesions could appear as a large alopecic patch with a central area of hyperpigmentation and multifocal erythematous macules, pustules, or crusts intermittently along the leading margin; this lesion could then appear arciform. Scaling may also occur at the leading margins of inflammation. The healing phase of a chronic lesion may appear as a patch of alopecia and hyperpigmentation with no other primary or secondary lesions, as they have spontaneously resolved or responded to therapy.

Because diseases and their lesions are evolutionary, the clinician must attempt to learn all the stages. The recognition of the different stages as well as the lesions becomes important when selecting areas to sample for diagnostic tests.

Distribution Patterns of Skin Lesions

The areas of skin involved with lesions or affected by symptoms of the disease help in determining the differential diagnosis, as most skin diseases have a typical distribution.[3] It is important to emphasize that the accurate determination of the distribution necessitates detection of all changes in the haircoat or the skin, the location of symptoms related to the disease, and the location of all primary and secondary lesions. An adequate determination of the distribution pattern can be achieved only by a thorough history and dermatologic examination; cursory examinations are often incomplete.

The study of skin diseases involves understanding the primary lesions that occur as well as the typical distribution patterns. Diseases less commonly present with atypical patterns. The combination of the type of lesions present and their distribution is the basis for developing a differential diagnosis. The distribution pattern may be very helpful by allowing clinicians to establish the differential diagnosis based on the region involved when animals have lesions and symptoms confined to certain regions (Table 2:4). In some instances, this regional pattern is such a major feature that it is a required aspect of the disease. The best examples are otitis externa, pododermatitis, and nasal dermatitis. Actually, these terms refer to skin disease of a specific region, give little more information, and certainly are not specific diagnoses.

Table 2:4 lists areas or parts of the body along with the common skin diseases that are most frequently localized or especially severe in those areas. The chart should be useful in the differential diagnosis. However, the clinician must also be aware that other diseases may occur in these regions and that diseases that often affect a certain region can also occur elsewhere and not involve the typical region. Therefore, regional evaluations aid in ranking differential diagnostic possibilities: they do *not* determine the diagnosis.

In many instances, the patterning that skin diseases take is unexplained. Recently, *homeobox genes* have received much attention.[41a] These genes are a family of regulatory proteins that

Table 2:4. Regional Diagnosis of Non-Neoplastic Dermatoses

Region	Common Disease	Less Common Disease
Head	Atopy	Feline leprosy
	Demodicosis	Juvenile cellulitis
	Dermatophytosis	Pemphigus erythematosus
	Facial fold intertrigo	Pemphigus foliaceus
	Feline food hypersensitivity	Sporotrichosis
	Folliculitis, bacterial	Sterile pyogranuloma syndrome
	Scabies, feline	Systemic lupus erythematosus
		Vasculitis
		Zinc-responsive dermatosis
Ear	Atopy	Alopecia, pattern
	Food hypersensitivity	Cold agglutinin disease
	Demodicosis	Frostbite
	Dermatomyositis	Melanoderma and alopecia of
	Dermatophytosis	Yorkshire terriers
	Fly dermatitis	Pinnal thrombovascular necrosis
	Otitis externa (see Chap. 18)	Solar dermatitis, feline
	Otodectic mange	Sterile eosinophilic pinnal folliculitis
	Scabies	Trombiculiasis
	Seborrhea, marginal (pinna)	Vasculitis and vasculopathy
Eyelid	Chalazion	Lupus erythematosus
	Demodicosis	Dermatomyositis
	Dermatophytosis	
	Distichiasis	
	Entropion	
	Folliculitis, bacterial	
	Hordeolum	
	Seborrheic blepharitis	
	Trichiasis	
Nasal planum	Discoid lupus erythematosus	Contact dermatitis
	Drug eruption	Dermatophytosis *(M. persicolor)*
	Erythema multiforme	Hereditary nasal pyogranuloma and
	Nasodigital hyperkeratosis	vasculitis (Scottish terriers)
	Pemphigus erythematosus	Sporotrichosis
	Pemphigus foliaceus	Sterile pyogranuloma syndrome
		Uveodermatologic syndrome
		Vitiligo
Lip	Demodicosis	Candidiasis
	Indolent ulcer, feline	Contact dermatitis (plastic, rubber)
	Lip fold intertrigo	Juvenile cellulitis
	Lupus erythematosus	Mucocutaneous bacterial pyoderma
	Muzzle furunculosis, bacterial	
	Oral papillomatosis, canine	
	Uveodermatologic syndrome	
	Vitiligo-like lesions	
Oral cavity (mucosal lesions)	Discoid lupus erythematosus	Bullous pemphigoid
	Eosinophilic granuloma, canine and	Candidiasis
	feline	Pemphigus vulgaris
	Eosinophilic plaque, feline	Systemic lupus erythematosus
	Erosions, chemical	Thallotoxicosis
	Erosions, viral, feline	
	Erythema multiforme	
	Fusospirochetal stomatitis	
	Gingival hypertrophy	
	Indolent ulcer, feline	
	Marginal gingivitis, ulcerative,	
	dental	
	Plasma cell stomatitis	
	Vegetative glossitis (foreign body)	

Table continued on following page

Table 2:4. Regional Diagnosis of Non-Neoplastic Dermatoses *Continued*

Region	Common Disease	Less Common Disease
Mucocutaneous junctions	Epitheliotropic lymphoma Erythema multiforme Mucocutaneous pyoderma Systemic lupus erythematosus Vitiligo	Bullous pemphigoid Candidiasis Idiopathic ulcerative dermatosis (collies and Shetland sheepdog) Pemphigus vulgaris Phaeohyphomycosis Thallotoxicosis Toxic epidermal necrolysis
Chin	Demodicosis Eosinophilic granuloma, feline Furunculosis, bacterial Juvenile cellulitis	Dermatophytosis *Malassezia* dermatitis
Neck	Atopy, feline Dermoid sinus Flea bite hypersensitivity, feline Injection reactions Food hypersensitivity, feline *Malassezia* dermatitis	Contact dermatitis (collars) Ulcerative dermatitis with linear subepidermal fibrosis, feline
Lower chest	Folliculitis, bacterial Sternal callus	Contact dermatitis *Pelodera* dermatitis
Axilla	Acanthosis nigricans Atopy Folliculitis, bacterial Food hypersensitivity *Malassezia* dermatitis	Bullous pemphigoid Contact dermatitis Erythema multiforme Idiopathic ulcerative dermatosis (collies and Shetland sheepdog) Pemphigus vulgaris
Back	Atopy Comedo syndrome, Schnauzers Flea bite hypersensitivity Folliculitis, bacterial Food hypersensitivity Hypothyroidism Psychogenic dermatitis or alopecia, feline Seborrhea, primary	Calcinosis cutis Cheyletiellosis Pediculosis
Trunk	Demodicosis, generalized Folliculitis, bacterial Hyperadrenocorticism Hypothyroidism Sebaceous adenitis	Hyperestrogenism, female Hyposomatotropism Panniculitis, sterile Sterile eosinophilic pustulosis Subcorneal pustular dermatosis Vitamin A–responsive dermatosis

Abdomen	Atopy, feline
	Eosinophilic plaque, feline
	Feline symmetric alopecia
	Folliculitis, bacterial
	Food hypersensitivity, feline
	Hyperadrenocorticism
	Impetigo
	Linear prepucial erythema
	Panniculitis, sterile
	Psychogenic alopecia and dermatitis,
	  feline
	Solar dermatitis, dog
	Trombiculiasis
		Bullous pemphigoid
		Calcinosis cutis
		Contact dermatitis (ventral
		  abdomen)
		Erythema multiforme
		Hookworm dermatitis
		Idiopathic ulcerative dermatosis
		  (collies and Shetland sheepdog)
		Mycobacteriosis, atypical, feline
		Pelodera dermatitis

Tail	Feline symmetric alopecia Flea bite hypersensitivity Hyperplasia of tail gland, stud tail Mechanical irritation (tail suckers)	Cold agglutinin disease Dermatomyositis Frostbite

Table 2:4. Regional Diagnosis of Non-Neoplastic Dermatoses *Continued*

Region	Common Disease	Less Common Disease
Tail *(Continued)*	Psychogenic dermatitis or alopecia, feline	
	Pyotraumatic dermatitis	
	Tip of tail trauma	
Anus	Anal sac disease	Bullous pemphigoid
		Food hypersensitivity
		Pemphigus vulgaris
		Perianal gland hyperplasia
Legs	Acral furunculosis, bacterial	Decubital ulcers
	Acral lick dermatitis	Feline leprosy
	Contact dermatitis	Lymphangitis, bacterial, fungal
	Demodicosis	Lymphedema
	Dermatophytosis	*Pelodera* dermatitis
	Elbow callus	
	Elbow callus pyoderma	
	Hygroma	
	Eosinophilic granuloma, feline	
	Scabies, canine	
	Tarsal fistulae, German shepherd	
Paws	Atopy	Acral mutilation
	Demodicosis	Collagen disease of German shepherd footpads
	Dermatophytosis	Contact dermatitis
	Digital pad hyperkeratosis	Hookworm dermatitis
	Food hypersensitivity	Leishmaniasis
	Interdigital foreign bodies	Mycetoma
	Malassezia dermatitis	Necrolytic migratory erythema
	Pemphigus foliaceus	*Pelodera* dermatitis
	Plasma cell pododermatitis, feline	Phaeohyphomycosis
	Sterile pyogranuloma syndrome	Tyrosinemia
	Trauma	Vitiligo (pads)
	Trombiculiasis	Zinc-responsive dermatosis
Claws	Hyperthyroidism, feline	Arteriovenous fistula
	Lupoid onychodystrophy	Bullous pemphigoid
	Paronychia	Leishmaniasis
	Bacterial	Onychomycosis
	Feline leukemia	Pemphigus foliaceus
	Traumatic	Pemphigus vulgaris
	Trauma	Systemic lupus erythematosus
		Vasculitis
		Vitiligo

influence pattern formation at many levels, and may be fundamental to the development of the many patterns used to diagnose skin diseases.

Differential Diagnosis

A differential diagnosis is developed on the basis of a compilation of the preceding information. The possible diagnoses should be considered in their proposed likely order of occurrence. This point is important as the first step in developing a cost-effective plan.

Developing a Diagnostic or Therapeutic Plan

Laboratory tests or therapies can be recommended on the basis of tentative diagnosis and differential diagnosis. If a strong tentative diagnosis is not determined from the history and the physical examination, the approach should be directed at the two or three most likely diagnoses. Client-veterinarian interaction is critical at this point. The client decides what is going to be done, but his or her decision is based on the clinician's recommendations. Therefore, the client needs to know the tentative or possible diagnoses, as well as expected costs and anticipated results of the diagnostic or therapeutic options proposed.

Diagnostic tests and laboratory procedures are useful whenever a definitive diagnosis cannot be made from the case history and clinical examination alone.[4] Laboratory procedures may confirm many clinical diagnoses and provide a logical basis for successful therapeutic management. They should be recommended on the basis of the most likely diagnosis and should not be randomly suggested or recommended just to be comprehensive. The cost effectiveness of each test should also be considered. In practice, it is often unacceptable to recommend numerous tests to screen for the long list of possible diagnoses in any given case. Instead, the results of recommended tests should confirm or rule out the diagnoses that the clinician deems most likely.

■ LABORATORY PROCEDURES

Surface Sampling

The lesions and pathologic changes of a skin disease are often readily available for study, and a variety of laboratory tests are based on this easy access to the skin's surface. A great deal of information may be obtained by studying microscopically materials collected from the hair and skin. Skin scraping, obtaining an acetate tape impression, and flea combing are all techniques to find microscopic ectoparasites. Hairs may be removed, and exudates may be collected and examined microscopically. Most of these techniques may be done in general clinical practice and rapidly add valuable information to a case work-up. However, practice and study may be necessary to maximize the benefits of many tests. The effort to learn these techniques is well worth the time. The alternatives are not to obtain this information, to do other more expensive and time-consuming tests, or to send samples to a laboratory, which adds cost and time delays.

Skin Scraping

Skin scraping is one of the most frequently used tests in veterinary dermatology and is recommended anytime the differential diagnosis includes microscopic ectoparasitic diseases. Its purpose is to enable the clinician to find and to identify small and microscopic ectoparasites. It is important to realize that, although testing may accurately confirm diseases, its sensitivity for ruling out a diagnosis depends on the disease and the aggressiveness of sampling. Skin scraping is most commonly used to verify or rule out the diagnosis of demodectic mange. It is also commonly used to try to establish the diagnosis of sarcoptic mange, *Cheyletiella* infestation, and some other ectoparasitic diseases, although it does not effectively rule out these diagnoses. The equipment needed to perform a skin scraping is mineral oil, a scalpel blade (with or without a handle) or a curet, microscope slides, coverslips, and a microscope.

Not all skin scrapings are made in the same way. Success in finding parasites is enhanced if the technique of scraping is adapted to the specific parasite that the clinician expects to find. The method of scraping for demodectic mites is different from that of scraping for sarcoptic mites. *Cheyletiella, Dermanyssus*, cat fur mites, and ear mites each necessitate a slightly different scraping technique.

No matter which type of scraping is made, a consistent, orderly examination of the collected material should be done until a diagnosis is made or all the collected material has been examined. It is easiest to start the examination at one end of the scraped material mixed with oil and move the microscope stage straight across the slide in either a horizontal or a vertical direction. At the end of the slide, the examination moves over one field of vision and goes back in the opposite direction. This is continued back and forth until all the scraped material on the slide has been examined.

The following discussions elaborate on the special techniques needed to enhance the effectiveness of scraping for specific parasites.

EXAMINATION FOR PARASITES

■ *Demodectic Mites.* Generally, multiple scrapings from new lesions should be obtained. The affected skin should be squeezed between the thumb and the forefinger to extrude the mites from the hair follicles. The obtained material is scraped up and placed on a microscope slide. It is helpful to apply a drop of mineral oil to the skin site being scraped, or to the scalpel blade or curet, to facilitate the adherence of material to the blade. Then, additional material is obtained by scraping the skin more deeply, until capillary bleeding is produced (Fig. 2:29). It is important that true capillary bleeding is obtained and not blood from laceration. This is especially true when scraping the paw or the interdigital area in cases of pododermatitis. Please note that the Chinese Shar Pei breed presents an unusual situation in which mites may be confined to the deep follicle, and even with good scrapes characterized by capillary bleeding, false-negative results may occur. In addition, skin scrapings may be negative in dogs with chronic pododemodicosis, wherein the paws are swollen, fibrotic, and granulomatous. Only skin biopsies are diagnostic in such cases.

Generally, two or three drops of mineral oil are added to the usual amount of scraped material on the microscope slide. The oil is mixed with the scraped material to obtain an even consistency. Placing a coverslip on the material to be examined ensures a uniform layer that is more readily examined. Lowering the condenser causes more light diffraction and contrast, resulting in easier recognition of the mites.

Diagnosis is made by demonstrating multiple adult mites, finding adult mites from multiple

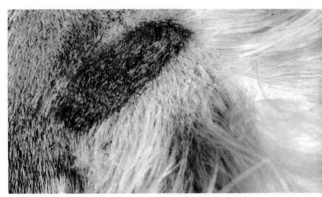

Figure 2:29. Capillary oozing indicating that an adequate depth was scraped for ruling out demodectic mange.

sites, or finding immature forms of mites (ova, larvae, and nymphs). When dogs are fractious or sites are difficult to scrape, another technique may be used. Hairs from the affected area can be plucked, placed in mineral oil on a slide, and examined. When the findings are positive, this technique precludes the need for deep skin scrapes. However, negative results of hair pluck examinations should not rule out the presence of *Demodex*.

It seems that skin scraping is a straightforward, easy laboratory procedure; however, the authors have encountered referred demodicosis cases in which false-negative skin scraping findings led to misdiagnosis or skin scrapings were not performed. Skin scrapings are advised in most cases of canine pyoderma and scaling and follicular disorders, because generalized demodicosis may be the primary disease. Skin scrapings should be performed whenever *Demodex* infection is among the primary differential diagnostic possibilities, the clinician is not certain of the diagnosis, or the dog does not adequately respond to the initial therapy. Dogs typically harbor only one species of mite, *Demodex canis*, whereas cats have two species, *D. cati* (which resembles the canine mite) and a second, unnamed species that is short and squat.

Scrapings taken from a normal dog, especially from the face, may contain an occasional adult mite. If one or two mites are observed, repeated scrapings should be done. Multiple positive results of scrapings from different sites should be considered abnormal. Observing whether the mites are alive (mouthparts or legs moving) or dead is of prognostic value while the animal is being treated. As a case of generalized *Demodex* infestation responds to treatment, the ratio of live to dead mites decreases, as does the ratio of eggs and larvae to adults. If this is not occurring, the treatment regimen should be re-evaluated.

■ *Canine Scabies Mites.* Canine sarcoptic mites, *Sarcoptes scabiei* (var. *canis*), reside within the superficial epidermis. However, because small numbers of mites are usually present, it is hard to find one. Multiple superficial scrapings are indicated, with emphasis on the pinnal margins and elbows. Skin that has not been excoriated, preferably skin with red raised papules and yellowish crusts on top, should be scraped (see Fig. 6:28 *B* and *C*). The more scrapings are performed, the more likely is a diagnosis. However, even with numerous scrapings, scabies cannot be ruled out because of negative results.

Extensive amounts of material should be accumulated in the scrapings and spread on microscope slides. Double-sized coverslips are sometimes useful. Alternatively, a second microscope glass slide may be used instead of a normal coverslip to compress the thick crusts. The clinician examines each field until a mite is found or all material has been examined; one mite is diagnostic. Dark brown, round or oval fecal pellets (Fig. 2:30) or ova from adult mites, if found, are also diagnostic. In difficult cases, it may be useful to accumulate an even larger amount of hair and keratin debris from scrapings. The material is placed in a warm solution of 10 per cent potassium hydroxide (KOH) for 20 minutes to digest keratin, and the mixture is then stirred and centrifuged. Mites are thus concentrated and can often be picked off the surface film and identified with a microscope.

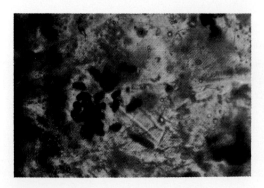

Figure 2:30. Fecal pellets of scabies mites.

■ *Feline Scabies Mites.*   The feline scabies mite, *Notoedres cati*, is much easier to find than the canine mite; otherwise, the diagnostic techniques described for canine scabies are appropriate. The best place to scrape is the head, the face, or the ears, in areas with crusts and scales.

■ *Cheyletiella Mites.*   *Cheyletiella* mites are relatively large compared with scabies mites and may even be seen with a magnifying glass. They look like small white scales that move, which is why the disease has been called ''walking'' dandruff. To examine for them microscopically, the clinician may obtain superficial scrapings, which are not as accurate as acetate tape impressions or flea-combing specimens. These mites may be difficult to demonstrate in some cases, especially in cats.

■ *Chigger Mites.*   The most common chigger mite is *Eutrombicula alfreddugesi.* These mites can be seen with the naked eye, especially easily on the concave surface of the pinna. They appear as bright orange objects adhering tightly to the skin or centered in a papule. They are easily recognized by their large size, relatively intense color, and tight attachment to the skin. They are often found around the external orifice of the ear canal but are not present in the canal. They should be covered with mineral oil and picked up with a scalpel blade. A true skin scraping is not needed. However, when removed from the host for microscopic examination, they should immediately be placed in mineral oil, or they may crawl away. Only the larval form is pathogenic, and these have only six legs.

■ *Poultry Mites.*   *Dermanyssus gallinae* is a mite that attacks poultry, wild and cage birds, and dogs and cats, as well as humans. It is red when engorged with blood; otherwise, it is white, gray, or black. When the animal shows evidence of itching and the history indicates exposure to bird or poultry housing, a skin scraping for this mite is indicated. One or two mites on the dog or cat may cause severe pruritus. The best place to find the mites is at excoriated sites.

The clinician collects the debris, scales, and crusts that harbor the mites. The materials are placed on a microscope slide, and several drops of mineral oil are added. The slide is covered with another glass slide instead of a coverslip. The two slides are squeezed together firmly to crush any crusted material. The acetate tape method of collection may be used successfully.

■ *Cat Fur Mites.*   *Lynxacarus radovsky* are mites that attach themselves to the external aspect of the hair shafts and therefore may be demonstrated microscopically by searching for salt-and-pepper hairs. The mites are usually located along the topline. A true superficial skin scraping can be made if the mites are suspected to be on the skin, but plucking affected hairs and examining them in a mineral oil preparation is usually diagnostic. The acetate tape impression method can also be used.

■ *Ear Mites.*   *Otodectes cynotis* mites are usually located in the external ear canal of dogs and cats. However, they may also be found on the skin, especially around the head, the neck, the rump, and the tail. They may be found by superficial scraping or acetate tape methods, such as described for *Cheyletiella* mites, and identified by microscopic examination.

Acetate Tape Impression

This alternative to skin scraping has been recommended to find superficial ectoparasites such as *Cheyletiella* mites, poultry mites, and cat fur mites. Clear, pressure-sensitive acetate tape (Scotch No. 602 [3M Co.] is a good type) is pressed to the hair surface and to the skin adjacent to parted hairs or in shaved areas. Superficial scales and debris are collected when one suspects cheyletiellosis or poultry mites. The tape is then stuck with pressure on a microscope slide and examined.

Flea Comb and Flotation

The recovery of *Cheyletiella* mites is enhanced with the flea-combing method. In this technique, large areas of the body are combed and the collected scale and debris are put in a fecal flotation solution. Material and scale that fall on the table or on a sheet of paper placed under the patient during combing should also be added to the flotation solution. A coverslip is applied to the surface of the flotation solution, is allowed to stand for 10 minutes, and then is transferred to a microscope slide and examined.

DEBRIS EXAMINATION OR FLOTATION

During examination of a pet, scabs and debris may readily be collected on the table surface. This may be enhanced by briskly rubbing the pet's skin and haircoat while the animal is standing on the table or over a piece of paper. This material may be collected and examined directly or mixed with a fecal flotation solution. Direct examination may find otherwise undetected flea dirt, flea eggs, or rarely, mites.

Hair Examination

Plucking hairs from the skin and examining them under the microscope is referred to as trichography and is helpful for diagnosing self-inflicted alopecia, dermatophytosis, color dilution alopecia, nutritional or congenital hair dysplasias, trichomycosis axillaris, trichorrhexis nodosa, anagen defluxion, telogen defluxion, endocrine alopecia, and pigmentary disturbances of hair growth. Hair examination may be beneficial in some cases of demodicosis or *Malassezia* dermatitis. Trichography is performed by grasping a small number of hairs with the fingertips or rubber-covered hemostats, epilating them completely, laying them in same orientation on a microscope slide with mineral oil, and examining them with the low-power objective of the microscope. If abnormalities are detected during scanning, closer examination will be necessary to categorize the defect.

Hairs will have either an anagen or telogen root (bulb). Anagen bulbs are rounded, smooth, shiny, glistening, often pigmented and soft, so the root may bend (Fig. 2:31 *A*). Telogen bulbs are club- or spear-shaped, rough-surfaced, nonpigmented, and generally straight (Fig. 2:31 *B*). A normal hair shaft is uniform in diameter and tapers gently to the tip (Fig. 2:31 *C*). Straight-coated animals have straight hair shafts while curly- or wavy-coated animals have twisted hair shafts. All hairs should have a clearly discernible cuticle, and a sharply demarcated cortex and medulla. Hair pigmentation depends on the coat color and breed of animal but should not vary greatly from one hair to the next in regions where the coat color is the same.

Normal adult animals have an admixture of anagen and telogen hairs, the ratio of which varies with season, management factors, and a variety of other influences (see Chap. 1). The anagen to telogen ratio can be determined by categorizing the bulbs from approximately 100 hairs. Since no well-established normal values are available, the authors rarely compute this ratio. However, estimation of this ratio can be valuable. No normal animal should have all of its hairs in telogen (Fig. 2:31 *D*); therefore, this finding suggests a diagnosis of telogen defluxion or follicular arrest (see Chap. 10). Inappropriate numbers of telogen hairs (e.g., mostly telogen during the summer, when the ratio should be approximately 50:50) suggest a diagnosis of a nutritional (see Chap. 16) or endocrine and metabolic disease (see Chap. 9).

Examination of the hair shaft follows bulbar evaluation. Hairs that are inappropriately curled, misshapen, and malformed (Fig. 2:31 *E*) suggest an underlying nutritional or metabolic disease. Hairs with a normal shaft that are suddenly and cleanly broken (Fig. 2:31 *F*) indicate external trauma from excessive licking or scratching or too vigorous grooming. Breakage of hairs with abnormal shafts can be seen in color dilution alopecia (Fig. 2:31 *G*) and other congenitohereditary disorders (see Chap. 11), trichorrhexis nodosa (see Chap. 10), trichomycosis axillaris

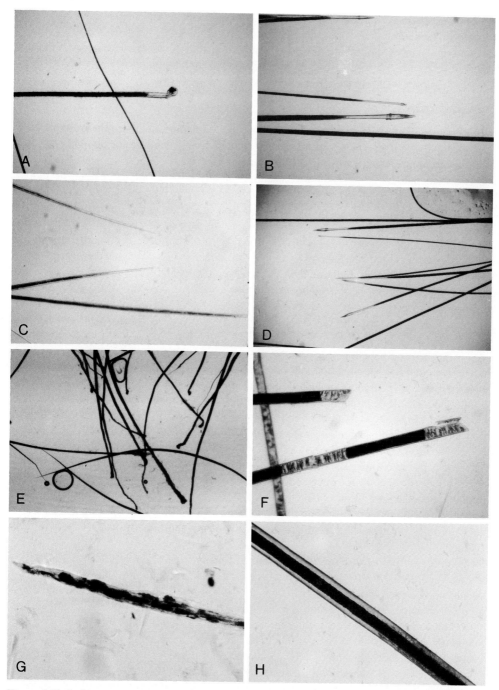

Figure 2:31. *A,* Anagen hair bulb from a cat. *B,* Telogen hair bulbs from a cat. *C,* The distal ends of normal hairs from a cat. Note the clearly defined cuticle, the distinct cortex and medulla, and the gradual tapering to the tip. *D,* Uniform telogenization of hairs from a cat with telogen defluxion. *E,* Misshapen and malformed hairs from a dog with severe nutritional deprivation. *F,* Cleanly fractured hairs from a cat with psychogenic alopecia. *G,* Hair from a blue dachshund showing pigmentary clumping, cortical bulging, and shaft fracture. *H,* Abrupt alteration in hair pigmentation from a dog taking procainamide. The drug caused lightening of the coat color.

(see Chap. 4), and dermatophytosis. Abnormalities in hair pigmentation that are not associated with color dilution alopecia have not been well studied. When unusual pigmentation is observed (Fig. 2:31 *H*), external sources (e.g., salivary staining, chemicals and topical medications, sun bleaching or conditions that influence the transfer of pigment to the hair shaft (e.g., drugs, nutritional imbalances, endocrine disorders, and idiopathic pigmentary disorders) must be considered.

Cytologic Examination

An enormous amount of vital diagnostic data can be obtained by microscopic examination of stained material, such as smears of tissues or fluids, during a clinical examination.[11] It is possible to accomplish this with minimal equipment and in less than 5 minutes. The cost is much less than that for a yeast culture, bacterial culture and sensitivity testing, or biopsy. Although the same information as obtained by these more expensive tests is not really gathered, microscopic examination often supplies sufficient data to narrow a differential diagnosis and develop a diagnostic plan.

The type of inflammatory, neoplastic, or other cellular infiltrate; the relative amount of protein or mucin; and the presence of acantholytic keratinocytes, yeasts, and bacteria can be determined by cytologic evaluation. It is the most common and most rewarding office test performed by the authors. The equipment includes a clean microscope slide, a coverslip, a stain, and a microscope.

Specimen Collection

Materials for cytologic examination can be gathered by a variety of techniques. Those most commonly used by the authors include direct smears, impression smears, swab smears, scrapings, and fine needle aspiration. In most situations, clipping the hair should be the only preparation of the surface. Scrubbing and applying alcohol or disinfectants are used only in areas where a fine needle aspirate of a mass lesion is to be done.

Direct smears are usually performed for fluid-containing lesions. A small amount of material is collected with the corner of a slide, the tip of a needle, or another sharp-edged object. The material is then smeared on the microscope slide.

Impression smears are often obtained when lesions are moist or greasy. This technique is also used after removing crusts, expressing fluid from lesions, or gently opening the surface of papules, pustules, or vesicles. The microscope slide is pressed directly against the site to be examined.

Swab smears are most often used to obtain specimens from draining tracts or sinuses, ear canals and interdigital webs, and dry crusty-surfaced lesions. The cotton-tipped applicator is moistened and inserted into the tract, the sinus, or the ear canal. For dry lesions and interdigital webs, the moistened cotton tip is rubbed briskly over the skin surface. After the lesion has been sampled, the cotton tip is rolled over the surface of the microscope slide.

Scrapings are used to sample underneath crusts, vesicles, and peeling stratum corneum. They may also be used to collect more cells from the cut surface of surgically removed biopsy specimens. The skin is scraped with a scalpel blade held at a 15- to 90-degree angle to the surface. The collected material is then gently wiped onto the surface of a microscope slide.

Fine needle aspiration is most commonly used to sample nodules, tumors, and cysts, although pustules, vesicles, or bullae may also be sampled this way. Fluid-filled lesions can be aspirated with 20- or 22-gauge needles and a 3-ml syringe. Firm lesions should be aspirated with 20-gauge needles and 6- or 10-ml syringes to obtain better suction. Fibrotic or dense masses may necessitate the use of an 18-gauge needle to get an adequate sample. The needle is introduced into the lesion, and then suction is gently applied by withdrawing the plunger of the syringe. Little withdrawing is necessary for fluid-filled lesions, and the material within the needle is sufficient. In mass lesions, the plunger is withdrawn one half to three fourths of the syringe volume. Suction is then interrupted while the needle is redirected into another area of the mass. Suction is again applied, and this procedure is repeated for a total of three or four times. Suction is then released, and the needle is withdrawn from the lesion. The syringe and the needle are then separated, air is introduced into the syringe, the needle is reattached, and the contents of the needle and hub are expelled onto the surface of a glass slide. The material is then streaked across the surface with another glass slide or the needle.

Stains

Collected materials are allowed to dry on the slide. Oily, waxy, or dry skin samples collected by direct impression or moistened cotton applicators should always be heat-fixed before staining. After the specimens are heat-fixed and dried, the slide is stained and examined microscopically. The stains of choice in clinical practice are the modified Wright's stain (Diff Quik) and new methylene blue. Diff Quik is a quick and easy Romanovsky-type stain. It gives less nuclear detail than the supravital stains such as new methylene blue stain. However, it allows better differentiation of cytoplasmic structures and organisms. Because this is most commonly what the practitioner is interested in with non-neoplastic skin diseases, the Diff Quik stain is preferred by the authors. When a neoplasm is suspected, two slides may be made and both stains used. A Gram stain is occasionally used to acquire more information on the identity of bacteria.

Cytologic Findings

Cytologic study is helpful to distinguish between bacterial skin infection and bacterial colonization, to determine the relative depth of infection, to determine whether the pustule contains bacteria or is sterile, to discover yeasts and fungi, to identify various cutaneous neoplasms, or to find the acantholytic cells of the pemphigus diseases.

Bacteria are a frequent finding in impression smears from skin and can be seen as basophilic-staining organisms in specimens stained with new methylene blue or Diff Quik. Although identification of the exact species of bacteria is not possible with a stain (as it is in a culture), it is possible to distinguish cocci from rods (Fig. 2:32 A and B) and often to institute appropriate and effective antibiotic therapy without performing a culture and antibiotic sensitivity testing. Generally, when cocci are seen they are *Staphylococcus intermedius*. If no bacteria are found in the stained fluid, the clinical condition is probably not a bacterial pyoderma. If neither granulocytes nor intracellular bacteria are seen, even large numbers of bacteria are not likely to be of etiologic significance.

It is also possible to obtain some clues as to the type of bacterial pyoderma or the underlying condition.[2] In general, deep infections have fewer bacteria present, with the vast majority being intracellular. In addition, deep infections have a mixed cellular infiltrate with large numbers of histiocytes, macrophages, lymphocytes, and plasma cells. The presence of these cells suggests that longer-term antibiotic therapy is necessary. Large numbers of intracellular and extracellular cocci are seen more commonly in cases of impetigo or in dogs with bacterial infections associated with iatrogenic or natural Cushing's disease.[2]

Direct impression smears are one of the most effective methods for detecting the presence of *Malassezia* (Fig. 2:32 D). Although *Malassezia pachydermatis* is an inhabitant of the skin in most normal dogs and cats, the yeast is difficult to find by examining direct impression smears and usually only 1 or 2 yeasts (rarely more than 20) are found when 1-cm^2 sections of slide are examined.[45] In a study done on skin with lesions, the presence of more than one yeast organism per high-power microscopic field was associated with certain diseases, such as seborrhea, or with previous antibiotic therapy.[46] Although the presence of more than one yeast per high-power field is not diagnostic of *Malassezia* dermatitis, the authors believe that this

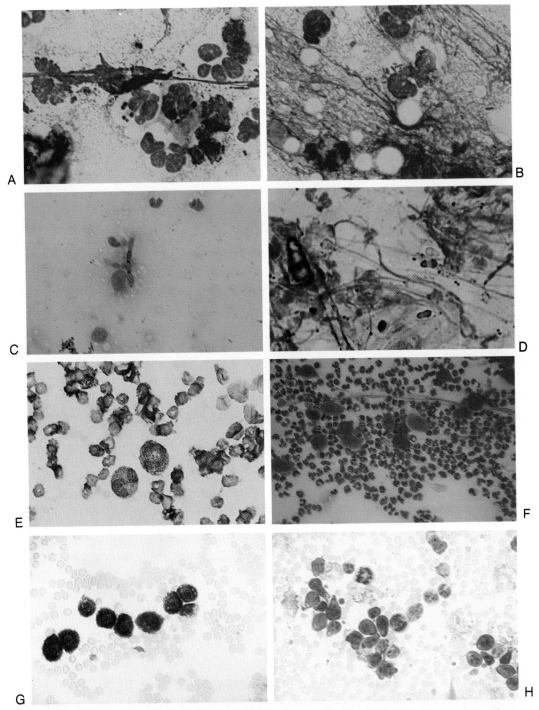

Figure 2:32. *A*, Degenerate neutrophils with phagocytosed cocci (*Staphylococcus* spp.) from a dog with pyoderma. *B*, Degenerate neutrophils with phagocytosed rods (*Pseudomonas* spp.) from a dog with otitis externa. *C*, Macrophage containing fungal hyphae from a cat with phaeohyphomycosis. *D*, Multiple *Malassezia* with neutrophils, keratinocytes, and cocci. Note variation in staining of *Malassezia. E*, Basophil and eosinophil from feline flea allergy dermatitis. *F*, Acantholytic cells and neutrophils from a dog with pemphigus foliaceus. *G*, Mast cells from a dog with a cutaneous mast cell tumor. *H*, Malignant lymphocytes from a dog with cutaneous lymphoma.

indicates that yeasts are present in abnormally high numbers and may be contributing to the pathologic changes seen.

Next, one looks for the cytologic response of the skin. Are there inflammatory cells (Fig. 2:32)? Are they eosinophils (Fig. 2:32 *E*), neutrophils, or mononuclear cells? If eosinophils are present, any extracellular bacteria seen probably represent colonization—not infection, and most likely an ectoparasitic or allergic disease is the primary problem. This finding can be especially helpful when evaluating dogs with suspected atopy or food hypersensitivity, as the presence of eosinophils strongly suggests that these diseases alone are not the cause of the skin disease. Conversely, cats with allergic skin disease frequently have tissue eosinophilia. If large numbers of eosinophils are seen in combination with degenerate neutrophils and intracellular bacteria, furunculosis is most likely present (free keratin and hair shafts serve as endogenous foreign bodies). It must be emphasized that eosinophils may be less numerous than expected or completely absent in inflammatory exudates from animals receiving glucocorticoids.

If neutrophils are present, do they exhibit degenerative or toxic cytologic changes, which suggest infection? If bacteria and inflammatory cells are found in the same preparation, is there phagocytosis? Are the bacteria ingested by individual neutrophils, or are they engulfed by macrophages and multinucleate histiocytic giant cells? Are there many bacteria, but few or no inflammatory cells, none of which exhibit degenerative cytologic changes or phagocytosis? When macrophages containing numerous clear cytoplasmic vacuoles are present, one should consider the possibility of a lipophagic granuloma such as is seen with panniculitis and foreign-body reactions.

Less commonly, cytologic examination allows the rapid recognition of (1) unusual infections (Fig. 2:32 *C*) (infections due to actinomycetes, mycobacteria, leishmania, and subcutaneous and deep mycoses); (2) sterile pustular dermatoses (pemphigus, sterile eosinophilic pustulosis, and subcorneal pustular dermatosis); (3) autoimmune dermatoses (pemphigus) (Fig. 2:32 *F*); and (4) neoplastic conditions (Fig. 2:32 *G* and *H*).

A synopsis of cytologic findings and their interpretation is presented in Table 2:5. Cytomorphologic characteristics of neoplastic cells are presented in Table 2:6.

Culture and Examination for Fungi

Identification of fungi that have been isolated provides important information for case management and for public health decisions (see Chap. 5). When agents causing subcutaneous or deep mycoses are suspected, the samples should be sent to a veterinary laboratory with appropriate mycology skills.[44] The propagation of many pathologic fungi, especially the agents of subcutaneous and deep mycoses, creates airborne health hazards. Additionally, examinations of the mycelial phase should be carried out in biological safety cabinets. For these reasons, the authors recommend that, in the general practice setting, fungal assessments be limited to direct tissue microscopic examination and culturing for dermatophytes. For other suspected fungal infections, samples should be collected and sent to an appropriate laboratory.

In general, for subcutaneous and deep mycotic infections, punch biopsies from the lesion are the best way to obtain a culture specimen. Pieces from the margin and the center of lesions, as well as any different-appearing lesions, should be submitted for laboratory analysis. Tissue samples may be placed in a bacteriologic transport medium and should reach the laboratory within 12 hours, although up to 24 hours is permissible. Refrigeration may be helpful to preserve some fungi but *Aspergillus* spp. and Zygomycetes are sensitive to cold. When these organisms are suspected, the sample should be kept at room temperature.

Direct examination for most nondermatophyte fungal organisms is acceptable as described under Cytologic Examination in this chapter. In general, the Diff Quik stain is suitable for many fungi, especially yeasts and *Histoplasma capsulatum*. Periodic acid–Schiff stain is useful but beyond the level of most general practice settings. India ink mixed with tissue fluid outlines the capsule of yeast and has been useful for identifying *Cryptococcus neoformans*. Clearing

Table 2:5. Cytologic Diagnosis From Stained* Smears

Finding	Diagnostic Considerations
Neutrophils	
Degenerate	Bacterial infection
Nondegenerate	Sterile inflammation (e.g., canine allergy, pemphigus, subcorneal pustular dermatosis, linear IgA dermatosis), irritants, foreign-body reaction
Eosinophils	Ectoparasitism, endoparasitism, feline allergy, furunculosis, eosinophilic granuloma, feline eosinophilic plaque, mast cell tumor, pemphigus, sterile eosinophilic folliculitis, sterile eosinophilic pustulosis
Basophils	Ectoparasitism, endoparasitism, feline allergy
Mast cells	Ectoparasitism, feline allergy, mast cell tumor (poorly stained with Diff Quik)
Lymphocytes, macrophages, and plasma cells	
Granulomatous	Infectious (especially furunculosis) versus sterile (e.g., foreign body, sterile granuloma syndrome, and sterile panniculitis)
Pyogranulomatous (many neutrophils too)	Same as for granulomatous
Eosinophilic granulomatous	Furunculosis, ruptured keratinous cyst, eosinophilic granuloma
Plasma cells	Plasma cell pododermatitis, plasmacytoma
Acanthocytes	
Few	Any suppurative dermatosis
Many	Pemphigus
Bacteria	
Intracellular	Infection
Extracellular only	Colonization
Yeast†	
Peanut shaped	*Malassezia* or rarely *Candida* dermatitis
Fungi	Fungal infection
Spores, hyphae	
Atypical or monomorphous cell population	
Clumped and rounded	Epithelial neoplasm
Individual, rounded, and numerous	Lymphoreticular or mast cell neoplasm
Individual, rounded or elongated, and sparse	Mesenchymal neoplasm

*Diff Quik or new methylene blue.
†Commonly seen, rarely pathogenic.

Table 2:6. Cytomorphologic Characteristics Suggestive of Malignancy

GENERAL FINDINGS	NUCLEAR FINDINGS	CYTOPLASMIC FINDINGS
Pleomorphism (variable cell forms)	Marked variation in size	Variable staining intensity, sometimes dark blue
Variable nucleus to cytoplasm ratios	Coarsely clumped, sometimes jagged chromatin	Discrete, punctate vacuoles
Variable staining intensity	Nuclear molding	Variable amounts
	Peripheral displacement by cytoplasmic secretions or vacuoles	
	Prominent, occasionally giant, or angular nucleoli	

samples with 10 per cent KOH as discussed for dermatophytes under Direct Examination in this chapter may help to identify hyphae of other fungi. When collecting samples for hyphal examination, one should not use gauze or cotton swabs because fibers may be mistaken for hyphae.

EXAMINATION FOR DERMATOPHYTES

In contrast to the case for other mycotic diseases, suspected cases of dermatophytosis and *Malassezia* infestation can readily be tested for in a general practice situation. To ascertain the cause of a dermatophytosis, proper specimen collection and isolation and correct identification of dermatophytes are necessary.

Wood's Lamp Examination

One aid in specimen collection is the Wood's lamp examination. The Wood's lamp is an ultraviolet light with a light wave of 253.7 nm filtered through a cobalt or nickel filter. The Wood's lamp should be turned on and allowed to warm up for 5 to 10 minutes, because the stability of the light's wavelength and intensity is temperature dependent. The animal should be placed in a dark room and examined under the light of the Wood's lamp. When exposed to the ultraviolet light, hairs invaded by *M. canis* may result in a yellow-green fluorescence in 30 to 80 per cent of the isolates. Hairs should be exposed for 3 to 5 minutes, as some strains are slow to show the obvious yellow-green color. The fluorescence is due to tryptophan metabolites produced by the fungus. These metabolites are produced only by fungi that have invaded actively growing hair and cannot be elicited from an in vitro infection of hair. To decrease the number of false-positive results, it is imperative that the individual hair shafts are seen to fluoresce. Fluorescence is not present in scales or crusts or in cultures of dermatophytes. Other less common dermatophytes that may fluoresce include *Microsporum distortum, M. audouinii,* and *Trichophyton schoenleinii.*

Many factors influence fluorescence. The use of medications such as iodine destroys it. Bacteria such as *Pseudomonas aeruginosa* and *Corynebacterium minutissimum* may fluoresce, but not with the apple green color of a dermatophyte-infected hair. Keratin, soap, petroleum, and other medication may fluoresce and give false-positive reactions. If the short stubs of hair produce fluorescence, the proximal end of hairs extracted from the follicles should fluoresce. These fluorescing hairs should be plucked with forceps and used for inoculation of fungal medium or for microscopic examination.

Specimen Collection

Accurate specimen collection is necessary to isolate dermatophytes. Hair is most commonly collected for the isolation of dermatophytes. When a Wood's lamp examination is positive, hairs that fluoresce are selected and removed with a forceps or a hemostat. When the Wood's lamp examination is negative, another means of collecting infected hair for culture is the toothbrush (MacKenzie) method. A sterile toothbrush is gently brushed through the animal's coat to accumulate hair and keratin debris. The toothbrush is then gently pressed onto the surface of the culture medium. The technique has proved especially valuable in detecting asymptomatic cats that may be carriers of *M. canis.*

Hair may also be collected from the margins of lesions. Whenever possible, one should select newly formed or actively expanding lesions that have not been recently medicated. The margins, as well as adjacent areas, are sampled. One should look for hairs that are broken or misshapen and associated with inflammation, scale, or crust. In long-haired breeds, the hairs can be shaved so that only 0.5 to 1 cm protrudes above the skin. However, if hairs are to be sampled from a lesion for fungal culture, it is valuable to clip excessive hair and gently clean the area. Patting the lesion clean with 70 per cent alcohol-impregnated gauze or cotton and then letting it air-dry decreases the occurrence of contaminants. The hairs obtained by these methods can be used for culture or microscopic examination. Some scales may also be collected, but one should avoid putting exudates or medications on the medium.

Claws

Claws and pads are frequently heavily contaminated with microorganisms and may have transient dermatophytes present. Therefore, before claws and pads are sampled, they need to be prepared with 70 per cent alcohol scrubs. The distal portion of the claws should be removed and discarded and samples then collected from the remaining claw. An alternative is to avulse or elevate pieces of claw and obtain the sample by scraping the concave aspect of the claw. Material from within the claw or the concave aspects should be collected whenever possible.

Hair, scale, and claw collected from suspected lesions can be placed onto culture medium and into mineral oil or clearing solution on a microscope slide for direct examination. Scrapings should never be placed in closed containers such as screw-capped tubes, which increase moisture and encourage the growth of contaminating bacteria and thus make it more difficult to isolate the dermatophytes. If the samples are to be transported and not immediately used, they may be placed in a clean envelope or a pill vial.

Direct Examination

The clinician should practice direct examination to become adept at identifying dermatophytes. Even the experienced clinician does not always obtain a diagnosis in cases of dermatophytosis. A negative direct examination finding does not rule out a diagnosis of dermatophytosis. Because most infections in animals are caused by ectothrix dermatophytes, clearing the hairs is not as necessary as it is for infections involving humans. The authors use only mineral oil to suspend hair with suspected dermatophytes. Others recommend clearing the keratin to visualize the hyphae and spores better. The hair, scales, and claw material may first be cleared by placing the specimens in several drops of 10 to 20 per cent KOH on a microscope slide. A coverslip is added, and the slide is gently heated for 15 to 20 seconds. One should avoid overheating and boiling the sample. Alternatively, the preparation may be allowed to stand for 30 minutes at room temperature. An excellent result is obtained if the mount is placed on the microscope lamp for gentle heating. The preparation is ready for examination in 15 to 20 minutes, and the structures are better preserved.

The following formula called chlorphenolac has been recommended as a replacement for the KOH solution in the digestion process to clear keratin: 50 gm of chloral hydrate is added to 25 ml of liquid phenol and 25 ml of liquid lactic acid. Several days may pass before the crystals go into solution, but when they do, no precipitate forms. The slide can be read almost immediately after hair and keratin are added to this chloral hydrate–phenol–lactic acid solution.

Examination of cleared, mineral oil–suspended, or stained scrapings from mycotic lesions may reveal yeasts, conidia, hyphae, or pseudohyphae. To find dermatophyte-infected hairs, one should look for fragmented pieces of hair that are larger in diameter than most hairs present. Generally, it is best to look near the hair bulbs and watch for distorted hairs. Dermatophyte-infected hairs appear swollen and frayed, irregular, or fuzzy in outline, and the clear definition between cuticle, cortex, and medulla is lost. It is also important to remember that dermatophytes do not form macroconidia in tissue. Any macroconidia seen represent saprophytes and have no known clinical significance. The hyphae of the common dermatophytes are usually uniform in diameter (2 to 3 μm), septate, and variable in length and degree of branching. Older hyphae are usually wider and may be divided into beadlike chains of rounded cells (arthroconidia).

In haired skin and scales from small animals, the branched septate hyphae of different dermatophytes may be identical to one another and necessitate isolation and culture for identification.

In an ectothrix invasion of hair, hyphae may be seen within the hair shaft, but they grow outward and show a great propensity to form arthroconidia in a mosaic pattern on the surface of the hair (Fig. 2:33 *A*). Large conidia (5 to 8 μm) in sparse chains outside the hairs are seen in *Microsporum gypseum* and *M. vanbreuseghemii* infections. Intermediate-sized conidia (3 to 7 μm) in dense chains are seen with *Trichophyton mentagrophytes*, *T. verrucosum*, and *T. equinum* infections.

An endothrix infection is characterized by conidia formation within the hair shaft (Fig. 2:33 *B*); the hair cuticle is not broken, but the hairs break off or curl. Endothrix invasion is rarely

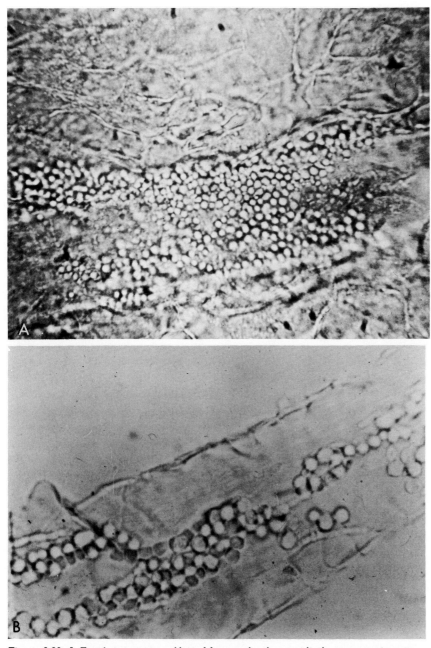

Figure 2:33. *A*, Ectothrix invasion of hair. Masses of arthroconidia form a mosaic pattern on the surface of the hair, and hyphae may penetrate the shaft. *B*, Endothrix invasion. Arthroconidia are within the hair shaft. (Courtesy C. Pinello.)

seen in animals but is typical of *Trichophyton tonsurans* infections in humans. The clinician should practice to develop the technique of direct examination for fungi. The best way to learn this technique is to find a highly Wood's lamp–positive *M. canis* infection in the cat. A large volume of positive hairs should be collected and kept in a loosely closed pill vial. Every few days, some hairs should be removed and examined until the affected hairs are rapidly recognized. After this is done, affected hairs should be mixed with normal hairs and the process repeated several times during the succeeding weeks. This type of practice greatly improves one's ability to locate dermatophyte-infected hairs by microscopic examination.

FUNGAL CULTURE

Sabouraud's dextrose agar and dermatophyte test medium (DTM) are traditionally used in clinical veterinary mycology for isolation of fungi; however, other media are available, although rarely used in general practice. DTM is essentially a Sabouraud's dextrose agar containing cycloheximide, gentamicin, and chlortetracycline as antifungal and antibacterial agents. The pH indicator phenol red has been added. Dermatophytes first use protein in the medium, with alkaline metabolites turning the medium from yellow to red (Fig. 2:34 *A*). When the protein is exhausted, the dermatophytes use carbohydrates, giving off acid metabolites. The medium changes from red to yellow. Most other fungi use carbohydrates first and proteins only later; they too may produce a change to red in DTM—but only after a prolonged incubation (10 to 14 days or longer). Consequently, DTM cultures should be examined daily for the first 10 days. Fungi such as *Blastomyces dermatitidis, Sporothrix schenckii, H. capsulatum, Coccidioides immitis, Pseudoallescheria boydii*, and some *Aspergillus* species may cause a change to red in DTM, so microscopic examination is essential to avoid an erroneous presumptive diagnosis.

Because cycloheximide is present in DTM, fungi sensitive to it are not isolated. Organisms sensitive to cycloheximide include *Cryptococcus neoformans*, many members of the Zygomycota, some *Candida* species, *Aspergillus* species, *P. boydii*, and many agents of phaeohyphomycosis. DTM may depress the development of conidia, mask colony pigmentation, and inhibit the growth of some pathogens. Therefore, it is valuable to place part of the specimen on plain Sabouraud's dextrose agar. In some cases, identification is more readily obtainable from the sample inoculated onto Sabouraud's dextrose agar. For this reason, a double plate containing one side of DTM and one of Sabouraud's dextrose agar has gained favor among many dermatologists. When bottles containing DTM are used, it may be difficult to get a toothbrush onto the medium surface. When bottles are used, it is also important to put the lid on loosely.

Skin scrapings, claws, and hair should be inoculated onto Sabouraud's dextrose agar and DTM. Desiccation and exposure to ultraviolet light hinder growth. Therefore, cultures should be incubated in the dark at 30°C with 30 per cent humidity. A pan of water in the incubator usually provides enough humidity. Cultures should be incubated for 10 to 14 days and should be checked daily for fungal growth. Proper interpretation of the DTM culture necessitates recognition of the red color change simultaneously with visible mycelial growth. False-positive results occur most commonly when the cultures are not observed frequently. As a saprophyte grows, it eventually turns the media red, thus emphasizing the importance of correlating the initial mycelial growth with the color change. Figure 2:34 illustrates the gross colony morphologic patterns of some common fungi.

IDENTIFICATION OF FUNGI

If a suspected dermatophyte is grown on culture, it should be identified. This necessitates collection of macroconidia from the mycelial surface. Generally, the colony needs to grow for 7 to 10 days before macroconidia are produced. Although colonies grown on DTM may provide adequate macroconidia, in some cases the colonies on the Sabouraud's dextrose agar may need to be sampled to find them. In occasional cases, especially with *Trichophyton* spp., no macro-

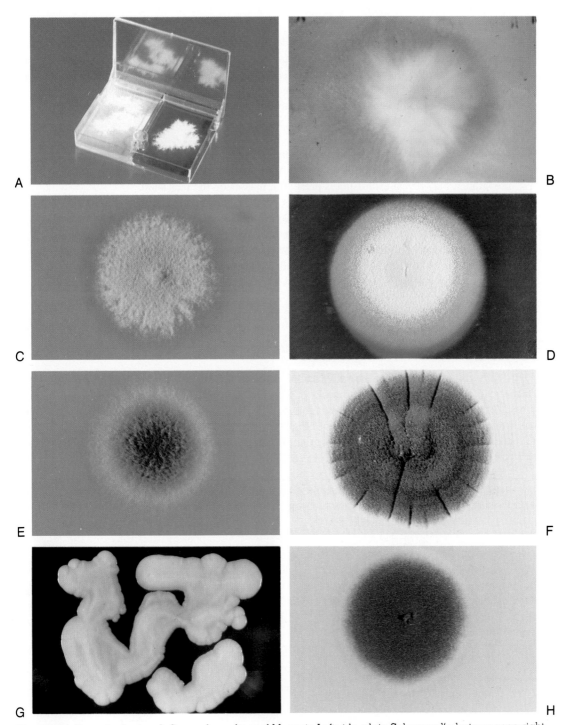

Figure 2:34. Fungal colonies. *A*, Seven-day culture of *M. canis*. Left side, plain Sabouraud's dextrose agar; right side, DTM medium. *B*, Gross colony of *M. canis*. *C*, Gross colony of *M. gypseum*. *D*, Gross colony of *T. mentagrophytes*. *E*, Gross colony of *Aspergillus*. *F*, Gross colony of *Penicillium*. *G*, Gross colony of *Candida albicans*. *H*, Gross colony of *Alternaria*. (*A, C, E, H*, courtesy C. Pinello. *B, D, F, G*, courtesy P. Jacobs.)

conidia are found. Subculturing these colonies on Sabouraud's dextrose agar or potato dextrose agar may facilitate sporulation. Alternatively, the sample may be sent to a diagnostic laboratory for identification.

The macroconidia are most readily collected by gently applying the sticky side of clear acetate tape (Scotch No. 602, [3M Co.]) to the aerial surface. The tape with sample is then placed onto several drops of lactophenol cotton blue that is on the surface of a microscope slide. A coverslip is placed over the tape and sample, and this is examined by microscopy.

Salient facts useful in identifying the three major dermatophytes (Figs. 2:34 and 2:35) are briefly described:

■ **Microsporum canis.** These lesions may show a yellow-green fluorescence. Hairs that fluoresce should be plucked for culture or microscopic examination. Examination of a KOH preparation may reveal arthrospores present in masses on the hair shaft.

■ *Colony Morphology.* On Sabouraud's dextrose agar, *M. canis* produces a white cottony- to woolly-appearing colony (see Fig. 2:34 *A* and *B*). With age, the colony becomes more powdery, has a central depressed area, and may show radial folds. The pigment on the undersurface of the colony is yellow-orange, becoming dull orange-brown. On potato dextrose agar, the pigment is lemon yellow.

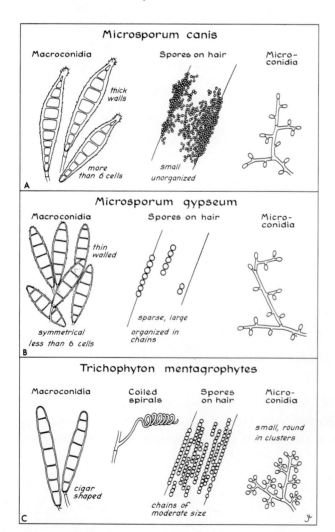

Figure 2:35. *A*, Characteristic microscopic morphology of *M. canis; B*, characteristic microscopic morphology of *M. gypseum; C*, characteristic microscopic morphology of *T. mentagrophytes.* The macroconidia and spirals are microscopic structures. The hair shafts are much larger.

■ *Microscopic Morphology.* *M. canis* usually forms abundant spindle-shaped macroconidia with thick echinulate walls. The echinulations (spines) are more pronounced at the terminal end, which often forms a knob. The macroconidia are composed of six or more cells (see Fig. 2:35 *A*). One-celled microconidia may be seen. Conidia develop best on rice agar medium and poorly or not at all on Sabouraud's dextrose agar.

■ *Diagnostic Criteria.* The distinctive macroconidia and the lemon yellow pigment are characteristic of *M. canis.*

■ **Microsporum gypseum.** Fluorescence is rare and, if present, is dull. The arthrospores on hair shafts are larger than those of *M. canis.*

■ *Colony Morphology.* Colonies are rapid growing with a flat to granular texture and a buff to cinnamon brown color (see Fig. 2:34 *C*). Sterile white mycelia may develop in time. The undersurface pigmentation is pale yellow to tan.

■ *Microscopic Morphology.* Echinulate macroconidia contain up to six cells with relatively thin walls (see Fig. 2:35 *B*). The abundant ellipsoid macroconidia lack the terminal knob present in *M. canis.* One-celled microconidia may be present.

■ *Diagnostic Criteria.* The abundant ellipsoid macroconidia and flat to granular texture of the colony are definitive features.

■ **Trichophyton mentagrophytes.** No fluorescence is seen with Wood's light. Ectothrix chains of arthroconidia may be observed on hair.

■ *Colony Morphology.* Colony morphologic characteristics are variable. Most zoophilic forms produce a flat colony with a white to cream-colored powdery surface (see Fig. 2:34 *D*). The color of the undersurface is usually brown to tan, but may be dark red. The anthropophilic form produces a colony with a white cottony surface.

■ *Microscopic Morphology.* The zoophilic form of *T. mentagrophytes* produces globose microconidia that may be arranged singly along the hyphae or in grapelike clusters. Macroconidia, if present, are cigar shaped with thin smooth walls (see Fig. 2:35 *C*). Some strains produce spiral hyphae, which may also be seen in other dermatophytes but are most characteristic of *Trichophyton.* Samples that show this change should be submitted to a diagnostic laboratory for identification.

■ *Diagnostic Criteria.* The colony morphologic characteristics, spiral hyphae, macroconidia, and microconidia are useful for identifying *T. mentagrophytes.* When grown on potato dextrose agar, *T. menta*grophytes does not produce a dark red pigment like that formed by *T. rubrum.* Strains of *T. mentagrophytes* are more apt to be urease positive than is *T. rubrum.* Because *T. rubrum* may be incorrectly identified as *T. mentagrophytes,* the above differential features are important.

Examination for Bacteria

In general practice, cytologic examination is the primary method used to identify the presence of pathogenic bacteria. Unusual lesions, nodular granulomatous lesions, and draining nodules should also be cultured. Bacterial culture and sensitivity testing are not routinely cost effective for the initial work-up of the case with a suspected bacterial pyoderma. Cytologic examination is the initial test of choice, and if intracellular cocci are seen, empirical antibiotic therapy for coagulase-positive staphylococci is warranted. When cytologic study reveals rod-shaped organisms, or when cocci are seen but appropriate empirical therapy is ineffective, bacterial culture and sensitivity testing are indicated. Veterinarians frequently take specimens for bacterial culture, but infrequently grow and identify the cultures in their own practice. Specimens should be collected for culture, properly prepared, and rapidly sent to a skilled microbiologist in a laboratory equipped to provide prompt, accurate identification and antibacterial sensitivities.

The selection of appropriate lesions for culturing is critical. Moist erosions and many crusts may be contaminated by bacteria, and cultures are not routinely recommended for these lesions. In cases with pustules, an intact pustule should be opened with a sterile needle. The pus collected on the needle should be transferred to the tip of a sterile swab. Papules may also be superficially punctured, and a relatively serous droplet of pus may be obtained. These superficial papular and pustular lesions should not be prepared at all, as false-negative cultures may result. With superficial cultures, a positive culture does not prove pathogenicity, and concurrent cytologic examination should be performed. This allows documentation of the intracellular location of bacteria, which confirms their role in eliciting an inflammatory response. In cases with furuncles, needle aspirates may be taken and cultured. When plaques, nodules, and fistulous tracts are to be cultured, the surface is disinfected and samples are taken aseptically by skin biopsy. The skin sample is placed in a culture transport medium and submitted to the laboratory, where it should be ground and cultured.

When unusual bacterial diseases such as mycobacteriosis, bacterial pseudomycetoma, actinomycosis, actinobacillosis, and nocardiosis are suspected, unstained direct smears and tissue biopsy specimens should be submitted. The laboratory should be informed of the suspected disorder.

Deep lesions, cellulitis, and nodular lesions may also be cultured for anaerobic bacteria. Again, tissue biopsy is preferred, and special transport media or equipment is necessary. A good diagnostic laboratory supplies material for sample transport.

Biopsy and Dermatohistopathologic Examination

Skin biopsy is one of the most powerful tools in dermatology.* However, maximization of the potential benefits of this tool necessitates enthusiastic, skilled teamwork between a clinician who has carefully selected, procured, and preserved the specimens and a pathologist who has carefully processed, perused, and interpreted the specimens. When the clinician and the pathologist truly work together, the skin biopsy can correctly reflect the dermatologic diagnosis in more than 90 per cent of cases.[34] However, despite this, skin biopsies are often not performed or are done relatively late in the diagnostic work-up. In other cases, the skin biopsy findings are unrewarding because of poor specimen selection, poor technique, or both. In many dermatologic cases, the differential diagnosis primarily includes diseases that can be diagnosed only by biopsy or other nonhematologic or serum laboratory tests. Yet the authors see numerous cases in which a variety of hematologic tests and cultures have been performed when the biopsy is the most cost-effective test to recommend to the client.

When the condition presented is not readily recognized, the skin biopsy is often the most informative test. Skin biopsy should not be regarded as merely a diagnostic aid for the difficult case or for the case that can be diagnosed only by biopsy. It is also helpful in establishing the group of diseases to consider. Even without a definitive diagnosis, a biopsy usually helps to guide the clinician in the appropriate diagnostic direction. It provides a permanent record of the pathologic changes present at a particular time, and knowledge of this pathologic finding

---

*See references 12, 15, 16, 18, 20, 22, 23, 31, 34, and 36 to 39.

stimulates the clinician to think more deeply about the basic cellular changes underlying the disease. Symptomatic therapies may also be directed on the basis of cytologic findings.

Although biopsies are helpful, it is still important for the clinician to remember that they only add information. The diagnosis is usually made by the clinician who correlates all the relevant findings of a case, not by the pathologist. The biopsy contributes to those findings; it does not replace a thorough history, physical examination, or other ancillary test results. Excellent textbooks on veterinary dermatopathology are now available.[17, 39a, 43]

WHEN TO BIOPSY

There are no definite rules on when to perform a skin biopsy. The following suggestions are offered as general guidelines. Biopsy should be performed on (1) all obviously neoplastic or suspected neoplastic lesions; (2) all persistent ulcerations; (3) any case that is likely to have the major diseases that are most readily diagnosed by biopsy (e.g., follicular dystrophy, zinc-responsive dermatosis, sebaceous adenitis, dermatomyositis, and immune-mediated skin disease); (4) a dermatosis that is not responding to apparently rational therapy; (5) any dermatosis that, in the experience of the clinician, is unusual or appears serious; (6) vesicular dermatitis; and (7) any suspected condition for which the therapy is expensive, dangerous, or sufficiently time consuming to necessitate a definitive diagnosis before beginning treatment.

In general, skin biopsy should be performed within 3 weeks for any dermatosis that is not responding to what appears to be appropriate therapy. This early intervention (1) helps to obviate the nonspecific, masking, and misleading changes due to chronicity, the administration of topical and systemic medicaments, excoriation, and secondary infection and (2) allows more rapid institution of specific therapy, thus reducing permanent disease sequelae (scarring, alopecia), the patient's suffering, and needless cost to the owner. Anti-inflammatory agents can dramatically affect the histologic appearance of many dermatoses. The administration of such agents, especially glucocorticoids, should optimally be stopped for 2 to 3 weeks before biopsy. If a secondary bacterial pyoderma is present, it is helpful to perform a biopsy after an appropriate course of systemic antibiotic therapy.

WHAT TO BIOPSY

The selection of appropriate biopsy sites is partly an art. Experienced clinicians often pick lesions and subtle changes that they suspect will show diagnostic changes. They are already aware of what histopathologic changes are helpful in making a diagnosis. They also know what types of changes may be expected to be found with certain clinical lesions. For example, pigmentary incontinence is a helpful histopathologic feature of lupus erythematosus. The clinician who knows this, and also knows that slate blue depigmenting lesions have that color because of dermal melanin (often from pigmentary incontinence), selects those sites for biopsy. One histologic criterion of lupus is likely to be present because the clinician knew the pathogenesis of that lesion.

If the disease is an unknown one or appears strange, a biopsy is important. If the distribution of lesions is unusual for the suspected disease, the clinician obtains biopsy specimens from the unusual areas, not just those typical of the suspected disease. It is also important to perform biopsy of areas representative of primary diseases and not just secondary complications. Many clinicians perform biopsy of secondary bacterial pyoderma lesions but not noninfected areas in cases with underlying allergy or keratinization disorders.

The histologic examination of the full spectrum of lesions present gives more information than does the examination of one lesion or stage. Therefore, the clinician should take multiple samples and obtain specimens from a variety of lesions. When primary lesions are present, a sample of at least one should be submitted to the laboratory. Fluid-filled lesions (pustules, vesicles) are often fragile and transient in canine and feline skin and, if present, should be sampled as soon as possible. If the suspected disease historically has pustules, having the patient return may allow sampling of the most appropriate lesions. In other cases, the patient may be hospitalized and be examined every 2 to 4 hours to find early intact lesions for biopsy. Most diseases that can be diagnosed by dermatopathologic examination have early, fully developed, and late changes. The greater the number of characteristic changes recognized, the more accurate the diagnoses are, and by selecting a variety of lesions, it is more likely that multiple characteristic changes are seen.

Multiple samples can document a pathologic continuum. Whenever possible, the clinician obtains biopsy specimens from the spontaneous primary lesions (macules, papules, pustules, vesicles, bullae, nodules, and tumors) and secondary lesions. Examination of crusts may sometimes add as much information as a biopsy of a papule. A greater number of biopsy specimens maximizes results.[18] However, in practice, clinicians are usually limited to three to five samples. Most important is that one learns from biopsy attempts. One should try to pay attention to what lesions are selected and what specimens give the best results. With practice, the clinician becomes more adept at selecting informative biopsy sites. Reading does not replace practice, attention to results, and experience, but it can help the clinician to achieve some proficiency in the art of maximizing the benefits of skin biopsy.

INSTRUMENTS REQUIRED

Biopsies are often performed simply and quickly with just local anesthesia. Two per cent lidocaine; a selection of punch biopsies of different sizes; Adson thumb forceps; iris or small, curved scissors; formalin vials; needles and suture material; needle holders; and gauze pads are the equipment that is needed for most cases. Occasionally, scalpel handles, blades, and large formalin vials may also be necessary.

HOW TO BIOPSY

In general, a 4- to 6-mm biopsy punch provides an adequate specimen. It is imperative not to include any significant amount of normal skin margin with punch biopsy specimens. Unless the person obtaining the biopsy specimen personally supervises the processing of the specimen in the tissue block, rotation in the wrong direction may result in failure to section the pathologic portion of the specimen. In general, when a punch biopsy specimen is received at the laboratory, it is cut in half through the center. Therefore, a macule, pustule, papule or small lesions should be centered in the biopsy specimen. If the lesion is to one side, only the normal tissue may be examined. The sample is also generally cut parallel to the growth of the hair (Fig. 2:36). In many laboratories, only half of the specimen is sectioned and processed; the other half is saved in case problems occur and new sections or blocks are needed. So even with deeper cuts, if the wrong half is blocked, the lesion may not be present. The clinician must also realize that, after fixation, erythema and color changes are not detectable by the pathologist who sections the sample. Small lesions such as papules and pustules may no longer be grossly visible.

It is important for the clinician to compare the pathologist's report with the description of the clinical lesion. If a pustule was observed clinically and the pathologist's report does not describe a pustule, it may have been missed. If a biopsied lesion is missed or the tissue is interpreted as normal, the clinician should explain this to the pathologist and obtain deeper sections to find the lesion.

It is also important for the clinician to be aware of what changes occur in the specimen after the biopsy. Autolysis starts to occur almost immediately after removal of the biopsy specimen. Therefore, it is important to place the newly acquired samples into appropriate fixatives (10 per cent neutral buffered formalin) immediately. This should be done for each sample; one should

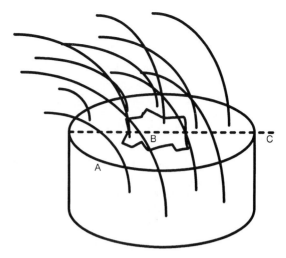

Figure 2:36. The diagram illustrates a punch biopsy. The margins of the biopsy *(A)* may appear relatively normal if a small lesion *(B)* is centered within the punch. The dotted line *(C)* demonstrates how most pathologists section the sample: The cut *(C)* parallels the angle of the hair growth.

not wait until all samples are taken before placing them in formalin. Punch biopsy specimens left under a hot surgery light have microscopically observable damage in less than 5 minutes.[15]

Excisional biopsy with a scalpel is often indicated (1) for larger lesions; (2) for vesicles, bullae, and pustules (the rotary and shearing action of a punch may damage the lesion); and (3) for suspected disease of the subcutaneous fat (punches often fail to deliver diseased fat).

Skin biopsy is usually easily and rapidly accomplished using physical restraint and local anesthesia.[19, 24] The sites are gently clipped (if needed); the veterinarian is careful not to remove surface keratin, and the surface is left untouched or gently cleaned by daubing or soaking with a solution of 70 per cent alcohol. The sites should *not* be prepared with other antiseptics (e.g., iodophors). Under no circumstances should biopsy sites be scrubbed. Such endeavors remove important surface pathologic changes and create iatrogenic inflammatory lesions.

After the surface has air-dried, the desired lesion is undermined with an appropriate amount, usually 1 to 2 ml, of local anesthetic (2 per cent lidocaine) injected subcutaneously. An exception to this procedure is made when disease of the fat is suspected, in which case regional or ring blocks or general anesthesia should be used, because injection into fat distorts the tissues. The local injection of lidocaine stings, and some animals object strenuously. The desired lesion is then punched or excised, including the underlying fat.

Great care should be exercised when manipulating the biopsy specimen, avoiding the use of forceps and instead using tiny mosquito hemostats, Adson thumb forceps, or the syringe needle through which the local anesthetic was injected. One cruciate (crisscross) suture effectively closes defects produced by 5- or 6-mm biopsy punches. One or two simple interrupted sutures may also be placed.

COMPLICATIONS OF SKIN BIOPSY

Complications after skin biopsy are rare. Caution should be exercised when performing biopsy on patients with bleeding disorders, including patients taking aspirin and anticoagulants. The administration of such medication should be stopped, if possible, for 1 to 2 weeks before biopsy. Problems with wound healing should be anticipated in patients with hyperadrenocorticism and hypothyroidism, in patients with various collagen defects (such as cutaneous asthenia), and in patients taking glucocorticoids or antimitotic drugs. The administration of such drugs should be stopped 2 to 3 weeks before biopsy, if possible. Wound infections are rare.

Caution should be exercised when injecting lidocaine, which may contain epinephrine, near extremities (ear tips, digits, and so forth); into patients with impaired circulation, cardiovascular disease, or hypertension; or into patients receiving phenothiazines, β-adrenergic receptor blockers, monoamine oxidase inhibitors (e.g., amitraz), or tricyclic antidepressants. Finally, one should be careful of the total amount of lidocaine injected into small kittens and puppies, because it can produce myocardial depression, muscle twitching, neurotoxicity, and death. One should not exceed a dose of 0.5 ml per kitten or puppy. Seizures have been induced when 0.5 ml of lidocaine has been injected subcutaneously on the head of small dogs or kittens.[2]

WHAT TO DO WITH THE BIOPSY SPECIMEN

Skin biopsy specimens should be gently blotted to remove artifactual blood. In most instances, the fixative of choice is 10 per cent neutral phosphate buffered formalin (100 ml of 40 per cent formaldehyde, 900 ml of tap water, 4 gm of acid sodium phosphate monohydrate, and 6.5 gm of anhydrous disodium phosphate). It is not stable and oxidizes to formic acid, which can be seen histologically by the formation of acid hematin in blood cells. Also, the ratio of formalin to tissue is important, with a minimum of 10 parts formalin to 1 part tissue being necessary for adequate rapid fixation. Freezing should also be avoided; this sometimes occurs when samples are mailed in the winter months.[15] This can be prevented by adding 95 per cent ethyl alcohol as 10 per cent of the fixative volume.

Fixation in formalin also causes sample shrinkage, which is not a problem with 4-mm and 5-mm punch biopsy specimens. Larger punch biopsy specimens and elliptic excisions should be placed epidermal side down on a piece of wooden tongue depressor or cardboard to minimize the artifacts induced by shrinkage. They should be gently pressed flat for 30 to 60 seconds to facilitate adherence. Placing the specimens on a flat surface allows proper anatomic orientation and prevents potentially drastic artifacts associated with curling and folding. The specimen and its adherent splint are then immersed in fixative within 1 to 2 minutes, because artifactual changes develop rapidly in room air.

Also, formalin rapidly penetrates only about 1 cm of tissue. Samples larger than 1 cm should be partially transected at 1-cm intervals. This most commonly becomes important when large nodules and tumors are excised and submitted for histopathologic evaluation.

The last critical consideration is deciding where to send a skin biopsy specimen. Obviously, the clinician wants to send it to someone who can provide the most information. The choices should be ordered as follows: (1) a veterinary pathologist specializing in dermatopathology, (2) a veterinary dermatologist with a special interest and expertise in dermatohistopathology, (3) a general veterinary pathologist, and (4) a physician dermatopathologist with a special interest in comparative dermatopathology.

The clinician frequently does not provide adequate information concerning skin biopsy specimens. The clinician and the pathologist are a diagnostic team, and an accurate diagnosis is more likely (and the patient is best served) when both members of the team do their part. A concise description of the history, the physical examination findings, the results of laboratory examinations and therapeutic trials, and the clinician's differential diagnosis should always accompany the biopsy specimen.

TISSUE STAINS

Hematoxylin and eosin stain is most widely used routinely for skin biopsies. In the laboratory of two of the authors (DWS and WHM), acid orcein–Giemsa (AOG) stain is also used regularly for skin biopsies. The routine use of AOG markedly reduces the need for ordering special stains (Table 2:7). Table 2:8 contains guidelines for the use of various special stains.

ARTIFACTS

Even the best dermatohistopathologist cannot read an inadequate, poorly preserved, poorly fixed, or poorly processed specimen.[12, 15, 18, 22, 23] Numerous artifacts can be produced by errors

Table 2:7. Staining Characteristics of Various Cutaneous Components with Acid Orcein–Giemsa Stain

Test Component	Color
Nuclei	Dark blue
Cytoplasm of keratinocytes	Blue-purple
Cytoplasm of smooth muscle cells	Light blue
Keratin	Blue
Collagen	Pink
Elastin	Dark brown to black
Mast cell granules	Purple
Some acid mucopolysaccharides	Purple
Melanin	Dark green to black
Hemosiderin	Yellow-brown to green
Erythrocytes	Green-orange
Eosinophil granules	Red
Cytoplasm of histiocytes, lymphocytes, and fibrocytes	Light blue
Cytoplasm of neutrophils	Clear to light blue
Cytoplasm of plasma cells	Dark blue to gray-blue
Amyloid	Sky blue to gray-blue
Hyaline	Pink
Fibrin and fibrinoid	Green-blue
Keratohyalin	Dark blue
Trichohyalin	Red
Bacteria, fungal spores, and hyphae	Dark blue
Serum	Light blue

Table 2:8. Staining Characteristics of Various Substances with Special Stains

Stain	Tissue and Color
van Gieson's	Mature collagen—red; immature collagen, keratin, muscle, and nerves—yellow
Masson trichrome	Mature collagen—blue; immature collagen, keratin, muscle, and nerves—red
Verhoeff's	Elastin and nuclei—black
Gomori's aldehyde fuchsin	Elastin, sulfated acid mucopolysaccharides, and certain epithelial mucins—purple
Oil red O*	Lipids—dark red
Sudan black B*	Lipids—green-black
Scarlet red*	Lipids—red
Gomori's or Wilder's reticulin	Reticulin, melanin, and nerves—dark brown to black
Periodic acid–Schiff	Glycogen, neutral mucopolysaccharides, fungi, and tissue debris—red
Alcian blue	Acid mucopolysaccharides—blue
Hale's colloidal iron	Acid mucopolysaccharides—blue
Toluidine blue	Acid mucopolysaccharides and mast cell granules—purple
Gomori's methenamine silver	Fungi—black
Gram's or Brown-Brenn	Gram-positive bacteria—blue Gram-negative bacteria—red
Fite's modified acid-fast	Acid-fast bacteria—red
Fontana's ammoniacal silver nitrate	Premelanin and melanin—black (hemosiderin usually positive too, but less intense)

*Require frozen sections of formalin-fixed tissue.

in site selection, preparation, technique in taking and handling and fixation and processing of skin biopsy specimens. It is important that the clinician and the pathologist be cognizant of these potentially disastrous distortions.

1. Artifacts due to improper site selection include excoriations and other physicochemical effects (e.g., maceration, inflammation, necrosis, and staining abnormalities caused by topical medicaments).

2. Artifacts due to improper preparation include inflammation, staining abnormalities, and removal of surface pathologic changes (from surgical scrubbing and the use of antiseptics), as well as collagen separation pseudoedema and pseudosinus formation (due to intradermal injection of local anesthetic).

3. Artifacts due to improper technique in taking and handling include pseudovesicles, pseudoclefts, and shearing (caused by a dull punch or poor technique); pseudopapillomas or pseudonodules, pseudosclerosis, pseudosinuses, pseudocysts, and lobules of sebaceous glands within hair follicles, on the skin surface, or both (squeeze artifacts due to intervention with forceps); marked dehydration, elongation, and polarization of cells and cell nuclei (due to electrodesiccation); and intercellular edema, clefts, and vesicles (due to friction).

4. Artifacts caused by improper fixation and processing include dermo-epidermal separation, intracellular edema, and fractures (due to autolysis); shrinkage, curling, and folding (due to failure to use wooden or cardboard splints); intracellular edema, vacuolar alteration, and multinucleate epidermal giant cells (from freezing); formalin pigment in blood vessels and extravascular phagocytes (due to the use of nonbuffered formalin); hardening, shrinkage, and loss of cellular detail (from alcohol in the fixative); poor staining and soft, easily displaced, and distorted tissue (with Bouin's solution); thick, fragmented sections (due to inadequate dehydration during tissue processing); pseudoacanthosis (in tangential sections associated with poor orientation of the specimen); and dermo-epidermal separation and displacement of dermal tissues into epidermis (attributable to cutting sections from dermis to epidermis).

■ THE VOCABULARY OF DERMATOHISTOPATHOLOGY

Dermatopathology is a specialty of medicine requiring many hours of training and many more of experience to master. It is beyond the scope of this book to train the student adequately in both dermatology and dermatopathology. However, because dermatopathologic examination is the single most valuable laboratory aid to the dermatologist, it is important to understand the vocabulary of the dermatopathologist.

Dermatohistopathology has a specialized vocabulary, because many of the histopathologic changes are unique to the skin. Unfortunately, as is true of most sciences, the dermatologic and general medical literatures abound with confusing and sometimes inappropriate dermatohisto-pathologic terms. The following discussion of terms is based on an amalgamation of such considerations as precision of definition, descriptive value, popular usage, historical precedent, and diagnostic significance in dermatohistopathology.[12, 21–23, 39]

Epidermal Changes

HYPERKERATOSIS

Hyperkeratosis is an increased thickness of the stratum corneum. It may be absolute (an actual increase in thickness, which is most common) or relative (an apparent increase due to thinning of the underlying epidermis, which is rare). The types of hyperkeratosis are further specified by the adjectives *orthokeratotic*, or anuclear (Fig. 2:37), and *parakeratotic*, or nucleated (Fig. 2:38). Orthokeratotic and parakeratotic hyperkeratoses are commonly, but less precisely, referred to as orthokeratosis and parakeratosis, respectively. Other adjectives commonly used to

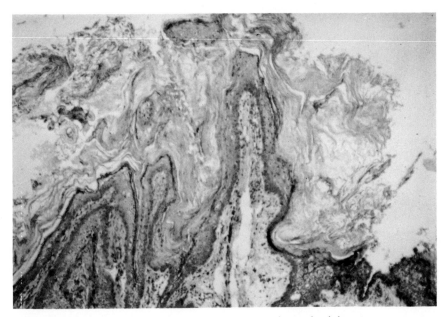

Figure 2:37. Marked orthokeratotic hyperkeratosis in a dog with ichthyosis.

Figure 2:38. Marked parakeratotic hyperkeratosis in a dog with necrolytic migratory erythema.

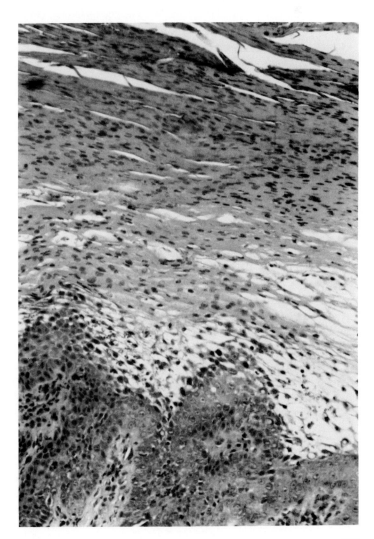

describe further the nature of hyperkeratosis include *basket weave* (e.g., dermatophytosis and endocrinopathic conditions), *compact* (e.g., lichenoid dermatoses and cutaneous horns), and *laminated* (e.g., ichthyosis).

Orthokeratotic and parakeratotic hyperkeratosis may be seen as alternating layers in the stratum corneum. This observation implies episodic changes in epidermopoiesis. If the changes are generalized, the lesions appear as horizontal layers. If the changes are focal, the lesion is a vertical defect in the stratum corneum. Orthokeratotic and parakeratotic hyperkeratosis are common, nondiagnostic findings in virtually any chronic dermatosis. They simply imply altered epidermopoiesis, whether inflammatory, hormonal, neoplastic, or developmental. However, diffuse parakeratotic hyperkeratosis suggests ectoparasitism, zinc-responsive dermatosis, lethal acrodermatitis, some vitamin A–responsive dermatoses, thallotoxicosis, generic dog food dermatosis, necrolytic migratory erythema, and occasionally dermatophytosis and dermatophilosis.

Focal parakeratotic hyperkeratosis overlying epidermal papillae (parakeratotic ''caps'') in which the subjacent dermal papillae are edematous (papillary ''squirting'') is seen in primary idiopathic seborrheic dermatitis of dogs.

Diffuse orthokeratotic hyperkeratosis suggests endocrinopathies, nutritional deficiencies, secondary seborrheas, and developmental abnormalities (ichthyosis, follicular dysplasia, and color dilution alopecia). Orthokeratotic hyperkeratosis that is disproportionately severe in hair follicles suggests vitamin A–responsive dermatosis, vitamin A deficiency, acne, Schnauzer comedo syndrome, follicular dysplasia, sebaceous adenitis, comedo nevus, and follicular cyst.

HYPOKERATOSIS

The decreased thickness of the stratum corneum, called *hypokeratosis*, is much less common than hyperkeratosis and reflects an exceptionally rapid epidermal turnover time, decreased cohesion between cells of the stratum corneum, or both. Hypokeratosis may be found in seborrheic and other exfoliative skin disorders. It may also be produced by excessive surgical preparation of the biopsy site or by friction and maceration in intertriginous areas.

HYPERGRANULOSIS AND HYPOGRANULOSIS

The terms *hypergranulosis* and *hypogranulosis* indicate, respectively, an increase and a decrease in the thickness of the stratum granulosum. Both entities are common and nondiagnostic. Hypergranulosis may be seen in any dermatosis in which there is epidermal hyperplasia and orthokeratotic hyperkeratosis (Fig. 2:39). Hypogranulosis is often seen in dermatoses in which there is parakeratotic hyperkeratosis, and is most easily appreciated in the footpads and the nasal planum.

HYPERPLASIA

An increased thickness of the noncornified epidermis due to an increased number of epidermal cells is called *hyperplasia*. The term *acanthosis* is often used interchangeably with hyperplasia. However, acanthosis specifically indicates an increased thickness of the stratum spinosum and may be due to hyperplasia (true acanthosis, which is the most common) or hypertrophy (pseudoacanthosis, which is uncommon). Epidermal hyperplasia is often accompanied by rete ridge formation (irregular hyperplasia resulting in pegs of epidermis that appear to project downward into the underlying dermis). Rete ridges are not found in normal haired skin of dogs and cats.

The following adjectives further specify the types of epidermal hyperplasia: (1) *irregular*— uneven, elongated, pointed rete ridges with an obliterated or preserved rete-papilla configuration; (2) *regular*—approximately evenly thickened epidermis (Fig. 2:40); (3) *psoriasiform*— approximately evenly elongated rete ridges, which are clubbed, fused, or both at their bases

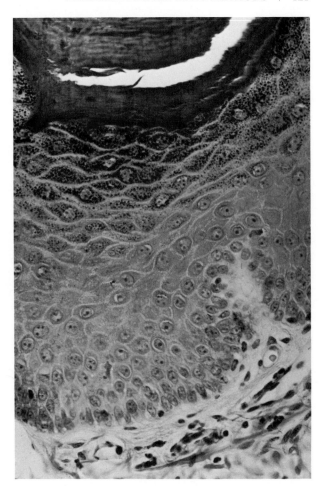

Figure 2:39. Hypergranulosis in a dog with ichthyosis.

(Fig. 2:41); (4) *papillated*—digitate projections of the epidermis above the skin surface (Fig. 2:42); and (5) *pseudocarcinomatous* (pseudoepitheliomatous)—extreme, irregular hyperplasia, which may include increased mitoses, squamous eddies, and horn pearls, thus resembling squamous cell carcinoma; however, cellular atypia is absent, and the basement membrane zone is not breached (Fig. 2:43). These five forms of epidermal hyperplasia may be seen in various combinations in the same specimen.

Epidermal hyperplasia is a common, nondiagnostic feature of virtually any chronic inflammatory process. The five types are generally useful descriptively but have little specific diagnostic significance. Pseudocarcinomatous hyperplasia is most commonly associated with underlying dermal suppurative, granulomatous, or neoplastic processes and with chronic ulcers. Papillated hyperplasia is most commonly seen with neoplasia, callosities, epidermal nevi, seborrheic dermatitis, and zinc-responsive dermatosis. Psoriasiform hyperplasia is most commonly seen with epitheliotropic lymphoma, psoriasiform-lichenoid dermatosis of English Springer spaniels, parapsoriasis, and chronically traumatized lesions (e.g., chronic allergy and acral lick dermatitis).

HYPOPLASIA AND ATROPHY

Hypoplasia is a decreased thickness of the noncornified epidermis due to a decrease in the number of cells. *Atrophy* is a decreased thickness of the noncornified epidermis due to a

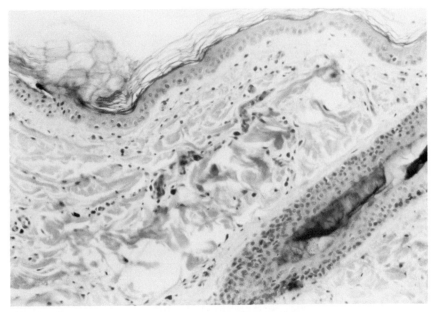

Figure 2:40. Regular epidermal hyperplasia in a dog with atopy.

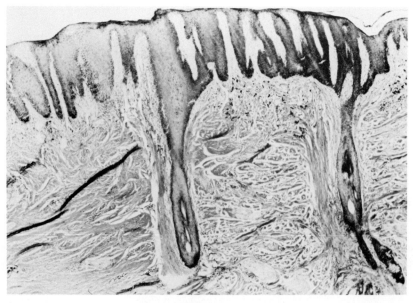

Figure 2:41. Psoriasiform epidermal hyperplasia in a dog with atopy.

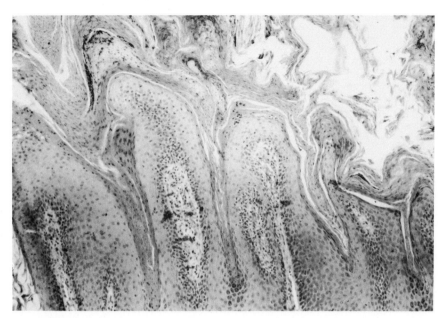

Figure 2:42. Papillated epidermal hyperplasia in a dog with zinc-responsive dermatosis. There is also diffuse parakeratotic hyperkeratosis.

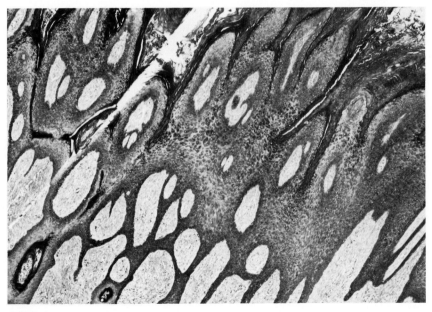

Figure 2:43. Pseudocarcinomatous epidermal hyperplasia in a dog with acral lick dermatitis.

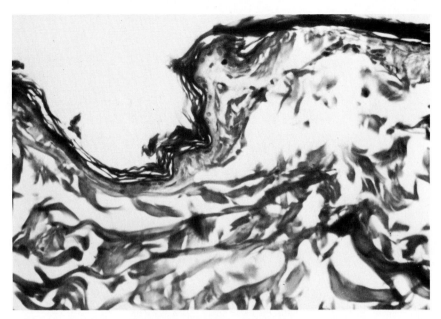

Figure 2:44. Epidermal atrophy in a dog with a sex hormone dermatosis.

decrease in the size of cells (Fig. 2:44). An early sign of epidermal hypoplasia or atrophy is the loss of the rete ridges in areas of skin where they are normally present (i.e., in the nonhaired skin of dogs and cats).

Epidermal hypoplasia and atrophy are uncommon in skin diseases of dogs and cats but are occasionally seen with hormonal (usually hyperadrenocorticism, rarely hypothyroidism), developmental (cutaneous asthenia, feline acquired skin fragility), and inflammatory (discoid lupus erythematosus, traction alopecia, dermatomyositis, vaccine-induced vasculitis) dermatoses.

NECROSIS, DYSKERATOSIS, AND APOPTOSIS

The term *necrosis* refers to the death of cells or tissues in a living organism and is judged to be present primarily on the basis of nuclear morphologic findings. The term *necrolysis* is often used synonymously with necrosis but actually implies a separation of tissue due to the death of cells (e.g., toxic epidermal necrolysis). Nuclear changes indicative of necrosis include *karyorrhexis* (nuclear fragmentation), *pyknosis* (nuclear shrinkage and consequent hyperchromatism), and *karyolysis* (nuclear ghosts). With all three necrotic nuclear changes, individual keratinocytes are characterized by loss of intercellular bridges, with resultant rounding of the cell, and a normal-sized or swollen eosinophilic cytoplasm. Necrosis is further specified by the adjectives *coagulation* (preservation of cell outlines, but loss of cell detail) or *caseation* (complete loss of all structural details, the tissue being replaced by a granular material containing nuclear debris).

Epidermal necrosis may be focal as a result of drug eruptions (Fig. 2:45), microbial infections, or lichenoid dermatoses or may be generalized as a result of physicochemical trauma (primary irritant contact dermatitis, burns, and thallotoxicosis), interference with blood supply (vasculitis, thromboembolism, subepidermal bullae, and dense subepidermal cellular infiltrates), or an immunologic mechanism (toxic epidermal necrolysis and erythema multiforme). Satellite cell necrosis (satellitosis) is characterized by necrosis of individual keratinocytes in association with contiguous (satellite) lymphoid cells (Fig. 2:46). Satellitosis is also seen in erythema multiforme and numerous uncommon dermatoses such as lupus erythematosus and graft-versus-host disease.

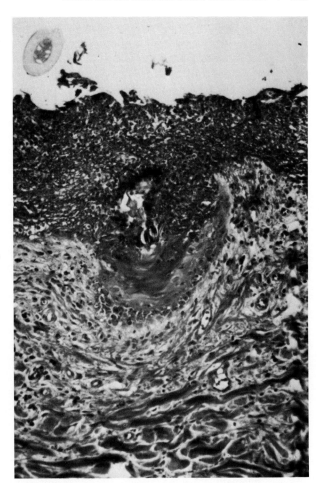

Figure 2:45. Full-thickness necrosis of the epidermis and outer root sheath of a hair follicle in a dog with erythema multiforme.

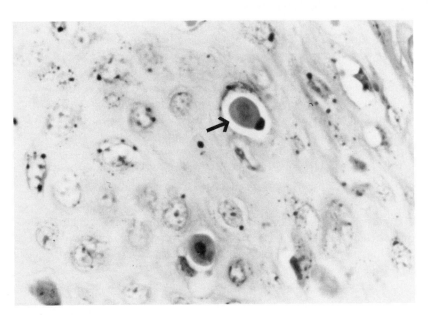

Figure 2:46. Satellite cell necrosis in a dog with erythema multiforme. Note the lymphocyte attached to a necrotic keratinocyte (*arrow*).

Dyskeratosis is a premature and faulty keratinization of individual cells (Fig. 2:47). The term is also used, although less commonly, to indicate a general fault in the keratinization process and thus in the state of the epidermis as a whole. Dyskeratotic cells are characterized by eosinophilic, swollen cytoplasm with normal or condensed, dark-staining nuclei. Such cells are difficult or impossible to distinguish from necrotic keratinocytes on light microscopic examination. The judgment usually depends on whether the rest of the epithelium is thought to be keratinizing or necrosing. This defect in keratinization may be seen in a number of inflammatory dermatoses (especially the lichenoid dermatoses, the pemphigus complex, zinc-responsive dermatoses, lethal acrodermatitis, some vitamin A–responsive dermatoses, and generic dog food dermatoses) and neoplastic dermatoses (especially papilloma, squamous cell carcinoma, keratoacanthoma, and warty dyskeratoma).

Apoptosis is a peculiar type of nuclear pyknosis and cytoplasmic fragmentation resulting from a programmed cell destruction as a countermeasure to mitotic cell multiplication.[43a] This intrinsic programming can be enhanced or inhibited by extrinsic stimuli. Apoptotic bodies (colloid bodies, hyaline bodies, filamentous bodies, ovoid bodies, and Civatte's bodies) are degenerate keratinocytes that appear as small, round to angular, homogeneous, eosinophilic bodies in the epidermis and hair follicle outer root sheath (Fig. 2:48). Apoptotic bodies are features of interface dermatoses, but they may be seen in very small numbers even in normal epithelium.

As can be appreciated from the above descriptions, the light microscopic distinction among keratinocytes that are necrotic, dyskeratotic, or apoptotic can be extremely difficult and is controversial. Thus, pathologists frequently use different terms to describe the same histopathologic finding. Fortunately for the clinician and the patient, the differential diagnosis is not, in most instances, radically altered by the choice of terms. Careful correlation of other histopathologic changes with the clinical findings overcomes the confusion of dermatohistopathologic semantics.

INTERCELLULAR EDEMA

Intercellular edema (spongiosis) of the epidermis is characterized by a widening of the intercellular spaces with accentuation of the intercellular bridges, giving the involved epidermis a spongy appearance (Fig. 2:49). Severe intercellular edema may lead to rupture of the intercellular bridges and the formation of spongiotic vesicles within the epidermis. Severe spongiotic vesicle formation may, in turn, cause blowout of the basement membrane zone in some areas, giving the appearance of subepidermal vesicles.

Intercellular edema is a common, nondiagnostic feature of any acute or subacute inflammatory dermatosis. Diffuse spongiosis, which also involves the outer root sheath of hair follicles, may be seen with feline eosinophilic plaque, feline eosinophilic granuloma, seborrheic dermatitis, *Malassezia* dermatitis, and zinc-responsive dermatoses. Spongiosis of the upper one half of the epidermis, which is overlaid by marked diffuse parakeratotic hyperkeratosis, is seen in necrolytic migratory erythema (hepatocutaneous syndrome). Spongiosis of the upper half of the epidermis with superficial epidermal necrosis may be seen with contact irritant dermatitis.

INTRACELLULAR EDEMA

Intracellular edema (hydropic degeneration, vacuolar degeneration, and ballooning degeneration) of the epidermis is characterized by increased cell size, cytoplasmic pallor, and displacement of the nucleus to the periphery of affected cells (Fig. 2:50). Severe intracellular edema may result in reticular degeneration and intraepidermal vesicles.

Intracellular edema is a common, nondiagnostic feature of any acute or subacute inflammatory dermatosis. Caution must be exercised not to confuse intracellular edema with freezing artifact, delayed fixation artifact, or the intracellular accumulation of glycogen that is seen in the outer root sheath of normal hair follicles and results from epidermal injury.

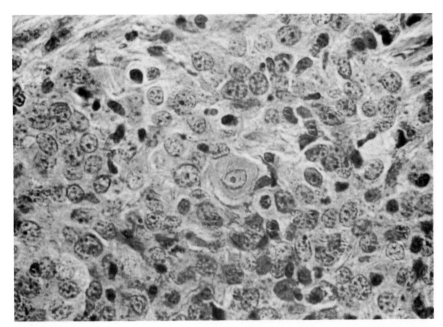

Figure 2:47. Dyskeratotic keratinocyte (center) in a dog with squamous cell carcinoma. (Courtesy J. D. Conroy.)

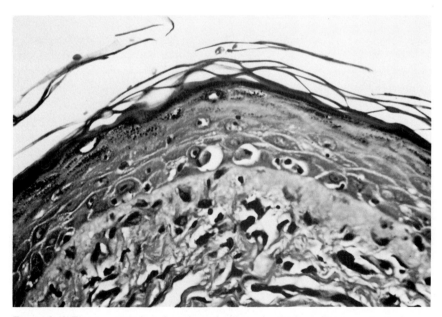

Figure 2:48. Two apoptotic basal epidermal cells and a thickened basement membrane zone in a dog with systemic lupus erythematosus.

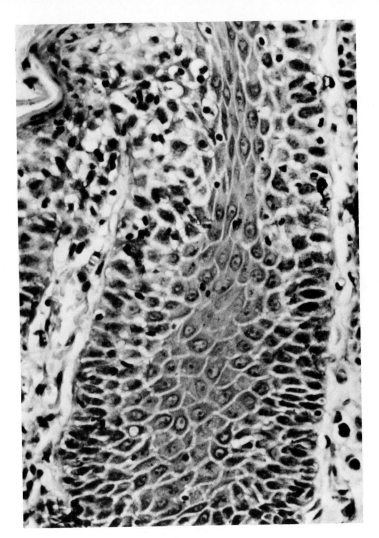

Figure 2:49. Spongiosis in a dog with contact dermatitis. There is also lymphocytic exocytosis.

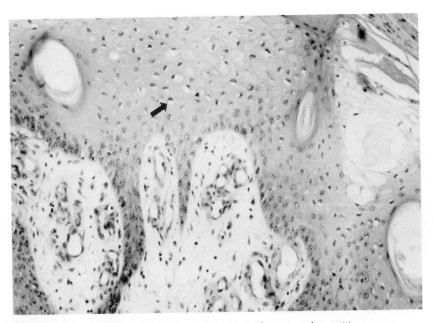

Figure 2:50. Intracellular edema (*arrow*) in a dog with contact dermatitis.

RETICULAR DEGENERATION

Reticular degeneration is caused by severe intracellular edema of epidermal cells in which the cells burst, resulting in multilocular intraepidermal vesicles in which septa are formed by resistant cell walls (Fig. 2:51). It may be seen with any acute or subacute inflammatory dermatosis, but especially dermatophilosis and acute contact dermatitis.

BALLOONING DEGENERATION

Ballooning degeneration (koilocytosis) is a specific type of degenerative change seen in epidermal cells and characterized by swollen eosinophilic to lightly basophilic cytoplasm without vacuolization, by enlarged or condensed and occasionally multiple nuclei, and by a loss of cohesion resulting in acantholysis (Fig. 2:52). Ballooning degeneration is a specific feature of viral infections.

HYDROPIC DEGENERATION

Hydropic degeneration (liquefaction degeneration or vacuolar alteration) of the basal epidermal cells describes intracellular edema restricted to cells of the stratum basale (Fig. 2:53). This process may also affect the basal cells of the outer root sheath of hair follicles. Hydropic degeneration of basal cells is usually focal but, if severe and extensive, may result in intrabasal or subepidermal clefts or vesicles owing to dermo-epidermal separation. Hydropic degeneration of basal cells is an uncommon finding and is usually associated with lupus erythematosus, idiopathic lichenoid dermatoses, drug eruptions, toxic epidermal necrolysis, erythema multiforme, dermatomyositis, hereditary lupoid dermatosis of German shorthaired pointers, and lichenoid keratoses.

ACANTHOLYSIS

A loss of cohesion between epidermal cells, resulting in intraepidermal clefts, vesicles, and bullae (Fig. 2:54), is known as *acantholysis* (dyshesion, desmolysis, or desmorrhexis). Free epidermal cells in the vesicles are called acantholytic cells (Fig. 2:55). This process may also

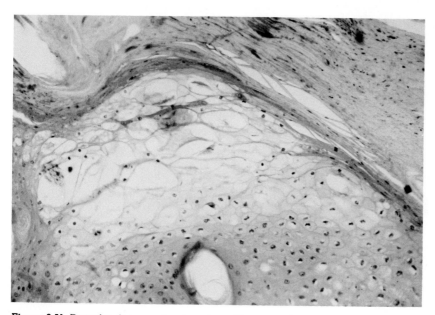

Figure 2:51. Reticular degeneration in a dog with contact dermatitis.

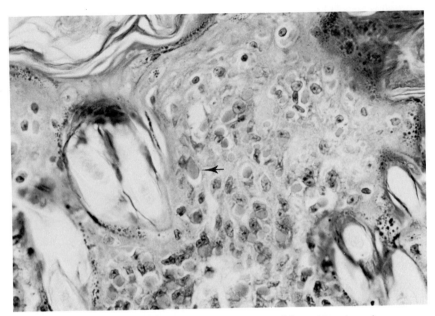

Figure 2:52. Hyperplasia and ballooning degeneration of the epidermis and intracytoplasmic inclusions (*arrow*) in a cat with feline poxvirus infection.

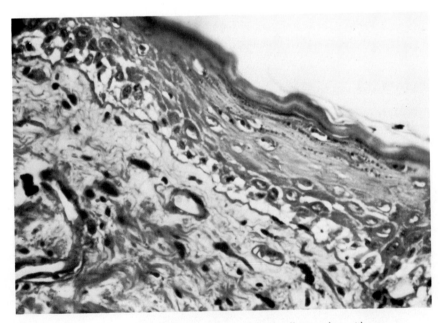

Figure 2:53. Hydropic degeneration of epidermal basal cells in a dog with epidermolysis bullosa simplex. (From Scott, D. W., Schultz, R. D.: Epidermolysis bullosa simplex in the collie dog. J. Am. Vet. Med. Assoc., 171:721, 1977.)

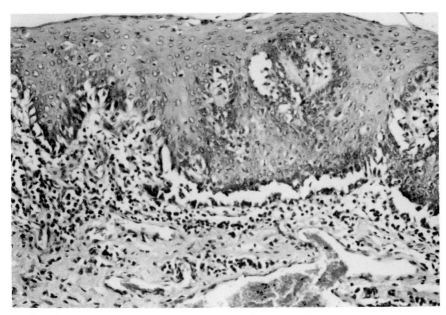

Figure 2:54. Acantholysis indicates a loss of cohesion between epidermal cells or adnexal keratinocytes or both that is due to degeneration or faulty formation of intercellular bridges (desmosomes). This leads to intraepidermal clefts, lacunae, vesicles, and bullae. It is seen here in a case of canine pemphigus vulgaris. This photomicrograph illustrates a suprabasilar cleft and intraepidermal vesicles containing acantholytic cells. (Courtesy A. A. Stannard.)

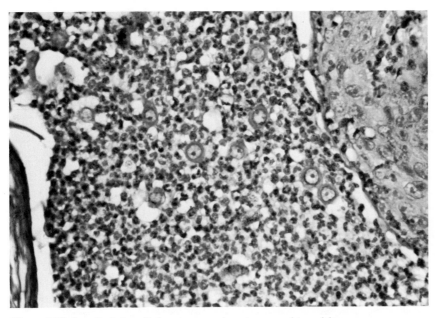

Figure 2:55. Acantholytic cells from a case of canine pemphigus foliaceus.

involve the outer root sheath of hair follicles and glandular ductal epithelium. Acantholysis is further specified by reference to the level at which it occurs (e.g., subcorneal, intragranular, intraepidermal, and suprabasilar).

Acantholysis is most commonly associated with the pemphigus complex due to autoantibodies against desmoglein or other cellular adhesion molecules. However, other causes of acantholysis are severe spongiosis (with any acute or subacute inflammatory dermatosis), ballooning degeneration (in viral infection), proteolytic enzymes released by neutrophils (in bacterial and fungal dermatoses and subcorneal pustular dermatosis) or eosinophils (in sterile eosinophilic pustulosis), developmental defects (benign familial chronic pemphigus), and neoplastic transformation (squamous cell carcinoma, actinic keratosis, and warty dyskeratoma).

EXOCYTOSIS AND DIAPEDESIS

The term *exocytosis* refers to the migration of inflammatory cells, erythrocytes, or both through the intercellular spaces of the epidermis (Fig. 2:56). Exocytosis of inflammatory cells is a common, nondiagnostic feature of any inflammatory dermatosis. When the condition involves eosinophils in combination with spongiosis, it is often referred to as *eosinophilic spongiosis* and may be seen in ectoparasitism, pemphigus, pemphigoid, sterile eosinophilic pustulosis, eosinophilic plaque, eosinophilic granuloma, and hypereosinophilic syndrome.

Diapedesis occurs when erythrocytes are present in the intercellular spaces of the epidermis. Diapedesis of erythrocytes implies loss of vascular integrity and may be seen whenever superficial dermal inflammation and vascular dilatation and engorgement are pronounced or when vasculitis or coagulation defects occur.

CLEFTS

The slitlike spaces known as *clefts* (lacunae), which do not contain fluid, occur within the epidermis or at the dermo-epidermal junction. Clefts may be caused by acantholysis or hydropic degeneration of basal cells (Max Joseph spaces, Fig. 2:57). However, they may also be caused by mechanical trauma and tissue retraction associated with obtaining, fixing, and processing biopsy specimens.

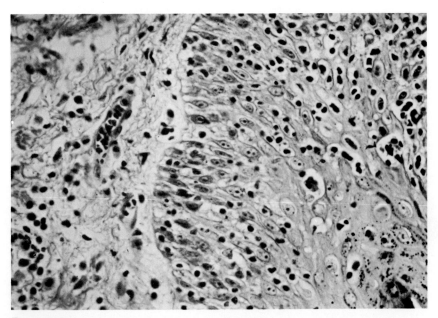

Figure 2:56. Exocytosis of leukocytes through the epidermis in a dog with scabies.

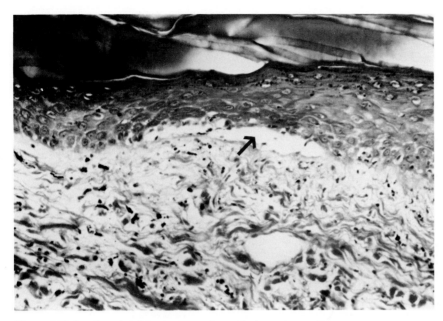

Figure 2:57. Intrabasal cleft (*arrow*) in a dog with dermatomyositis.

Artifactual dermo-epidermal separation is fairly commonly observed at the margin of a biopsy specimen. In general, only tissue weakened through the dermal-epidermal junction will separate in this manner during processing. Thus, this "usable artifact" may be valid evidence of basal cell or basement membrane damage. Spurious separation is characterized by clefting at different anatomic sites within the same specimen, and evidence of tissue trauma (e.g., torn cytoplasm and fibers, bare cellular nuclei).

MICROVESICLES, VESICLES, AND BULLAE

Microvesicles (Fig. 2:58), vesicles, and bullae are microscopic and macroscopic, fluid-filled, relatively acellular spaces within or below the epidermis. Such lesions are often loosely referred to as *blisters*. These lesions may be caused by severe intercellular or intracellular edema, ballooning degeneration, acantholysis, hydropic degeneration of basal cells, subepidermal edema, or other factors resulting in dermo-epidermal separation (e.g., the autoantibodies in bullous pemphigoid). Microvesicles, vesicles, and bullae may thus be further described by their location as subcorneal, intragranular, intraepidermal, suprabasilar, intrabasal, or subepidermal. When these lesions contain larger numbers of inflammatory cells, they are referred to as *vesicopustules*.

MICROABSCESSES AND PUSTULES

Microabscesses and pustules are microscopic or macroscopic intraepidermal and subepidermal cavities filled with inflammatory cells (Fig. 2:59), which can be further described on the basis of location and cell type as follows:

(1) *Spongiform pustule of Kogoj* (Fig. 2:60) is a multilocular accumulation of neutrophils within and between keratinocytes, especially those of the stratum granulosum and the stratum spinosum, in which cell boundaries form a spongelike network. It is seen in microbial infections and occasionally in canine subcorneal pustular dermatosis, linear IgA dermatosis, and superficial suppurative necrolytic dermatitis of Schnauzers.

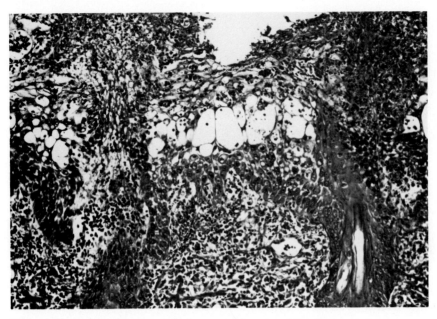

Figure 2:58. Epidermal microvesicles in a cat with eosinophilic plaque.

(2) *Munro's microabscess* (Fig. 2:61) is a small, desiccated accumulation of neutrophils within or below the stratum corneum, which is seen in microbial infections, seborrheic disorders, and psoriasiform-lichenoid dermatosis of English Springer spaniels.

(3) *Pautrier's microabscess* (Fig. 2:62) is a small, focal accumulation of abnormal lymphoid cells, which is seen in epitheliotropic lymphomas.

(4) *Eosinophilic microabscess* is a lesion seen in ectoparasitism, eosinophilic granuloma, eosinophilic folliculitis, sterile eosinophilic pustulosis, bullous pemphigoid, the pemphigus complex, feline allergy, and occasionally with *Malassezia* dermatitis.

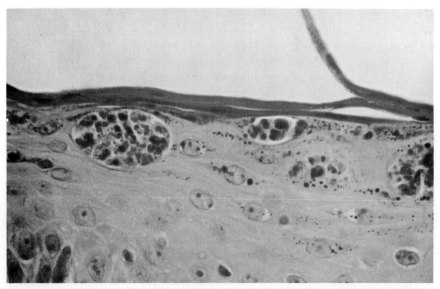

Figure 2:59. Microabscesses are observed in many dermatoses. This photomicrograph illustrates microabscesses containing many eosinophils located within the epidermis. (Courtesy J. D. Conroy.)

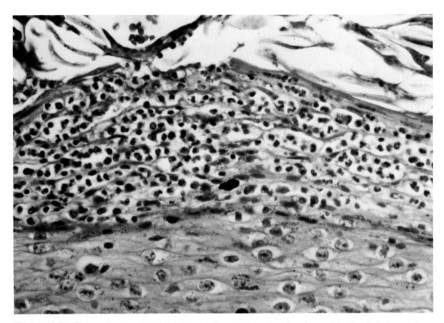

Figure 2:60. Spongiform microabscess in the epidermis of a dog with staphylococcal folliculitis.

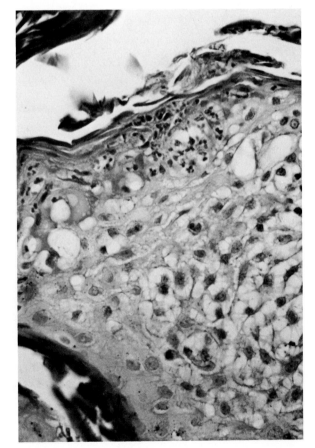

Figure 2:61. Munro's microabscess in the superficial epidermis of a dog with seborrheic dermatitis.

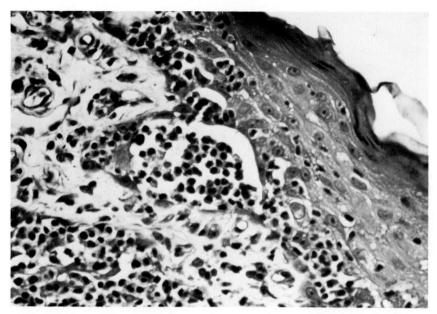

Figure 2:62. Pautrier's microabscess in the lower epidermis of a dog with epitheliotropic lymphoma.

HYPERPIGMENTATION

Hyperpigmentation (hypermelanosis) refers to excessive amounts of melanin deposited within the epidermis and often concurrently in dermal melanophages. Hyperpigmentation may be focal or diffuse and may be confined to the stratum basale or present throughout all epidermal layers (Fig. 2:63). It is a common, nondiagnostic finding in chronic inflammatory and hormonal dermatoses as well as in some developmental and neoplastic disorders. Hyperpigmentation

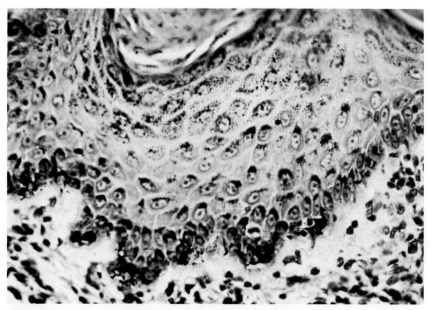

Figure 2:63. Epidermal melanosis (hyperpigmentation) in a dog with acanthosis nigricans.

must always be cautiously assessed with regard to the patient's normal pigmentation. Hyperpigmentation of sebaceous glands with extrusion of linear melanotic casts into hair follicle lumina is seen with follicular dysplasias.

HYPOPIGMENTATION

Hypopigmentation (hypomelanosis) refers to decreased amounts of melanin in the epidermis. The condition may be associated with congenital or acquired idiopathic defects in melaninization (e.g., leukoderma and vitiligo), the toxic effects of certain chemicals (e.g., monobenzyl ether of dihydroquinone in rubbers and plastics) on melanocytes, inflammatory disorders that affect melaninization or destroy melanocytes, hormonal disorders, and dermatoses featuring hydropic degeneration of basal cells (e.g., lupus erythematosus). In the hypopigmented dermatoses associated with hydropic degeneration of basal cells, the underlying superficial dermis usually reveals pigmentary incontinence.

CRUST

The consolidated, desiccated surface mass called *crust* is composed of varying combinations of keratin, serum, cellular debris, and often microorganisms. Crusts are further described on the basis of their composition: (1) *serous*—mostly serum, (2) *hemorrhagic*—mostly blood, (3) *cellular*—mostly inflammatory cells, (4) *serocellular* (exudative)—a mixture of serum and inflammatory cells (Fig. 2:64), and (5) *palisading*—alternating horizontal rows of orthokeratotic to parakeratotic hyperkeratosis and pus (e.g., in dermatophilosis and dermatophytosis).

Crusts merely indicate a prior exudative process and are rarely of diagnostic significance. However, crusts should always be closely scrutinized, because they may contain the following important diagnostic clues: (1) dermatophyte spores and hyphae, (2) the filaments and coccoid elements of *Dermatophilus congolensis*, and (3) large numbers of acantholytic keratinocytes (in pemphigus complex). Bacteria and bacterial colonies are common inhabitants of surface debris and are of no diagnostic significance.

The presence of yeasts in surface debris is more difficult to interpret. Yeasts (*M. pachydermatis*) are occasionally seen in surface debris and may be of no diagnostic significance.[32, 33]

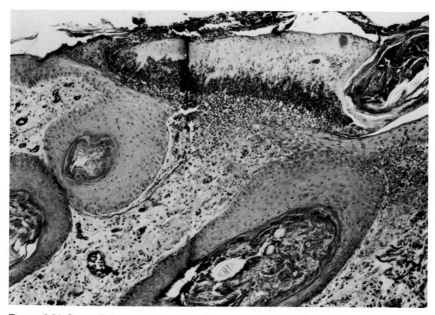

Figure 2:64. Serocellular crust in a cat with primary irritant contact dermatitis.

However, the pathologist and the clinician should always carefully consider the potential importance of yeast in contributing to dermatitis. Histopathologically, the presence of surface yeasts accompanied by subjacent epidermal parakeratotic hyperkeratosis, spongiosis, and lymphocytic exocytosis is a reaction pattern that strongly suggests that these organisms are contributing to the clinical dermatitis.

DELLS

Dells are small depressions or hollows in the surface of the epidermis. They are usually associated with focal epidermal atrophy and orthokeratotic hyperkeratosis. Dells may be seen in lichenoid dermatoses, especially in lupus erythematosus.

EPIDERMAL COLLARETTE

The term *epidermal collarette* refers to the formation of elongated, hyperplastic rete ridges at the lateral margins of a pathologic process that appear to curve inward toward the center of the lesion. Epidermal collarettes may be seen with neoplastic, granulomatous, and suppurative dermatoses.

HORN CYSTS, PSEUDOHORN CYSTS, HORN PEARLS, AND SQUAMOUS EDDIES

Horn cysts (keratin cysts) are multiple, small, circular cystic structures that are surrounded by flattened epidermal cells and that contain concentrically arranged lamellar keratin. Horn cysts are features of hair follicle neoplasms and basal cell tumors. *Pseudohorn cysts* are illusory small cystic structures formed by the irregular invagination of a hyperplastic, hyperkeratotic epidermis. They are seen in numerous hyperplastic or neoplastic epidermal dermatoses.

Horn pearls (squamous pearls) are focal, circular, concentric layers of squamous cells showing gradual keratinization toward the center, often accompanied by cellular atypia and dyskeratosis. Horn pearls are features of squamous cell carcinoma and pseudocarcinomatous hyperplasia.

Squamous eddies are whorl-like patterns of squamoid cells with no atypia, dyskeratosis, or central keratinization. Squamous eddies are features of numerous neoplastic and hyperplastic epidermal disorders.

EPIDERMOLYTIC HYPERKERATOSIS

Epidermolytic hyperkeratosis (granular degeneration) is characterized by (1) perinuclear clear spaces in the upper epidermis, (2) indistinct cell boundaries formed either by lightly staining material or by keratohyalin granules peripheral to the perinuclear clear spaces, (3) a markedly thickened stratum granulosum, and (4) orthokeratotic hyperkeratosis. It is seen in certain types of ichthyosis, epidermal nevi (Fig. 2:65), actinic keratoses, seborrheic keratoses, papillomas, keratinous cysts, and squamous cell carcinoma.

EPIDERMAL MAST CELLS

Mast cells are frequently seen within the epidermis and the outer root sheath of the hair follicle in biopsy specimens from cats with inflammatory dermatoses (Fig. 2:66).[30] They are most commonly found in diseases of allergic or immune-mediated origin, especially those with tissue eosinophilia.

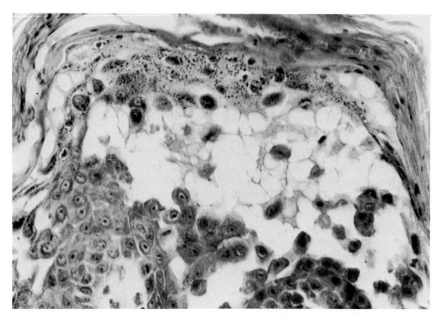

Figure 2:65. Epidermolytic hyperkeratosis (granular degeneration) in a dog with epidermal nevus.

Dermal Changes

COLLAGEN CHANGES

Dermal collagen is subject to a number of pathologic changes and may undergo the following: (1) *hyalinization*—a confluence and an increased eosinophilic, glassy, refractile appearance, as seen in chronic inflammation and connective tissue diseases; (2) *fibrinoid degeneration*—deposition on or replacement with a brightly eosinophilic fibrillar or granular substance resembling fibrin, as seen in connective tissue diseases; (3) *lysis*—a homogeneous, eosinophilic,

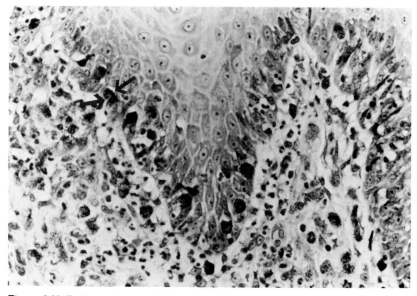

Figure 2:66. Epidermal mast cells (*arrows*) in a cat with flea bite hypersensitivity.

complete loss of structural detail, as seen in microbial infections and ischemia; (4) *degeneration*—a structural and tinctorial change characterized by slight basophilia, granular appearance, and frayed edges of collagen fibers, as seen in canine and feline eosinophilic granuloma; (5) *dystrophic mineralization*—deposition of calcium salts as basophilic, amorphous, granular material along collagen fibers, as seen in hyperadrenocorticism; (6) *atrophy*—thin collagen fibrils and decreased fibroblasts, with a resultant decrease in dermal thickness, as seen in hormonal dermatoses; and (7) *disorganization* and *fragmentation*—cutaneous asthenia.

FIBROPLASIA, DESMOPLASIA, FIBROSIS, AND SCLEROSIS

The term *fibroplasia* refers to the formation and development of fibrous tissue in increased amounts and is often used synonymously with granulation tissue. The condition is characterized by a fibrovascular proliferation in which the blood vessels with prominent endothelial cells are oriented roughly perpendicular to the surface of the skin (Fig. 2:67). The new collagen fibers, with prominent fibroblasts, are oriented roughly parallel to the surface of the skin. Edema and inflammatory cells are constant features of fibroplasia. *Desmoplasia* is the term usually used when referring to the fibroplasia induced by neoplastic processes.

Fibrosis is a later stage of fibroplasia in which increased numbers of fibroblasts and collagen

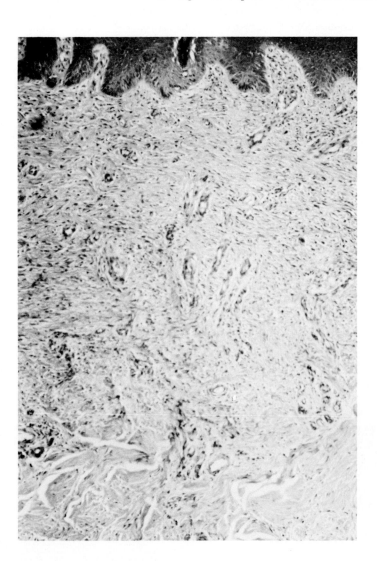

Figure 2:67. Fibroplasia in a dog subsequent to vascular infarct.

fibers are the characteristic findings. Little or no inflammation is present. Alignment of collagen fibers in vertical streaks seen as elongated, thickened parallel strands of collagen in the superficial dermis, perpendicular to the epidermal surface, is found in chronically rubbed, licked, or scratched skin, such as that with acral lick dermatitis and hypersensitivity reactions. *Sclerosis* (scar formation) may be the end point of fibrosis, in which the increased numbers of collagen fibers have a thick, eosinophilic, hyalinized appearance, and the number of fibroblasts is greatly reduced.

SOLAR ELASTOSIS

Solar elastosis appears in H & E–stained sections as a tangle of indistinct amphophilic fibers, often in linear bands running approximately parallel to the surface epidermis, within the superficial dermis. With Verhoeff or acid orcein–Giemsa stains, the tangled, thickened, elastotic material is clearly seen. Solar elastosis is a rare manifestation of ultraviolet light–induced skin damage in dogs and cats.

PAPILLOMATOSIS, VILLI, AND FESTOONS

Papillomatosis refers to the projection of dermal papillae above the surface of the skin, resulting in an irregular undulating configuration of the epidermis. Often associated with epidermal hyperplasia, papillomatosis is also seen with chronic inflammatory and neoplastic dermatoses. Papillomatosis and papillate epidermal hyperplasia are often present with seborrheic dermatitis and zinc-responsive dermatoses.

Villi are dermal papillae, covered by one or two layers of epidermal cells (Fig. 2:68), that project into a vesicle or bulla. Villi are seen in pemphigus vulgaris and warty dyskeratoma and occasionally in actinic keratosis and squamous cell carcinoma.

Festoons are dermal papillae, devoid of attached epidermal cells, that project into the base of a vesicle or a bulla. They are seen in bullous pemphigoid, epidermolysis bullosa, and drug-induced pemphigoid.

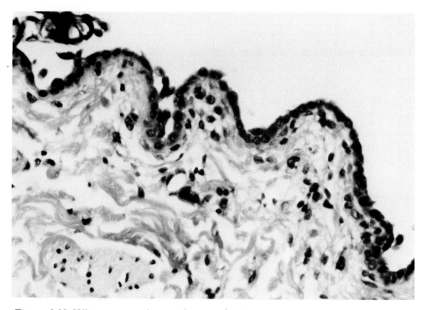

Figure 2:68. Villi in a cat with pemphigus vulgaris.

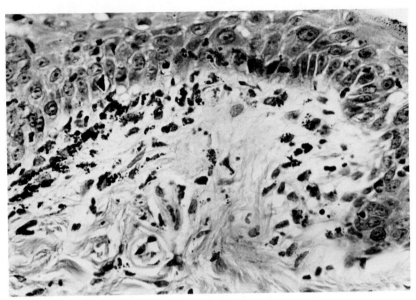

Figure 2:69. Pigmentary incontinence in a dog with discoid lupus erythematosus.

PIGMENTARY INCONTINENCE

Pigmentary incontinence refers to the presence of melanin granules that are free within the subepidermal and perifollicular dermis and within dermal macrophages (melanophages) (Fig. 2:69). Pigmentary incontinence may be seen with any process that damages the stratum basale and the basement membrane zone, especially with hydropic degeneration of basal cells (lichenoid dermatoses, lupus erythematosus, dermatomyositis, and erythema multiforme). In addition, melanophages may be seen, especially in a perivascular orientation, in chronic noninflammatory conditions in which melanin production is greatly increased.

EDEMA

Dermal edema is recognized by dilated lymphatics (not visible in normal skin), widened spaces between blood vessels and perivascular collagen (perivascular edema), or widened spaces between large areas of dermal collagen (interstitial edema). The dilated lymphatics and widened perivascular and interstitial spaces may or may not contain a lightly eosinophilic, homogeneous, frothy-appearing substance (serum). A scattering of vacuolated macrophages may be seen in the interstitium in chronic severe dermal edema.

Dermal edema is a common, nondiagnostic feature of any inflammatory dermatosis. Severe edema of the superficial dermis may result in subepidermal vesicles and bullae, necrosis of the overlying epidermis, and predisposition to artifactual dermo-epidermal separation during the handling and processing of biopsy specimens. Severe edema of the superficial dermis may result in a vertical orientation and stretching of collagen fibers, producing the gossamer (web-like) collagen effect seen with erythema multiforme and severe urticaria.

MUCINOSIS

Mucinosis (myxedema, mucoid degeneration, myxoid degeneration, or mucinous degeneration) is characterized by increased amounts of an amorphous, stringy, granular, basophilic material that separates, thins, or replaces dermal collagen fibrils and surrounds blood vessels and appendages in sections stained with hematoxylin and eosin (Fig. 2:70). Only small amounts of

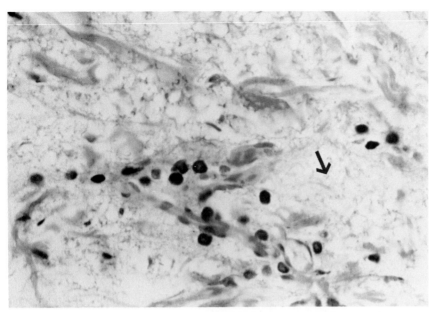

Figure 2:70. Dermal mucinosis (arrow) and scattered mast cells in a Chinese Shar Pei with idiopathic mucinosis.

mucin are ever visible in normal skin, mostly around appendages and blood vessels. Mucin is more easily demonstrated with stains for acid mucopolysaccharides, such as Hale's iron and Alcian blue stains. Mucinosis may be seen as a focal (usually perivascular) change in numerous inflammatory, neoplastic, and developmental dermatoses. Diffuse mucinosis may be seen with hypothyroidism, acromegaly, lupus erythematosus, dermatomyositis, various idiopathic mucinoses, and the normal skin of the Chinese Shar Pei.

Mucin may also be seen in the epidermis and hair follicle outer root sheath in cats with alopecia mucinosa and dermatoses associated with numerous eosinophils (e.g., eosinophilic plaque, eosinophilic granuloma, allergies), and in dogs with discoid lupus erythematosus.

GRENZ ZONE

This marginal zone of relatively normal collagen separates the epidermis from an underlying dermal alteration (Fig. 2:71). A grenz zone may be seen in neoplastic and granulomatous disorders.

FOLLICULAR CHANGES

Follicular epithelium is affected by most of the histopathologic changes described for the epidermis. Follicular (poral) keratosis, plugging, and dilatation are common features of such diverse conditions as inflammatory, hormonal, and developmental dermatoses. Excessive *trichilemmal keratinization* (flame follicles) is seen with endocrine and developmental disorders (Fig. 2:72).[29] *Perifolliculitis, folliculitis*, and *furunculosis* (penetrating or perforating folliculitis) refer to varying degrees of follicular inflammation. *Follicular atrophy* refers to the gradual involution, retraction, and occasionally miniaturization that are characteristic of hormonal and nutritional dermatoses.

Hair follicles should be examined closely to determine the phase of the growth cycle. *Telogenization*, a predominance of telogen hair follicles, is characteristic of hormonal dermatoses and states of telogen defluxion as associated with stress, disease, and drugs. *Follicular*

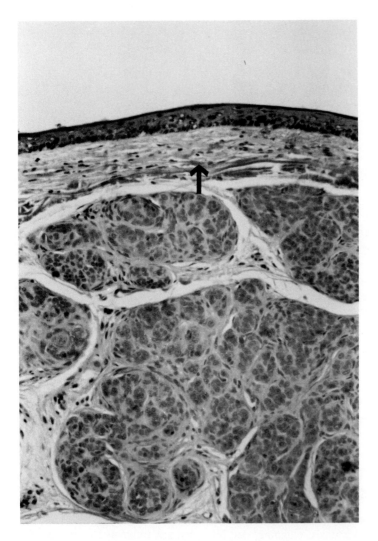

Figure 2:71. Grenz zone of superficial dermal collagen (*arrow*) separating epidermis from underlying neoplasia.

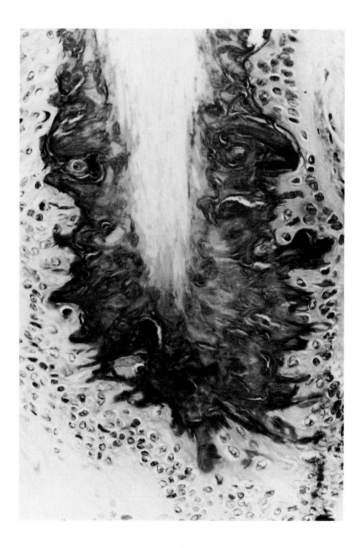

Figure 2:72. Flame follicle (excessive trichilemmal keratinization) in a dog with hypothyroidism.

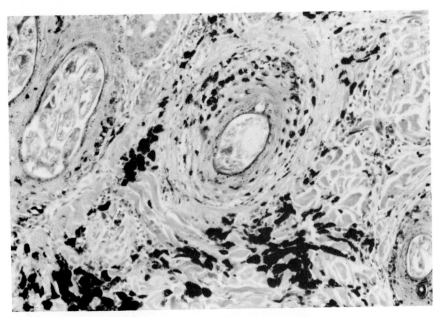

Figure 2:73. Perifollicular melanosis in a dog with generalized demodicosis.

dysplasia refers to the presence of incompletely or abnormally formed hair follicles and hair shafts and is seen in developmental abnormalities such as hypotrichosis and color dilution alopecia.

Perifollicular melanosis (Fig. 2:73) is a common finding in canine demodicosis and follicular dysplasia.[14] Perifollicular fibrosis is seen in chronic folliculitis, canine dermatomyositis, and granulomatous sebaceous adenitis. Dystrophic basement membrane zone and subsequent trans-epithelial elimination of mineral is seen in the calcinosis cutis of hyperadrenocorticism and as a senile change in dogs, especially Poodles and Bedlington terriers.[18, 35] The finding of large numbers of cocci or yeasts in noninflamed hair follicles in dogs almost always indicates the presence of clinically relevant bacterial or yeast infection.[32, 33]

GLANDULAR CHANGES

Sebaceous and apocrine sweat glands may be affected in various dermatoses. Sebaceous glands may be involved in many suppurative and granulomatous inflammations (sebaceous adenitis). In dogs and cats, an idiopathic granulomatous sebaceous adenitis may be characterized by complete absence of sebaceous glands in the late stages. They may become atrophic (reduced in number and size, with pyknotic nuclei predominating) or cystic in hormonal and developmental dermatoses, in occasional chronic inflammatory processes, and as a senile change. Sebaceous glands may also become hyperplastic in chronic inflammatory dermatoses, sebaceous gland nevi, and senile nodular sebaceous hyperplasia. Sebaceous gland atrophy and hyperplasia must always be cautiously assessed with regard to the area of the body from which the skin specimen was taken.

Apocrine sweat glands are commonly involved in suppurative and granulomatous dermatoses (hidradenitis) (Fig. 2:74). Periapocrine accumulation of plasma cells is commonly seen in acral lick dermatitis, chronic infections, and lichenoid dermatoses. The apocrine sweat glands may become dilated or cystic in many inflammatory, developmental, and hormonal dermatoses; in apocrine cystomatosis; and with senile changes. The light microscopic recognition of apocrine gland atrophy is moot, because dilated apocrine secretory coils containing flattened epithelial cells are a feature of the normal postsecretory state.

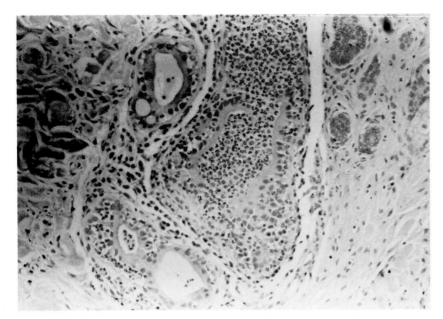

Figure 2:74. Suppurative hidradenitis in a dog with staphylococcal furunculosis.

VASCULAR CHANGES

Cutaneous blood vessels exhibit a number of histologic changes, including dilatation (ectasia), endothelial swelling, hyalinization, fibrinoid degeneration, vasculitis, thromboembolism, and extravasation (diapedesis) of erythrocytes (purpura).

Subcutaneous Fat Changes

The subcutaneous fat (panniculus adiposus, or hypodermis) is subject to the connective tissue and vascular changes described above. It is frequently involved in suppurative and granulomatous dermatoses. In addition, subcutaneous fat may exhibit its own inflammatory changes (panniculitis or steatitis) without any significant involvement of the overlying dermis and epidermis. This occurs in sterile nodular panniculitis, feline nutritional steatitis, infectious panniculitis (especially atypical mycobacteriosis and bacterial and dermatophytic pseudomycetoma), bacterial endocarditis, subcutaneous fat sclerosis, and erythema nodosum. Subcutaneous fat may atrophy in various hormonal, inflammatory (wucher atrophy), and idiopathic dermatoses. Fat micropseudocyst formation and lipocytes containing radially arranged needle-shaped clefts are seen with subcutaneous fat sclerosis.

Miscellaneous Changes

■ ***Thickened Basement Membrane Zone.*** Thickening of the basement membrane zone appears as focal, linear, homogeneous, eosinophilic bands below the stratum basale on light microscopic examination (Fig. 2:75). The basement membrane zone is better demonstrated with periodic acid–Schiff stain. Thickening of the basement membrane zone is a feature of lichenoid dermatoses, especially lupus erythematosus.

■ ***Subepidermal Vacuolar Alteration.*** Subepidermal vacuolar alteration is characterized by multiple small vacuoles within or immediately below the basement membrane zone, giving the

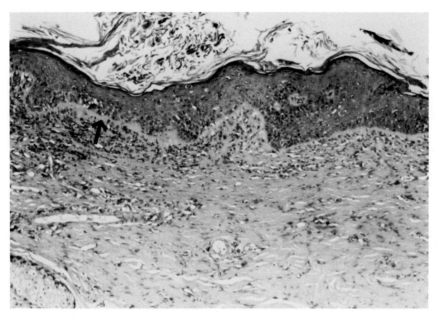

Figure 2:75. Focal thickening of the basement membrane zone (*arrow*) in a dog with systemic lupus erythematosus.

appearance of subepidermal bubbles. These "subepidermal bubblies" are seen in bullous pemphigoid, lupus erythematosus, and occasionally, overlying dermal fibrosis and scar.

■ *Papillary Squirting.* Papillary squirting is present when superficial dermal papillae are edematous and contain dilated vessels and when the overlying epidermis is also edematous and often contains exocytosing leukocytes and parakeratotic scale. Squirting papillae are a feature of seborrheic dermatitis and zinc-responsive dermatoses.

■ *Dysplasia.* The term *dysplasia* refers to a faulty or abnormal development of individual cells, and it is also commonly used to describe abnormal development of the epidermis or hair follicle as a whole. Dysplasia may be a feature of neoplastic, hyperplastic, and developmental dermatoses.

■ *Anaplasia.* *Anaplasia* (atypia) is a feature of neoplastic cells, in which there is a loss of normal differentiation and organization.

■ *Metaplasia.* *Metaplasia* refers to a change in the type of mature cells in a tissue into a form that is not normal for that tissue (e.g., osseous metaplasia in the skin of a patient with hyperadrenocorticism). Through metaplasia, a given cell may exhibit epithelial, mesothelial, or mesenchymal characteristics, regardless of the tissue of origin.

■ *Nests.* *Nests* (theques) are well-circumscribed clusters or groups of cells within the epidermis or the dermis (Fig. 2:76). Nests are seen in some neoplastic and hamartomatous dermatoses, such as melanomas and melanocytomas.

■ *Lymphoid Nodules.* Lymphoid nodules are rounded, discrete masses of primarily mature lymphocytes (Fig. 2:77). They are often found perivascularly in the deep dermis, the subcutis, or both. Lymphoid nodules are most commonly recognized in association with immune-mediated dermatoses, dermatoses with tissue eosinophilia, and panniculitis.[28] They are also

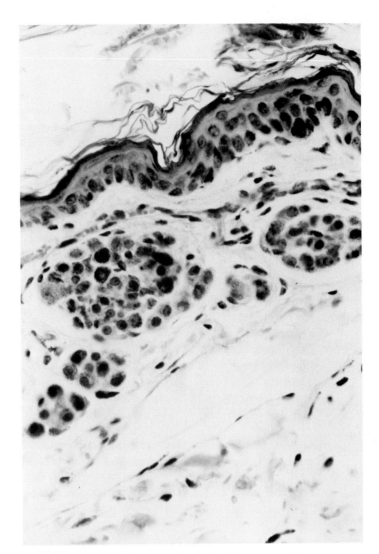

Figure 2:76. Nests of neoplastic melanocytes in a cat with melanocytoma.

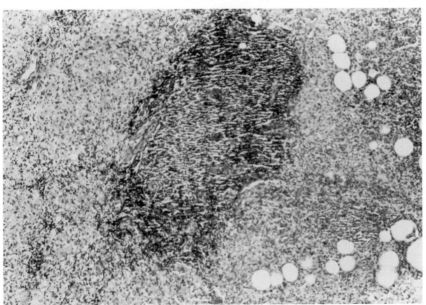

Figure 2:77. Lymphoid nodule in a cat with idiopathic sterile panniculitis.

prominent in insect bite granuloma (pseudolymphoma), postinjection panniculitis, and some feline mast cell tumors.

■ *Multinucleate Epidermal Giant Cells.* Multinucleate epidermal giant cells are found in viral infections and in a number of nonviral and non-neoplastic dermatoses characterized by epidermal hyperplasia, dyskeratosis, chronicity, or pruritus.

■ *Squamatization.* *Squamatization* refers to the replacement of the normally cuboid or columnar, slightly basophilic basal epidermal cells by polygonal or flattened, eosinophilic keratinocytes. It may be seen in lichenoid tissue reactions.

■ *Flame Figure.* A flame figure is an area of altered collagen surrounded by eosinophils and eosinophilic granules (Fig. 2:78). In chronic lesions, the eosinophil content decreases, histiocytes increase in number, and palisading granulomas may be formed. Flame figures may be seen in canine and feline eosinophilic granuloma, sterile eosinophilic pustulosis, and insect or arthropod bite reactions.

■ *Transepidermal Elimination.* Transepidermal elimination is a mechanism by which foreign or altered constituents can be removed from the dermis (Fig. 2:79). The process involves unique morphologic alterations of the surface epidermis or the hair follicle's outer root sheath, which forms a channel and thereby facilitates extrusion. Transepidermal elimination may be seen in foreign-body reactions, calcinosis cutis, calcinosis circumscripta, and perforating dermatitis of cats.

■ *Dunstan's Blue Line.* The overlying stratum corneum is lifted and subtended at its point of attachment to the underlying epidermis by degenerate nuclear debris and staphylococci. As such, the stratum corneum seems to be separating in the direction of a "blue line." This is most commonly seen in superficial staphylococcal infections.

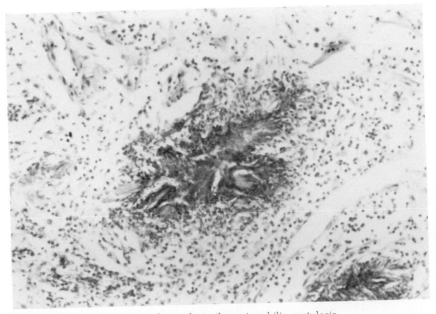

Figure 2:78. Flame figure in a dog with sterile eosinophilic pustulosis.

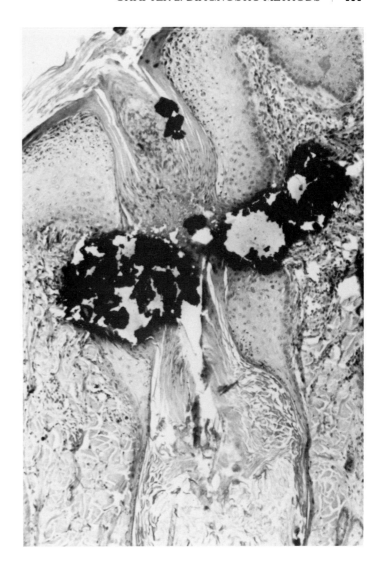

Figure 2:79. Transepidermal elimination of mineral through the outer root sheath of a hair follicle in a dog with spontaneous hyperadrenocorticism.

Confusing Terms

NECROBIOSIS

Necrobiosis is the degeneration and death of cells or tissue followed by replacement. Examples of necrobiosis are the constant degeneration and replacement of epidermal and hematopoietic cells. The term necrobiosis has been used in dermatohistopathology to describe various degenerative changes in collagen found in canine and feline eosinophilic granuloma and in human granuloma annulare, necrobiosis lipoidica, and rheumatoid and pseudorheumatoid nodules. The use of the term necrobiosis to describe a pathologic change is inappropriate and confusing, both histologically and etymologically, and should be discouraged. It is better to use the more specific terms described under Collagen Changes in this chapter.

NEVUS AND HAMARTOMA

A *nevus* is a circumscribed developmental defect in the skin. Nevi may arise from any skin component or combination of components. Nevi are hyperplastic. The term nevus should never be used alone, but always with a modifier such as epidermal, vascular, sebaceous, and collagenous.

Hamartoma literally means a tumor-like proliferation of normal or embryonal cells. A hamartoma is a macroscopic hyperplasia of normal tissue elements, and the term is often used synonymously with nevus. However, the term hamartoma may be applied to hyperplastic disorders in any tissue or organ system, whereas the term nevus is restricted to the skin.

Cellular Infiltrates

Dermal cellular infiltrates are described in terms of (1) the types of cells present and (2) the pattern of cellular infiltration. In general, cellular infiltrates are either monomorphous (one cell type) or polymorphous (more than one cell type). Further clarification of the predominant cells is accomplished by modifiers such as lymphocytic, histiocytic, neutrophilic, eosinophilic, and plasmacytic.

Cellular infiltrations usually have one or more of the following basic patterns: (1) perivascular (angiocentric—located around blood vessels), (2) perifollicular and periglandular (appendagocentric, periappendageal, periadnexal—located around follicles and glands), (3) lichenoid (assuming a bandlike configuration that parallels the overlying epidermis and surrounds epidermal appendages), (4) nodular (occurring in basically well-defined groups or clusters at any site), and (5) interstitial or diffuse (scattered lightly or solidly throughout the dermis). The types of cells and patterns of infiltration present are important clues in the diagnosis of many dermatoses.

■ DERMATOLOGIC DIAGNOSIS BY HISTOPATHOLOGIC PATTERNS

In 1978, A. B. Ackerman published a textbook on the histopathologic aspects of inflammatory dermatoses in humans.[12] The essence of this book was histopathologic diagnosis by pattern analysis, that is, first categorizing inflammatory dermatoses by their appearance on the scanning objective of the light microscope and then zeroing in on a specific diagnosis, whenever possible, by the assimilation of fine details gathered by low- and high-power scrutiny. Pattern analysis has revolutionized veterinary dermatohistopathology and made the reading of skin biopsy specimens much simpler and more rewarding (for the pathologist, the clinician, and the patient).[16, 18, 34, 38, 39] However, as with any histologic method, pattern analysis works only when clinicians supply pathologists with adequate historical and clinical information and biopsy specimens most representative of the dermatoses being sampled.

In a retrospective study of skin biopsies from cats with inflammatory dermatoses,[34] pattern analysis was shown to be a useful technique. The specific clinical diagnosis was established in about 40 per cent of the cases and was included in a reaction pattern–generated differential diagnosis in another 50 per cent of the cases. A single reaction pattern was found in 75 per cent of the cases, and mixed reaction patterns (two or three different patterns) in 25 per cent of the cases. Mixed reaction patterns were usually caused by single etiologic factors or by a coexistence of two or three different dermatoses.

Perivascular Dermatitis

In perivascular dermatitis, the predominant inflammatory reaction is centered on the superficial or deep dermal blood vessels, or both. Perivascular dermatitis is subdivided into three types on the basis of accompanying epidermal changes: (1) pure perivascular dermatitis (perivascular dermatitis without significant epidermal changes), (2) spongiotic perivascular dermatitis (perivascular dermatitis with prominent spongiosis), and (3) hyperplastic perivascular dermatitis (perivascular dermatitis with prominent epidermal hyperplasia).

Superficial perivascular dermatitis is by far the most common form of perivascular dermatitis (Fig. 2:80 *A*). The usual causes are hypersensitivity reactions (to inhalants, dietary constituents, drugs, contact allergens, and so forth), ectoparasitisms, dermatophytosis, nutritional deficiencies, seborrheic disorders, and contact dermatitis. Deep perivascular dermatitis (Fig. 2:80 *B*) is less common and may be seen with systemic disorders (systemic lupus erythematosus, septicemia, hypereosinophilic syndrome, viral infections, and canine systemic histiocytosis) or severe local reactions (vasculitis, discoid lupus erythematosus, cellulitis, eosinophilic plaque, and tick bite reactions).

Any perivascular dermatitis containing numerous eosinophils should first be suspected of representing ectoparasitism or endoparasitism. In the cat, tissue eosinophilia is commonly seen with hypersensitivity disorders (reactions to inhalants or dietary constituents).[34] Focal areas of epidermal edema, eosinophilic exocytosis, and necrosis (epidermal "nibbles") suggest ectoparasitism. Numerous eosinophils are also seen in the hypereosinophilic syndrome and occasionally in zinc-responsive dermatoses.

Diffuse orthokeratotic hyperkeratosis with perivascular dermatitis suggests endocrinopathy, nutritional deficiencies, developmental abnormalities (ichthyosis, follicular dysplasia, and color dilution alopecia), and secondary seborrheic disorders. Disproportionate follicular orthokeratotic hyperkeratosis in concert with perivascular dermatitis suggests vitamin A–responsive dermatosis, vitamin A deficiency, acne, Schnauzer comedo syndrome, follicular dysplasia, sebaceous adenitis, comedo nevus, and follicular cyst. Diffuse parakeratotic hyperkeratosis in combination with perivascular dermatitis suggests zinc-responsive dermatosis, generic dog food dermatosis, ectoparasitism, lethal acrodermatitis, some vitamin A–responsive dermatoses, thallotoxicosis, canine necrolytic migratory erythema, and occasionally, dermatophytosis and dermatophilosis.

Focal parakeratotic hyperkeratosis (parakeratotic caps) may be seen with ectoparasitism, seborrheic disorders, dermatophytosis, and dermatophilosis. When parakeratotic caps are combined with papillary squirting, seborrheic dermatitis is likely. Perivascular dermatoses accompanied by vertical streaking of collagen, sebaceous gland hyperplasia, or both suggest chronic

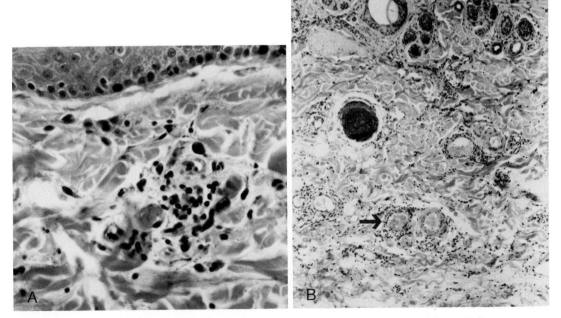

Figure 2:80. Perivascular dermatitis. *A,* Superficial perivascular dermatitis in a dog with atopy. *B,* Deep perivascular dermatitis (*arrow*) in a cat with atopy.

pruritus (rubbing, licking, or chewing), such as that seen with hypersensitivity reactions and acral lick dermatitis.

Pure Perivascular Dermatitis

The most likely diagnoses include hypersensitivity reactions (to inhalants, dietary constituents, or drugs), urticaria, and dermatophytosis.

Spongiotic Perivascular Dermatitis

Spongiotic perivascular dermatitis is characterized by prominent spongiosis and spongiotic vesicle formation. Severe spongiotic vesiculation may cause blowout of the basement membrane zone, resulting in subepidermal vesicles. The epidermis frequently shows varying degrees of hyperplasia and hyperkeratosis. The most likely diagnoses include hypersensitivity reactions, contact dermatitis, ectoparasitisms, dermatophytosis, *Malassezia* dermatitis, dermatophilosis, viral infection, and eosinophilic plaque. Diffuse spongiosis, in which the outer root sheath of the hair follicle is also involved, suggests eosinophilic plaque, eosinophilic granuloma, seborrheic dermatitis, *Malassezia* dermatitis, and zinc-responsive dermatosis. Marked spongiosis and intracellular edema of the upper one half of the epidermis with overlying diffuse parakeratotic hyperkeratosis are seen with necrolytic migratory erythema.

Hyperplastic Perivascular Dermatitis

Hyperplastic perivascular dermatitis is characterized by varying degrees of epidermal hyperplasia and hyperkeratosis, with little or no spongiosis. This is a common, nondiagnostic, chronic dermatitis. It is frequently seen with hypersensitivity reactions, contact dermatitis, diseases of altered keratinization, ectoparasitisms, indolent ulcer, and acral lick dermatitis. Psoriasiform perivascular dermatoses are unusual and may represent chronic contact dermatitis, chronic hypersensitivity reactions, acral lick dermatitis, psoriasiform-lichenoid dermatosis of English Springer spaniels, necrolytic migratory erythema, and dermatophytosis. The most common cause of psoriasiform perivascular dermatitis in dogs is epitheliotropic lymphoma.

Interface Dermatitis

In interface dermatitis, the dermo-epidermal junction is obscured by hydropic degeneration, lichenoid cellular infiltrate, or both (Fig. 2:81).[26] Apoptotic bodies, satellite cell necrosis, and pigmentary incontinence are commonly seen. The hydropic type of interface dermatitis is seen with drug eruptions, lupus erythematosus, toxic epidermal necrolysis, erythema multiforme, dermatomyositis, hereditary lupoid dermatosis of German shorthaired pointers, idiopathic ulcerative dermatosis of collies and Shetland sheepdogs, graft-versus-host reactions, and various vasculitides and vasculopathies.

The lichenoid type is seen with drug eruptions, lupus erythematosus, pemphigus, pemphigoid, erythema multiforme, Vogt-Koyanagi-Harada–like syndrome, idiopathic lichenoid dermatoses, lichenoid keratoses, psoriasiform-lichenoid dermatosis of English Springer spaniels, and epitheliotropic lymphoma. The bandlike cellular infiltration of lichenoid tissue reactions consists predominantly of lymphocytes and plasma cells. If nearby ulceration or secondary infections exist, numerous neutrophils may be present. Uniquely, the lichenoid infiltrate of uveodermatologic syndrome has numerous large histiocytes, which contain lightly sprinkled melanin. A lichenoid tissue reaction with many eosinophils suggests an insect or arthropod bite reaction (e.g., scabies and cheyletiellosis) or a drug eruption. Small numbers of eosinophils are also a feature of psoriasiform-lichenoid dermatosis of English Springer spaniels. Focal thickening or smudging of the basement membrane zone suggests lupus erythematosus and dermatomyositis.

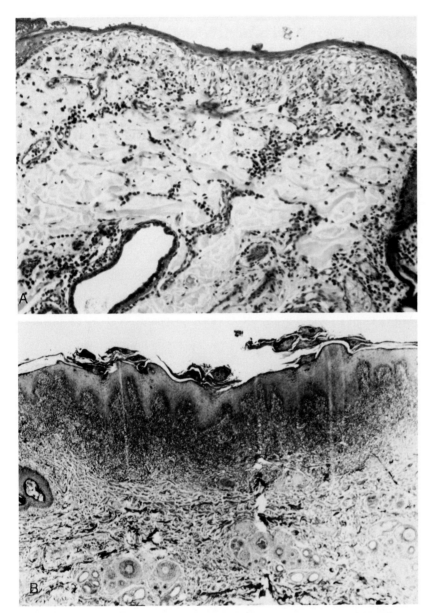

Figure 2:81. Interface dermatitis. *A*, Hydropic interface dermatitis in a dog with systemic lupus erythematosus. *B*, Lichenoid interface dermatitis in a dog with idiopathic lichenoid dermatitis.

Vasculitis

Vasculitis is an inflammatory process in which inflammatory cells are present within and around blood vessel walls and there are concomitant signs of damage to the blood vessels (e.g., degeneration and lysis of vascular and perivascular collagen, swelling and necrosis of endothelial cells, extravasation of erythrocytes, thrombosis, effacement of vascular architecture, and fibrinoid degeneration) (Fig. 2:82). Vasculitides are usually classified on the basis of the dominant inflammatory cell within vessel walls, the types being neutrophilic, eosinophilic, and lymphocytic. Fibrinoid degeneration is rare in canine and feline cutaneous vasculitides. Biopsy specimens from animals with vasculitis sometimes do not reveal visually inflamed vessels, but rather the hallmarks of vasculitis: unexplained areas of purpura and leukocytoclasis, wedge-shaped areas of necrosis, and areas of fading appendages (a loss of structural detail, especially in hair follicles). Serial sections or repeated biopsy may be necessary to visualize the actual vasculitis.

Neutrophilic vasculitis, the most common type, may be leukocytoclastic (associated with karyorrhexis of neutrophils, resulting in "nuclear dust"). This is seen in connective tissue disorders (lupus erythematosus, rheumatoid arthritis, and dermatomyositis), allergic reactions (drug eruptions, infections, and reactions to toxins), polyarteritis nodosa, canine staphylococcal hypersensitivity, Rocky Mountain spotted fever, and canine leishmaniasis; hereditary nasal pyogranuloma and vasculitis of Scottish terriers; as an idiopathic disorder; and occasionally with plasma cell pododermatitis. Neutrophilic vasculitis may also be nonleukocytoclastic, as seen with septicemia and thrombophlebitis from intravenous catheters' causing thromboembolism. Exceptions to these rules may be seen, such as in the case of allergic vasculitides, which may be leukocytoclastic or nonleukocytoclastic.

Lymphocytic vasculitis is rare, and may be seen in drug eruptions, vaccine-induced panniculitis, dermatomyositis, familial vasculopathy of German shepherds, and as an idiopathic disorder.

Eosinophilic vasculitis is very rare, and is seen with insect- and arthropod-induced lesions, feline eosinophilic granuloma, and mast cell tumor.

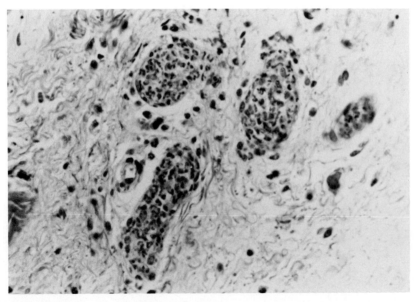

Figure 2:82. Vasculitis. Leukocytoclastic vasculitis in a dog with idiopathic cutaneous vasculitis.

Interstitial Dermatitis

Interstitial dermatitis is characterized by the infiltration of cells between collagen bundles (in the interstitial spaces) of the dermis (Fig. 2:83). The infiltrate is poorly circumscribed, is mild to moderate in intensity, and does not obscure the anatomic features of the skin. When the superficial dermis is primarily involved and the overlying epidermis is normal, urticaria is likely. When the superficial dermis is primarily involved and the epidermis is hyperplastic, the most likely causes are staphylococcal infection (numerous neutrophils), dermatophytosis (numerous neutrophils), yeast dermatitis (numerous lymphocytes), and ectoparasitism, especially scabies and flea bite hypersensitivity (numerous eosinophils). When the superficial and deep dermis are involved, likely diagnoses include bacterial or fungal infection (numerous neutrophils, macrophages, or both), early eosinophilic plaque (numerous eosinophils), and early plasma cell pododermatitis (numerous plasma cells).

Nodular and Diffuse Dermatitis

Nodular dermatitis denotes discrete clusters of cells. Such dermal nodules are usually multiple but may occasionally be large and solitary (Fig. 2:84). In contrast, *diffuse dermatitis* denotes a cellular infiltrate so dense that discrete cellular aggregates are no longer easily recognized and the anatomy of the skin is no longer easily visualized (Fig. 2:85).

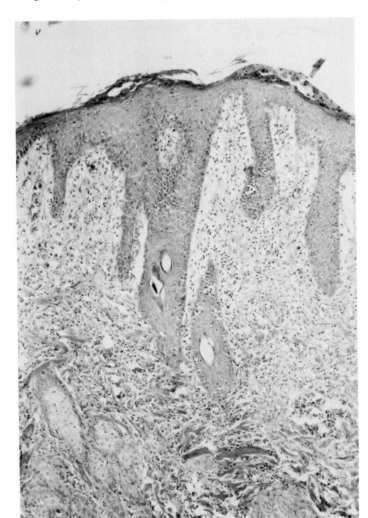

Figure 2:83. Interstitial dermatitis in a cat with food hypersensitivity. Note that the anatomic structures are still readily identified. There are also focal areas of perifolliculitis.

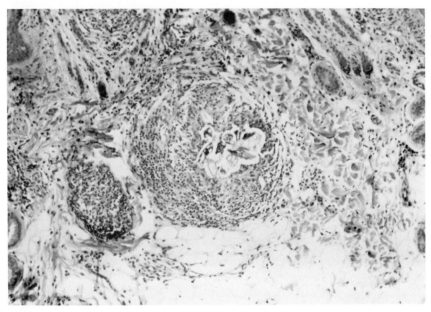

Figure 2:84. Nodular dermatitis. Dermal nodule with *Demodex* mites in the center in a dog with generalized demodicosis.

Granulomatous inflammation represents a heterogeneous pattern of tissue reactions in response to various stimuli. There is no simple, precise, universally accepted way to define granulomatous inflammation. A commonly proposed definition of granulomatous inflammation is as follows: a circumscribed tissue reaction that is subacute to chronic in nature and is located about one or more foci, in which the histiocyte or the macrophage is a predominant cell type. Thus, granulomatous dermatitis may be nodular or diffuse, but not all nodular and diffuse

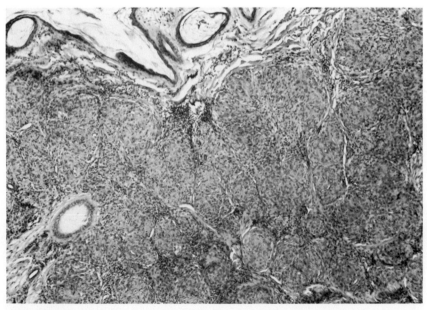

Figure 2:85. Diffuse dermatitis. Diffuse granulomatous dermatitis in a dog with sarcoidal granulomas.

dermatoses are granulomatous. Nongranulomatous diffuse dermatoses include eosinophilic plaque, plasma cell pododermatitis, and cellulitis. Pseudolymphoma (insect or arachnid bites; drug reactions; idiopathic) is an example of a nongranulomatous nodular dermatitis. Granulomatous infiltrates that contain large numbers of neutrophils are frequently called pyogranulomatous. The most common causes of nodular pyogranulomatous dermatitis in dogs are furunculosis and ruptured keratinous cysts.

Cell Types

Nodular dermatitis and diffuse dermatitis are often associated with certain unusual inflammatory cell types.

Foam cells are histiocytes with elongated or oval vesicular nuclei and abundant, finely granular, eosinophilic cytoplasm with ill-defined cell borders. They are called *epithelioid* because they appear to cluster and adjoin like epithelial cells.

Multinucleate histiocytic giant cells (Fig. 2:86) are histiocytic variants that assume three morphologic forms: (1) Langhans-type (nuclei form a circle or semicircle at the periphery of the cell), (2) foreign body–type (nuclei are scattered throughout the cytoplasm), and (3) Touton-type (nuclei form a wreath that surrounds a central, homogeneous, amphophilic core of cytoplasm, which is in turn surrounded by abundant foamy cytoplasm). In general, these three

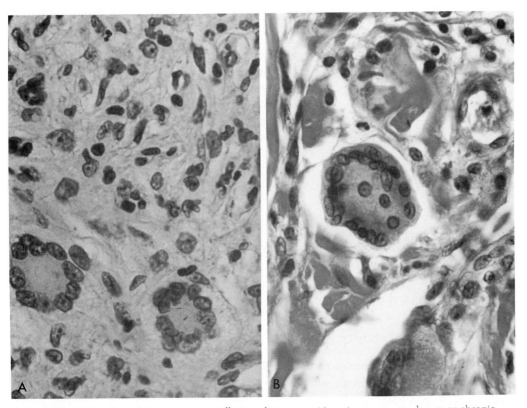

Figure 2:86. Multinucleate histiocytic giant cells are often present in cutaneous granulomas or chronic inflammations localized around foci of irritation. However, one should understand that identification of any one type of giant cell is not diagnostic alone. Several types may be found in a single section, and all are "foreign body" in character. Their different structure is probably related to the physiochemical nature of the foreign material. *A,* Touton-type giant cell. There is a complete ring of nuclei around a "ground glass" center, and all are enclosed within a vacuolated cytoplasm. The photomicrograph is from a human xanthoma. (Courtesy J. D. Conroy.) *B,* Langhans-type giant cell. The peripheral rim of nuclei is arranged in a horseshoe fashion.

forms of giant cells have no diagnostic specificity, although numerous Touton-type cells are usually seen with xanthomas.

Characterization

Certain general principles apply to the examination of all nodular and diffuse dermatitides. The processes that should be used are (1) polarizing foreign material, (2) staining for bacteria and fungi, and (3) culturing. In general, microorganisms are most likely to be found near areas of suppuration and necrosis.

Nodular and diffuse dermatitis may be characterized by predominantly neutrophilic, histiocytic, eosinophilic, or mixed cellular infiltrates. Neutrophils (dermal abscess) often predominate in dermatoses associated with bacteria, mycobacteria, actinomycetes, fungi, *Prototheca*, and foreign bodies. Histiocytes may predominate in the chronic stage of any of the entities just listed, in xanthomas, in canine histiocytosis (cutaneous and systemic), and in the sterile pyogranuloma-granuloma syndrome. Eosinophils may predominate in feline and canine eosinophilic granuloma, in certain parasitic dermatoses (insect and arachnid bite reactions, dirofilariasis, and dracunculiasis), and in locations where hair follicles have ruptured. Mixed cellular infiltrates are most commonly neutrophils and histiocytes (in pyogranuloma), eosinophils and histiocytes (in eosinophilic granuloma), or a combination.

Plasma cells are common components of nodular and diffuse dermatitis of dogs and cats and are of no particular diagnostic significance. They are commonly seen around glands and follicles in chronic infections. Periapocrine accumulations of plasma cells are also commonly seen in acral lick dermatitis and lichenoid dermatoses. Hyperactive plasma cells may contain eosinophilic intracytoplasmic inclusions (Russell bodies). These accumulations of glycoprotein are largely globulin and may be large enough to push the cell nucleus eccentrically.

Granulomas may be subclassified as tuberculoid, sarcoid, and palisading. Tuberculoid granulomas have a central zone of neutrophils and necrosis surrounded by histiocytes and epithelioid cells, which are in turn surrounded by giant cells, followed by a layer of lymphocytes, and finally an outer layer of fibroblasts. These are seen in tuberculosis, atypical mycobacteriosis, and feline leprosy (Fig. 2:87). Sarcoid granulomas have "naked" epithelioid cells (unaccompanied by surrounding inflammation and fibrosis), as seen in foreign-body reactions or canine sarcoid granuloma (Fig. 2:88). In palisading granulomas, the histiocytes are aligned like staves around a central focus of collagen degeneration (in canine and feline eosinophilic granuloma [Fig. 2:89]); fibrin (in rheumatoid nodule); lipids (in xanthoma); or parasite, fungus, or other foreign material (e.g., calcium, as in dystrophic calcinosis cutis and calcinosis circumscripta [Fig. 2:90]). Granulomas and pyogranulomas that track hair follicles and result in large, vertically oriented (sausage-shaped) lesions are typical of the sterile pyogranuloma–granuloma syndrome.

Reactions to ruptured hair follicles are a common cause of nodular and diffuse pyogranulomatous dermatitis, and any such dermal process should be carefully scrutinized for keratinous and epithelial debris and should be serially sectioned to rule out this possibility.

Intraepidermal Vesicular and Pustular Dermatitis

Vesicular and pustular dermatitides show considerable microscopic and macroscopic overlap, because vesicles tend to accumulate leukocytes early and rapidly. Thus, vesicular dermatitides in dogs and cats frequently appear pustular or vesicopustular, both macroscopically and microscopically.

Intraepidermal vesicles and pustules (Fig. 2:91) may be produced by intercellular or intracellular edema (in any acute to subacute dermatitis reaction), ballooning degeneration (in viral infections), acantholysis (due to the autoantibodies of pemphigus, the proteolytic enzymes from neutrophils in microbial infections and subcorneal pustular dermatosis, and the proteolytic

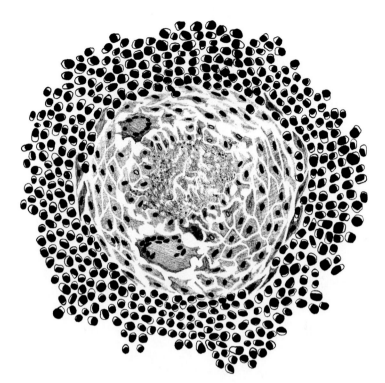

Figure 2:87. Tuberculoid granuloma. (From Ackerman, A. B.: Histologic Diagnosis of Inflammatory Diseases. Lea & Febiger, Philadelphia, 1978, p. 398.)

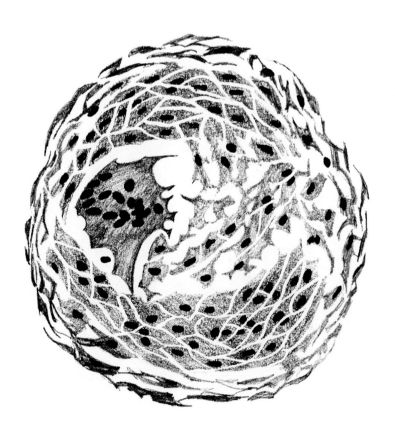

Figure 2:88. Sarcoid granuloma. (From Ackerman, A. B.: Histologic Diagnosis of Inflammatory Diseases. Lea & Febiger, Philadelphia, 1978, p. 408.)

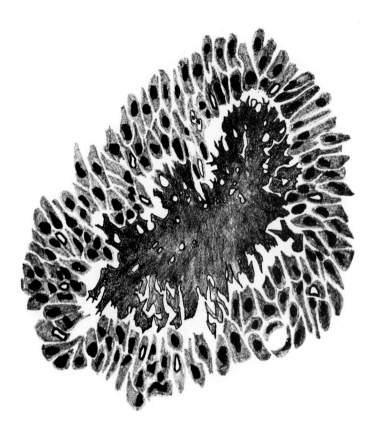

Figure 2:89. Palisading granuloma. (From Ackerman, A. B.: Histologic Diagnosis of Inflammatory Diseases, Lea & Febiger, Philadelphia, 1978, p. 416.)

Figure 2:90. Foreign-body granuloma. (From Ackerman, A. B.: Histologic Diagnosis of Inflammatory Diseases, Lea & Febiger, Philadelphia, 1978, p. 436.)

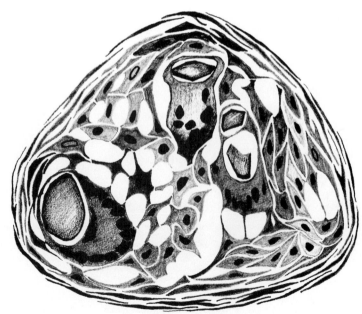

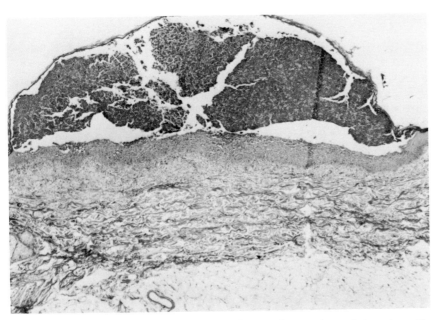

Figure 2:91. Intraepidermal pustular dermatitis. Large subcorneal pustule in a dog with pemphigus foliaceus.

enzymes from eosinophils in sterile eosinophilic pustulosis), and hydropic degeneration of basal cells (in lupus erythematosus, erythema multiforme, toxic epidermal necrolysis, dermatomyositis, and drug eruptions). It is useful to classify intraepidermal vesicular and pustular dermatitides as to their anatomic level of occurrence within the epidermis (Table 2:9).

Subepidermal Vesicular and Pustular Dermatitis

Subepidermal vesicles and pustules (Fig. 2:92) may be formed through hydropic degeneration of basal cells (in lupus erythematosus, erythema multiforme, dermatomyositis, drug eruption, and toxic epidermal necrolysis), dermo-epidermal separation (in bullous pemphigoid, drug eruption, and epidermolysis bullosa), severe subepidermal edema or cellular infiltration (especially in urticaria, cellulitis, vasculitis, ectoparasitism, and dermal erythema multiforme), and severe intercellular edema, with blowout of the basement membrane zone (in spongiotic perivascular dermatitis). Concurrent epidermal and dermal inflammatory changes are important diagnostic clues (Table 2:9). Caution is warranted when examining older lesions, as re-epithelialization may cause subepidermal vesicles and pustules to assume an intraepidermal location. Such re-epithelialization is usually recognized as a single layer of flattened, elongated basal epidermal cells at the base of the vesicle or pustule.

Perifolliculitis, Folliculitis, and Furunculosis

Perifolliculitis denotes the accumulation of inflammatory cells around a hair follicle. Strictly defined, perifolliculitis necessitates the exocytosis of these cells into the follicular epithelium (Fig. 2:93). However, the term is often used more loosely to describe those commonly occurring superficial perivascular dermatitides in which the perifollicular vascular plexus is preferentially involved. It has been suggested that the term *mural folliculitis* be used to describe lesions in which the wall of the follicle is targeted. *Folliculitis* implies the accumulation of inflammatory cells within follicular lumina (Fig. 2:94). *Furunculosis* (penetrating or perforating

Table 2:9. Histopathologic Classification of Intraepidermal and Subepidermal Pustular and Vesicular Diseases

Anatomic Location*	Other Helpful Findings
Intraepidermal	
SUBCORNEAL	
Microbial infection	Neutrophils, microorganisms (bacteria, fungi), ± mild acantholysis, focal necrosis of epidermis, ± follicular involvement
Canine subcorneal pustular dermatosis	Neutrophils, ± moderate acantholysis
Canine sterile eosinophilic pustulosis	Eosinophils, ± follicular involvement
Pemphigus foliaceus	Marked acantholysis, neutrophils and/or eosinophils, ± follicular involvement
Pemphigus erythematosus	Marked acantholysis, neutrophils and/or eosinophils, ± follicular involvement, ± lichenoid infiltrate
Canine linear IgA dermatitis	Neutrophils, ± mild acantholysis
Systemic lupus erythematosus	Neutrophils, ± mild acantholysis, interface dermatitis
Leishmaniasis	Neutrophils, ± microorganism
Superficial suppurative necrolytic dermatitis of Schnauzer	Neutrophils, epithelial necrosis
INTRAGRANULAR	
Pemphigus foliaceus	Marked acantholysis, granular ''cling-ons,'' neutrophils and/or eosinophils, ± follicular involvement
Pemphigus erythematosus	Marked acantholysis, granular ''cling-ons,'' neutrophils and/or eosinophils, ± lichenoid infiltrate, ± follicular involvement
INTRAEPIDERMAL	
Pemphigus vegetans	Marked acantholysis, eosinophils, papillomatosis
Epitheliotropic lymphoma	Atypical lymphoid cells, Pautrier's microabscesses
Viral dermatoses	Ballooning degeneration, ± inclusion bodies, ± acantholysis
Spongiotic dermatitis	Eosinophilic spongiosis suggests ectoparasitism, pemphigus, pemphigoid, canine sterile eosinophilic pustulosis
Necrolytic migratory erythema	Diffuse parakeratosis, marked edema of upper epidermis
SUPRABASILAR	
Pemphigus vulgaris	Marked acantholysis, ± follicular involvement
INTRABASAL	
Lupus erythematosus	Interface dermatitis, ± thickened basement membrane zone, ± dermal mucinosis
Dermatomyositis	Interface dermatitis, ± thickened basement membrane zone, ± dermal mucinosis, ± perifollicular fibrosis
Erythema multiforme	Interface dermatitis, marked single-cell necrosis of keratinocytes
Toxic epidermal necrolysis	Full-thickness coagulation necrosis of epidermis, little or no inflammation
Graft-versus-host disease	Interface dermatitis
Hereditary lupoid dermatosis of German shorthaired pointer	Interface dermatitis
Idiopathic ulcerative dermatitis of collie and Shetland sheep dog	Interface dermatitis
Subepidermal	
Bullous pemphigoid	Subepidermal vacuolar alteration, variable inflammation
Epidermolysis bullosa	Little or no inflammation, ± hydropic degeneration
Lupus erythematosus	Interface dermatitis, ± thickened basement membrane zone, ± dermal mucinosis
Dermatomyositis	Interface dermatitis, ± thickened basement membrane zone, ± dermal mucinosis, ± perifollicular fibrosis
Erythema multiforme	Interface dermatitis, marked single-cell necrosis of keratinocytes
Toxic epidermal necrolysis	Full-thickness coagulation necrosis of epidermis, little or no inflammation
Severe subepidermal edema or cellular infiltration	
Severe spongiosis	Spongiotic vesicles
Burns	Necrosis of epidermis and superficial dermis

*Drug eruptions can mimic virtually all of these reaction patterns.

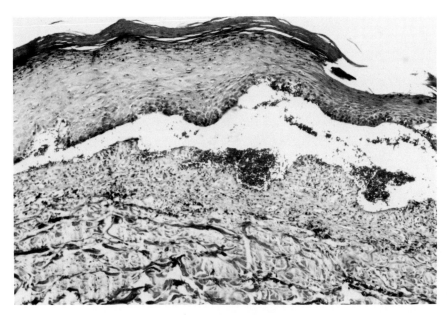

Figure 2:92. Subepidermal vesicular dermatitis. Subepidermal vesicle in a dog with bullous pemphigoid.

folliculitis) signifies hair follicle rupture (Fig. 2:95). Obviously, perifolliculitis, folliculitis, and furunculosis usually represent a pathologic continuum and may all be present in the same specimen. Follicular inflammation is a common gross and microscopic finding, and one must always be cautious in assessing its importance. It is a common secondary complication in pruritic dermatoses (e.g., hypersensitivities and ectoparasitism), seborrheic dermatoses, and hormonal dermatoses. Thus, a thorough search (histologically and clinically) for underlying causes is mandatory.

Follicular inflammation may be caused by bacteria, fungi, and parasites (*Demodex* spp. and *Pelodera strongyloides*) and, rarely, by atopy, food hypersensitivity, and seborrheic dermatitis. The folliculitides associated with bacteria, fungi, and parasites are usually suppurative initially, whereas those occasionally associated with atopy, food hypersensitivity, and seborrheic dermatitis are predominantly spongiotic perifolliculitides (with small numbers of exocytosing mononuclear cells, neutrophils, or both). Any chronic folliculitis, particularly if there is furunculosis, can become pyogranulomatous or granulomatous.

Regardless of the initiating cause, furunculosis is frequently associated with moderate to marked tissue eosinophilia. The significance of this finding is unknown, but it may represent a foreign-body reaction (e.g., to keratin). Eosinophilic folliculitides are occasionally seen. In dogs, these may be idiopathic (sterile eosinophilic pustulosis or sterile eosinophilic pinnal folliculitis) or arthropod or insect induced (eosinophilic furunculosis of the face). In cats, sterile eosinophilic folliculitis may be seen as a focal pathologic change with hypersensitivity reactions (atopy, food hypersensitivity, and flea bite hypersensitivity), eosinophilic plaque, and eosinophilic granuloma.[34]

Mural folliculitis is a feature of pemphigus, and any significant degree of acantholysis mandates a consideration of this disorder. Mononuclear mural folliculitis suggests epitheliotropic lymphoma. Likewise, the outer root sheath of the hair follicle may be involved in the hydropic degeneration and lichenoid cellular infiltrates of lupus erythematosus, erythema multiforme, drug eruption, and idiopathic lichenoid dermatoses.

Alopecia areata is characterized initially by a perifolliculitis, in which lymphocytes surround (like a "swarm of bees") the inferior segment of the hair follicle. A mild perifolliculitis

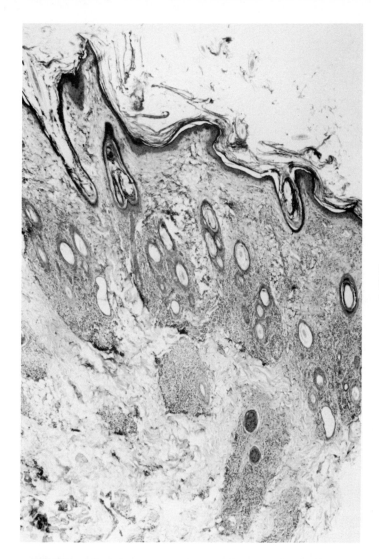

Figure 2:93. Perifolliculitis. Perifollicular pyogranulomas in a dog with visceral leishmaniasis.

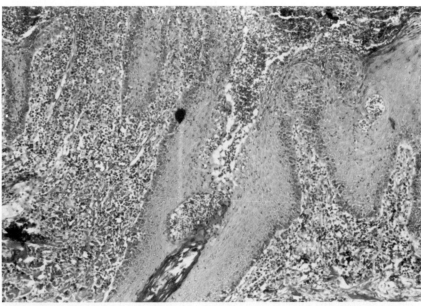

Figure 2:94. Folliculitis. Folliculitis in a dog with sterile eosinophilic pustulosis.

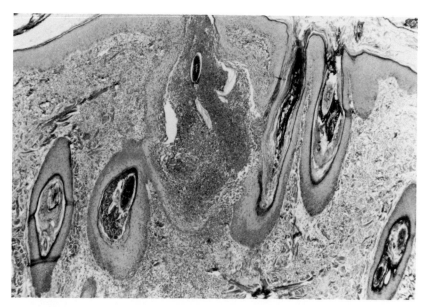

Figure 2:95. Furunculosis. Follicular rupture in a dog with staphylococcal furunculosis.

associated with marked mucinosis of the outer root sheath is seen with alopecia mucinosa. Perifollicular fibrosis is seen with chronic folliculitides, dermatomyositis, and chronic granulomatous sebaceous adenitis. Perifollicular melanosis can occasionally be seen with numerous folliculitides, but is most characteristic of canine demodicosis.[14] Necrotizing folliculitis is a rare manifestation of drug eruption. Granulomatous sebaceous adenitis and canine leishmaniasis produce an apparent perifolliculitis (until closer inspection reveals minimal or no exocytosis of the outer root sheath) and an inflammatory process centered on sebaceous glands.

Fibrosing Dermatitis

Fibrosis marks the resolving stage of an intense or insidious inflammatory process, and it occurs mainly as a consequence of collagen destruction. Fibrosis that is histologically recognizable does not necessarily produce a visible clinical scar. Ulcers that cause damage to collagen in the superficial dermis only do not usually result in scarring, whereas virtually all ulcers that extend into the deep dermis inexorably proceed to fibrosis and clinical scars.

Fibrosing dermatitis (Fig. 2:96) follows severe insults of many types to the dermis. Thus, fibrosing dermatitis alone is of minimal diagnostic value, other than for its testimony to antecedent injury. The pathologist must look carefully for signs of the antecedent process, such as furunculosis, vascular disease, foreign material, lymphedema, lupus erythematosus, dermatomyositis, acral lick dermatitis, and morphea. In cats, an uncommon chronic ulcerative dermatitis is characterized by linear subepidermal fibrosis, which extends peripheral to the ulcer.

Panniculitis

The panniculus is commonly involved as an extension of dermal inflammatory processes, especially of suppurative and granulomatous dermatoses. Likewise, there is usually some deep dermal involvement in virtually all panniculitides.

Panniculitis is conveniently divided on an anatomic basis into the lobular type (primarily involving fat lobules), the septal type (primarily involving interlobular connective tissue septa),

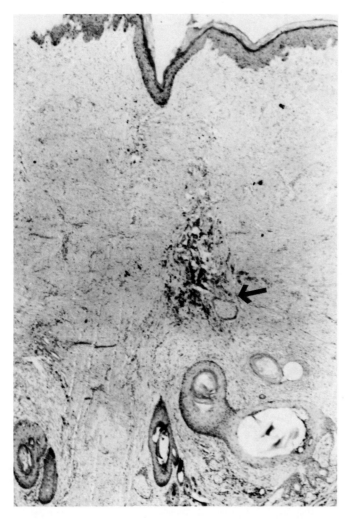

Figure 2:96. Fibrosing dermatitis. Dermal fibrosis after follicular rupture in a dog with staphylococcal furunculosis. Note orphaned sebaceous gland and pigmentary incontinence (*arrow*).

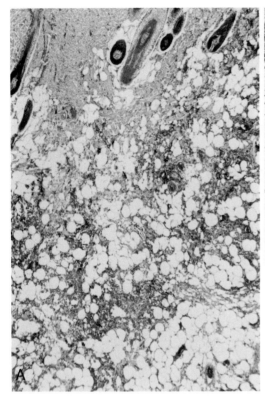

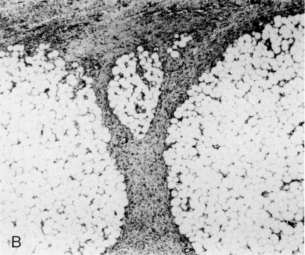

Figure 2:97. Panniculitis. *A*, Lobular panniculitis in a cat with idiopathic sterile panniculitis. *B*, Septal panniculitis in a cat with idiopathic sterile panniculitis.

and the diffuse type (both anatomic areas involved) (Fig. 2:97). Patterns of panniculitis appear to have little diagnostic or prognostic significance in dogs and cats, and all three patterns may be seen in a single lesion from the same patient.[27] Neither does the cytologic appearance (pyogranulomatous, granulomatous, suppurative, eosinophilic, lymphoplasmacytic, or fibrosing) appear to have much diagnostic or prognostic significance.[27] Most panniculitides, regardless of the cause, look histologically similar.

In dogs, diffuse panniculitis is the most common pattern, and septal panniculitis is most often found in cats. As with nodular and diffuse dermatitis, polarization, the use of special stains, and cultures are usually indicated. Septal panniculitis is seen with vasculitides and erythema nodosum. A rare form of canine panniculitis, one associated with lupus erythematosus (lupus profundus or lupus erythematosus panniculitis), is characterized by lymphoplasmacytic septal to lobular panniculitis, with septal vasculitis, numerous lymphoid nodules, mucinosis, and often an overlying interface dermatitis. Similar microscopic lesions occur at the sites of previous vaccinations (especially rabies) or drug injections. Feline subcutaneous fat sclerosis is characterized by marked septal fibrosis, fat micropseudocyst formation, and lipocytes that contain radially arranged, needle-shaped clefts.

Atrophic Dermatosis

Atrophic dermatosis is characterized by varying degrees of epithelial and connective tissue atrophy (Fig. 2:98). The most common disorders in this category are endocrine, nutritional, and developmental dermatoses; telogen defluxion; and postclipping follicular arrest. Atrophic dermatoses show variable combinations of the following histopathologic changes:[17, 25] diffuse orthokeratotic hyperkeratosis, epidermal atrophy, follicular keratosis, follicular atrophy, telogenization of hair follicles, excessive trichilemmal keratinization (flame follicles),[29] epithelial melanosis, and sebaceous gland atrophy. Inflammatory changes are frequent and potentially

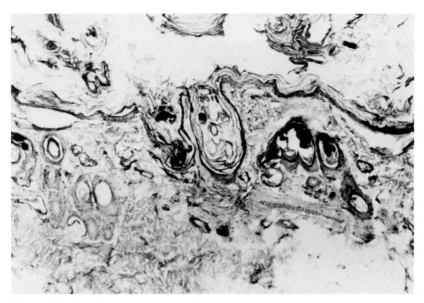

Figure 2:98. Atrophic dermatosis in a dog with hyposomatotropism.

misleading in the atrophic dermatoses and reflect the common occurrence of secondary bacterial infection, seborrhea, or both with these disorders. Findings suggestive of specific endocrinopathies include diffuse mucinosis (hypothyroidism), dystrophic mineralization (hyperadrenocorticism), hypertrophied or vacuolated arrector pili muscles (hypothyroidism), decreased dermal elastin (hyposomatotropism and hyperadrenocorticism), dermal atrophy (hyperadrenocorticism and hyposomatotropism), and absence of arrector pili muscles (hyperadrenocorticism). Adrenal sex hormone abnormalities seem to produce a unique combination of atrophic dermatosis and follicular dysplasia.

Findings suggestive of nutritional disorders include misshapen, corkscrew hairs and small hairs. Developmental disorders (hypotrichosis, follicular dysplasia, and color dilution alopecia) are characterized by follicular dysplasia and anomalous deposition of melanin. Telogen defluxion is characterized by diffuse telogenization of hair follicles with no other signs of cutaneous atrophy. Postclipping follicular arrest is characterized by diffuse catagenization (occasionally telogenization) of hair follicles with no other signs of cutaneous atrophy. In the chronic stage, alopecia areata is characterized by follicular atrophy, as well as by ''orphaned'' cutaneous glands and arrector pili muscles. In the chronic stage, granulomatous sebaceous adenitis may have complete absence of sebaceous glands, a feature not usually seen with endocrine and nutritional dermatoses. The acquired skin fragility syndrome of cats is characterized by striking atrophy and attenuation of dermal collagen.

Mixed Reaction Patterns

Because skin diseases have a pathologic continuum, reflecting various combinations of acute, subacute, and chronic changes, and because animals can have more than one dermatosis at the same time, it is common for one or two biopsy specimens from the same animal to show two or more reaction patterns. For instance, it is common to see an overall pattern of perivascular dermatitis (due to hypersensitivity reactions or ectoparasitism) or atrophic dermatosis (due to endocrinopathy) with a subordinate, focal pattern of folliculitis, furunculosis, or intraepidermal pustular dermatitis (due to secondary bacterial infection). Likewise, one can find multiple patterns from one or two biopsy specimens from an animal with a single disease (e.g., vasculitis, diffuse necrotizing dermatitis, and fibrosing dermatitis in a patient with necrotizing vasculitis). Mixed reaction patterns (two or three patterns) were found in about 25 per cent of the biopsy specimens from cats with inflammatory dermatoses.[34]

Invisible Dermatoses

Generations of dermatohistopathologists have struggled with biopsy specimens from diseased skin that appear normal under the microscope. Because normal skin is rarely included in biopsy specimens in clinical practice, one must assume that some evidence of disease is present. From the perspective of the dermatohistopathologist, the invisible dermatoses are clinically evident skin diseases that show a histologic picture resembling normal skin.[13] Technical problems must be eliminated, such as sampling errors that occur when normal skin on an edge of the biopsy specimen has been sectioned and the diseased tissue has been left in paraffin.

When confronted with an invisible dermatosis, the dermatohistopathologist should consider the following possible disorders and techniques for detecting them: dermatophytosis (special stain for fungi in keratin); ichthyosis (removal of surface keratin); psychogenic alopecia; pigmentary disturbances such as hypermelanoses and hypomelanoses, including lentigo and vitiligo; amorphous deposits in the superficial dermis (Congo red stain for amyloid deposits); urticaria; urticaria pigmentosa (toluidine blue stain for mast cells); connective tissue disorder (cutaneous asthenia); and various nevi.

Conclusion

A skin biopsy can be diagnostic, confirmatory, and helpful, or it can be inconclusive, depending on the dermatosis; the selection, handling, and processing of the specimen; and the skill of the histopathologist.

The dermatopathologist has no right to make a diagnosis of nonspecific dermatitis or inflammation. Every biopsy specimen is a sample of some specific process, but the visible changes may be noncharacteristic and may not permit a diagnosis.[23]

The clinician should never accept the terms ''nonspecific changes'' and ''nonspecific dermatitis.'' Many pathologic entities that are now well recognized were once regarded as nonspecific. Recourse to serial sections (the key pathologic changes may be focal), special stains, second opinions, and further biopsies may be necessary.

■ SPECIAL PROCEDURES

In the past decade, a number of techniques have been developed for studying biopsy specimens. These techniques were usually advanced to allow the identification of special cell types. Examples of such procedures include immunofluorescence testing, electron microscopy, enzyme histochemistry, and immunocytochemistry. The latter two procedures have not yet been extensively investigated in small animal dermatology but should become increasingly used and invaluable diagnostic tools in the future.

Immunofluorescence testing is not routinely done in veterinary medicine (see Chap. 8). Biopsy specimens for immunofluorescence testing must be carefully selected and either snap-frozen or placed in Michel's fixative. Electron microscopy is best performed on small specimens (1 to 2 mm in diameter) fixed in 3 per cent glutaraldehyde. Enzyme histochemistry is performed on frozen sections or on tissues fixed in 2 per cent paraformaldehyde, dehydrated in acetone, and embedded in glycol methacrylate (Table 2:10). Immunocytochemistry may be performed on formalin-fixed, routinely processed tissues (e.g., immunoperoxidase methods) or on frozen sections (e.g., lymphocyte markers), depending on the substance being studied (Table 2:10).

Molecular biological techniques (in situ hybridization, polymerase chain reaction) are having an impact on many different aspects of medicine.[44a] In the realm of infectious agents, these nucleic acid probes are enhancing diagnostic capabilities, avoiding the need of culturing

Table 2:10. Examples of Markers for the Identification of Cell Types

Marker	Cell Type
Enzyme Histochemical	
α-Naphthyl acetate esterase	Monocyte, histiocyte, Langerhans' cell, plasma cell
Chloroacetate esterase	Neutrophil, mast cell
Acid phosphatase	Monocyte, histiocyte, plasma cell
Alkaline phosphatase	Neutrophil, endothelial cell
β-Glucuronidase	Histiocyte, T lymphocyte, plasma cell
Adenosine triphosphatase	Histiocyte, plasma cell, B lymphocyte, endothelial cell
5′-Nucleotidase	Endothelial cell
Nonspecific esterase	Monocyte, histiocyte, Langerhans' cell
Lysozyme	Monocyte, histiocyte
α$_1$-Antitrypsin	Monocyte, histiocyte, mast cell
Chymotrypsin-like protease	Mast cell
Dipeptidyl peptidase II	Mast cell
Immunohistochemical	
Cytokeratin	Squamous and glandular epithelium, Merkel's cell
Vimentin	Fibroblast, Schwann cell, endothelial cell, myoepithelial cell, lipocyte, smooth muscle, skeletal muscle, mast cell, plasma cell, melanocyte, lymphocyte, monocyte, histiocyte, Langerhans' cell
Desmin	Skeletal muscle, smooth muscle
Neurofilament	Axon cell bodies, dendrites
S100 protein	Melanocyte, Schwann cell, Langerhans' cell, myoepithelial cell, sweat gland acini and ducts, lipocyte, macrophage
Myoglobin	Skeletal muscle
Factor VIII–related antigen	Endothelial cell
Ulex europaeus agglutinin I	Endothelial cell
Leukocyte common antigen	Leukocyte
Peanut agglutinin	Histiocyte
Myelin basic protein	Schwann cell
Neuron-specific enolase	Schwann cell, Merkel's cell
Laminin	Basement membrane
Leu and OKT (various numerical designations)	Lymphocytes (various developmental and functional types)
CD1	Langerhans' cell
CD3	T lymphocyte

infectious agents for the purpose of diagnosis, allowing earlier detection of infection, and permitting the detection of latent infections.

REFERENCES

General

1. Alhaidari, Z.: Les lésions élémentaires dermatologiques. Prat. Méd. Chirurg. Anim. Cie. 23:101, 1988.
2. Griffin, C. E. G.: Unpublished observations.
3. Scott, D. W.: Examination of the integumentary system. Vet. Clin. North Am. (Small Anim. Pract.) 11:499, 1981.
4. Shearer, D.: Laboratory diagnosis of skin disease. In Pract. 13:149, 1991.

Age

5. Bourdeau, P.: Dermatologie du jeune carnivore. Point Vét. 21:439, 1989.
6. Bourdeau, P.: Eléments de dermatologie du chien et du chat vieillessants. Point Vét. 22:255, 1990.
7. Foil, C. S.: The skin. In: Hoskins, J. D. (ed.). Veterinary Pediatrics. W. B. Saunders Co., Philadelphia, 1990, p. 359.
8. Halliwell, R. E. W.: Skin diseases of old dogs and cats. Vet. Rec. 126:389, 1990.

Breed

9. Ihrke, P. J., Franti, C. E.: Breed as a risk factor associated with skin diseases in dogs seen in northern California. Calif. Vet. 39(5):13, 1985.
10. Scott, D. W., Paradis, M.: A survey of canine and feline skin disorders seen in a university practice: Small Animal Clinic, University of Montreal, Saint-Hyacinthe, Quebec (1987–1988). Can. Vet. J. 31:830, 1990.

Cytologic Examination

11. Perman, V., et al.: Cytology of the Dog and Cat. American Animal Hospital Association, South Bend, IN, 1979.

Biopsy and Dermatopathologic Examination: The Vocabulary of Dermatohistopathology

12. Ackerman, A. B.: Histopathologic Diagnosis of Inflammatory Skin Diseases. Lea & Febiger, Philadelphia, 1978.
13. Brownstein, M. H., Rabinowitz, A. D.: The invisible dermatoses. J. Am. Acad. Dermatol. 8:579, 1983.
14. Cayatte, S. M., et al.: Perifollicular melanosis in the dog. Vet. Dermatol. 3:165, 1992.
15. Dunstan, R. W.: A user's guide to veterinary surgical pathology laboratories or, why do I still get a diagnosis of chronic dermatitis even when I take a perfect biopsy? Vet. Clin. North Am. (Small Anim. Pract.) 20:1397, 1990.
16. Goldschmidt, M. H.: Small animal dermatopathology: 'What's old, what's new, what's borrowed, what's useful.' Semin. Vet. Med. Surg. (Small Anim.) 2:162, 1987.
17. Gross, T. L., Ihrke, P. J.: The histologic analysis of endocrine-related alopecia in the dog. In: von Tscharner, C., Halliwell, R. E. W. (eds.). Advances in Veterinary Dermatology, Vol. 1. Baillière-Tindall, Philadelphia, 1990, p. 77.
18. Gross, T. L. et al.: Veterinary Dermatopathology. A Macroscopic and Microscopic Evaluation of Canine and Feline Skin Disease. Mosby Year Book, St. Louis, 1992.
19. Henfrey, J. I., et al.: A comparison of three local anaesthetic techniques for skin biopsy in dogs. Vet. Dermatol. 2:21, 1991.
20. Langham, R. F., Schirmer, R. G.: Value of histopathologic examination in diagnosis of dermatologic disorders of small animals. J. Am. Vet. Med. Assoc. 153:1754, 1968.
21. Leider, M., Rosenblum, M.: A Dictionary of Dermatological Words, Terms, and Phrases. McGraw-Hill Book Co., New York, 1968.
22. Lever, W. F. Schaumburg-Lever, G.: Histopathology of the Skin VII. J. B. Lippincott Co., Philadelphia, 1990.
23. Mehregan, A. H.: Pinkus' Guide to Dermatohistopathology IV. Appleton-Century-Crofts, New York, 1986.
24. Robinson, J. K.: Fundamentals of Skin Biopsy. Year Book Medical Publishers, Chicago, 1986.
25. Scott, D. W.: Histopathologic findings in the endocrine skin disorders of the dog. J. Am. Anim. Hosp. Assoc. 18:173, 1982.
26. Scott, D. W.: Lichenoid reaction in the skin of dogs: Clinicopathologic correlations. J. Am. Anim. Hosp. Assoc. 20:305, 1984.
27. Scott, D. W., Anderson, W. I.: Panniculitis in dogs and cats: A retrospective analysis of 78 cases. J. Am. Anim. Hosp. Assoc. 24:551, 1988.
28. Scott, D. W.: Lymphoid nodules in skin biopsies from dogs, cats, and horses with non-neoplastic dermatoses. Cornell Vet. 79:267, 1989.
29. Scott, D. W.: Excessive trichilemmal keratinization (flame follicles) in endocrine skin disorders of the dog. Vet. Dermatol. 1:37, 1990.
30. Scott, D. W.: Epidermal mast cells in the cat. Vet. Dermatol. 1:65, 1990.
31. Scott, D. W.: Veterinary dermatohistopathology: What's new and exciting? Adv. Dermatol. 6:289, 1991.
32. Scott, D. W.: Bacteria and yeast on the surface and within non-inflamed hair follicles of skin biopsies from dogs with non-neoplastic dermatoses. Cornell Vet. 82:371, 1992.
33. Scott, D. W.: Bacteria and yeast on the surface and within non-inflamed hair follicles of skin biopsies from cats with non-neoplastic dermatoses. Cornell Vet. 82:379, 1992.
34. Scott, D. W.: Analyse du type de réaction histopathologique dans le diagnostic des dermatoses inflammatoires chez le chat: Étude portant sur 394 cas. Point Vét. 26:57, 1994.
35. Seaman, W. J., Chang, S. H.: Dermal perifollicular mineralization of toy poodle bitches. Vet. Pathol. 21:122, 1984.
36. von Bomhard, D.: Histopathologie von nicht-tumorosen Hauterkrankungen des Hundes und der Katze. Kleintierpraxis 31:391, 1986.
37. von Tscharner, C., Hauser, B.: Pathologie der Haut. Kleintierpraxis 26:449, 1981.
38. Yager, J. A., Wilcock, B. P.: Skin biopsy: Revelations and limitations. Can. Vet. J. 29:969, 1988.
39. Yager, J. A., Scott, D. W.: The skin and appendages. In: Jubb, K. V. P., et al. (eds.). Pathology of Domestic Animals IV, Vol. 1. Academic Press, New York, 1993, p. 531.
39a. Yager, J. A., Wilcock, B.P.: Color Atlas and Text of Surgical Pathology of the Dog and Cat. Dermatopathology and Skin Tumors. Wolfe Publishing, London, 1994.

Miscellaneous

40. Bevier, D. E.: In: Von Tschaner, C., Halliwell, R. E. W. (eds.). Advances in Veterinary Dermatology, Vol. 1. Baillière-Tindall, Philadelphia, 1990, p. 126.
41. Brignac, M. M., et al.: Microscopy of color mutant alopecia. Proc. Am. Acad. Vet. Dermatol. Am. Coll. Vet. Dermatol. 4:14, 1988.
41a. Brown, W. M., Stenn, K. S.: Homeobox genes and the patterning of skin diseases. J. Cutan. Pathol. 20:289, 1993.
42. Doubleday, D. W.: Who is Nikolsky and what does his sign mean? J. Am. Acad. Dermatol. 16:1054, 1987.
43. Goldschmidt, M. H., Shofer, F. S.: Skin Tumors of the Dog and Cat. Pergamon Press, New York, 1992.
43a. Haake, A. R., Polakowska, R. R.: Cell death by apoptosis in epidermal biology. J. Invest. Dermatol. 101:107, 1993.
44. Jang, S. S., Biberstein, E. L.: Laboratory diagnosis of fungal and algal infections: Grune LE (ed). Infectious Diseases of the Dog and Cat. W. B. Saunders Co., Philadelphia, 1990, pp. 639–648.
44a. Jaworsky, C.: The molecular diagnosis of infection. J. Cutan. Pathol. 20:508, 1993.
45. Kennis, R. A.: Quantitation and topographical analysis of Malassezia organisms in normal canine skin. Proc. Am. Acad. Vet. Dermatol. Am. Coll. Vet. Dermatol. 9:23, 1993.
46. Plant, J. D., et al.: Factors associated with and prevalence of high *Malassezia pachydermatis* numbers on dog skin. J. Am. Vet. Med. Assoc. 201:879, 1992.

Dermatologic Therapy

■

Chapter Outline

■ CLIENT COMPLIANCE

The successful treatment of skin disorders depends to a large extent on the client. In addition to supplying the necessary historical information to make a diagnosis, the client administers most prescribed therapies. The successful management of many dermatologic diseases necessitates long-term or lifelong therapy, often involving more than one medicament. The client must also give the medications correctly at the proper intervals and for the proper duration.

Many animals are referred to the authors after the correct diagnosis was made and appropriate treatment was recommended, but the pet failed to respond because of improper execution by the owner. Excellent diagnosticians often have poor results if they are not able to interact with clients effectively, because this often leads to failure in compliance. These failures may occur for a variety of reasons. Understanding the possible reasons for poor compliance, recognizing when treatment failures occur, and developing corrective measures is an art that the successful clinician develops.

The reasons for poor client compliance include the following: (1) failure of the client to understand the importance of giving the treatment; (2) lack of education of the client regarding the proper treatment; (3) improper frequency of or interval between medication applications; (4) faulty application, which can take multiple forms (Table 3:1); (5) inadequate duration of

Table 3:1. Reasons for Improper Treatment Application

Reason	Examples
Incorrect dosage	Not giving the prescribed dose
	Improperly diluting topical products
	Adding to food bowl, resulting in incomplete intake
Interactions with other substances	Giving drugs with food that should be given on an empty stomach
Incorrect frequency	Giving TID drugs with breakfast, lunch, and dinner and not closer to q8h
Improper duration	Not leaving shampoo on long enough
Failure to apply to the proper site	Dipping for scabies but not treating the ears and face
	Only treating the external ear canal and failing to treat the pinna with topical steroid in allergic otitis externa
Application that does not reach the skin	Failing to have dip penetrate the haircoat
	Not shaving the hair in thick-coated, long-haired pets
Failure to understand the application method	Rinsing dips out of the haircoat

therapy; (6) client's lack of time or labor-intensive treatment; (7) disagreeable cosmetic appearance or odor of treatment; (8) perceived danger of treatment; (9) premature discontinuation of treatment because of perceived lack of efficacy; and (10) discontinuation of treatment because it was too difficult or not tolerated by the pet. Many of these problems are avoidable if the clinician or the veterinary assistants adequately explain the treatment plan.

It is important to make the client aware of potential problems, and these possible difficulties should be discussed before clients leave the office. The authors encounter numerous cases wherein the clients have unused treatments at home. This is particularly true of flea products; because the treatment was too labor-intensive or the treatment appeared ineffective, the client discontinued it. The successful clinician tries to prevent these treatment failures. For example, if clients do not or cannot dip their cats, a flea collar, although normally considered less effective than a properly applied dip, becomes relatively more efficacious. The best flea dip ever invented never works sitting on a shelf. Some clients may not readily admit that a treatment will be too difficult or unacceptable, and therefore, alternatives may not be offered.

Another major factor influencing client compliance is the use of multiple therapeutic agents. Often, the best management of a dermatologic disease, particularly a chronic one, is a therapeutic regimen or plan that entails the use of multiple products. This makes education of the client more difficult and time consuming, as well as potentially more confusing. Despite these problems, the best long-term control is often achieved by using such a plan versus a single medicament.

■ CARE OF NORMAL SKIN AND HAIRCOAT

The veterinarian is vitally concerned with the health of the patient's skin and is often consulted by clients regarding preventive care as well as the optimal maintenance of the normal skin and haircoat. Most commonly, questions about the healthy pet's skin and hair relate to nutrition, skin and coat supplements, ectoparasite control (see Chap. 6), bathing, and shedding. Additionally, the veterinarian may be queried about optimal grooming. Many veterinary practices offer medicated baths and dips as well as routine bathing.

Although the skin reflects the animal's general health, many vigorous, healthy, normal pets have unkempt haircoats—mainly because of neglect or the client's lack of knowledge regarding proper grooming. Keeping the haircoat free from mats and removing the shedded undercoat allows more appropriate thermoregulation and discourages irritation and secondary bacterial infection. Therefore, it is valuable for the veterinarian to be familiar with routine grooming equipment as well as general skin and hair care.

Because most veterinarians are not groomers, questions regarding grooming and especially haircut styles are usually handled more appropriately by a qualified groomer. Styles change, and variations in clipping can enhance or mask aspects of conformation that affect the animal's appearance. These nuances of style are the province of owners, breeders, handlers, and commercial grooming establishments. However, most clients expect veterinarians to know about grooming and groomers' tools. Much of the following discussion is presented as background for students or information that can be transmitted to clients.[4, 173, 219]

Routine Grooming Care

Dog and cat breeds have many different coat types, so generalization about grooming details is difficult.[4, 154, 173, 219] A few important principles can be emphasized—the most critical being the frequency of care. When a schedule of grooming is found to suffice for keeping the pet looking sharp, it should be followed conscientiously. It is better to spend a few minutes grooming regularly than many hours sporadically.

Excessive shedding of hair into the house environment is greatly decreased by routine grooming. Products have been marketed that claim to reduce shedding. The substantiation of these claims appears to relate more to the instructions for use than to the active ingredients.

Recommended use of these products involves extensive brushing before and after each weekly bath. Properly performed brushing, 15 to 30 minutes weekly, greatly decreases the amount of hair shed into the environment, regardless of which shampoo is used.

Because the client must be motivated to perform grooming regularly, making it easy is important. If proper facilities, effective tools, and a cooperative patient are combined, the task of grooming becomes tolerable or even enjoyable. A solid, convenient table with a nonskid surface and a grooming post with a neck or body sling are helpful. Grooming is facilitated if performed in a quiet area without distractions. A grooming stand with a chair is helpful but not necessary.

The proper grooming tools should be clean and in good repair. Comb, brush, claw clipper and file, towels, cotton balls, and cotton-tipped swabs (Q-Tips) are the vital implements needed for most breeds. Shampoo, hair-conditioning rinses, ear-cleaning solution, and flea dips are also necessary. Specialized tools (see below) are essential for grooming and conditioning some coats.

The animal and its training can greatly affect the ease of grooming. Regular habits of good behavior during grooming, established early in life, result in cooperation. Most properly trained pets either enjoy or tolerate well their grooming care.

Prospective owners should contemplate grooming problems before purchasing a pet. If time and expense are likely to be obstacles, one should not choose a pet from a longhaired, wiry- or woolly-coated breed, but instead select a short-coated animal that is easy to groom. An owner should perform simple daily or weekly grooming chores but should periodically take advantage of a professional grooming service. The grooming needs of five typical coat types are discussed below.

Grooming Tools

Various grooming implements are needed (Fig. 3:1); the number and type depend on the breed and the coat type. Books that cover the fine points of grooming individual breeds can be obtained from bookstores and pet shops.[154, 219]

■ *Clipping Implements.* Electric clippers designed for small animals are best and are also available in cordless, rechargeable battery models. They should have changeable heads or a selection of different-sized blades. Clippers should be held gently on the skin surface and moved slowly. The moving parts should be clean, sharp, and well lubricated. If the blades become hot, are forced, or are pointed down at the skin, severe irritation and burns may result. The delicate skin of the genital, eye, and ear regions is most susceptible. Irritation and folliculitis may occur when dull blades pull anagen hairs from the follicle. This may also occur in the ear canal if hairs are plucked.

Clipping against the ''lay'' of the hair produces a shorter cut with any blade than cutting with the lay of the hair. Clipping blades are numbered—the larger the number, the closer the cut is made to the skin and the more hair is removed. The No. 40 blade produces a shaven appearance when used against the hair. Only a slight stubble is left when it is used with the lay of the hair. The No. 15 blade also cuts closely. No. 10 blades leave enough hair to show the natural color of the coat. Two blades (Nos. 10 and 15) have general purpose uses, especially around the face, the feet, and the ears of many breeds. The No. 7 blade leaves hair about 0.62 cm (¼ inch) long, and No. 5 leaves about 1.25 cm (½ inch). These latter blades (Nos. 5 and 7) are used for machine clipping wiry-coated breeds. Machine clipping makes all hairs the same length but leaves the dead hair in place—not a desirable practice. Often, owners of terrier breeds prefer stripping the haircoat in contrast to clipping. Clipper blades (Oster) are available that leave 2.5 cm (1 inch) or 3.75 cm (1½ inch) of coat intact.

Dogs should be carefully introduced to the clipper during the first session. The owner can be helpful by training the dog at home. By holding an electric razor near the dog and rubbing it

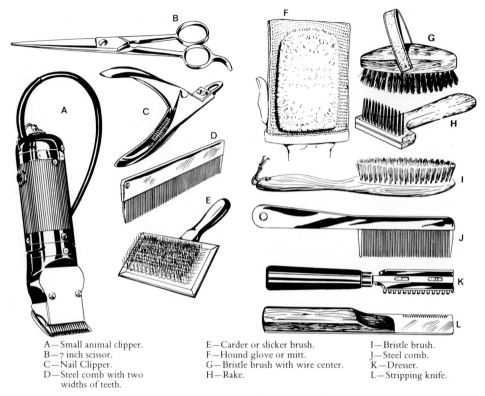

A—Small animal clipper.
B—7 inch scissor.
C—Nail Clipper.
D—Steel comb with two
    widths of teeth.

E—Carder or slicker brush.
F—Hound glove or mitt.
G—Bristle brush with wire center.
H—Rake.

I—Bristle brush.
J—Steel comb.
K—Dresser.
L—Stripping knife.

Figure 3:1. Grooming implements. (From Miller, D.: Know How to Groom Your Dog. By permission of Pet Library Ltd., a subsidiary of Sternco Industries, Inc., New York City.)

over the dog's coat several times daily, owners can help the dog to become accustomed to its vibration and noise. Gentle firmness and frequent short breaks for relaxation are necessary during the actual clipping sessions.

Shears are often used in conjunction with a comb. Barber scissors about 17.5 cm (7 inches) long with blunt tips are used to trim long hairs and whiskers around the eyes, the ears, the face, and the feet. They are often needed to remove mats and tags. Thinning shears have one solid blade and one serrated blade, so that large bulky coats can be thinned without obvious signs. It is well to insert the shears deeply under the surface of the coat to avoid destroying the external color of coats in which the undercoat and the outer coat are different colors.

A mat and tangle splitter slices mats so they can be removed more easily, leaving some hair, as compared with clippers, which remove all hair.

■ *Combing Implements.* Combs should have rounded teeth to avoid scratching the skin. To perform efficiently, combs should always be inserted to their full depth into the coat. Different tooth spacing is needed for each coat type. Metal, plastic, and bone combs are available. The material is not as important as the design. Forced combing or pulling at tangled mats extracts live and dead hairs and can easily ruin a coat or produce irritation and secondary bacterial infection of the skin.

The rake is especially useful in hacking through the heavy mats in a badly tangled coat. The rake has a single row of long metal teeth set at right angles to the handle. It can inflict wounds, especially inside the hock and thigh, and should be used with utmost care. It can also pull live hair needlessly and thus produce irritations.

A carder is a square board with a short handle. It has bent, fine-wire teeth set close together.

The teeth are placed near the skin, and the carder is twisted outward from the skin. This loosens the coat and removes dead hair and some of the smaller hair mats.

Brushes may be used in the same way on long coats. If the hair is meant to stand away from the skin, the hair should be brushed (with short strokes) against its natural growth. Smooth-coated dogs should be brushed with the lay of the hair. Some groomers believe that nylon or synthetic bristles accumulate static electricity and cause hair breakage. They prefer natural pig bristles or soft wire brushes. Brushes for longer coats have wider-spaced, longer bristles that are firmly set into the rubber-base handle. Excessive brushing breaks hair and pulls it out. Except on short coats, surface brushing is not effective. The hair mats from the skin outward, while the surface looks fine. The hair should be combed or brushed from the skin in small amounts at a time. Concentrating on small areas by holding the hair back and making parts right down to the skin facilitates brushing.

Hound gloves have a palm consisting of boar hair, wire, or fiber bristles. They are used on short-haired dogs to remove the dead undercoat and to give polish to the outer coat.

Stripping combs are also referred to as dressers. They may have a razor blade encased in serrated teeth or may be merely a serrated metal blade attached to a wooden handle. These instruments are used to help pull out dull, dead hair. Hair is grasped between the thumb and the comb and removed with a twisting motion. Chalk is sometimes used on the coat to make it easier to grip the hair firmly. If the hair is grasped between the thumb and the forefinger and extracted, the process is called *plucking*. The purpose of stripping and plucking, as applied to terrier-type breeds whose coats are "blown" (loose, or "ripe"), is to remove the telogen hairs but retain the anagen hairs. When these animals are clipped, both types of hairs are shortened. Although machine clipping is fast, it is obviously much less desirable.

Hand toweling is used to rub out dead hairs, to stimulate skin circulation, and to give a gloss or glow to the hair. It should be used on only short-coated breeds, or there may be increased tangles.

Cleaning the Skin

The normal skin surface film contains excretory products of skin glands and keratinocytes, corneocytes, bacteria and dirt, pollen, grains, and mold spores. Excessive amounts of these, together with altered or abnormal fatty acids, serum, red blood cells, proteinaceous exudates, degenerating inflammatory cells, and the byproducts of their degradation as well as bacterial degradation are found in the surface film of abnormal skin. To promote health, the skin and coat should be groomed to minimize these accumulations. If proper skin and coat care is neglected, skin irritation may result, or accumulations of debris may adversely affect a skin disease that is already present.

PREPARATION FOR BATHING

Before dogs are bathed, the haircoat should be brushed out and the claws should be clipped or filed to keep them short. With frequent filing, the quick recedes and the claw can be maintained properly. Also, one should check between the toes for foreign objects and remove hair under the foot between the pads. Care should be exercised when using scissors between pads. Clippers are safer, as they are less apt to produce lacerations. If the dog's coat is unkempt and severely matted, the tags and mats should be cut out before they are wet; otherwise, the mats become set and are more difficult to remove.

The anal sacs should be palpated and expressed, if necessary, before bathing so any soilage can be removed during the bath. One should place cotton over the anus and, with the thumb on one side of the anus and the fingers on the other side, press forward and together to express the sacs. A more complete expression of sac contents can be performed by inserting a gloved finger into the rectum to express each sac separately.

The ears should also receive attention and care before the animal is bathed. The ears are carefully examined, as well as cleaned and dried thoroughly if necessary (see Chap. 18). Some terriers and Poodles may have large amounts of hair growing in the ear canals. Excessive hair should be plucked from the external ear canal in dogs prone to ear problems, as it may allow cerumen accumulation and contribute to irritation. The process of plucking may cause irritation in normal ears and should be used only when it is deemed necessary on the basis of the history and examination of the ear canal. Antibacterial and anti-inflammatory medication should be instilled in the ear canal after the plucking is complete and the canal is clean and dry. Pledgets of cotton may be placed firmly in each ear before bathing to block the entrance of soap and water. After the bath, the cotton is removed or, if none was applied, a drying agent is put into the ear canal.

In the past, it has been recommended to apply ointments or oils to eyes as a protection against inadvertent entry of irritants. This should *not* be done because the oil vehicle makes rinsing an irritant from the eye more difficult. This is especially true of lipid-soluble irritants, which may cause more damage if applied to an eye pretreated with an oil or an ointment. Nothing should be applied to the eyes, and if an irritant (e.g., dip and soap) enters the eye, it should immediately be rinsed with fresh water.

HAIR CARE PRODUCTS

■ *Shampoos.* Shampoos should remove external dirt, grime, and sebum and leave the hair soft, shiny, and easy to comb. To accomplish this, they should lather well, rinse freely, leave no residue, cause no eye damage, and remove soil rather than natural oils. Some shampoos still have a soap base, but most shampoos are surfactants or detergents with a variety of additives that function as thickeners, conditioners, lime soap dispersants, protein hydrolysates, and perfumes. Dozens of products are on the market.

Many clients are familiar with pH-balanced shampoos for human use. The same promotion of pH adjusting for canine shampoos has been recommended. The canine skin is approximately neutral with a pH of 7 to 7.4, which is different from that of human skin. Therefore, human pH-adjusted shampoos are not optimal for canine use. Theoretically, pH products temporarily affect the electrostatic charges in the surface lipid bilayer and could alter the normal barrier effect. However, the clinical relevance or the documentation of alterations in barrier function related to the pH of a shampoo is lacking in veterinary medicine.

Soap shampoos work well in soft water. In hard water, they leave a dulling film of calcium and magnesium soap on the hair unless special lime-dispersing agents are added to bind calcium, magnesium, and heavy metal ions.

Detergent shampoos are synthetic surfactants, usually salts of lauryl sulfate. They do not react with hard water, but they tend to be harsher cleaning agents than soap. This disadvantage is partially overcome by various additives. Satisfactory detergents to use as shampoos for normal coats tend to dry the coat and contain few additives to counter the detergent effect. Conditioners should be used after detergents. Glycol, glyceryl esters, lanolin derivatives, oils, and fatty alcohols are considered superfattening or emollient additives that prevent the complete removal of natural oils or tend to replace them. They also give the hair more luster and, as lubricants, make it easier to comb.

■ *Conditioners.* Hair conditioners have two main purposes: (1) to reduce static electricity so that coarse hair does not snarl or become flyaway and (2) to give body to limp or thin hair. Normal hair maintains electric neutrality. However, if clean, dry hair is in a low-humidity environment or is brushed excessively, it picks up increased negative electric charges. Adjacent hairs that are similarly charged repel one another and produce the condition known as flyaway. Conditioners or cream rinses are cationic (positively charged) surfactants or amphoteric materials that neutralize the charge and eliminate flyaway. They are slightly acidic, which hardens keratin and removes hard water residues. They also contain a fatty or oily component that adds a film to provide luster. Thus, these products make hair lie flat and comb easily, but they do not provide the body or fluff that some coats require.

Protein conditioners, or body builders, contain oil and protein hydrolysates. Oils add luster, whereas protein hydrolysates coat the hair and make it seem thicker. This may be a slight advantage in hair with a dried, cracked, outer cuticle layer, but the effect is actually minimal. Only a thin film is added, so hair is not strengthened. If the protein is added to a shampoo rather than used separately, most of it is washed away during rinsing, further reducing the effect.

BATHING

The dog is placed in a raised tub and is wet completely with warm water. A shower spray hose makes bathing easier and rinsing much faster. A bland nonmedicated, moisturizing or hypoallergenic shampoo should be used for most dogs. The shampoo is applied to the neck and topline of the dog. More water is added, and a vigorous lather is worked up. Some owners apply excessive amounts of shampoo when the product is applied right from the bottle. This is wasteful and can lead to skin irritation because it is difficult to rinse the heavy concentration of shampoo. Predilution of the shampoo in 5 to 10 parts of water can help to eliminate this problem.

The lather should be rubbed into short-haired dogs but squeezed into long coats, as rubbing may mat the long hair excessively. One can work a small rubber brush back and forth through the coat to clean the skin and remove any foreign materials from the hair. In some short-coated breeds, especially Doberman pinschers and Dalmatians, washing against the normal hair growth may induce a postbathing folliculitis.

The dog's face should be washed and rinsed carefully. Gently placing a finger over the eyes keeps the eyelids closed and helps to prevent shampoo or rinse water from entering the eyes. A washcloth is also useful to control lather and keep soap from the dog's eyes.

The entire coat is rinsed thoroughly. A second lather and rinse may be needed to wash the dog until the water runs off clear. Thorough rinsing is essential. If the outer coat is rinsed but soap is left close to the skin, irritation results. This is most commonly seen in areas that tend to be overlooked or difficult to rinse, such as heavily feathered caudal thighs, and axillary, groin, periscrotal, ventral tail, and interdigital areas. The haircoat should be rinsed until clear, detergent-free water runs off. In general, except when short-coated breeds are washed or unless medicated shampoos necessitating longer contact times are used, the rinsing takes longer than the cleaning phase of bathing. The hair should squeak as it is rinsed. Vinegar, lemon, or bleaching rinses are not recommended, except for special problems. However, a small amount of dog or cat coat conditioner or oil can be added to water for the last rinse and adds gloss to the coat. Flea dips may also be necessary in some cases and usually can be mixed with the conditioner.

The coat should be squeezed to eliminate water and the dog wrapped in a towel and lifted from the tub to a table. All animals should be protected from chilling and hypothermia during a bath and for several hours afterward, until thoroughly dry. Short-coated dogs can be toweled almost dry and then lightly brushed and kept confined or calm until dry.

Dogs with medium-length and long coats may be blotted with towels until only damp and then brushed. Alternatively, they may be placed in a stream of warm air and the coat can be combed, brushed, and fluffed as needed to accomplish the desired effect.

The frequency of a grooming routine depends on the breed and the individual animal's needs. In normal dogs not getting dirty, the bathing may be as infrequent as every few months. Dogs prone to normal dog odor that is noticeable to the client may require much more frequent bathing, as often as weekly. If normal dogs are bathed frequently, once monthly or more frequently, conditioners or oil rinses are advisable. The frequency of bathing needed in dogs with skin disease is generally much greater than that in normal dogs.

Dry baths are sometimes used to avoid the drying influence of water baths, especially in dogs with long coats. Talc, boric acid powder, or special products available at pet stores are dusted into the coat and then thoroughly brushed out. With careful application, the coat is left relatively clean and lustrous. However, dry baths are good for only a quick cosmetic cleanup. Powder cleaners are actually inefficient; they dry the coat and increase its static electricity. They should not be used for routine cleaning, as they do not replace bathing. Shampoo and water baths are still the most effective way to clean the coat thoroughly.

Grooming Needs of Individual Coat Types

For grooming purposes, dogs' coats can be divided into five types: the long coat, the silky coat, the nonshedding curly coat, the smooth coat, and the wiry coat.[4] Special grooming greatly enhances the appearance of each dog, but it must have a good natural coat and good conformation for the best effect. The ability to grow a coat depends largely on inherited factors.

Long Coat

Typical breeds include Newfoundlands, German shepherds, collies, Old English sheepdogs, Siberian huskies, Samoyeds, and Welsh corgis. Necessary implements for grooming them include a rake, a bristle or wire brush, and regular and fine Resco combs. A rake should be used to remove dead hair. The coat should be combed and brushed forward over the top and sides and backward over the flanks. A fine comb is necessary for the hair under the chin and the tail and behind the ears.

Silky Coat

Typical breeds include spaniels, Afghan hounds, Maltese and Yorkshire terriers, setters, Lhasa apsos, and Pekingese. Necessary implements include wire brushes; medium and fine steel combs; bristle brushes; Oster clipper with blades Nos. 7, 10, and 15; Duplex stripping knife; and barber scissors. Although all long coats need frequent regular brushing, silky coats in addition require fairly frequent bathing to prevent mats and skin irritation. It may be necessary to use oils or conditioners to keep the hair soft and lubricated and to prevent snarls and hair breakage. Dry hair tends to respond to static electricity by matting. To brush out these coats, the hair can be lifted with the hand and combed or brushed down until it is free from snarls to the level of the skin. Spaniels grow two or three coats per year and should be stripped or clipped about every 3 months.

Nonshedding Curly or Woolly Coat

Typical breeds include Poodles, Bedlington terriers, and Kerry blue terriers. Necessary implements include Oster clipper with blades Nos. 7A, 10, and 15; natural bristle brush; fine, medium, and coarse steel combs; and scissors. The three breeds listed above are usually clipped every 4 to 8 weeks for best appearance, although some owners may wish to allow the haircoat to be kept long. The puppies should be exposed to grooming from 8 weeks of age so that they accept the clippers. The first clip should be when the dog is between 8 and 12 weeks of age, when just the face, feet, and tail are shaved. Scissors should be used cautiously under the tail, as that skin is tender and easily irritated by clippers. A soothing lotion, such as Vaseline Intensive Care lotion and Nivea Creme, should be applied to areas of possible abrasion.

Because dead and loose hairs from these coats are mostly secondary hairs that become enmeshed in the coat, neglect causes a felt matting. All dead hair must be completely combed out before bathing. Therefore, routine care of this group includes daily to at least weekly use of combs and wire brushes or carders to prevent mats.

Smooth Coat

Typical breeds include the hounds, the retrievers, dachshunds, Dalmatians, beagles, whippets, Doberman pinschers, smooth terriers, and boxers. Necessary implements include only a hound glove or a rubber hound brush and scissors. The scissors are used to trim off the tactile hairs on the face or to shape the fringes on the tail, the ears, and the brisket. The coat can be rubbed to shiny sleekness using the hound glove or towels. This also removes dead hairs.

Wiry Coat

Typical breeds include wire-haired Fox terriers, Welsh terriers, Airedale terriers, Lakeland terriers, Schnauzers, and Sealyham terriers. Necessary implements include the Oster clipper blades Nos. 7, 10, and 15; a Duplex stripping knife; a slicker brush; fine and medium steel combs; a hound glove; and barber scissors. Pups of these breeds should be started on a grooming routine at 4 months of age by trimming the head, the ears, and the tail. As adults, they require machine clipping every 6 to 8 weeks or hand stripping about every 12 weeks.

There are some groomers, showers, and breeders of wiry-coated dogs that believe clippers should *never* be used on the body of animals being shown, because it softens the coat by removing the coarse guard hairs.[173] Supposedly, the change may be permanent, and dogs such as Miniature Schnauzers may be ruined for future showing.[173] Hand stripping should be done only when the coat is ready. New hair should not be stripped, except to keep the dog tidy. The fingers can best be used to pluck excessive hair from the vicinity of the eyes.

Corded Coat

The Komondor and the Puli, two Hungarian breeds, have a corded coat. Necessary implements are few. Only mild shampoo, diluted 10:1 with water before application (so it can be rinsed out easily); a heavy-duty water spray; and a heavy-duty dryer are required. Dogs with corded coats should *never* be clipped or combed. They are rarely washed or groomed in any way. These dogs have a thick double coat that forms naturally into tassel-like cords described as ''controlled matting.'' Sometimes, puppies' coats must be teased with a comb to encourage the formation of even cording. The cording is usually complete when the dogs are 1 to 2 years old, and the adult coat does not shed. Pulis may be shown corded or with the coat brushed out. Komondors are shown only corded. If the coats become dirty, bathing can be done carefully. One should always use dilute shampoo. It is squeezed into the coat—not brushed or rubbed vigorously. The animal is thoroughly rinsed with large volumes of warm water sprayed into the coat with pressure to lift and float out the dirt and shampoo. Thorough rinsing is essential. The coat is not rubbed dry with towels or combs but is dried with warm air blowers. It is best to handle these coats like a good wool sweater. Water is squeezed out by hand, and the coat is allowed to drip dry. This takes a long time. Nothing ruins these coats faster than grooming. Dogs with corded coats should always be referred to knowledgeable professional groomers or handlers for proper coat care; it should not be done by the owner.

Special Grooming Problems

Mats can usually be teased apart and combed out if they are small. Small mats behind the ears and under the legs can be cut off. Larger mats can be slit with a scissors, a knife, or a mat and tangle splitter and then teased apart with one or two teeth of a comb. Some badly neglected long-coated cats or dogs may have an almost complete covering of felt matting. The only solution to some of these unfortunate cases is general anesthesia and complete, close clipping. Extreme care is necessary to avoid cutting or irritating the skin. Sometimes, the teeth of a comb can be slipped between the mat and the skin to serve as a shield so that the mat can be safely scissored away.

Tar or paint embedded in the coat may be difficult to remove. Small deposits should be allowed to harden and then cut off. Tar masses can be soaked in vegetable oil or an emollient oil with a surfactant for 24 hours (and bandaged if needed) to soften the tar, and then the entire mass can be washed out with soap and water. One should *never* use paint removers or organic solvents such as kerosene, turpentine, and gasoline to remove tar or paint. They are irritating and toxic and may produce severe caustic burns. Ether may be used carefully for small areas. Clipping the tar or paint-coated hair is often the simplest procedure if the cosmetic appearance is not paramount.

Odors about a coat usually originate from places such as the mouth, the ears, the feet, and the perineum. These areas should be checked and washed carefully. Most detergents remove the typical odors that dogs pick up. In many cases, the odor is an indication of skin disease (often, superficial bacterial pyoderma or *Malassezia* dermatitis) that may not be noted by the owner. In other cases, excessive lipid accumulation is present and degreasing agents such as benzoyl peroxide and tar may be useful. A variety of commercial rinses may be applied, or the coat may be rinsed with a dilute chlorophyll solution or dilute sodium hypochlorite (in a white animal only). Highly scented dressings and sprays are objectionable to many people and do not reliably mask odors. The odor of skunks can be greatly ameliorated with bathing with soap and water and rinsing with a dilute ammonia-water solution (5 to 10 ml [1 to 2 tsp] of household ammonia in 1 L [1 qt] of water). A tomato juice soak is effective but messy. After the dog dries, the odor is gone, but when wet, the hair may have a faint skunk scent for several weeks.

Rarely, dogs are presented for severe *body odor* that seems to emanate from their entire body. Physical examination fails to reveal any visible abnormalities. Typically, these dogs' malodor responds transiently (24 hours) to a variety of shampoos and rinses. The authors have had the best results with long-term once-daily antibiotic therapy with lincomycin, erythromycin, or cephalosporins. Some dogs respond better with twice-weekly vinegar-water (equal parts of each) rinses, but the faint odor of vinegar disturbs some owners. The cause of this condition is unknown, and it is lifelong.

Clipping is beneficial when topical treatment will be used. Clipping permits thorough cleaning, adequate skin contact, and a more economical application of the desired medicament. In many cases, complete removal of the coat may be preferred, but usually, clipping the local area suffices. This should be done neatly to avoid disfigurement. If the hair over the involved area is clipped closely (against the grain with a No. 40 clipper), while a border around this is clipped less closely (with the grain), the regrowth of hair more quickly blends the area into the normal coat pattern.

Clipping should always be discussed with the owner to obtain approval. This contact is especially important when treating show animals or those with long coats, such as Yorkshire terriers, Old English sheepdogs, and Afghan hounds. The corded breeds such as Pulis and Komondors take years to regrow clipped cords; therefore, clipping should be avoided unless absolutely necessary. All needless clipping should be avoided. During clipping, a vacuum cleaner can be used to remove all loose hair and debris. Shampoo therapy may be an acceptable alternative to clipping in some cases. It may remove surface lipids and clean the skin and hair enough that topical dips are able to be effectively applied to the skin surface. In other cases, the desired active ingredients may be incorporated into the shampoo formulation.

Comments on Grooming Cats

In general, the grooming implements used for dogs serve adequately for cats. However, special applications are outlined here. There is absolutely no substitute for routine daily grooming or for grooming every second or third day. Cats detest bathing and dematting and can be most resentful of rough treatment. Even when cats are petted, many of them slip away afterward to rearrange their haircoat thoroughly by licking and grooming themselves.

GROOMING NEEDS OF VARIOUS COAT TYPES

From the grooming standpoint, cats have three types of coats—the shorthaired, single coat; the shorthaired, double coat; and the long coat.

The shorthaired, single coat is typified by Siamese, Burmese, Havana brown, Rex, Korat, and domestic shorthair cats. These cats can be bathed in shampoo and water, quickly dried to avoid chilling, and brushed and combed against the coat to remove dead hair. Final brushing is with the hair. A fine metal comb and natural boar bristle brush are the only implements needed.

The shorthaired, double coat is typified by Abyssinian, Manx, Russian blue, and American shorthair cats. The double coat is composed of two sets of hair. The long guard hair gives the coat its color, and the dense, short undercoat provides warmth. Both sets of hair are essential in these breeds. The basic coat care of this group is similar to that used for single coats, except that caution must be employed because overgrooming can destroy the coat. Loss of the long guard hairs may give the coat a patchy or moth-eaten appearance.

The longhaired coat is typified by Persians and Himalayans. Several sizes of metal combs and a boar bristle brush are necessary for grooming these breeds. The kittens should be started with grooming at 4 weeks of age.

Older kittens and adults can be bathed with mild shampoo and water. They can be placed on a slanted window screen in a tub. Cats feel secure on the wire and stay put, yet water passes through easily. They are rinsed well and dried quickly with a towel and warm air blower. This fluffs the coat and gives it body. One should not bathe cats frequently and not within 2 weeks preceding a show. Cats almost never require bathing.

Mats tend to form behind the ears and under the chin, the legs, and the tail. The skin under the mat becomes irritated. Mats can be prevented by daily combing and brushing.

Some breeders dry-clean the coats with powder or talc sprinkled into the coat and carefully brushed out with a motion up and away from the body. This is rarely a satisfactory grooming method. If powder is left in the hair, it resembles unsightly dandruff and is highly objectionable.

The ruff or tail of a long-haired cat is never clipped. The eyes and nasal area should be cleaned to remove exudates that may accumulate.

SPECIAL FELINE GROOMING PROBLEMS

A cat's claws should be clipped only if necessary. They soon grow out again and are honed sharply.

Cats' ears are much less prone to infection than are dogs' ears, but they should always be checked and cleaned if needed. Young cats are especially predisposed to ear mite infections.

The large supracaudal organ on the dorsal surface of the tail is a mass of hyperactive sebaceous glands that may cause trouble if neglected. Breeders call the problem *stud tail*, although it occurs in both sexes. A waxy, unsightly accumulation builds up in the area if proper hygiene is neglected. The exudate can be removed by applying powder to soak it up, by applying a thin oil to soften it, or by sponging the area with alcohol or detergents as solvents. The oil can usually be brushed or washed off with shampoos satisfactorily. Periodic cleaning should prevent any future problem.

■ TOPICAL THERAPY

Topical therapy has always played a large role in dermatology because of the obvious access to the affected tissue.[9, 113, 173, 228, 230a, 231] In the past, topical therapy was used for treating localized lesions and ectoparasite infestations. In the last 10 years, topical applications have become even more prominent in treating skin disease. Undoubtedly, this growth in topical therapy reflects multiple factors, which may include (1) the development of more products, better delivery systems, and active ingredients; (2) the reduction in systemic absorption or effects and adverse reactions; and (3) the recognition of the adjunctive and synergistic effects in the overall management of numerous skin diseases. These factors are also the advantages that topical therapy offers to the clinician and the pet owner.

There are disadvantages, however. In general, topical therapy is much more time consuming and labor-intensive than is systemic therapy. Understanding the proper use and application of topical therapy is also important, and therefore, client education and client compliance become harder to achieve. Localized adverse reactions not seen with systemic therapy may occur, most commonly irritant reactions. Topical therapy is often adjunctive, and it may significantly increase the cost of the overall therapeutic plan. Some topical agents may be so costly that their use is limited to localized lesions. On the other hand, appropriate topical therapy may greatly reduce the need for systemic therapy. The clinician needs to consider the potential benefits and disadvantages, the client's preferences, and the patient's needs when deciding on the use of topical therapy.

When a clinician elects to use topical therapy, several factors must be considered. First and foremost is, what is the purpose or desired result of the topical therapy? Is this the sole therapy, or is it adjunctive to other nontopical therapies? What type of delivery system best facilitates obtaining the desired result? What active ingredients are used for this purpose? And, as previously discussed, patient and client considerations are paramount. Table 3:2 lists the most common delivery systems and formulations of active ingredients used in veterinary dermatology. The amount of use for each type of product relative to the others is based solely on the authors' opinions and clinical impressions.

Factors That Influence Drug Effects on the Skin

Topical medications consist of active ingredients incorporated in a vehicle that facilitates application to the skin. In selecting a vehicle, one must consider the solubility of the drug in the vehicle, the rate of release from the vehicle, the ability of the vehicle to hydrate the stratum corneum, the stability of the active agent in the vehicle, and the interactions (chemical and physical) among the vehicle, the active agent, and the stratum corneum. The vehicle is not always inert, and many have important therapeutic effect.

When topical medications are used, one basic question is whether the drug penetrates the skin and, if so, how deeply. Absorption is highly variable, and most drugs penetrate only 1 to 2 per cent after 16 to 24 hours.[72] However, even in the same vehicle, similar drugs may vary dramatically in their absorption.[69] This was exemplified in a study with three organophosphate

Table 3:2. Topical Formulations and Relative Efficacy of Incorporated Active Agents

Topical Formulations	Astringent	Emollient	Anti-seborrheic	Anti-pruritic	Anti-bacterial	Anti-mycotic	Anti-parasitic	Anti-inflammatory	Ultraviolet Screen
Shampoo	X	XX	XXXX	XX	XXX	X	XX	X	—
Rinse	X	XXXX	—	XX	X	XXX	XXXX	X	—
Powder	—	—	—	X	X	?	X	X	—
Lotion	XXX	X	X	XXX	XX	XX	—	XXX	X
Spray	XX	XXX	XX	XXX	X	X	XXX	XX	X
Cream or ointment	—	X	X	XX	XXX	X	—	XXX	XXXX
Gels	—	—	X	—	XX	X	—	—	—

*Relative use based on authors' opinions and clinical impressions: — = not used; X = infrequently used or use associated with lower efficacy; XX = occasionally used; XXX = commonly used and tend to be efficacious; and XXXX = preferred formulation for that class of active ingredients.

insecticides applied topically in three different vehicles.[92] With only one organophosphate (parathion) of the three tested, the vehicle dimethyl sulfoxide (DMSO) increased absorption from 4 to 5 per cent up to 15 to 30 per cent. In some cases (e.g., insecticides), the absorbability greatly influences the potential for side effects.

Clinical efficacy and absorption are not synonymous; absorption is only one factor in efficacy. Some drugs in an insoluble form in the vehicle have only a surface effect. Absorption of drugs through the skin involves many variables. There are physiochemical factors related to the topical formulation and biological factors.[9] The physiochemical factors involve the interactions between the drug and the vehicle, the drug and the skin, and the vehicle and the skin. Some of these factors are determined by the concentration of the drug, the drug's movement between the vehicle and the skin, and the diffusion coefficient.

1. The concentration of the drug and its solubility in the vehicle affects absorption. The package label gives the percentage of drug concentration, not the percentage of solubility. In addition to concentration, the solubility of the drug and the solubilizing capacity of the vehicle affect drug absorption. In general, poor solubility and excessive solubilizing capacity decrease the rate of absorption.[9] Usually, ointment vehicles for topical corticosteroids increase solubility and drug delivery, so systemic effects after topical use are more common—and potentially dangerous.
2. The drug must move from the vehicle through the skin barrier to be effective. The solubility of the drug in the horny layer relative to its solubility in the vehicle is described by the partition coefficient. The concentration of the drug in the barrier, not in the vehicle, is what determines the diffusion force. Increased lipid solubility favors drug penetration, because the stratum corneum is lipophilic.
3. The *diffusion coefficient* is a measure of the extent to which the barrier interferes with the drug's mobility. The stratum corneum is unsurpassed as an unfavorable environment for drug penetration. Physical disruption of the epidermal barrier by the use of lipid solvents, keratolytic agents, or cellulose tape stripping of the top layers of cells increases the potential for absorption. DMSO facilitates cutaneous penetration of some substances. Moisture and occlusive dressings enhance percutaneous absorption as well. Large molecular size results in poor mobility and poor absorption.

Temperature and hydration of the skin can affect the interaction among the drug, the vehicle, and the skin. Hydration probably plays a greater role than temperature in affecting absorption. In general, permeability to drugs increases as the hydration of the stratum corneum increases.[9]

Biological factors also affect drug absorption. The body region treated greatly influences absorption. In humans, tremendous variation was shown, with the amount of hydrocortisone being absorbed varying, in descending order, on the scrotum, the forehead, the forearm, and the plantar foot.[72] Age is an important factor, with newborns having greater absorption than adolescents, who have greater absorption than adults. Obviously, the health and condition of the skin is important, as inflamed, abraded, or otherwise damaged skin often absorbs more drug. Blood flow also affects absorption. Greater blood flow favors increased systemic absorption.

Hydrotherapy

Water is often overlooked as a therapeutic agent, especially when it is applied with a shampoo, as a rinse, or as a component of many lotions. Hydrotherapy may be used to moisten the stratum corneum, to dry out the epidermis, to cool or heat the skin, to soften surface crusts, and to clean the skin. Increased effects occur by adding other agents (see Topical Active Ingredients in this chapter).

Water may be applied as a wet dressing or in baths. Frequent periodic renewal of wet dressings (15 minutes on, several hours off) prolongs the effect; but if more continuous therapy or occlusive coverings are used, the skin becomes overly moistened, the skin temperature rises, and undesirable maceration occurs. This is less likely to happen if the wet dressings are left open.

Hydrotherapy can hydrate or dehydrate the skin, depending on how it is managed. The application of loose, damp gauze compresses for 15 minutes and then removal for 1 hour promote evaporation of water from the gauze and from the subadjacent skin surface and are drying to the underlying tissues. If water is maintained on the skin surface constantly by wet towels, soaks, or baths, the skin hydrates as water is taken up by keratin and hair. If a film of oil is applied immediately after soaking (occlusive rinses), evaporation of water (transpiration) is hindered and the skin retains moisture.

The water may be cool or above body temperature. Whirlpool baths, with or without detergents and antiseptics added, make gentle, effective cleaning possible. These treatments may be used to remove crusts and scales, to clean wounds and fistulae, to rehydrate skin, to reduce pain and pruritus, and to provide prophylaxis for patients prone to decubital problems, urine scalds, and other ills. Ten to 15 minutes of therapy once or twice daily is adequate. The patients should be toweled and placed in an air stream drier to dry. Other topical medications can be applied later, if needed.

In hydrotherapy, moisture is the specific agent, and various additives change its actions only slightly, but add their own effects. Astringents, antipruritics, moisturizers, parasiticides, and antibiotics are common additives. In general, water treatment removes crusts, bacteria, and other debris and greatly reduces the possibility of secondary infection. It promotes epithelialization and allays the symptoms of pain and burning. Cool water is antipruritic. It also softens keratin. The suppleness and softness of the skin are due to its water content, not to the oils on the surface.[173] Dryness of the skin is recognized when any one of the following is present: roughness of the surface, scaliness, inflexibility of the horny layer, and fissuring with possible inflammation.

Normal skin is not a waterproof covering but is constantly losing water to the environment by transpiration (Fig. 3:2 *A*). This loss depends on body temperature, environmental temperature, and relative humidity. The stratum corneum, composed of corneocytes and an intercellular matrix lipid bilayer, is the major deterrent to water loss. The lipids of this layer are derived from phospholipids and lipids secreted by the keratinocytes as they migrate to the stratum corneum and from sebum. Dry skin may result from excessive transpiration of water (Fig. 3:2 *B*).

Sebum on the skin or externally applied lipid films tend to make the surface feel smoother. The flexibility of keratin is directly related to its moisture content. The amount of water that the horny layer receives from the epidermis and the transepidermal loss are major factors determining moisture content. The transepidermal loss from the stratum corneum partially depends on the environment, especially the relative humidity. Water content of the horny layer can be increased by applying occlusive dressings or agents to prevent loss (Fig. 3:2 *D*), by adding water with baths or wet dressings (Fig. 3:2 *C*), or by using hygroscopic medications to attract water.

Topical Formulations

Active medications may be applied to the skin by a variety of delivery systems. These different delivery systems include, but are not limited to, the following formulations: shampoos; rinses; powders; lotions; sprays; creams, emulsions, and ointments; and gels. Each type of formulation has advantages and disadvantages that the clinician should consider when selecting a topical medication. Besides incorporating active ingredients, each type of formulation contains ingredients that act as the vehicle for delivering the active agents. These vehicles may also have certain therapeutic, irritant, or cosmetic effects, making the overall formulation more or less desirable. In general, vehicles contain ingredients to adjust the pH, to stabilize the active agents,

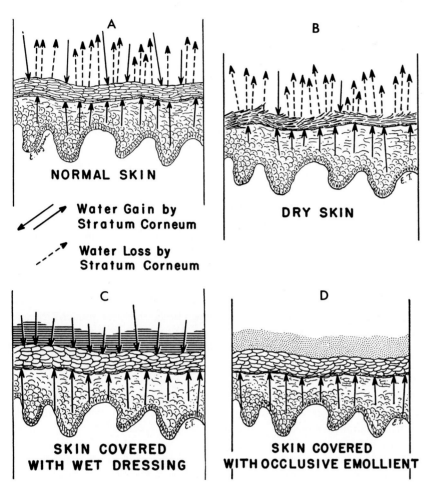

Figure 3:2. *A*, Water exchange through the stratum corneum of normal skin in equilibrium with the environment. Water is being received from the underlying tissues and from the environment. In addition, water is being lost to the environment, and there is a net transfer from the underlying tissues to the environment. *B*, Water exchange through the stratum corneum of skin that has been transferred from a high to a low environmental humidity. The water loss to the environment is temporarily increased and that received from the environment is decreased. The stratum corneum becomes dehydrated, because the amount of water it can receive from the underlying tissues is limited. *C*, Water exchange through the stratum corneum when the skin is covered with a wet dressing. The stratum corneum hydrates, because water is being received both from the underlying tissues and the external water. *D*, Water exchange through the stratum corneum when the skin is covered with an occlusive emollient. The stratum corneum hydrates, because water is being received from the underlying tissues and water loss to the environment is prevented. (From Frazier, E. N., Blank, I. H.: A Formulary for External Therapy of the Skin. Charles C Thomas, Springfield, IL, 1954.)

to prolong the effects of the active ingredients, to promote the delivery of the active agents to the skin surface or into or through the stratum corneum, and to make the product cosmetically pleasing (e.g., fragrance). The selection of the topical formulation depends on a variety of factors, most notably, the surface area to be treated, the need for residual activity, the presence of hair in the area to be treated, and the nature of lesion (e.g., moist or dry).

The active ingredients are often available in a variety of different formulations and delivery systems. In general, they have the same basic activity regardless of the formulation, but their ease of use, cost, and efficacy for the desired purpose are affected by the formulation and the method of application. The following categories of active agents are used: astringents, or drying agents; emollients and moisturizers; antiseborrheics; antipruritics; antibacterials; antifungals; antiparasitics; anti-inflammatory agents; and ultraviolet screens. The discussion describes first the different delivery systems and then the types of active ingredients.

SHAMPOOS

Medicated shampoos contain additional ingredients that enhance or add other actions to that of the shampoo. The active drugs have a limited contact time because they are removed during the rinsing of the shampoo base. Some medicaments may have enough opportunity for effect or for limited absorption during a prolonged shampoo, and their addition may be justified (e.g., insecticides, salicylic acid, sulfur, tar, and antiseptics). Medicated shampoos are valuable in that they may be used for diseases involving large areas of the body or localized lesions.

Efficacy is determined by proper use as well as active ingredients. It is imperative that products be applied properly, left on for sufficient contact time, and then properly rinsed. Education of the client regarding their use is an important element and time well spent. The client should be instructed to use a clock to determine the correct contact time because subjective assessments are often inadequate. Contact time starts after the shampoo is applied, not when the bath begins. More severely affected regions should be the first areas to be shampooed. Sometimes, problem areas benefit from a second lathering before the final rinse.

Pharmaceutical companies provide a multitude of medicated shampoos, which often have specific indications and contraindications. It is important to become familiar with a few (perhaps one of each type) and to understand thoroughly the ingredients and their concentration and actions. Choosing the mildest or most client-pleasing shampoo that produces the desired actions often increases compliance. Strong shampoos can be harmful as well as helpful.

The clinician must evaluate the whole animal when selecting active ingredients, and some animals may benefit from the simultaneous use of different products. Although one shampoo may be recommended for the whole body, another shampoo may be applied to a more localized region. The case of an Irish setter with idiopathic seborrhea with truncal scaling, dry coat, and localized patches of comedones with pyoderma and alopecia on the ventral chest (Fig. 3:3) is an example. A topical antiseborrheic containing sulfur and salicylic acid may be preferred for most of the body, but may not be potent enough for the ventral region. A benzoyl peroxide shampoo may be used on just the ventral thorax because of its superior antibacterial and follicular flushing effect.

Medicated shampoos are often classified on the basis of their primary activity or function.

1. Antiparasitic shampoos are commonly used, but in general, they are *not* as efficacious as antiparasitic rinses. Their main use is for quick removal of fleas in puppies, kittens, and debilitated animals. They are often ineffective for adequate long-term flea control. The most common ingredients are pyrethrins and synthetic pyrethroids.

2. Antiseborrheic shampoos usually contain salicylic acid, sulfur, and tar in various combinations and strengths. Sebbafon, SebaLyt, Sebolux, and Micro Pearls sulfur–salicylic acid shampoos contain sulfur and salicylic acid. LyTar and Allerseb-T contain tar, sulfur, and salicylic acid. Adams sulfur shampoo contains only sulfur in a shampoo vehicle. Nu Sal T contains salicylic acid, and Clear Tar contains only tar.

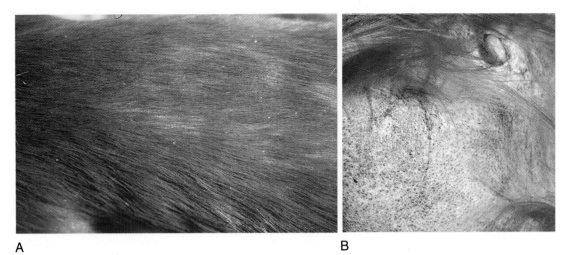

A   B

Figure 3:3. *A.* Irish setter with primary idiopathic seborrhea. There is fine white scaling on the trunk, which would respond well to a sulfur and salicylic acid shampoo. *B.* Ventral thorax has an area of comedones and pyoderma, which would respond better to a benzoyl peroxide shampoo.

    3. Antibacterial shampoos contain disinfectants or antibiotics such as chlorhexidene, benzoyl peroxide, iodine, ethyl lactate, triclosan, and sulfur. One study showed that benzoyl peroxide is a more effective prophylactic agent against *Staphylococcus intermedius* than is chlorhexidene, iodine, or triclosan.[125] Another clinical study showed similar results for treating superficial pyoderma with either benzoyl peroxide or ethyl lactate shampoo. Forty-five per cent of 18 dogs with superficial pyoderma were successfully treated (without other therapy) by bathing, with 10-minute contact time, three times per week.[122] Other ingredients with less effect include quaternary ammonium compounds and phenols (both *not* to be used in cats), alcohols, and parabens.

    4. Antimycotic shampoos are used mainly as adjunctive therapy for dermatophytosis (to achieve a quick decrease of contagion) and *Malassezia* dermatitis. They have been recommended as sole therapy for *Malassezia* dermatitis.[145] However, in the authors' experience, they have limited efficacy and work best as adjunctive therapy or as a preventive to decrease the recurrence rate.

    5. Antipruritic or anti-inflammatory agents, such as 1 per cent hydrocortisone (Cortisoothe), 0.01 per cent fluocinolone (FS shampoo), 2 per cent diphenhydramine (Histacalm), 1 per cent pramoxine (Relief), colloidal oatmeal (Epi-Soothe), and moisturizers (HyLyt* efa and Allergroom), are seen in a variety of shampoo formulations. In general, they are adjunctive treatments and are not effective as the sole therapy unless they are used every 1 to 2 days. This high frequency of use is usually not acceptable to owners.

       The topical fluocinolone shampoos have been shown *not* to be systemically absorbed in the dog.[17, 281] Controlled studies of their efficacy are lacking. In a preliminary open clinical trial, a 0.01 per cent fluocinolone acetonide product caused a beneficial response in 25 per cent of dogs with generalized pruritus.[281] The nonshampoo glucocorticoids offer a residual effect because they are not rinsed and often deliver higher concentrations of active ingredients.

    For localized or regional applications, many topical formulations other than shampoos and rinses may be used.

RINSES

Rinses are made by mixing concentrated solutions or soluble powders with water. They are usually poured, sponged, or sprayed onto the animal's body. Similar to the case with shampoos, they may be used to treat large areas of the body. Rinses are generally a cost-effective and efficacious method to deliver topical active ingredients such as moisturizers, antipruritic agents, parasiticides, and antifungal agents.

Rinses that dry on the pet's skin leave a residual layer of active ingredients and therefore have more prolonged effects than application by shampoo therapy. Rinses are often used after a medicated or cleaning shampoo. If the active ingredient to be applied is lipid dispersed, shampooing may remove the normal surface lipids and decrease the longevity of the active ingredients. In these situations, adding a small amount of safflower oil or lipid-containing moisturizer may help to prolong the effect. This is most commonly recommended for lipid-soluble (petroleum distillate–based) parasiticidal agents.

Rinses are the authors' preferred method of delivery for most topical medications, other than antibacterials and antiseborrheics, that require whole-body coverage.

POWDERS

Powders are pulverized organic or inorganic solids that are applied to the skin in a thin film. In some cases, they are made to be added to water for use as a rinse, to liquids to form "shake lotions," or to ointments to form pastes. Some powders (talc, starch, zinc oxide) are inert and have a physical effect; other powders (sulfur) are active ingredients that have a chemical or antimicrobial effect. Powders are used to dry the skin and to cool and lubricate intertriginous areas. Most often, powders are used with parasiticidal agents (flea powders) and locally with anti-inflammatory agents (Neo-Predef powder). Some powders may contain antimicrobials for use on localized lesions and, although not yet available in the United States, an enilconazole powder has shown promise for the treatment of dermatophytosis.

The affected skin should be cleaned and dried before the powder is applied. Powder build-up or caking should be avoided, but if it occurs, wet compresses or soaks can gently remove the excess. On long-coated animals, a fine powder is used as a retention vehicle for insecticides and fungicides. Powders dry the coat and skin and may accumulate in the environment, making them less desirable for whole-body use. Some owners find powders irritating to their own respiratory mucosa. The authors use powders infrequently and prefer other delivery systems.

LOTIONS

Lotions are liquids in which medicinal agents are dissolved or suspended. Some are essentially liquid powders, because when the liquid evaporates, a thin film of powder is left on the skin. Lotions tend to be more drying (because of their water or alcohol base) than liniments, which have an oily base. Newer lotions tend to use more propylene glycol and water with less or no alcohol. Drying, cooling lotions contain alcohol, whereas soothing, moisturizing lotions usually do not. These medications tend to be cooling, antipruritic, and drying (depending on the base).

Lotions are vehicles for active ingredients such as sulfur (Adams sulfur lotion), 1 per cent hydrocortisone with aluminum acetate (Hydro-B 1020 [Butler], Hydro-Plus [Phoenix]), 0.1 per cent betamethasone valerate (Valisone), 1 per cent pramoxine (Relief), 1 per cent diphenhydramine with calamine and camphor (Caladryl), malaleuca, and aloe vera. The liquid preparations can be applied repeatedly, but they should not be allowed to build up. In general, lotions are indicated for acute oozing dermatoses and are contraindicated in dry, chronic conditions. They are most often used to deliver localized treatment with astringents and antipruritic, anti-inflammatory, and antifungal agents. They occasionally carry ultraviolet screens and antiseborrheic agents.

SPRAYS

A variety of topical lotions are available in pump spray bottles. Most commonly, they are used when relatively larger body areas are to be treated and when the product needs to be applied to only the haircoat or small, nonhaired areas. Rinses may also be applied by pump spray bottles, but if skin contact is needed, thorough soaking through the haircoat is required. Sprays are most commonly used with emollients or moisturizers that are lightly applied and then rubbed into the coat, antiparasitic agents (particularly those with repellent activity), and antipruritic agents for local lesions.

Antipruritic sprays contain agents such as 1 per cent hydrocortisone (Cortispray), 2 per cent diphenhydramine (Histacalm), 1 per cent pramoxine, *Hamamelis* extract with menthol (Dermacool), and tar (LyTar). Sprays are also frequently used to apply astringents and anti-inflammatory agents, such as 1 per cent hydrocortisone with aluminum acetate. Occasionally, sprays are used for antifungal agents and the application of ultraviolet screens to the inguinal region. Sprays are valuable for local application to interdigital webs, ventral paws, and concave pinnae.

CREAMS, EMULSIONS, AND OINTMENTS

Creams and ointments lubricate and smooth skin that is roughened. They form a protective covering that reduces contact with the environment, and certain occlusive types may reduce water loss. They also transport medicinal agents into follicular orifices and keep drugs in intimate contact with the horny layer. Creams and ointments are mixtures of grease or oil and water that are emulsified with high-speed blenders. Emulsifiers, coloring agents, and perfumes are added to improve the physical characteristics of the product. Pastes are highly viscous ointments into which large amounts of powder are incorporated. Although pastes may be tolerated on slightly exudative skin (the powder takes up water), in general, creams and ointments are contraindicated in oozing areas.

A wide variation in characteristics of the products is determined by the relative amount and melting point of the oils used. This can be illustrated by comparing cold cream and vanishing cream. Cold cream is mostly oil with a little water. The oils have a low melting point, so when the water evaporates a thick, greasy film is left on the skin. A vanishing cream, on the other hand, is mostly water with oils that have a high melting point. When the water evaporates, a thin film of fat is left on the skin. This waxlike film does not feel greasy. Urea added to creams also decreases the greasy feel and, as a hygroscopic agent, helps to moisturize the stratum corneum.

Emulsions are oily or fatty substances that have been dispersed in water. As a group, they have a composition between that of lotions and ointments. Emulsions are thicker than lotions but thinner than ointments. They are similar to creams, which for the most part, have replaced their use in small animal practice. Emulsions are of two types: oil dispersed in water, and water dispersed in oil. Although both types are used as vehicles, the former dilutes with water, loses water rapidly, and therefore is cooling. The latter type dilutes with oil and loses its water slowly. In both cases, after the water evaporates, the action of the vehicle on the skin is no different from that of the oil and emulsifying agent alone. Thus, the characteristics of the residual film are those of the oily phase of the vehicle.

These bases are commonly used as vehicles for other agents. They have the advantage of easy application, give mechanical protection, and are soothing, antipruritic, and softening. The more oily creams and ointments tend to be occlusive, which facilitates hydration of the stratum corneum and often increases penetration of incorporated active ingredients. The disadvantage of their use in the hairy skin of animals is that they are occlusive, greasy, heat-retaining, and messy, and also may produce a folliculitis because of occlusion of pilosebaceous orifices. These types of medication should be applied with gentle massage several times daily to maintain a thin film on the skin. Thick films are wasteful, occlusive, and messy to surroundings. An obvious film of ointment left on the skin surface means that too much has been applied.

Water-washable ointment bases such as polyethylene glycol (Carbowax 1500) can be readily removed with water. Oily bases are not freely water washable. It is important for the clinician to understand the uses and advantages of these types of bases because the total effect on the skin is caused by the vehicle as well as its active ingredient.

Hydrophobic oils (e.g., mineral oil and sesame oil) mix poorly with water. They contain few polar groups (—OH, —COOH, and so on). These oils contact the skin, spread easily, and are often incorporated into emulsion-type vehicles. Because they are hydrophobic, it is difficult for water to pass through a film of these oils, and they are occlusive. They retain heat and water, and thick films of the more viscid forms are messy and may get on articles in contact with the pet.

Hydrophilic oils are miscible with water. They contain many polar groups, and those oils with the greatest number are most soluble in water. Although they are ointments only in regard to their physical characteristics, the polyethylene glycols are alcohols that are readily miscible with water. Polymers with a molecular weight greater than 1000 are solid at room temperature, but a slight rise in body temperature causes melting to form an oily film. (Carbowax 1500 is such a product.) It mixes with skin exudates well, is easily washed off with water, and is less occlusive than other bases.

The use of creams, emulsions, and ointments is limited to localized, relatively small lesions. Most commonly, they are used with antimicrobial, anti-inflammatory, and ultraviolet radiation–blocking agents. For areas needing moisturization or keratolytic effects, they are often the most efficacious delivery system, but their application is usually limited to localized areas such as nasal planum, paws, and elbows.

GELS

Gels are topical formulations composed of combinations of propylene glycol, propylene gallate, disodiumethylenediamine tetraacetate, and carboxypolymethylene, with additives to adjust the pH. They act as a clear, colorless, thixotropic base and are greaseless and water miscible. The active ingredients incorporated in commercially used bases of this type are completely in solution.

Gels are being more widely used, because despite their oily appearance, they can be rubbed into the skin completely and do not leave the skin with a sticky feeling. Gels are relatively preferable to creams and ointments because they pass through the haircoat to the skin and are not messy. Most commonly, they are used for localized lesions for which antimicrobial or antiseborrheic effects are desired.

The most common ingredient is benzoyl peroxide for areas of bacterial pyoderma and follicular hyperkeratosis (such as acne) or areas of comedones. (Examples of gels used in veterinary medicine with benzoyl peroxide are OxyDex and Pyoben.) However, because they are cosmetically tolerated better than creams and ointments, their use is expanding to include virtually any ingredient that can be stabilized in a gel form. KeraSolv is a keratolytic, humectant gel for hyperkeratotic conditions such as nasal hyperkeratosis.

Topical Active Agents

ASTRINGENTS

Astringents precipitate proteins and, in general, do not penetrate deeply. These agents are drying and decrease exudations. They are indicated in acute, subacute, and some chronic exudative dermatoses.

Vegetable astringents include tannins from oak trees, sumac, or blackberries; they are especially recommended for more potent action. Tan Sal (5 per cent tannic acid and 5 per cent salicylic acid, in 70 per cent alcohol) is a potent astringent and should not be used more than once on the same lesion (it may cause irritation or sloughing).

Aluminum acetate solution (Burow's solution) is available commercially as Domeboro. It is drying, astringent, antipruritic, and mildly antiseptic. The solution is usually diluted 1:40 in cool water, and soaks are repeated three times daily for 30 minutes. (One packet of powder, or one tablet, is added to 0.5 L [1 pt] or 1 L [1 qt] of water.) It is tolerated better than tannins and does not stain. It tends to be used more frequently than other astringents.

Silver nitrate 0.25 per cent solution may be applied to moist, weeping, denuded areas as an antiseptic, coagulant, and stimulating agent. It should be used frequently and sparingly. It stains the skin.

Potassium permanganate 1:1000 to 1:30,000 solution (1-grain tablet or 5 ml [1 tsp] to 15 ml [1 tbsp] of crystals per 1 L [1 qt] of water) may be applied in fresh preparations for soaks or irrigations. It is astringent, antiseptic, and antimicrobial and toughens and stains the skin.

EMOLLIENTS AND MOISTURIZERS

Emollients are agents that soften or soothe the skin; *moisturizers* increase the water content of the stratum corneum. Both types of drugs are useful in hydrating and softening the skin.

Many of the occlusive emollients are actually oils (safflower, sesame, and mineral oil) or contain lanolin listed below. These emollients decrease transepidermal water loss and cause moisturization. These agents work best if applied immediately after saturation of the stratum corneum with water. For maximal softening, the skin should be hydrated in wet dressings, dried, and covered with an occlusive hydrophobic oil. The barrier to water loss can be further strengthened by covering the local lesion with plastic wrap under a bandage. Nonocclusive emollients are relatively ineffective in retaining moisture.

1. Vegetable oils—olive, cottonseed, corn, and peanut oil
2. Animal oils—lard, whale oil, anhydrous lanolin (wool fat), and lanolin with 25 to 30 per cent water (hydrous wool fat)
3. Hydrocarbons—paraffin and petrolatum (mineral oil)
4. Waxes—white wax (bleached beeswax), yellow wax (beeswax), and spermaceti

Hygroscopic agents are moisturizers that work by being incorporated into the stratum corneum and attracting water. These agents, such as propylene glycol, glycerin, colloidal oatmeal, urea, sodium lactate, and lactic acid, may also be applied between baths. Both occlusive and hygroscopic agents are found in a variety of veterinary spray and rinse formulations, which are more effective than shampoo bases. A liposome-based humectant technology (Micro Pearls cream rinse) was shown to be superior to a traditional humectant emollient (Humilac) for the treatment of dry skin in dogs.[240]

ANTISEBORRHEICS

The seborrheic complex comprises important and somewhat common skin diseases, such as primary seborrhea (in Cocker and Springer spaniels, Irish setters, and Doberman pinschers), secondary seborrhea (accompanying atopy, scabies, and demodicosis), Schnauzer comedo syndrome, and tail gland hyperplasia.[124] Topical antiseborrheic therapy is the primary mode of treatment for these diseases. Other primary scaling disorders such as sebaceous adenitis, vitamin A–responsive dermatosis, and some follicular dysplasias may benefit from adjunctive therapy with antiseborrheics, which speed the response to the primary treatment.

Antiseborrheics can be applied as ointments, creams, gels, and lotions, but the most popular form for hairy skin is the antiseborrheic shampoo or the humectant rinse. Antiseborrheics are commercially available in various combinations. The clinician must decide which combination of drugs to use and needs to know each drug's actions and concentrations. Ideal therapeutic response depends on the correct choice, but individual patient variation does occur. For dry and scaly seborrhea (seborrhea sicca), a different preparation is needed than for oily and greasy seborrhea (seborrhea oleosa). Sulfur, for instance, is useful in dry seborrhea but is not a good degreaser. Benzoyl peroxide, on the other hand, degreases well but can be too keratolytic and drying for dry, brittle skin. The following discussion may help the clinician to understand the differences and uses and to help distinguish the correct medication from among the myriad of commercially available pharmaceuticals.

Antiseborrheic drugs include keratolytics and keratoplastics. Keratolytic agents facilitate decreased cohesion among corneocytes, desquamation, and shedding, resulting in a softer stratum corneum and removal of scale. They do not dissolve keratin. Keratoplastic agents improve the keratinization and abnormal epithelialization that is present in keratinization disorders. The complete mechanism of these effects is not known, although some keratoplastic agents (particularly tar) are believed to normalize epidermal proliferation by decreasing deoxyribonucleic acid (DNA) production with a resultant decrease in the mitotic index of the epidermal basal cells. Follicular flushing is a term used to describe agents that help to remove follicular secretions, to remove bacteria, and to decrease follicular hyperkeratosis.

The most common ingredients in antiseborrheic products include tars, sulfur, salicylic acid, benzoyl peroxide, and selenium sulfide. They are usually applied in shampoo formulations. Other less commonly used ingredients are reserved for localized lesions or specialized situations. These ingredients, urea, lactic acid at high concentration, 3 per cent or greater concentration of salicylic acid, dioctyl sodium sulfosuccinate, and tretinoin, are usually found in lotions, gels, and creams.

Sulfur is both keratoplastic and keratolytic. Sulfur is also antibacterial, antifungal, antiparasitic, and antipruritic; is a mild follicular flushing agent; but is *not* a good degreaser. It is available in ointments in concentrations from 2 to 10 per cent. Its most popular form is in shampoos, such as Adams sulfur shampoo, SebaLyt, Sebolux, and Micro Pearls sulfur–salicylic acid shampoo. It is also mixed with tar in products such as LyTar and Allerseb-T. The smaller the sulfur particles are (colloidal are smaller than precipitated), the greater is the efficacy. The best keratolytic action occurs when sulfur is incorporated in petrolatum. This is in sharp contrast to the findings with salicylic acid, which produces its effect faster when employed in an emulsion base.

The keratolytic effect of sulfur results from its superficial effect on the horny layer and the formation of hydrogen sulfide. The keratoplastic effect is caused by the deeper action of the sulfur on the basal layer of the epidermis and by the formation of cystine. Shampoo formulations with 0.5 to 2 per cent sulfur are most commonly prescribed in scaly disorders and some superficial bacterial pyodermas. Ten per cent precipitated sulfur in lotions or ointments may intensify epidermal peeling and is useful for locally seborrheic and intertriginous dermatoses. Sulfur rinses (2 to 5 per cent) may be used effectively for fungal and some parasitic infections. The antibacterial, antifungal, and antiparasitic effects of sulfur have been attributed to the formation of pentathionic acid and hydrogen sulfide.

Salicylic acid (0.1 to 2 per cent) is keratoplastic and exerts a favorable influence on the new formation of the keratinous layer. It is also mildly antipruritic and bacteriostatic. It is a common ingredient in most of the antiseborrheic shampoos previously listed. In stronger concentrations (3 to 6 per cent), it acts as a keratolytic agent (Keralyt 6 per cent), causing shedding and softening of the stratum corneum. When salicylic acid is combined with sulfur, it is believed that a synergistic effect occurs. A common combination is a 2 to 6 per cent concentration of each drug. In human dermatologic practice, a 40 per cent salicylic acid plaster is used to treat calluses and warts.

Tar preparations are derived from destructive distillation of bituminous coal or wool. Birch tar, juniper tar, and coal tar are crude products listed in order of increasing capacity to irritate. Coal tar solution (5, 10, or 20 per cent) produces a milder, more readily managed effect. Coal tar solution contains only 20 per cent of the coal tar present in coal tar extract or refined tar. Most pharmaceutical preparations for dermatologic use have been highly refined to decrease the staining effect and the strong odor. In this refining process, some of the beneficial effects of tar are lost, and its potential carcinogenic danger is also decreased. Unadulterated tar lotions have no place in small animal practice because of their toxicity and tendency to cause local irritation. Cats are especially sensitive to coal tar. All tars are odiferous, potentially irritating and photosensitizing, and carcinogenic. Some tars may stain light-colored coats. In one of the author's (DWS) experience, tars are the most irritating topical antiseborrheic medications in veterinary dermatology, and he does not use tar-containing topical preparations.

Tar shampoos are widely used, however, and seem to be helpful in managing seborrhea. They are keratolytic, keratoplastic, and mildly degreasing. They include LyTar, Mycodex tar and sulfur, and Allerseb-T.

Popular veterinary ointments that make use of some of the principles just listed include those containing cetyl alcohol, coal tar, and sulfur as well as salicylic acid in an emulsion base (Pragmatar), sulfur ointment, ichthammol ointment, zinc oxide, and thuja.

Benzoyl peroxide (2.5 to 5 per cent) is keratolytic, antibacterial, degreasing, antipruritic, and follicular flushing. It is metabolized in the skin to benzoic acid, which lyses intercellular substance in the horny layer to account for its keratolytic effect. It is available as a 5 per cent gel (OxyDex and Pyoben) and as a 2.5 to 3 per cent shampoo (OxyDex, Pyoben, and Micro Pearls benzoyl peroxide shampoo). It is not a stable ingredient and should not be repackaged, diluted, or mixed with other products. Additionally, reputable brands should be used, as poor products have short shelf lives, little activity, or increased irritation potential. Because of its potent degreasing action, benzoyl peroxide excessively dries out normal skin with prolonged use, and it is generally contraindicated in the presence of dry skin.[230] A study showed that benzoyl peroxide combined with a liposome-based humectant technology (Micro Pearls benzoyl peroxide shampoo) eliminates or minimizes this drying effect.[241] Other side effects of 2.5 to 3 per cent benzoyl peroxide include contact dermatitis (less than 10 per cent of patients) and bleaching of hair and clothing. It has skin tumor–promoting activity in laboratory rodents, but no skin tumor–initiating activity has been documented in any other species.[241]

ANTIPRURITICS

Antipruritic agents attempt to provide temporary relief of itching but are not usually satisfactory as sole therapy because of their short duration of effect. As adjunctive therapy or for small localized areas of pruritus, they can be more beneficial. Some antipruritic agents listed here have other actions and are discussed elsewhere in this chapter. Table 3:3 lists some veterinary nonsteroidal, topical, antipruritic agents. In general, antipruritics give relief from itching by means of five methods:

1. Decreasing the pruritic load by depleting, removing, or inactivating pruritic mediators. For example, astringents denature proteins and high-potency corticosteroids deplete cutaneous mast cells. Shampoos or cleaners can also remove surface irritants, bacteria, pruritogenic substances, and allergens that are on the surface of the skin waiting to be absorbed and to contribute to the pruritic load.
2. Substituting some other sensation, such as heat and cold, for the itch. This may also help by raising the pruritic threshold. Heat initially lowers the pruritic threshold, but if the heat is high enough and is applied for a sufficient duration, the increased itching or burning sensation abates and induces a short-term antipruritic effect. Cooling tends to decrease pruritus. Examples of such agents are menthol 0.12 to 1 per cent, camphor 0.12 to 5 per cent, thymol 0.5 to 1 per cent, heat (warm soaks or baths), and cold (ice packs) or cool wet dressings.
3. Protecting the skin from external influences such as scratching, biting, trauma, temperature changes, humidity changes, pressure, and irritants. This can be done with bandages or any impermeable protective agents.
4. Anesthetizing the peripheral nerves by using local anesthetics such as benzocaine, tetracaine, lidocaine, benzoyl peroxide, and tars. These products generally have short actions, and in cases of chronic pruritus, resistance often occurs.

Table 3:3. Useful Nonsteroidal Topical Agents for Pruritic Dogs and Cats

Product	Active Ingredients or Action	Form	Manufacturer
Spot Application			
Caladryl	1% diphenhydramine hydrochloride, 8% calamine, camphor	Lotion	Parke-Davis
Dermacool	*Hamamelis* extract, menthol	Spray	Allerderm/Virbac
Domeboro	Aluminum sulfate, calcium acetate	Soak	Miles
Histacalm	2% diphenhydramine	Spray	Allerderm/Virbac
Ice	Water-cold	Pack	Nature!
PTD lotion	2% benzyl alcohol, 0.05% benzalkonium chloride, *Hamamelis* distillate	Lotion	Veterinary Prescription
Relief	1% pramoxine	Spray, lotion	DVM
Total Body Application			
Allergroom	Moisturizing, hypoallergenic	Shampoo	Allerderm/Virbac
HyLyt*efa	Moisturizing, hypoallergenic	Shampoo	DVM
Epi-Soothe	Colloidal oatmeal	Shampoo	Allerderm/Virbac
Histacalm	2% diphenhydramine	Shampoo	Allerderm/Virbac
Micro Pearls cream rinse	Humectant, hypoallergenic	Rinse	EVSCO
HyLyt*efa	Moisturizing, hypoallergenic	Rinse	DVM
Water	Water	Soak	Nature!
Aveeno	Colloidal oatmeal	Soak	Rydelle
Epi-Soothe	Colloidal oatmeal	Soak	Allerderm/Virbac
Relief	1% pramoxine	Shampoo, rinse	DVM

5. Using specific biochemical agents, such as topical glucocorticoids, antihistamines, and moisturizers.

Most potent glucocorticoids, administered systemically and topically, are helpful, because of their anti-inflammatory effect, but they are not without risk (see p. 206). Hydrocortisone 0.5 to 2 per cent is safest for topical use and could be considered an antipruritic agent because, at these concentrations, it has mild anti-inflammatory effects. The fluorinated corticosteroids are more potent and penetrate better but with greater risk of systemic absorption and both local or systemic adverse effects. Antihistamines administered systemically are occasionally useful, but when applied topically, they have even less efficacy. They may be helpful as a component of a combination product, such as 1 per cent diphenhydramine with calamine and camphor (Caladryl). Some topical antihistamines were shown to cross the stratum corneum and may exert their antihistaminic effect after topical application.[21, 104] Topical anesthetics may be partially effective, but they may be toxic (causing methemoglobinemia) or have sensitizing potentials (phenol 0.5 per cent; tetracaine and lidocaine 0.5 per cent).[45a, 295] Also, their duration of effect is short and becomes even less when used frequently and repetitively. Veterinary products with these types of agents are Histacalm shampoo (2 per cent diphenhydramine), Histacalm spray (2 per cent diphenhydramine), Relief shampoo, spray, rinse, and lotion (1 per cent pramoxine), and Dermacool (*Hamamelis* extract and menthol).

Cool wet dressings are often helpful, and in general, any volatile agent provides a cooling sensation that might be palliative. This is the basis for using menthol (1 per cent), thymol (1 per cent), and alcohol (70 per cent) in antipruritic medications. In addition, menthol has a specific action on local sensory nerve endings. Cool water baths alone or accompanied by Burow's solution (aluminum acetate) soaks (Domeboro) or colloidal oatmeal (Aveeno and Epi-Soothe) may be helpful for hours to days.

ANTIMICROBIAL AGENTS

No group of drugs is employed more widely than are antimicrobial agents. The terminology used to describe the actions of drugs on microbes is somewhat confusing because of discrepancies between strict definitions of terms and their general usage. *Antiseptics* are substances that kill or prevent growth of microbes (the term is used especially for preparations applied to living tissue). *Disinfectants* are agents that prevent infection by destruction of microbes (the term is used especially for substances applied to inanimate objects). Antiseptics and disinfectants are types of *germicides*, which are agents that destroy microbes. Germicides may be further defined by the appropriate use of terms such as *bactericide, fungicide,* and *virucide.*

In a discussion of such heterogeneous compounds as antimicrobials, some method of classification is desirable. Because the compounds are so varied with respect to chemical structure, mechanism of action, and use, too strict a classification may be more confusing than elucidating. The following discussion is a compromise.

The antiseptic agents are listed with brief comments so that their purposes can be appreciated when they are recognized as ingredients in proprietary formulations. The use of some of these agents is described elsewhere in the text.

■ *Alcohols.*   These act by precipitating proteins and dehydrating protoplasm. They are bactericidal (not sporicidal), astringent, cooling, and rubefacient. However, they are irritating to denuded surfaces and are generally contraindicated in acute inflammatory disorders. Seventy per cent ethyl alcohol and 70 to 90 per cent isopropyl alcohol are the most effective concentrations and are bactericidal within 1 to 2 minutes at 30°C.

■ *Propylene Glycol.*   This is a fairly active antibacterial and antifungal agent. A 40 to 50 per cent concentration is best. It and polyethylene glycol are primarily used at concentrations of less than 50 per cent as vehicles for other powerful antimicrobial agents. In dilute solution, propylene glycol has few humectant properties because it is hygroscopic. In a 60 to 75 per cent solution, it denatures and solubizes protein and is keratolytic.

■ *Phenols and Cresols.*   Agents such as hexachlorophene, resorcinol, hexylresorcinol, thymol, and picric acid act by denaturing microbial proteins. They are also antipruritic and somewhat antifungal. They may be added at low levels as preservatives in some products. At higher antimicrobial levels, they are irritating, are toxic (hexachlorophene),[190a] and currently have few legitimate uses on the skin. Phenols and cresols are contraindicated in cats.

■ *Chlorhexidine.*   Chlorhexidine is a phenol-related biguanide antiseptic and disinfectant that has excellent properties: it is *highly effective* against many fungi, viruses, and most bacteria, except perhaps some *Pseudomonas* and *Serratia* strains. It appears that a 1 per cent concentration of chlorhexidine is needed for a good anti-*Malassezia* effect. It is nonirritating, rarely sensitizing, not inactivated by organic matter, and persistent in action; and it is effective in shampoo, ointment, surgical scrub, and solution formulations containing 0.5 to 2 per cent concentrations of chlorhexidine diacetate or gluconate. A 0.05 per cent dilution in water is an effective, nonirritating solution for wound irrigation. This agent is safe for cats.

■ *Halogenated Agents*

■ *Iodine.*   This is one of the oldest antimicrobials. Elemental iodine is the active agent (its mechanism is unknown). It is rapidly bactericidal, fungicidal, virucidal, and sporicidal. Older products such as tincture of iodine (2 per cent iodine and 2 per cent sodium iodide in alcohol) and Lugol's iodine solution (5 to 7 per cent iodine and 10 per cent potassium iodide in water) are irritating and sensitizing, especially in cats, and should no longer be used.

Currently the only commonly used iodines are the ''tamed'' iodines (iodophors) because of their lower level of irritation or sensitization. Povidone-iodine (Betadine)—iodine with polyvinylpyrrolidone, which slowly releases iodine to tissues—has a prolonged action (4 to 6 hours), is nonstinging and nonstaining, and is not impaired by blood, serum, necrotic debris, or pus. A study using a povidine-iodine shampoo showed efficacy, although less than that of benzoyl peroxide as a prophylactic agent against *S. intermedius*.[125] A newer tamed iodine, polyhydroxydine (Xenodine) at 1 per cent, is reportedly superior in efficacy against gram-positive and gram-negative organisms to povidine-iodine solutions or tincture of iodine. Even tamed iodines can be drying to the skin, staining to light-colored haircoats, and especially irritating to scrotal skin and the external ear.

■ *Sodium Hypochlorite and Chloramines.*   These are effective bactericidal, fungicidal, sporicidal, and virucidal agents. Their action is thought to be due to liberation of hypochlorous acid. Fresh preparations are needed. Sodium hypochlorite 5.25 per cent (Clorox) diluted with water 1:10 (modified Dakin's solution) is usually well tolerated. The presence of organic material greatly reduces the solution's antimicrobial activity. It is most often recommended as an antifungal agent or disinfectant. It can be irritating to cats.

■ *Oxidizing Agents.*   Hydrogen peroxide is a weak germicide that acts through the liberation of nascent oxygen (e.g., 3 per cent hydrogen peroxide used in dilute water solution). It has limited usefulness for skin disease, although it is used as an ear-flushing agent and for cleaning minor skin wounds, partly for its effervescent activity.

Potassium permanganate acts as a bactericidal, astringent, and fungicidal agent (especially against *Candida* spp.). Its action is thought to involve liberation of nascent oxygen. This agent stings and stains, and it is inhibited by organic material. The staining is particularly a problem.

Benzoyl peroxide is a potent, broad-spectrum antibacterial agent that has keratolytic, antipruritic, degreasing, and follicular flushing action.[230, 241] It is a potent oxidizing agent, which reacts with biological materials. The resultant benzoyl peroxy radicals interact with hydroxy and sulfoxy groups, double bonds, and other substances. This allows the benzoyl peroxide to disrupt microbial cell membranes. It is irritating in fewer than 10 per cent of the animals treated.

Benzoyl peroxide is available as a 5 per cent gel and a 2.5 or 3 per cent shampoo (OxyDex, SulfOxydex, Pyoben, and Micro Pearls benzoyl peroxide shampoo), which is an excellent adjunct to antibiotic therapy for superficial and deep bacterial pyodermas. In a shampoo formulation, it was superior to chlorhexidine, complexed iodine, and triclosan for prophylaxis against *S. intermedius*.[125] It is often recommended in seborrheic disorders, particularly cases that are greasy or have follicular plugs, follicular casts, or comedones.

One should not use generic or more concentrated formulations (e.g., 5 per cent shampoo or 10 per cent gel) on animals, as stability may be compromised and the higher concentrations are more often irritating. Even at 2.5 or 3 per cent concentrations, it is drying and occasionally irritating, especially in dogs with allergic skin disease. Repackaging should not be done, as improper packaging may affect stability of the product. A commercial benzoyl peroxide shampoo containing liposome-based humectant technology (Micro Pearls benzoyl peroxide shampoo) can be used even on dogs with dry skin without exacerbating the dryness.[241]

■ *Surface-Acting Agents.*   These agents in the form of emulsifiers, wetting agents, or detergents act by altering energy relationships at interfaces, thus disrupting or damaging cell membranes. They also denature proteins and inactivate enzymes. The most commonly used examples are the cationic detergents (quaternary ammonium compounds), especially benzalkonium chloride (Zephiran chloride). Benzalkonium chloride is a broad-spectrum antibacterial agent (not effective against *Pseudomonas* spp.). However, anionic soaps inactivate it, and it is toxic to cats, producing skin and muscle necrosis.[231]

Silver salts precipitate proteins and interfere with bacterial metabolic activities. They are antibacterial and astringent but irritating, staining, stinging, and escharotic (e.g., silver nitrate 0.5 per cent). Silver sulfadiazine is useful to treat superficial burns. At 1 per cent concentration, it was effective, and superior to sodium hypochlorite, for the treatment of experimentally induced *Pseudomonas* spp. otitis externa.[277]

■ *Ethyl Lactate.* Ten per cent ethyl lactate is an excellent antibacterial agent that is well tolerated.[91a] Being very liposoluble, it rapidly penetrates hair follicles and sebaceous glands, where it is hydrolyzed by bacterial lipases to form lactic acid and ethanol. The lactic acid and ethanol kill bacteria, and the ethanol is degreasing and comedolytic. Ethyl lactate has recently been released in the United States (Etiderm [Allerderm/Virbac]).

■ *Sulfur.* The bacteriostatic factor in sulfur is thought to be pentathionic acid. Sulfur is used in a 1 to 10 per cent concentration. It is also an effective fungicide and parasiticide, which are its major uses.

■ *Antibiotics.* Many potent antibacterial agents are available in topical form. The most commonly used are mupirocin, neomycin, gentamicin, bacitracin, polymyxin B, gramicidin, nitrofurazone, and thiostrepton. Important considerations for some of these agents are as follows: (1) mupirocin is not systemically absorbed, but is still more effective than other topical agents for penetrating and treating deeper bacterial pyodermas, and it has poor activity against gram-negative infections; (2) neomycin has more potential for allergic sensitization than do most topicals, and sensitivity is variable for gram-negative organisms; (3) polymyxin B and bacitracin in combination may be effective for gram-negative as well as gram-positive organisms; however, they are rapidly inactivated by purulent exudates and do not penetrate well; and (4) nitrofurans may be sensitizing, and plasma and blood inhibit their action.

Often, topical antibiotics are formulated with other ingredients, most commonly glucocorticoids. There are numerous antibiotic-steroid combinations (Gentocin spray, Neo-Aristovet, Neo-Synalar, Neo-Polycin-HC, Tresaderm, and Panalog). These are occasionally indicated in chronic, dry, lichenified, secondarily infected dermatoses (seborrhea complex and allergic dermatoses) and pyotraumatic dermatitis and are commonly indicated in otitis externa. Several clinical and bacteriologic trials in humans showed that these antibiotic-steroid combinations were superior to either agent alone. However, there is some evidence that, in canine bacterial otitis externa, this clinical improvement does not always correlate with negative cultures.[151]

ANTIMYCOTIC AGENTS

Local therapy of dermatophytoses in dogs and cats is not always effective.[171] The heavy haircoat and the organisms' habitat deep in the hair follicle often make contact with topical agents incomplete. Topical agents tend to be more effective in short-coated animals, for localized alopecic lesions, or in long-haired animals that have been clipped. Clipping the hair and using liquid, low surface tension vehicles are helpful in obtaining more penetration. Some patients have thick keratin scales, and keratolytic agents may promote good contact.

Powder vehicles are of little value with the older active agents, although work with newer agents is encouraging. Creams, emulsions, and ointments are useful on only glabrous areas. Iodine solutions are fungicidal but may be highly irritating (especially in cats) if used repeatedly, and they stain coats. Iodochlorhydroxyquin in a cream form (Vioform), however, is a nonirritating form of iodine. Sodium hypochlorite solution (5.25 per cent stock solution) can be diluted to 1:10 and used safely on all animals; commercial lime sulfur solutions diluted to 2 per cent are also effective. Chlorhexidine is an excellent antifungal agent and is available as a solution, ointment, and shampoo. Tolnaftate, which is effective on the glabrous skin of humans, is not effective on the hairy skin of dogs and cats.

Dermatophyte infections may be self-limited and heal spontaneously, thus making some treatments appear efficacious. Even dogs with generalized dermatophytosis may experience self-cure as shown by a study in which three of five dogs improved with an inert oral treatment.[149] This small study concluded that, if a significant improvement is not seen within 4 weeks of diagnosis, topical, and possibly parenteral, treatment should be begun. A different situation exists in cats, particularly in long-haired cats, in cats with generalized disease, or in multiple-cat households. Topical treatment should be started immediately.[68, 149]

The following is a concensus of the authors regarding current effective topical antifungals. The most common active antimycotic agents found in creams, emulsions, ointments, or lotions for localized use include haloprogin (Halotex), econazole nitrate (Spectazole), miconazole nitrate (Micatin and Conofite), clotrimazole (Lotrimin and Veltrim), and ketoconazole (Nizoral). Nystatin suspension, amphotericin B suspension or cream, clotrimazole, econazole, and miconazole are useful for *Candida* infections. Nystatin is effective against yeast only (e.g., Panalog ointment and Nystatin cream). Thiabendazole (Tresaderm) is effective for dermatophytes and some *Malassezia*. Topical enilconazole has been highly successful in the treatment of canine nasal aspergillosis and, in some parts of the world, is labeled for veterinary use in dermatophytosis (see Chap. 5).[113, 254]

To use for generalized cases, to decrease contagion, and to treat animals with undetected lesions or asymptomatic carriers, shampoos and rinses are most commonly used. In these cases, the active agents generally employed include povidine-iodine, chlorhexidine, lime sulfur, sodium hypochlorite, miconazole, and ketoconazole. A study evaluated the ability of the following solutions to kill dermatophyte-infected hair when used as a rinse twice weekly: chlorhexidine 25 ml/L, lime sulfur 30 ml/L, povidone-iodine 42 ml/L, sodium hypochlorite 50 ml/L, and enilconazole 20 ml/L.[294] A shampoo formulation containing ketoconazole, which was rinsed off, was also tested. Lime sulfur and enilconazole rinses killed the fungus in 1 week, and chlorhexidine and povidine-iodine solutions in 2 weeks. Ketoconazole shampoo and sodium hypochlorite needed 4 weeks of use before killing the fungus. Doubling the concentration did not increase the speed of killing the fungus. Captan did *not* kill the fungus.

ANTIPARASITIC AGENTS

Numerous products are available for use on dogs and cats, and this aspect of topical therapy is the subject of much research owing to the tremendous economic potential.[140] As a result, product formulations rapidly change. The demand for less toxic, more environmentally safe, and more efficacious products has produced not just new formulations but many new active agents as well. The active ingredients are primarily incorporated into rinses, shampoos, sprays, and powders. They are designed for use against fleas on animals, in the environment, or both. Some ingredients are incorporated into creams, lotions, ointments, and even roll-on or wipe-on (mousse or lotion) formulations.

This group of active ingredients has also generated much research into newer, innovative methods of delivery. This is exemplified by the development of focal treatment sources that disperse throughout the coat (supposedly related to lipid solubility), as is seen with some flea collars and products for spot liquid application. Examples are Ex-Spot and Defend, wherein the topical application of the vehicle and active agent (permethrin) in one to two spots disperses to give total body coverage.

Other developments such as microencapsulation and photostabilization are directed at increasing residual activity. Microencapsulation of most insecticides prolongs their effective action from 1 day to 4 weeks or longer. This process suspends the insecticide in microcapsules that are inactive while suspended in liquid. When sprayed onto a surface, they become active as they dry and small amounts of insecticide keep moving up to the surface of the capsules. Only the surface layer is exposed to ultraviolet light and the environment. Oral intake does not appear to break down the capsules. Some microcapsules may also adhere to the exoskeleton of parasites that contact them. The insecticide is then absorbed through the parasite's chitin with toxic effect. These features impart several excellent qualities to these types of product. They have lower oral and cutaneous median lethal doses, with increased residual activity in killing parasites. Their biggest disadvantage is generally a lower percentage of kills, which may be erratic during the residual period depending on environmental factors.[114] Also, these products do not have any quick-kill or knockdown power unless mixed with some active solution. Some insecticide products provide a mix of microencapsulated pyrethrins and natural pyrethrins for quick knockdown and prolonged effect (Sectrol).

Many antiparasitic agents would be highly toxic if applied in a vehicle that promoted absorption, or in a form that enabled the animal to ingest quantities by licking the medication. Cats are especially prone to licking habits and are particularly susceptible to toxic reactions with chlorinated hydrocarbons and organophosphate products.

It is critical that clinicians prescribe topical and environmental antiparasitic agents within the bounds of label indications. Most insecticides are registered by the U.S. Environmental Protection Agency (EPA), and extralabel use, either for the species treated or in the concentration, method, or frequency of application, is illegal. Failure to follow label indications is not condoned or allowed, and the practitioner is not protected by the argument that it is a standard acceptable practice. These products are not regulated by the U.S. Food and Drug Administration (FDA). Many of these products, if improperly used, pose environmental dangers. Even the disposal of insecticidal products is facing regulation, and it is possible that, as a profession, veterinarians will be severely limited in their ability to use or prescribe, or may be required to be licensed to use, these agents to ensure that safe practices are followed.

Topical antiparasitic therapy is primarily directed against ectoparasites that feed or live on dogs and cats. When treating parasitic dermatosis, it is critical that the parasite; its life cycle, epidemiology, and natural behavior; and the pathogenesis of the disease that it is causing be considered. Topical therapy may be just one aspect of an overall treatment plant or the sole therapy prescribed.[74] Proper application becomes critical if it is the sole therapy. Specific protocols or treatment for diseases attributable to each parasite are described in Chapter 6. This discussion is an overview of active agents that are incorporated into various delivery systems and formulations.

■ *Sulfur.*   With the emphasis on newer, more effective drugs, it is sometimes forgotten that sulfur and its derivatives are excellent and safe parasiticides. The commercial lime sulfur solution (LymDyp) is safe for dogs and cats and is an inexpensive, effective treatment of infestations of several types of mites, as well as being fungicidal, bactericidal, keratolytic, and antipruritic. Adams sulfur lotion and 10 per cent sulfur ointment USP are other forms of sulfur medications. Sulfur is a natural parasiticide that is relatively nontoxic and environmentally safe.

In general, sulfur shampoo is *not* an effective antiparasitic agent. Its major drawback is the foul odor. It also stains jewelry and temporarily discolors hair, especially white hair. It is drying, but only rarely irritating when used at a 2 per cent concentration. (A 2 to 5 per cent lime sulfur solution is effective against *Sarcoptes, Notoedres, Cheyletiella,* chiggers, fur mites, and lice.) Contrary to common belief, sulfur is *not* an effective flea repellent, either topically or systemically. Sulfur is most commonly used as an antiparasitic agent for the treatment of canine and feline scabies and cheyletiellosis.

■ *Pyrethrin.*   This agent is a volatile oil extract of the chrysanthemum flower. It contains six active pyrethrins that are contact poisons and have a fast knockdown action and flushing action on insects, but no residual activity. It is rapidly inactivated by ultraviolet light. Pyrethrins, because of their low toxicity, rapid inactivation, and lack of tissue residue and build-up, are relatively environmentally safe, although still toxic to fish and bees. For clients concerned with chemicals, the use of pyrethrins may be more acceptable, as this is an organic natural insecticide.

There is no cholinesterase suppression. Pyrethrin demonstrates a rapid kill but low toxicity, and the low concentration of 0.06 to 0.4 per cent is effective *if* synergized with 0.1 to 2 per cent piperonyl butoxide, which forms a stable complex with cytochrome P450, thus limiting the metabolism of pyrethrins in insects.[70a] Cats may develop central nervous system (CNS) signs in response to piperonyl butoxide, but otherwise toxicity is low. Pyrethrins are effective against fleas, *Otodectes*, flies, lice, and mosquitos. Effective use for fleas usually necessitates daily application as a spray or a rinse unless microencapsulators or ultraviolet light stabilizers are added to the formulation. Such products include Sectrol and Adams flea and tick 14 day mist.

■ *Rotenone.*   This natural organic compound is derived from the root of the *Derris* plant. It is similar to pyrethrins in having low toxicity, rapid action, and quick degradation. It is available mixed with pyrethrin for use as a rinse or a shampoo for dogs and cats (Durakyl) and is used in some products that are safe for puppies and kittens.

■ *Pyrethroids.*   These synthesized chemicals are modeled after pyrethrin and include D-trans-allethrin, resmethrin, tetramethrin, D-phenothin, fenvalerate, and permethrin.[70a] In action and toxicity, they are relatively comparable, although not identical, to pyrethrin. They produce a quick kill that is improved by the addition of a synergist and pyrethrin. Some of the early pyrethroids degrade on exposure to ultraviolet light, so there is little or no residual activity. Some pyrethroids are relatively photostable compared with pyrethrin.

One of the most popular pyrethroid agents is permethrin, which is found in numerous products with a wide variety of delivery systems. Part of permethrin's desirability is its low toxicity (except in cats, so only limited low-concentration formulas are approved in this species), relative stability on exposure to ultraviolet light, and potential for use as a repellent. As with pyrethrins, the synthetic pyrethroids are often combined with other active agents, particularly repellents.

■ *Chlorinated Hydrocarbons.*   These dangerous insecticides have become outdated and re-placed by safer products. They persist in the environment and animal tissue for long times (for years, in some cases). Representatives of this group are dichlorodiphenyltrichloroethane (DDT), lindane, chlordane, dieldrin, and methoxychlor. This class of compounds is tightly restricted or their use is prohibited. There is no indication for their use in dogs and cats, as safer alternatives exist.

■ *Cholinesterase Inhibitors.*   Two kinds of cholinesterase inhibitors are available, carbamates and organophosphates. They were once the mainstay of insect control. However, with the advent of safer products and better alternative treatment regimens, their use on pets is decreas-ing. They are still valuable for environmental treatment in cases of infestation of fleas and other insects or arachnids.

■ *Carbamates.*   These products are typified by carbaryl (Sevin) and are safe for dogs and cats in 3 to 5 per cent concentrations in powders (Diryl) and 0.5 to 2 per cent concentrations in sprays and dips. Carbaryl should be avoided on pets with white hair, as long-term use may turn the coat golden yellow. Although lower concentrations may be used on kittens and puppies older than 6 weeks, it is probably safer to use only pyrethrin until these animals are several months old.

A flea colony bred from a newly collected strain of Florida fleas was compared with commercially available fleas (which had been reared away from the natural environment for the past 20 years) in susceptibility to insecticides. The Florida fleas were more tolerant to bendiocarb (Ficam), malathion, and carbaryl as compared with the strain raised commercially.[55] This more susceptible commercial strain was most commonly used for flea product efficacy tests in the past.

Bendiocarb is a carbamate used by exterminators for premises flea control. Propoxur (Sendran) is relatively insoluble in water, but it is used in collars and powders because of its rapid knockdown and reasonable residual effect.

■ *Organophosphates.* The most toxic insecticides in use are organophosphates. They are potent cholinesterase inhibitors, and a cumulative effect may be seen if animals are exposed to similar insecticides in another preparation or in lawn and garden applications. None of this group should be used on kittens, and most are also dangerous to adult cats. Malathion is different in some respects from the rest of the group. It provides a quick insect knockdown, and it can be used carefully on adult cats. The main use of this class is for fleas and ticks. They are generally effective for *Cheyletiella* and lice, but are not routinely effective for treating scabies. Some of the commonly used organophosphates are the following:

1. Chlorfenvinphos (Supona and Dermaton) is used for fleas and ticks or premises sprays. It is not a good scabicide.
2. Chlorpyrifos (Dursban) is still popular for sprays and dips for fleas on dogs, as well as environmental treatment. Fleas are especially sensitive to even low levels of chlorpyrifos.[55] It is used by commercial exterminators and has been microencapsulated for a long residual effect (Duratrol). Chlorpyrifos has the advantage, compared with most organophosphates, in having a relatively high median lethal dose, which, coupled with the low concentrations effective in flea killing, allows a good margin of safety.
3. Diazinon is popular for premises use for fleas and ticks. It has a long residual effect, and insects do not easily become resistant. It is available in powder, liquid, and microencapsulated forms.
4. Dichlorvos (Vapona) has been used in fly strips and flea collars. It has fast knockdown but little residual action.
5. Phosmet (Paramite dip) is used for flea control on mature dogs and cats. It is not a reliable scabicide.

■ *Insect Growth Regulators (IGRs).* These are natural chemicals in insects that control early stages of their metabolism, morphogenesis, and reproduction.[70a] Final maturation and pupation of flea larvae proceed only in the presence of appropriate levels or absence of the IGR for that stage of larval growth. Methoprene (Precor) and fenoxycarb are the two currently available topical agents with biochemical activities that mimic those of the natural IGR. Application of methoprene or fenoxycarb to the premises by spray or fogger prevents maturation of pupal fleas if they are exposed to it. Methoprene is sensitive to ultraviolet light, so that it has little value outdoors. Another problem with both products is the difficulty in delivering the product deep into rugs, cracks, and recessed places where the larvae are developing.

Additionally, IGRs do not affect the adult flea, so that results are delayed for several weeks. This is corrected by simultaneous spraying or mixing with insecticides that kill adult fleas. The finding that makes these IGRs attractive for topical therapy is their effect on eggs. Because many or most flea eggs are laid on the pet, a topical formulation with residual activity may expose the eggs to the IGR left on the pet's coat. It is now known that both methoprene and fenoxycarb, if applied to newly laid eggs, cause death and failure of the eggs to hatch. Because eradication of the flea eggs is a major and previously poorly accomplished component of flea control, these products offer an excellent opportunity to attack this stage of the life cycle. Newer IGRs offer promise in that affected adult fleas lay eggs that cannot develop normally. Currently, these are primarily systemic drugs.

■ *Formamidines.* These newly formulated acaricidal agents act by inhibition of monoamine oxidase. Amitraz (Mitaban), the veterinary form, is available as a rinse and as a collar for tick control. The amitraz collar is *not* effective for canine demodicosis. The rinse is effective against

Demodex, Cheyletiella, Otodectes, Sarcoptes, and *Notoedres,* but not against fleas. Its primary use is for canine demodicosis (see Chap. 6). The drug is unstable and rapidly oxidizes on exposure to air or sunlight, so it is important not to use expired product or to divide the contents of a bottle for use on different days. Oxidized product may have increased toxicity.

Its other actions include α-adrenergic agonism and prostaglandin inhibition. Side-effects of treatment often include transient sedation and pruritus, hypothermia, bradycardia, hypotension, and hyperglycemia. The vehicle, xylene, is thought to contribute to toxicity problems.[100, 282] Amitraz dips are used at different strengths and frequencies in various parts of the world. The protocol approved in the United States and Canada is the *least* effective for chronic canine demodicosis (see Chap. 6).

■ *Repellents.* Although these chemicals are capable of keeping insects away, they necessitate frequent application—often, every few hours depending on temperature, humidity, the density of insects, the movement of the animal, and the drying effect of the wind. For control of fleas, some products only need daily or alternate-day application. Spray repellents are the primary form for flea control because large areas must be treated frequently. Compounds with repellent action include pyrethrin, permethrin, diethyltoluamide (DEET), ethohexadiol, dimethyl phthalate, butoxypropylene glycol, MGK-264, and ingredients in Avon's Skin-So-Soft bath oil (some believe the fragrance). Amitraz has been effective in repelling ticks and is available in a tick collar formulation.

ANTI-INFLAMMATORY AGENTS

Cold dressings are among the simplest and safest agents that reduce inflammation. However, topical glucocorticoid preparations are used most commonly and effectively to reduce inflammation. There is little evidence to suggest that they have caused dissemination of cutaneous infections, but if they are used in the presence of known infections, specific antibacterial or antifungal agents should be added to the preparation.

In high concentration, in abraded skin, or under occlusive dressings, these corticosteroids are absorbed. They rarely produce serious untoward clinical effects if used short term. However, Moriello[171a] found that short-term application (7 days) of topical otic products (Panalog and Tresaderm) can adversely affect the adrenocortical response to exogenous corticotropin (adrenocorticotropic hormone [ACTH]). Marked adrenocortical suppression was still present 14 days after therapy was discontinued. These products also produced elevations in routinely monitored liver enzyme test results (e.g., serum alkaline phosphatase and leucine aminotransferase activity). Similarly, Zenoble and Kemppainen[300] reported that the daily application of triamcinolone, fluocinonide, or betamethasone to the skin of normal dogs for 5 days produced suppression of adrenocortical responses to ACTH, which persisted for 3 to 4 weeks after the last application. Finally, Glaze and co-workers[79] reported that daily application of ophthalmic preparations containing glucocorticoids also suppressed adrenocortical responses to ACTH and produced elevations in hepatic enzyme activity in normal dogs. It may be concluded that topical glucocorticoids should not be considered innocuous drugs.[233]

Local effects, including atrophy, scaling, comedones, alopecia, and pyoderma, may occur even without systemic effects (Fig. 3:4). They maintain a pool in the skin, enough that once-daily application may suffice to continue the topical effect. Topical glucocorticoid therapy should follow similar principles as for systemic therapy. That is, the administration of potent drugs should be twice daily to stop inflammation, then tapered to once daily and, finally, if the drugs are still effective and long-term treatment is expected, the treatment is changed to less potent topical agents for maintenance therapy and alternate-day administration is used whenever possible. *People handling these medications should wear gloves to prevent exposure and toxic effects.*

The fluorinated steroids are more potent, penetrate better, and thus are more effective. Table

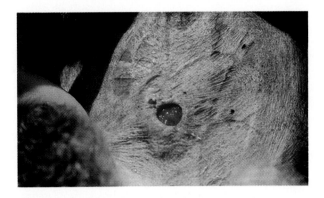

Figure 3:4. Long-term administration of topical glucocorticoids resulted in a thin atrophic epidermis and dermis, comedones, and pyoderma.

3:4 lists therapeutic concentrations of several topical glucocorticoids and provides brand name examples.

MISCELLANEOUS TOPICAL AGENTS

■ *Vitamin A Acid.* A 0.05 per cent concentration of retinoic acid (tretinoin [Retin-A]) is popular in human dermatology (used for treating acne, decreasing wrinkles, and treating

Table 3:4. Relative Anti-Inflammatory Potencies of Selected Topical Glucocorticoids*

Agent	Brand Name	Manufacturer
GROUP I		
Betamethasone dipropionate, 0.05% cream, ointment	Diprolene	Schering
Clobetasol propionate, 0.05% cream, ointment	Temovate	Glaxo Derm
Diflorasone diacetate, 0.05% ointment	Psorcon	Dermik
GROUP II		
Betamethasone dipropionate, 0.05% ointment	Diprosone	Schering
Desoximetasone, 0.25% cream, ointment	Topicort	Hoechst-Roussel
Fluocinonide, 0.05% cream, ointment	Lidex	Dermik
GROUP III		
Betamethasone valerate, 0.1% ointment	Valisone	Schering
Triamcinolone acetonide, 0.5% cream	Kenalog	Westwood-Squibb
GROUP IV		
Fluocinolone acetonide, 0.025% ointment	Synalar	Syntex
Fluocinolone acetonide, 0.1% solution	Synotic†	Syntex
Triamcinolone acetonide, 0.1% ointment	Vetalog†	Solvay
GROUP V		
Betamethasone valerate, 0.1% cream, lotion	Valisone	Schering
Fluocinolone acetonide, 0.025% cream	Synalar†	Syntex
Triamcinolone acetonide, 0.1% cream, lotion	Kenalog	Westwood-Squibb
GROUP VI		
Desonide, 0.05% cream	Tridesilon	Miles
Fluocinolone acetonide, 0.01% shampoo	FS shampoo	Hill
GROUP VII		
Dexamethasone, 0.1% cream	Decaderm	MSD
Dexamethasone, 0.04% spray	Decaspray	MSD
Hydrocortisone, 1 and 2.5% cream, ointment	Hytone	Dermik
Hydrocortisone, 1% spray	Cortispray†	DVM
Hydrocortisone, 1% spray	Dermacool-HC†	Allerderm/Virbac
Hydrocortisone, 1% spray	Hydro-Plus†	Phoenix
Hydrocortisone, 1% spray	Hydro-10 mist†	Butler
Hydrocortisone, 1% spray	PTD-HC†	VRx
Hydrocrotisone, 1% shampoo	Cortisoothe	Allerderm/Virbac

*Group I is most potent; Group VII is least potent.
†Veterinary label.

ichthyosis). It is relatively expensive but has been used in dogs and cats for acne and some localized keratinization disorders.[123] The gel form at 0.01 per cent concentration is initially used, as it is less irritating than 0.025 per cent. It increases the epidermal turnover time and reduces the cohesiveness of keratinocytes. Local irritation is a significant problem for many people and cats (e.g., with Retin-A).

■ *Urea.* Urea has hygroscopic and keratolytic actions that aid in normalizing the epidermis, especially the quality of the stratum corneum. The application of urea in a cream or an ointment base has a softening and moisturizing effect on the stratum corneum and makes the vehicle feel less greasy. It acts as a humectant in concentrations of 2 to 20 per cent; however, in concentrations above that level, it is keratolytic. That action is a result of the solubilization of prekeratin and keratin and the possible breakage of hydrogen bonds that keep the stratum corneum intact.

Humilac contains both urea and lactic acid, and it can be used as a spray or rinse. To make a rinse, 5 capfuls of Humilac are added to 1 L (1 qt) of water. The mixture is rinsed over the dog's coat and allowed to dry. KeraSolv contains 6 per cent salicylic acid, 5 per cent urea, and 5 per cent sodium lactate. It is a potent keratolytic used to treat nasal hyperkeratosis, calluses, ear margin dermatosis, and acne.[124]

■ *α-Hydroxyacids 2 to 10 Per Cent.* These include lactic, citric, pyruvic, glutamic, glycolic, and tartaric acids. They have been effective in modulating keratinization, especially in human ichthyosis (related to biosynthesis of mucopolysaccharides).

■ *Fatty Acids.* These are keratolytic and fungistatic. Examples are caprylic, propionic, and undecylenic acids. The best of these (although it is weak) is undecylenic acid (e.g., Desenex). Topical fatty acids are also used to treat essential fatty acid deficiency. Topical sunflower oil, which is high in linoleic acid, decreased transepidermal water loss in seborrheic dogs.[36]

■ *Propylene Glycol.* This agent is primarily used as a solvent and a vehicle. At higher concentrations, it may occasionally cause irritation or sensitization. It is an excellent lipid solvent and defats the skin; however, its chief value is probably the ability to enhance percutaneous penetration of drugs. Propylene glycol is also a potent and reliable antibacterial agent. For most dermatologic cases, it can be used in concentrations of 30 to 40 per cent. Higher concentrations are particularly helpful in hyperkeratotic conditions, and 75 per cent propylene glycol spray is effective in managing sebaceous adenitis (see Chap. 17).

Dimethyl Sulfoxide (DMSO)

DMSO is a simple, hygroscopic, organic solvent.[29] Because it is freely miscible with lipids, organic solvents, and water, it is an excellent vehicle. When exposed to the air, concentrated solutions take in water to become hydrated at 67 per cent. Stronger concentrations tend to cross the skin barrier better. DMSO penetrates skin (within 5 minutes), mucous membranes, and the blood-brain barrier, as well as cell, organelle, and microbial membranes. Unlike most solvents, DMSO achieves penetration without membrane damage. It facilitates absorption of many other substances across membranes, especially corticosteroids. On a cellular level, DMSO and steroids exert a synergistic effect.

DMSO has properties of its own as a cryoprotective, radioprotective, anti-ischemic, anti-inflammatory, and analgesic agent. It also has variable antibacterial, antifungal, and antiviral properties, depending on the concentration (usually 5 to 50 per cent) and the organism involved. Although its mechanism of action is incompletely understood, the systemic toxicity and teratogenicity of this solvent in its pure form are considered low. Toxicity may be of concern, depending on the dose, the route of administration, the species, and the individual animal's reaction. Impurities or combinations with other agents may make DMSO dangerous as a result of its ability to enhance transepidermal absorption. Industrial forms of DMSO should never be used for medical purposes, because the contained impurities are absorbed and may be toxic.

At present, DMSO has FDA approval in the United States only for musculoskeletal problems in horses and as a vehicle for a topical otic product (fluocinolone acetonide [Synotic]). When approved, potential uses might include topical application to cutaneous ulcers, burns, open wounds, and skin grafts; reduction of exuberant granulation tissue; and treatment of acral lick dermatitis. One formula shown to be safe and useful contains Burow's solution, hydrocortisone, and 90 per cent DMSO.[153] Equal parts of 90 per cent DMSO and Hydro-B 1020 (1 per cent hydrocortisone and 2 per cent Burow's solution in a water and propylene glycol base) are mixed. The formulation is applied daily to benefit patients with pyotraumatic dermatitis and acral lick dermatitis.

Topical Sunscreens

A dense haircoat protects most small animals from excessive exposure to sunlight. In some dogs, the skin is pigmented, which also protects from ultraviolet radiation damage. However, whenever nonpigmented, unhaired skin is exposed to sunlight, solar damage may occur. Predisposed areas include the ear tips in white cats, the glabrous abdomen in Dalmatians and bull terriers, and hairless areas. Some animals respond with hyperpigmentation, whereas other animals do not have hyperpigmentation but may have sunburn or solar dermatitis.

Protection from the sun can be attained by staying indoors from 10 AM to 4 PM, by tanning the skin (a process of building up pigmentation and mild acanthosis and hyperkeratosis), and by using topical or oral sunscreens.[184] Topical sunscreens may act physically or chemically. In chemical screens, aminobenzoic acid or benzophenone derivatives act to absorb ultraviolet rays. They are clear, cosmetically acceptable lotions or gels.

Physical sunscreens include chemicals such as zinc oxide and titanium dioxide, which reflect and scatter light by forming an opaque barrier. These barrier types are available in many colors (Bullfrog brand), including black, which some owners prefer for use on noses. They also are water resistant and are not as easily removed by the pet. These agents are messy, especially in long haircoats. Topical sunscreens are rated for efficiency by a sun protective factor (SPF) number. Numbers 2 to 4 are mild blockers, 8 to 10 give moderate protection, and 15 or higher gives blockage. For use in animals, water-resistant sunscreens with an SPF of 15 or greater should be used. These numbers are only guides, because the frequency and thickness of application, temperature, humidity, the potency of light exposure, the patient's sensitivity, and many other factors modify results.

Usually, sunscreen needs to be applied three or four times a day for greatest effectiveness. A common misconception is that if the animal licks the area after application, the sunscreen is removed. Although this is true for the physical blockers (e.g., zinc oxide), it is a minimal problem with chemical blockers, as these products are absorbed into the skin, and pool within the stratum corneum to produce a reservoir of protection. Chemical blockers are *not* effective if no epithelium is present (e.g., on ulcers).

■ PHYSICAL THERAPY

The use of heat, cold, light, and radiation therapy for the treatment of skin disorders is not new, but advances have made the therapies more specific and more effective. Freezing, heat, electricity, and laser light are presented as surgical techniques at the end of this chapter.

Photochemotherapy

Photochemotherapy uses light waves to excite or increase the energy of a photosensitive drug that causes a selective cytotoxic effect on tumors. The drug is a hematoporphyrin derivative

(Photofrin-V).[275] The drug has a much greater affinity for tumor tissue than for surrounding normal cells. Light is effective on only a few layers of surface cells, except red-range lights, which can penetrate as much as 1 to 2 cm. The light source is a laser system that produces a red laser beam that passes through low-attenuation fiberoptic tracts. These are directed through 19-gauge needles into the appropriate areas of tumor. Treatment takes about 20 minutes, and repeated exposures are no problem. Patients should be kept out of sunlight for 3 to 4 weeks, as they are systemically photosensitized.

Approximately 50 per cent of tumors respond completely, and an additional 30 per cent show partial responses.[275] The most favorable results were obtained in patients with malignant melanoma, fibrosarcoma, mast cell tumor, adamantinoma, and synovial cell sarcoma. Mixed responses were seen in animals with squamous cell carcinoma, adenocarcinoma, leiomyosarcoma, and hemangiopericytoma.

Hyperthermia

Local current-field radiofrequency is used to produce enough heat in a local superficial area to cause tissue necrosis. Two groups have used a temperature of 50°C for 30 to 60 seconds to treat feline tumors.[85a, 111a, 173] The heat was controlled to affect only the tumor and 2 to 3 mm of surrounding normal tissue. Results were much better with lesions less than 5 mm in diameter by 2 mm deep. In these cases, approximately 70 per cent of the tumors completely regressed, and an additional 20 per cent partially regressed. With larger tumors, the results were much poorer. Favorable responses were obtained with squamous cell carcinomas, fibrosarcomas of cats, and hepatoid gland tumors of dogs. There were no serious side-effects. This therapy should not be used on the pinna of the ear, as it may cause necrosis and sloughing.

Hyperthermia has also been used for topical treatment of localized dermatophytosis. By using the same system and producing heat of 50°C for 30 seconds in an area 4 mm deep by 1 cm in diameter, successful results were achieved after only one treatment. For large lesions, the heat probe was moved sequentially to new areas of 1 cm in diameter until the whole lesion was treated. Fluorescence disappeared within 48 hours, and healing was complete in 2 to 6 weeks. Hyperthermia was considered the treatment of choice for localized dermatophytosis. However, this type of therapy necessitates anesthesia, is cumbersome, is impractical with widespread lesions, and has not been corroborated by other investigators.

Heat is also used in electrosurgical procedures, such as fulguration, to destroy tissue.

Radiation Therapy

Radiation therapy has important benefits in the treatment of skin tumors, carefully selected cases of feline indolent ulcer, and canine acral lick dermatitis. Because not all cells are equally sensitive to radiation, these rays act selectively. Cells that divide rapidly, such as carcinoma cells, basal cells of the hair papilla, and vascular endothelial cells, are damaged more easily than those of the remaining skin. X-ray beams that are filtered through aluminum or copper sheets to remove soft rays penetrate deeply into the tissues because of their short wavelengths. Radiation delivered at about 80 kV with little or no filtration (0.5 mm of aluminum) has longer wavelengths, and its energy is dissipated superficially.

Before considering radiation therapy for a patient, the clinician must be certain of the following:

1. The treatment has good potential for benefit and little potential for harm.
2. Safer forms of therapy were not effective.
3. Relative cost of this therapy is acceptable.

4. Proper, safe equipment and facilities are available so that
   a. The exact dose can be administered.
   b. The patient can be anesthetized or restrained for therapy without exposure of personnel.
   c. Proper shielding of unaffected parts is provided.
5. Adequate records are kept for future reference.

If these points can be accomplished, radiation therapy may be considered.

In superficial skin diseases, such as feline indolent ulcer and canine acral lick dermatitis, radiation has been reported to be helpful, although other therapies are usually tried initially. In general, these cases should be referred to a radiologist. The usual dosage is 300 to 500 R.

Hepatoid gland tumors are highly sensitive to radiation. Benign lesions (hyperplasia and adenoma) receive 1000 to 2000 R; malignant lesions (adenocarcinoma) should receive 2000 to 4000 R.

Transmissible venereal tumors also are exquisitely radiosensitive, so this method is an excellent treatment. A dose of 1000 to 2000 R produces complete remission.

Mast cell tumors are usually radiosensitive, but multiple sites and rapid extension complicate the treatment problems. The usual dose is 2000 to 4000 R.

Squamous cell carcinoma may be sensitive, but some tumors are highly resistant. If surgical excision is not possible, 3000 to 4000 R may be beneficial.

Malignant melanoma should be removed surgically by wide excision. Because it metastasizes early, secondary palliative radiation may be temporarily useful. The dose is 3000 to 4000 R.

Fibrosarcoma should be treated surgically if possible, but palliative radiation therapy (3000 to 4000 R) may be used adjunctively.

Neurofibrosarcomas are highly resistant to radiation therapy.

■ SYSTEMIC THERAPY

Systemic Nonsteroidal Antipruritic or Nonsteroidal Anti-Inflammatory Agents

In practice, one is often presented with a pruritic or inflammatory dermatosis that is not microbial or parasitic. In other cases, even though a specific cause (e.g., scabies) is determined, symptomatic antipruritic or anti-inflammatory therapy may be desired.[132] Systemic glucocorticoids are most commonly prescribed. However, although glucocorticoids are highly effective in managing these cases and many hypersensitivity disorders, the frequent occurrence of side-effects of variable severity stimulates continual investigations for alternative drugs or methods that will allow an avoidance or reduction in the dose of glucocorticoid.[28, 159, 233, 249, 250] Reasons for electing nonsteroidal agents include (1) unacceptable acute, or chronic glucocorticoid side-effects; (2) immunosuppressed patients (e.g., cats with feline leukemia virus or feline immunodeficiency virus infections); (3) patients with infectious diseases (viral, fungal, and bacterial); (4) patients with other diseases in which glucocorticoids may be contraindicated (diabetes mellitus, pancreatitis, renal disease, and neoplasia); and (5) pet owners who do not want to use glucocorticoids in their animals. A variety of unrelated nonsteroidal drugs may be utilized.

Scott and Buerger[236] used a supplement that contained omega-3/omega-6 fatty acids (DVM DermCaps), three different antihistamines (chlorpheniramine, diphenhydramine, hydroxyzine), an antibiotic (erythromycin), and aspirin in an open study of nonsteroidal anti-inflammatory agents in the management of 45 cases of canine pruritus. Thirty-two dogs had atopy or flea bite hypersensitivity, and 13 dogs had idiopathic nonseasonal pruritus. As a group, the six drugs controlled itching in 40 per cent of the cases, and there was improvement in another 15 per cent. However, side-effects were seen in 46 per cent of the cases, being severe enough in 33

Table 3:5. Results of a Study of Nonsteroidal Anti-Inflammatory Agents in 45 Cases of Canine Pruritus

Drug	Dosage	Number Controlled	Number Improved	Number with Side-Effects
Chlorpheniramine	4 mg q8h	4	4	12
Diphenhydramine	25–50 mg q8h	3	7	7
Hydroxyzine	2.2 mg/kg q8h	3	8	7
Erythromycin	11 mg/kg q8h	2	4	4
EPA formula	1 cap/9 kg q8h	5	5	4
Aspirin	25 mg/kg q8h	1	4	2

Data from Scott, D.W., Buerger, R.G.: Nonsteroidal anti-inflammatory agents in the management of canine pruritus. J. Am. Anim. Hosp. Assoc. 24:425, 1988.

per cent of the dogs to cause treatments with one or more of the drugs to be halted. Good to moderate improvement of pruritus was obtained for each medication (Table 3:5). Subsequent studies, several of which were placebo-controlled and double-blind studies, show that options other than systemic glucocorticoids are available. The majority of the work has evaluated three main classes of drugs: antihistamines, fatty acids, and psychotropic agents.

ANTIHISTAMINES

Histamine is a potent chemical mediator that has variable actions, depending on what receptors and tissues are stimulated. The effects of histamine can be blocked in three ways: by physiologic antagonists, such as epinephrine; by agents that reduce histamine formation or release from mast cells and basophils; and by histamine receptor antagonists. The latter are commonly used.

First-generation (classic, or traditional) antihistamines are H_1 blockers. However, not all the effects of histamine are blocked by H_1 blockers. The use of antihistamines in managing canine and feline pruritic diseases has been promoted for many years. Although their efficacy was previously controversial, the past several years have seen the publication of multiple studies documenting their efficacy. It is often recommended that their use is primarily for atopic disease or other diseases in which immediate hypersensitivity and mast cell degranulation are important; however, several studies have included treatment of pruritus due to multiple causes.[165, 180, 182a, 182b, 250] Because the antihistamines are metabolized by the liver, they should be used with caution in patients with hepatic disease. In addition, their anticholinergic properties contraindicate their use in patients with glaucoma, gastrointestinal atony, and urinary retentive states. Some antihistamines are teratogenic in various laboratory animals. No information on teratogenicity is available for dogs and cats; however, this issue should be considered before treating pregnant bitches and queens. Finally, the efficacy of antihistamines is notoriously unpredictable and individualized in a given patient. Thus, the clinician may try several antihistamines before finding the one that is beneficial for a given patient.

Antihistamines block the physiologic effects of histamine. At least three different types of histamine receptors have been recognized. However, in general, the H_1-receptor antagonists are utilized in small animal dermatology. This is because H_1 receptors are primarily responsible for pruritus, increased vascular permeability, release of inflammatory mediators, and recruitment of inflammatory cells.[257] In addition to their histamine-blocking action, H_1-receptor antagonists have therapeutic value because of their sedative, antinausea, anticholinergic, antiserotoninergic, and local anesthesic effects. Some, such as hydroxyzine, astemazole, and cetrizine, may also inhibit mast cell degranulation. Most of the second-generation, or nonsedating, antihistamines block mediator release to some degree.[257] However, the effects may differ with the variable being evaluated (i.e., different results may occur with various sources of mast cells, basophils, or eosinophils). Variable results may also occur depending on the method used to induce cellular responses such as immunoglobulin E (IgE)–induced release or nonantibody inducers.[257] Cetrizine, a second-generation antihistamine, is particularly effective in blocking the allergen-induced late-phase cutaneous reaction and decreasing the influx of eosinophils in response to allergens.[22]

A number of open uncontrolled or open controlled comparative studies have been reported.[156, 160, 165, 236, 251] These indicated that the first-generation antihistamines, chlorpheniramine (0.4 mg/kg q8h), diphenhydramine (2 mg/kg q8h), and hydroxyzine (2 mg/kg q8h), may each be effective in up to 10 per cent of the dogs with allergic pruritus.

In cats with allergic pruritus, chlorpheniramine (2 to 4 mg/cat q12h) was reported to be effective in 70 per cent of the cases.[167] Results of an open clinical trial indicated that clemastine (0.1 mg/kg q12h) was effective in 50 per cent of cats with allergic pruritus.[166]

A double-blind placebo-controlled study in 30 dogs revealed that the placebo was totally ineffective, whereas clemastine fumarate (Tavist) at 0.05 mg/kg every 12 hours was effective in 30 per cent of the cases.[182a] Two other open clinical trials confirmed the effectiveness of clemastine in dogs.[160, 182b] Trimeprazine tartrate (Temaril) at 0.12 mg/kg every 12 hours was effective in only 3 per cent of dogs with allergic pruritus. Cyproheptadine hydrochloride (Periactin) at 0.1 mg/kg every 12 hours and terfenadine (Seldane) at 5 mg/kg every 12 hours were ineffective in double-blind placebo-controlled studies.[245, 246]

Antihistamines may also be used to act synergistically with, or reduce required doses of glucocorticoids.[182a, 249, 250] In one study, the addition of trimeprazine to ongoing, alternate-day prednisone regimens in allergic dogs allowed an average 30 per cent reduction in the prednisone dosage in 75 per cent of the patients.[182a] Antihistamines can also be used synergistically with other nonsteroidal anti-inflammatory agents that work by different mechanisms.[182b, 249, 250, 251, 252] In one open clinical trial, dogs that responded to neither chlorpheniramine nor a fatty acid–containing supplement (DVM Derm Caps) when these were administered as individual drugs were given the same two drugs in combination.[251] Approximately 30 per cent of the dogs responded well. Similarly, 50 per cent of the cats that responded neither to chlorpheniramine nor to DVM Derm Caps liquid when these were administered individually responded well when the two drugs were used in combination.[252]

Second-generation (nonsedating) antihistamines are also H_1 blockers. But, because they are poorly lipid soluble and minimally cross the blood-brain barrier, they exert much less sedative action and anticholinergic effects than do first-generation antihistamines. For some reason, second-generation antihistamines have not been useful in dogs to date. Terfenadine (Seldane) at 5 mg/kg every 12 hours,[246] astemizole (Hismanal) at 0.25 mg/kg every 24 hours,[182a] and loratadine (Claritin) at 10 mg/kg every 24 hours[98] were all ineffective in dogs with allergic pruritus.

H_2-receptor blockers may have a role in modifying the cutaneous inflammatory response. Cimetidine hydrochloride (Tagamet) and ranitidine, which is more powerful and longer acting, are available for clinical use, but are not approved by the FDA for small animals. H_2 antihistamines (cimetidine) should not be given alone because they inhibit the negative feedback that histamine exerts on mediators released by mast cells, thus potentially exacerbating an inflammatory dermatosis.[7] The combination of H_1 and H_2 blockers counteracts the action of any circulating histamine by blocking all of the available histamine receptors. H_1 and H_2 antagonists have no effect on the receptor sites of each other.

Cimetidine is not a first-line drug in human dermatology, but it is used in combination with H_1 antihistamine for urticarial, allergic, and immunologic dermatoses when other therapy fails. It has also been used as an antipruritic in dermatoses related to systemic disorders and as an immunorestorative in cases of T cell lymphoma, epitheliotropic lymphoma, mycosis fungoides, and candidiasis.[7] In a study of 15 dogs with allergic skin disease, cimetidine alone was helpful in only one dog, and no dog responded better to the combination of H_2 (cimetidine) and H_1 (diphenhydramine) blockers than to the H_1 blocker alone.[156]

Cimetidine appears safe for dogs and cats at a dosage of 5 to 10 mg/kg orally every 6 to 8 hours.[49] It may be useful in some cases of chronic recurrent pyoderma with pruritus.[204] Much more evaluation remains to be done in small animal dermatology, however.

FATTY ACIDS

Fatty acids have been recommended for many years as dietary supplements to improve the sheen and luster of the hair.[2, 60] However, their use for treating inflammatory diseases has been the subject of much debate and research.[155, 159, 287] It is now impossible for the small animal clinician to practice without some knowledge of fatty acids. Fatty acids are long carbon chains with a methyl group at one end. Polyunsaturated fatty acids have multiple double bonds. The numeric formulas used to identify fatty acids give the number of carbon atoms, followed by the number of double bonds, then the location of the first double bond from the methyl group. Therefore, the formula for linoleic acid (18:2N-6) means there are 18 carbons and 2 double bonds, with the first occurring at the sixth carbon atom from the methyl end of the molecule.

The fatty acids that have the first double bond three carbon molecules away from the methyl group are the omega-3 (N-3) series. The omega-6 (N-6) series of polyunsaturated fatty acids have the first double bond six carbons from the methyl group. These two complete series of fatty acids cannot be synthesized by dogs and cats, and therefore the 18-carbon molecule (linoleic and linolenic acid) must be supplied in the diet. They are referred to as essential fatty acids for this reason. The essential fatty acids most important in cutaneous homeostasis are linoleic acid (18:2N-6) and linolenic acid (18:3N-3) in the dog. In the cat, arachidonic acid (20:4N-6) is also an essential fatty acid. Dihomo-γ linolenic acid (DGLA) (20:3N-6) and eicosapentaenoic acid (EPA) (20:5N-3) can be synthesized in the animal from linoleic acid and linolenic acid, respectively.

The synthesis of fatty acids involves the action of various desaturase enzymes, which insert double bonds into the chain. Other enzymes referred to as elongases add additional carbon molecules to the existing chain. The presence of these specific enzymes varies in different groups or species of animals and may also differ in individuals with certain diseases. The best example of this is Δ-6-desaturase deficiency in atopic humans. Also, the skin is deficient in desaturase enzymes. Therefore, when local accumulation of linoleic acid, γ-linolenic acid (18:3N-6), or DGLA occur, they cannot be metabolized to arachidonic acid locally. DGLA competes with arachidonic acid for cyclooxygenase and lipoxygenase enzymes. This competitive inhibition, in addition to the effects of their metabolic byproducts, is believed to be the mechanism for anti-inflammatory action of fatty acid therapy, which in general, involves modification of leukotriene and prostaglandin synthesis and activity. However, fatty acids are also important for other reasons.

Fatty acids are valuable components of cell membranes but also have extracellular function in the skin. They are responsible for the luster of the normal haircoat and the smoothness of the skin. Linoleic acid is particularly important, because only it supplies the proper conditions for the water permeability functions of the intercellular lipid bilayer of the skin (see Chap. 1).

Metabolic byproducts are important in promoting or inhibiting inflammation. This is especially true of arachidonic acid metabolites. Arachidonic acid is stored in cells in an unavailable form until it is released by the action of phospholipase A_2. Arachidonic acid metabolites have been identified in many cell types, besides mast cells, that participate in hypersensitivity reactions (neutrophils, eosinophils, lymphocytes, monocytes, macrophages, keratinocytes, and vascular endothelial cells).

The effects of prostaglandins on the skin include alteration of vascular permeability, potentiation of vasoactive substances such as histamine, modulation of lymphocyte function, and potentiation of pain and itch. Prostaglandins and leukotrienes potentiate each other. The effects of leukotrienes on the skin are to alter vascular permeability, to activate neutrophils, to modify lymphocyte function, and to cause potent neutrophil and eosinophil chemotaxis.[81] Manipulation of fatty acid metabolism by using the shared enzyme system to inhibit formation competitively of some of the above substances seems possible.

It was shown that dogs with seborrhea sicca have abnormally low cutaneous levels of linoleic acid.[36] Additionally, these dogs have increased levels of cutaneous oleic acid. Oleic acid is believed to be substituted in phospholipid membranes when there is a relative deficiency of linoleic acid. However, serum linoleic levels in the seborrheic dogs were normal and they were not receiving a diet deficient in essential fatty acids. Despite normal serum levels, treatment with oral sunflower oil reversed the cutaneous abnormalities. Sunflower oil, which is 78 per cent linoleic acid, was added to the diet at 1.5 ml/kg/day.[36] Safflower oil is also a good source of linoleic acid and has been recommended at 0.5 ml/kg/day.[287]

An omega-6 and omega-3 fatty acid–containing product (DVM Derm Caps) was effective in a small number of Cocker spaniels with idiopathic seborrhea, but was of no benefit in West Highland white terriers with epidermal dysplasia or in Springer spaniels with psoriasiform-lichenoid dermatosis.[173] Another interesting study showed that seborrheic dogs have abnormal transepidermal water loss, and this may be corrected by topical application of linoleic acid.[35] The suggestion that topical application may be more effective than oral administration was raised. Studies to determine the most efficacious, cost-effective, and client-acceptable way to treat dogs with dry skin deficient in linoleic acid are being awaited. The dose used in the study of topical application would have made dogs too greasy for most clients.

Now that the value of linoleic acid in the diet is well established for seborrheic dogs, it is important that clinicians counsel clients accordingly. Besides the possibility of adding linoleic acid sources to the diet, the proper handling of dog food should also be considered. Overcooking foods may decrease the levels of linoleic acid. Allowing rancidity to occur by improper or prolonged storage or inadequate levels of antioxidants is another consideration. In general, dry foods should be kept at room temperature, out of direct light, in non–lipid-permeable or nonabsorbing containers and not stored open for longer than 1 month. To ensure adequate levels of linoleic acid, supplementation with 5 ml (1 tsp) of sunflower or safflower oil per 240 ml (8 oz) dry dog food should be sufficient. This may not be effective in cases in which maldigestion, malabsorption, or abnormal fatty acid metabolism is occurring.

A possible example is the atopic dog. Although these dogs have relatively normal triglyceride levels, the absorption of fats were shown to be abnormal.[284] This study suggested that abnormal lipid absorption or metabolism is present in atopic dogs, and possibly response to fatty acid supplements relates to countering this abnormal function. Another clinical situation that may lead to dry skin is the use of a fat-restricted diet in obese dogs or dogs with pancreatitis. Because caloric intake is restricted with low-fat diets, a relative fatty acid deficiency could occur.

As previously mentioned, the use of fatty acids as antipruritic or anti-inflammatory agents in dogs and cats has been the subject of numerous studies.* The proposed mechanism, besides the inhibition of arachidonic acid metabolism, relates to metabolic byproducts of fatty acid metabolism. Supplements used for pruritus usually contain one or both of γ-linolenic acid and EPA. γ-Linolenic acid is found in relatively high concentrations in evening primrose, borage, and black currant oils. It is elongated to DGLA, which directly competes with arachidonic acid as a substrate for cyclooxygenase and 15-lipoxygenase. The result of DGLA metabolism is the formation of prostaglandin E_1 and 15-hydroxy-8,11,13-eicosatetraenoic acid, both of which are believed to have anti-inflammatory effects.[287]

EPA, which is usually supplied by using cold water marine fish oils, also competes as a substrate for cyclooxygenase and 5- and 15-lipoxygenase. The metabolism of EPA by the lipoxygenase enzymes results in the formation of leukotriene B_5 and 15-hydroxyeicosapentaenoic acid. These two products are believed to inhibit leukotriene B_4, which is a potent pro-inflammatory mediator. This mechanism was reviewed by White,[287] and Figure 3:5 demonstrates the interactions of γ-linolenic acid, EPA, and arachidonic acid.

---

*See references 26, 27, 137, 162, 163, 182b, 220, 236, 243, and 252.

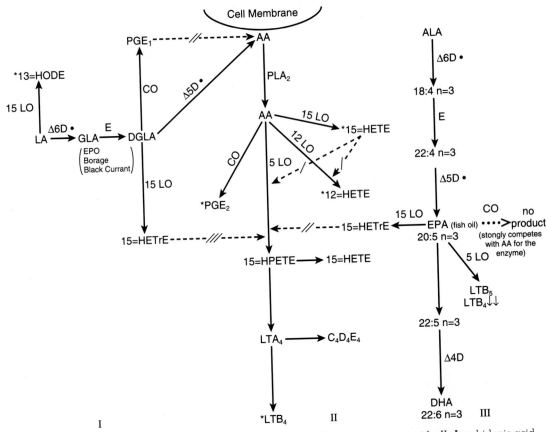

Figure 3:5. *I*, N-6 fatty acid metabolism with production of anti-inflammatory eicosanoids. *II*, Arachidonic acid cascade with production of proinflammatory eicosanoids. *III*, N-3 fatty acid metabolism with production of anti-inflammatory eicosanoids. 13-HODE, 13-hydroxyoctadecadienoic acid; PG, prostaglandin; E, elongase; Δ-6-D, Δ-6-desaturase; LA, linoleic acid; GLA, γ-linolenic acid; EPO, evening primrose oil; DGLA, dihomo-γ-linolenic acid; AA, arachidonic acid; ALA, α-linolenic acid; EPA, eicosapentaenoic acid; DHA, docosahexaenoic acid; DES, desaturase; PLA$_2$, phospholipase A$_2$; CO, cyclooxygenase; LO, lipoxygenase; HETE, hydroxyeicosatetraenoic acid; HPETE, hydroperoxyeicosatetraenoic acid; HEPE, hydroxyeicosapentaenoic acid; 15-HETrE, 15-hydroxy-8,11,13-eicosatrienoic acid; LT, leukotriene. * indicates arachidonic acid–derived eicosanoids identified in inflammatory skin disease; → indicates inhibitory or anti-inflammatory eicosanoid (number of slash lines indicates degree of inhibition). (From White, P.: Essential fatty acids: Use in management of canine atopy. Comp. Cont. Educ. 15:451, 1993.)

The use of fatty acids for atopic disease and chronic pruritus has been extensively studied. The beneficial effect has been documented in multiple double-blind or placebo-controlled studies.[26, 27, 134, 138, 220, 221, 243] In addition, multiple open uncontrolled studies have been published. In five separate clinical trials in North America, DVM Derm Caps were effective in 11 to 27 per cent of the allergic dogs treated.[162, 164, 182b, 236, 243] In cats, omega-6 and omega-3 fatty acid–containing products have been effective in more than 50 per cent of allergic patients.[95, 96, 96a, 163] How well fatty acids work depends on many variables, with 10 to 80 per cent of atopic animals realizing varying degrees of clinical improvement. The benefit is maximized if other contributing diseases such as food hypersensitivity, flea bite hypersensitivity, bacterial pyoderma, and *Malassezia* dermatitis are controlled. Overall, it is probably safe to inform clients that about 20 per cent of the dogs, and about 50 per cent of the cats, with allergic pruritus, experience improvement. There is also evidence that higher doses of γ-linolenic acid enhance the results. The additional dosage has not been completely determined, but may be 4 to 10 times the recommended dose.[26, 27, 96, 134, 220, 221] Another factor that may be important is the type of diet the animal is receiving. Dogs receiving lower-fat diets may respond better to the supplements.[96]

Although the benefits of these products are clear, which fatty acid, which combination of fatty acids, what ratio of omega-6 to omega-3, and what dose of these agents is most effective remains inconclusive. Several studies compared different types of supplements. In one study evaluating four different supplements, no one product was effective in all cases and response could not be predicted.[243] Failure to respond to one product does not preclude a favorable response to another product. This study suggested that a perfect dose and type or blend of fatty acids cannot be discovered. Therefore, multiple trials may be best. In the dog, various doses (up to three times the manufacturer's recommendation) of only omega-6 fatty acids have not been effective in controlling pruritus.[137, 220] With recommended doses of omega-3 fatty acids, canine allergic pruritus was not controlled.[137] However, large doses (up to seven times those usually given) of omega-3 fatty acids effectively controlled pruritus in 30 to 60 per cent of the dogs.[134] Whereas twice the manufacturer's dose of an omega-6 and omega-3 fatty acid–containing product was no more effective than the recommended dose,[251] other studies reported that 2 to 10 times the recommended dose may be necessary to control allergic pruritus in dogs.[26, 27]

Another area that still needs investigation is the importance or effect of combining the fatty acids with other elements such as vitamins and minerals and cofactors. Some manufacturers and authors[138] have claimed that the right combination of cofactors maximizes the beneficial effects. Controlled studies to determine this and what cofactors are most important have not yet been presented. In one double-blind study, a fatty acid product containing cofactors was no more effective than products that did not contain cofactors.[243] Other formulations claim to improve fatty acid absorption such as by miscillization. Again, controlled studies are needed. How long one should try a product has also not been definitively determined. Although some dogs and cats show a favorable response within 1 to 2 weeks, an adequate therapeutic trial might necessitate between 9 and 12 weeks.*

Although fatty acids may be solely effective for controlling pruritus and inflammation in some animals, their roles in synergistic therapy should be considered. Little has been done to study their synergistic role, but it has been suggested that they should frequently be tried in combination with other antipruritic agents for managing allergic pruritus.[86] A synergistic effect was documented between fatty acids and antihistamines.[182b, 249–252] A synergistic effect with glucocorticoids was also described.[155, 182a, 249, 250]

The risks and side-effects of fatty acid supplementation are few. The most serious, although rarely reported, side-effect is pancreatitis.[86] With large doses, an increase in weight or diarrhea may also be seen. With supplements containing fish oil, some clients have reported an unpleasant odor or increased eructation (''fish breath'').

A beneficial role of fatty acids has been documented, and they play an important role in managing pruritic dogs and cats. Because of their low potential for risk and their good potential for benefit, trial therapy is often warranted. Their exact role, indications, and optimal use still need to be elucidated. In addition, the practitioner is presented with numerous different formulations and products from which to choose. Until more studies are done, it is best to use products with proven efficacy (DVM Derm Caps) and develop one's own clinical intuition about effectiveness and indications.

PSYCHOTROPIC AGENTS

A variety of drugs that are known for their CNS effects are also being used to treat a number of diseases characterized by pruritus.[112] These drugs include tricyclic antidepressants and nar-

---

*See references 26, 27, 36, 96, 96a, 134, 138, 159, 163, 182b, and 243.

cotic antagonists. Tricyclic antidepressants are serotonin and norepinephrine uptake inhibitors, and some of them, such as amitriptyline and doxepin, are potent H_1 blockers. These drugs can also induce cardiac arrhythmias, lower the seizure threshold, and enhance monamine oxidase inhibitor toxicity, in addition to having the metabolic results and side-effects that are inherent with first-generation antihistamines. Amitriptyline hydrochloride (Elavil) at 1 mg/kg every 12 hours was effective in 16 per cent of the allergic dogs treated,[165] whereas doxepin hydrochloride (Sinequan) at 1 mg/kg every 8 hours was ineffective.[182a] Anecdotal reports indicate that the serotonin uptake inhibitor fluoxetine hydrochloride (Prozac at 1 mg/kg q24h) is effective in 30 per cent of dogs with allergic pruritus.[98, 180, 256] One open study also suggested that it may be effective for acral lick dermatitis.[256]

Endorphins may also play a role in perpetuating or inducing pruritic behavior such as excessive grooming. Feline psychogenic alopecia and canine acral lick dermatitis are two syndromes characterized by excessive self-licking. Studies using endorphin blockers demonstrated some efficacy. In cats with feline psychogenic alopecia, naloxone injected subcutaneously (1 mg/kg) resulted in improvement in four of five treated cats.[297] Another study in dogs with acral lick dermatitis showed that the endorphin blocker naltrexone (2.2 mg/kg q24h) was helpful in 70 per cent of the cases treated.[288a]

MISCELLANEOUS ANTIPRURITIC OR ANTI-INFLAMMATORY AGENTS

Various agents with different anti-inflammatory properties have been used in allergic dogs. The following agents were of no benefit: acetylsalicylic acid,[236] doxycycline,[237] papaverine,[237] vitamin C,[164] and zinc.[156]

It was reported that oxatomide—a mast cell stabilizer—was effective at 15 to 30 mg every 12 hours for controlling pruritus in allergic cats.[98, 193]

Systemic Antibiotics

Systemic antibiotic agents are used for bacterial skin diseases, whether primary or secondary, that are not treatable with topical therapy. Because the overwhelming majority of canine skin infections are caused by coagulase-positive *S. intermedius*, antibiotics that affect these bacteria and concentrate in the skin are of primary interest. Occasionally, *Proteus* spp., *Pseudomonas* spp., and *Escherichia coli* are involved as secondary invaders in deeper soft tissue infections. In cats, the primary bacteria are *Pasteurella multocida* and β-hemolytic streptococci.[231] Thus, the penicillins and ampicillins are frequently effective antibiotics for cats.

Proper antibiotic use necessitates that the antibiotic inhibit the specific bacteria, preferably in a bactericidal manner. Bacteriostatic drugs may also be effective as long as the host is not immunocompromised. The drug should have a narrow spectrum, so that it produces little effect on organisms of the natural flora of the skin or the intestinal tract (for oral medications). The antibiotic should be inexpensive, should be easily given (orally, if it is to be prescribed for home use) and absorbed, and should have no adverse effects.

The most important factors influencing the effectiveness of antibiotics are the sensitivity of the bacteria and the distribution to the skin in effective levels of activity at the infection site. Only about 4 per cent of the cardiac output of blood reaches the skin, compared with 33 per cent that reaches muscle.[11] This variation is reflected in the relative distribution of antibiotics among organs. In studies of the different regions of skin, the levels of penicillin-type antibiotic in the hypodermis reached about 60 per cent, and dermal-epidermal junction levels reached about 40 per cent, of the peak serum levels in dogs.[11] Cephalexin levels in dog skin are only 20 to 40 per cent of those in plasma.[111]

Although the epidermis is relatively avascular, studies on skin infections showed that the systemic route of therapy is better than the topical route for all but the most superficial infections. The stratum corneum is a major permeability barrier to effective topical drug penetration. These facts led to the inescapable conclusion that the skin is one of the most difficult tissues in which to obtain high antibiotic levels.

Factors that may reduce the effectiveness of a therapeutic plan are the following:

1. The organism is resistant to the antibiotic, and because most *S. intermedius* produce β-lactamase, antibiotics resistant to this should be selected.
2. The dosage is inadequate to attain and then maintain inhibitory concentrations in the skin.
3. The organism may be surviving inside macrophages where it is not exposed to most antibiotics' effect.
4. The organism is within a necrotic center or protected by a foreign body such as a hair fragment.
5. The organism is walled off by dense scar tissue.
6. The duration of therapy is inadequate to eradicate the infection.

Antibiotic sensitivity of *S. intermedius* isolated from canine pyodermas varies depending on the use of antibiotics in the region. In general, penicillins, ampicillin, amoxicillin, tetracycline, and nonpotentiated sulfonamides are poor antibiotic choices and should not be prescribed. When antibiotics have been given previously, the frequency of susceptibility to the above antibiotics, as well as erythromycin and lincomycin, decreases.[117, 122] There may also be other interesting variables. In the United States, about 60 per cent of coagulase-positive *Staphylococcus* spp. isolates are resistant to amoxicillin and ampicillin, whereas in the United Kingdom, only about 5 per cent are resistant.[144] However, studies have shown that previous antibiotic use did not significantly alter the resistance to oxacillin, trimethoprim-sulfadiazine, amoxicillin-clavulanate, cephalothin, and ormetoprim-sulfadimethoxine.[37, 71, 91, 105, 106, 117, 239] This and other factors suggest that culture and sensitivity tests should be performed in chronic, refractory cases of pyoderma to guide selection of the most effective drug. However, for initial infections, be they superficial or deep, direct smears and evaluation of modified Wright-type stain or other quick stains of exudates usually provide adequate information to start rational therapy immediately.[105, 106, 173]

Dosage is a critical question. Although some clinicians believe that intermittent dosage and fluctuating blood levels are satisfactory therapy (especially for penicillin-type drugs), the authors believe that constant, high blood levels are imperative. Antibiotic combinations are usually unnecessary. Antibiotics that are well absorbed and that distribute well to tissues are desirable. Chloramphenicol, a trimethoprim-sulfonamide combination, and amoxicillin-clavulanate distribute well to superficial tissues, whereas lincomycin, erythromycin, and the synthetic penicillins do not. These characteristics must be matched against the spectrum of activity, the route and ease of dosage, the cost, and the resistance factors when decisions are made on the drug choice.

Antibiotics must be given in maximal dose for at least 14 to 21 days for superficial infections and for 30 to 60 days in more complex infections. Clinical trials showed that the necessary duration of antibiotic therapy varies from 17 to 91 days.[181, 239, 244] Selection of antibiotics for pyoderma based on its chronicity and the type of case has been recommended.[122] The antibiotics that are commonly used on the basis of this scheme for skin infections and their dosages are listed in Table 3:6. In this scheme, appropriate antibiotics to consider when treating first-occurrence pyoderma include clindamycin, erythromycin, tylosin, and lincomycin.[96b, 194, 244]

Refractory or recurrent pyodermas are usually treated with chloramphenicol, ormetoprim-sulfadimethoxine, or trimethoprim-sulfadiazine. In cases with resistant staphylococci, or when long-term or pulse therapy is required for chronic recurrent pyoderma, amoxicillin-clavulanate, cephalosporins, and oxacillin are most commonly prescribed. In certain cases of unusually resistant staphylococci and in infections in which *Pseudomonas* or *Proteus* is encountered (especially otitis externa or otitis media), enrofloxacin is often used.

Table 3:6. Common Oral Antibiotic Regimens Used in Dermatology

Drug	Dosage (mg/kg)	Frequency (h)
First-occurrence pyoderma:		
Chloramphenicol	50	8
Clindamycin	5.5	12
Erythromycin	15	8
Lincomycin	22	12
Tylosin	20	12
Recurrent cases with previous antibiotic treatment:		
Ormetoprim-sulfadimethoxine	55 on day 1, 27.5 on subsequent days	24
Trimethoprim-sulfadiazine	15–30	12
or		
Trimethoprim-sulfamethoxazole	15–30	12
Enrofloxacin	2.5	12
Enrofloxacin	5	24
Plus all antibiotics listed for long-term use		
Long-term use:		
Amoxicillin–potassium clavulanate	13.75	12
Cefadroxil	22	12
Cephalexin	22–33	12
Cloxacillin	10	6
Oxacillin	20	8
Scarred pyoderma and interdigital granuloma:		
Clindamycin*	11	12
Enrofloxacin	2.5	12
Enrofloxacin	5	24
Rifampin† (in conjunction with cephalexin or oxacillin)	5	24
Gram-negative rod pyodermas and otitis:		
Enrofloxacin	2.5–5	12
Enrofloxacin	5–10	24

*Resistance is common and may preclude use.
†Toxicity, especially liver disease, is a significant risk and monitoring is recommended.

Another special situation arises with certain cases of excessively scarred deep pyodermas. In these cases, exemplified by chronic interdigital pyoderma and some callus or pressure point pyodermas, rifampin may be prescribed.[1, 222] However, because of the rapid emergence of resistant strains of bacteria, rifampin should be used in combination with another β-lactamase–resistant antibiotic. Rifampin has the unusual advantage of being able to penetrate tissues extremely well, even going intracellularly. This unique ability to penetrate tissues and cells so well, along with the usual sensitivity of susceptible staphylococci to small concentrations of the drug, makes rifampin an effective antibiotic.[1] However, it is not without risk, and hepatotoxicity is a primary concern when it is used in dogs.

In rare situations, such as septicemia associated with deep pyoderma or severe *Pseudomonas* or other gram-negative rod infections, injectable aminoglycosides may be needed.[122] In these cases, gentamicin 2.2 mg/kg subcutaneously or intramuscularly every 8 hours or amikacin 10 mg/kg subcutaneously every 12 hours is usually given. Many of these drugs can be used sequentially with good effect. In general, they should not be used in combination simultaneously. Another rare indication for unusual antibiotic therapy is feline mycobacterial infections (see Chap. 4). The drug clofazimine was useful in treating feline leprosy. Clofazimine has both antimycobacterial and anti-inflammatory effects.[174] It was well tolerated for up to 9 months when given at a dosage 2 to 3 mg/kg orally every 24 hours.

Patients should be weighed, and medications should be administered in full dose at specified intervals for the optimal length of time. It is extremely hard to reach effective antibiotic levels in the skin. A common mistake is to administer a lower dose because the optimal dose is not available in an oral preparation (e.g., a dog weighing 16 kg should receive 350 mg of cephalexin q12h, but is given 250 mg q12h instead of 500 mg q12h). When treating skin infections with oral antibiotics, it is *always* better to overdose than to underdose.

No drug is without potential hazard, but the most commonly prescribed antibiotics are relatively safe. Virtually all the antibiotics occasionally cause vomiting or diarrhea. Drug reactions are uncommon but occur more frequently with sulfonamides than with cephalosporins. If one wishes to decrease the risk of drug reactions, alternative antibiotics may be given. The Doberman pinscher is at higher risk for drug reactions to sulfonamides, and these drugs should be used with great caution in this breed. Some Doberman pinschers seem to have a genetic predisposition to a sulfadiazine-induced type III hypersensitivity reaction (immune complex disease) and nonseptic polyarthritis.[6, 77]

Comments about other possible antibiotic-related side-effects deserve attention. Enrofloxacin should not be used in young growing dogs because it may damage articular cartilage. Chloramphenicol commonly causes an asymptomatic, mild, reversible anemia in dogs when given for longer than 2 to 3 weeks. In cats, however, chloramphenicol may cause severe hematopoietic toxicity and should be used with great care in that species. Thus, in cats, the dose is repeated once every 12 hours for only 1 week. Erythromycin is more likely to produce vomiting initially. Administering it with food may help, or an antiemetic may be given concurrently during the first 2 days of therapy. Rifampin causes hepatotoxicity in some cases, and monitoring liver function is recommended if treatment goes longer than 10 days. Long-term use of many sulfonamides (but apparently *not* ormetoprim-sulfadimethoxine) often produces keratoconjunctivitis sicca.

Systemic Antifungal Agents

The most common indication for systemic antifungal therapy is generalized dermatophytosis. Griseofulvin is still the systemic antifungal agent of choice in these cases. However, if it has caused complications or is otherwise contraindicated, ketoconazole or itraconazole may be acceptable alternatives. For *Malassezia* infections, griseofulvin is not effective and ketoconazole is the drug of choice. Other regimens or treatments may be necessary for the less commonly encountered mycotic infections (see Chap. 5). Newer antifungals, particularly the triazole compounds, are becoming available, but in general, they still have not been shown to be preferred over griseofulvin for routine use. The two drugs receiving the most attention are itraconazole and fluconazole.

■ *Griseofulvin.* Griseofulvin is a fungistatic antibiotic obtained by fermentation from several species of *Penicillium*. Its antifungal activity results from the inhibition of cell wall synthesis, nucleic acid synthesis, and mitosis. This agent is primarily active against growing cells, although dormant cells may be inhibited from reproducing.[97] After oral administration, the drug may be detected in the stratum corneum. The highest concentrations are in the outermost layers and the lowest are in the basal layers. The drug is secreted in sweat and is deposited in keratin precursor cells and remains tightly bound during the differentiation process. Consequently, new growth of hair or claws is the first to be free from disease. Holzworth[99] suggested that animals (cats) be given griseofulvin for several days before clipping, so that unaffected hair grows out and most of the affected hair is clipped away. Otherwise, cats with generalized disease should be clipped at least twice.

Griseofulvin is in a state of flux in the skin, and, consequently, a dosage administered once or twice daily is needed to maintain constant blood levels. This drug is indicated for only dermatophyte infections *(Microsporum* and *Trichophyton)*. It is not generally effective topically or against yeasts *(Candida* and *Malassezia)*.

Griseofulvin is variably and incompletely absorbed from the gastrointestinal tract. Therefore, not all animals respond at the lower end of the dosage levels. If a poor response is seen, the dosage may have to be increased. It should be given with a fatty meal to enhance absorption. Griseofulvin has a disagreeable taste, and nausea may be seen. Dividing daily doses increases absorption and reduces nausea. The particle size of the drug also affects absorption, and this influences the dosage. There are two common forms, a microsize crystal Fulvicin-U/F, (Schering) given in a dosage of 25 to 60 mg/kg every 12 hours (most common initial dose is 25 mg/kg q12h) and ultramicrosize Gris-PEG in polyethylene glycol (Herbert), given in a dosage of 2.5 to 15 mg/kg every 12 hours. This difference is important to recognize or toxicities may result. Idiosyncratic toxic reactions, particularly bone marrow suppression, have been reported.[97] In problem cases, the dosage of microsize griseofulvin can be increased to at least 120 mg/kg/day with reasonable safety. One author recommended that kittens younger than 12 weeks of age not receive griseofulvin, although some clinicians use it in kittens as young as 6 weeks.[171] Gris-PEG should not be given to kittens younger than 6 weeks of age. Kunkle and Meyer[119] gave cats 110 to 145 mg/kg daily for 11 weeks without any signs of clinical, hematologic, or hepatic toxicity. They concluded that abnormalities developing with the use of high-dose griseofulvin therapy may be an idiosyncratic reaction found in only a few cats.[119] Adverse reactions to griseofulvin may be more common and severe in Persians, Himalayans, Siamese, and Abyssinians.[171]

Griseofulvin is a potent teratogen; therefore, it is absolutely contraindicated in pregnant animals. The most common problem is gastrointestinal upsets that resolve when administration of the drug is discontinued. Anemia, leukopenia, depression, ataxia, and pruritus have also been reported. They supposedly regress when the drug is withdrawn, although fatal reactions may occur. Hemograms every 2 weeks and careful observation are advisable during therapy to monitor those blood variables and the early onset of toxicity. The bone marrow reactions occur more commonly in cats with feline immunodeficiency virus infection, and screening before therapy is indicated.[255]

Griseofulvin does have anti-inflammatory and immunomodulatory properties and is known to suppress delayed-type hypersensitivity reactions and irritant reactions in the skin.[44] These properties can lead to important clinical misinterpretations. The authors have seen dogs and cats whose inflammatory skin diseases (e.g., bacterial pyoderma and pemphigus foliaceus) showed significant improvement while the animals were receiving large doses of griseofulvin for presumed dermatophytosis.

■ *Ketoconazole.* Ketoconazole (Nizoral [Janssen]) is a synthetic fungal imidazole derivative that is active against many fungi and yeasts, including dermatophytes, *Candida, Malassezia,* and numerous dimorphic fungi responsible for systemic mycoses.[94, 170, 201] It acts by inhibiting the synthesis of ergosterol, the main membrane lipid of fungal cells. With decreased ergosterol levels, the cell is unable to maintain membrane integrity, and the results are increased permeability, cell degeneration, and death. This effect is delayed, and the onset of action of ketoconazole takes 5 to 10 days. Consequently, in serious cases of systemic fungal disease, amphotericin B, which acts rapidly, is often used in combination with ketoconazole to compensate for this initial delay.

Ketoconazole is insoluble in water but soluble in dilute acid solutions, and increased gastric acidity promotes absorption. When it is given with food, especially tomato juice, absorption is enhanced. It should not be given with gastric antacids, drugs such as cimetidine, or anticholinergics. Although ketoconazole is not approved for use in dogs and cats in the United States, there are many reports of its use with suggested dosages and frequencies of administration varying from 2.5 to 40 mg/kg given every 24 hours to every 12 hours, respectively. In the authors' experience, 10 mg/kg every 24 hours is effective in more than 90 per cent of cases. For systemic mycoses, higher dosages (30 to 40 mg/kg/day) are more commonly needed. Because ketoconazole does not readily enter the CNS, a dosage of 40 mg/kg every 24 hours is commonly necessary for life-threatening CNS and nasal mycoses. Recommended doses for *Malassezia* dermatitis vary from as low as 2.5 mg/kg to 10 mg/kg every 12 hours. One report indicated that 10 mg/kg every 12 hours was routinely effective but that 7.5 mg/kg every 12 hours was effective in only 80 per cent of cases.[146] The authors and many other clinicians had excellent results with 10 mg/kg every 24 hours (see Chap. 5).

Although this agent is relatively well tolerated, canine side-effects occur, including inappetence, pruritus, alopecia, and a reversible lightening of the haircoat.[170] It also enhances the effects of anticoagulants and increases the blood levels of cyclosporine and antihistamines, and its concentration may be decreased if it is given concurrently with rifampin. At dosages higher than 40 mg/kg/day, there were anorexia, nausea, and increased liver enzyme levels. Cats are more sensitive and more frequently have anorexia, fever, depression, vomiting, diarrhea, and neurologic abnormalities; therefore, lower doses or even alternate-day therapy may be necessary. Cholangiohepatitis has also been seen in cats treated with ketoconazole.[90, 170, 177] Ketoconazole may be teratogenic. In dosages of 10 to 30 mg/kg/day, it suppressed basal cortisol concentration and response to ACTH, suppressed serum testosterone concentrations, and increased serum progesterone concentrations in dogs.[175] When administration of the drug is halted, a sharp rebound of testosterone levels occurs. In therapeutic use, one should be aware of the possible effect on libido and breeding effectiveness in male animals and the possibility of inducing or exacerbating prostate disease, as well as the potential for managing prostate disease, mammary carcinoma, and spontaneous hyperadrenocorticism.[32] Ketoconazole also has various immunomodulatory effects, including suppression of neutrophil chemotaxis and lymphocyte blastogenic responses, inhibition of 5-lipoxygenase activity, and inhibition of leukotriene production.[130, 215, 283]

In veterinary medicine, ketoconazole is effective in the treatment of dermatophytosis, candidiasis, *Malassezia* dermatitis, blastomycosis, coccidioidomycosis, histoplasmosis, and cryptococcosis (see Chap. 5).[83, 187] In addition, it may be effective in some cases of mycetoma, phaeohyphomycosis, zygomycosis, sporotrichosis, alternariosis, aspergillosis, and prototheccosis (see Chap. 5). In humans and experimental animals, it produced good results in candidiasis, dermatophytosis, histoplasmosis, and paracoccidioidomycosis; moderate results with coccidioidomycosis, chromomycosis, and aspergillosis; but poor results with mycetomas, aspergillomas, and phaeohyphomycoses.[269] Ketoconazole is often prescribed in combination with amphotericin B for systemic infections, because the antifungal activity of both seems to be enhanced.

■ *Iodides.* Iodides are given orally in daily doses of saturated solutions. They have a disagreeable taste and may cause nausea and iodism, especially in cats. Iodism may manifest as vomiting, diarrhea, depression, and anorexia. In dogs, ocular and nasal discharge, scaling, and a dry haircoat may be seen. Other signs that have been described in cats include twitching, hypothermia, and cardiovascular failure. Although iodides are widely distributed in the body, their mechanism of action is unknown because they have no efficacy against fungal organisms in vitro. Iodides are anti-inflammatory agents by virtue of their ability to quench toxic oxygen metabolites and inhibit neutrophil chemotaxis.[168]

Iodides are highly effective in the treatment of sporotrichosis. A supersaturated solution of potassium iodide is used. Dogs are given 40 mg/kg orally every 12 hours with food. Cats are given 20 mg/kg every 12 to 24 hours with food.

■ *Itraconazole.* Itraconazole (Sporonox [Janssen]) is a triazole, similar to imidazole derivatives, but contain three nitrogens on the azole ring. It is used orally for the systemic treatment of mycoses at 10 to 20 mg/kg every 24 to 48 hours (see Chap. 5).[38] It is more efficacious than ketoconazole. Susceptible organisms include dermatophytes, *Candida* spp., *Malassezia*, those causing many intermediate and deep mycoses, *Aspergillus*, and the protozoans *Leishmania* and *Trypanosoma*. The drug is given orally and produces higher tissue levels than the corresponding peak plasma levels. Itraconazole is bound to keratinocytes and is secreted in sweat and sebum.

Toxicity studies in dogs showed that, even at a dosage of 40 mg/kg/day for 90 days, there were no reactions. Although it is not recommended during pregnancy owing to teratogenic effects at high dosages, there were no detectable teratogenic effects at 10 mg/kg/day. In cats, 50 to 100 mg/kg/day produced some side-effects, which appeared to be dose dependent. Anorexia, nausea, and hepatotoxicity were primarily seen and usually resolved after drug withdrawal.

■ *Fluconazole.* Fluconazole (Diflucan [Roerig]) is another synthetic triazole that is given orally at 2.5 to 5 mg/kg every 24 hours in the dog. It is relatively poorly bound to plasma protein and penetrates CNS and saliva well. This feature makes it more desirable for treating fungal meningitis and oral candidiasis.

■ *Amphotericin B.* Amphotericin B (Fungizone [Apothecon]) is a fungicidal antibiotic that disrupts fungal (and bacterial) cell membranes by binding with ergosterol. It also binds to mammalian cell membranes and therefore is relatively toxic. Amphotericin B is most effective for blastomycosis, histoplasmosis, coccidioidomycosis, cryptococcosis, and candidiasis: in the first three diseases, when combined with ketoconazole, and in the last two, when combined with flucytosine. These combination protocols are used to take advantage of the prompt action of amphotericin B and to reduce its toxicity. Problems of therapy include nephrotoxicity (especially in dehydrated and hyponatremic animals), anemia, phlebitis, and hypokalemia.[216]

Organisms tend to develop resistance to the drug. Amphotericin given systemically must be given intravenously dissolved *only* in 5 per cent dextrose and water. A reasonable dosage for dogs is 0.5 mg/kg on alternate days and for cats, which are more sensitive, 0.15 mg/kg. Treatment with this drug is dangerous and complicated, and clinicians are advised to consult other references for specific guidelines.[83, 170, 216]

■ *Flucytosine.* Flucytosine (Ancobon [Roche]) is an orally administered fluorinated pyramidine that has been useful against *Candida, Cryptococcus, Aspergillus,* and some fungi associated with phaeohyphomycosis. Fungal cells are susceptible if they convert flucytosine to fluorouracil, which interferes with DNA synthesis. Resistant, mutant organisms emerge regularly and rapidly in the presence of the drug, which is why it is combined with amphotericin B. The oral dosage is 60 mg/kg every 8 hours, but it is used as a second-line treatment, when more effective drugs, such as the imidazole and thiazole derivatives, are not available or are not well tolerated. As a single agent, flucytosine rarely produces side-effects. Hematologic, gastrointestinal, and hepatic toxicities are reported. Fixed drug eruptions on the scrotum of dogs and toxic epidermal necrolysis have also been seen by the authors.

Systemic Antiparasitic Agents

A variety of oral, topical, or parenterally given products are available that produce either blood levels or cutaneous levels of the active agents. The advantages of these products are their relative ease of administration and the certainty of their reaching the whole body. The diffuse and certain distribution make this type of product especially valuable in eliminating mites in long-coated animals. The disadvantages are the relative risks and the use of parasitic poisons internally to kill ectoparasite infestations. There is also the risk of additive toxicity if the pet is exposed to other topical insecticides. Another potential difficulty is the duration of effective blood levels between treatments. Fortunately, the newer generations of systemic parasiticidal agents are not similar to the poisons of the past.

Two main mechanisms for presentation to parasites occur with systemic products. The original products, such as cythioate and fenthion, produce a level of active agent in the blood, so that when a flea bites, it ingests a toxic dose. In this situation, the allergic host is still exposed to the saliva and any antigens it contains.[136] Therefore, this type of product is best for nonallergic patients. The other mechanism is incorporation or secretion into the epidermis or surface emulsion, as typified by permethrin.

The use of systemic agents should be approached with knowledge regarding the parasite to be treated and, most importantly, the biology of the parasite. For example, feeding habits of the parasite may influence efficacy, as shown in a study by Dryden.[50] Female fleas, owing to their ingestion of larger quantities of blood, are more effectively killed by cythioate than are male fleas.[50] Systemic agents are particularly valuable in treating obligate parasites such as *Sarcoptes, Notoedres, Cheyletiella,* and *Demodex* mites. They are valuable as adjunctive therapy for nonobligate parasites, such as fleas, because they are generally not effective as a sole therapeutic agent. The mechanism of action of the drug, the route of parasitic exposure, the duration of effective tissue or exposure levels, and the biology of the parasite must all be considered when using systemic antiparasitic agents.

SYSTEMIC ORGANOPHOSPHATES

■ *Cythioate.* Cythioate (Proban [Miles]) is a popular, orally administered organophosphate that has been heavily promoted to dog owners. It is marketed in a 1.6 per cent solution or in 30-mg tablets for oral use. The dosage of 3 mg/kg twice weekly for weeks apparently has a wide margin of safety.[67b] However, severe overdosing sharply decreases serum cholinesterase levels without clinical signs. The levels return to normal 42 days after medication administration is halted.[226] In the United States, cythioate is not licensed for use in the cat. It is, however, frequently and safely used in cats at a dosage of 1.5 mg/kg given orally twice weekly.[16, 37a, 67b] However, this extralabel use should not be recommended in the United States.

Several problems may cause concern. Effective blood levels are maintained for only 6 to 12 hours after oral administration and an increase in dose frequency may produce toxicity. Administration to dogs with heartworms or liver disorders may be dangerous. The use of cythioate in animals with flea bite hypersensitivity does not stop the cause of the hypersensitivity reaction, and the flea burden in the environment must be controlled.

■ *Fenthion.* Fenthion is a highly toxic, stable organophosphate. It is primarily poured on large animals to eradicate *Hypoderma* larvae. It is an oily liquid with a disagreeable odor. In the past, it was used for flea control on dogs and cats in the United States in the form of a nonapproved product (Spotton [Miles]).[136] Mason and colleagues[147] showed in a field study that an optimal canine dosage of 20 mg/kg every 14 to 21 days was safe and highly effective. Although it decreased serum cholinesterase levels significantly, they were essentially reactivated after 14 days.[227]

The legal and only recommended form of fenthion (Pro-Spot) has been approved for dogs with a recommended dosage of 8 mg/kg repeated every 14 days.[10, 14] It is applied to the skin at the base of the skull or between the shoulders. Regrettably, the approved dosage (8 mg/kg) of this product is much lower than the optimal dosage (20 mg/kg), as determined by field trials. The benefit of this treatment is controversial, and this may partly reflect whether the drug is used at recommended or higher levels. In the authors' experience, adequate flea control with this approved product is maintained for only 5 to 7 days after application, necessitating either extra label use of the product, or the use of other flea control measures during the second week after application. Significant toxicity is seen after a dosage of 90 mg/kg every 14 days for three doses; death occurs after a single dose of 270 mg/kg.[140] Fenthion has also been used for flea control in cats (6.2 mg/kg applied to the back of the neck), although it has not been approved for this usage.[67a]

Use of fenthion has been controversial, as unintentional toxicity may occur and it has unpredictable effects. Additionally, there are reports of human intoxication following handling of fenthion or pets recently treated with the nonapproved product (Spotton). As with cythioate, exposure to other cholinesterase-inhibiting products (powders, sprays, dips, and premise sprays) may lead to toxicity, even when usually safe recommended dosages of either product are used. Fenthion is dangerous to patients and owners. Nonapproved fenthion (Spotton) should not be used in small animals.

PERMETHRIN "SPOT-ON"

Permethrin (Ex-Spot and Defend [Pitman-Moore]) is available as a topical concentrated (65 per cent) formula. It is licensed as a topical parasiticide but may have some systemic effect via percutaneous diffusion. However, it does not always have a complete systemic effect. Many anecdotal reports of incomplete control with just one or two spot applications, as directed on the package, have been received by the authors. Clients and veterinarians have noted fleas confined to areas (e.g., distal limbs and face) distant from the treated sites, and reported improved efficacy when a recommended dose is divided into smaller amounts and applied in a greater number of spots.

SYSTEMIC ENDECTOCIDES

These parasiticides were developed from macrocyclic lactones produced by the fermentation of various actinomycetes.[20, 24] This class of drugs includes avermectins (e.g., ivermectin), milbemycin, and moxidectin. Currently, the two products used in veterinary dermatology are ivermectin and milbemycin. Both at least partly act by potentiating the release and effects of γ-aminobutyric acid (GABA). GABA is a peripheral neurotransmitter in susceptible nematodes, arachnids, and insects.[20] In mammals, GABA is limited to the CNS. Because these drugs do not cross the blood-brain barrier in most adult animals, they are relatively safe and have a wide margin between efficacy and mammalian toxicity. The current known exception is the collie breed of dog, which often seems to lack the effectiveness of the blood-brain barrier in inhibiting access of these drugs, when used at higher dosages necessary to treat some arachnid infestations. In general, these drugs are effective for nematodes, microfilaria, lice, fur mites, *Otodectes*, *Sarcoptes*, *Notoedres*, *Cheyletiella*, and *Demodex*.

■ ***Ivermectin.*** Ivermectin (Ivomec [MSDAGVET]) is a derivative of avermectin B from fermentation products of *Streptomyces avermitilis*.[179, 263] This drug is noted for activity against nematodes, microfilaria, and *Sarcoptes*, *Cheyletiella*, *Notoedres*, and *Otodectes* mites.[179, 263] Although in the past ivermectin was not shown to be efficacious for *Demodex* with the treatment protocols that had been effective for other ectoparasites (e.g., 0.2 to 0.4 mg/kg, subcutaneously, weekly for up to 8 weeks),[253] reports confirm the efficacy of ivermectin when administered orally at 0.3 to 0.6 mg/kg/day (see Chap. 6).[182, 183] It has also been advocated as beneficial for treating *Demodex* infestation when used concurrently with topical amitraz. In these cases, it is dosed at 0.25 mg/kg subcutaneously every 7 to 14 days.[120] However, the long-term benefits of this combination of drugs have yet to be conclusively demonstrated. One author (CEG) found it to be effective in cases that were amitraz treatment failures.[90]

Ivermectin does not affect trematodes and cestodes, because GABA is not involved in neurotransmission in those species. Parasite paralysis is the main action of ivermectin, but it also suppresses reproduction. Ticks are not killed, but their egg production and molting are suppressed.

Ivermectin can be given parenterally or orally with good absorption. Ivermectin is rapidly absorbed orally and persists in the tissues for prolonged periods. This is important because it does not have a rapid killing effect on susceptible parasites. Ivermectin is approved in the United States only for dogs at a low monthly dosage (0.06 mg/kg orally) for heartworm prophylaxis (Heartgard 30 [MSDAGVET]). Neither this dosage nor this frequency of administration is effective against ectoparasites. Experimental reports indicate that single oral or subcutaneous doses of 0.2 mg/kg are effective for canine and feline scabies and *Otodectes* infestations.[20, 24, 70, 140, 173, 179] Ivermectin (Ivomec) has been administered subcutaneously to dogs and cats (0.3 mg/kg, repeated in 3 weeks) for the successful treatment of canine and feline cheyletiellosis.[179]

The use of ivermectin in a collie, Shetland sheepdog, or any dog resembling a collie is contraindicated. The authors (DWS and WHM) also believe that Old English sheepdogs should be included in this group. In addition, ivermectin should not be administered to puppies younger than 3 months of age, because toxicity may be seen in *any* breed. Ivermectin should *not* be used concurrently with other GABA-potentiating drugs (e.g., diazepam). The vehicle has no effect on toxicity of the oral dosage form,[185] and injectable doses of 1/200 of the lethal dose for beagles killed collies sensitive to the drug. Collies that died had high levels of ivermectin in the CNS. Signs of toxicity advanced from ataxia, depression, mydriasis, tremors, recumbency, and vomiting to death.[196] Some animals respond to supportive care, but picrotoxin is the only drug with the potential to reverse the toxicity.[20] No adverse effects on spermatogenesis, fertility, or reproductive performance were seen when ivermectin was given to male beagles at 0.6 mg/kg orally per month for eight treatments.[45]

Ivermectin also has apparent anti-inflammatory properties. The authors have seen many dogs, whose ultimate dermatologic diagnosis was atopy, food hypersensitivity, or bacterial pyoderma, that had marked reduction in pruritus or decreased visible inflammation for 3 to 7 days after receiving ivermectin. Ivermectin has been shown to have immunomodulatory effects, especially at the level of T cells, in mice.[23]

Ivermectin toxicosis is rare in cats (usually seen in kittens), develops within 1 to 12 hours after administration of the drug, and is characterized by abnormal behavior, ataxia, lethargy, weakness, recumbency, apparent blindness, coma, and death.[130a]

■ *Milbemycin.*   Milbemycin (Interceptor [Ciba-Geigy]) is derived from fermentation products of *Streptomyces hygroscopicus*. It is similar to ivermectin in activity with the notable addition of efficacy in amitraz-resistant generalized canine demodicosis.[76, 161, 199] An oral dosage of 0.5 mg/kg every 24 hours may be effective, but improved results were seen with 1 mg/kg every 24 hours.[161] Similar to the case with ivermectin, some collies are sensitive to milbemycin[280] at dosages of 5 mg/kg or higher. Because dosages of 1 to 2 mg/kg have not been reported to cause adverse reactions, milbemycin is probably safe for use in collies with generalized demodicosis. Two of the authors (DWS and WHM) have found milbemycin to be very effective in the treatment of canine scabies (2mg/kg orally, once weekly for three treatments).

CHITIN SYNTHESIS INHIBITORS

Another approach to flea destruction is the use of chitin synthesis inhibitors.[24a, 70a, 98a] Chitin is a major component of the flea exoskeleton. This class of drugs prevents the normal production of chitin, which is needed for insect embryogenesis and hatching. The first of this type of product is a systemic drug that is absorbed by the flea when it feeds. Lufeneron (Ciba-Geigy), a benzoyl urea, is dosed orally at 10 to 15 mg/kg once monthly. Eggs laid by fleas that feed on an adequately treated dog fail to hatch or new larvae fail to molt.

■ IMMUNOMODULATING AGENTS

The immune system plays a role in virtually any inflammatory and possibly some noninflammatory skin diseases. Numerous drugs exert all or part of their action by interfering or interacting with some aspect of the patient's immune response. Therefore, any scheme that tries to classify drugs by their effect on the immune system is obviously greatly oversimplified and numerous crossovers occur. However, for the clinician, it is sometimes helpful to consider drugs by their overall influence on the immune system as it relates to proposed causes of certain types of dermatologic diseases. Considering the difficulty encountered with oversimplification, the authors still believe that it is appropriate to look broadly at immunomodulating drugs in several ways.

Hyposensitization is the process of decreasing the hypersensitive (allergic) response of an animal to the exposure of an allergen. *Immunorestoration* is the use of drugs or biological agents to restore a more normal immune response. *Immunostimulation* is the use of drugs or biological agents to stimulate a protective immune response. *Immunosuppressive* agents are drugs that are used to treat autoimmune skin diseases, as well as diseases classified as immune-mediated owing to inappropriate immune responses. *Anti-inflammatory* agents are drugs or agents used to decrease tissue inflammation.

Many biological and synthetic immunomodifiers, adjuvants, and drugs with both specific and nonspecific effects on immunity have been investigated.[8, 57, 206, 259, 261] Many new therapies are in the developmental stage. Many of these agents and products were discovered as being a regulatory component of normal immune responses and are being investigated for their potential therapeutic uses. However, it appears likely that important gains of the next decade will come from the sphere of immunomodulation. When the mechanism of actions of the many immunomodulating agents are more completely understood, specific sequential combinations can be used to achieve desired clinical results.

Hyposensitization

Hyposensitization is a biological therapy typically used for atopic patients. It involves giving multiple increasing doses of antigens (allergens) that the animal is sensitive to parenterally. The classic explanation of the beneficial effects is the blocking antibody theory. This theory proposes that the patient responds by forming allergen-specific IgG antibodies against each specific antigen. These circulating antibodies are protective because they bind with invading allergens before those allergens reach tissue-fixed, allergen-specific IgE or IgGd. This blocking antibody theory is only a partial explanation of hyposensitization, because other mechanisms are proposed, such as a decrease in cellular sensitivity or a long-term diminution of the reaginic antibody available to sensitize mediator-releasing cells (tolerization). Hyposensitization therapy methods are covered in Chapter 8, in the discussion on canine atopy.

Immunorestoration

The concept of restoring a dysfunctional or failing immune system has many parallels with treatment of other organ systems in the body. The most obvious in immunology relate to immunoglobulin replacement, interferon therapy, administration of thymic hormones, and bone marrow and fetal liver transplantation. In addition, T cell–produced soluble mediators, such as lymphokines and interleukins, transmit growth and differentiation signals among immunocytes.

Immunoglobulins have long been used for passive immunization of patients with primary and secondary humoral immunodeficiency disorders. Immune and hyperimmune serum globulins have been used in a variety of primary B cell deficiencies (agammaglobulinemia) and secondary immunodeficiencies (burns, exfoliative dermatitis, and chronic lymphocytic leukemia) of humans, but the expense and frequent occurrence of adverse reactions are major concerns.

Levamisole (Levasole [Pitman-Moore]) is a synthetic chemical derivative of tetramisole, first introduced as a broad-spectrum anthelmintic. It acts directly on lymphocytes, macrophages, and granulocytes to modify their mobility, secretion, and proliferation. Its exact mechanism of action is unknown, but its effects are most pronounced in increasing the number and function of T lymphocytes in aged, diseased, or immunocompromised hosts.[31, 270] There is no effect on B cells or antibody production, and the drug does not increase immune responses above normal levels.

Although levamisole is a potent anthelmintic, it is not toxic to bacteria, viruses, protozoa, fungi, or tumor cells. It may increase the protective effect of some vaccines and stabilize tumor remission. Its potentiating effects are enhanced by the parallel administration of a primary stimulus such as an antigen. In humans, no effect is observed in young people, but in older people, the drug restores to normal levels a variety of immunologic functions. Levamisole has been used in humans with rheumatic, hypersensitivity, and neoplastic diseases, but the adverse effects of granulocytopenia, skin hypersensitivity, gastrointestinal disturbances, and immune suppression have made it a less desirable agent. Canine toxicity was reported after its use in a case of dirofilariasis at a dosage of 12 mg/kg every 24 hours.[169] The dog experienced ataxia, diarrhea, dyspnea, salivation, bradycardia, and stupor but responded within 4 days to treatment with the administration of atropine, isoproterenol, and glycopyrrolate and supportive care. Levamisole is also a potential cause of cutaneous drug eruption, erythema multiforme, and toxic epidermal necrolysis in dogs.

In veterinary immunology, it may be useful for chronic or recurrent infections involving skin or soft tissues and in primary and secondary immunodeficiency states.[15, 204] The dosage is critical, because levamisole has a so-called window effect: doses that are higher or lower than optimum may produce immunosuppression rather than stimulation. Clinicians presently use 2.2 mg/kg orally repeated three times weekly.

Thiabendazole (Mintezol [MSD]) may be used as an immunorestorative, in a manner somewhat similar to levamisole, in dosages of 5 to 10 mg/kg orally three times weekly.[204]

Interferon is a natural, broad-spectrum antiviral glycoprotein that is species specific and produced by virtually all nucleated animal cells.[13a, 260] Three types are known: alpha, produced by monocytes; beta, produced by fibroblasts; and gamma, produced by T cells. When a cell is invaded by a virus, it responds by synthesizing and releasing interferon. The interferon binds to the surface of uninfected neighboring cells and stimulates them to produce a group of protective proteins that inhibit viral reproduction in a manner that is not fully understood. Interferon also activates macrophages and increases the destructive capacity of cytotoxic T cells and natural killer cells. It inhibits the division of cells, including some tumor cells. Although the therapeutic potential of interferon is promising, all types are pyrogenic, and there are many serious side-effects.

Thymic hormones are peptides that circulate in peripheral blood and are important in the development and maintenance of the immune system.[13, 271] Thymosin and its thymic fractions control the maturation and differentiation of T cells, and thus their normal function. With aging, there is decreased production of thymic hormones and an associated increased frequency of autoantibodies. These changes lead to increased susceptibility to infections, decreased resistance to tumor growth, and increased incidence of autoimmune diseases.[261] It is anticipated that thymic hormones may have future therapeutic relevance in problems of the aged and in management of some of the disease states common to that group of patients.[260, 261]

Immunostimulation

Immunostimulation describes therapies that theoretically normalize a deficient immunologic response status or enhance the patient's immunologic response. In veterinary dermatology, the most common indication for this type of therapy is recurrent staphylococcal infection. In general, it is speculative how these drugs work and what specific immunodeficiency the patient has, if any. In the vast majority of dermatologic cases treated with immunostimulants, the immunologic defect, if any, is probably relatively limited, because these dogs do not generally have severe immunosuppression. This is evidenced by their usual ability to survive and do well with intermittent antibiotic therapy, their lack of disease in other organ systems, and their lack of unusual susceptibility to other infectious agents (viral, protozoal, fungal, and so forth).

However, certain exceptions, including genetic diseases such as IgA deficiency, do exist. It is interesting to note that these proven immunologic disorders usually have symptoms other than skin disease, and for some of these, the typical immune stimulants are not effective in their management. Even in IgA deficiency, which is considered a relatively more common cause of immunodeficiency in the dog, treatment with staphage lysate can ameliorate the symptoms without normalizing the serum IgA levels.[93]

In practice, the use of immunostimulants is practical and helpful if certain principles are considered. The most important is that other diseases and causes of the patient's disease should be ruled out. Because the most common use of immunostimulants in dogs is for chronic, recurrent, staphylococcal pyoderma, these cases should first have other causes, such as hypo-thyroidism, Cushing's disease (endogenous or iatrogenic), allergic diseases, ectoparasite infestations, and keratinization disorders, ruled out or adequately controlled. It is often stated that immunostimulants are not efficacious in these diseases and are primarily indicated for idiopathic recurrent pyoderma.[15, 19, 48]

The next factor to consider is the relative need. If a dog needs antibiotics only intermittently, such as every 2 to 3 months, the use of immunostimulation therapy should be questioned. This decision can also be based on cost effectiveness. For small dogs that respond well to low levels of antibiotic pulse or maintenance therapy, the cost of immunostimulants may far exceed that for the antibiotics, which in most cases, are not associated with adverse effects. In evaluating the rational use and cost effectiveness of immunostimulants, the clinician should also consider that these agents are usually employed as adjunctive therapy. In most cases, the administration of immunostimulants only decreases the frequency of antibiotic use, but does not eliminate their use.

More than 50 immunostimulants have been described for use in veterinary medicine.[15] However, in routine clinical practice, only several are commonly utilized. This discussion is limited to more commonly used agents.

Staphylococcus phage lysate (staphage lysate) is an injectable solution made from the lysis of Cowan Types I and II *Staphylococcus aureus* by bacteriophage. The final solution contains bacterial antigenic components as well as virulent bacteriophage and medium components. Efficacy for treating superficial staphylococcal pyoderma in dogs has been documented in a double-blind, placebo-controlled trial.[47] This study showed that 33 per cent more of the dogs responded well with antibiotics and staphage lysate as compared with those responding to antibiotics and placebo.

A variety of treatment protocols have been recommended. In the controlled study, dogs were given 0.5 ml subcutaneously twice weekly. Other clinicians use 1 ml subcutaneously once weekly. Side-effects or adverse reactions are infrequent. It is believed to work by stimulating T lymphocytes, activating phagocytic cells, enhancing primary immune responses, and elevating immunoglobulin levels. Although it does stimulate immunoglobulin production in the dog, staphage lysate does not normalize depressed serum IgA levels, nor does it increase levels of IgG antibody to *S. intermedius*.[46, 48, 93] It does normalize deficient IgM levels.[46, 93] Staphage lysate did stimulate lymphocyte blastogenesis in dogs with bacterial pyoderma.[211]

Bacterial antigens may be useful in recurrent staphylococcal skin infections.[195, 198, 204] However, there is much debate about their effectiveness and method of action.[140, 204, 285] Cell wall antigens, particularly protein A and peptidoglycan, may be the most important immunostimulating components and may also act as hyposensitizing agents. Autogenous bacterins are expensive and have not been highly effective. However, in some cases that fail to respond to other immunostimulants, autogenous bacterins have been effective. *S. aureus* bacterin-toxoid (Staphoid A-B [Burroughs Wellcome]) is a cell wall antigen and toxoid mixture (both α and β toxins) from whole cultures of *S. aureus* (phage Types I, III, and V), which are inactivated in formalin. This product is used in cases of bacterial hypersensitivity, according to the dosage schedule in Table 3:7, with 67 to 88 per cent success.[195]

Propionibacterium acnes in a killed suspension (Immunoregulin [ImmunoVet]) is available as an immunostimulant for recurrent canine bacterial pyoderma. Initial reports suggested giving intravenous injections twice weekly for 2 weeks, then once weekly until improvement is seen, with once-monthly injections for maintenance. More than 50 per cent of the cases were said to be in complete remission, according to the manufacturer. In one study, placebo-controlled dosages of 0.03 to 0.07 ml/kg biweekly intravenously were used to treat chronic recurrent bacterial pyoderma. The Immunoregulin was used in conjunction with antibiotic therapy and, reportedly, improved the results.[19] Tinsley and Taylor[278] reported on its use in the successful management of a multicentric malignant mast cell tumor in a dog. The results in other field

Table 3:7. Staphoid A-B Dosage Schedule

Day	Intradermal (ml)	Subcutaneous (ml)	Total Dosage (ml)
1	0.1	0.15	0.25
2	0.1	0.40	0.50
3	0.1	0.65	0.75
4	0.1	0.90	1.00
5	0.1	1.15	1.25
12	0.1	1.40	1.50
19	0.1	1.65	1.75
26	0.1	1.90	2.00
Monthly	0.1	1.90	2.00

reports on tumors and bacterial pyoderma have been equivocal or disappointing.[15, 204] Additional work is needed to evaluate this product properly in small animal dermatology.

Other treatments that have been reported as helpful in treating chronic pyoderma include ketoconazole, cimetidine, and cimetidine-hydroxyzine combination.[122, 208] The cost of recommended dosage for cimetidine (5 to 10 mg/kg q12 h) may be prohibitive.[122] No controlled studies have been reported that document their efficacy, but when other treatments have been ineffective, their use should be considered.

Immunosuppression

The drugs used to treat immune-mediated skin diseases are generally referred to as immunosuppressive agents. However, for some of these drugs, their exact mechanism is unknown. They may act in methods different from those of the more classic immune-suppressive agents. They are considered together because, whatever their mechanism of action, they share the feature of being beneficial to manage the immune-mediated skin diseases. Glucocorticoids are the most common class of drugs used as immunosuppressive agents. They are discussed elsewhere in this chapter. However, many other drugs are used in practice and some are effective only in specific diseases (Table 3:8).

Cyclophosphamide

Cyclophosphamide (Cytoxan [Bristol-Meyers]) is an alkylating agent that is used alone or in combination with chemotherapy for the treatment of various neoplasms, as well as for its immunosuppressive activity in nonmalignant diseases and organ transplants.[204, 264] It acts to revert mitosis by interference with DNA replication and ribonucleic acid (RNA) translation. Able to kill cells in all phases of the cell cycle, this type of cytotoxic drug is more effective in slow-growing tumors than are phase-specific drugs that act during only a specific time of the cell cycle. It is most effective against rapidly dividing cells. Lymphocytes are especially sensitive to cyclophosphamide. The drug is immunosuppressive to both the humoral and cell-mediated immune systems, but it is more effective against B cells than against T cells. Cyclophosphamide suppresses antibody production. Maximal effect is seen if the drug is given shortly after the antigenic stimulus, when it suppresses primary and secondary humoral responses.

Major toxic sequelae include sterile hemorrhagic cystitis, bladder fibrosis, teratogenesis, infertility, alopecia, nausea, inflammation of the gastrointestinal tract, increased susceptibility to infections, and depression of the bone marrow and hematopoietic systems. Its effects should be monitored with periodic hemograms and urinalysis.

Clinical indications include lymphoreticular neoplasms, for which the drug is best combined

Table 3:8. Immunosuppressive Drugs and Indications

Drug	Induction Dose	Indications
Glucocorticoids		Short-term use in severe cases of autoimmune disease
Prednisone	2.2–6.6 mg/kg q24h	
Prednisolone	2.2–6.6 mg/kg q24h	
Triamcinolone	0.2–0.6 mg/kg q24h	
Dexamethasone	0.2–0.6 mg/kg q24h	
Cyclophosphamide	1.5–2.5 mg/kg q48h	Undesirable for long-term use, short-term use only in severe cases
Azathioprine	1.5–2.5 mg/kg q24h (low dose in dogs >30 kg; high dose in dogs <15 kg)	All immune-mediated disorders; not for use in cats
Chlorambucil	0.1–0.2 mg/kg q24–48h (in cats, usually 0.2 mg/kg q48 h)	All, but especially feline diseases
Cyclosporine	10–20 mg/kg q24h	All
Chrysotherapy		
Aurothioglucose	1 mg/kg IM	Feline pemphigus foliaceus; plasma cell stomatitis; plasma cell pododermatitis; canine pemphigus complex (second choice)
Auranofin	3–6 mg q24h	
Dapsone	1 mg/kg q8h (in dogs)	Subcorneal pustular dermatosis; leukocytoclastic vasculitis; dermatitis herpetiformis
Sulfasalazine	22–44 mg/kg q8h	Subcorneal pustular dermatitis; vasculitis
Vitamin E	100–400 mg q12h	Discoid lupus erythematosus; pemphigus erythematosus; epidermolysis bullosa
Tetracycline and/or niacinamide	In dogs >10 kg: 500 mg q8h each In dogs <10 kg: 250 mg q8h each	Discoid lupus erythematosus; pemphigus erythematosus
Sun avoidance		Discoid lupus erythematous, pemphigus erythematosus, systemic lupus erythematosus

with corticosteroids or vincristine. It can be given with high doses of glucocorticoids to achieve remission of severe cases of immune-mediated diseases such as systemic lupus erythematosus, vasculitis, pemphigus complex, bullous pemphigoid, idiopathic thrombocytopenia, hemolytic anemia, gammopathies, and rheumatoid arthritis.[204, 264] The potential for hemorrhagic cystitis and bladder fibrosis makes this drug less desirable for long-term use than azathioprine or chlorambucil. The dosage for neoplasms is 50 mg/m² of body surface area for 4 days, then off 3 days; repeat each week. For immunosuppression, the oral dosage is 1.5 to 2.5 mg/kg every other day.

Azathioprine

Azathioprine (Imuran [Burroughs Wellcome]) is a synthetic modification of 6-mercaptopurine that can be given orally or by injection.[18a, 204] However, for skin diseases, the oral route is usually used. It is metabolized to 6-mercaptopurine, which interferes with DNA and RNA metabolism. Azathioprine primarily affects rapidly proliferating cells, with its greatest effects on cell-mediated immunity and T lymphocyte–dependent antibody synthesis. Primary antibody synthesis is affected more than secondary antibody synthesis. Azathioprine is preferred over 6-mercaptopurine because it has a more favorable therapeutic index.

Even so, it is a potent drug with potential toxicities, which include anemia, leukopenia, thrombocytopenia, vomiting, hypersensitivity reactions (especially of the liver), pancreatitis, elevated serum alkaline phosphatase levels, skin rashes, and alopecia. The most common significant side-effect is diarrhea, which may be hemorrhagic. This often responds to dose reductions or temporary discontinuation of the drug.[88] More than 90 per cent of the cases experience anemia and lymphopenia, but usually not to the degree that treatment needs to be discontinued. It has also been suggested that patients not responding to therapy that are not lymphopenic and otherwise tolerate the drug should have their dose of azathioprine increased.[88] Long-term therapy is associated with the development of demodicosis, recurrent bacterial pyoderma, or dermatophytosis in at least 10 per cent of cases.[88]

Patients should be monitored initially every 2 weeks with complete blood counts and platelet counts.[88, 204] After the patient's condition is stable, monitoring can be tapered to once every 4 months. If other symptoms occur, or at least yearly, a chemistry panel should also be run. Hepatitis and pancreatitis are the major conditions to monitor with chemistry panels.

In small animals, azathioprine may be beneficial for pemphigus complex, bullous pemphigoid, and both types of lupus erythematosus, as well as other autoimmune and immune-mediated disorders.[204] It is most commonly used in cases of canine pemphigus foliaceus that do not respond to glucocorticoids. Azathioprine is usually not used alone but is combined with systemic glucocorticoids. After remission is achieved, the dosages of both drugs are tapered, but initially, unless side-effects are a problem, the glucocorticoid dosage is tapered to levels approaching 1 mg/kg every 48 hours. The oral dosage of azathioprine for dogs is 1.5 to 2.5 mg/kg every 24 hours until clinical response is achieved, and then it is continued every other day for a month or longer. Slow tapering down to as little as 1 mg/kg every 72 hours may be achieved. Slow tapering to the lowest dose possible decreases side-effects and the expense of therapy. Corticosteroids can be given on the alternate days when azathioprine is not given.

Cats are susceptible to azathioprine toxicity (including fatal leukopenia and thrombocytopenia), and this drug should be used *very* cautiously, if at all, in this species.[18, 18a]

Chlorambucil

Chlorambucil (Leukeran [Burroughs Wellcome]) is an orally administered alkylating agent.[204] Compared with other alkylating agents, it is slow acting and less toxic. Although serious toxicity is rare at usual doses, myelosuppression is possible. Consequently, patients should initially be monitored with hemograms every 2 to 4 weeks.

Chlorambucil may be useful in the pemphigus complex, bullous pemphigoid, discoid and systemic lupus erythematosus, immune-mediated vasculitis, and cold agglutinin disease, as well as in lymphocyte and plasma cell malignancies.[204] It is particularly valuable in cats because azathioprine is relatively more toxic. It is most commonly combined with a glucocorticoid and, occasionally, with azathioprine. Chlorambucil may be used to replace cyclophosphamide if hemorrhagic cystitis develops during the use of that drug. The oral dosage in dogs and cats is 0.1 to 0.2 mg/kg every 24 to 48 hours.[202, 204, 205]

Cyclosporine

Cyclosporine (Sandimmune [Sandoz]) is a fat-soluble cyclic polypeptide metabolite of the fungus *Tolypocladium inflatum gams*.[204, 206] It is effective in preventing human organ transplantation rejection.[178] In animal models, it has been used with similar excellent results.[286] It has also been evaluated for the treatment of immune-mediated skin diseases and epitheliotropic lymphoma in animals.[206] Cyclosporine has low cytotoxicity relative to its immunosuppressive potency. It blocks the proliferation of activated T lymphocytes by inhibiting interleukin-2 (IL-2), gene activation, and messenger RNA transcription. Another important mechanism may be the inhibition of T cell surface receptors.

A high incidence of nephrotoxicity and hepatic toxicity is seen in people. Dogs may experience gingival hyperplasia and papillomatosis, vomiting, diarrhea, bacteriuria, bacterial skin infection, anorexia, nephropathy, bone marrow suppression, and a lymphoplasmacytoid dermatosis.[204, 206] Cats are reported to have only minor side-effects, although they may be more susceptible to viral infections.[85, 204, 206]

The clinical indications for cyclosporine therapy are organ transplantation and inhibition of delayed-type hypersensitivity reactions of many immune-mediated diseases. It is used in pemphigus foliaceus and immune-mediated myasthenia gravis, thyroiditis, neuritis, uveitis, and arthritis. Initial studies in dogs and cats with immunologic dermatoses such as pemphigus foliaceus, pemphigus erythematosus, and discoid lupus erythematosus have shown cyclosporine by itself to be rarely effective.[204, 206] Cyclosporine has been ineffective in the treatment of canine and feline epitheliotropic lymphoma (mycosis fungoides).[206]

The oral dosage for dogs and cats is 10 to 20 mg/kg daily, the dose for cats being divided and given twice daily.[126, 204] Variable absorptions may occur among individuals and from day to day, so it is possible that dosages of 10 mg/kg/day may be effective. After a response is seen, tapering to as low as 10 mg/kg every 48 hours may be effective.[206] As this is an expensive drug, the reduction to the lowest effective levels is usually important. Additionally, the expense and marginal efficacy usually limit its use to cases of treatment failure with or adverse reaction to alternative treatments.

Other Immunomodulatory Agents

CHRYSOTHERAPY

Chrysotherapy is the use of gold as a therapeutic agent. Gold compounds are capable of modulating many phases of immune and inflammatory responses, but the exact mechanisms of this effect are unknown.[173, 229] Gold is available in two dosage forms, which have dissimilar pharmacokinetics: the oral compound auranofin (Ridaura [SmithKline Beecham]) and the parenteral compound aurothioglucose (Solganal [Schering]). Neither form is approved for use in dogs and cats, but their distribution, metabolism, and actions have been established in humans and laboratory animals. Studies in humans show that the oral forms are 25 per cent absorbed and attain blood levels with a 21-day half-life, but only small amounts can be detected in tissues and skin.[276] In a few clinical trials in dogs with immune-mediated dermatoses, the results with oral gold were equivocal, but no adverse side-effects were observed.[288] The parenteral form is 100 per cent absorbed but has only a 6-day half-life in blood. It is 95 per cent protein bound and is well distributed to cells of the mononuclear phagocytic system, liver, spleen, bone marrow, kidneys, and adrenal glands. Much lower levels are detected in skin.

In humans, gold may act at several levels of the inflammatory and immune response. Auranofin appears to have an additional immunomodulating action, but both oral and parenteral golds inhibit bacteria, the first component of complement, and the epidermal enzymes that may be responsible for blister formation in pemphigus. Both also reduce the release of inflammatory mediators, such as lysosomal enzymes, histamine, and prostaglandin, and interfere with immunoglobulin-synthesizing cells.

Toxic effects are worrisome in humans, because 33 per cent of patients have some adverse reaction, although 80 per cent of these are minor. Most common are skin eruptions, oral reactions, proteinuria, and bone marrow depression. During the induction phase, a hemogram and urinalysis should be checked weekly, and monthly thereafter.[61, 229] Three cases of fatal toxic epidermal necrolysis were reported in dogs that had been treated with Solganal for 3 to 9 months.[115] This may be enhanced by previous or concurrent administration of azathioprine.[173, 204] Solganal-related erythema multiforme has been seen in both dogs and cats by the authors.

Parenteral gold (aurothioglucose) has been reported to be effective for the treatment of cases of canine and feline pemphigus that were unresponsive to glucocorticoids.[205, 229, 289] It has been useful for the treatment of canine bullous pemphigoid and feline plasma cell pododermatitis.[150, 173, 204] Although most adverse reactions develop late in therapy, it is suggested that a small test dose of 1 mg be given intramuscularly to patients with less than 10 mg of body weight and that 5 mg be given to larger patients in the first week. Dosage is increased to 1 mg/kg intramuscularly weekly until remission occurs. If no response is seen after 12 weeks of therapy, the dosage can be increased to 1.5 to 2 mg/kg.[204] After remission, one dose is given every 2 weeks, and then once monthly for several months. It is advisable to halt medication administration eventually for observation, because some patients go into complete remission, whereas other animals can be maintained on a reduced dosage. Two points of caution: (1) the treatment takes 6 to 12 weeks for full effect to occur, so that other medication—typically glucocorticoids—should be maintained, if needed, at full dosage until this lag period is passed; and (2) gold compounds should not be administered simultaneously with other cytotoxic drugs (such as azathioprine and cyclophosphamide), as toxicity is thereby enhanced.

The oral form of gold (auranofin) has been used in only a few dogs with pemphigus (at 3 to 6 mg/day) with little success. In addition, this oral form is expensive.

Gold is seldom the first-choice drug for pemphigus. Patients are usually started on a glucocorticoid regimen, with cyclophosphamide or azathioprine added to reduce the steroid dosage. In cases with excessive side-effects, gold is a logical second choice. It may be especially useful in cats.[150, 204]

SULFONES AND SULFONAMIDES

■ *Dapsone.* Dapsone (dapsone tablets, [Jacobus]) is an anti-inflammatory, antibacterial chemical (4,4'-diaminodiphenyl sulfone). It inhibits the action of lysosomal enzymes; neutrophil chemotaxis; degranulation of mast cells; synthesis of IgG, IgA, and prostaglandin; activation of the alternative complement pathway; and T cell responses.[299] It is an antioxidant scavenger and also inhibits proteases. Dapsone is useful in various diseases characterized by accumulations of neutrophils. It is often effective for vasculitis with lupus erythematosus or systemic lupus erythematosus–like disorders in humans. In these cases, the human dosage regimen starts low and rapidly builds to 150 mg/day. This dosage is held until response occurs and then is gradually decreased and stopped after 4 to 10 months. In many cases, there is no relapse. Treatment with dapsone is also effective in human leprosy, dermatitis herpetiformis, subcorneal pustular dermatosis, and some cases of pemphigus, pemphigoid, and rheumatoid arthritis.

In dogs, dapsone has been used with benefit in cases of subcorneal pustular dermatosis, leukocytoclastic vasculitis, linear IgA dermatosis, and pemphigus foliaceus and erythematosus.[234] Dapsone is most useful in the first two diseases, although not all cases were controlled. In the last three diseases, only about half the cases showed benefit. However, in some cases of pemphigus that were successfully treated with immunosuppressive combinations (such as azathioprine with corticosteroids), the addition of dapsone permitted lowering the dose of the corticosteroid.

Dapsone is not approved for use in dogs and cats in the United States, but reports suggest a dosage of 1 mg/kg every 8 hours orally for 2 to 4 weeks until lesions clear, and then a reduction of the frequency of administration to every 12 or 24 hours. The maintenance dosage should be further reduced to every 48 hours once or twice weekly, or even stopped, because toxicity is somewhat dose related.

Potential toxicity can be serious. During induction, mild anemia, leukopenia, and moderate elevations of serum alanine aminotransferase levels may be expected, but do not necessitate stopping treatment if the animal remains clinically normal. Blood dyscrasias, thrombocytopenias, skin reactions, and hepatic toxicity can be serious.[127] Patients should be monitored every 2 weeks during induction therapy with hemograms and platelet counts, blood urea nitrogen determination, urinalysis, and serum alanine aminotransferase determination. Cats are especially susceptible to dapsone toxicity, with hemolytic anemia and various neurotoxicities reported.

■ *Sulfasalazine.* Sulfasalazine (Azulfidine [Pharmacia]) is converted in the colon to sulfapyridine 5-aminosalicylate, which has anti-inflammatory action.[234] The dosage is 10 to 20 mg/kg every 8 hours orally.[208, 234] The dosage may be reduced or even changed to every other day, while maintaining clinical remission. A serious side-effect with long-term administration is the production of keratitis sicca. Thus, tear production should be checked regularly. In one report, two dogs with subcorneal pustular dermatosis were managed satisfactory with sulfasalazine after becoming refractory to dapsone.[234] Sulfasalazine has also been used successfully in the management of vasculitis.[63, 204]

TETRACYCLINE AND NIACINAMIDE

The combination of tetracycline and niacinamide has been recommended for the treatment of discoid lupus erythematosus and pemphigus erythematosus in dogs. Reported results are variable, but 25 to 65 per cent of cases have an excellent response.[203, 292] The precise mechanism of action is unknown. However, tetracyclines possess various anti-inflammatory and immunomodulatory properties, including suppression of in vitro lymphocyte blastogenic transformation and antibody production, suppression of in vivo leukocyte chemotactic responses, inhibition of the activation of complement component 3, inhibition of lipases and collagenases, and inhibition of prostaglandin synthesis.[103] Niacinamide has been shown to block antigen-IgE–induced histamine release in vivo and in vitro, prevent degranulation of mast cells, inhibit phosphodiesterases, and decrease protease releases.[293]

The initial dosage for dogs weighing more than 10 kg is 500 mg of tetracycline and 500 mg of niacinamide given every 8 hours. If a favorable response is seen, the dosage may be decreased to every 12 hours and then to every 24 hours. Although no studies have been reported, one author (CEG) noted that this combination may have shown benefit when used concurrently with vitamin E or glucocorticoids. It was also reported that tetracycline alone may be beneficial in treating discoid lupus erythematosus.[203] Side-effects are uncommon, although vomiting, diarrhea, and anorexia have been reported.[203] One author (CEG) also saw two cases of anorexia with increased liver enzyme activity that resolved with discontinuation of therapy. In one case, tetracycline administration was continued, suggesting that the niacinamide was responsible for the adverse reactions.

PENTOXIFYLLINE

Pentoxifylline (Trental [Hoechst-Roussel]) is a methylxanthine derivative that produces a variety of physiologic changes at the cellular level.[217a] Immunomodulatory effects include increased leukocyte deformability and chemotaxis, decreased leukocyte responsiveness to IL-1 and TNF-α, inhibition of T and B lymphocyte activation, and decreased natural killer cell activity. In humans, these effects are beneficial in the treatment of peripheral vascular disease, vasculitis, and contact hypersensitivity. The drug also affects wound healing and connective tissue disorders through increased production of collagenase and decreased production of collagen, fibronectin, and glycosaminoglycans. Pentoxifylline has been used in veterinary medicine for the treatment of canine familial dermatomyositis (see Chap. 11).

ANTIMALARIALS

Several antimalarials have been useful for the treatment of humans with discoid lupus erythematosus, dermatomyositis, polymorphous light eruption, solar urticaria, and scleroderma.[107] There are also anecdotal reports of response with cutaneous leishmaniasis, cutaneous cryptococcosis, epidermolysis bullosa, and lymphocytic skin infiltrations.[272] Antimalarials may have future use in problem cases involving animals with such diseases.

Their specific mode of action is unknown, but the drugs stabilize lysosomal membranes and thus are anti-inflammatory. They inhibit protein synthesis, viral replication, and cell-mediated immunity. They do not affect the development of primary or secondary antibody response but do inhibit complement. Consequently, they may inhibit the formation of immune complexes, which explains their effectiveness in systemic lupus erythematosus and related autoimmune disorders. The drugs are seldom used alone for first-line therapy and, in humans, are usually given with salicylates or small doses of corticosteroids. Side-effects are numerous, the most serious affecting the eyes.

The drugs most commonly used in humans are quinacrine hydrochloride (Atabrine hydrochloride [Winthrop]), chloroquine (Aralen [Winthrop]), and hydroxychloroquine sulfate (Plaquenil sulfate [Winthrop]). Their place in veterinary dermatology has yet to be determined, although anecdotal reports suggested that the antimalarials may be beneficial in canine lupus erythematosus.[173] No case reports or studies supporting their efficacy have been reported.

Sun Avoidance

The immune-mediated diseases discoid lupus erythematosus and pemphigus erythematosus are often aggravated by exposure to sunlight. Sunlight has also been suggested to play a role in systemic lupus erythematosus, pemphigus complex, and bullous pemphigoid. At least in discoid lupus erythematosus, sun avoidance may make a dramatic difference in the severity of disease and, owing to its low expense and lack of side-effects, it should be recommended whenever possible.

■ NUTRITIONAL FACTORS

Nutritional factors that influence the skin are exceedingly complex (see Chap. 16). However, a variety of treatments use nutritional supplements. In most situations, these treatments entail high doses that most likely have other metabolic or pharmacologic effects than just meeting nutritional requirements. In most cases other than those discussed in Chapter 16, the success of these treatments is probably not related to nutritional deficiency. The most common agents used in nutritional therapies are fatty acids, vitamins, and minerals. Fatty acids as therapeutic agents were previously discussed. Although anecdotal reports suggested that vitamin C was useful for the treatment of allergic dogs, a clinical trial failed to support such claims.[164] B vitamins have also been purported to be effective flea repellents, but multiple controlled studies failed to document any efficacy.[12] Vitamin A and E do appear useful in specific syndromes and are discussed. Mineral therapy is also often recommended to clients. Sulfur, once believed to be an effective flea repellent, was shown not to be efficacious.[262] The one mineral that is useful to treat specific syndromes is zinc.

Vitamin A (retinol) must be available to cats, because they cannot convert β-carotene. In addition to its use for normal growth and differentiation of keratinocytes, vitamin A has important roles in the biosynthesis of mucopolysaccharides, labilization of lysosomal enzymes, inhibition of abnormal keratinization proliferation, suppression of size and function of sebaceous glands, modulation of neutrophil and macrophage function, and synthesis of prostaglandin.[43] It has been useful in large doses for treating a specific follicular keratosis called vitamin A–responsive dermatosis (see Chap. 13). An oral daily dosage of 1000 IU/kg is suggested, although higher dosages can be given initially, with lower dosages later in the course of therapy. Normal nutritional maintenance dosage approximates 100 IU/kg/day, and the toxic dosage is approximately 20,000 IU/kg daily.

Vitamin E is a fat-soluble natural antioxidant that is a mild antagonist to leukotriene formation. Therefore, one might more appropriately consider it an anti-inflammatory agent. Vitamin E has been used in the treatment of discoid lupus erythematosus, pemphigus erythematosus, epidermolysis bullosa, and acanthosis nigricans with variable results.[204, 242] Its mechanism of action in these immune-mediated skin diseases is unknown. The recommended dosage of *dl*-α-tocopherol acetate is 100 to 400 mg per animal twice daily for at least 30 to 60 days before its effect is seen. Excessive supplementation with fatty acids (especially unsaturated) may make vitamin E less available and may produce pancreatitis. Oral vitamin E was found to be of no value in treating dogs with allergic skin disease.[156]

Vitamin E has also been recommended for the treatment of generalized canine demodicosis, because low serum levels of vitamin E were found in that disease.[65, 66] However, in another study in which serum levels, not treatment, were evaluated there was no statistical difference in serum levels in dogs with pyoderma, demodicosis, or demodicosis with pyoderma.[78]

Zinc is an important factor in many enzyme systems; it is necessary for normal growth, keratinization, metabolism of protein and carbohydrate, and normal immune function.[118] In puppies fed zinc-deficient diets, there is T cell hypoplasia of the lymph nodes, spleen, and thymus.[218] Anecdotal comments have suggested it for treating burns, seborrhea, and recurrent bacterial pyoderma, as well as for stimulating wound healing.

Zinc has been effective in treating two specific dermatoses. One results from a probable genetic defect that is characterized by decreased intestinal absorption of zinc. This includes a disease seen in Siberian huskies and Malamutes (see Chap. 16) and carriers of lethal acrodermatitis of bull terriers (see Chap. 11). The other is a zinc-responsive dermatosis in dogs (often puppies) that are fed diets with excessive ingredients that interfere with zinc absorption or diets truly zinc deficient. This latter situation was reported with the syndrome generic dog food dermatosis (see Chap. 16). The ingredients calcium phytate (vegetable fiber and soybean meal), iron, tin, and copper in excess interfere with zinc absorption. This interference provides a classic example of how excessive use of nutritional supplements with a multitude of ingredients may do more harm than good.

Oral administration of zinc usually causes rapid resolution of the skin lesions. However, other investigators reported that, in zinc-related dermatoses of Siberian huskies and bull terriers (genetic problem), zinc sulfate is effective only if given intravenously.[296] A dosage of 10 to 15 mg/kg is given intravenously every week for 4 to 6 weeks (without adverse effects) and then used as needed for maintenance. In the first type of disorder, supplementation may be needed for life, whereas in the second case, after the patient responds, zinc supplements can be halted if the dietary imbalances are corrected.

Several zinc salts are effective. Dosages are variable and those given are the initial doses that should be tried. Zinc sulfate is inexpensive and available in 200-mg tablets and 220-mg capsules. It is dosed at 10 mg/kg every 24 hours or divided every 12 hours.[121] Zinc methionine (Zinpro) is said to be better absorbed, and therefore a dosage of 4 mg/kg/day is appropriate. Zinc gluconate is also satisfactory, although usually only available in smaller-sized tablets such as 20 mg. It is dosed at 5 mg/kg every 24 hours or divided and given every 12 hours. More research is needed to determine the efficacy of different methods of zinc administration. In addition, some cases respond at only doses much higher than the recommended initial dose. Oral administration of zinc was found to be of no value in treating dogs with allergic skin disease.[156]

■ SYNTHETIC RETINOIDS

Retinoids refer to all the chemicals, natural or synthetic, that have vitamin A activity. Synthetic retinoids are primarily retinol, retinoic acid, or retinal derivatives or analogs. They have been developed with the intent of amplifying certain biological effects while being less toxic than their natural precursors. More than 1500 synthetic retinoids have been developed and evaluated.[123, 191] Different synthetic drugs, all classed as synthetic retinoids, may have profoundly different pharmacologic effects, side-effects, and disease indications. With all the retinoid research being conducted, there will undoubtedly be many new discoveries and uses in the near future. To date, the biggest deterrent to their use is expense.

Naturally occurring vitamin A is an alcohol, all-*trans* retinol. It is oxidized in the body to retinal and retinoic acid. Each of these compounds has variable metabolic and biological activities, although both are important in the induction and maintenance of normal growth and differentiation of keratinocytes. Only retinol has all the known functions of vitamin A. Currently, two compounds are being used clinically in veterinary dermatology: isotretinoin (13-

cis-retinoic acid; Accutane [Roche]), synthesized as a natural metabolite of retinol, and etretinate (Tegison [Roche]), a synthetic retinoid. Etretinate will soon be unavailable for humans, because it is being replaced by acitretin, which is a carboxylic acid metabolically active metabolite of etretinate. Acitretin is less toxic owing to a shorter terminal elimination half-life of 2 days versus etretinate's 100 days. Etretinate is stored in body fat and has been found in trace amounts up to 3 years after cessation of therapy.[186]

Because of their numerous pharmacologic effects, retinoids are being used in the management of numerous diseases in humans. The long list includes such diverse diseases as acne, gram-negative folliculitis, hidradenitis suppurativa, the ichthyoses, multiple forms of psoriasis, a variety of cutaneous neoplasms, epidermal nevi, subcorneal pustular dermatosis, discoid lupus erythematosus, and acanthosis nigricans.[56, 186] The biological effects of retinoids are numerous, but their ability to regulate proliferation, growth, and differentiation of epithelial tissues is their major benefit in dermatology. However, retinoids also affect proteases, prostaglandins, humoral and cellular immunity, and cellular adhesion and communication.[186]

Isotretinoin is usually dosed at 1 to 3 mg/kg every 24 hours and appears to be indicated in diseases that require alteration or normalization of adnexal structures, although some epidermal diseases may respond.[123] Diseases in which isotretinoin has been reported to be effective in veterinary dermatology include Schnauzer comedo syndrome,[123] sebaceous adenitis (particularly early in the disease in Poodles and Vizslas or shorthaired breeds),[123, 191, 265] ichthyosis,[123] feline acne,[123] epitheliotropic lymphoma,[123, 191, 291] keratoacanthoma,[123, 191, 291] and sebaceous gland hyperplasias and adenomas.[191] Isotretinoin has been ineffective for primary idiopathic seborrhea of Cocker spaniels and Basset hounds and epidermal dysplasia of West Highland white terriers.[62, 123, 191] It was also ineffective in the treatment of preneoplastic and squamous cell carcinoma lesions in cats.[58]

Toxicity of isotretinoin in the dog and cat appears to be less of a problem than in humans.[123, 191] In the dog, conjunctivitis, hyperactivity, pruritus, pedal and mucocutaneous junction erythema, stiffness, vomiting, diarrhea, and keratoconjunctivitis may be seen. Laboratory abnormalities that are generally not associated with clinical signs include hypertriglyceridemia, hypercholesterolemia, and increased levels of alanine aminotransferase, aspartate aminotransferase, and alkaline phosphatase.[123, 191] In cats, conjunctivitis, diarrhea, anorexia, and vomiting have been the major side-effects seen.[90, 123, 191] These side-effects may be transient or self-limited with discontinuation or decrease in dose of the drug. With long-term use, skeletal abnormalities, including cortical hyperostosis, periosteal calcification, and long bone demineralization, are a concern.[56, 123, 186, 191] All retinoids are potent teratogens.

Etretinate is believed to be indicated for disorders of epithelial or follicular development or keratinization. Most commonly, etretinate is given at 1 mg/kg every 24 hours. Etretinate is reportedly effective for primary idiopathic seborrhea of Cocker and Springer spaniels,[90, 123, 191, 192] Golden retrievers, Irish setters, and some mixed breeds. It has not been effective in West Highland white terriers, Basset hounds, or collies.[123, 191] However, one author (CEG) saw some partial responses in West Highland white terriers after secondary *Malassezia* dermatitis was controlled. Although the use is more controversial, etretinate may also be effective in sebaceous adenitis.[90, 191] In contrast to one report, the author (CEG) notes favorable response to etretinate in Akitas with sebaceous adenitis.

Ichthyosis has also been reported to respond to etretinate. In dogs, solar dermatosis and squamous cell carcinoma were reported to improve.[143a, 191] Follicular dysplasias such as color dilution alopecia may also respond, with less scaling and partial hair growth.[87] Keratoacanthomas may also respond, although it appears that isotretinoin is more effective.[87]

Toxicity with etretinate is similar to that seen with isotretinoin. In humans, etretinate is considered safer for long-term use because of a lower propensity for producing skeletal abnormalities. However, it is considered more of a teratogen and should be used only in spayed females, breeding males, or female dogs that will not be used for breeding. Teratogenicity may persist even 2 years after cessation of therapy.[186, 191, 192] Monitoring for both synthetic retinoids includes pretreatment measurement of tear production, hemogram, chemistry profile, and urinalysis. This is repeated in 1 to 2 months and, if no problems are detected, then repeated only as deemed necessary.[191, 192] Because experience with increased triglyceride levels shows that they normalize when animals are receiving low-fat diets, it is recommended that dogs being given etretinate may benefit from changing to such a diet.[191, 192]

■ HORMONAL AGENTS

Hormonal agents are often used in the management of cutaneous diseases. In many instances, they are prescribed for reasons other than a documented hormonal deficiency and responses may not reflect replacement therapy. Although they have been used for many years, there is still much that is not known. Often, indications for use and dosages are determined empirically.

Glucocorticoid Hormones

Glucocorticoid hormones have potent effects on the skin, and they profoundly affect immunologic and inflammatory activity.[233, 235] The major effects believed important in counteracting allergic inflammatory reactions are presented in Table 3:9 and have been reviewed.[223] In addition, fibroblastic activity is reduced, synthesis of histamine is delayed, and complement is inhibited. Antibody production is not stopped but may be decreased. At pharmacologic levels, glucocorticoids block the action of phospholipase A_2 on cell membranes, which results in inhibition of the arachidonic acid cycle. This action is probably one of the more clinically relevant actions in decreasing inflammation. Glucocorticoid response to inflammatory stimuli is nonspecific: it is the same whether it is a response to infection, trauma, toxin, or immune complex deposition. The drug must reach the local site of inflammation to be effective, and the degree of response and cellular protection from injury is proportionate to the concentration of glucocorticoid in the inflamed tissue. Thus, dosages and dose intervals should vary with the patient's specific needs.

Several other factors influence the tissue glucocorticoid effect. One is the relative potency of the drug. Synthetic compounds made by adding methyl or fluoride groups to the basic steroid molecule increase the potency and the duration of action. Another factor is the effect of protein binding. Only free glucocorticoid is metabolically active. Many synthetics are poorly protein bound, which partly explains their relatively high potency at low doses.

Corticosteroid-binding globulin is a specific glycoprotein that binds glucocorticoids, but it has a relatively low binding capacity. When large doses of glucocorticoids are administered, its capacity is exceeded, and albumin becomes the protein used for binding. Animals with low

Table 3:9. Anti-Inflammatory Actions of Glucocorticoids

Effects on eosinophils:	Decrease formation in bone marrow
	Induce apoptosis and inhibit prolongation of eosinophil survival and function from IL-3 and IL-5
Effects on lymphocytes and monocytes:	Reduce number of lymphocytes and monocytes that bear low affinity IgE and IgG receptors
	Decrease lymphocyte production of IL-1, 2, 3, 4, 5, 6 and IFN-γ
	Inhibit release of IL-1 and TNF-α from monocytes
Effects on mast cells:	May decrease number of mast cells
Inhibition of phospholipase A_2:	Decrease production of arachidonic acid metabolites
	Decrease production of platelet-activating factor
Decreased vascular permeability:	Mechanism unknown
Reversal of reduced β-adrenergic responsiveness:	Part of this effect is by increasing the number of β-adrenergic receptors expressed on cell surface

serum albumin levels have a lower binding capacity, and the excessive unbound glucocorticoid becomes freely available, increasing toxicity.[89, 223] In addition, the route of administration and water solubility affect the duration of action. Oral glucocorticoids, given as the free base or as esters, are rapidly absorbed. Parenteral glucocorticoids are usually esters of acetate, diacetate, phosphate, or succinate. Acetate and diacetate are relatively insoluble, resulting in slow release and prolonged absorption. The phosphates and succinates are water soluble and are rapidly absorbed. As a result, parenteral glucocorticoids produce continuous low levels of glucocorticoid for days (water soluble) or weeks (water insoluble). The effect produces significant adrenal suppression, a problem that can be diminished by giving short-acting glucocorticoids orally every other day.

Many of the desirable properties of glucocorticoids can be responsible for adverse effects if present in excess or at the wrong time. In addition, adverse effects may relate to the numerous other effects that glucocorticoids have on carbohydrate, protein, and lipid metabolism. It is imperative to make an accurate diagnosis so that the need for and the type, duration, and level of glucocorticoid therapy can be determined. Except in the case of hypoadrenocorticism, glucocorticoids do not correct a primary deficiency, but act symptomatically or palliatively. The anti-inflammatory and immunosuppressive actions desired for one therapeutic need may facilitate the establishment or spread of concomitant infections or parasitic diseases. Animals treated with glucocorticoids tend to experience bacterial infections of the skin and the urinary and respiratory systems.[89, 233]

■ *Indications.* The major indications for glucocorticoid therapy are hypersensitivity dermatoses (flea bite hypersensitivity, atopy, and food hypersensitivity), pyotraumatic dermatitis (''hot spot''), contact dermatitis (irritant or hypersensitivity reactions), and immune-mediated dermatoses (pemphigus, pemphigoid, and lupus erythematosus). Whenever possible, their use should be short term (less than 3 months). Glucocorticoids are usually only *part* of the management employed for most dermatoses, and the clinician must control or minimize other predisposing, precipitating, and complicating factors to keep the glucocorticoids in their proper perspective, which is to use them (1) as infrequently as possible, (2) at as low a dose as possible, (3) in alternate-day regimens whenever possible, and (4) only when other less hazardous forms of therapy have failed or could not be employed.[108, 110, 233, 235]

■ *Administration.* For dermatoses, glucocorticoids are usually administered orally, by injection (intramuscularly, subcutaneously intralesionally, and intravenously), topically, or in some combination thereof. In any given patient, the decision as to which route or routes to employ depends on various factors.

Of the systemic routes, oral administration is preferred because (1) it can be more closely regulated (a daily dose is more precise than with a repository injection; the drug can be rapidly withdrawn if undesirable side-effects occur), and (2) it is the *only* safe, therapeutic, physiologic way to administer glucocorticoids for more long-term therapy.[40, 89, 109, 172, 233, 235]

Injectable glucocorticoids are usually administered intramuscularly or subcutaneously. Although most injectable glucocorticoids are licensed for only intramuscular use, many clinicians administer them subcutaneously. The reasons purported for choosing the subcutaneous route are (1) there are few patient objections (and fewer pet owner crises), and (2) it is clinically as effective as intramuscular administration.[233]

There is a theoretical preference for using the intramuscular route in the obese patient, because subcutaneous deliveries could be sequestered in fat tissue. However, the major reason for using the intramuscular route (other than the liability or legal issue) is to decrease the occurrence of local atrophy. Although this problem may be more common in humans, it also occurs in the dog. Local areas of alopecia, pigmentary changes, and epidermal and dermal atrophy are more commonly induced by subcutaneous injection (Fig. 3:6). These reactions are

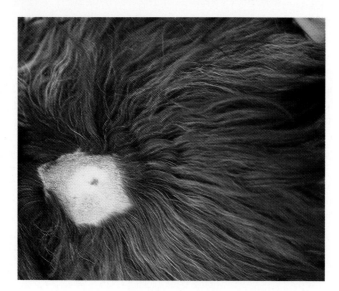

Figure 3:6. Atrophy from a subcutaneous steroid injection.

noninflammatory and atrophic in contrast to most other injection reactions. Yorkshire and Silky terriers, Lhasa apsos, Poodles, and Shih tzus may be predisposed to this reaction.[90]

An excellent injectable anti-inflammatory glucocorticoid is methylprednisolone acetate (Depo-Medrol). Clinically, dogs are given doses of 1.1 mg/kg, subcutaneously or intramuscularly, and the effect may last for 1 week to 6 months. Other commonly used injectable glucocorticoids are presented in Table 3:10.

Intralesional injections of glucocorticoids are often thought of as local, intracutaneous therapy, devoid of any systemic effect. Intralesional therapy is employed for solitary or multiple cutaneous lesions, but it has systemic effects, some of which can be serious. The major indications for intralesional use are acral lick dermatitis, histiocytomas, sterile granulomas, eosinophilic granulomas, feline indolent ulcers, and proliferative otitis externa. In general, triamcinolone acetonide is the glucocorticoid of choice for intralesional therapy.

Intravenous use for dermatologic indications is primarily limited to regimens of pulse therapy for immune-mediated dermatoses. In addition to the intravenous route, high dosages are used. In a study, dogs were hospitalized and given 11 mg/kg of methylprednisolone sodium

Table 3:10. Injectable Glucocorticoids for Use in Pruritic Dogs and Cats

| Agent | Brand Name | Company | Manufacturer's Regimen | |
			Dose	Route*
Betamethasone	Betasone	Schering	0.2–0.4 mg/kg in dog	IM
Dexamethasone	Azium	Schering	0.25–1 mg/dog	IM
			0.125–0.5 mg/cat	IM
Dexamethasone	Voren	Bio-Ceutic	0.25–1 mg/dog	IM
			0.125–0.5 mg/cat	IM
Flumethasone	Flucort	Syntex	0.06–0.25 mg/dog	IM or SC
			0.03–0.125 mg/cat	IM or SC
Methylprednisolone	Depo-Medrol	Upjohn	2–40 mg/dog	IM
			10–20 mg/cat	IM
Triamcinolone	Vetalog	Solvay	0.1–0.2 mg/kg in dog	IM or SC
			0.1–0.2 mg/kg in cat	IM or SC
Prednisone	Meticorten	Schering	0.5 mg/kg q24h	IM
	Prednisolone acetate	Generic	0.5 mg/kg q24h	IM

*IM, intramuscular; SC, subcutaneous.

succinate intravenously in 250 ml of 5 per cent dextrose and water during a 1-hour period for 3 consecutive days.[290] The reported advantages of glucocorticoid pulse therapy include immediate symptomatic relief, avoidance of side-effects seen with high-dose oral administration of glucocorticoids, and the ability to lower the dosage or discontinue the use of oral glucocorticoids after the pulse therapy. The side-effects seen with intravenous pulse therapy, such as cardiac arrhythmias, pancreatitis, diabetes mellitus, and gastric or duodenal ulcers, are enough of a concern, although not routinely observed, to limit this form of therapy to animals with severe disease.[107a, 290]

■ *Choosing a Glucocorticoid.* The choice of a glucocorticoid may be difficult. One cannot establish a single rule or set of rules that apply to all patients with a given glucocorticoid-responsive dermatosis. Factors that must be considered include the duration of therapy, the personality of the patient, the personality and reliability of the owner, the response of the patient to the drug, the response of the patient's *disease* to the drug, and other considerations specific to the patient or the disease.

The personality of the patient can significantly influence the choice of glucocorticoid; witness the attempts to administer pills to the obstreperous cat that is a blur of fur, fangs, and claws. Likewise, the reliability of the owner can be the deciding factor; there are owners who cannot, or will not, give oral medicaments to their pets. However, for long-term use even in these situations, the risk of injectable glucocorticoids overrides these drawbacks.

The clinician learns, by history or personal experience, that some glucocorticoids do not seem to work as well as others in certain patients. However, the claim that injectable glucocorticoids are needed in some cases and that oral glucocorticoids are not effective is rarely accurate. In the majority of these cases, ineffective oral dosages were used or tapered too fast. A common mistake is to give an injection then go immediately to a low alternate-day oral dose.[90, 233] In some cases, the problem probably reflects dosage, absorption, and metabolic differences.

As a corollary, the clinician notes that, in some patients, a glucocorticoid that was previously satisfactory apparently loses its effectiveness. For example, in an atopic dog that initially did well when given prednisolone, the prednisolone seemed to lose its effect. Subsequently, the dog responded well to equipotent doses of orally administered triamcinolone. In most cases, after a variable length of time, the clinician is able to return to managing the atopy successfully with prednisolone. This well-recognized but poorly understood phenomenon is called *steroid tachyphylaxis*.[51, 233] However, in most clinical cases referred to dermatology specialists for the development of steroid resistance or steroid tachyphylaxis, the real problem is the development of concurrent disorders.[86, 233] In such cases, secondary bacterial pyoderma, *Malassezia* dermatitis, increased exposure to fleas, or reactions to ongoing topical therapy are often the reasons for failure of previously effective glucocorticoid regimens.

Finally, the clinician may discover, by history or personal experience, that a patient can receive certain glucocorticoids without significant adverse effects, but not other glucocorticoids. Hence, a dog may develop colitis or behavioral changes with prednisolone but not with methylprednisolone, dexamethasone, or triamcinolone. In some cases, switching to methylprednisolone or triamcinolone may have a relative steroid-sparing effect. A lower dose than the prednisolone equivalent may be effective for that disease in that animal. In some cases, signs of iatrogenic Cushing's disease or marked liver enzyme activity elevations greatly improve on the alternative glucocorticoid alternate-day regimen.[86]

■ *Therapeutic Dosage.* Optimal therapeutic doses have not been scientifically determined for *any* canine or feline dermatosis. Presently espoused anti-inflammatory, antipruritic, antiallergic, or immunosuppressive glucocorticoid doses have been determined through years of clinical experience. Moreover, it is imperative to remember that every patient is unique and that glucocorticoid therapy must be individualized. Recommended glucocorticoid doses are only guidelines.

The two most commonly used oral glucocorticoids are prednisolone and prednisone. For all practical purposes, these two drugs are identical (the choice of one or the other is usually based on cost). However, prednisone must be converted in the liver to prednisolone, the active form. Dosage recommendations in this text are based on prednisolone (prednisone) equivalents. Table 3:11 contains information on approximate equipotent dosages of other oral glucocorticoids.

Physiologic doses of glucocorticoids are those that approximate the daily cortisol (hydrocortisone) production by normal individuals. In dogs, daily cortisol production has been reported to be 0.2 to 1 mg/kg/day.[235] No such information is available for cats. Pharmacologic doses of glucocorticoids exceed physiologic requirements. Significantly, any pharmacologic dose of glucocorticoid, no matter how large or small, may suppress the hypothalamic-pituitary-adrenal axis.[233, 247, 266]

Clinicians usually talk in terms of anti-inflammatory versus immunosuppressive doses of glucocorticoids. A commonly used anti-inflammatory (as in allergic dermatoses) induction dosage of oral prednisolone in dogs is 1.1 mg/kg every 24 hours. However, in severe allergy, such as the dog with flea allergy that has numerous fleas, a higher dosage of 1.75 to 2 mg/kg/day may often be needed.[86] For maintenance, the dosage should be lowered as much as possible and optimally ends up at less than 0.25 to 0.5 mg/kg every 48 hours. For immune-mediated diseases, the initial dosage is usually 2.2 mg/kg every 24 hours. If the dog fails to respond, this may be raised to as high as 6.6 mg/kg every 24 hours. Two of the authors (DWS and WHM) administer oral glucocorticoids only once daily and find no loss of clinical efficacy, but a definite reduction in side-effects. A commonly used immunosuppressive maintenance dosage for dogs is 1.1 mg of prednisolone per kilogram every other morning.

In general, compared with dogs, cats require about twice the dose of glucocorticoid orally for induction and maintenance therapy.[40, 173, 230, 233, 235] Resistance of cats to glucocorticoid effects may relate to their decreased number of glucocorticoid receptors.[284a] It is probable that the diurnal rhythm of dogs and cats is not dramatic, and timing dosages to morning or evening hours is less important than was previously thought. It is important, however, to maintain the 24-hour alternate-day freedom from medication so that adrenal suppression and chronic side-effects are minimized.

■ *Regimen.* Glucocorticoid regimens vary with the nature of the dermatosis, the specific glucocorticoid being administered, and the use of induction versus maintenance therapy.

Table 3:11. Relative Potency and Activity of Oral Glucocorticoids

Drug	Equivalent Dose (mg)	Duration of Effect (h)	Alternate-Day Therapy*
SHORT ACTING			
Cortisone	25	8–12	NAS
Hydrocortisone	20	8–12	NAS
INTERMEDIATE ACTING			
Prednisone	5	24–36	P
Prednisolone	5	24–36	P
Methylprednisolone	4	24–36	P
LONG ACTING			
Flumethasone	1.3	36–48	
Triamcinolone	0.5†	36–48	A‡
Dexamethasone	0.5	36–54	‡
Betamethasone	0.4	36–54	

*NAS, Not acceptable for short duration; P, preferred; A, alternative selection for alternate-day therapy.

†Previous publications stated dosages often equivalent to those of methylprednisolone. No studies on clinical effects are available, and this value represents the authors' clinical impression.

‡May be useful on every-third-day regimen.

In general, dermatoses necessitating anti-inflammatory doses of oral glucocorticoid need smaller doses and shorter periods of daily induction therapy to bring about remission, as compared with dermatoses necessitating immunosuppressive doses. Anti-inflammatory induction doses are usually given for 2 to 6 days, whereas immunosuppressive induction doses are often administered for 4 to 10 days. Initially, the doses are given every 24 hours or divided and given every 12 hours for 2 to 4 days then the total daily dose is given every 24 hours. This is continued until signs of disease are markedly decreased or in remission. After this point, tapering to maintenance therapy begins.

Maintenance therapy with oral glucocorticoid is best accomplished with prednisolone, prednisone, or methylprednisolone on an alternate-day basis.[41, 233, 235, 247] Oral triamcinolone is often effective in managing prednisone-responsive cases at doses approximately 10 to 20 per cent of the prednisone dose (on a milligram basis).[89, 233] According to the standard published glucocorticoid potency equivalency, this is significant steroid-sparing effect. However, because triamcinolone suppresses the hypothalamic-pituitary-adrenal axis for 24 to 48 hours, it is best given every 72 hours.

With alternate-day therapy, the daily dose of glucocorticoid used for successful induction therapy is given as a single massive dose, usually every other morning for dogs and every other evening for cats. Some clinicians (DWS and WHM) begin alternate-day therapy as soon as remission is achieved with induction therapy.[233, 235] Other investigators gradually reduce one alternate-day dose until no drug is given, while the other alternate-day dose remains at the induction dose.[89] For maintenance therapy, the alternate-day dose is reduced by 50 per cent, every 1 to 2 weeks, until the lowest satisfactory maintenance dose is achieved. This regimen does not eliminate adrenal atrophy, but it is less severe and its onset is delayed. *It is the only dosage system that should be used for long-term therapy of steroid-responsive diseases in small animals.*

In some animals, alternate-day glucocorticoid therapy can be extended to every third or fourth day. Rarely, anti-inflammatory alternate-day glucocorticoid therapy with the preferred prednisolone, prednisone, or methylprednisolone is not successful. In these cases, the clinician has three therapeutic options (assuming that glucocorticoid therapy is all that can be done): (1) to administer prednisolone, prednisone, or methylprednisolone on a *daily* basis, informing the owner of the inevitability of iatrogenic hyperglucocorticoidism; (2) to switch to a more potent oral glucocorticoid on an alternate-day basis; or (3) to switch to injectable glucocorticoids. Although the more potent oral glucocorticoids are usually satisfactory for alternate-day therapy unless given at low doses, they do not spare the hypothalamic-pituitary-adrenal axis (because of potency and duration of effect). They may occasionally be employed with few or no significant side-effects, especially in cats.[86, 233] Clinically, the most satisfactory agents in this respect appear to be triamcinolone and dexamethasone. Because of factors related to the patient and the owner, not the disease, some animals may be satisfactorily managed with only injectable glucocorticoids.

Intramuscular or subcutaneous glucocorticoid therapy is usually fine for acute, short-term diseases that necessitate a single injection. Additionally, animals that need only three or four injections per year probably do not have significant side effects. However, for dermatoses that need long-term maintenance therapy, injectable glucocorticoids are usually not satisfactory. It has been shown that a single intramuscular injection of methylprednisolone acetate (Depo-Medrol) is capable of altering adrenocortical function in dogs for at least 5, and up to 10, weeks.[108] In other studies, a single intramuscular injection of triamcinolone acetonide (Vetalog) was capable of altering adrenocortical function in dogs for up to 4 weeks.[109, 247]

Intralesional injections of glucocorticoids are usually repeated every 7 to 10 days until the dermatosis is in remission (usually two to four treatments) and then given as needed.

■ **Side-Effects.** The side-effects in dogs associated with systemic glucocorticoid therapy are numerous.[235, 247] In contrast, cats appear relatively tolerant to this therapy. Because of the diverse effects of glucocorticoids on protein, lipid, and carbohydrate metabolism; endocrine function; fluid balance; and host defense mechanisms, it is expected that their use is associated with many side-effects. Sequelae may appear with any duration or form of glucocorticoid therapy. In most cases, the side-effects seen with short-term therapy may also be seen with long-term therapy, but are not generally major health problems. The exceptions are the acute sequelae of high-dose therapy. These include gastrointestinal ulceration, perforation, myopathy, and pancreatitis. These side-effects most commonly occur with dosages at or greater than 2.2 mg/kg/day of prednisone (or equipotent doses of other glucocorticoids).

The other side-effects that are not related to treatment duration include polyuria, polydipsia, polyphagia (which may lead to weight gain), behavioral changes (depression, hyperactivity, and aggression), panting, and diarrhea. Most of these side-effects are somewhat dose related. However, the disease being treated may not be controllable at a dosage that does not produce the undesired results. In general, these side-effects are minimized with low-dose, alternate-day therapy, or may occur on only the day of treatment. Switching types of glucocorticoid may also eliminate these sequelae.

Long-term therapy is associated with many more side-effects and particularly side-effects leading to poor health or disease. Of major concern is the increased risk of infections. A variety of bacterial infections may be seen but the most common are bacteriuria, pyoderma, septicemia, and respiratory infections. Generalized demodicosis or *Malassezia* dermatitis may also occur. Cutaneous and subcutaneous changes that may commonly be seen include dry poor coat, dry scaly skin, fat redistribution, and an increase in lipomas or their size. In more susceptible dogs, or dogs receiving higher dosages, alopecia, thin skin, hypotonic skin, calcinosis cutis, atrophic remodeling of scars, comedones, and milia-like follicular cysts may occur alone or in combination.

Musculoskeletal abnormalities that occur may go unrecognized as glucocorticoid side-effects. Osteoporosis, muscle atrophy, and weak ligaments may result from the glucocorticoid effects of protein catabolism, fibroblast inhibition and decreased intestinal calcium absorption. Although no studies have documented an association, it has been suggested that dogs receiving long-term glucocorticoid therapy are at higher risk for ligament damage, particularly cruciate rupture.[273]

The alteration in metabolism may lead to hyperlipidemia and steroid hepatopathy. Endocrine changes induced may include adrenal gland suppressions, then atrophy, diabetes mellitus, decreased thyroid hormone synthesis, and increased parathyroid hormone levels. Significant side-effects with appropriate anti-inflammatory systemic glucocorticoid regimens are uncommon in dogs, occurring in less than 10 per cent of the animals treated. However, with immunosuppressive regimens, the frequency and the severity of glucocorticoid side-effects escalate alarmingly, and less than 50 per cent of the dogs so treated can be satisfactorily managed.[233, 238]

It must be emphasized that alternate-day therapy with prednisolone is not a panacea. Occasionally, some dogs cannot be successfully managed with such therapy without developing iatrogenic hyperglucocorticoidism.[233, 235, 238] This probably reflects differences in serum protein levels, receptor levels, or absorption, metabolism, or clearance of glucocorticoid in those individuals. Additionally, occasional dramatic individual variation is observed in susceptibility to acute or chronic glucocorticoid side-effects;[233, 235] therefore, (1) one can see various degrees of iatrogenic hyperglucocorticoidism after as little as 3 weeks to as long as 7 years of therapy, and (2) one may see only calcinosis cutis or full-blown Cushing's syndrome as an individual dog's manifestation of hyperglucocorticoidism.[232, 233, 235, 247]

Although clinically effective doses of systemic glucocorticoids in cats are usually twice those needed in dogs, significant side-effects are rare.[231, 233, 235, 247] Polydipsia, polyuria, polyphagia, a tendency for weight gain, depression, and diarrhea are occasionally seen. Significant iatrogenic hyperglucocorticoidism has been produced in cats only after the weekly subcutaneous administration of methylprednisolone acetate for 10 weeks. Obviously, such therapy would never be either employed or indicated in clinical situations.

Significant side-effects after intralesional glucocorticoid therapy have not been reported in dogs and cats. Local cutaneous atrophy and local inflammatory reactions (presumably due to crystalline material left at the injection site) are rarely seen. These side-effects, as well as panniculitis, sterile abscesses, necrosis, and pigmentary disturbances, are well recognized in humans.[80, 142, 266]

A potentially much more significant side-effect of intralesional therapy is systemic hyperglucocorticoidism.[173, 233] Normal dogs given subconjunctival injections of methylprednisolone acetate had suppressed adrenocortical responses to exogenous ACTH for 9 to 20 days.[173] Additionally, dogs that received intracutaneous or subconjunctival injections of methylprednisolone or betamethasone were unresponsive to intradermal histamine and skin test allergens for up to 4 weeks. The health significance of such findings in dogs is unknown. Certainly such medications could influence interpretation of results of hematologic, adrenal function, and intradermal allergy skin tests.

■ *Evaluation.* Evaluation of the results during glucocorticoid therapy is important. When appropriate systemic anti-inflammatory glucocorticoid therapy is given to an otherwise healthy dog or cat, the risks are minimal. The risks associated with immunosuppressive doses are of greater concern, especially because the medication is usually prescribed for serious or life-threatening diseases, which will probably be treated for the rest of the animal's life. Significant concurrent dysfunction of major organ systems also drastically increases the risks. Some owners balk at the expense, the risk, and the unpleasant side-effects or at the complex therapy protocol, and they refuse treatment. Occasionally, the clinician may be forced to choose between using drugs that may not be in the animal's best long-term interest or performing euthanasia at the owner's request.

When long-term systemic therapy is started, owners should be instructed to observe their animals closely and to report immediately any significant side-effects. A physical checkup is advised every 6 to 12 months. Periodic urinalysis and urine cultures may be needed to recognize urinary tract infections that are not clinically apparent. Serum chemistry screens are advised every 12 to 24 months before more medication is dispensed. The ACTH response test is useful in animals with suspected iatrogenic Cushing's disease. Marked suppression indicates that other attempts at lowering the dosage should be made, because major problems are inevitable. Dogs receiving appropriate long-term, alternate-day steroid therapy usually have mildly to moderately suppressed adrenocortical responses to ACTH and elevated serum alkaline phosphatase levels, but are otherwise clinically normal.

Thyroid Hormones

Thyroid hormones are indicated as replacement therapy for primary, secondary, and tertiary hypothyroidism; for adjunctive management of some canine bacterial pyodermas and of some idiopathic canine seborrhea syndromes; and for treatment of feline symmetric alopecia (feline endocrine alopecia).[212, 213] The administration of thyroid hormones induces varying degrees of hair growth in normal dogs as well as in dogs and cats with various nonthyroid dermatoses.

The metabolically active thyroid hormones are L-thyroxine (T_4), which is the main secretory product of the thyroid gland, and L-triiodothyronine (T_3), which is three to five times more potent than T_4 and secreted in small amounts by the thyroid gland. T_4 acts as a prohormone, being deiodinated by peripheral tissues to the more potent T_3, as needed. In dogs, 40 to 60 per cent of T_3 is derived this way.[64] This control mechanism safeguards against T_3 deficiency in critical tissues. In addition, the liver and the kidneys can concentrate thyroid hormone and may exchange hormone rapidly with the plasma, if necessary. As is true of many other hormones, only thyroid hormones that are unbound (to protein) are metabolically active. In dogs, only about 0.1 per cent of total serum T_4 and 1 per cent of serum T_3 are free. The plasma half-life of T_4 is 10 to 16 hours, whereas that of T_3 is 5 to 6 hours. These figures reflect plasma disappearance and do not indicate the duration of biological half-life.

Thyroid Supplementation in Dogs

Dogs are thought to absorb only 10 to 50 per cent of an oral dose of levothyroxine (synthetic T_4), whereas absorption of liothyronine (synthetic T_3) may be much higher.[59] In peripheral tissues, conversion of T_4 to T_3 may be impaired by starvation, surgery, diabetes mellitus, and other acute and chronic illnesses such as infectious liver and renal disease. These nonthyroidal illnesses produce a syndrome called the *euthyroid sick syndrome*, characterized by low blood levels of T_3 and T_4 (see Chap. 9). This may be an adaptive mechanism to limit the catabolic state of illness or malnutrition. Low laboratory-derived hormone levels in this syndrome or in drug-induced T_3 and T_4 reductions do not constitute an indication for thyroid hormone supplementation.

There are four types of thyroid hormone medications. Only two are recommended for use in dogs and cats. Crude preparations from desiccated thyroid tissue (thyroid USP) and synthetic thyroid hormone combinations that are intended to mimic the normal T_4 to T_3 ratio in humans should not be used.

Synthetic levothyroxine (T_4) is the medication of choice for canine hypothyroidism. It is the main natural secretory substance produced and, by virtue of being the prohormone, provides the hormone replacement in a physiologic manner. It also aids in the proper feedback for thyrotropin (thyroid-stimulating hormone) release and is inexpensive. Some clinicians recommend that brand name products be used (Table 3:12) and that generic products be avoided. Products may vary in actual content of active hormone, but the variation from batch to batch is less with proprietary (brand name) products.[212–214] Therefore, if an animal is adequately regulated on a given proprietary product, it likely stays regulated with refills of the same product. Generic products may fluctuate much more from batch to batch.

The initial oral dosage is 0.02 mg/kg every 12 hours. If postpill testing after 4 to 6 weeks of therapy reveals insufficient serum levels, or if the animal is not clinically responding after 12 weeks, the dosage may be increased. In most cases, the recommended dosage is effective. Dogs that have clinically responded to the every-12-hour regimen can usually be maintained with 0.02 mg/kg every 24 hours.[213, 214] Because the dosage is proportional to the metabolic rate, a better schedule might be 0.5 mg/m² of body surface area. However, definitive studies are needed.

Table 3:12. Synthetic Brands of Thyroid Supplements for Use in Dogs and Cats

Product	Manufacturer
LEVOTHYROXINE (T_4)	
Levoid	Nutritional Control Products
Levothroid	Rorer
Levoxine	Daniels
Noroxine	Vortech
Soloxine	Daniels
Synthroid	Boots-Flint
Thyro-Form	Vet-a-mix
Thyro-Tab	Vet-a-mix
LIOTHYRONINE (T_3)	
Cytobin	Norden
Cytomel	SmithKline Beecham
Tertroxin	Pitman-Moore
Cyronine	Major

Synthetic liothyronine (T_3) is the active intracellular hormone, but it should not usually be given for routine treatment of hypothyroidism, as it bypasses the normal physiologic and cellular regulatory pathways. In addition, it is more expensive than levothyroxine. Because it has a short half-life, even administration at short intervals tends to produce frequent high peaks of the drug, which favors toxicity; it may be indicated in so-called poor converters—those rare individuals who cannot convert T_4 to T_3. Oral dosage, if needed, would be 4 to 6 μg/kg every 8 hours or perhaps every 12 hours.

Response to therapy with either of the above medications is seen as increased activity and mental alertness in 10 to 14 days; hair regrowth is often observed at 4 to 6 weeks, but 4 to 5 months are necessary for complete regrowth; reduction in hyperpigmentation is noted in 3 to 6 months; and reduction of recurrent bacterial pyoderma often occurs in 3 to 4 months. In general, some clinical improvement should be seen after 4 to 6 weeks of therapy.[212, 213]

Although these clinical evaluations are the best measure of successful replacement, there may be equivocal responses that should be studied by measuring serum hormone levels. T_3 is primarily intracellular and difficult to measure, and a protocol is not well delineated. T_4, however, can be measured by the postpill test. This should be done only when the animal is in a steady state, having been receiving regular medication for at least 14 days. However, owing to changes in metabolism, most authors recommend waiting 4 to 6 weeks. One author (CEG) prefers testing at 10 to 14 days, as a steady state of more than 5 plasma half-lives should be obtained. Dogs with low levels at this dosage and time have generally only lower levels as their metabolism increases. This regimen is recommended so that the client does not spend 12 weeks giving an incorrect dose. If one waits 6 weeks, a favorable response (not complete) should already be noted in most cases and, if not, the dosage should be raised for the next 6 weeks. Failure to respond at this point requires further postpill testing, and if an adequate dose is present, the diagnosis should be questioned.

For dogs receiving adequate, once-daily medication, testing just before daily medication is given should show normal or low-normal serum T_4 levels. Animals receiving twice-daily medication should be checked 4 to 6 hours after receiving a dose, when the serum levels should be in the high-normal range or slightly higher. If there are not high-normal T_4 levels, the dosage should be increased and testing should be repeated 1 month later, if no clinical response is noted.

Complications with therapy involve medication for patients with concurrent cardiac or adrenal insufficiencies or thyrotoxicosis. Initiating T_4 medication may rapidly increase tissue metabolism and exhaust the cardiac reserve of a marginally coping heart or may exacerbate an adrenal crisis. For patients with cardiac disease, T_4 is started at one fourth the recommended dosage and increased slowly to full dosage by 4 weeks.[212, 213] Patients with hypoadrenocorticism should have glucocorticoid therapy instituted before T_4 replacement. Thyrotoxicosis is rare in dogs but may be evidenced by polyuria and polydipsia, nervousness, aggressiveness, panting, diarrhea, tachycardia, pyrexia, and pruritus. One should perform a postpill serum T_4 determination, stop the medication, and reinstitute medication at a lower dose after clinical status improves.

Feline Thyroid Supplementation

The dosage of levothyroxine for cats is 0.05 to 0.20 mg per cat daily.[64] The dosage of liothyronine in cats is initially 20 μg per cat twice daily. This may be increased gradually by increments of 10 μg every 3 days to a maximal dosage of 50 μg twice daily.[275a] In cats, the major indications for thyroid supplementation are postthyroid ablation for hyperthyroidism and feline symmetric alopecia. For feline symmetric alopecia, liothyronine is the treatment of choice. In treatment for feline symmetric alopecia, hair regrowth is obvious between 4 and 10 weeks.[274a] Signs of iatrogenic hyperthyroidism in the cat are rare. In one report, 1 of 26 liothyronine-treated cats developed a soft systolic murmur and ventricular premature beats that resolved on discontinuation of T_3 supplementation.[275a]

Growth Hormone

Growth hormone (GH) deficiency can be divided into two groups; primary GH deficiency, and GH deficiency secondary to conditions such as hypothyroidism, hyperadrenocorticism, and zinc deficiency. In the secondary forms, treatment of the primary cause produces a normalization of GH secretory responses.[54] There are two potential indications for GH therapy: pituitary dwarfism and hyposomatotropism in the mature dog (see Chap. 9).

GH is expensive and difficult to obtain. It also is a regulated drug owing to human abuse. Therefore, treatments should be administered only in the clinic. Besides these problems, side-effects occur. In addition, recurrences usually occur within 6 to 30 months, necessitating retreatments during the lifetime of the dog. Some cases of adult-onset hyposomatotropism in dogs may spontaneously resolve without treatment. Some authors currently advise against the use of GH,[209] whereas other investigators (including CEG) strongly discourage its use. Human GH is active in phylogenetically lower animals such as dogs. Nonprimate GH preparations (feline, bovine, canine, porcine, and ovine) are immunologically interrelated, and all except ovine appear to be effective for small animal therapy. Genetically engineered GH is also available and appears effective in dogs.

If treatment must be given, it is by subcutaneous injections. A protocol for GH therapy that appears to be associated with a lower incidence of diabetes mellitus has been proposed.[209] This dosage is 0.1 IU/kg given three times a week for 6 weeks. In the past, other protocols were used. For pituitary dwarfism, 10 IU of bovine GH, or 2 IU of porcine GH, was given three times a week for 4 to 6 weeks. For hyposomatotropism in mature dogs (pseudo-Cushing's disease), either of the above products was given every other day for 10 injections. For dogs less than 14 kg of body weight, the dose was 2.5 IU per injection, and for those more than 14 kg of body weight, it was 5 IU per injection. Using this latter protocol, one author (CEG) noted one dog that became a permanent diabetic and another dog that temporarily became diabetic.

With successful therapy, hair growth should be evident in 4 to 6 weeks. Usually, alopecia develops again, then GH treatment may be repeated. Some dogs may become unresponsive, perhaps because antibodies develop against GH, which decrease its biological activity.

Therapy with GH involves some risks. Diabetes mellitus may develop, although it may resolve when treatment is halted. Acromegaly may be produced, or patients may experience anaphylaxis during retreatment. Treatment should be initally monitored with weekly blood glucose determinations.

Sex Hormones

Sex hormone replacement therapy is an enigma.[157, 158] Most hormones are present in both sexes, and their levels in blood fluctuate markedly during the day. The available assays are expensive and often unsatisfactory, in part because there are many compounds related to one hormone, and the assay systems typically measure only one compound.

In addition, androgens and estrogens are produced by the adrenal glands and gonads, or by peripheral conversion. Abnormalities of sex hormone tissue receptors and sex hormone binding–globulin may markedly affect the biological availability of hormones (more than 90 per cent of sex steroids are protein bound and inactive.).[157] All the doses of sex hormones given in this discussion are empirical. Please refer to Chapter 9 and to the references for more detailed information.

Estrogens

Estrogens are steroid hormones produced by the aromatization of androgens in the ovarian granulosa cells, in the zona reticularis of the adrenal gland, and peripherally at local sites (hair follicle dermal papilla) from circulating androgens. In addition, one type of estrogenic compound may be interconverted to another form at peripheral sites.[75, 102, 157, 197] The three main estrogenic compounds in decreasing order of potency are estradiol, estrone, and estriol. They bind weakly to sex hormone–binding globulin and to albumin. Cutaneous effects are variable by species, but in the dog, they appear to cause decreased epidermal mitosis, decreased epidermal thickness, and sebaceous gland and subcutaneous atrophy at high doses.[224] Estrogens are not required for hair growth and actually prolong telogen, decrease the rate and thickness of hair shaft production, and may cause alopecia. In the dog, alterations in density of estrogen receptors may cause hyperestrogenic changes in the absence of increased serum levels of estrogen.[53] This may occur more readily in the flank region.

Estrogen therapy is indicated in estrogen-responsive dermatosis of female dogs, and has been used in a repository injectable form at a 1:20 ratio with testosterone for the treatment of feline acquired symmetric alopecia. In dogs, diethylstilbestrol can be given orally at 0.02 mg/kg, up to 1 mg total dose, by various protocols. Induction schedules range from daily for a 3- or 4-week cycle, then stop a week, and repeat the cycle, to dosing every other day or twice weekly until clinical response is seen, which usually occurs in 6 to 12 weeks.[158, 210] After induction therapy, the frequency of administration is gradually decreased to a minimum, typically once or twice weekly.[212] Initial hair regrowth should be evident in 2 to 4 weeks, with complete response in 2 to 3 months. The treatment should not be continued for more than 3 months if there is no response.

Complications of estrogen therapy include induction of estrus, bone marrow suppression in dogs (anemia, leukopenia, and thrombocytopenia),[274] hepatotoxicity, and nymphomania. Cats are highly sensitive to estrogens, and lethal effects are common with a total dose of 10 mg of diethylstilbestrol, even when the hormones are administered over several weeks. In intact female animals, the possibility of abortion or pyometra should be considered, whereas in male animals, prostatic hyperplasia may result.

Androgens

Androgens are steroid hormones produced in the testicle by interstitial cells, in the ovary by the theca cells, and in the zona reticularis of the adrenal gland. The interstitial (Leydig) cells produce, in increasing order of potency, dihydroepiandrosterone, androstenedione, testosterone (the major form), and dihydrotestosterone. Androgens are potent anabolic agents; they promote protein production and increase epidermal mitosis, collagen and dermal ground substance production, and melanization. Sebaceous, scent, and perianal glands are also stimulated by androgens. Their effects on hair may be paradoxical, depending on interconversion, aromatization to estrogens, and relative density of tissue receptors. However, in general, they stimulate hair growth but inhibit the initiation of the anagen phase.

Androgens are indicated in hypoandrogenism of male dogs, and some cases of the following diseases respond: estrogen-responsive dermatosis of female dogs,[210] hypogonadism of the intact male dog,[210] adrenal sex hormone imbalances, adult onset hyposomatotropism,[224] and feline acquired symmetric alopecia. Methyltestosterone administered orally at 0.5 to 1 mg/kg up to a total maximal dose of 30 mg every 48 hours is most commonly used. Testosterone propionate aqueous suspension in propylene glycol or alcohol or in oil can be given intramuscularly once weekly at doses of 0.5 to 1 mg/kg, or it may be given at 2 mg/kg intramuscularly every 4 to 16 weeks.[212] The latter drug can be given intramuscularly once to cats with feline acquired symmetric alopecia at a total dose of 12 mg. It is often combined with 0.6 mg of repository stilbestrol or 0.5 mg of repository estradiol. Successful treatment produces significant regrowth of hair within 2 to 3 months.

Complications include aggressive behavior, greasy hair coat, prostatic hypertrophy, and hepatotoxicity. It is advisable to have baseline liver profiles before initiating therapy and to monitor them monthly the first 3 months.[210, 214] In addition, cats receiving testosterone may spray urine the first few days.

Progestagens

Progestagens are steroid hormones produced by the ovarian corpus luteum and adrenal zona reticularis. They are precursors of the other metabolically active steroid hormones (androgens, estrogens, glucocorticoids, and mineralocorticoids). They bind minimally to sex hormone–binding globulin but more to albumin and corticosteroid-binding globulin. Cushing's disease or steroid therapy may increase available free progestagens. Both progesterone and 17-hydroxyprogesterone are metabolically active and bind to progestogen receptors and weakly to androgen receptors. They suppress release of gonadotropin and ACTH and induce GH release in part by action on the hypothalamus and limbic system. Hair effects may be species variable because they have little effect in rodents but may cause retention in anagen phase in women and dogs and induce alopecia in the cat. Medroxyprogesterone acetate causes alopecia in the dog and cat. Progestagens interfere with 5-α-reductase and, at least in the cat, appear to have glucocorticoid effects. Progestational compounds have been used rather indiscriminately in the management of behavioral disorders and the treatment of a variety of nonspecific inflammatory dermatoses, especially in cats.

Two synthetic progestagens are used in small animal dermatology and have similar effects. They can often be used interchangeably, although in some cases one product is better than the other.[176]

Megestrol acetate (Ovaban [Schering] and Megace [Bristol-Meyers]) is an oral drug originally marketed to suppress canine estrus and still not approved in the United States for feline dermatoses. It has potent anti-inflammatory effects, especially in cats, but in the typical dose, produced more severe and longer-lasting adrenal suppression than did anti-inflammatory doses of prednisolone.[143] It has also been blamed for the development of diabetes mellitus, but one study showed no change in glucose tolerance curves after 3 weeks of therapy with megestrol acetate.[143] The dosage of megestrol acetate in dogs with behavioral dermatoses is 2 to 4 mg/kg daily. For induction therapy in cats, the dosage is 2.5 to 5 mg per cat every other day, declining to 2.5 to 5 mg every 7 to 14 days for maintenance. This is a potent drug with serious toxic potential, and it should not be used if alternative therapy is available.

Medroxyprogesterone acetate (Depo-Provera [Upjohn]) is an injectable repository progestogen. Repository progesterone in oil is also available. Because progestagens can have serious side-effects, injectable long-lasting dosage forms should be used only if the short-acting (and thus, safer) oral products present problems of administration. Dosages are 50 to 100 mg per cat and 20 mg/kg for dogs. These are repeated only if needed in 3 to 6 months.

Clinical use of the above progestagens has been empirical, and much of the rationale revolves around behavior modification to prevent self-trauma and the progestagens' anti-inflammatory effect. In dogs, boredom-related dermatoses or obsessive-compulsive disorders may be ameliorated with this treatment. Thus, flank sucking, acral lick dermatitis, tail biting, and foot licking are some of its typical indications. Canine hormonal alopecias that do not respond to other hormone therapy may benefit from a short course and low dosage of megestrol acetate.[116] In cats, progestogen therapy may benefit indolent ulcers, eosinophilic plaques, and eosinophilic granulomas, but especially alopecias that are due to licking and chewing. It has been helpful in feline acquired symmetric alopecia and feline hyperesthesia syndrome.[116] Because it has antiandrogen effects, it has been advocated for tail gland hyperplasia (stud tail) in male cats and for feline acne.

Several major side-effects must be considered when progestogen therapy is contemplated. Decreased spermatogenesis, development of pyometra, and postponement of estrus may be seen. GH levels increase, and acromegaly may develop. Mammary gland fibroadenomatous hyperplasia is seen in both intact and neutered male and female cats and has little correlation with the dose of medication or the frequency of administration. Some cases regress when treatment is halted, but in others, the mammary tissue ulcerates and neoplasms may develop, necessitating surgical removal. Diabetes mellitus has been reported in cats being treated with megestrol acetate.[188] Some cats require insulin, but usually, the disorder is transient and spontaneously regresses. Behavioral abnormalities are common. Often, the animals are more affectionate and slightly lethargic and have polydipsia and polyphagia. Consequently, they gain weight. The most serious side-effect is adrenocortical suppression, which occurs with even low doses and persists for many weeks, probably because of the long half-life of the progestagens.[152] This suppression is a major reason to avoid these drugs.

Other Sex Hormone Therapies

The gonadotropins and prolactin are adenohypophyseal hormones that are stimulated by hypothalamic releasing factors and that regulate endogenous sex hormones. They are involved in complex interhormonal reactions, and specifically targeted effects are not possible. These compounds are not used in routine dermatology practice; however, it has been speculated that they may play an important role in some acquired alopecias (see Chap. 9).

Hormone-Modulating Agents

The recognition of alopecic syndromes with suspected hormonal interactions and adrenal disease without hyperglucocorticoidism has led to the attempted use of another group of drugs. These drugs modify hormone production (most often, steroid hormones) or interfere with receptor actions. To date, the most obvious and commonly used of these drugs is mitotane (Lysodren [Bristol-Meyers]), which is the treatment of choice for pituitary-dependent hyperadrenocorticism in dogs. However, low-dose mitotane, ketoconazole, aminoglutethimide, and tamoxifen citrate have been tried in small numbers of dogs with adrenal sex hormone disorders and other sex hormone dermatoses.[90, 207, 225] In general, these drugs interfere with steroid hormone production or block estrogen or progesterone receptors. The use of mitotane to treat hyperadrenocorticism is extensively covered elsewhere (see Chap. 9).

The use of mitotane to treat adrenal-origin sex hormone abnormalities involves administering a lower dosage, 15 to 25 mg/kg every 24 hours for 5 days. Maintenance dosages of 15 to 25 mg/kg every 7 to 14 days were then given. Post-ACTH administration cortisol levels were monitored, with attempts to regulate the levels at just below the normal expected value. Hair regrowth was seen in 10 of 12 dogs with suspected adrenal sex hormone dermatoses.[207]

■ ORAL SUNSCREENS

Oral sunscreens are chemicals such as β-carotene and chloroquine that quench free radicals and stabilize membranes. They have not been proved to prevent sunburn in people but have been useful in cases of light-induced dermatosis.[133, 222] A β-carotene derivative has been used in cats and dogs to reduce phototoxicity (see Chap. 15). Canthaxanthin (β,β-carotene-4,4'-dione) is a red-orange pigment found in plants and other sources. The safety of this product has been challenged. Side-effects include orange-brown skin, brick red stools, crystalline gold deposits on the retinae, orange plasma, and lowered amplitudes on electroretinograms. The usual maximal dosage for humans is 25 mg/kg daily, but some companies recommend four 30-mg capsules once daily (Golden Tan, Orobronze). In toxicity studies of dogs, the long-term and short-term lethal dose is greater than 10,000 mg/kg.

■ SKIN SURGERY

Skin surgery can be an important part of small animal dermatology. Many new developments have been seen, from skin biopsies for diagnosis to cryosurgery for specialized procedures. It is essential to know what equipment is needed and to be able to use the equipment properly. Cold steel surgery, cryosurgery, laser surgery, and electrosurgery are discussed in this chapter. Biopsy techniques are covered in Chapter 2.

Dermatologists recommend plastic surgery for the correction of anatomic defects causing dermatoses of facial, tail, vulva, and lip folds. Skin grafting (pinch, strip, mesh, and pedicle grafts) is useful to repair defects of skin of the extremities where tumors or lesions such as acral lick dermatitis have been removed surgically. Plastic repair of ear flaps and the external ear canal may be helpful in correcting associated dermatologic or cosmetic problems. Plastic surgery techniques are not discussed in this chapter, but information on them can be found in references.[25, 258, 267]

Cold Steel Surgery

Excision of small tumors and other lesions is a minor procedure that can often be done on an outpatient basis, but is usually better performed if the animal is held in the hospital for several hours. This enables the practitioner to use tranquilization, sedation, or general anesthesia as needed to promote control and relaxation of the patient. Cases requiring extensive surgery with plastic repair procedures and grafts need an operating room with complete aseptic routine. Even minor cases, however, must be handled with proper preparation, sterile instruments, and other measures to accomplish a scrupulously clean operation.

The dermatologist who employs surgical treatment of human diseases usually performs minor techniques on skin that is relatively hairless; therefore, the cosmetic effects are crucial. Most procedures appear complex because avoidance of scarring is a primary consideration. In veterinary dermatology, the clinician should, of course, avoid disfigurement; but because of the dense pelage, small scars are relatively unimportant.

With any surgical procedure, it is necessary to clip the hair closely, wash the unbroken skin surface carefully until it is clean using a surgical scrub solution such as 1 per cent chlorhexidine diacetate (Nolvasan [Fort Dodge]) or 0.75 per cent povidone-iodine (Betadine [Purdue Frederick]), and rinse thoroughly. The skin is defatted by wiping the surface in a circular fashion from the center outward, using sterile swabs soaked in 70 per cent alcohol. The skin can then be sprayed or swabbed with 0.5 per cent solution of chlorhexidine diacetate or, as a second choice, 1 per cent solution of povidone-iodine. The surgical site is then ready to drape. If a mast cell tumor is suspected, one should avoid a rough surgical preparation, which could trigger the release of vasoactive substances.

Basic instruments needed for skin surgery are in the average emergency or spay pack. The following additional instruments are useful for the delicate work in many skin surgical procedures:

1. Bard-Parker handles and blades, Nos. 10, 11, and 15
2. Small curved mosquito hemostats
3. Allis' tissue forceps
4. Skin hooks (sharp single prong)
5. Iris forceps (mouse toothed)
6. Olsen-Hegar needle holder with suture scissors
7. Skin punches, sizes 1 to 9 mm
8. Small automatic skin retractor

The lesions should be outlined by elliptic scalpel incisions that extend through the skin. The specimen or lesion is dissected free from the underlying tissue with scissors, hemostats, or both. Healing and final results are better if the long-axis incisions are oriented parallel to the tension lines shown in Figure 3:7. For closure, nylon sutures such as Vetafil produce good approximation with minimal scarring. Many quality suture materials are available, and the exact selection is a matter of personal preference. Swaged-on needles can further reduce the chance of infection and result in smaller scars. In routine cases with small incisions, the sutures can be removed in 10 to 14 days.

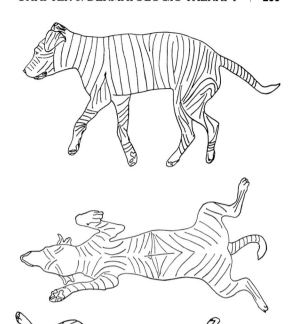

Figure 3:7. Composite drawing of the lateral, ventral, and dorsal aspects of a dog to show skin tension lines (based on six cases). (From Irwin D. H. G.: Tension lines in the skin of the dog. J. Small Anim. Pract. 7:593, 1966.)

Cryosurgery

Cryosurgery is the controlled use of freezing temperatures to destroy undesirable tissue, while doing minimal damage to surrounding healthy tissue. In general, cryosurgery is the most useful for small localized skin lesions treated on an outpatient basis. It does not cure where a blade does not cure, but it is sometimes more convenient. The anal and oral areas are preferred sites for cryosurgery, and it is indicated in selected cases of acral lick dermatitis. Specific conditions in which cryosurgery may be indicated include perianal fistulae, oral tumors, rectal tumors, nasal mucosal tumors, tail gland hyperplasia, feline indolent ulcers, and acral lick dermatitis. In the nasal, oral, and rectal areas where surgical access and hemostasis are difficult, cryosurgery has advantages. In large lesions of acral lick dermatitis that cannot be removed by cold steel surgery, cryosurgery offers a favorable alternative to skin grafting. For readers who are seriously considering using cryosurgery, excellent references are available.[258, 298]

The discussion of cryosurgery includes basic principles, freezing agents, cryosurgical units, and dermatologic indications.

BASIC PRINCIPLES

The lethal effect of subzero temperatures on cells depends on five factors:

1. Type of cell being frozen
2. Rate of freezing
3. Final temperature (must be at least $-20°C$)
4. Rate of thawing
5. Repetition of the freeze-thaw cycle

Cell damage is more severe with rapid freezing, slow thawing, and three freeze-thaw cycles. A final temperature of $-70°C$ is reached at the surface of the probe with nitrous oxide equipment, so that it can cool only a limited mass of tissue below the required $-20°C$, thereby restricting its application to small, superficial lesions. A final temperature of $-185°C$ can be reached at the tissue junction using liquid nitrogen. This enables the forming of a larger ice ball of tissue and allows larger areas to be effectively frozen.

A spray of liquid nitrogen offers the most effective way to freeze large tumor masses but also presents the greatest potential hazard if used carelessly. One advantage is that the base or periphery of a mass can be frozen first, by careful spraying around a delineated area extending 3 to 5 mm beyond the visible edge. The remaining tissues within this frozen "stockade" can be treated by spraying in ever-decreasing circles. Used with care, the spray may prevent the escape of malignant cells into the circulation, and it enables the operator to form superficial, solid frozen plaques on the surface without damaging deeper structures. In contrast, a probe must freeze a hemisphere as deep as the visible radius. It is important to use needle thermocouples at the deep margins of the tissues to be frozen to monitor the effect and to prevent excessive damage to normal tissue.

In human dermatology practice, it is common to apply liquid nitrogen with an ordinary cotton applicator stick, which is dipped into the container of liquid and touched to the lesion, frequently a small tumor or wart. The applicator stick is touched intermittently to the lesion until the desired area and depth are frozen. Dermatologists with experience in using this method get good results. The pain is minimal and well tolerated by most patients without local anesthesia.

Many soft tissues, especially glandular tissues, are particularly susceptible to freezing. On the other hand, bone, fascia, tendon sheath, perineurium, and the walls of large blood vessels are fairly resistant. A knowledge of relative tissue susceptibility is of great practical importance.

To ensure that no cells escape destruction, the freeze-thaw cycle should be repeated two times or more. Thawing usually takes one and a half to two times as long as freezing. Freezing is accomplished much more rapidly during the second and third freeze, because circulation to the target area has been compromised.

It has been speculated that useful immunologic effects are possible with cryosurgery. When a cell mass is frozen and left to die in situ, membrane lipoprotein complexes, and hence antigen-antibody complexing and receptor sites, are inevitably disrupted or altered. They are probably not totally destroyed. The nucleus may remain relatively intact. Thus, for a short time, antigenicity may be enhanced. Enough antigen is released systemically to produce a strong specific immunologic response that may kill escaped cells of the same tumor species.

After cryosurgery of canine skin tissue, histopathologic changes occur in an orderly progression of edema, erythema, infiltration of inflammatory cells, tissue necrosis, sloughing, repair by granulation, and re-epithelialization.[33]

Advantages

Cryosurgery has the following advantages:

1. Lesions can be removed in areas where the skin is so tight or the lesion so large that closure with sutures is impossible. Large lesions of acral lick dermatitis or tumors on the lower portions of the leg are examples.
2. In cases in which conventional excision surgery would produce shock or excessive blood loss, cryosurgery results in minimal hemorrhage. This is particularly effective in old or debilitated patients. Scarring is slight, and the cosmetic effect is good.
3. Selective destruction of diseased or neoplastic skin is possible with little damage to normal tissue. Chances of the spread of tumor cells from premalignant lesions are reduced.
4. Cryosurgery has a possible immunotherapeutic effect on malignant neoplasms.

Disadvantages

Cryosurgery has the following disadvantages:

1. The surgeon performing cryosurgery must be experienced and needs postgraduate training. Without specialized knowledge and skill, undesirable sequelae can result.
2. The necrosis and sloughing of frozen tissue are visually unpleasant and malodorous for 2 to 3 weeks after cryosurgery.
3. Regrowth of depigmented, white hair on the surgery site sometimes leaves a cosmetic defect.
4. Vital structures surrounding the frozen lesion may be damaged. This applies especially to blood vessels, nerves, tendons, ligaments, and joint capsules. For example, in cryosurgery for multiple perianal fistulae, fecal incontinence can result if the anal sphincter is damaged. Freezing of bone can result in pathologic fractures.
5. Large blood vessels frozen during cryosurgery for tumor removal may start bleeding 30 to 60 minutes later, when postoperative attention has been relaxed, or several hours later when the animal is at home. Air embolism is possible if sprays are used on open vessels.
6. Cryosurgery is contraindicated for mast cell tumors.

FREEZING AGENTS

Liquid nitrogen and nitrous oxide are the agents of choice in veterinary medicine. Carbon dioxide and Freon have also been used, but not commonly by veterinarians.

Liquid nitrogen is the most popular freezing agent in cryosurgery. It is a clear, colorless, odorless liquid. It is not flammable and produces a temperature of $-195.8°C$ ($-320.5°F$). It can usually be obtained from the medical supply companies that sell oxygen or from welding gas suppliers. Liquid nitrogen is delivered in various-sized vacuum-insulated Dewar's flasks. It can easily be poured from the flask into the cryosurgical unit. When small quantities are sufficient, physicians keep liquid nitrogen in ordinary quart insulated (Thermos) bottles that are refilled as needed by the supplier. If not agitated, it remains active in the insulated container for about 2 days. Liquid nitrogen can be kept active for a limited time. Usually, 1 month is the maximum, if the original container is opened several times.

Nitrous oxide is the second most popular freezing agent and is most effective for removing small tumors (less than 3 cm) or for treating superficial skin lesions. It requires cryosurgical units specifically designed for its use. Applied with probes, it produces a temperature of $-89°C$ ($-138°F$). Although it is more expensive on a unit basis than is liquid nitrogen, there is no waste, and nitrous oxide is readily available in veterinary hospitals that use gas anesthesia (halothane, nitrous oxide, and oxygen). One large tank can be used for many months, because it is usually connected directly to the unit and is not poured, as is liquid nitrogen.

CRYOSURGICAL UNITS

Cryosurgical units deliver the freezing action by spray or probe. Some units (smaller, hand-held bottles) are designed to spray the gas only. Other units have both spray and probe attachments.

Some cryosurgery units deliver gas to a probe that is held against the tissue or inserted into crevices, fistulae, or other tracts to be destroyed. Cryoprobes use the Joule-Thompson effect: rapid expansion of the gas under pressure provides low freezing temperatures. This is the method used with nitrous oxide. A great variety of probes are available, each for a different purpose. They can be round, flat, curved, pointed, or needle sharp. A special probe has even been devised for anal sac destruction.

There is a trend toward the use of the spray units. Some units look like modified insulated (Thermos) bottles with a spraying tip at the top. A mixture of liquid and vaporized liquid nitrogen is sprayed directly on the area to be treated. Different spray devices deliver different mixtures of liquid nitrogen, vapor, and liquid. This can vary from 15 per cent vapor and 85 per cent liquid to 55 per cent vapor and 45 per cent liquid. The higher the percentage of liquid in the spray, the lower is the temperature, and the more potent is the freeze.

DERMATOLOGIC INDICATIONS

Cryosurgery differs in many ways from cold steel surgery and electrosurgery. Although it has specific uses, it is never a total replacement for conventional surgery. Proponents of cryosurgery believe that it has an excellent place in small animal practice, but knowledge, skill, and experience are necessary for best results. Detractors may have used the technique for the wrong conditions or without proper training, consequently experiencing poor results or complications. Some clinicians were once enthusiastic about cryosurgery but now use it less frequently. As improved units are manufactured, some designed especially for veterinary surgery, the practitioner will find it easier to select the proper cryosurgical apparatus and use it effectively.

Podkonjak reported a series of dermatologic problems treated with cryosurgery. The success rate after one treatment was 86 per cent, and after one or more treatments, 93 per cent. Cases included melanoma, squamous cell carcinoma, fibrosarcoma, papilloma, basal cell tumor, hemangioma, histiocytoma, and trichoepithelioma. Also treated were follicular cysts, nonhealing ulcers, granulation tissue, proliferative tissue in the external ear canal, tail gland hyperplasia, perianal fistulae, and perianal adenomas.[190]

■ *Tumors.* Cryosurgery does not and should not replace conventional surgery. However, scalpel surgery is difficult or impossible to use in some situations.

■ *Oral Cavity.* Access to the oral cavity by means of conventional surgical instruments may be difficult, and hemorrhage may be hard to control. Cryosurgery is a simple and more effective method of therapy. It is an alternative in treating recurrent tumors, for cases in which other surgical procedures have failed, and especially for malignant neoplasms. Oral cavity squamous cell carcinomas may respond well to cryosurgery. Gingival epulis can be frozen, and sloughing occurs without need for hemostasis.

■ *Anal Area.* The main advantage of cryosurgery in managing anal tumors, especially perianal adenomas, is that it involves less risk of damaging the anal sphincter or the vital anal nerve supply. In general, though, careful cold steel surgery is still the preferred method of removing perianal adenomas.

■ *Acral Lick Dermatitis.* Cryosurgery is indicated in acral lick dermatitis when the lesion is so large that the skin cannot be stretched for suturing after surgical excision. Skin grafting has been used successfully, but only by practitioners highly skilled in plastic surgery. It is difficult to keep dogs from damaging the grafted area, because it is their favorite place to lick. Freezing the large lick lesion destroys the thickened skin, which is then replaced by granulation tissue that is covered by normal epithelium from the wound margins. Because cryosurgery temporarily deadens the sensory nerves, there is less licking and less chance for recurrence at the same site for up to 6 months. Care must be taken not to freeze the underlying bone. To have complete control of the depth of freezing, it is essential to insert thermocouples under the lesion. After the lesion heals, the resulting scar and white hair are seldom objectionable in these difficult cases. Regrettably, recurrences are the rule, usually within 6 to 12 months.

■ *Multiple Perianal Fistulae.* Perianal fistulae are difficult to treat by any method, but favorable results have been described using cryosurgery. This method of therapy for perianal fistulae reached a high level of popularity in the late 1970s, but some veterinary surgeons are now returning to the use of surgical excision. The number of lengthy cryosurgical procedures (two or more) and the frequent recurrences of fistulae are two reasons that it has lost favor. In addition, the occurrence of anal strictures is high. Anal sac removal is always recommended before cryosurgery. However, the anal sac area is usually difficult to see because of surrounding scar and granulation tissue. Every attempt must be made to avoid the complication of fecal incontinence, which can be a greater problem.

Laser Surgery

Laser surgery is highly successful in some branches of medicine, but its place in dermatology is still unclear.[25, 258] It is not a first-line choice in human disorders, except in the treatment of angiomas. Otherwise, laser surgery is reserved for instances when other treatments are not helpful. The technique has been useful in treating warts, vascular lesions, and extensive superficial skin tumors, but questions need to be considered about when to treat the condition, the age of the patient, and the potential for scarring. Standardization of treatments is necessary for humans, and as this modality becomes more available for animals, the issue must also be resolved for them. In veterinary medicine, laser therapy has been reported to be useful in certain cases of feline indolent ulcer and eosinophilic granuloma, acral lick dermatitis, excessive granulation tissue, and skin tumors of the eyelid, pinna, and tail.[30]

Electrosurgery

Just as heat cautery was replaced by electrocautery, the latter has been improved by modern electrosurgery.[25, 258] However, electrocautery equipment is still used to destroy tissue and to control hemorrhage by means of specialized tips that are heated to a bright cherry red, producing incandescent heat. The healing of tissue after the use of electrocautery is like that after a third-degree burn. This is not discussed further, because the newest electrosurgical units are more efficient. High-frequency electrosurgical units are capable of cutting, cutting and coagulation, desiccation (Fig. 3:8), fulguration (Fig. 3:9), and coagulation (Fig. 3:10). An electrosurgical unit can be extremely useful in small animal dermatology.[84]

The main advantages of electrosurgery are (1) reduction of surgery time, (2) reduction of total blood loss, (3) ease of coagulation when ligature application is difficult, and (4) reduction of foreign material left in the wound. The disadvantages are (1) improper use, leading to greater tissue damage; (2) presence of necrotic tissue within a wound; (3) delay in wound healing; (4) reduced early tensile strength of wound, up to 40 days after surgery; (5) decreased resistance

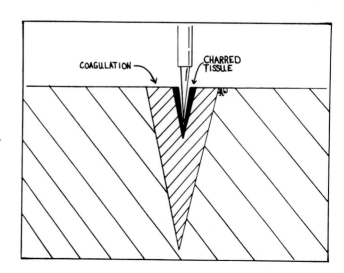

Figure 3:8. Desiccation. This technique is used for dehydration and deliberate destruction of tissue. (From Greene, J. A., Knecht, C. D.: Electrosurgery. Vet. Surg. 9:29, 1980.)

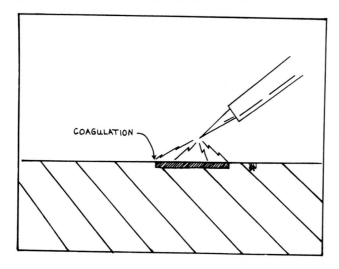

COAGULATION

Figure 3:9. Fulguration. This technique is used for superficial dehydration or coagulation of the tissue. (From Greene, J. A., Knecht, C. D.: Electrosurgery. Vet. Surg. 9:29, 1980.)

to infection; (6) greater scar width on the skin; and (7) inability to suture most electrosurgical wounds.

The greatest practical use of electrosurgery is for the removal of small pedunculated gingival or skin tumors. However, the procedure frequently makes histopathologic interpretation of the mass impossible. Broad-based tumors are best removed with a blade. Next in value is hemostasis during both conventional surgery and electrosurgery. The newest electrosurgical units generate currents that perform cutting and coagulation functions simultaneously.

MECHANISM AND INSTRUMENTATION

Electrosurgery uses electric currents to destroy tissues selectively. Electrosurgery is possible because electric current of greater than 10,000 Hz passes through the body without causing pain or muscle contractions, whereas the tissues and fluid of the body have electric impedance. Low frequencies (3000 Hz) result in pain and muscle contractions. At moderate frequencies (3000 to 5000 Hz), heat is produced, which causes tissue damage. Heat production is directly related to the power and concentration of the current delivered, the duration of application to the tissue, and the resistance of the tissue.

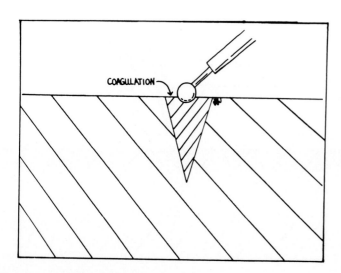

COAGULATION

Figure 3:10. Coagulation. This is the sealing of small blood vessels. The electrode is left in contact with the tissue until a deep white coagulum is formed. (From Greene, J. A., Knecht, C. D.: Electrosurgery. Vet. Surg. 9:29, 1980.)

With a biterminal electrosurgical unit, current passes from the unit to the active electrode in the handpiece and through the body. The current is conducted over a large surface area, which reduces resistance and current density, and it leaves the patient through the (indifferent) electrode or patient ground plate and returns to the unit. This plate should be as large as possible and covered with electrode paste or alcohol-soaked sponges to prevent secondary heating and burns.

The waveform of the current produced by the electrosurgical unit determines the tissue effect. Continuous, undamped sine waves are used for cutting but have poor hemostatic qualities. Interrupted or damped sine waves have poor cutting properties but achieve excellent hemostasis. Modulated, pulsed sine waves produce simultaneous cutting and coagulation.

An electric unit that produces a square wave was developed. When the waves are continuous, cutting without coagulation is possible; when the pulses of square waves are interrupted, coagulation without cutting results; and when a combined waveform is produced, both cutting and coagulation are possible.

The currents are generated by a spark gap, by radio tubes, or by battery-operated electrolysis machines. The machines range from inexpensive office units to high-priced hospital models. A unit in the medium price range is practical and versatile enough for use in most veterinary hospitals. Two main types of current are used: spark gap and electronic currents. These are converted from ordinary 110 V house current by a high-frequency generator in the electrosurgical unit. In all cases, it is mandatory for the patient to be grounded to the machine.

TECHNIQUES

■ *Cutting (Electroincision).* Bipolar cutting current is produced in a spark gap machine by increasing the frequency of successive wave trains.

■ *Cutting Without Coagulation.* Of any electrosurgical method, cutting without coagulation makes an incision with the least damage to surrounding tissue. It can be done in relatively nonvascular tissues. When simultaneous hemostasis is needed, however, a combination of cutting and coagulation gives the most satisfactory results.

■ *Desiccation.* Electrodesiccation is the application of a monopolar electric current (short spark) of high frequency and high tension to diseased or neoplastic tissue (see Fig. 3:8). The tissue is dried up by the current.

In dermatology, electrodesiccation can be combined with curettage. If a biopsy is required, the lesions can first be removed surgically by shaving the dome-shaped portion above the skin level (shave biopsy). This can be done with a scalpel blade held parallel to the skin or with small curved scissors with the convex surface toward the skin. The tissue remaining below the surface is then destroyed by desiccation and removed by curettage. Such electrodesiccation and curettage are especially useful for removing many sebaceous adenomas, perianal adenomas, fibrovascular papillomas, nevi, actinic keratoses, seborrheic keratoses, and small basal cell tumors.

■ *Coagulation.* Electrocoagulation is used to seal small blood vessels by boiling the vessels' endothelial cells with the current from the ball-like probe (see Fig. 3:10).

There are two methods of applying coagulation. One is to touch the electrode (ball) directly to the small blood vessel until the vessel wall shrinks and the hemorrhage is stopped by the tissue coagulation. The other method is to grasp the small blood vessel with a hemostat, which is then touched with the electrode (a flat probe is best) and the current is turned on with the foot switch. It is important to be sure that a good seal of the vessel is produced by either method, because new hemorrhage results from insufficient coagulation of the vessel walls.

■ *Fulguration.* Electric fulguration is the destruction of tissue by electric sparks generated by a high-frequency current (see Fig. 3:9). Direct fulguration occurs when the metal point of the probe is connected to the uniterminal of the high-frequency unit and a spark of electricity is directed to the tissue to be treated. Electrosurgical units capable of fulguration usually have a special probe into which the handpiece is inserted. Some units use the same handpiece, whereas others have special fulguration handpieces that cannot be plugged into cutting or coagulation plugs. Fulguration is used for destruction of superficial warts and tumors. Without need to touch the lesion, the current dehydrates and coagulates the tissue at the same time. This tissue does not need curettage but is allowed to slough. Most fulguration probes have a sharp point.

■ *Electrolysis.* Electric epilation of hair can be done by battery-operated units or electrosurgical units that can be used at low power. The probe must be a special tiny wire of such small diameter that it can be introduced into the hair follicle. With skill and experience, and under magnification, epilation can be accomplished. A too-low current allows epilated hair to grow back, whereas a current that is too high or an application that is too long can cause scarring. This method has been used for the removal of cilia in trichiasis and distichiasis (eyelid diseases, see Chap. 18).

Wounds

HEALING

Veterinary dermatologists perform minor surgical procedures and manage ulcers and other skin defects. Therefore, a basic understanding of wound healing is essential. In addition to the discussion that follows, more in-depth information can be found in the references.[42, 128, 129]

Wound healing is divided into three overlapping series of events: (1) inflammation, (2) new tissue formation, and (3) matrix remodeling. These stages progress along a continuum, and they may overlap considerably. An incised wound begins to heal by 5 to 8 days, with re-establishment of epidermal continuity and a proliferation of connective tissue from the papillary layer of the dermis. Thus, healing occurs in a "dished," or inverted, configuration until the production of underlying connective tissue pushes the epithelium up into an everted position (Fig. 3:11). (The major cell, matrix, and mediator components of wound healing are presented in Table 3:13.)

In the inflammatory stage, the immediate reaction to a full-thickness skin loss is for the normal elasticity of skin and muscle tension to enlarge and distort the defect. Vessels contract and constrict for 5 to 10 minutes to limit hemorrhage to the injured area, resulting in more widespread leakage of plasma constituents. Infiltrating neutrophils attempt to clear the area of

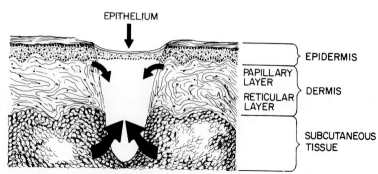

Figure 3:11. General pattern of wound healing. The wound epithelializes, with most of the connective tissue proliferating from the subcuticular areas upward into the wound *(large arrows)*. A smaller amount of connective tissue proliferates from the papillary layer of the dermis into the wound *(small arrows)*. The reticular layer of the dermis takes part in producing connective tissue to fill the intradermal area. (From Swaim, S. F.: Surgery of Traumatized Skin. W. B. Saunders Co., Philadelphia, 1980, p. 71.)

Table 3:13. Major Components of Wound Healing

Inflammation

CELLS	MATRIX	ENZYME CASCADES
Neutrophils	Fibrin	Hagemen factor pathways
Endothelial cells	Fibronectin	Coagulation
Mast cells		Fibrinolysis
Platelets		Complement

New Tissue Formation

CELLS	MATRIX	MEDIATORS*
Keratinocytes	Fibrin	PDGF
Macrophages	Fibronectin	FGF
		EGF
Endothelial cells	Collagen Types I or III	TGF-α
Fibroblasts	Hyaluronic acid	TGF-β

Matrix Remodeling

CELLS	MATRIX	MEDIATORS*
Keratinocytes	Basement membranes	TGF-β
Endothelial cells	Laminin	Collagenase
Fibroblasts	Type IV collagen	Other proteases
	Heparin sulfate	
	Type VI collagen	Glycosidases
	Chondroitin sulfate	
	Dermatan sulfate	

*PDGF, platelet-derived growth factor; FGF, fibroblast growth factor; EGF, epidermal growth factor; TGF, transforming growth factor.

foreign particles, especially bacteria. Peripheral blood monocytes are progressively attracted, are activated, and become macrophages. Macrophages, like platelets, produce growth factors critical for the initiation of granulation tissue formation. Blood vessel disruption leads to extravasation of blood constituents. Platelet aggregation and blood coagulation initiate the early phase of inflammation. Clot formation within vessel lumina effects hemostasis and within the surrounding connective tissue provides a substrate for cell migration into the wound space. Mediators released as a consequence of blood coagulation, complement pathways, and cell activation (or death) cause the influx of inflammatory leukocytes and increase the permeability of undamaged adjacent vessels. The mechanisms dispose of microorganisms, foreign material, and devitalized tissue, and set the stage for wound repair.

The new tissue formation stage proceeds quickly when clots, necrotic tissue, and other barriers to healing are removed from the wound. During this stage, the following processes occur: re-epithelialization, fibroplasia and wound contraction, and neovascularization (Fig. 3:12). In simple wounds, fibroblast proliferation and capillary infiltration start by the third to the fifth day. In open wounds, evidence of these processes is recognized as granulation tissue. Fibroblasts are most active in a wound for 14 to 21 days, and they advance along lines of fibrin within a clot and along capillaries that are growing into a wound. At first, the fibrin, fibroblasts, and new collagen fibers are vertically oriented in a wound, but after about 6 days, they are horizontally aligned, parallel to the wound surface.

The fibroblasts secrete various glycoproteins that constitute the ground substance of the wound. Collagen synthesis by the fibroblasts begins on the fourth or fifth day, and the tiny fibrils bond together into larger fibers that become ever stronger and less soluble. As sufficient collagen is formed, the number of fibroblasts in the wound decreases, marking the end of the

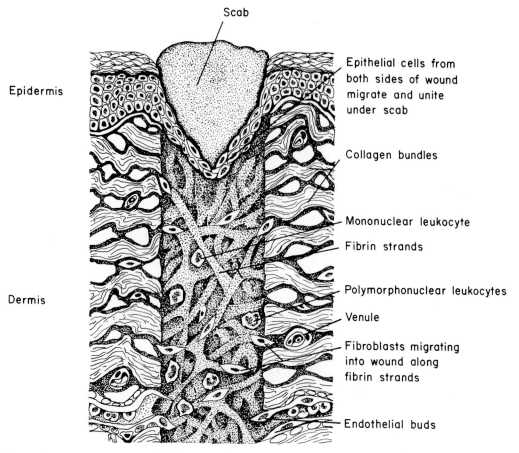

Figure 3:12. Early new tissue formation stage of wound healing. (From Swaim, S. F.: Surgery of Traumatized Skin. W. B. Saunders Co., Philadelphia, 1980, p. 78.)

repair stage. Elastic fibers play little part in wound repair, which explains the lack of scar elasticity.

Capillary infiltration of the healing wound is important to ensure optimal oxygen supply for the fibroblasts. Without optimal oxygen tension, fibroblasts cannot synthesize collagen adequately. The capillaries are a major part of the bright red granulation tissue that appears in open wounds from 3 to 6 days after injury. In small wounds, this occurs beneath a scab and is not visible. The proliferating capillaries form loops, or "knuckles," that give the wound a granular surface. The new vessels anastomose freely and differentiate progressively into arterioles and venules (Fig. 3:13). Lymphatic vessels develop in a similar manner, but a little later in the healing process.

Epithelial proliferation and migration are the first obvious signs of rebuilding and repair. Re-epithelialization of the epidermal defect begins within 24 hours after injury and continues during granulation tissue formation. Peripheral epidermal and infundibular hair follicle keratinocytes participate in the repair. An intense epidermal reaction occurs up to 5 mm back from the wound edge, and the number of epidermal cell layers dramatically increases. The cells lose their firm attachment to the underlying dermis, and they flatten and extend outward and downward over the incised dermis in a leapfrog fashion.

In simple wounds with clean, close approximation of edges, the defect may be covered by epithelium in 24 hours. In larger wounds, granulation tissue must form before wound epithelialization can start, and the process may take days or even weeks to complete (Fig. 3:14). If hair follicles are damaged, they participate in healing because the ends of the cut follicles are deep in the dermis and closer to the depth of the wound (Fig. 3:15). The new epithelium has a smooth undersurface with weak attachment to the connective tissue, so it is easily traumatized and may be knocked from a healing wound. With the passage of time, new sebaceous glands and hair follicles may regenerate by differentiation of migrating cells.

Wound contraction is the reduction in size of an open wound as a result of centripetal movement of the whole-thickness skin that surrounds the lesion. Contraction can be useful in loose skin, because it decreases the size of the wound that must be covered with epithelium. Over joints and in areas of tight skin, contractures can cause deformities. Contracture takes place between 5 and 45 days after injury. It is thought to result from a pulling action by modified fibroblasts in granulation tissue that take some of the characteristics of smooth muscle cells. These cells are called *myofibroblasts*, and they are also capable of producing collagen.

The matrix remodeling stage is a period of consolidation, strengthening, and remodeling of the wound (Fig. 3:16). In a fresh wound, a lag phase occurs (4 to 5 days), during which there is little gain in wound strength. The initial strength is due to the fibrin clot, adhesive forces of epithelialization, coagulation of protein in the wound, and ingrowth of capillaries, fibroblasts, and collagen fibrils. The amount of collagen increases rapidly during the first 3 weeks of healing, and then reaches a state of equilibrium. Over a long time, maturation and remodeling take place by cross-linkage and changes in the physical weave of the collagen fibers. The strength of skin and fascia increases but always remains 15 to 20 per cent weaker than surrounding normal tissue. All repair activity is confined to an area within approximately 15 mm of the wound.

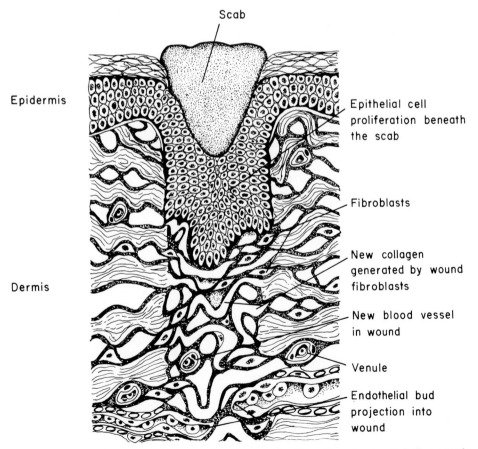

Scab

Epidermis

Epithelial cell proliferation beneath the scab

Fibroblasts

New collagen generated by wound fibroblasts

Dermis

New blood vessel in wound

Venule

Endothelial bud projection into wound

Figure 3:13. Later new tissue formation stage of wound healing. (From Swaim, S. F.: Surgery of Traumatized Skin. W. B. Saunders Co., Philadelphia, 1980, p. 80.)

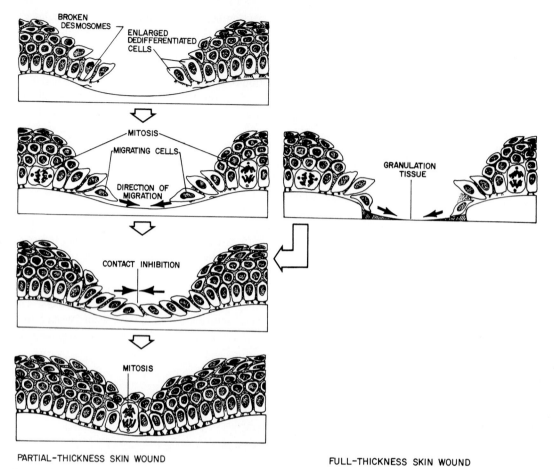

Figure 3:14. Basic processes of epithelial proliferation and migration. (From Swaim, S. F.: Surgery of Traumatized Skin. W. B. Saunders Co., Philadelphia, 1980, p. 84.)

Initially, scar tissue is vascular and cellular and appears pink and raised. As maturation occurs, the scar becomes white, hard, and flattened.

The following general factors are often considered to enhance or hasten wound healing: young age, administration of anabolic steroids, administration of topical and systemic vitamin A, ambulation of the patient, warm environment, and general good health. Ultrasound therapy has been reported to benefit wound healing when connective tissue is needed.[3] Although it increases inflammation and delays epithelialization, it stimulates fibroblast and collagen production and enhances vascularization of granulation tissue.

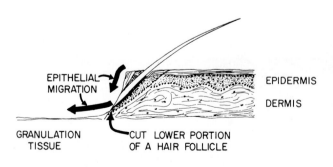

Figure 3:15. Hair follicle contribution to wound epithelialization. The edge of the wound that is situated in the direction of hair flow becomes oblique (forms an obtuse angle) with the wound. The cut lower parts of the hair follicles lie 1 to 2 mm closer to the wound center than does the epidermal edge. Epithelialization occurs from the ends of the cut follicles and from the epidermal edge. (From Swaim, S. F.: Surgery of Traumatized Skin. W. B. Saunders Co., Philadelphia, 1980, p. 85.)

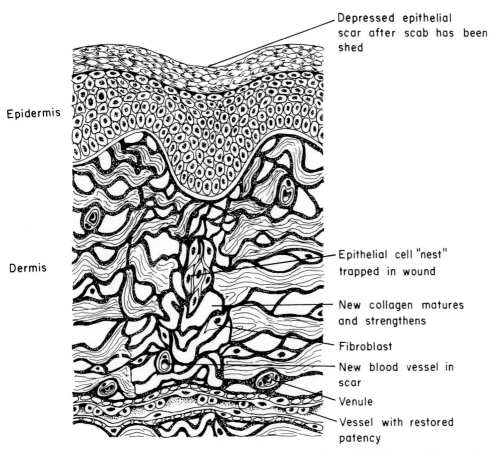

Epidermis

Dermis

Depressed epithelial scar after scab has been shed

Epithelial cell "nest" trapped in wound

New collagen matures and strengthens

Fibroblast

New blood vessel in scar

Venule

Vessel with restored patency

Figure 3:16. Mature remodeling stage of wound healing. (From Swaim, S. F.: Surgery of Traumatized Skin. W. B. Saunders Co., Philadelphia, 1980, p. 88.)

Factors that generally delay or are detrimental to wound healing, in addition to the poor health factors mentioned above, include obesity and old age, steroids and steroid-related factors, denervation, the presence of foreign bodies, infection, devitalized tissue, dead space, insulin deficiency, hypoproteinemia, anemia, hypovolemia, malnutrition, shock, increased catabolic rate, movement of the wound, neoplasia, tissue anoxia, radiation and cytotoxic drugs, seromas and hematomas, edema, cold temperatures, excessive trauma, and exposure during surgery. Nutritional deficiencies (especially of vitamins A, K, E, and C; the B complex; and zinc) are also detrimental to wound healing.

MANAGEMENT

Epidermal Abrasions

Margins of an abraded area are shallow and usually involve only the epidermis. Centrally, the defect may extend into the dermis. Initially, the injury fills with a blood clot and necrotic debris that dehydrate to form a scab. The epidermal adnexa may be injured, but they remain and regenerate. In partial-thickness wounds, they are the major source for re-epithelialization. The only care needed is initial gentle cleaning, allowing the scab to form, and protection from infection and trauma while the epidermal cells slide under the scab to re-epithelialize the exposed dermis.

Contaminated Wounds

The early time after a wound is called the "golden period"—an interval of about 6 hours during which prophylactic antibiotics are effective. The first aid for wounds should involve only covering the wound with moist, dry, clean, nonadhering material to control bleeding and to minimize contamination until definitive care can be provided.

For proper care, it may be necessary to use sedation or anesthesia, if allowed by the status of the patient. Otherwise, flushing the wound with 1 per cent lidocaine or using regional anesthesia may be sufficient for proper wound manipulation. Prophylactic antibiotics are completely effective for only up to 3 hours after trauma, and therefore systemic agents should be given first. One of the cephalosporins and gentamicin provide broad, effective coverage. The wound can be filled with a water-soluble gel (such as K-Y jelly) to protect it from further contamination while the area is prepared for surgery. Mineral oil or petroleum jelly can be applied to clippers to cause the hair to adhere to the blades while the area is being clipped. A vacuum is used to collect and direct debris away from the wound. The skin is prepared with chlorhexidine surgical scrub and gently cleaned with alcohol wipes. The clinician should then thoroughly irrigate the wound with large volumes of sterile saline or chlorhexidine solution 0.05 per cent to remove the gel and all foreign particles such as hair, dirt, and clotted blood.

Chlorhexidine is preferred to povidone-iodine solution, because it has a wide spectrum of antibacterial effectiveness, immediately reduces the bacterial flora, and has a residual effect as a result of binding to the stratum corneum so tightly that it cannot be removed with alcohol.[268] In the above dilution, it is nonirritating and does not delay healing. Systemic absorption, toxicity, and inactivation by organic matter are not a problem. However, if the tympanic membrane is ruptured, chlorhexidine solution should not be used in the external ear canal, because it may cause ototoxicity.

Clay is by far the most deleterious of the soil contaminants. Pressure lavage (10 psi) applied with an 18-gauge needle and 30-ml syringe or 70 psi pulsating pressure lavage, as provided with a dental water pick may be used to decontaminate the wound. These pressures have not been found to spread infection.

The wound can then be draped and explored for special problems. Layered debridement and sharp dissection are used to remove devitalized or severely traumatized tissue. Wound closure is made with properly placed sutures to approximate skin and to obliterate dead spaces. Proper placement of drains, if needed, and bandaging as appropriate complete the initial treatment.

Decubital Ulcers

Debilitated, paralyzed patients have poor circulation, and their immobility allows pressure between bony prominences and their bedding to restrict circulation further to a local tissue area. The area becomes red, and a punched-out ulcer develops later. The ulcer may have a gray fibrous coating with surrounding necrotic tissue.

Prevention by providing frequent turning, gentle massage, flexion of muscles and joints, and placing the patient on a waterbed is most important. After it has developed, the ulcer is treated by cleaning with 0.05 per cent chlorhexidine solution to remove necrotic tissue, pus, and debris. The ulcer should be covered with moist occlusive bandages or a nonadherent film, and protected from pressure by "doughnut" rings or bandage rolls. Although mild antibacterial dressings are often useful initially, the application of a live yeast cell derivative and phenylmercuric nitrate in shark liver oil (Preparation H [Whitehall]) ointment increases oxygen utilization and collagen formation in tissues, and it increases wound healing. It also lubricates and protects the ulcer. When the patient becomes mobile, the ulcers heal spontaneously.

REFERENCES

1. Ackerman, L.: Cutaneous bacterial granuloma (botryomycosis) in five dogs: Treatment with rifampin. Mod. Vet. Pract. 68:404, 1987.

2. Ackerman, L.: Nutritional supplements in canine dermatoses. Can. Vet. J. 28:29, 1987.
3. Al-Sadi, H. I.: Effects of ultrasonic therapy on wound healing. Canine Pract. 11:50, 1984.
4. American Kennel Club: The Complete Dog Book, 17th ed. Howell House, New York, 1985.
5. Anderson, R. K.: Canine pododermatitis. Comp. Cont. Educ. 2:361, 1980.
6. Angarano, D. W., MacDonald, J. M.: Efficacy of cefadroxil in the treatment of bacterial dermatitis in dogs. J. Am. Vet. Med. Assoc. 194:57, 1989.
7. Aram, H.: Cimetidine in dermatology. Int. J. Dermatol. 26:161, 1987.
8. Aram, H.: Colchicine in dermatologic therapy. Int. J. Dermatol. 22:566, 1983.
9. Arndt, K. A., et al.: The pharmacology of topical therapy. In: Fitzpatrick T. B., et al. (eds.). Dermatology in General Medicine, 4th ed. McGraw-Hill Book Co., New York, 1993, p. 2837.
10. Arther, R. G., Cox, D. D.: Evaluating the efficacy of fenthion for control of fleas on dogs. Vet. Med. (S.A.C.) 80:28, 1985.
11. Ayliffe, T. R.: Penetration of tissue by antibiotics. Br. Vet. Dermatol. Newsl. 5:233, 1980.
12. Baker, N. F., Farver, T. B.: Failure of brewer's yeast as a repellent to fleas on dogs. J. Am. Vet. Med. Assoc. 183:212, 1983.
13. Bardana, E. J.: Recent developments in immunomodulatory therapy. J. Allergy Clin. Immunol. 75:423, 1985.
14. Barnes, L. E.: Adapting the use of fenthion to special cases. Vet. Med. (S.A.C.) 81:492, 1986.
15. Barta, O.: Immunoadjuvant therapy. In: Kirk, R. W., Bonagura, J. D. (eds.). Kirk's Current Veterinary Therapy XI. W. B. Saunders Co., Philadelphia, 1992, p. 217.
16. Battistella, M. W.: Evaluating the safety of cythioate for feline flea control. Vet. Med. (S.A.C.) 81:475, 1986.
17. Beale, K. M., et al.: A study of long term administration of FS shampoo in dogs. Proc. Annu. Memb. Meet. Am. Acad. Vet. Dermatol. Am. Coll. Vet. Dermatol. 9:36, 1993.
18. Beale, K. M.: Azathioprine toxicity in the domestic cat. In: Von Tscharner, C., Halliwell, R. E. W. (eds.). Advances in Veterinary Dermatology, Vol. 1. Baillière-Tindall, Philadelphia, 1990, p. 457.
18a. Beale, K. M.: Azathioprine for treatment of immune-mediated diseases of dogs and cats. J. Am. Vet. Med. Assoc. 53:1236, 1992.
19. Becker, A. M., et al.: *Propionibacterium acnes* immunotherapy in chronic recurrent canine pyoderma: An adjunct to antibiotic therapy. J. Vet. Intern. Med. 3:26, 1989.
20. Bennett, D. G.: Clinical pharmacology of ivermectin. J. Am. Vet. Med. Assoc. 189:100, 1986.
21. Bernstein, J. E., et al.: Inhibition of histamine induced pruritus by topical tricyclic antidepressants. J. Am. Acad. Dermatol. 5:582, 1981.
22. Bierman, C. W., et al.: Effect of H_1 receptor blockade on late cutaneous reactions to antigen: A double-blind controlled study. J. Allergy Clin. Immunol. 87:151, 1991.
23. Blaldey, B. R., Rousseaux, C. G.: Effect of ivermectin on the immune response in mice. Am. J. Vet. Res. 52:593, 1991.
24. Blagburn, B. L., et al.: Anthelmintic efficacy of ivermectin in naturally parasitized cats. Am. J. Vet. Res. 48:670, 1987.
24a Blagburn, B. L., et al.: Efficacy dosage titration of lufenuron against developmental stages of fleas (*Ctenocephalides felis felis*) in cats. Am. J. Vet. Res. 55:98, 1994.
25. Bojrab, M. J.: Current Techniques in Small Animal Surgery, 3rd ed. Lea & Febiger, Philadelphia, 1990.
26. Bond, R., Lloyd, D. H.: A double blind comparison of olive oil and a combination of evening primrose oil and fish oil in the management of chronic atopy. Vet. Rec. 131:558, 1992.
27. Bond, R., Lloyd, D. H.: Randomized single-blind comparison of an evening primrose oil and fish oil combination and concentrates of these oils in the management of canine atopy. Vet. Dermatol. 3:215, 1992.
28. Bourdeau, P., Paragon, B. M.: Alternatives aux corticoides en dermatologie des carnivores. Rev. Méd. Vét. 168:645, 1992.
29. Brayton, C. F.: Dimethyl sulfoxide (DMSO), a review. Cornell Vet. 76:61, 1986.
30. Breen, P. T.: Lasers in dermatology. In: Kirk, R. W. (ed.). Current Veterinary Therapy X. W. B. Saunders Co., Philadelphia, 1989, p. 580.
31. Brunner, C. J., Muscoplat, C. C.: Immunomodulatory effects of levamisole. J. Am. Vet. Med. Assoc. 176:1159, 1980.
32. Bruyette, D. S., Feldman, E. C.: Efficacy of ketoconazole in the management of spontaneous canine hyperadrenocorticism. Resident's forum, University of California, Davis, 1987.
33. Bushby, P. A., et al.: Microscopic tissue alterations following cryosurgery of canine skin. J. Am. Vet. Med. Assoc. 173:177, 1978.
34. Bussieras, J., et al.: Le traitment des teignes des carnivores domestiques au moyen de dérivatives récents de l'imidazole. Prat. Méd. Chirurg. Anim. Cie. 19:152, 1984.
35. Campbell, K. L., Kirkwood, A. R.: Effect of topical oils on transepidermal water loss in dogs with seborrhea sicca. In: Ihrke, P. J., et al. (eds.). Advances in Veterinary Dermatology Vol. 2. Pergamon Press, New York, 1993, p. 157.
36. Campbell K. L., et al.: Effects of oral sunflower oil on serum and cutaneous fatty acid concentration profiles in seborrheic dogs. Vet. Dermatol. 3:29, 1992.
37. Carlotti, D., Ovaert, P.: Utilisation de l'association amoxycilline acide clavalonique dans le traitement de pyodermites du chien. Prat. Méd. Chirurg. Anim. Cie. 23:519, 1988.
37a. Carlotti, D. N., Delahaut, M. P.: Le Contrôle parasitaire autour du chien atteint de D.A.P.P.: intérêt du cythioate chez les chats congénères. Prat. Méd. Chirurg. Anim. Cie. 27:543, 1992.
38. Cauwenbergh, G., et al.: Pharmacokinetic profile of orally administered intraconazole in human skin. J. Am. Acad. Dermatol. 18:263, 1988.

39. Chalmers, S. A.: Evaluation of ketoconazole in the treatment of canine and feline dermatophytosis. Proc. Annu. Memb. Meet. Am. Acad. Vet. Dermatol. Am. Coll. Vet. Dermatol. 5:15, 1989.
40. Chastain, C. B., Ganjam, V. K.: Clinical Endocrinology of Companion Animals. Lea & Febiger, Philadelphia, 1986.
41. Chastain, C. B., Graham, C. L.: Adrenocortical suppression in dogs on daily and alternate day prednisolone administration. Am. J. Vet. Res. 40:936, 1979.
42. Clark, R. A. F.: Cutaneous wound repair. In: Goldsmith, L. A. (ed.). Physiology, Biochemistry, and Molecular Biology of the Skin II. Oxford University Press, Oxford, 1991.
43. Cytil, E.: Vitamin A and the skin. In: Goldsmith, L. A. (ed.). Biochemistry and Physiology of the Skin. Oxford Press, New York, 1983.
44. D'Arcy, P., et al.: The anti-inflammatory action of griseofulvin in experimental animals. J. Pharm. Pharmacol. 12:659, 1960.
45. Daurio, C. P., et al.: Reproductive evaluation of male beagles and the safety of ivermectin. Am. J. Vet. Res. 48:1755, 1987.
45a. Davis, J. A., et al.: Benzocaine-induced methemoglobinemia attributed to topical application of the anesthetic in several laboratory animal species. Am. J. Vet. Res. 54:1322, 1993.
46. DeBoer, D. J., et al.: Clinical and immunological responses of dogs with recurrent pyoderma to injections of staphylococcus phage lysate. In: Von Tscharner, C., Halliwell, R. E. W. (eds.). Advances in Veterinary Dermatology, Vol. 1. Baillière-Tindall, Philadelphia, 1990, p. 335.
47. DeBoer, D. J., et al.: Evaluation of a commercial staphylococcal bacterin for management of idiopathic recurrent pyoderma in dogs. Am. J. Vet. Res. 51:636, 1990.
48. DeBoer, D. J., Pukay, B. P.: Workshop report 2. Recurrent pyoderma and immune stimulants. In: Ihrke, P. J., et al. (eds.). Advances in Veterinary Dermatology II. Pergamon Press, New York, 1993, p. 443.
49. DeNovo, R. C.: Therapeutics of gastrointestinal diseases. In: Kirk, R. W. (ed.). Current Veterinary Therapy IX. W. B. Saunders Co., Philadelphia, 1986, p. 862.
50. Dryden, M. W.: Differential activity of cythioate against female and male *Ctenocephalides felis* on cats. Am. J. Vet. Res. 53:801, 1992.
51. duVivier, A., Stoughton, R. B.: Tachyphylaxis to the action of topically applied corticosteroids. Arch. Dermatol. 111:581, 1975.
52. Edney, A. T. B., Smith, P. M.: Study of obesity in dogs visiting veterinary practices in the United Kingdom. Vet. Rec. 118:391, 1986.
53. Eigenmann, J. E., et al.: Estrogen-induced flank alopecia in the female dog: Evidence for local rather than systemic hyperestrogenism. J. Am. Anim. Hosp. Assoc. 20:621, 1984.
54. Eigenmann, J. E.: Growth hormone–deficient disorders associated with alopecia in the dog. In: Kirk, R. W. (ed.). Current Veterinary Therapy IX. W. B. Saunders Co., Philadelphia, 1986, p. 1015.
55. El Gazzar, L. M., et al.: J. Econ. Entomol. 79:132, 1986.
56. Ellis, C. N., Voorhees, J. J.: Etretinate therapy. J. Am. Acad. Dermatol. 16:267, 1987.
57. Esterly, N. B., et al.: The effect of antimicrobial agents on leukocyte chemotaxis. J. Invest. Dermatol. 70:51, 1978.
58. Evans, A. G., et al.: A trial of 13-*cis*-retinoic acid for treatment of squamous cell carcinoma and preneoplastic lesions of the head in cats. Am. J. Vet. Res. 46:2553, 1985.
59. Evinger, J. V., Nelson, R. W.: The clinical pharmacology of thyroid hormones in the dog. J. Am. Vet. Med. Assoc. 185:314, 1984.
60. Fadok, V. A.: Nutritional therapy in veterinary dermatology. In: Kirk, R. W. (ed.). Current Veterinary Therapy IX. W. B. Saunders Co., Philadelphia, 1986, p. 591.
61. Fadok, V. A.: Thrombocytopenia and hemorrhage associated with gold salt therapy for bullous pemphigoid in a dog. J. Am. Vet. Med. Assoc. 181:261, 1982.
62. Fadok, V. A.: Treatment of canine idiopathic seborrhea with isotretinoin. Am. J. Vet. Res., 47:1730, 1986.
63. Fadok, V. A., Barrie, J.: Sulfasalazine responsive vasculitis in the dog: A case report. J. Am. Anim. Hosp. Assoc. 20:161, 1984.
64. Ferguson, D. C.: Thyroid hormone replacement therapy. In: Kirk, R. W. (ed.). Current Veterinary Therapy IX. W. B. Saunders Co., Philadelphia, 1986, p. 1018.
65. Figueiredo, C.: Vitamin E serum contents, erythrocyte and lymphocyte counts, PCV and Hg determinations in normal dogs, dogs with scabies and dogs with demodicosis. Proc. Annu. Memb. Meet. Am. Acad. Vet. Dermatol. Am. Coll. Vet. Dermatol., 1985.
66. Figueiredo, C., et al.: Clinical evaluation of the effect of vitamin E in the treatment of generalized canine demodicosis. In: Ihrke, P. J., et al. (eds.). Advances in Veterinary Dermatology, Vol. 2. Pergamon Press, New York, 1993, p. 247.
67. Fine, R. M.: Physiologic effects of systemic corticosteroids in dermatology. Cutis 11:217, 1973.
67a. Fisher, M. A., et al.: Efficacy of fenthion against the flea, *Ctenocephalides felis*, on the cat. J. Small Anim. Pract. 34:434, 1993.
67b. Fisher, M. A., et al.: Efficacy of cythioate against fleas on dogs and cats. Vet. Dermatol. 1:46, 1989.
68. Foil, C. S.: Dermatophytosis. In: Griffin, C. E., et al. (eds.). Current Veterinary Dermatology. Mosby Year Book, St. Louis, 1993, p. 22.
69. Fledman, R. J., Maibach, H. I.: Regional variation in percutaneous penetration of C^{14} cortisol in man. J. Invest. Dermatol. 48:181, 1967.
70. Franc, M., et al.: Studies on the therapy of otacariasis of cats with ivermectin. Rev. Méd. Vét. 136:681, 1985.
70a. Franc, M.: La lutte contre les puces dans l'environnement. Pract. Méd. Chirurg. Anim. Cie. 28:235, 1993.

71. Frank, L. A., Kunkle, G. A.: Comparison of the efficacy of cefadroxil and generic and proprietary cephalexin in the treatment of pyodermas in dogs. J. Am. Vet. Med. Assoc. 203:530, 1993.
72. Franz, T. J.: Kinetics of cutaneous drug penetration. Int. J. Dermatol. 22:499, 1983.
73. Fredenberg, M. F., Malkinson, F. S.: Sulfone therapy in the treatment of leukocytoclastic vasculitis. J. Am. Acad. Dermatol. 16:772, 1987.
74. Fridinger, T. L.: Designing the ultimate weapon against fleas. Vet. Med. (S.A.C.) 79:1151, 1984.
75. Frieden, I. J., Price, V. H.: Androgenetic alopecia. In: Thiers, B. H., Dobson, R. L. (eds.). Pathogenesis of Skin Disease. Churchill Livingstone, New York, 1986.
76. Garfield, R. A., Reedy, L. M.: The use of oral milbemycin oxime (Interceptor) in the treatment of chronic generalized canine demodicosis. Vet. Dermatol. 3:231, 1992.
77. Giger, U., et al.: Sulfadiazine-induced allergy in six Doberman pinschers. J. Am. Vet. Med. Assoc. 186:479, 1985.
78. Gilbert, P. A., et al.: Serum vitamin E levels in dogs with pyoderma and generalized demodicosis. J. Am. Anim. Hosp. Assoc. 28:407, 1992.
79. Glaze, M. R., et al.: Ophthalmic corticosteroid therapy: Systemic effects in the dog. J. Am. Vet. Med. Assoc. 192:73, 1988.
80. Goette, D. K., Odom, R. B.: Adverse effects of corticosteroids. Cutis 23:477, 1979.
81. Goldyne, M. E.: Leukotrienes: Clinical significance. J. Am. Acad. Dermatol. 10:659, 1984.
82. Greaves, M. W.: Pharmacology and significance of nonsteroidal anti-inflammatory drugs in the treatment of skin diseases. J. Am. Acad. Dermatol. 16:751, 1987.
83. Greene, C. E. (ed.): Clinical Microbiology and Infectious Diseases of the Dog and Cat. W. B. Saunders Co., Philadelphia, 1984.
84. Greene, J. A., Knecht, C. D.: Electrosurgery: A review. Vet. Surg. 9:327, 1980.
85. Gregory, C. R., et al.: Response to isoantigens and mitogens in the cat: Effects of cyclosporine A. Am. J. Vet. Res. 48:126, 1987.
85a. Grier, R. L., et al.: Hyperthermic treatment of superficial tumors in cats. J. Am. Vet. Med. Assoc. 177:227, 1980.
86. Griffin, C. E.: Canine atopic disease. In: Griffin, C. E., et al. (eds.). Current Veterinary Dermatology. Mosby Year Book, St. Louis, 1993, p. 99.
87. Griffin, C. E.: Open forum—Etretinate—How is it being used in veterinary dermatology? Derm. Dialog. Spring/Summer 1993.
88. Griffin, C. E.: Pemphigus foliaceus: Recent findings on the pathophysiology and results of treatment. Proceedings, The University of Edinburgh, 1993, p. 85.
89. Griffin, C. E.: Systemic glucocorticoid therapy in veterinary medicine. Presentation, Am. Acad. Vet. Dermatol., New Orleans, March, 1986.
90. Griffin, C. E.: Unpublished observations.
91. Guaguère, E., Marc, J. P.: Utilisation de la céfalexine dans le traitement des pyodermites. Prat. Méd. Chirurg. Anim. Cie. 24:124, 1989.
91a. Guaguère, E., Picard, G.: Utilization de la céfalexine et du lactate d'ethyle dans le traitement des pyodermites canines. Pract. Méd. Chirurg. Anim. Cie. 25:547, 12990.
92. Gyrd-Hansen, N., et al.: Percutaneous absorption of organophosphorus insecticides in pigs—The influence of different vehicles. J. Vet. Pharmacol. Ther. 16:174, 1993.
93. Hall, I.: In DeBoer and Pukay. Workshop report 2. Recurrent pyoderma and immune stimulants. In: Ihrke, P. J., et al. (eds.). Advances in Veterinary Dermatology II. Pergamon Press, New York, 1993, p. 443.
94. Harris, R., et al.: Orally administered ketoconazole: Route of delivery to the human stratum corneum. Antimicrob. Agents Chemother. 24:876, 1983.
95. Harvey, R. G.: Management of feline miliary dermatitis by supplementing the diet with essential fatty acids. Vet. Rec. 128:326, 1991.
96. Harvey, R. G.: A comparison of evening primrose oil and sunflower oil for the management of papulocrustous dermatitis in cats. Vet. Rec. 133:571, 1993.
96a. Harvey, R. G.: Effect of varying proportions of evening primrose oil and fish oil on cats with crusting dermatosis (''miliary dermatitis''). Vet. Rec. 133:208, 1993.
96b. Harvey, R. G., et al.: A comparison of lincomycin hydrochloride and clindamycin hydrochloride in the treatment of superficial pyoderma in dogs. Vet. Rec. 132:351, 1993.
97. Helton, K. A., et al.: Griseofulvin toxicity in cats: Literature review and report of seven cases. J. Am. Anim. Hosp. Assoc. 22:453, 1986.
98. Heripret, D.: Les antiprurigineux non steroidiens. Prat. Méd. Chirurg. Anim. Cie. 28:73, 1993.
98a. Hink, W. F., et al.: Evaluation of a single oral dose of lufenuron to control flea infestations in dogs. Am. J. Vet. Res. 55:822, 1994.
99. Holzworth, J.: Diseases of the Cat. W. B. Saunders Co., Philadelphia, 1987.
100. Hsu, W. H., Schaffer, D. D.: Effects of topical application of amitraz on plasma glucose and insulin concentrations in dogs. Am. J. Vet. Res. 49:130, 1988.
101. Hubbell, S. J.: Personal communication, 1982.
102. Hubert, B., Olivry, T.: Sex hormones and the skin of domesticated carnivores. Eur. J. Comp. Anim. Pract. 2:41, 1991. (Reprinted.)
103. Humbert, P., et al.: The tetracyclines in dermatology. J. Am. Acad. Dermatol. 25:691, 1991.
104. Humphreys, F., Shuster, S.: The effect of topical dimethindene maleate on wheal reactions. Br. J. Clin. Pharmacol. 23:234, 1987.
105. Ihrke, P. J.: Antibiotic therapy in canine skin disease—Dermatologic therapy III. Comp. Cont. Educ. 11:177, 1980.

106. Irhke, P. J.: Antibacterial therapy in dermatology. In: Kirk, R. W. (ed.). Current Veterinary Therapy IX. W. B. Saunders Co., Philadelphia, 1986, p. 566.

107. Isaacson, D., et al.: Antimalarials in dermatology. Int. J. Dermatol. 21:379, 1982.

107a. Jeffers, J. G.: Diabetes mellitus induced in a dog after administration of costicosteroids and methylprednisolone pulse therapy. J. Am. Vet. Med. Assoc. 199:77, 1991.

108. Kemppainen, R. J., et al.: Adrenocortical suppression in the dog after a single dose of methylprednisolone acetate. Am. J. Vet. Res. 42:822, 1981.

109. Kemppainen, R. J., et al.: Adrenocortical suppression in the dog given a single intramuscular dose of prednisone or triamcinolone acetonide. Am. J. Vet. Res. 42:204, 1982.

110. Kemppainen, R. J.: Principles of glucocorticoid therapy in nonendocrine disease. In: Kirk, R. W. (ed.). Current Veterinary Therapy IX. W. B. Saunders Co., Philadelphia, 1986, p. 954.

111. Kietzmann, M., et al.: Vertraglichkeif and pharmakokinetik von cefalexin (cefaseptin dragees) beim hund. Kleintierpraxis 35:390, 1990.

111a. Kobay, M. J., and Jones, B. R.: Local current yield radiofrequency hyperthermia for the treatment of superficial skin tumors in cats. New Zealand Vet. J. 31:173, 1983.

112. Koblenzer, C. S.: Pharmacology of psychotropic drugs useful in dermatologic practice. Int. J. Dermatol. 32:162, 1993.

113. Koch, H. J., Vercelli, A.: Workshop report 3: Shampoos and other topical therapies. In: Ihrke, P. J., et al.: Advances in Veterinary Dermatology. Vol. 2. Pergamon Press, Oxford, 1993, p. 409.

114. Koehler, et al.: Residual efficacy of insecticides applied to carpet for control of cat fleas. J. Econ. Entomol. 79:1063, 1986.

115. Kummel, B.: Treatment of autoimmune disease. Derm. Dialog. 4:2, 1985.

116. Kunkle, G. A.: Progestagens in dermatology. In: Kirk, R. W. (ed.). Current Veterinary Therapy IX. W. B. Saunders Co., Philadelphia, 1986, p. 601.

117. Kunkle, G. A.: Sensitivity of staphylococcal isolates in canine pyoderma. Proceedings, Am. Acad. Vet. Dermatol., Phoenix, March 19, 1987, p. 6.

118. Kunkle, G. A.: Zinc responsive dermatoses in dogs. In: Kirk, R. W. (ed.). Current Veterinary Therapy VII. W. B. Saunders Co., Philadelphia, 1980, p. 472.

119. Kunkle, G. A., Meyer, D. J.: Toxicity of high doses of griseofulvin in cats. J. Am. Vet. Med. Assoc. 191:322, 1987.

120. Kwochka, K. W.: Canine demodicosis. In: Kirk, R. W. (ed.). Current Veterinary Therapy IX. W. B. Saunders Co., Philadelphia, 1986, p. 531.

121. Kwochka, K. W.: Primary keratinization disorders of dogs. In: Griffin, C. E., et al. (eds.). Current Veterinary Dermatology, Mosby Year Book, St. Louis, 1993, p. 176.

122. Kwochka, K. W.: Recurrent pyoderma. In: Griffin, C. E., et al. (eds.). Current Veterinary Dermatology. Mosby Year Book, St. Louis, 1993, p. 3.

123. Kwochka, K. W.: Retinoids and vitamin A therapy. In: Griffin, C. E., et al. (eds.). Current Veterinary Dermatology. Mosby Year Book, St. Louis, 1993, p. 203.

124. Kwochka, K. W.: Symptomatic topical therapy of scaling disorders. In: Griffin, C. E., et al. (eds.). Current Veterinary Dermatology. Mosby Year Book, St. Louis, 1993, p. 191.

125. Kwochka, K. W., Kowalski, J. S.: Prophylactic efficacy of four antibacterial shampoos against *Staphylococcus intermedius* in dogs. Am. J. Vet. Res. 52:115, 1991.

126. Latimer, K. S., et al.: Effects of cyclosporin A administration in cats. Vet. Immunol. Immunopathol. 11:161, 1986.

127. Lees, G. E., et al.: Fatal thrombocytopenic hemorrhagic diathesis associated with dapsone administration to a dog. J. Am. Vet. Med. Assoc. 174:49, 1979.

128. Lees, M. J., et al.: Factors influencing wound healing: Lessons from military wound management. Comp. Cont. Educ. 11:8550, 1989.

129. Lees, M. J., et al.: Second-intention wound healing. Comp. Cont. Educ. 11:857, 1989.

130. Lesher, J. L., Chalker, D. K.: Response of the cutaneous lesions of Reiter's syndrome to ketoconazole. J. Am. Acad. Dermatol. 13:161, 1985.

130a. Lewis, D.T., et al: Ivermectin toxicosis in a kitten. J. Am. Vet. Med. Assoc. 205:584, 1994.

131. Lewis, L. D.: Cutaneous manifestations of nutritional imbalances. Lecture notes, 1982.

132. Lichtenstein, J., et al.: Nonsteroidal anti-inflammatory drugs. Their use in dermatology. Int. J. Dermatol. 26:80, 1987.

133. Lober, C. W.: Canthaxanthin: The "tanning" pill. J. Am. Acad. Dermatol. 13:660, 1985.

134. Logas, D.: Double-blind crossover study with high-dose eicosapentaenoic acid supplementation for the treatment of canine allergic pruritus. Proc. Annu. Memb. Meet. Am. Acad. Vet. Dermatol. Am. Coll. Vet. Dermatol. 9:37, 1993.

135. Long, P. G.: Sulfones and sulfonamides in dermatology today. J. Am. Acad. Dermatol. 1:479, 1979.

136. Lorenz, M.: Managing flea-allergy dermatitis—2: Should you use systemic therapy to control flea allergy dermatitis? Vet. Med. (S.A.C.) 79:1148, 1984.

137. Lloyd, D. H., Thomsett, L. R.: Essential fatty acid supplementation in the treatment of canine atopy. A preliminary study. Vet. Dermatol. 1:41, 1989.

138. Lloyd, D. H.: Essential fatty acids and skin disease. J. Small Anim. Pract. 30:207, 1989.

139. Lueker D. C., Kainer, R. A.: Hyperthermia for the treatment of dermatomycoses in dogs and cats. Vet. Med. (S.A.C.) 76:658, 1981.

140. MacDonald, J. M., Miller, T. A.: Parasiticide therapy in small animal dermatology. In: Kirk, R. W. (ed.). Current Veterinary Therapy IX. W. B. Saunders Co., Philadelphia, 1986, p. 571.

141. MacDonald, K. R., et al.: Remission of staphylococcal dermatitis by autogenous bacteria therapy. Can. Vet. J. 13:45, 1972.

141a. MacEwen, E. G.: Approaches to cancer therapy using biological response modifiers. Vet. Clin. North Am. (Small Anim. Pract.) 15:667, 1985.

142. Maibach, H. I., Stoughton, R. B.: Topical corticosteroids. Med. Clin. North Am. 57:1253, 1973.

143. Mansfield, P. D., Kemppainen, R. J.: Effects of megestrol acetate treatment on glucose concentration and insulin response to glucose administration in cats. J. Am. Anim. Hosp. Assoc. 22:515, 1986.

143a. Marks, S. L., Song, M. D., et al.: Clinical evaluation of etretinate for the treamtent of canine solar induced squamous cell carcinoma and preneoplastic lesions. J. Am. Acad. Dermatol. 27:11, 1992.

144. Marshall, A. B.: Antibiotic therapy of small animal dermatitis. Br. Vet. Dermatol. Newsl. 5:2, 1980.

145. Mason, K. V.: Clinical and pathophysiologic aspects of parasitic skin diseases. In: Ihrke, P. J., et al. (eds.). Advances in Veterinary Dermatology, Vol. 2. Pergamon Press, New York, 1993, p. 177.

146. Mason, K. V., Stewart, L. J.: Workshop report 1. *Malassezia* canine dermatitis. In: Ihrke, P. J., et al. (eds.). Advances in Veterinary Dermatology Vol. 2. Pergamon Press, New York, 1993, p. 399.

147. Mason, K. V., et al.: Fenthion for flea control on dogs under field conditions: Dose response efficacy studies and effect on cholinesterase activity. J. Am. Anim. Hosp. Assoc. 20:591, 1984.

148. McLain, N.: Personal communication, 1987.

149. Medleau, L., Chalmers, S. A.: Resolution of generalized dermatophytosis without treatment in dogs. J. Am. Vet. Med. Assoc. 201:1891, 1992.

150. Medleau, L., et al.: Ulcerative pododermatitis in a cat: Immunofluorescent findings and response to chrysotherapy. J. Am. Anim. Hosp. Assoc. 18:449, 1982.

151. Merchant, S.: Quantitative and qualitative analysis of bacteria and yeast from normal canine ears. Proc. Annu. Memb. Meet. Am. Acad. Vet. Dermatol. Am. Coll. Vet. Dermatol. 4:12, 1988.

152. Middleten, D. J., et al.: Suppression of cortisol responses in cats during metestrol acetate and prednisolone therapy. Can. J. Vet. Res. 51:60, 1987.

153. Miele, J. A., Krakowha, S.: Quantitative aspects of binding of canine serum immunoglobulins and *Staphylococcus aureus* protein A. Am. J. Vet. Res. 42:2065, 1981.

154. Miller, D.: Know How to Groom Your Dog. Pet Library Ltd., New York.

155. Miller, W. H., Jr.: Fatty acid supplements as anti-inflammatory agents. In: Kirk, R. W. (ed.). Current Veterinary Therapy X. W. B. Saunders Co. Philadelphia, 1989, p. 563.

156. Miller, W. H., Jr.: Non-steroidal anti-inflammatory agents in the management of canine and feline pruritus. In: Kirk, R. W. (ed.). Current Veterinary Therapy X. W. B. Saunders Co., Philadelphia, 1989, p. 566.

157. Miller, W. H., Jr.: Gonadal aberration in a Keeshond. Dermatol. Reports 1:1, 1982.

158. Miller, W. H., Jr.: Sex hormone–related dermatoses in dogs. In: Kirk, R. W. (ed.). Current Veterinary Therapy X. W. B. Saunders Co., Philadelphia, p. 595.

159. Miller, W.H., Jr., Scott, D.W.: Medical management of chronic pruritus. Comp. Cont. Educ. 16:449, 1994.

160. Miller, W. H., Jr., et al.: A clinical trial on the efficacy of clemastine in the management of allergic pruritus in dogs. Can. Vet. J. 34:25, 1993.

161. Miller, W. H., Jr., et al.: Clinical efficacy of milbemycin oxime in the treatment of generalized demodicosis in the adult dog. J. Am. Vet. Med. Assoc. 203:1426, 1993.

162. Miller, W. H., Jr., et al.: Clinical trial of DVM Derm Caps in the treatment of allergic disease in dogs: A nonblinded study. J. Am. Anim. Hosp. Assoc. 25:163, 1989.

163. Miller, W. H., Jr., et al.: Efficacy of DVM Derm Caps Liquid in the management of allergic and inflammatory dermatoses of the cat. J. Am. Anim. Hosp. Assoc. 29:37, 1993.

164. Miller, W. H., Jr., et al.: Investigation on the antipruritic effects of ascorbic acid given alone and in combination with a fatty acid supplement to dogs with allergic skin disease. Canine Pract. 17(5):11, 1992.

165. Miller, W. H., Jr., et al.: Nonsteroidal management of canine pruritus with amitriptyline. Cornell Vet. 82:53, 1992.

166. Miller, W. H., Jr., Scott, D. W.: Clemastine fumarate as an antipruritic agent in pruritic cats: Results of an open clinical trial. Can. Vet. J. 35:502, 1994.

167. Miller, W. H., Jr., Scott, D. W.: Efficacy of chlorpheniramine maleate for the management of allergic pruritus in cats. J. Am. Vet. Med. Assoc. 197:67, 1990.

168. Miyachi, Y., Niwa, Y.: Effects of potassium iodide, colchicine, and dapsone on the generation of polymorpho-nuclear leukocyte–derived oxygen intermediates. Br. J. Dermatol. 107:209, 1982.

169. Montgomery, R. D., Pidgeon, D. L.: Levamisole toxicity in a dog. J. Am. Vet. Med. Assoc. 189:684, 1986.

170. Moriello, K. A.: Ketoconazole: Clinical pharmacology and therapeutic recommendation. J. Am. Vet. Med. Assoc. 188:303, 1986.

171. Moriello, K. A.: Management of dermatophyte infections in catteries and multiple households. Vet. Clin. North Am. (Small Anim. Pract.) 20:1457, 1990.

171a. Moriello, K. A., et al.: Adrenocortical suppression associated with topical otic administration of glucocorticoids in dogs. J. Am. Vet. Med. Assoc. 193:329, 1988.

172. Mulnix, J. A.: Corticosteroid therapy in the dog. Proceedings, Am. Anim. Hosp. Assoc., annual meeting, 1977.

173. Muller, G. H., et al. (eds.): Small Animal Dermatology, 4th ed. W. B. Saunders Co., Philadelphia, 1989.

174. Mundell, A. C.: New therapeutic agents in veterinary dermatology. Vet. Clin. North Am. (Small Anim. Pract.) 20:1541, 1990.

175. Nachreiner, W. R., et al.: Ketoconazole-induced changes in selected canine hormone concentrations. Am. J. Vet. Res. 47:2504, 1986.

176. Noxon, J. O.: Progestational compounds in dermatology. Presentation, Am. Acad. Vet. Dermatol., New Orleans, March, 1986.

177. Noxon, J. O.: Ketoconazole therapy in canine and feline cryptococcosis. J. Am. Anim. Hosp. Assoc. 22:179, 1986.
178. Page, E. H., et al.: Cyclosporine A. J. Am. Acad. Dermatol. 14:785, 1986.
179. Paradis, M.: Ivermectin in small animal dermatology. In: Kirk, R. W. (ed.). Current Veterinary Therapy X. W. B. Saunders Co., Philadelphia, 1989, p. 560.
180. Paradis, M., Bettenay, S.: Nonsteroidal antipruritic drugs in small animals. In: Ihrke, P. J., et al. (eds.): Advances in Veterinary Dermatology, Vol. 2. Pergamon Press, New York, 1993, p. 429.
181. Paradis, M., et al.: Efficacy of enrofloxacin in the treatment of canine bacterial pyoderma. Vet. Dermatol. 1:123, 1990.
182. Paradis, M., Laperriere, E.: Efficacy of daily ivermectin treatment in a dog with amitraz-resistant, generalized demodicosis. Vet. Dermatol. 3:85, 1992.
182a. Paradis, M., et al.: Further investigations on the use of nonsteroidal and steroidal antiinflammatory agents in the management of canine pruritus. J. Am. Anim. Hosp. Assoc. 27:44, 1991.
182b. Paradis, M., et al.: The efficacy of clemastine (Tavist), a fatty acid–containing product (DVM Derm Caps), and the combination of both products in the management of canine pruritus. Vet. Dermatol. 2:17, 1991.
183. Paradis, M., Ristic, Z.: Efficacy of daily ivermectin in dogs with generalized demodicosis. Proc. Eur. Soc. Vet. Dermatol. 10:59, 1993.
184. Pathak, M. A.: Sunscreens, topical and systemic approaches for protection of human skin against harmful effects of solar radiation. J. Am. Acad. Dermatol. 7:285, 1982.
185. Paul, A. J., et al.: Clinical observations of collies given ivermectin orally. Am. J. Vet. Res. 48:684, 1987.
186. Peck, G. L., Di Giovanna, J. S.: Retinoids. In: Fitzpatrick, T. B., et al. (eds.). Dermatology in General Medicine 4th ed. McGraw-Hill Book Co., San Francisco, 1993.
187. Pentlarge, V. W., Martin, R. A.: Treatment of cryptococcosis in three cats using ketoconazole. J. Am. Vet. Med. Assoc. 188:536, 1986.
188. Peterson, M. E., et al.: Insulin-resistant diabetes mellitus associated with elevated growth hormone concentrations following megestrol acetate treatment in a cat. Proceedings, American College of Veterinary Internal Medicine, 1981, p. 63.
189. Plewig, G., Schopf, E.: Anti-inflammatory effects of antimicrobial agents: An in vivo study. J. Invest. Dermatol. 65:532, 1975.
190. Podkonjak, K. R.: Veterinary cryotherapy—2. Vet. Med. (S.A.C.) 77:183, 1982.
190a. Poppenga, R. H., et al.: Hexachlorophene toxicosis in a litter of Doberman pinschers. J. Vet. Diagn. Invest. 2:129, 1990.
191. Power, H. T., Ihrke, P. J.: Synthetic retinoids in veterinary dermatology. Vet. Clin. North Am. (Small Anim. Pract.) 20:1525, 1990.
192. Power, H. T. Personal communication.
193. Prost, C.: Les dermatoses allergiques du chat. Prat. Méd. Chirurg. Anim. Cie. 28:151, 1993.
194. Prost, C., Arfi, L.: Utilisation de la lincomycine dans le traitement des pyodermites du chien. Prat. Méd. Chirurg. Anim. Cie. 28:495, 1993.
195. Pukay, B. P.: Treatment of canine bacterial hypersensitivity by hyposensitization with Staphylococcus aureus bacterin-toxoid. J. Am. Anim. Hosp. Assoc. 21:479, 1985.
196. Pulliam, J. D., et al.: Investigating ivermectin toxicity in collies. Vet. Med. (S.A.C.) 80:30, 1985.
197. Randall, V. A., et al.: Mechanism of androgen action in cultured dermal papilla cells derived from human hair follicles with varying responses to androgens in vivo. J. Invest. Dermatol. 78:865, 1992.
198. Reedy, L. M.: The role of staphylococcal bacteria in canine dermatology. Proceedings, Am. Anim. Hosp. Assoc., annual meeting, April, 1982.
199. Reedy, L. M.: Results of a clinical study with an oral antiparasitic agent in generalized demodicosis. Proc. Annu. Memb. Meet. Am. Coll. Vet. Derm. Am Acad. Vet. Derm. 7:43, 1991.
200. Regnier, A., et al.: Adrenocortical function and plasma biochemical values in dogs after subconjunctival treatment with methylprednisolone acetate. Res. Vet. Sci. 32:306, 1982.
201. Restrepo, A. K., et al.: First international symposium on ketoconazole. Rev. Infect. Dis. 2:519, 1980.
202. Rhodes, K. H., Shoulberg, N.: Chlorambucil: effective therapeutic option for the treatment of feline immune-mediated dermatoses. Feline Pract. 20:5, 1992.
203. Rosenkrantz, W. S.: Discoid lupus erythematosus. In: Griffin, C. E., et al. (eds.). Current Veterinary Dermatology. Mosby Year Book, St. Louis, 1993, p. 149.
204. Rosenkrantz, W.: Immunomodulating drug in dermatology. In: Current Veterinary Therapy X: Small Animal Practice. W. B. Saunders Co., Philadelphia, 1989, p. 570.
205. Rosenkrantz, W. S.: Pemphigus foliaceus. In: Griffin, C. E., et al. (eds.). Current Veterinary Dermatology. Mosby Year Book, St. Louis, 1993, p. 141.
206. Rosenkrantz, W. S., et al.: Clinical evaluation of cyclosporine in animal models with cutaneous immune-mediated disease and epitheliotropic lymphoma. J. Am. Anim. Hosp. Assoc. 25:377, 1989.
207. Rosenkrantz, W. S., Griffin, C. E.: Lysodren therapy in suspect adrenal sex hormone dermatoses. Proceedings, Second World Congress of Veterinary Dermatology, Montreal, 1992.
208. Rosser, E.: Recurrent pyodermas. Proc. Annu. Memb. Meet. Am. Coll. Vet. Dermatol. Am. Acad. Vet. Dermatol. Phoenix, March, 1987.
209. Rosser, E. J.: Growth hormone–responsive dermatosis. In: Griffin, C. E., et al. (eds.). Current Veterinary Dermatology. Mosby Year Book, St. Louis, 1993, p. 288.
210. Rosser, E. J.: Sex hormones. In: Griffin, C. E., et al. (eds.). Current Veterinary Dermatology. Mosby Year Book, St. Louis, 1993, p. 292.
211. Rosser, E.: Staphphage lysate. Proc. Annu. Memb. Meet. Am. Coll. Vet. Dermatol. Am. Acad. Vet. Dermatol. Las Vegas, 1982.

212. Rosychuk, R. A. W.: Hormone therapy in veterinary dermatology. Presentation, Am. Acad. Vet. Dermatol., New Orleans, March, 1986.
213. Rosychuk, R. A. W.: Management of hypothyroidism. In: Kirk, R. W. (ed.). Current Veterinary Therapy VIII. W. B. Saunders Co., Philadelphia, 1983, p. 869.
214. Rosychuk, R. A. W.: Personal communication.
215. Rowan-Kelly, B., et al.: Modification of polymorphonuclear leukocyte function by imidazoles. Int. J. Immunopharmacol. 6:389, 1984.
216. Rubin, S. I.: Nephrotoxicity of amphotericin B. In: Kirk, R. W. (ed.). Current Veterinary Therapy IX. W. B. Saunders Co., Philadelphia, 1986, p. 1142.
217. Rubin, S. I.: Nonsteroidal anti-inflammatory drugs, prostaglandin, and the kidneys. J. Am. Vet. Med. Assoc. 188:1065, 1986.
217a. Samlaska, C. P., et al.: Pentoxifylline. J. Am. Acad. Dermatol., 30:603, 1994.
218. Sanechi, R. K., et al. Extracutaneous histologic changes accompanying zinc deficiency in pups. Am. J. Vet. Res. 46:2120, 1985.
219. Saunders, B.: How to Trim, Groom, and Show Your Dog. Howell House, New York, 1967.
220. Scarff, D. H., Lloyd, D. H.: Double blind, placebo controlled, crossover study of evening primrose oil in the treatment of canine atopy. Vet. Rec. 131:97, 1992.
221. Scarff, D. H., et al. A multicenter placebo-controlled practitioner study to investigate the effect of evening primrose oil in canine atopic dermatosis. In: Von Tscharner, C., Halliwell, R. E. W. (eds.). Advances in Veterinary Dermatology, Vol. 1. Baillière-Tindall, Philadelphia, 1990, p. 481.
222. Schauder, S., Ippen, H.: Photodermatoses and light protection. Int. J. Dermatol. 21:241, 1982.
223. Schleimer, R. P.: Glucocorticosteroids. In: Middleton, E., et al. (eds.). Allergy Principles and Practice. Mosby Year Book, St. Louis, 1993.
224. Schmeitzel, L. P.: Endocrinology Review. Am. Acad. Vet. Dermatol., residents review session, 1992.
225. Schmeitzel, L. P., Parker, W.: Workshop report 13. Growth hormone and sex hormone alopecia. In: Ihrke, P. J., et al. (eds.). Advances in Veterinary Dermatology II. Pergamon Press, New York, 1993, p. 451.
226. Schmidt, J. A., et al.: Assessing the safety of long-term cythioate therapy. Vet. Med. (S.A.C.) 79:1159, 1984.
227. Schmidt, J. A., et al.: Safety studies evaluating the effect of fenthion on cholinesterase concentrations. Vet. Med. (S.A.C.) 80:21, 1985.
228. Schwartzman, R. M.: Topical dermatologic therapy. In: Kirk, R. W. (ed.). Current Veterinary Therapy VI. W. B. Saunders Co., Philadelphia, 1977, p. 506.
229. Scott, D. W.: Chrysotherapy (gold therapy). In: Kirk, R. W. (ed.): Current Veterinary Therapy VIII. W. B. Saunders Co., Philadelphia, 1983, p. 448.
230. Scott, D. W.: Clinical assessment of topical benzoyl peroxide in treatment of canine skin diseases. Vet. Med. (S.A.C.) 74:808, 1979.
230a. Scott, D. W.: Topical cutaneous medicine, or "Now what should I try?" Proc. Am. Anim. Hosp. Assoc. 46:89, 1979.
231. Scott, D. W.: Feline dermatology 1900–1978. J. Am. Anim. Hosp. Assoc. 16:331, 1980.
232. Scott, D. W.: Hyperadrenocorticism. Vet. Clin. North Am. (Small Anim. Pract.) 9:3, 1979.
233. Scott, D. W.: Rational use of glucocorticoids in dermatology. In: Bonagura, J. (ed.). Kirk's Current Veterinary Therapy XII. W. B. Saunders Co., Philadelphia, 1995.
234. Scott, D. W.: Sulfones and sulfonamides in canine dermatology. In: Kirk, R. W. (ed.). Current Veterinary Therapy IX. W. B. Saunders Co., Philadelphia, 1986, p. 606.
235. Scott, D. W.: Systemic glucocorticoid therapy. In: Kirk, R. W. (ed.). Current Veterinary Therapy VII. W. B. Saunders Co., Philadelphia, 1980, p. 988.
236. Scott, D. W., Buerger, R. G.: Nonsteroidal anti-inflammatory agents in the management of canine pruritus. J. Am. Anim. Hosp. Assoc. 24:425, 1988.
237. Scott, D. W., Cayatte, S. M.: Failure of papaverine hydrochloride and doxycycline hyclate as antipruritic agents in pruritic dogs: Results of an open clinical trial. Can. Vet. J. 34:164, 1993.
238. Scott, D. W., et al.: Observations on the immunopathology and therapy of canine pemphigus and pemphigoid. J. Am. Vet. Med. Assoc. 180:48, 1982.
239. Scott, D. W., et al.: The combination of ormetoprim and sulfadimethoxine in the treatment of pyoderma due to *Staphylococcus intermedius* infection in dogs. Canine Pract. 18(2):29, 1993.
240. Scott, D. W., et al.: A clinical study on the efficacy of two commercial veterinary emollients (Micro Pearls and Humilac) in the management of winter-time dry skin in dogs. Cornell Vet. 81:419, 1991.
241. Scott, D. W., et al.: A clinical study on the effect of two commercial veterinary benzoyl peroxide shampoos in dogs. Canine Pract. 19:7, 1994.
242. Scott, D. W., et al.: Canine lupus erythematosus. II. Discoid lupus erythematosis. J. Am. Anim. Hosp. Assoc. 19:481, 1983.
243. Scott, D. W., et al.: Comparison of the clinical efficacy of two commercial fatty acid supplements (EfaVet and DVM Derm Caps), evening primrose oil, and cold water marine fish oil in the management of allergic pruritus in dogs: A double-blinded study. Cornell Vet. 82:319, 1992.
244. Scott, D. W., et al.: Efficacy of tylocine for the treatment of pyoderma due to *Staphylococcus intermedius* infection in dogs. Can. Vet. J. (accepted 1994).
245. Scott, D. W., et al.: Failure of cyproheptadine hydrochloride as an antipruritic agent in allergic dog: Results of a double-blinded, placebo-controlled study. Cornell Vet. 82:247, 1992.
246. Scott, D. W., et al.: Failure of terfenadine as an antipruritic agent in atopic dogs: Results of a double-blinded, placebo-controlled study. Can. Vet. J. 35:286, 1994.

247. Scott, D. W., Green, C. E.: Iatrogenic secondary adrenocortical insufficiency in dogs. J. Am. Anim. Hosp. Assoc. 10:555, 1974.
248. Scott, D. W., Walton, D. U.: Clinical evaluation of oral vitamin E for the treatment of primary acanthosis nigricans J. Am. Anim. Hosp. Assoc. 21:345, 1985.
249. Scott, D. W., Miller, W. H., Jr.: Medical management of allergic pruritus in the cat, with emphaisis on feline atopy. J. So. Afr. Vet. Ass. 64:103, 1993.
250. Scott, D. W., Miller, W. H., Jr.: Nonsteroidal anti-inflammatory agents in the management of canine allergic pruritus. J. S. Afr. Vet. Assoc. 64:52, 1993.
251. Scott, D. W., Miller, W. H., Jr.: Nonsteroidal management of canine pruritus: Chlorpheniramine and a fatty acid supplement (DVM Derm Caps) in combination, and the fatty acid supplement at twice the manufacturer's recommended dosage. Cornell Vet. 80:381, 1990.
252. Scott, D. W., Miller, W. H., Jr.: The combination of an antihistamine (chlorpheniramine) and an omega-3/omega-6 fatty acid–containing product (DVM Derm Caps Liquid) for the management of pruritic cats: Results of an open clinical trial. N. Z. Vet. J. (accepted 1994)
253. Scott, D. W., Walton, D.: Experiences with the use of amitraz and ivermectin for the treatment of generalized demodectic mange in the dog. J. Am. Anim. Hosp. Assoc. 12:203, 1985.
253a. Serra, D. A., White, S. D.: Oral chrysotherapy with auranofin in dogs. J. Am. Vet. Med. Assoc. 194:1327, 1989.
254. Sharp, N.: Personal communication, 1987.
255. Shelton, G. H., et al.: Severe neutropenia associated with griseofulvin therapy in cats with feline immunodeficiency virus infection. J. Vet. Intern. Med. 4:317, 1990.
256. Shoulberg, N.: The efficacy of fluoxetine (Prozac) in the treatment of acral lick and allergic-inhalant dermatitis in canines. Proc. Annu. Memb. Meet. Am. Acad. Vet. Dermatol. Am. Coll. Vet. Dermatol. 6:31, 1990.
257. Simon, F. E., Simon, K. J.: Antihistamines. In: Middleton, E., et al. (eds.). Allergy Principles and Practice. Mosby Year Book, St. Louis, 1993.
258. Slatter, D. H. (ed.): Textbook of Small Animal Surgery, 2nd ed. W. B. Saunders Co., Philadelphia, 1993.
259. Sloan, J. B., Lotlani, K.: Iontophoresis in dermatology. J. Am. Acad. Dermatol. 15:671, 1986.
260. Smalley, R. V., Borden, E. C.: Interferon: Current status and future directions of this prototypic biological. Springer Semin. Immunopathol. 9:73, 1986.
261. Solomon, S. E.: Drugs and the immune system. In: Katzung, B. G. (ed.): Basic and Clinical Pharmacology, 2nd ed. Lange Medical Publishers, Los Altos, CA, 1984.
262. Song, M.: Fleas and Flea Control. The Prof. Library Series. AAHA, 1993.
263. Song, M.D.: Using ivermectin to treat feline dermatoses caused by external parasites. Vet. Med. 86:498, 1991.
264. Stanton, M. E., Legendre, A. M.: Effects of cyclophosphamide in dogs and cats. J. Am. Vet. Med. Assoc. 188:1319, 1986.
265. Stewart, L. J., et al.: Isotretinoin in the treatment of sebaceous adenitis in two Vizslas. J. Am. Anim. Hosp. Assoc. 27:65, 1991.
266. Storrs, F. J.: Use and abuse of systemic corticosteroid therapy. J. Am. Acad. Dermatol. 1:95, 1979.
267. Swaim, S. F.: Surgery of Traumatized Skin: Management and Reconstruction in the Dog and Cat. W. B. Saunders Co., Philadelphia, 1980.
268. Swaim, S. F., Lee, A. H.: Topical wound medications: A review. J. Am. Vet. Med. Assoc. 190:1588, 1987.
269. Symoens, J., et al.: An evaluation of two years of clinical experience with ketoconazole. Rev. Infect. Dis. 2:674, 1980.
270. Symoens, J., Rosenthal, M.: Levamisole in the modulation of the immune response: The current experimental and clinical state. J. Reticuloendothel. Soc. 21:2176, 1977.
271. Sztein, M. B., Goldstein, A. L.: Thymic hormones—A clinical update. Springer Semin. Immunopathol. 9:1, 1986.
272. Tannenbaum, L., Tuffanelli, D. L.: Antimalarial agents. Arch. Dermatol. 116:587, 1980.
273. Tarvin, G., Lenehan, T.: Personal communication, 1993.
274. Teske, E.: Estrogen-induced bone marrow toxicity. In: Kirk, R. W. (ed.): Current Veterinary Therapy IX. W. B. Saunders Co., Philadelphia, 1986, p. 495.
274a. Thoday, K. L.: Differential diagnosis of symmetric alopecia in the cat. In: Kirk, R. W. (ed): Current Veterinary Therapy IX. Philadelphia: W. B. Saunders, 1986, p. 546.
275. Thoma, R. E., et al.: Phototherapy: A promising cancer therapy. Vet. Med. (S.A.C.) 78:1693, 1983.
275a. Thoday, K. L.: Aspects of feline symmetric alopecia. In: Von Tocharner, C., and Halliwell, R. E. W. (eds.): Advances in Veterinary Dermatology, Vol. 1. Baillière-Tindall, London, 1990, p. 47.
276. Thomas, I.: Gold therapy and its indications in dermatology. J. Am. Acad. Dermatol. 16:845, 1987.
277. Thomas, M. L.: Development of a bacterial model for canine otitis externa. Proc. Annu. Memb. Meet. Am. Acad. Vet. Dermatol. Am. Coll. Vet. Dermatol. 6:28, 1990.
277a. Thuong-Nguyen, V., et al.: Inhibition of neutrophil adherence to antibody by dapsone: A possible therapeutic mechanism of dapsone in the treatment of IgA dermatoses. J. Invest. Dermatol. 100:349, 1993.
278. Tinsley, P. E., Taylor, D. O.: Immunotherapy for multicentric malignant mastocytoma in a dog. Mod. Vet. Pract. 68:225, 1987.
279. Tolman, E. L., et al.: The arachidonic acid cascade and skin disease. In: Stone, J. (ed.). Dermatology Immunology and Allergy. C. V. Mosby, St. Louis, 1985.
280. Tranquilli, W. J., et al.: Assessment of toxicosis induced by high-dose administration of milbemycin oxime in collies. Am. J. Vet. Res. 52:1170, 1993.
281. Trettien, A.: Workshop Report 13: Shampoos and other topical therapy. In: Von Tscharner, C., Halliwell, R. E. W. (eds.). Advances in Veterinary Dermatology, Vol. 1. Baillière-Tindall, Philadelphia, 1990, p. 434.

282. Turnbull, G. J.: Animal studies in the treatment of poisoning by amitraz and xylene. Hum. Toxicol. 2:579, 1983.

283. Van Cutsen, J., et al.: The antiinflammatory effects of ketoconazole. J. Am. Acad. Dermatol. 25:257, 1991.

284. Vanden Broek, A. H. M., Simpson, J. W.: Fat absorption in dogs with atopic dermatitis. In: von Tschanner, Hallwell, R. E. W. (eds): Advances in Veterinary Dermatology, Vol. 1. Baillière-Tindall, Philadelphia, 1990, p. 155.

284a. Vanden Broek, A.H.M., Stafford, W.L.: Epidermal and hepatic glucocorticoid receptors in cats and dogs. Res. Vet. Sci. 52:312, 1992.

285. Weiss, R. C.: Immunotherapy for feline leukemia using staphylococcal protein A for heterologous interferons: Immunopharmacologic actions and potential use. J. Am. Vet. Med. Assoc. 192:681, 1988.

286. White, J. V.: Cycylosporin: Prototype of a T-cell selective immunosuppressant. J. Am. Vet. Med. Assoc. 189:566, 1986.

287. White, P.: Essential fatty acids: Use in management of canine atopy. Comp. Cont. Educ. 15:451, 1993.

288. White, S.: Oral gold therapy. Derm. Dialog. 5:2, 1986.

288a. White, S. D.: Treatment of acral lick dermatitis with endorphin blocker haltrexone. Proc. Annu. Memb. Meet. Am. Acad. Vet. Dermatol. Am. Coll. Vet. Dermatol. 4:37, 1988.

289. White, S.: Report: Gold therapy. Am. Anim. Hosp. Assoc., annual meeting, Las Vegas, April, 1982.

290. White, S. D., et al.: Corticosteroid (methylprednisolone sodium succinate) pulse therapy in five dogs with autoimmune skin disease. J. Am. Vet. Med. Assoc. 191:1121, 1987.

291. White, S. D., et al.: Isotretinoin and etretinate in the treatment of benign and malignant cutaneous neoplasia and in sebaceous adenitis of longhaired dogs. Proc. Annu. Memb. Meet. Am. Acad. Vet. Dermatol. Am. Coll. Vet. Dermatol. 7:101, 1991.

292. White, S. D., et al.: The efficacy of tetracycline and niacinamide in the treatment of autoimmune skin disease in 20 dogs. Proc. Annu. Memb. Meet. Am. Acad. Vet. Dermatol. Am. Coll. Vet. Dermatol. 6:43, 1990.

293. White, S. D., et al.: Use of tetracycline and niacinamide for treatment of autoimmune skin disease in 31 dogs. J. Am. Vet. Med. Assoc. 200:1497, 1992.

294. White-Weithers, N.: Evaluation of topical therapies for the treatment of dermatophytosis in dogs and cats. Proc. Annu. Memb. Meet. Am. Acad. Vet. Dermatol. Am. Coll. Vet. Dermatol. 9:29, 1993.

295. Wilkie, D. A., Kirby, R.: Methemoglobinemia associated with dermal application of benzocaine cream in a cat. J. Am. Vet. Med. Assoc. 192:85, 1988.

296. Willemse, T.: Intravenous $ZnSO_4$ for zinc related dermatoses in Siberian huskies. Derm. Dialog. 5:1, 1986.

297. Willemse, T., et al.: Feline psychogenic alopecia and the role of the opioid system. In: Von Tscharner, C., Halliwell, R. E. W.: Advances in Veterinary Dermatology, Vol. 1. Baillière-Tindall, Philadelphia, 1990, p. 195.

298. Withrow, S. J., (ed.): Symposium on cryosurgery. Vet. Clin. North Am. (Small Anim. Pract.) 10:753, 1980.

299. Wozel, G., Barth, J.: Current aspects of modes of action of dapsone. Int. J. Dermatol. 27:547, 1988.

300. Zenoble, R. D., Kemppaainen, R. J.: Adrenocortical suppression by topically applied corticosteroids in healthy dogs. J. Am. Vet. Med. Assoc. 191:685, 1987.

4

Bacterial
Skin
Diseases

■

Chapter Outline

■ CUTANEOUS BACTERIOLOGY AND NORMAL DEFENSE MECHANISMS

The skin forms a protective barrier, without which life would be impossible. The defense has three components: physical, chemical, and microbial.[68a, 90, 126] Hair forms the first line of physical defense to protect against the contact of pathogens with the skin. It may also harbor bacteria, especially staphylococci.[3, 34, 147] However, the relatively inert stratum corneum forms the basic physical defense layer. Its tightly packed keratinized cells are permeated by an emulsion of sebum and sweat and intercellular cement substance. The emulsion is concentrated in the outer layers of keratin, where some of the volatile fatty acids vaporize, leaving a fairly impermeable superficial sebaceous crust.[89, 96, 101] Together, the cells and the emulsion function as an effective physical barrier. The emulsion provides a chemical barrier to potential pathogens in addition to its physical properties. Fatty acids, especially linoleic acid, have potent antibacterial properties. Water-soluble substances in the emulsion include inorganic salts and proteins that inhibit bacteria.

The skin is viewed as an immune organ that plays an active role in the induction and maintenance of immune responses, which can be beneficial or detrimental.[157] Specific components include epidermal Langerhans' cells, dermal dendrocytes, keratinocytes, skin-seeking T lymphocytes, mast cells, and the endothelium of postcapillary venules. Various cytokines, complement, and immunoglobulins IgA, IgG, IgG_1, IgG_{2a}, IgG_{2b}, IgG_{2c}, IgM, and IgE are found in the emulsion layer and contribute to the skin's immunologic function.[89, 90, 130, 157] Many individual components of this complicated system have antimicrobial effects, so the normal skin should be viewed as an organ that is resistant to infection.

The normal skin microflora also contributes to skin immunity. Bacteria are located in the superficial epidermis and in the infundibulum of the hair follicles, where sweat and sebum provide nutrients.[89, 136, 137] The normal flora is a mixture of bacteria that live in symbiosis, probably exchanging growth factors. The flora may change with different cutaneous environments. These are affected by factors such as heat, pH, salinity, moisture, albumin level, and fatty acid level. The close relationship between the host and the microorganisms enables bacteria to occupy microbial niches and to inhibit colonization by invading organisms. In addition, many bacteria (*Bacillus* spp., *Streptococcus* spp., and *Staphylococcus* spp.) are capable of producing antibiotic substances, and some bacteria can produce enzymes (e.g., β-lactamase) that inhibit antibiotics.

Bacteria cultured from normal skin are called normal inhabitants and are classified as resident or transient, depending on their ability to multiply in that habitat.[80, 81] Residents successfully multiply on normal skin. A variety of studies have been performed to identify the normal flora of the skin of dogs and cats. Site and temporal variation have been observed, but differences in methodology make direct comparison of the various studies difficult. In general, most studies report the following findings on resident and transient organisms.

Resident Organisms

Micrococcus sp.; coagulase-negative staphylococci, especially *Staphylococcus epidermidis* and *S. xylosus*; α-hemolytic streptococci; and *Acinetobacter* sp. are normal residents of dogs' skin.[33, 109, 155] It has been suggested that *Propionibacterium* sp. also be included in the list.[67] Debate exists as to whether *Staphylococcus intermedius* belongs in the list of resident or of transient flora.[3, 4, 92] Because this organism is frequently isolated from the hair and skin of normal dogs, resident status is probably appropriate.

The dog's resident staphylococcal flora appears to be acquired from its dam in the neonatal period.[4] Regional variation in the number of organisms at any one body site occurs with moist areas (chin, interdigital web, and abdomen) typically more heavily colonized. The anal, nasal, and oral mucocutaneous sites are important sites of carriage of *S. intermedius*.[5, 48] Staphylococci can be isolated from both hair and its underlying skin. The numbers of *S. intermedius* on the hair and skin appear equal, while coagulase-negative staphylococci are higher in number on hairs.

The resident flora of cats includes *Micrococcus* sp.; coagulase-negative staphylococci, especially *Staphylococcus simulans*; α-hemolytic streptococci; and *Acinetobacter* sp.[109, 132] In one study, 50 per cent of the cultures were negative.[81] Coagulase-positive staphylococci, including both *Staphylococcus aureus* and *S. intermedius*, are also commonly isolated from normal skin and should be considered residents.[34, 47, 103] Household cats have a higher frequency of isolation of coagulase-negative *(S. capitis, S. epidermidis, S. haemolyticus, S. hominis, S. sciuri,* and *S. warneri)* and coagulase-positive *(S. aureus* and *S. intermedius)* organisms as compared with the case in cattery cats, suggesting that these organisms may be transferred from humans.

Transient Organisms

Transient organisms may be cultured from the skin but are of no significance unless they become involved in a pathologic process as secondary invaders. These organisms do not multiply on the normal skin of most animals. Transients of the dog include *Escherichia coli, Proteus mirabilis, Corynebacterium* sp., *Bacillus* sp., and *Pseudomonas* sp., whereas β-hemolytic streptococci, *E. coli, P. mirabilis, Pseudomonas* sp., *Alcaligenes* sp., *Bacillus* sp., *Staphylococcus* sp. (coagulase positive), *Staphylococcus* spp. (coagulase negative, other than *S. simulans)* are found in the cat.

The primary skin pathogen of dogs, and probably cats, is *S. intermedius*. Some strains produce slime, which may increase their virulence.[75] Because of incomplete laboratory identification in the past, all coagulase-positive staphylococci were routinely reported as *S. aureus*.[14, 114] Taxonomic studies have shown that the genus *Staphylococcus* can be divided into at least 10 coagulase-negative species and three coagulase-positive species *(S. aureus, S. intermedius,* and *S. hyicus)*. *S. intermedius* isolates from dogs and cats produce protein A as do *S. aureus* isolates from people.[36, 57] The presence of protein A in these isolates could contribute to the pathogenesis of staphylococcal infections of animals by acting as a cell wall adhesin, as occurs in humans.[96] Transepidermal penetration of protein A may also be important in allergy.[100]

There has been speculation about the means by which only a small number of a vast array of bacteria in the environment are able to colonize or infect the skin. The potent cleaning forces of dilution, washout, drying, and desquamation of surface cells prevent many organisms from colonizing the skin. It is now recognized that bacterial adhesion is a prerequisite to colonization and infection.[59, 96, 126] Bacterial adhesion correlates with bacterial virulence, tissue tropism, and host susceptibility to infecting agents. Many bacteria possess surface adhesion molecules, such as lipoteichoic acid, which binds to specific receptor molecules on cell walls (fibronectin) to fix the organisms to the host. Protein A, for example, is thought to act as an adhesin for staphylococcal organisms to the skin of atopic people and possibly dogs. Certain strains of bacteria seem to adhere better to certain regions of the host, and this may play a great part in the variable virulence that is often observed. Much more investigation needs to be done to explain the potential of this mechanism of infection.

Other organisms from the transient group may be pathogenic in rare cases.[29, 49] Gram-negative organisms tend to flourish in moist, warm areas and to predominate when medications depress the gram-positive flora. Cats infrequently develop pyoderma but commonly have subcutaneous abscesses. Because these are often from bite wounds, the mouth flora of the cat is an important factor. It includes *Pasteurella multocida*, β-hemolytic streptococci, *Corynebacterium* spp., *Actinomyces* spp., *Bacteroides* spp., and *Fusobacterium* spp.

Anaerobic bacteria are usually abundant in gastrointestinal secretions; therefore, fecal contamination is a cause of soft tissue infections due to these organisms. Anaerobic bacteria isolated from dog and cat infections include *Actinomyces* spp., *Clostridium perfringens, Clostridium* sp., *Peptostreptococcus anaerobius, Bacteroides melaninogenicus, Bacteroides* sp., and *Fusobacterium necrophorum, Fusobacterium* sp., and *Propionibacterium* sp.[12, 52, 94, 118] They are usually found in granulomas, cellulitis, abscesses, fistulae, and other soft tissue wounds, but they may also be cultured from more superficial pyoderma, otitis, or stomatitis cases.[51] The aminoglycosides such as gentamicin are notoriously ineffective in therapy for anaerobic bacterial infections. Metronidazole is usually highly effective.

Antibacterial sensitivity for obligate anaerobic bacteria has been rated as follows:[12, 13, 70] Ninety per cent or more are sensitive to ampicillin, amoxicillin, carbenicillin, chloramphenicol, and clindamycin; 75 to 90 per cent are sensitive to cephalosporin, lincomycin, and penicillin G (except *Bacteroides* spp., which are resistant to penicillin, ampicillin, and cephalothin); 50 to 75 per cent are sensitive to tetracycline and erythromycin; less than 25 per cent are sensitive to gentamicin.

Staphylococci are among the most resistant of the non–spore-forming organisms. They resist dehydration, are relatively heat resistant, and tolerate antiseptic medications better than the vegetative forms of most bacteria. Many strains produce one or several toxins. These may cause tissue necrosis at the point of infection. Repeated injections of heat-killed staphylococci protect rabbits against otherwise fatal doses of *S. aureus*. Bacterins may be valuable in combating chronic infections in dogs and cats.

The numbers of resident bacteria on the skin tend to vary with individuals; some animals have many organisms, whereas others have few. The number per individual may remain constant, unless disturbed by antibacterial treatment or changes in climate. More bacteria are found on the skin in warm, wet weather than in cold, dry weather.[126] Moist, intertriginous areas tend to have large numbers, and individuals with oily skin have higher counts. Total counts of aerobic organisms on normal skin ranged from 10^0 to 10^3 organisms/cm^2, and similar counts from seborrheic skin ranged from 10^3 to 10^7/cm^2.[71]

Disease states influence the species and numbers of bacteria present. In seborrheic skin, coagulase-positive staphylococci predominate.[71] This is also true in most pyodermas and in most other bacterial infections of the skin. In patients with various dermatoses (atopy, seborrheic dermatitis, and allergic and irritant contact dermatitis in humans), increased numbers of resident bacteria are found in all areas of the skin, not just in the affected areas.[80] Compared with dogs that are normal, dogs with dermatoses have a more prolific growth of aerobic organisms, a greater number of sites carrying coagulase-positive staphylococci, and a higher number of gram-negative microorganisms. Thus, these animals are heavily colonized with potentially pathogenic bacteria, a fact to consider when providing basic therapy for the primary dermatosis.

Microorganisms isolated from an intact lesion such as a pustule are evidence of infection, not colonization. Colonization means that a potential pathogen is living on the skin or in a lesion but that its presence is causing no reaction in the host. The problem in evaluating a pyoderma culture is to separate secondary colonization from secondary infection. The presence of many degenerate neutrophils and phagocytosed bacteria is direct evidence of a host reaction and is compatible with infection. Infection can be determined by direct smears of lesion exudates, which may be more informative than cultures.

■ SKIN INFECTIONS

The staphylococcal organisms, the primary isolates from skin infections in dogs and cats, are not particularly virulent and thus any skin infection should be considered a sign of some underlying cutaneous, metabolic, or immunologic abnormality. Traditionally, skin infections are classified as either primary or secondary to reflect the absence or the presence of an underlying cause.

Secondary infections are by far the most common and result from some cutaneous, immunologic, or metabolic abnormality. Secondary infections may involve organisms other than staphylococci, tend to respond slowly or poorly to treatment if the underlying problem is ignored, and recur unless the cause is resolved. Virtually any skin condition described in this text can predispose to infection, but allergic, seborrheic, or follicular disorders are the most common causes of infection. Interestingly, infection appears to be relatively uncommon in the autoimmune disorders.[119] This may be due to the presence of high cutaneous levels of cytokines which have antimicrobial properties.

Allergic dogs are especially prone to infections because of the damage that they do to their skin while itching, the corticosteroids that they often receive, and possibly some immunologic abnormalities that are associated with their allergic predisposition. When their skin becomes infected, the level of pruritus increases quickly and does not respond well to corticosteroid administration. Antibiotic treatment resolves the lesions of infection and reduces but does not eliminate the pruritus.

Seborrheic animals have greatly increased numbers of bacteria on their skin surface, which can colonize an epidermal or follicular defect and cause infection. They also contribute to the alteration of the surface lipid layer to one that can induce inflammation. In this latter situation, the patches of seborrheic dermatitis cause the animal to itch and induce true infection in these areas. Superficial infections result in significant scaling during their development and resolution. It can sometimes be difficult to decide whether the seborrhea induced the infection or vice versa. Scaling caused by infection decreases quickly with antibiotic therapy. If seborrheic signs are still pronounced after 14 to 21 days of antibiotic treatment, the animal should be evaluated for an underlying seborrheic disorder.

Follicular inflammation, obstruction, degeneration, or a combination of these predisposes the follicle to bacterial infection. Inflammatory causes are numerous, but demodicosis and dermatophytosis are most commonly implicated. Follicular obstruction occurs as part of generalized seborrhea, in focal seborrheic disorders (e.g., feline acne and Schnauzer comedo syndrome), sebaceous adenitis, follicular dysplasias and other congenital disorders of the follicle, and endocrine disorders. Follicular degeneration can be caused by all of the above plus alopecia areata. In cases of follicular infection, examination of skin scrapings for demodicosis and evaluations for dermatophytes (e.g., trichogram and fungal culture) are always recommended. After those tests, the skin biopsy is most useful because pathologic changes are too deep to be appreciated with the naked eye. The inflammation associated with the secondary bacterial infection can mask some of the histologic features of the predisposing disease, thus it is best to resolve the infection first and then perform the skin biopsy.

The most common metabolic causes of skin infection are hypothyroidism and hyperadrenocorticism (iatrogenic or spontaneous), but diabetes mellitus, other endocrine skin disorders, and other systemic metabolic problems (e.g., hyperlipidemia) must also be considered. These disorders predispose to infection by their impact on the animal's immune system and the changes they induce in the hair follicle. In most instances, the number of infected follicles is small compared with the number that are visually abnormal (e.g., hyperkeratotic and hairless), so the index of suspicion for an underlying metabolic disorder should be high.

The classification of primary infection is more problematic. Primary infections are described as those that occur in otherwise healthy skin, are staphylococcal with rare exception, and are cured by appropriate antibiotic therapy. This definition overlooks the tendency for the infection to recur. It is common to examine a dog for a skin infection and find no historical or physical abnormality to explain the infection. Is this a primary infection, an infection secondary to some transient insult to the skin, or an infection secondary to some as yet undefined underlying problem? The key to the primacy of the infection is its tendency to recur. Infections that resolve with no residual skin disease and do not recur with regularity or within a reasonable period (e.g., 3 to 6 months) could be considered primary infections. If the infection recurs early, the animal has some subclinical skin disease or an immunologic abnormality.

■ IMMUNODEFICIENCIES

Immunodeficiencies are classified as either primary or acquired. Primary immunodeficiencies are congenital and are usually inherited. In these animals, infections develop early in life for no apparent reason. Infections of the respiratory, gastrointestinal, urogenital, and integumentary systems are most common. In some cases, the skin infection follows a known insult (e.g., flea bites) but is far out of proportion in severity to the insult. Depending on the nature and severity of the immunodeficiency, the infection may or may not respond to treatment as expected. If response is seen, relapse weeks to months after the discontinuation of treatment can be expected. A variety of primary immunodeficiencies have been described in dogs, and those with associated skin infection are listed in Table 4:1.

Acquired immunodeficiencies are common complications of many serious systemic illnesses.[38, 77] Because the immunodepression follows the underlying disease, there is no age, breed, or sex predilection for these acquired immunologic disorders. The best known examples of acquired immunodeficiency disease are associated with viral infections, especially feline leukemia virus and feline immunodeficiency virus. In most other conditions, the signs of the primary illness predominate and precede those of the immunodepression. Examples in which the skin looks normal or nearly so before the infection include adult-onset demodicosis (see Chap. 7), hypothyroidism (see Chap. 9), and hyperadrenocorticism (see Chap. 9).

■ TREATMENT OF SKIN INFECTIONS

Satisfactory resolution of a skin infection necessitates that the cause of the infection be identified and corrected and that the infection receive proper treatment. If the cause of the infection persists, either the response to treatment is poor or the infection recurs shortly after treatment is discontinued. If the cause is resolved but inappropriate treatment for the infection is given, the infection persists and worsens.

Skin infections can be treated topically, systemically, surgically, or by some combination of these. Most infections of dogs and cats are too widespread or too deep to be resolved with topical treatment alone, but judicious topical therapy can make the patient more comfortable

Table 4:1. Primary Immunodeficiencies of Dogs

Disease	Breeds Involved	Mechanisms of Defect	References
Phagocytic Defect			
Cyclic hematopoiesis	Collie, Pomeranian, Cocker spaniel	Blockade of bone marrow release	30
Granulocytopathy	Doberman pinscher, Irish setter, Weimaraner	Bactericidal defect in neutrophils	17, 37, 121
Granulocytopathy	Irish setter	Reduced granulocyte adherence	63, 143
Humoral Defect			
Complement deficiency	Brittany spaniel	Absence of C3	15
Transient hypogammaglobulinemia	Many	Delayed development of functioning humoral system	61
Selective IgM deficiency	Doberman pinscher	Low IgM levels	117
Selective IgA deficiency	Many	Low IgA levels	21, 42, 117
Cell-Mediated Defect	Bull terrier, Weimaraners, others	T cell dysfunction	56, 72, 107, 125
Combined Immunodeficiency	Basset hound	B cell and T cell dysfunction	60, 73

and hasten its response to antibiotics. Topical treatment can take considerable time and effort on the owner's part and can irritate the skin if the products are too harsh. Surgery alone can be useful with focal lesions or can be performed as an adjunct to other treatments. Management must be individualized.

Topical treatment is aimed at removing tissue debris from the skin surface and superficial portion of the hair follicle, reducing or eliminating the surface bacterial population on and around the lesions, and encouraging drainage. These goals can be accomplished with a variety of products and delivery systems. Agents commonly used include chlorhexidine, hexachlorophene, povidone-iodine, ethyl lactate, and benzoyl peroxide.[9, 84, 86, 91, 113] These agents usually are applied in soak solutions or via shampoos.

Superficial infections are best treated with antibacterial shampoos. The manipulation of the skin during its application and the vehicle of the shampoo removes tissue debris, which allows better contact between the antiseptic and the bacteria. When four commercial antibacterial shampoos were studied, none could completely sterilize the skin but all significantly reduced the bacterial population.[84] Benzoyl peroxide was the most effective, followed by chlorhexidine acetate. Another study demonstrated equal efficacy of benzoyl peroxide and ethyl lactate, with fewer adverse reactions to the latter.[9] Product selection depends on the preferences of the owner and the clinician and the condition of the animal's skin. Benzoyl peroxide products can be irritating and should be avoided in animals with severely inflamed or sensitive skin. A thorough bath with a 10- to 15-minute shampoo contact time is indicated at the beginning of treatment. The timing to the next bath depends on the severity of the infection, the cause of the infection, and the speed of the animal's response to the antibiotics used. Some clinicians request that the client bathe the animal at a set interval, typically every third to seventh day, whereas other clinicians give the client guidelines for when a bath is indicated and let the client decide when to bathe. If the client is not overzealous, the latter method is most appropriate because it treats the animal on the basis of its needs.

In the case of deep draining infections, the hair in the area must be clipped to prevent the formation of a sealing crust and to allow the topical agents to contact the diseased tissues. Although shampooing is beneficial, soaks are more appropriate at the onset of treatment. Hydrotherapy loosens and removes crusts, decreases the number of surface bacteria, promotes epithelialization, and helps to lessen the discomfort associated with the lesions. With warm water soaks, the vascular plexus opens, which may allow better distribution of the systemic antibiotic. For widespread infection, tub soaks with or without whirlpool are most appropriate. Antiseptics such as chlorhexidine and povidone-iodine are added for additional antibacterial activity. Chlorhexidine has been most effective but may retard wound healing.[86] If there are draining lesions on a foot or distal limb, the area can be soaked in a bucket. For these lesions, a mildly hypertonic drawing solution of magnesium sulfate (2 tbsp/qt or 30 ml/L of warm water) can be beneficial. Because hydrotherapy hydrates the epithelium, excessively soaked skin macerates easily and may become infected more easily. As the antibiotic therapy progresses, drainage should decrease. When little drainage is noted after a soak, the frequency of soaking should be decreased or stopped entirely. Typically, soaking is done for 3 to 7 days.

Multiple studies on the antibiotic sensitivity of *S. intermedius* from dogs have been conducted and, although some marked intercontinental differences have been noted, the sensitivity of this organism remains fairly predictable and stable. In early studies on skin isolates, in vitro sensitivity was excellent (>90 per cent) to oxacillin and cephalosporin; good (75 to 90 per cent) to chloramphenicol, erythromycin, and lincomycin; fair (50 to 75 per cent) to potentiated sulfa drugs; and poor (<50 per cent) to penicillin, ampicillin, and tetracycline.[69, 95] Since those studies were published, the sensitivity data have remained basically unchanged, except that newer studies classify the potentiated sulfas as agents with good to excellent sensitivity.* Clavulanated amoxicillin, enrofloxacin, and tylosin have become available, and all have excel-

*See references 6, 33, 35, 62, 83, 102, 105, 111, 115, and 138.

lent sensitivity.[35, 112, 138a] Clindamycin appears to have the same sensitivity spectrum and clinical efficacy as lincomycin.[67a]

Data for cats are much more limited. Current studies on coagulate-positive staphylococci show excellent sensitivity to cloxacillin, cephalosporin, chloramphenicol, erythromycin, potentiated sulfas, and clavulanated amoxicillin; good sensitivity to clindamycin; fair sensitivity to tetracycline; and poor sensitivity to penicillin and amoxicillin.[103, 104, 149] Efficacy data for enrofloxacin are unavailable, but it appears to have excellent sensitivity.

For the previously untreated staphylococcal infection, antibiotic selection can be done on an empirical basis or via the results of culture and sensitivity testing. This latter option is not available in many cases because intact primary lesions are not available and culture and sensitivity testing may not be cost effective in small to medium-sized dogs. Culture and sensitivity testing usually costs the client $20 or more, delays treatment for 48 hours or longer, and does not always accurately predict in vivo efficacy. Because of these shortcomings and the stable sensitivity of canine staphylococci, the authors do not recommend the culturing of previously untreated staphylococcal infections unless the patient is known to have adverse reactions to the commonly used drugs or the course of treatment is to exceed 21 days. With long courses of treatment, especially in large dogs, sensitivity testing can be cost effective if it indicates that the isolate from the patient is sensitive to an inexpensive antibiotic.

Antibiotic selection is not so straightforward in cases in which the empirically selected antibiotic is not effective or when the infection recurs shortly after treatment is discontinued. If the empirically selected antibiotic has only good sensitivity, most clinicians empirically select another drug with an excellent sensitivity. If this new drug fails to be effective, one must carefully evaluate whether the owner is complying with the treatment regimen and whether the skin is truly infected. If no reason for this poor response can be found, sensitivity testing is mandatory.

More commonly, the clinician is faced with the problem of antibiotic selection in recurring infections. Most studies show that drugs with excellent sensitivity (clavulanated amoxicillin, oxacillin, cephalosporin, and enrofloxacin) maintain their efficacy in recurrences, but that the in vitro sensitivity to the other antibiotics decreases and becomes unpredictable. Some clinicians empirically select one of the excellent drugs, whereas other clinicians perform sensitivity testing in all cases. Either position can be argued, and each case should be managed on its own merits.

If cytologic study or culture shows a mixed infection, sensitivity testing is mandatory because the sensitivity of nonstaphylococcal organisms is not always predictable. If all organisms are sensitive to a safe, reasonably inexpensive drug, that drug should be used. Occasionally, no one drug fits the sensitivity profile of all organisms or the singular drug is too toxic or expensive for long-term use. If the infection contains *S. intermedius*, as most do, the initial antibiotic selection should be aimed at that organism. Eradication of the staphylococcal component may make the microenvironment unfavorable for the growth of the other organisms. If the antistaphylococcal antibiotic improves but does not resolve the infection, alternative drugs must be used.

After an antibiotic has been selected, it should be dispensed at the correct dosage, administered at the appropriate dosage interval, and be used for a sufficient period. Dosages for the antibiotics routinely used in treating staphylococcal infections are given in Chapter 3. Most drugs used are veterinary prescription items and have detailed pharmacologic data to support the suggested dosage. Some investigators believe that the dosage for clavulanated amoxicillin should be 22 mg/kg every 12 hours versus the recommended 13.75 mg/kg every 12 hours[85] and many clinicians dispense trimethoprim-sulfadiazine at 30 mg/kg every 12 hours versus the recommended 30 mg/kg every 24 hours or 15 mg/kg every 12 hours.[105] The authors believe that these higher dosages are unnecessary in most dogs and increase the cost of treatment. Some animals do not respond completely at the suggested dosage because of irregularities in drug distribution and metabolism or because the minimal inhibitory concentration for the organism in question cannot be achieved at the standard dosage. In these uncommon cases, dosage increases are appropriate.

With the exception of the potentiated sulfa drugs, for which once-daily treatment is recommended, all orally administered antibiotics need to be given twice to three times daily. More correctly, they must be given every 8 to 12 hours on a regular schedule. Most owners can administer drugs every 12 hours, but work schedules usually preclude the regular administration of drugs at 8-hour intervals. If the owner's lifestyle does not allow regular administration every 8 hours, another drug should be selected.

The most commonly recognized cause of the inability to resolve a skin infection or for its relapse days after the treatment is discontinued is an insufficient course of treatment. Although textbooks and clinical experience can suggest appropriate courses of treatment, each animal responds at its own rate and must be treated until its infection is resolved. Resolution means that all lesions have healed both on the surface and in the deeper tissues. Surface healing is easy to determine by visual inspection, but deep healing is much more difficult to assess and necessitates palpation of the lesions.

Intercurrent corticosteroid administration confounds the problem greatly. Corticosteroids decrease visual and palpable inflammation, which is the key sign in determining when an infection is resolved. An inflamed hair follicle is still infected, whereas one that looks and feels normal is probably healed. With intercurrent corticosteroid use, it is impossible to determine whether the antibiotic resolved the inflammation, and therefore the infection, or whether the corticosteroid is masking the infection. If an individual animal requires both antibiotics and corticosteroids, the corticosteroid administration should be discontinued at least 7 days before the final evaluation of the infection.

In infections of the intact hair follicle, deep tissues rarely become inflamed enough to be detected by palpation, so infection could still be present when the surface has healed. To prevent relapses because of this inapparent infection, it is recommended that antibiotic treatment be continued for 7 days after surface healing. In deeper infections, surface healing is misleading and antibiotic treatment must be continued after the dermal inflammation is gone. Deep lesions always heal on the surface well before the deep infection is resolved. Because some small, nonpalpable nidi of infection can persist even when the tissues feel normal by palpation, antibiotic treatment should be continued for 7 to 21 days after the tissues return to apparent normalcy. The time to resolution dictates the length of postnormalcy treatment.

Ideally, the clinician should re-examine all animals to determine when true healing has occurred. This is impractical in many instances and is not absolutely necessary in the case of more superficial infections. As long as the owner is an astute observer and treats the animal after clinical normalcy is present, most infections can be resolved without re-examination. Re-examination is mandatory for animals with deep infections. Owners cannot tell when the deep infection is resolved and always underestimate the need for antibiotics. Some clinicians schedule examinations every 14 days, whereas other clinicians examine the animal only when the owner reports that the lesions have healed. The approach is individualized for best results.

Deep infections are problematic for both the client and the clinician. With follicular rupture and damage to the dermal tissues, the inflammation tends to be pyogranulomatous and endogenous foreign bodies (keratin, hair shafts, and damaged collagen) are usually found in the dermis. During the first 2 to 4 weeks of antibiotic treatment, the lesion improves dramatically and then apparently stops responding. If treatment is stopped at this point, any ground gained is lost because it is unlikely that the deep infection is resolved. The rapid initial improvement is due to the resolution of the pyogenic component of the infection, but the granulomatous component remains and responds much more slowly. As long as there is slow, steady improvement, the antibiotic administration should be continued, even if the course of treatment approaches 12 weeks or longer. With long-term treatment, most lesions resolve completely, but the healing of some lesions reaches a certain point and improves no further. In these cases, the tissues never return to palpable normalcy because of resultant fibrosis, the presence of sterile endogenous foreign bodies in the dermis, or walled off nidi of infection. Skin biopsies can be both helpful and misleading. If infection is seen, the need for additional treatment is documented. If none is seen, the question remains as to whether some infection is present in areas that do not undergo biopsy. If the lesion does not improve at all with 2 to 3 weeks of additional antibiotic treatment, one must assume that the infection is resolved and stop treatment. If infection is present, the lesion begins to worsen again in 2 to 21 days.

Relapses are common in skin infections, either because the current infection was not treated appropriately or because the underlying cause of the infection was not identified or resolved. The timing to relapse is important. If new lesions appear within 7 days of the termination of treatment, it is likely that the infection was not resolved. More intense treatment is necessary. If the relapse occurs weeks to months after the last treatment, the animal has some underlying problem that must be resolved.

Management of Chronic Recurrent Skin Infections

Despite diligent diagnostic and therapeutic measures, some dogs have recurrent or nearly constant skin infections. The infection responds to prolonged treatment but recurs within weeks of drug withdrawal. Some of these dogs have a documented immunodeficiency, whereas other dogs appear normal with the currently available tests or cannot be tested. Poorly managed or poorly responsive allergic skin diseases must also be considered. These infections recur frequently, but the allergic pruritus damages the skin and predisposes to infection. This is especially true if corticosteroids are being used.

Immunomodulation can be considered in dogs with an immunodeficiency. The hope is that this type of treatment will make the animal's immune responsiveness more normal. It does not make a normal immune system hyperresponsive, so it has little or no benefit when the skin infections are due to weak skin and not a weak immune system. These treatments cannot resolve any pre-existing infection, but it is hoped that they can prevent or minimize further relapses.[85, 107] The agents are given concurrently with an appropriate antibiotic until the infection is completely resolved. If the animal has received a sufficient course of treatment with the immunomodulator by the time that the infection is resolved, the administration of the antibiotic is discontinued at that point while that of the modulator is continued. The success of treatment depends on the time to, and severity of, any relapse. If no relapses occur, treatment was a complete success. Because it is difficult to normalize the immune system completely, many animals that undergo successful treatment do have other episodes of infection, but these are widely spaced, are less severe, and respond rapidly to antibiotic therapy. In many dogs, no response is seen.

Chemical modulation with levamisole or cimetidine has received attention for treatment of recurrent skin infections, but no published reports offer specific details on the efficacy of either product.[45, 85] Levamisole, when administered at 2.2 mg/kg every other day, is thought to modulate the cell-mediated immune system and may be of some benefit in approximately 10 per cent of dogs with idiopathic recurrent infections.[71a] At this dosage, side-effects are rare but include drug eruption, gastrointestinal irritation (vomiting and diarrhea), and blood dyscrasias. Because histamine receptors are found on the cell surface of many mononuclear cells, histamine can affect cellular function.[157] Cimetidine, an H_2-receptor antagonist, may inhibit histamine-influenced immunosuppression. For dogs, dosages between 6 and 10 mg/kg every 8 hours are suggested and side effects are rarely reported. If either of these drugs helps to prevent relapses, it is continued for the life of the patient at the dosages indicated above. The cost of the cimetidine may be prohibitive, especially in large dogs.

Various bacterial products have received wide use in dogs with recurrent pyodermas. Autogenous staphylococcal bacterins, *Staphylococcus aureus* phage lysate (Staphage Lysate [SPL] [Delmont Laboratories]), and *Propionibacterium acnes* (Immunoregulin [Immunovet]) are the most commonly used preparations. The exact mechanism of action of these products in dogs is unknown, but it seems to focus on improving cell-mediated immunity with subsequent impact on nonspecific and humoral immunity.[44, 45, 85] No studies have been published in which dogs with recurrent pyodermas have been given all three preparations on a rotating basis to determine which is most effective. Placebo-controlled studies with SPL and Immunoregulin have been conducted, but none with autogenous products has been reported.

Autogenous staphylococcal vaccines are prepared from cultures taken from the dog's skin and thus contain the specific strain of *S. intermedius* causing the infection. Although some reports indicate widespread use of these autogenous bacterins,[10] few detailed reports on their efficacy are available. When some dogs with deep pyoderma[107] or staphylococcal blepharitis[27] were given 1 ml on a weekly basis, good to excellent response was seen. The authors are also aware of many cases in which no response was noted. One dog treated by one of the authors (WHM) became sensitive to the bacterin and experienced urticaria and anaphylaxis.

Immunoregulin is licensed for intravenous use only and can cause a necrotizing dermatitis if it is given subcutaneously or intramuscularly. It is given every third to fourth day for 2 weeks then weekly until the condition is resolved or stabilizes. Maintenance doses are given as needed, usually once monthly. When 28 dogs with recurrent skin infections were given either Immunoregulin or a placebo for 12 weeks, the rate of cure in the Immunoregulin-treated group was much better: 80 per cent versus 38.5 per cent.[11] Because the dogs were given antibiotics concurrently with the immunomodulator and details on relapses were not available, it is difficult to determine the efficacy of the product.

SPL was first developed for use in humans and contains components of *S. aureus*.[43-45, 85, 123] It is licensed for use in dogs by subcutaneous injection. Dosage schedules vary, but most investigators administer 0.5 ml twice weekly for 10 to 12 weeks. If response is seen, maintenance injections are given every 7 to 14 days. If a partial response is seen to the 0.5-ml dosage, gradual increases to 1.5 ml (the maximal dosage suggested by the manufacturer) may improve the responses. When 21 dogs with recurrent superficial pyoderma were given either SPL or a placebo for 18 weeks, 10 of 13 dogs (77 per cent) given the SPL had a good response, whereas 3 of 8 (46 per cent) in the placebo group had a good response.[43] Responders did have subsequent infections, but they were reported to be less severe with the SPL treatment and could resolve spontaneously.

This information suggests that immunomodulation may be of some benefit in carefully selected cases. If the recurrent infections are due to skin disease and not immunodeficiency, response beyond that seen with a placebo should not be expected. These agents are expensive and not innocuous, thus casual usage should be discouraged. Because cats rarely have recurrent skin infections other than abscesses associated with fighting, no data are available on the safety and efficacy of these products in cats. One author (WHM) has treated one cat with SPL given at 0.5 ml once weekly and saw positive results with no adverse reactions.

When the dog's recurrent pyoderma is due to an unresolvable skin disease, usually an allergic disorder, or fails to respond to immunomodulation, control can usually be achieved with long-term antimicrobial therapy. Topical antibacterial shampoos are usually insufficient and may be detrimental if the shampoos irritate or macerate the skin. Antibiotics are necessary. Because the drug is given for a prolonged period, only drugs with a wide margin of safety should be used. Most cases are treated with a cephalosporin, oxacillin, clavulanated amoxicillin, or enrofloxacin. Lincomycin and erythromycin are safe for long-term administration, but bacterial resistance usually precludes their use.

Antibiotics can be administered to these dogs on a recurrent episodic basis or continually. If the interinfection interval is 2 months or longer, episodic administration is most appropriate. At the first sign of infection, the drug is given at full therapeutic levels until the infection is resolved and then for an additional 7 to 14 days. When the infections recur shortly after the drug administration is discontinued, long-term treatment is indicated.[85] The dog is first treated with the full therapeutic dosages for 7 to 14 days after clinical remission, and then therapy is changed to a suboptimal or pulse regimen. No data are available to suggest that one method is more effective or less likely to cause side effects, so the protocol selected should be tailored to the patient's needs. The pulse method involves the administration of full therapeutic dosages for 7 days, with none given for the next 7 days. Depending on the animal's response, the interval with no treatment could be extended to 10 to 21 days.

A variety of suboptimal protocols are used. To clarify the discussion, let us say that the full therapeutic dosage of the drug of choice for the patient is 500 mg every 12 hours. After the infection is resolved, some investigators administer 500 mg every 24 hours, whereas others administer 500 mg every 12 hours every other day. If the patient's infection does not recur, additional reductions may be indicated. The investigators who use once-daily therapy often reduce the daily dosage to 250 mg or maintain the 500-mg dosage but administer it less often (e.g., every 48 or 72 hours). When the drug is not administered on a daily basis, the treatment interval is extended to every third or fourth day. After the lowest level of treatment is determined, the animal is maintained with that protocol for life or until it becomes ineffective. Long-term antibiotic administration is expensive, especially for large dogs, but has surprisingly few side effects. Concerns for the development of resistant staphylococci, plasmid transfer of resistance to other organisms, superinfections with yeast or other fungal organism (with the possible exception of *Malassezia*), or drug intoxications have not been realized. However, these concerns are valid, so this type of treatment should be undertaken only as a last resort.[22]

■ SURFACE BACTERIAL INFECTIONS

Pyotraumatic dermatitis occurs in two histopathologic patterns. One, clinically referred to as acute moist dermatitis, is a superficial, ulcerative inflammatory process caused by trauma (see Chap. 15). The other pattern, pyotraumatic folliculitis, is a deep suppurative folliculitis (see later discussion). Intertrigo, or skin fold dermatitis, is a surface irritation and inflammation caused by frictional trauma of skin rubbing against skin (see Chap. 15).

■ SUPERFICIAL BACTERIAL INFECTIONS (SUPERFICIAL PYODERMAS)

Superficial pyodermas are bacterial infections that involve the epidermis and follicular epithelium. They include impetigo, mucocutaneous pyoderma, superficial bacterial folliculitis, and dermatophilosis.

Impetigo

Impetigo is characterized by subcorneal pustules that affect sparsely haired areas of the skin.

CAUSE AND PATHOGENESIS

Impetigo is a bacterial disease that is invariably caused by coagulase-positive *Staphylococcus* organisms. It affects young dogs before or at the time of puberty. It is not contagious. Many cases in puppies occur for no apparent reason, whereas in other puppies the infection is secondary to parasitism, viral infections, a dirty environment, immune-mediated disease, or poor nutrition. Bullous impetigo is most often associated with hyperadrenocorticism, diabetes mellitus, hypothyroidism, or other debilitating diseases, and in these cases other bacteria such as *Pseudomonas* sp. and *E. coli* may be present.[109]

A superficial pustular dermatitis has been described in kittens in association with overzealous "mouthing" by the queen. Cultures revealed *Pasteurella multocida* or β-hemolytic streptococci.[132]

CLINICAL FEATURES

Small superficial pustules that do not involve hair follicles are found primarily, but not exclusively, in the glabrous areas of the inguinal and axillary regions in dogs (Fig. 4:1 *A*). They are not painful and rupture easily, leaving a peripheral epidermal collarette or honey-colored crust adherent to the skin. Pruritus is uncommon and, if present, usually indicates follicular involvement, and therefore not a true impetigo. This is a relatively benign problem that often heals spontaneously and may be noted only incidentally. In kittens, lesions are found mostly on the back of the neck, the head, and the withers. In bullous impetigo, the nonfollicular pustules are large and flaccid (Fig. 4:1 *B*), and large sheets of superficial epidermis may be seen to peel away. Coagulase-positive staphylococci are usually cultured from the lesions. Diagnosis is made by the history and the clinical appearance and by documentation of the bacterial cause by direct smears and stains or by cultures of the pustular exudate. Histopathologic findings show nonfollicular subcorneal pustules (Fig. 4:2). Bacteria may or may not be seen within the pustules.

CLINICAL MANAGEMENT

Impetigo may regress spontaneously, but therapy can hasten the healing process. When the lesions are few and widely separated, topical antibiotic or antibacterial creams or water-miscible ointments such as mupirocin and chlorhexidine can be effective.[20a] Typically, the lesions are too numerous to make this form of therapy practical, and bathing with antibacterial shampoos, such as chlorhexidine, ethyl lactate, and benzoyl peroxide, is indicated. The skin of puppies and kittens is easily irritated, and benzoyl peroxide should be used carefully. The affected areas are washed daily or on alternate days until healing occurs, typically in 7 to 10 days. Rarely are systemic antibiotics necessary, but if needed, a 10- to 14-day course is usually sufficient unless there is an intercurrent superficial folliculitis. It is desirable to check health management procedures to eliminate debilitating factors that may have influenced the onset of the disorder.

Impetigo-like lesions in unusual locations (e.g., facial) in puppies or in mature dogs necessitate more careful consideration and may carry a more guarded prognosis, because immunosuppression and other serious disorders mentioned above may be involved in the pathogenesis. Bullous impetigo usually responds rapidly to the administration of appropriate antibiotics and treatment of the underlying disease.

Mucocutaneous Pyodermas

Mucocutaneous pyoderma occurs in dogs and affects primarily the lips and perioral skin.[71b] Its etiology is unknown.

CLINICAL FEATURES

Dogs of any age, breed, or sex can be affected. German shepherd dogs and German shepherd crosses may be at greater risk. The first noticeable change is symmetric swelling and erythema of the lips, especially at the commissures. Crusting follows and can lead to fissuring and erosion. Exudate may be present beneath the crusts, especially ventral to the lips. Similar lesions may be seen at the nares, the vulva, the prepuce, or the anus. Depigmentation of the lips can be seen in chronic cases.

The lesions are tender, and the dogs rub the areas and resent examination and palpation of the area. Mucocutaneous pyoderma does not originate in lip folds but can coexist with lip fold dermatitis.

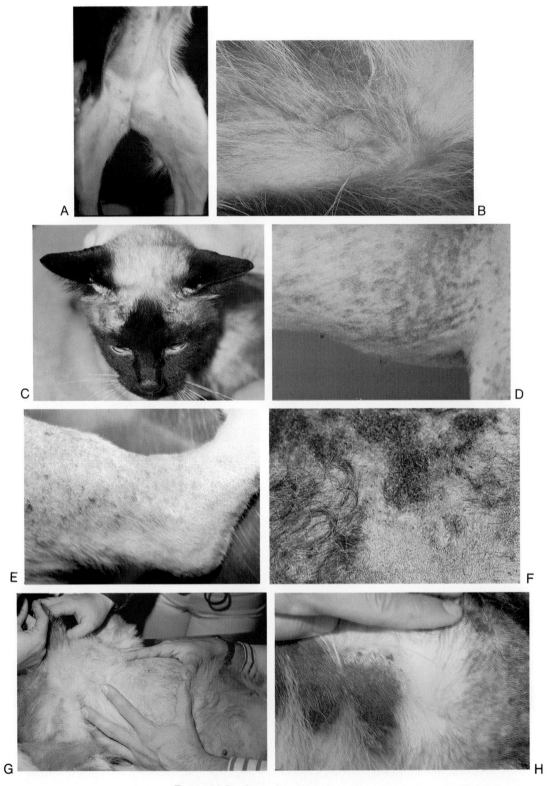

Figure 4:1 *See legend on opposite page*

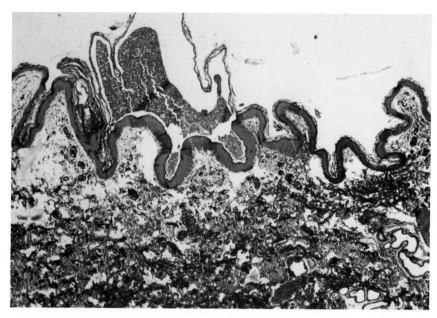

Figure 4:2. Staphylococcal impetigo in a dog. Note nonfollicular subcorneal pustule.

DIAGNOSIS

Mucocutaneous pyoderma is reported to be visually distinctive.[71b] Differential diagnostic possibilities include discoid lupus erythematosus, lip fold intertrigo, zinc-responsive dermatosis, early pemphigus foliaceus or erythematosus, and drug eruption.

Diagnosis is by clinical examination and skin biopsy. Histopathologic study shows epidermal hyperplasia with superficial pustulation and crusting. In the dermis, a dense, predominately plasmacytic, lichenoid dermatitis is seen. The dermal-epidermal interface is not obscured. Similar but milder inflammatory changes may be seen around appendages in biopsy specimens of haired skin.

CLINICAL MANAGEMENT

The condition responds to topical or systemic antibacterial therapy. For topical treatment, the surrounding hairs should be clipped and then the areas gently washed with benzoyl peroxide or some other suitable antibacterial shampoo. After the lesions are cleaned, a light film of a 2 per cent mupirocin ointment (Bactoderm [Smith Kline Beecham]) is applied. The areas are treated daily for 14 days and then once to twice weekly. In severe cases, systemic antibiotics are necessary for 3 to 4 weeks.

After the lesions have resolved, treatment can be discontinued, but relapses are common. For relapsing cases, normalcy can be maintained by an individualized topical program or, more rarely, maintenance administration of systemic antibiotics.

Figure 4:1. *A,* Multiple erythematous papules, pustules, and crusts on the abdomen of a dog with impetigo. *B,* Large, flaccid pustule of bullous impetigo in an old dog with immunodeficiency. *C,* Staphylococcal folliculitis on face and ears of Siamese cat. *D,* Lateral thorax of a Shar Pei with superficial folliculitis. Note the moth-eaten appearance. *E,* Superficial folliculitis on the lateral leg. Note the follicular pattern. *F,* Active erythematous papules and oozing at the periphery of chronic hyperpigmented plaques in a dog with superficial staphylococcal folliculitis. *G,* Multiple annular areas of erythema and alopecia in a dog with superficial staphylococcal folliculitis. *H,* Annular, coalescing areas of alopecia and hyperpigmentation with peripheral erythema and crust in a dog with superficial staphylococcal folliculitis.

Superficial Bacterial Folliculitis

A common clinical presentation is infection confined to the superficial portion of the hair follicle.

CAUSE AND PATHOGENESIS

In most cases, superficial folliculitis in dogs is caused by *S. intermedius,* although other staphylococcal species and other bacteria may be involved. Organisms may be introduced by local trauma, by bruising or scratching, or as an infection resulting from contamination due to dirty coats or poor grooming, seborrhea, parasitic infestation (especially demodicosis), hormonal factors, local irritants, or allergies. The three most common etiologic agents in canine folliculitis are staphylococci, dermatophytes, and demodectic mites. Superficial folliculitis may progress to deep folliculitis, furunculosis, and even cellulitis.

Folliculitis may or may not be pruritic, and if it is pruritic, its intensity can vary. It is not clear why these two types of folliculitis exist, or even if the two syndromes (pruritic and nonpruritic) are separate dermatoses. The clinical lesions, described histopathologic findings, and levels of antistaphylococcal IgE antibodies[64a] are identical for both types, the only difference between the two being the pruritus. A few cases may be due to bacterial hypersensitivity (so-called pruritic superficial pyoderma).[108a] Because staphylococcal folliculitis can be pruritic, and because so many pruritic dermatoses (e.g., hypersensitivities and ectoparasitisms) are frequently complicated by secondary staphylococcal folliculitis, it is crucial and apt to ask, ''Is it a rash that itches or an itch that rashes?'' Often, the answer is determined only by training the client to observe the skin before and during the next recurrence.

CLINICAL FEATURES

The primary feature of folliculitis, regardless of the cause, is a tiny, inflammatory pustule with a hair shaft protruding from the center. The typical pustule may be difficult to find, because pustular lesions are transient in dogs and cats, especially when the patient is pruritic. More common lesions are follicular papules (earliest lesion), which may or may not be crusted; epidermal collarettes; hyperpigmentation; excoriation; and alopecia (see Fig. 4:1 *D* to *F*). Annular areas of alopecia, erythema, scaling, crusting, and hyperpigmentation—the so-called bull's eye or target lesions (see Fig. 4:1 *G* and *H*)—are highly suggestive, but many vesicular and highly inflammatory processes that begin from a point (e.g., impetigo and pemphigus foliaceus) may produce similar circular lesions.

Superficial folliculitis has neither a specific distribution pattern nor a characteristic clinical presentation. Because staphylococcal infections are typically secondary to external or internal skin damage, the localization of the infection depends on the predisposing cause. With external trauma (e.g., laceration and fleas), the infection is initially localized in the area of trauma. With underlying systemic disorders, truncal lesions predominate. In either case, the infection can spread to involve wider areas, especially if the lesions are pruritic. In chronic cases, most of the skin can be involved.

The clinical lesions depend on density and length of the hairs in the involved area. In glabrous areas, the papulopustular lesions described above are easily seen. In haired skin, these lesions are not appreciated unless the hair is clipped away. In short-coated dogs, the first sign of superficial folliculitis is a dishevelment of the coat in the involved area, with small groups of hairs tufting together and rising above the skin's surface. These early lesions are often confused with urticaria. With time, the hairs fall out of the infected follicles and the dog is left with multiple, small areas of alopecia (see Fig. 4:1 *D*). The exposed skin is usually inflamed, but in the Shar Pei and dogs with darkly pigmented skin, the hairless areas look nonreactive, which can lessen the suggestion of bacterial folliculitis. With increasing chronicity, the alopecic areas enlarge to give the dog a moth-eaten look. Adjacent lesions can coalesce to form large areas of inflamed skin,[71c] which can be confused with dermatophytosis and a variety of other conditions. Careful inspection of the periphery of the hairless area usually shows an inflamed epidermal collarette and more typical lesions of superficial folliculitis. In chronic cases, the coalescence can be so advanced that the dog looks like it has an endocrine alopecia. However, the approximately annular appearance of the alopecic areas and the discrete borders between alopecic and haired areas are highly suggestive of follicular inflammation or dysplasia.

Superficial folliculitis in long-coated dogs is much more insidious, especially when the lesions are not pruritic. The first sign is usually a loss of luster of the hairs in the involved area with increased shedding. The area may or may not be seborrheic. With time, the scaling increases or becomes apparent and the hair loss increases so that the hypotrichosis is obvious. Coincidental with the increasing hair loss is the recognition of underlying skin lesions. Collies and Shetland sheepdogs can have large, approximately symmetric areas of alopecia over the trunk, resembling endocrine hair loss. Careful inspection of the margins of the alopecic areas reveals erythema, scaling, and epidermal collarettes.

Superficial folliculitis is rare in cats.[104, 132–135, 149] The most common presentation is a crusted papular eruption (miliary dermatitis), which is clinically indistinguishable from the other crusted papular lesions of cats. Some cats have annular areas of alopecia, scaling, and crusting over the head and neck (see Fig. 4:1 *C*), which is more commonly produced by dermatophytosis or demodicosis.

DIAGNOSIS

With adequate visualization of the lesions, the clinical diagnosis of superficial folliculitis is usually straightforward. The papular or pustular lesion has a follicular orientation. Because most cases of superficial folliculitis in the dog are staphylococcal in origin, it is likely that the patient being examined has a pyoderma. However, this is not absolute because follicular inflammation (folliculitis) is also seen in a number of conditions, including demodicosis, dermatophytosis, and a variety of immune-mediated skin disorders such as pemphigus foliaceus. To confuse the issue further, an inflamed hair follicle is easily infected such that it is common to see a secondary staphylococcal folliculitis superimposed on some other folliculopathy.

To confirm the diagnosis of bacterial superficial folliculitis, diagnostic tests must be performed. Skin scrapings and fungal techniques (hair examination and fungal culture) should be performed to rule out the other common causes of folliculitis and exudative cytologic specimens should be evaluated. The pus should contain cocci, neutrophils in varying stages of maturity, and most importantly, evidence of bacterial phagocytosis.

If no exudate is available or if the cytologic examination shows bacterial infection but the distribution and nature of the lesions suggests that the infection was caused by some other inflammatory folliculopathy, skin biopsies are necessary to define the problem. The histopathologic study of bacterial folliculitis shows a neutrophilic exudate within the hair follicles (Fig. 4:3). Bacteria may or may not be seen within the infected follicles. If a biopsy is done on chronic nonpustular lesions, one often finds superficial interstitial dermatitis, perifolliculitis, perifollicular fibrosis, or intraepidermal neutrophilic microabscesses.

Because skin infections rarely occur spontaneously in dogs and cats, the diagnostic effort should not stop at the identification of staphylococcal folliculitis. The most important question to be answered is, "Why is the skin infected?" The history and physical examination become important here. If there is any evidence of antecedent pruritus or skin disease before the pyoderma developed, the diagnostic effort needs to continue to define the underlying cause of the infection. In many cases, especially when the pyoderma is chronic and the lesions are pruritic, the history and the physical examination are of minimal use. Here, one is faced with

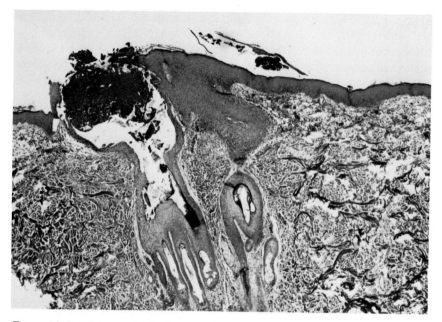

Figure 4:3. Staphylococcal folliculitis in a dog. Note cellular exudate within hair follicle.

the choice of performing other diagnostic tests (e.g., routine laboratory screening, endocrine testing, and allergy testing) or simply treating the infection appropriately.

Obviously, the specifics of the case dictate the best course of action, but if the animal has never been adequately treated for a superficial staphylococcal folliculitis, it is probably best to resolve the infection. It is not unusual for dogs with chronic widespread superficial folliculitis to return to clinical normalcy and remain normal after the infection is resolved. Obviously, the cause of the pyoderma in those cases was transient. If the animal's uninfected skin is abnormal or if the pyoderma recurs within 3 months of the cessation of treatment, the animal has some other disease that must be diagnosed and treated to prevent further relapses. Careful review of the history and the physical examination findings after antibiotic treatment directs the diagnostic effort.

CLINICAL MANAGEMENT

A superficial folliculitis in an immunologically normal animal heals fairly rapidly with a typical course of treatment of 21 to 28 days. In the case of recurrent infections, it is not uncommon for the lesions to heal more slowly, so longer courses of treatment can be expected.

Dermatophilosis

Dermatophilosis (cutaneous streptotrichosis) is an actinomycotic disease that produces a superficial, crusted dermatitis caused by *Dermatophilus congolensis*. It is rare in small animals.[1, 23, 28, 106]

CAUSE AND PATHOGENESIS

The organism is a gram-positive coccus that has not been found in the environment and therefore is thought to come from only carrier animals, usually farm animals.[23, 106] The clinical disease often develops shortly after the rainy season begins and is uncommon in dry climates.

Moisture that releases the infectious zoospores is an essential initiating factor. Affected animals usually have skin defects from ectoparasites, minor trauma, maceration, inflammation, or infection. Thus, the organism is usually a secondary invader that is easily found by stained smears or cultures. These are motile organisms that eventually form flagellated zoospores. That form is highly resistant and may persist in affected crusts for several years. The motile cocci are chemotropically attracted toward carbon dioxide diffusing from the surface of the skin. There, they germinate to produce a filament that invades the living epidermis and proliferates within it, causing the production of typical crusts.[88]

CLINICAL FEATURES

This is a rare disease in small animals, but it may be more common than is realized in moist, warm climates such as northern Australia, New Zealand, and the southeastern United States. It should be suspected in cases of acute moist dermatitis, chronic folliculitis, seborrheic dermatitis, and other crusted dermatoses in which excessive moisture is present. It has been noted to affect dogs[1, 122] and cats,[1, 23, 106, 132] and one report suggests that the fox is the only natural canine host.[122]

Lesions may involve all parts of the hairy or glabrous skin, and in cats, the organism has been isolated from soft tissue fistulae and granulomatous lesions of the lymph nodes, the mouth, and the bladder. With skin lesions, the crusts are usually concentrated on the dorsal back and over the scapula and lateral thigh. The face, the ears, and the feet may also be affected, and pain is evident, as the animals appear to be unhappy and are disinclined to move around.

Local lesions may start as erythematous papules and pustules, with crusts that occasionally thicken and expand to several centimeters in diameter. They may be isolated, circular lesions or may coalesce into larger areas. The classic lesion is an exudative, purulent dermatitis below raised tufts of hair and crusts. In early lesions, these crusts and the embedded hairs are easily removed (''paintbrush'' lesions) to reveal greenish pus on an oval, bleeding, ulcerated surface. The healing lesions are characterized by dry crusts, scaling, hyperpigmentation, and alopecia.

DIAGNOSIS

The purulent exudate or crushed crusts can be made into a direct smear and stained with Giemsa's, Wright's, or Gram's stain or Diff Quik. The organisms can be difficult to identify but appear as two to six parallel rows of gram-positive cocci that look like railroad tracks (Fig. 4:4).

For isolation and culture of the organisms, crusts are ground with sterile distilled water and let stand for 30 minutes. The inoculum is taken from the top of the water mixture and placed in antibiotic-enriched (polymyxin B) media. Many media, such as blood agar, are satisfactory, but Sabouraud's agar and MacConkey's agar should be avoided. Growth of a rough colony (later becoming smooth) occurs in 3 days, but organisms are small at first and may be missed in the midst of contaminants. With a scanning electron microscope, the colony appears as a mass of fine meshed filaments that become striated and divide into segments (cocci).

Skin biopsy of the affected skin is diagnostic and is especially useful in chronic cases in which the exudative cytologic findings are often negative. Histopathologic study shows a hyperplastic superficial perivascular dermatitis or perifolliculitis-folliculitis with a palisading crust of orthokeratotic-parakeratotic hyperkeratosis and leukocytes. Organisms are usually easily demonstrated within the keratin on hematoxylin and eosin (H & E), acid orcein–Giemsa, or Brown-Brenn stains.

Differential diagnosis should include seborrheic dermatitis, pustular dermatitis (impetigo, subcorneal pustular dermatosis, and pemphigus foliaceus), acute moist dermatitis, staphylococcal folliculitis, dermatophytosis, and zinc-responsive dermatosis.

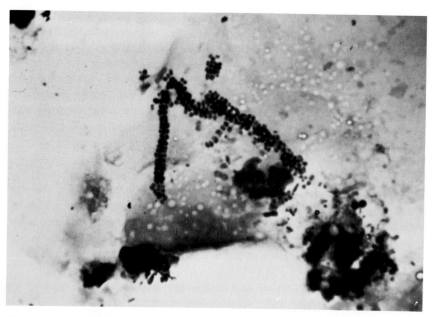

Figure 4:4. Dermatophilosis. Note branching chains of cocci ("railroad tracks") characteristic of *D. congolensis* in this direct smear of pus.

CLINICAL MANAGEMENT

With elimination of the primary inciting factors, many cases of dermatophilosis resolve spontaneously. This involves removing the moisture, parasites, or trauma that may be present.

The *Dermatophilus* organism should be eliminated from the skin. Because it does not thrive in an acid pH, topical therapy and good skin hygiene are useful. Crust removal and disposal are essential. Daily soaks with povidone-iodine or lime-sulfur solution given for 1 week and repeated weekly for 3 to 4 weeks are helpful. The systemic use of antibiotics is most effective and should be the primary focus of treatment. The organism is usually sensitive to ampicillin, cephalosporin, cloxacillin, lincomycin, tetracycline, tylosin, and high doses of penicillin. It is resistant to erythromycin, novobiocin, sulfonamides, polymyxin B, and low doses of penicillin.

Therapy with tetracycline or high levels of penicillin for 7 to 10 days is usually adequate. Positive cultures can often be obtained from the skin of healed animals for 7 to 8 months and up to 15 months, an important factor in recurrence of the disease.[1]

■ DEEP BACTERIAL INFECTIONS (DEEP PYODERMAS)

Deep pyodermas are serious bacterial infections that involve tissues deeper than the hair follicle. They invade the dermis and often the subcutaneous tissue as well. They can cause systemic signs of illness and often heal with scarring.

Deep pyodermas do not occur spontaneously in normal dogs and cats. There is always a cause of the infection, and successful treatment mandates the identification of the predisposing problem. When the infection remains localized to a small area, external trauma (e.g., laceration, penetrating wound, animal bite, and foreign body) is the most likely cause. When lesions are discrete but widely disseminated over the body, involve an entire region of the body (e.g., the rump), or are generalized, the animal has some additional disease that must be identified.

Deep skin infections are generally the continuation of a superficial infection or superficial folliculitis. The infection goes deeper into the follicles and breaks through the follicular wall to produce furunculosis or an infection of the dermis and subcutis. The infection follows tissue planes and may extend to the surface, producing multiple fistulae, or move deeper to invade subcutaneous and fatty tissues, producing cellulitis and panniculitis. The terminology for the condition depends on the location of the most obvious lesion, which may be called folliculitis and furunculosis, dermal fistulae, or cellulitis and panniculitis. Virtually any disease discussed in this text can be complicated by a deep staphylococcal infection.

In most instances, the infection remains confined to the hair follicle or progresses deeper at a gradual pace. In some cases, the progression is explosive. Factors that predispose to deep pyoderma include host immunoincompetence, severe follicular or dermal damage done by the primary disease (e.g., severe demodicosis), trauma (pressure, intense licking or chewing, and scratching) to the infected area, and inappropriate treatment of a superficial infection with an inefficient antibiotic, a corticosteroid, or both. In addition, many infections have distribution patterns that reflect areas of the body most subject to surface trauma. The basic pathogenesis of several common clinical syndromes is the same: deep folliculitis, furunculosis, and cellulitis; pyotraumatic folliculitis; nasal folliculitis and furunculosis; muzzle folliculitis and furunculosis; pedal folliculitis and furunculosis; German shepherd dog folliculitis, furunculosis, and cellulitis; acral lick furunculosis; anaerobic cellulitis; and subcutaneous abscesses.

Deep Folliculitis, Furunculosis, and Cellulitis

Deep folliculitis is a follicular infection that breaks through the hair follicle to produce furunculosis and cellulitis.

CAUSE AND PATHOGENESIS

Folliculitis and furunculosis start as a surface or follicular infection of bacterial, fungal, or parasitic cause. If there is a generalized distribution, one should suspect causes such as generalized demodicosis (see Fig. 7:21 *D*), generalized dermatophyte infection (see Fig. 5:1 *D*), drug eruptions, endocrine abnormalities, seborrhea, and immunosuppression. Bacteria present are usually *S. intermedius*, but deep skin infections are more apt to have secondary infections from *Proteus* sp., *Pseudomonas* sp., and *E. coli*.

Histologic examination of biopsy samples may be useful in understanding the mechanism, etiology, and state of development of the folliculitis and furunculosis syndrome. Folliculitis is an exceedingly common gross and microscopic finding in dogs. Because it is often a secondary development, a thorough search for an underlying cause is mandatory. Folliculitis associated with bacteria, fungi, or parasites is usually suppurative initially. The occasional case associated with atopy, food hypersensitivity, or seborrheic dermatitis is usually spongiotic and mononuclear. Any chronic folliculitis, especially if there is furunculosis, can become granulomatous or pyogranulomatous (Fig. 4:5). Furunculosis, regardless of cause, is usually associated with a tissue eosinophilia, which is assumed to suggest the presence of a foreign body (keratin or hairs). The absence of tissue eosinophilia with furunculosis usually implies immunosuppression, especially that due to concurrent glucocorticoid therapy or demodicosis.

CLINICAL FEATURES

The nature of the initial lesions depends on the number of follicles involved in the area, the depth and severity of the follicular involvement, and various host factors, especially its immunocompetence. Infection of one or a few contiguous follicles induces discrete papular lesions of varying size, whereas simultaneous involvement of many follicles causes poorly demarcated areas of alopecia, tissue swelling, and inflammation. The severity of the infection can be estimated by the coloration and size of the lesions. Large dark red to violescent lesions are more severely involved (Fig. 4:7 *D*) than those that are smaller, more superficial, or more pinkish (Fig. 4:6 *H*).

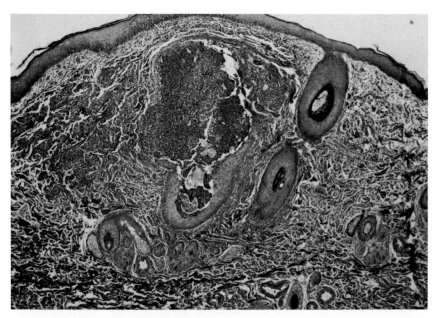

Figure 4:5. Staphyloccal furunculosis in a dog. Note follicular rupture with resultant pyogranulomatous dermal reaction around hair follicle.

The progression of the initial lesions is variable. Papular lesions soften to form deep pustules that ulcerate centrally and usually crust over. Before ulceration, hemorrhagic bullae may be seen. The larger lesions become more inflamed, become darker in color, and usually develop one or more fistulae that discharge exudate to the surface, where it crusts. Some of the severely infected larger areas become necrotic before fistulae develop and are irregular ulcers in the skin, which may or may not crust. If the infected area is traumatized (by pressure or pruritus), the speed and severity of progression is accelerated and the normal perilesional skin often becomes involved.

Lesions of folliculitis and furunculosis can occur wherever there are hair follicles but tend to be most common over pressure points or on the trunk. In short-coated dogs, the lesions described above are easily recognized. In long-coated dogs, the long hairs surrounding the infection entrap the exudate and tissue debris and encourage the development of large crusted lesions. The severity of the skin lesions in these crusted regions cannot be appreciated until the hair and crust are removed.

Bacterial folliculitis and furunculosis are rare in the cat (see Fig. 4:7 A). When they appear, follicular papules and pustules are usually located on the face and head (see Fig. 4:1 C) or over the dorsum in a flea bite hypersensitivity pattern. Cultures from these lesions have most commonly grown staphylococci, both coagulase positive and coagulase negative, and occasionally β-hemolytic streptococci and *P. multocida*. Feline chin folliculitis and furunculosis may be seen as a secondary infection complicating cases of feline acne (see Chap. 13).

Figure 4:6. *Folliculitis*—deep pyodermas. *A*, Pyotraumatic folliculitis and furunculosis on the cheek and neck of a dog. *B*, Nasal folliculitis (pyoderma) of a Pointer's nose. Pustules and crusts are typical of painful lesions. *C*, Nasal folliculitis (pyoderma) showing pustules on dorsum of the nose. *D*, Pododermatitis (interdigital pyoderma) showing pustules and draining fistulae. *E*, Pododermatitis (interdigital pyoderma) with severe edema, cellulitis, and draining sinuses. *F*, Lateral rump and thigh of a German shepherd with furunculosis. *G*, Rump, thigh, and trunk of a German shepherd with furunculosis. Note flea bite hypersensitivity type of distribution pattern. *H*, Rump of a Springer spaniel with deep folliculitis and furunculosis.

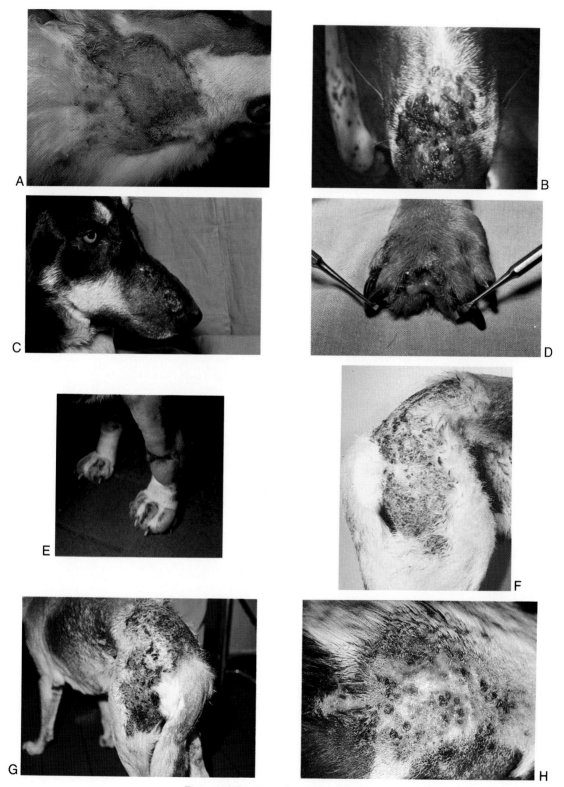

Figure 4:6 *See legend on opposite page*

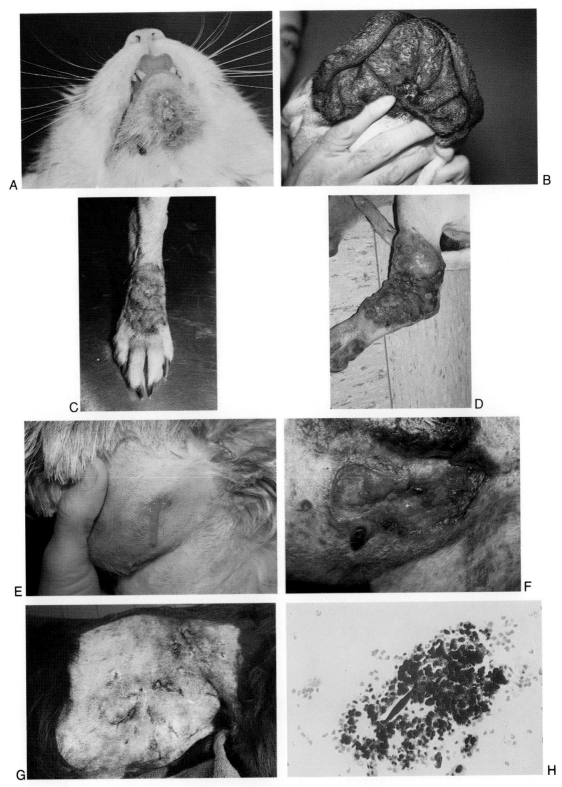

Figure 4:7 *See legend on opposite page*

CLINICAL MANAGEMENT

Although bacteremia and sepsis are apparently uncommon sequelae of a deep pyoderma, these serious debilitating infections necessitate careful, thorough, long-term treatment. Identification and resolution of the underlying cause is essential for a complete response. Most animals require a minimum of 4 to 6 weeks of treatment to resolve the visible lesions. Resolution of palpable lesions may necessitate treatment for 12 weeks or longer. Because of the seriousness of these infections, many investigators continue antibiotic administration for a full 14 days after clinical healing.

Pyotraumatic Folliculitis

Clinicians have long recognized that not all cases of pyotraumatic dermatitis (acute moist dermatitis or hot spots) respond to therapy rapidly and completely. One study reported a series of cases and discovered that they could be classified histologically into two groups.[120] In one group, the lesion did not have a large bacterial component. It was a superficial, ulcerated, inflammatory process of undetermined cause and pathogenesis (true pyotraumatic dermatitis or acute moist dermatitis) that responded readily to simple cleaning and corticosteroid administration (see Chap. 15; also see Fig. 15:9 F).

The second group also had superficial ulceration but, in addition, had deep suppurative and necrotizing folliculitis and occasional furunculosis (see Fig. 4:6 A). Clinically, this type of lesion is thickened, plaquelike, and surrounded by satellite papules and pustules. Lesions are especially common on the cheek and the neck. Numerous gram-positive cocci were present in the deep follicles, and it was common to observe panniculitis and hidradenitis with a neutrophilic infiltrate. The authors of this study speculated that the folliculitis was merely a complicating factor in some cases of pyotraumatic dermatitis. Alternatively, the infection could have been the primary event that induced the self-trauma. There was a strong tendency for young dogs to be affected; this pattern was observed in 70 per cent of the Golden retrievers and St. Bernards presumed to have pyotraumatic dermatitis but in only 20 per cent of all other breeds. Labrador retrievers and Newfoundlands are also commonly affected. These cases represent true local pyodermas.

Treatment of pyotraumatic folliculitis should include early administration of a systemic antibiotic effective against *S. intermedius*. It should be continued for 7 to 10 days beyond clinical cure. Local clipping, cleaning, and applying agents such as Burow's solution, chlorhexidine soaks, and calamine lotion daily are often helpful. Elizabethan collars may be indicated, but chemical sedation or analgesia is rarely necessary. Glucocorticoid administration is contraindicated.

Nasal Folliculitis and Furunculosis

Bacterial nasal folliculitis and furunculosis (nasal pyoderma) is an uncommon, painful, localized deep infection of the bridge of the nose and the area around the nostrils (see Fig. 4:6 B and C). It is most common in the German shepherd, bull terrier, collie, Pointer, and hunting-type (dolichocephalic) breeds. The cause is unknown, but the disorder may start from rooting or other local trauma. The onset is rapid, and with proper therapy, the course is short (14 to 21 days). Lesions start as papules and pustules, but deep folliculitis and furunculosis soon develop.

Figure 4:7. *A,* Furunculosis of the chin in a cat with feline acne. *B,* Muzzle furunculosis in a dog. *C,* Acral furunculosis in a dog. *D,* Severe pyogranulomatous furunculosis and fistulae on the hock of a dog. *E,* Draining abscess in the neck region of a dog (area has been clipped). *F,* Clostridial cellulitis and necrosis associated with mastitis. *G,* Bacterial pseudomycetoma (botryomycosis) on dog trunk. Area has been clipped to show nodules and draining tracts. *H,* Canine bacterial pseudomycetoma. Gram's stain of cutaneous discharge shows a tissue grain containing clumps of gram-positive cocci.

Self-trauma, which is common, worsens the lesions rapidly. The deep infection produces scarring, which can be aggravated by overly vigorous cleaning or topical therapy.

The differential diagnostic possibilities can be extensive, depending on the number and size of the lesions and the degree of self-trauma. With multiple, coalescent, crusted papular lesions, the primary differential diagnostic possibilities include pemphigus (foliaceus or erythematosus), lupus erythematosus, drug eruption, and dermatomyositis. When lesions are more discrete and papular to nodular, the primary differential diagnostic considerations include foreign body, other furuncular disorders (demodicosis; dermatophytosis, especially that due to *Trichophyton mentagrophytes* or *Microsporum gypseum*; and nasal eosinophilic folliculitis and furunculosis), sterile pyogranuloma syndrome, and early juvenile cellulitis.

Clinical management should include a careful consideration of underlying causes, especially if the examination of smears and cultures are negative for bacteria or fungi. The bacterial infections are usually secondary. Appropriate systemic antibiotics should be given in full dosage for 7 to 10 days beyond clinical cure. Gentle topical therapy with wet soaks using Burow's solution or chlorhexidine, three times daily for 10 minutes, is excellent. This must be applied gently to prevent further trauma to the tender, inflamed tissues. The use of Elizabethan collars and sedation are rarely needed to alleviate pain and prevent self-induced trauma during the first few days of treatment.

Muzzle Folliculitis and Furunculosis

This is a chronic inflammatory disorder of the chin and lips of young dogs (canine acne) characterized by a deep folliculitis and furunculosis (see Fig. 4:7 *B*). It is almost exclusively a disorder of short-coated breeds, such as boxers, Doberman pinschers, English bulldogs, Great Danes, Weimaraners, Mastiffs, Rottweilers, and German shorthaired pointers.

The cause of this syndrome is unknown, but it is clear that bacterial involvement is secondary. The initial lesions are hairless follicular papules of varying size, which histopathologically are characterized by marked follicular keratosis, plugging, dilatation, and perifolliculitis. Bacteria cannot be seen or isolated, and there is no response to systemic antibiotics. With time, the papules enlarge, ulcerate, and may discharge a seropurulent exudate. At this stage, a suppurative folliculitis or furunculosis is present and antibiotic treatment often improves but does not completely resolve the problem.

In previous editions of this text, it was suggested that the initial sterile follicular changes were triggered by the influence of androgens on acne-prone skin.[109] Although hormones may play some role in this problem, they cannot be solely responsible for it. If androgenic effects were paramount, all dogs, regardless of coat length, would be equally susceptible and male dogs should be overrepresented. No detailed studies on this condition have been published, but the authors have recognized it in neutered male and female animals and almost never see it in long-coated dogs.

The authors speculate that local trauma and possibly some undetermined genetic predisposition plays a central role in the development of the initial sterile lesions. Many short-coated dogs do not have muzzle folliculitis, even among the breeds predisposed to this disorder. Those who do may be more genetically susceptible to the disorder. During play, puppies frequently rub their muzzles and chins on hard, rough surfaces. Long hairs protect the underlying skin, but short hairs offer little protection and could break off below the skin's surface, inflaming the follicle and leaving the pilar canal open to bacterial invasion. Further trauma aggravates the condition and effectively seals off the pilar canal such that sterile or secondarily infected furunculosis occurs. After one infected furuncle develops, more can be expected.

Treatment depends on the severity and the chronicity of the problem. Early on, the lesions are few and are sterile. With modification of behaviors that traumatize the chin (e.g., chewing bones and chasing balls over carpeted surfaces) and frequent cleanings, the process can be arrested and the lesions heal slowly. Benzoyl peroxide products (shampoo or gel) are commonly used for cleaning because they also reduce the surface bacterial population and keep the hair follicle open. The chin is first treated on a daily basis and then as needed. These products should not be overused, as they can be irritating and increase the follicular inflammation. If the gel is used, the owner should be cautioned that the product can bleach carpets, furniture, and other fabrics. In cases that continue to worsen despite these measures, the administration of corticosteroids can be beneficial. If the lesions are not too deep, a potent cream or gel (e.g., betamethasone valerate) applied three or four times daily, rapidly decreases the follicular inflammation. For cases of deep lesions, the authors find that fluocinolone in dimethyl sulfoxide (Synotic) is beneficial. After the follicular inflammation is resolved, the use of the steroid should be gradually decreased and stopped.

Advanced cases are usually infected and necessitate a long (4- to 6-week) course of an appropriate antibiotic. Because deep infections heal with scarring, the chin is easy to traumatize, and endogenous foreign bodies (e.g., keratin and hair shafts) are typically found deep in these lesions, the antibiotic treatment does not resolve the entire condition. After the infection is resolved, the use of topical corticosteroids may be necessary to prevent the development of new lesions.

Pedal Folliculitis and Furunculosis

Pododermatitis (interdigital pyoderma) is an inflammatory, multifaceted disease complex that affects the feet of dogs.[98, 131, 148]

CAUSE AND PATHOGENESIS

The cause of this disease is often unknown, but in no cases are the resulting lesions cysts. The disease is complex and may be frustrating to diagnose and treat.[98] Local etiologic factors may be common and relatively easy to find and correct. These include foreign bodies (e.g., foxtails, awns, thorns, wood slivers, and seeds) and local trauma. When a single foot is affected, a foreign body, local injury, or neoplasia should be suspected, especially if there is only one interdigital fistula. The feet are subject to great variety and intensity of trauma, the front feet more so than the rear. Hunting or field dogs commonly have bruises from stones, stubble, and briars. Animals working in sticky substances may accumulate masses of sand, stone, tar, and hair that initiate injury. Contact with irritant chemicals, fertilizers, or weed killers may also cause trouble. Clipper burns from grooming procedures, irritation from housing on wire or rough stones, and inflammation from contact, inhalant, or food hypersensitivities have all initiated pododermatitis. Any of these factors may cause intense licking, which accentuates the irritation.

Fungal infections associated with pododermatitis include dermatophytosis, *Malassezia* dermatitis, candidiasis, mycetoma, sporotrichosis, blastomycosis, and cryptococcosis. These are reasonably rare but should be suspected in cases that are refractory to usual antibiotic therapy. Bacterial infections are always secondary and can include a wide variety of organisms. Bacterial hypersensitivity may be a complication (see Chap. 8).

Parasitic pododermatitis is particularly common, with demodicosis being its most troublesome cause. Every case of chronic interdigital pyoderma must be evaluated carefully for demodectic mites. Biopsy may be necessary to make the diagnosis of parasitic pododermatitis in chronically inflamed and fibrosed feet. It is often missed by other diagnostic techniques (e.g., skin scrapings). Other parasites involved may include *Pelodera strongyloides, Ancylostoma* spp., and *Uncinaria stenocephala*. Ticks and chiggers favor the interdigital webs and may initiate inflammation.

Psychogenic dermatitis may be manifested as excessive licking of the feet by high-strung, nervous individuals, especially Poodles, terriers, and German shepherds.

Sterile pyogranulomas may occur on the feet. The cause is unknown, but they are most common in smooth, short-coated breeds such as English bulldogs, dachshunds, Great Danes, and boxers (see Chap. 17). Osteomyelitis or local neoplasms more characteristically involve a single foot.

Cases of pododermatitis that involve several feet, are recurrent or refractory to treatments, and are nonpruritic may be caused by an inherited or acquired immunodeficiency. Pododermatitis may also be the only clinical sign of hypothyroidism or demodicosis with secondary suppression of cell-mediated immunity. One report suggested that the flat foot and the scoop-shaped web of breeds like the Pekingese and some terriers predispose the area to folliculitis and pedal dermatitis.[150]

Cases of pododermatitis with significant footpad involvement (hyperkeratosis and ulceration) may have an autoimmune basis (pemphigus, pemphigoid, or lupus erythematosus) or may be a manifestation of drug eruption, zinc-responsive dermatitis, necrolytic migratory erythema, or canine distemper.

In spite of all these possibilities, a substantial number of cases are idiopathic, recurrent bacterial infections. These can be exceedingly frustrating to manage.

CLINICAL FEATURES

Pododermatitis may affect dogs of any age, sex, or breed, but males of short-coated breeds, such as the English bulldog, Great Dane, Bassett hound, mastiff, bull terrier, boxer, dachshund, Dalmatian, German shorthaired pointer, and Weimaraner, are more commonly represented. Longer-coated breeds that are commonly affected include German shepherd, Labrador retriever, Golden retriever, Irish setter, and Pekingese. The front feet are more often affected, but one or all four feet may be involved.

Affected tissue may be red and edematous with nodules, ulcers, fistulae, hemorrhagic bullae, and a serosanguineous or seropurulent exudate (see Fig. 4:6 *D*). The feet may be grossly swollen (see Fig. 4:6 *E*). Pitting edema of the metacarpal and metatarsal areas can be marked. The skin may be alopecic and moist from constant licking, and varying degrees of pain, pruritus, and paronychia may be present. The pain may produce lameness. In some cases, the interdigital nodules are nontender and unresponsive to treatment and may be scars from previous lesions. Although the regional lymph nodes are enlarged, other systemic signs seldom occur.

DIAGNOSIS

A careful history and physical examination findings provide the diagnosis of pododermatitis. Because of the complex pathogenesis, all cases for which a cause is not quickly and easily discerned should undergo multiple skin scrapings, exudative cytologic study, fungal culture, bacterial culture and antibiotic sensitivity tests, and a representative skin biopsy. The direct smear may provide early clues of the cause by establishing the presence or the absence of neutrophils or phagocytosed bacteria and their staining property, or by showing large numbers of eosinophils, mycetoma or pseudomycetoma grains, yeast, or largely mononuclear cell exudate. Radiographs may also be needed to identify bony changes and opaque foreign bodies. In some instances, an evaluation of the immune status might be indicated and should include hemogram, serum immunoglobulin quantitation, and thyrotropin (thyroid-stimulating hormone) response, and low-dose dexamethasone suppression tests.

Histopathologic studies are essential to document foreign bodies (including free hair shafts or keratin in the tissue), bacteria, parasites, fungi, and neoplasia and to evaluate the cellular response. Special stains may be needed. In general, the histologic response is that of perifolliculitis, folliculitis, or furunculosis; with the last, a nodular to diffuse pyogranulomatous inflammation is common.

CLINICAL MANAGEMENT

Pododermatitis can be a frustrating problem, because it is often self-perpetuating. Lesions heal with scarring, which makes the foot more susceptible to future infections. Delays in treatment of the infection and its cause increase the scarring potential so the diagnostic and therapeutic effort should be maximal in these cases.

If the lesions are draining, foot soaks for 10 to 15 minutes twice daily are indicated until the drainage stops. Antibiotic treatment is prolonged, and 8- to 12-week courses are not unusual. Palpation is critical in monitoring these patients, as the surfaces of these lesions heal weeks before the deep lesions are resolved. Lesions that are tender on palpation are likely still infected. As long as dermal lesions are present and are becoming smaller, treatment should be continued.

Cases with advanced disease at the onset of treatment have varying degrees of scarring of the digital and interdigital skin and may have sterile dermal granulomas due to endogenous foreign bodies. Protection of the foot via restricting the animal's activity or having the animal wear boots can help prevent future infections. Focal areas of scarring or individual dermal granulomas may be amenable to surgical removal.

Some cases, especially those in which the infection includes secondary gram-negative organisms, are resistant to medical treatment alone. Surgical débridement of all the devitalized tissue may make medical treatment more effective. In severe cases, fusion podoplasty in which all disease is removed and the digits are joined together can be beneficial.[141]

German Shepherd Dog Folliculitis, Furunculosis, and Cellulitis

This is a idiopathic deep pyoderma of German shepherd dogs or German shepherd crosses.[79, 107, 123, 154] Affected dogs have deep skin infections, which resolve slowly and recur frequently. Often, there is no definable cause of the infection or, if one is defined (e.g., flea infestation),[79, 123] the severity of the infection is well out of proportion to the stimulus.

CAUSE AND PATHOGENESIS

This condition has been studied extensively in the Netherlands and, other than a familial predisposition (possibly autosomal recessive),[153] no cause of this susceptibility to deep infection could be found. Immunohyporeactivity of the nonspecific, phagocytic, and humoral immune systems could not be documented and bacterial hypersensitivity was not causal.[152] Flea bite hypersensitivity was seen in some dogs but would have to be considered an aggravating rather than causal factor. Another large study documented an underlying hypothyroidism in some dogs and most (12 of 17) had clinical or historical evidence of flea infestation or flea bite hypersensitivity.[79] In another two dogs, an underlying cell-mediated immunodeficiency was documented, but a similar investigation in another four dogs could not duplicate these results.[107] A study of 12 dogs showed that 10 dogs had an allergic dermatitis or hypothyroidism that triggered the infection.[123] Two dogs had no other skin disease but had a documented cell-mediated immunodeficiency.

These dogs probably have an inherited immunoincompetence that makes them susceptible to deep infection. Because these dogs do not experience infections of other organ systems and skin infection until middle age, they must have some degree of immunocompetence. With an insult to their skin (e.g., flea bite hypersensitivity) or immune system (e.g., hypothyroidism), they decompensate and develop a disproportionately severe pyoderma. Some dogs decompensate for no known reason, which suggests that the immunodeficiency can worsen with advancing age. Dogs in this latter group require lifelong treatment, whereas the other dogs may remain infection free if the triggering disease is resolved.

CLINICAL FEATURES

The disease almost exclusively affects middle-aged German shepherd dogs and is not sex specific or influenced by gonadal status. A familial history is occasionally given. In most dogs, the lesions are pruritic, and the pruritus usually stops after the infection is resolved. The distribution pattern is typical, with the rump, back, ventral abdomen, and thighs being affected in all cases. Because most affected dogs have fleas at examination and the initial distribution is typical of flea bite hypersensitivity, most of these dogs are presumed to have a flea allergy and are treated with corticosteroids. Some animals have more generalized lesions spreading to the chest and the neck. The front legs, the head, and the ears are usually much less involved.

Lesions are initially follicular in origin with clusters of papules, pustules, erosions, and crusts followed by ulcers, fistulae, furunculosis, alopecia, and hyperpigmentation (see Figs. 4:6 *F* and *G*). The lesions in haired skin are heavily crusted and the presence, depth, and severity of the infection in these areas cannot be appreciated until the crusts are removed. There may be a great deal of excoriation from the pruritus. Some animals have a secondary seborrhea, and cellulitis is evident in deeper infections. Peripheral lymphadenopathy is common. Animals with the disorder are usually in general good health, although there may be weight loss, poor appetite, and pyrexia. The lesions are usually painful, especially when the crusts are removed.

The course of the disease is long and stormy, with frequent stages of partial healing and exacerbation. This is usually produced by improper selection or inadequate dosage of antibiotics and inadequate duration of treatment, the concurrent use of corticosteroids, or failure to resolve predisposing factors.

DIAGNOSIS

The physical examination, coupled with exudative cytologic study, confirms the diagnosis of deep pyoderma but does not document this syndrome. The diagnosis of this syndrome is made by the exclusion of other causes of deep pyoderma (e.g., demodicosis and allergy), by the disproportionate severity of the infection if the dog has not received corticosteroids, or by repeated relapses.

All routine diagnostic tests are indicated in these dogs, as is an evaluation for thyroid disorders. If the lesions are pruritic and the pruritus does not stop with elimination of the infection, an evaluation for allergy should be performed. When all of these are determined to be noncontributory, an immunocompetency evaluation should be considered.

Skin biopsies are useful to determine underlying causes and to document the severity of the tissue damage. In one series of cases, histopathologic examination of skin biopsy tissues revealed folliculitis, furunculosis, and cellulitis as the most common findings.[79] Perifollicular pyogranulomatous inflammation was often seen, which supports the follicular origin of the disease. Only a few biopsy specimens showed the large number of eosinophils expected in furunculosis. Another report described the histopathologic findings in 23 cases in the Netherlands, which had hyperkeratosis, acanthosis, and a poorly demarcated, predominantly proliferative dermatitis.[154] Dermal edema was observed, with an exudate composed predominantly of neutrophils and mononuclear cells. In only four cases was the subcutis involved.

CLINICAL MANAGEMENT

Because many cases have an intercurrent allergic disorder or hypothyroidism, every effort should be made to identify and resolve this triggering event. If the predisposing disease is ignored, the animal's response to treatment will be poor or the infection will recur shortly after the antibiotics are withdrawn.

Clipping and topical therapy are essential in this disease. Twice-daily soaks or the use of whirlpool baths helps to remove any crusts, improves drainage, and makes the patient more comfortable. Long-term antibiotic administration is necessary, with 6- to 10-week courses not uncommon. It is imperative that the drug be given at the correct dosage and frequency after clinical cure has occurred. Because these dogs are prone to experience disproportionately severe infection, premature termination of therapy guarantees a severe relapse.

With resolution of the infection and the triggering event, many of these dogs stay infection free for long periods. The owners must be made aware that their dog is susceptible to skin infections. Any irregularities in the dog's management or grooming should be corrected, and the owners should be instructed to seek prompt attention whenever any skin lesions occur.

Some dogs experience relapse each time that antibiotics are withdrawn. These dogs probably have a cell-mediated immunodeficiency[107, 123] and may respond to immunomodulation. Most require lifelong antibiotic therapy.

Acral Lick Furunculosis

Acral lick dermatitis (see Chap. 14) is well recognized in dogs and has a variety of causes. Cytologic or histologic evidence of infection is found in many cases, especially those with an ulcerated surface. What is unclear is whether the infection preceded the dog's licking of the area or was superimposed on some underlying condition.

CLINICAL FEATURES

Acral lick lesions are typically found on the distal portion of a front limb but can be seen on a hind leg or on multiple limbs. The clinical appearance varies with the chronicity of the lesion and the amount of trauma to the area. Typically, the lesion is firm, raised, hairless, hyperpigmented at the periphery, and eroded or ulcerated centrally (see Fig. 4:7 C). In some cases, there is significant tissue destruction with exposure of underlying tendons or bone.

DIAGNOSIS

Infection should be suspected in all acral lick lesions, especially if the surface is ulcerated. This suspicion can be confirmed by biopsy or, in many cases, by exudative cytologic examination. For correct cytologic evaluation, the surface of the lesion should be scrubbed to remove all debris and surface bacteria. After the surface has dried, the lesion is squeezed firmly between the thumb and the forefinger until drops of seropurulent or serohemorrhagic exudate appear on the surface. This material is examined cytologically. This is painful, so the dog should be muzzled or tranquilized.

In many cases, evidence of infection (e.g., intracellular bacteria within phagocytic cells) is found, and staphylococci are the primary organisms seen. In some cases, gram-negative organisms are co-infectors. If gram-negative organisms are seen, a culture should be performed, preferably from tissue taken via sterile biopsy technique. Culture of the discharge expressed by manual pressure can be misleading because it may contain contaminating but not infecting organisms.

In some cases, no bacteria are seen cytologically or no exudate can be expressed. In these cases, infection can be proved or disproved by biopsy or by a therapeutic trial with antibiotics. If the latter course is chosen, a broad-spectrum drug should be used for a minimum of 21 days before response is estimated.

CLINICAL MANAGEMENT

In acral lick furunculosis, the clinician is faced with the problem of determining the cause of the infection and the treatment of a deep, fibrosing infection. With solitary lesions, the cause of the infection is often a transient insult to the skin, which is not evident when the animal is presented for treatment. Unless the history, physical examination findings, and exudative cytologic study suggest some underlying problem, it may be best to resolve the infection first and then to determine whether the diagnostic effort should go forward. With lesions on multiple limbs, transient trauma can be discounted, and a complete diagnostic evaluation should be performed, especially for allergy or hypothyroidism.

Soaks, especially with magnesium sulfate, and prolonged courses of antibiotics are necessary in acral lick furunculosis. The minimal course of treatment is 8 weeks, and some cases necessitate many months of treatment. Because of the need for long-term treatment, potentiated sulfa drugs should not be used. Most clients notice remarkable improvement within the first 3 weeks and then comment either that the lesion is getting no better or that the rate of improvement is much slower. Because these lesions are fibrotic at the onset of treatment, antibiotic administration should not be expected to resolve the lesion completely. Treatment is continued until no further improvement is detected by the clinician, not the client, and then for an additional 2 weeks. If, at the end of the treatment, the area is more fibrotic and hairless or if the animal continues to traumatize the area, the diagnostic effort must go forward.

The key to successful management of acral lick furunculosis is early and vigorous intervention. The more chronic the infection is, the poorer is the prognosis for a complete resolution. Large lesions heal incompletely and are covered by a thin, hairless, fragile epithelial layer. Because these lesions are often found over joints or in areas that are traumatized during normal activities, the area probably will be damaged in the future, which could trigger another infection. If there is significant tissue destruction at first presentation, or after the infection is resolved, amputation of the limb may be indicated.

Anaerobic Cellulitis

Cellulitis is a severe, deep, suppurative infection in which the area of infection is poorly defined and tends to dissect through tissue planes.[1] There may be extensive edema, and the skin is often friable, darkly discolored, and devitalized.[58] The weakened tissues may be sloughed or removed easily in the process of treatment so that the affected areas may appear to be more extensive during treatment then before it is initiated.

In small animals, anaerobic cellulitis typically follows bite wounds, traumatic puncture wounds, or foreign body introduction but can be a sequela to surgery, trauma, burns, or malignancy.[39, 118] Poor management of indwelling catheters can predispose to *Serratia* infection.[8] In humans, diabetes mellitus, corticosteroid administration, or immunodeficiency predisposes to anaerobic infection, and these factors are probably important in animals.

Anaerobic infections are characterized by rapid progression, poor demarcation, massive tissue edema and swelling, and necrosis (see Fig. 4:7 *F*). The wounds often, but not uniformly, have a putrid smell and are crepitant if the organism is a gas producer (*Clostridium* spp. and *Bacteroides* spp.).[51, 52, 58] Depending on the organism, toxins may be produced and cause profound systemic signs.

The presumptive diagnosis of anaerobic cellulitis can be made by the presence of the clinical signs described above. Exudative cytologic examination that yields neutrophilic and polybacterial findings is supportive. Cultures can be performed to isolate the anaerobe but are probably not necessary because the organisms have a fairly predictable sensitivity. Facultative anaerobes are of more concern because the sensitivity of these organisms can be limited and unpredictable.

Surgery is indicated to drain the exudate, remove necrotic tissue, and remedy tissue hypoxia. Hyperbaric oxygen treatment can be beneficial but is usually not available.[116] Systemic antibiotics should be administered until the infection is resolved and then for an additional 7 to 14 days. Penicillins (penicillin G, amoxicillin, and clavulanated amoxicillin) are the drugs of choice. Other useful antibiotics include clindamycin, chloramphenicol, cephalosporins, and metronidazole.[1, 51]

Subcutaneous Abscesses

Subcutaneous abscesses are uncommon in the dog but occur frequently in cats. In dogs, abscesses can be due to bite wounds, abscessed teeth, or foreign bodies (see Fig. 4:7 *E*), whereas bite wounds are most common in cats. Bacteria from claw or fang are injected under the skin when it is punctured during a cat fight. The wound is small and seals rapidly; a local infection develops in 2 to 4 days. Some bite wounds are handled well by the cat's normal defense mechanisms. Those that abscess are most commonly found around the tail base and the neck and shoulders. Abscess from bite wounds is one of the most common cat diseases handled in a small animal practice. Untreated, the abscess may rupture, drain, and heal during 2 to 3 weeks. However, the treatment of choice is liberal surgical drainage and thorough flushing of the area with saline, hydrogen peroxide, or chlorhexidine solution, together with high doses of penicillin or amoxicillin systemically for 5 to 7 days. These antibiotics effectively cover the organisms normally found in the cat's mouth and in abscesses (*P. multocida*, fusiform bacilli, β-hemolytic streptococci, and *Bacteroides* spp.). In dogs, the same treatment procedure is used, but antibiotic selection must be based on the cytologic or cultural identity of the organism.

Castration of intact male cats has been a helpful preventive measure, resulting in either rapid or gradual decline in fighting and roaming behavior to 80 to 90 per cent of the cats so treated.[66]

Recurrent or nonhealing feline abscesses should prompt a consideration of immunosuppression (feline leukemia virus infection or feline immunodeficiency virus infection), and other infectious agents (*Actinomyces* spp., *Nocardia* spp., *Yersinia pestis*, and mycobacteria), mycoses, or sterile panniculitis. *Rhodococcus (Corynebacterium) equi*, which is resistant to penicillin and tetracycline, was isolated from a feline abscess.[68] Many anaerobic organisms can be found in feline abscesses.[132–135] *Mycoplasma*-like organisms (see L-Form Infections, this chapter) have been isolated from cats with chronic subcutaneous abscesses.[26, 74]

Bacterial Pseudomycetoma

Bacterial pseudomycetoma (cutaneous bacterial granuloma or botryomycosis) is a chronic, suppurative, granulomatous disease caused by nonbranching bacteria. They form grains of compact colonies in tissues that are surrounded by pyogranulomatous inflammation.[2, 144] Bacterial pseudomycetoma is common in many species but is rarely reported, probably because it is misdiagnosed or overlooked. The causative bacteria are usually coagulase-positive staphylococci, but in some cases other bacteria, alone or associated with staphylococci, may be responsible. There may be *Pseudomonas* sp., *Proteus* sp., *Streptococcus* sp., and *Actinobacillus* sp. In cases involving dogs and cats, multiple organisms can be found.[144]

Most cases are initiated by local trauma from bites or other wounds, and some are associated with a foreign body. There may also be muscle or bone involvement. The granuloma develops because a delicate balance exists between the virulence of the organisms and the response of the host. The host is able to isolate and contain the infection but is unable to eradicate it. This may also be a type of bacterial hypersensitivity, or the grain formation may be associated with the formation of a polysaccharide slime coating[75] produced by the bacteria or with a glycoprotein covering resulting from a localized antigen-antibody reaction on the surface of the microorganisms.

Clinically, the lesions appear as firm, solitary or multiple nodules with draining fistulae (see Fig. 4:7 *G*). The purulent exudate may have small white granules similar to grains of sand (Fig. 4:8; also see Fig. 4:7 *H*). Special bacterial and fungal stains are necessary to differentiate the granules from those found in actinomycosis, nocardiosis, or mycetomas.

Histopathologically, there is a nodular to diffuse dermatitis or nodular to diffuse panniculitis, with tissue granules surrounded by a granulomatous to pyogranulomatous infiltrate of histiocytes, plasma cells, lymphocytes, neutrophils, and multinucleate histiocytic giant cells (see Fig.

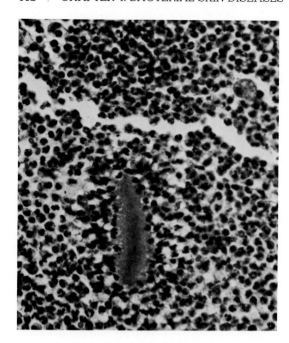

Figure 4:8. Bacterial pseudomycetoma. Pyogranulomatous dermatitis with central tissue grain.

4:8 *B*). The edges of the bacteria masses (granules) may show clubbing and may stain brightly eosinophilic with H & E (Hoeppli-Splendore material). The bacteria are best demonstrated with Gram's tissue stain or Brown-Brenn stain.

Differential diagnosis must include actinomycosis, nocardiosis, eumycotic mycetoma, systemic mycoses, dermatophytic pseudomycetoma, foreign body reactions, and chronic bacterial abscesses. Because of the variable prognoses and therapeutic formats, it is imperative that a specific diagnosis be made.

Simple systemic antibiotic therapy is usually not adequate. Frequent relapses are the rule. Therapy is essentially limited to complete surgical excision, because the granulomatous mass is relatively impermeable to antibiotics.[2, 144] Appropriate postsurgical antibiotic therapy is essential.

Mycobacterial Granulomas

Mycobacteria can be divided into three groups: obligate pathogens such as *Mycobacterium tuberculosis* and *M. lepraemurium*, which do not multiply outside vertebrate hosts; facultative pathogens, which normally exist as saprophytes in the environment but sporadically cause disease; and environmental saprophytes, which almost never cause disease.[1, 93] Mycobacteria and the disease syndromes they cause can be further classified as follows:

1. True tuberculosis mycobacteria. *M. tuberculosis*, both bovine and human types, cause small animal tuberculosis in endemic areas. They are photochromogenic and slow growers, and if injected into guinea pigs, cause death in 6 to 8 weeks; opportunistic mycobacteria do not (see discussion that follows).
2. Leprosy mycobacteria. *M. lepraemurium* causes rat leprosy, which is possibly transmitted to small animals. It is scotochromogenic and grows with great difficulty in the laboratory. Many acid-fast organisms are usually found in histologic sections (see Feline Leprosy in this chapter).
3. Opportunistic mycobacteria. These can be divided into groups according to their rate of growth and pigment production. One group of slow-growing organisms (longer than 7 days) is nonchromogenic and pathogenic only to cold-blooded animals. Another group

of slow-growing mycobacteria of this group include *M. kansasii, M. marinum, M. ulcerans,* and *M. avium* and are facultative pathogens. The fast-growing (2 to 3 days, or less than 7 days) mycobacteria in the atypical, or opportunistic, group include *M. fortuitum, M. chelonei, M. thermoresistible, M. xenopi, M. phlei,* and *M. smegmatis.* Organisms may be scattered through tissues so that a careful search must be made for them. They are often found in small vacuoles in the granulomatous tissue (see Opportunistic Mycobacterial Granulomas in this chapter).

Natural water may be teaming with saprophytic mycobacteria, including some that are facultative or opportunistic pathogens. These can produce infection after contamination when predisposing factors are present. In attempts to isolate and to identify individual species, decontamination of saprophytes from cultures, differentiation by biochemical tests, and immunodiffusion analysis are difficult.[1]

CUTANEOUS TUBERCULOSIS

The incidence of cutaneous tuberculosis of dogs and cats decreased with the decrease of the disease in humans and cattle, but may be becoming more prevalent owing to an increasing frequency in humans.[139] It is a rare disease in most parts of the world unless pets experience a high degree of exposure.[1, 25, 31, 46, 87] Animals that live where there are large numbers of people (restaurants or public places), have close contact with an infected owner (e.g., sleeping in the sick person's room), or are fed a variety of unprocessed meat or milk from areas of endemic disease, have an increased chance of infection. Although both dogs and cats are susceptible to both *M. tuberculosis* and *M. bovis,* there appears to be a higher incidence of *M. bovis* infection in cats.[46] Dogs and cats are relatively resistant to *M. avium* (a slow-growing environmental saprophyte), but cases have been reported.[25, 73a, 139a] Siamese cats may be predisposed.[73a] The predominant lesions in small animals are respiratory and digestive, but there can be some skin lesions. In cats, clinical signs may be insidious, and because diagnostic tests are unreliable, epidemiologic data are of questionable validity.[132, 139]

Clinical Features

Cutaneous lesions are single or multiple ulcers, abscesses, plaques, and nodules. Nodules may be in the skin or adherent to subcutaneous tissues. They fail to come to a head and may discharge a thick, yellow to green pus with an unpleasant odor. The lesions are most common on the head, the neck, and the limbs. Patients usually appear sick; they have anorexia, weight loss, fever, and lymphadenopathy.[1, 25, 31, 46]

Diagnosis

Diagnosis is by history, physical examination, radiography, biopsy, culture, bacille Calmette-Guérin or purified protein derivative test (in dogs),[1] serologic testing, or lymphocyte blastogenesis test (in cats).[78] Biopsy specimens may show a nodular to diffuse dermatitis due to pyogranulomatous inflammation (with necrosis and caseation), rare multinucleate histiocytic giant cells and mineralization, and few to many acid-fast organisms. Smears or biopsy do not differentiate between true tuberculosis and opportunistic mycobacterial granulomas. Injection of cultures into guinea pigs causes death in 6 to 8 weeks, but not if the organism is nontuberculous.

Bacille Calmette-Guérin or purified protein derivative (250 tuberculin units/0.1 ml) prepared for humans can be used to test dogs for tuberculosis. Intradermal injection (0.1 ml of purified protein derivative or 0.1 to 0.2 ml of bacille Calmette-Guérin) is best performed on the inner surface of the pinna and is read at 48 to 72 hours (no sooner). Erythema that resorbs by that time is a negative test result. Severe erythema with central necrosis progressing to ulceration at 10 to 14 days is significant. Ulceration after 18 to 21 days may occur in normal dogs. This testing is unreliable in the cat.

Clinical Management

Although combination chemotherapy has been shown to be effective in treating canine tuberculosis, most dogs are euthanized because of the seriousness of their disease or because of public health concerns. Dogs and cats with *M. tuberculosis* or *M. bovis* can be transient point sources of infection for humans or other animals. Because *M. avium* is an abundant environmental saprophyte, public health concerns are of less significance.

FELINE LEPROSY

Feline leprosy is a granulomatous, nodular, cutaneous infection associated with an acid-fast organism that is difficult to culture.

Cause and Pathogenesis

Feline leprosy is caused by a mycobacterium, which has not been completely characterized owing to difficulties in culture techniques. *M. lepraemurium* may or may not be the etiologic agent.[1, 97, 110, 128] Guinea pigs injected with homogenized fresh tissue from spontaneous feline cases are resistant, but rats and mice develop typical local cutaneous and lymph node lesions with demonstrable mycobacteria. In addition, many of the experimental rats develop a generalized granulomatous mycobacterial disease.[128] *M. lepraemurium* injections cause no lesions in cats but produce characteristic lesions of murine leprosy in rats. Local lesions appear in cats 2 to 5 months after experimental injections of tissue from naturally occurring lesions. The long incubation time is consistent with the higher incidence of diagnosis (50 per cent of the cases) in western Canada during the winter months after exposure in the summer. Live *M. leprae* (leprosy bacillus of humans) has been found in mosquitoes, fleas, and ticks, so it may also be possible for feline leprosy to be transmitted by these vectors. However, the natural mode of infection is unknown. The disease has been reported in New Zealand, Australia, Great Britain, France, the Netherlands, the United States, and Canada.

Human leprosy is closely associated with immunodeficiency, but the immunologic status of cats with feline leprosy is largely unknown. One experimental cat, which was affected naturally several years previously, failed to have lesions when inoculated with a homogenate of infectious tissue.[128] McIntosh inoculated five affected cats intradermally with lepromin.[97] Those with tuberculoid leprosy reacted positively, whereas those with lepromatous leprosy had reactions that were negative. Lymphocyte stimulation assays were normal in all cats.

In human leprosy, the type of tissue reaction is thought to be a reflection of the immune status of the host. Similar types of reactions are seen in feline leprosy. In refractory individuals that can mount a cell-mediated response, a tuberculoid granulomatous reaction results, with few (if any) bacilli present. Susceptible individuals, on the other hand, respond with a lepromatous granuloma and a huge number of bacteria are present.

Clinical Features

Lesions are single or multiple cutaneous nodules, which may or may not be ulcerated. Lesions are most common on the head or extremities. There may be abscesses or fistulae that show no signs of healing (Fig. 4:9 *A*) but do not spread. Lesions also have been found on the nasal, buccal, and lingual mucosae. Regional lymphadenopathy is often seen, but without local pain or systemic illness. There is no sex prevalence, but two thirds of cases occur in cats 1 to 3 years of age.

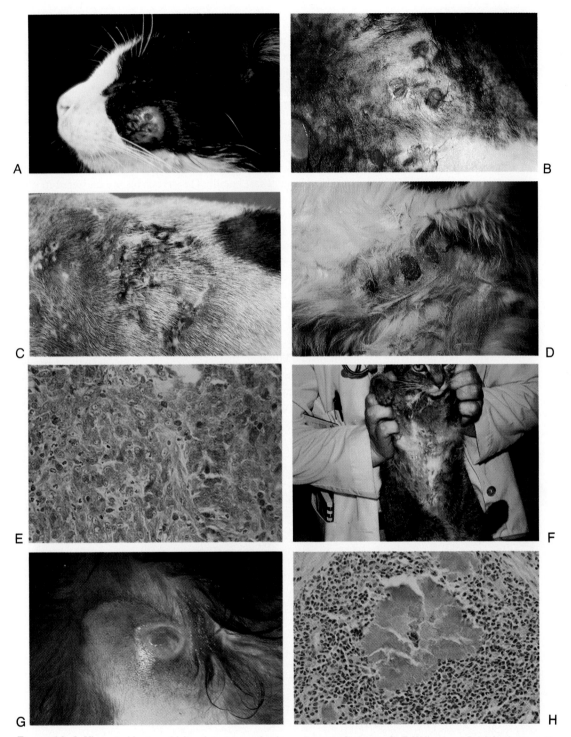

Figure 4:9. *A*, Ulcerated lesion of feline leprosy on the face of a cat. (Courtesy G. T. Wilkinson.) *B*, Multiple necrotic granulomatous lesions on the body of a cat associated with *M. fortuitum* infection. *C*, Soft tissue infection with draining fistulae on the thorax of a dog with atypical mycobacterial granulomas due to *M. chelonei*. (Courtesy G. A. Kunkle.) *D*, Atypical mycobacteriosis (with panniculitis) on the abdomen of a cat. *E*, Feline atypical mycobacteriosis. Note numerous acid-fast organisms within dermal macrophages (Fite-Faraco stain). *F*, Cutaneous nocardiosis (with panniculitis) in a cat. *G*, Nonhealing ulcer with suppurative discharge over the shoulder of a dog with actinomycosis. *H*, Actinomycosis. Eosinophilic (Hoeppli-Splendore phenomenon) tissue grain (sulfur granule) in pyogranulomatous dermatitis.

Diagnosis

Diagnosis is made on the basis of history, physical examination results, and the finding of acid-fast bacilli in direct smears and biopsy specimens (Ziehl-Neelsen stain or Fite-Faraco modification). Tissue homogenates should be cultured on the surface of 1 per cent Ogawa egg yolk medium[1] and also inoculated into guinea pigs to eliminate the diagnosis of tuberculosis.

Histopathologic examination may reveal two types of reactions. One is the tuberculoid response with caseous necrosis and relatively few organisms, and the organisms are often only in the areas of necrosis. These epithelioid granulomas are usually surrounded by zones of lymphocytes, which are also commonly aggregated around vessels (Fig. 4:10). The second type reaction (lepromatous leprosy) is a granuloma composed of solid sheets of large foamy macrophages containing significant numbers of acid-fast bacilli. The organisms are clustered in globi in a parallel stacking arrangement. Multinucleate histiocytic giant cells often contain bacilli, and lymphocytes and plasma cells may surround vessels (Fig. 4:11). Many polymorphonuclear leukocytes may be present and may cause the lesion to resemble a pyogranuloma.

Differential diagnostic considerations include tuberculosis; granulomas due to opportunistic mycobacteria or foreign bodies; mycotic infections such as kerion, mycetoma, and phaeohyphomycosis; chronic bacterial infection; and neoplasms such as mast cell tumors, carcinomas, and lymphoreticular tumors.

Clinical Management

Surgical excision is the treatment of choice when there are solitary or circumscribed lesions. When surgery fails or is impractical, chemotherapy with dapsone, rifampin, or clofazimine may or may not be successful.[99] Clofazimine appears to be most promising and is associated with the fewest side effects.[110] Currently, the drug is administered orally at a dosage of 2 to 3 mg/kg

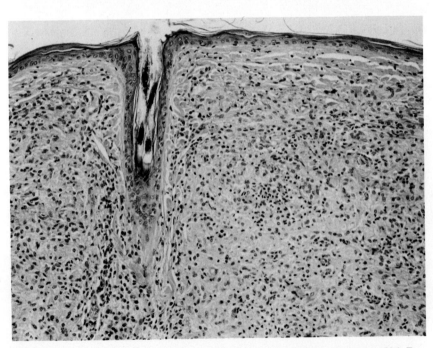

Figure 4:10. Granulomatous inflammation of dermis in a cat. Epidermis intact (H & E stain). (From Schiefer, B., et al.: A disease resembling feline leprosy in western Canada. J.A.V.M.A. 165:1085, 1974.)

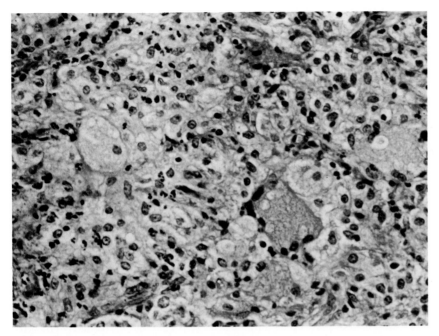

Figure 4:11. Histiocytes with foamy cytoplasm and giant cells (H & E stain). (From Schiefer, B., et al.: A disease resembling feline leprosy in western Canada. J.A.V.M.A. 165:1085, 1974.)

daily until all signs of disease are gone and then for an additional 6 to 12 weeks. Side effects appear to be few (elevated serum alanine aminotransferase activity) and dose related.

The public health significance of feline leprosy has not been determined.

OPPORTUNISTIC MYCOBACTERIAL GRANULOMAS

Opportunistic mycobacterial granulomas (atypical mycobacterial granulomas) in dogs and cats can be caused by several atypical mycobacteria that are facultative pathogens. The disease is characterized by chronicity, resistance to antibiotics and antituberculous drugs, and possible spontaneous resolution.

Cause and Pathogenesis

Organisms reported to cause cutaneous granulomas in dogs and cats include *Mycobacterium fortuitum, M. chelonei, M. phlei, M. xenopi, M. thermoresistible,* and *M. smegmatis.** Because *M. fortuitum* and *M. chelonei* share several metabolic characteristics and are facultative pathogens that produce similar clinical signs, they may be referred to as the *M. fortuitum-chelonei* complex. The disease has been reported most commonly in cats (perhaps because infection may be introduced through cat bite wounds), but cases in dogs have been recorded.[1, 64, 82]

These mycobacteria are ubiquitous, free-living organisms that are usually harmless and are commonly found in nature. They are found in the soil, but they especially favor water tanks, swimming pools, and sources of natural water.[93] After injury or injection, animals can have chronic subcutaneous abscesses and fistulae due to these organisms. The history of cases of these granulomas in humans commonly cites instances of the disease following a contaminated injection or an infected wound.

*See references 1, 50, 64, 82, 99, 108, 140, 142, 146, and 151.

Clinical Features

After contaminated injection, infection of a wound, or other trauma, the lesion develops slowly during a period of weeks. The course is prolonged, and lesions often have been present as nonhealing wounds for several months. Chronic soft tissue abscessation occurs, with ulcers and draining fistulae (see Fig. 4:9 *B* and *C*).

Lesions can occur anywhere but are most common in the cat in the caudal abdominal or inguinal region (see Fig. 4:9 *D*) or in the lumbar region. The lesions may or may not be painful, and regional lymph nodes are not always enlarged. Systemic illness, such as fever and anorexia, is rarely observed, and the animal feels well.

Diagnosis

Diagnosis is made by finding acid-fast organisms in smears, cultures, or biopsy specimens (see Fig. 4:9 *E*). The organism is often difficult to demonstrate. Smears made from fine needle aspirates of closed lesions are more likely to contain detectable organisms than are those made from exudates or tissue samples.[140] Cultures usually grow rapidly and should be made on blood agar, Löwenstein-Jensen medium, or Stonebrink's medium at 37°C (98.6°F).[1] Because cultures and biochemical tests for positive identification may be complex, the laboratory handling the cultures should be informed that a mycobacterial infection is suspected.

Histopathologic examination may be helpful. There is a nodular to diffuse dermatitis, panniculitis, or both due to pyogranulomatous inflammation. Stains such as Ziehl-Neelsen or Fite-Faraco modification should be used, and a careful search may be needed to find organisms. They are often clumped in the center of a clear vacuole and surrounded by clusters of neutrophils within the mature granuloma (Fig. 4:12). Alcohol processing in paraffin embedding may cause the acid-fast organism to stain poorly.[146] Using rapid Ziehl-Neelsen stain or snap-freezing the formalin-fixed tissues with subsequent acid-fast stain enables the bacilli to be seen.

Clinical Management

The prognosis in opportunistic mycobacterial infection is always guarded, especially in cats. Although spontaneous resolution of the lesions can occur after months to years of disease, most cases need treatment. There are reports of noncutaneous infections by opportunistic mycobacteria[142]; however, most infections remain a strictly cutaneous problem at the site of inoculation.

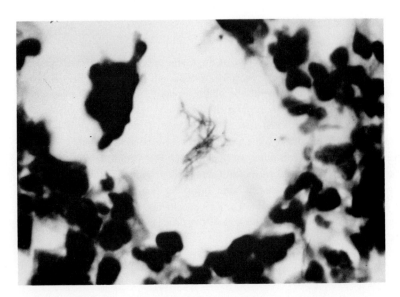

Figure 4:12. Atypical mycobacteriosis. Acid-fast organisms in the center of a clear vacuole in pyogranulomatous panniculitis. (Courtesy T. L. Gross.)

Accordingly, wide surgical excision of the diseased tissue should be considered and may be curative. When surgery is impractical or there is a postsurgical relapse, chemotherapy should be considered.

Opportunistic mycobacteria do not respond to antitubercular drugs, and sensitivity to conventional antibiotics varies among and within the various species of organisms.[1] For maximal efficacy, sensitivity data should be requested during culturing and drug selection should be based on those data. When sensitivity data are not available, response may be seen to kanamycin, gentamicin, amikacin, chloramphenicol, tetracyclines, potentiated sulfa drugs, and enrofloxacin.[1, 99, 140] The most successful drugs in cats appear to be doxycycline (5 mg/kg q12h)[1] and enrofloxacin (5 mg/kg q24h).[140] The drug should be administered until all clinical signs of disease are gone and then for an additional 4 to 6 weeks.

Actinomycosis

Actinomycosis is a rare pyogranulomatous or suppurative disease of many species caused by *Actinomyces* organisms. *A. odontolyticus, A. viscosus, A. meyeri,* and *A. hordeovulneris* have been suggested as being causative.[1, 18] They are gram-positive, non–acid-fast, catalase-positive, filamentous anaerobic rods that are opportunistic, commensal inhabitants of the oral cavity and the bowel.[1, 19, 76, 132] Infection occurs from trauma and contamination of penetrating wounds, especially those involving foreign bodies such as awns and quills.[65] Hunting or field dogs in southern climates are most commonly affected. It takes from months to 2 years for signs to develop after the injury; however, organisms can be found in the exudate within 2 weeks. The typical clinical lesion is a subcutaneous swelling or abscess of the head or neck, thoracic, paralumbar, or abdominal region (see Fig. 4:9 *G*). The lesion is usually tender and may or may not have draining tracts. Paralumbar lesions are usually a direct extension from retroperitoneal involvement. Other forms include osteomyelitis and empyema. Draining tracts (mycetoma-like) may discharge a thick, yellowish gray or thin, hemorrhagic, foul-smelling exudate that may or may not contain yellow sulfur granules.

Diagnosis is by anaerobic culture, direct smears of fine needle aspirates, and biopsy using special stains (Gram's, Brown-Brenn, or Gomori's methenamine silver). No method is completely reliable and cytologic study appears to be most effective.[76] Histopathologic examination reveals a nodular to diffuse dermatitis, panniculitis, or both due to suppurative or pyogranulomatous inflammation (Fig. 4:13). Tissue grains (sulfur granules) are present in approximately 50 per cent of cases. The granules are basophilic and often have a clubbed, eosinophilic periphery (Hoeppli-Splendore material) (see Fig. 4:9 *H*). The gram-positive, non–acid-fast, filamentous, occasionally beaded organisms are found within the granules, but they are not easily seen in ordinary H & E preparations. Actinomycosis must be differentiated from nocardiosis, a disease that it closely resembles.

The most successful treatment involves surgical excision or debulkment with a long course of antibiotics. High-dose penicillin is the optimum empirical treatment of choice.[1] Other drugs that may or may not be effective include ampicillin, cephalosporins, chloramphenicol, and tetracycline.[145] The treatment must continue for at least 1 month after complete remission and usually lasts 3 to 4 months. Prognosis is guarded with relapses reported to vary from 15 to 42 per cent.[76]

Actinobacillosis

Actinobacillosis is a rare disease of several animal species caused by *Actinobacillus lignieresii.*[1] It resembles actinomycosis in many of its cutaneous manifestations, but the causative organism is a gram-negative, aerobic coccobacillus that does not survive for a long time outside the host animal. It is a commensal organism found in the mouth of many animals, and clinical lesions often follow bite wounds or injuries around the face and mouth. Infection develops during weeks to months, and its course is long.

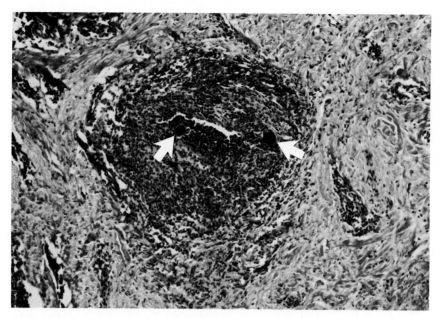

Figure 4:13. Actinomycosis in a dog. Note focal pyogranuloma with two tissue grains (arrows).

Clinical features include single or multiple thick-walled abscesses of the head, the neck, the mouth, and the limbs.[24] They discharge a thick, white to green, odorless pus with soft yellow granules. Diagnosis is made on the basis of aerobic cultures of pus, direct smears, or biopsy of affected tissues.

Histopathologic examination reveals a nodular to diffuse dermatitis, panniculitis, or both due to suppurative or pyogranulomatous inflammation. Tissue grains (sulfur granules) are usually present. The grains are basophilic and usually surrounded by eosinophilic Hoeppli-Splendore material. Special stains (Gram's or Brown-Brenn) are required to demonstrate the gram-negative organisms.

Clinical management includes surgical extirpation or drainage and curettage. Sodium iodide (20 mg/kg or 0.2 ml/kg of 20 per cent solution, orally q12h) and high doses of streptomycin or sulfonamides have been suggested for therapy. The organism is also usually sensitive to tetracycline and chloramphenicol. The course is long, and the prognosis is guarded.[24]

Nocardiosis

Nocardiosis is a rare disease characterized by pyogranulomatous and suppurative infection of the skin, the lungs or by widespread dissemination, caused by *Nocardia* spp.[1, 55, 76] The organisms involved, including *N. asteroides, N. brasiliensis*, and *N. caviae*, are common soil saprophytes that produce infection by wound contamination, inhalation, and ingestion, particularly in immunocompromised animals. Nocardia are gram-positive, partially acid-fast, branching filamentous aerobes. Except for *N. brasiliensis*, they have worldwide geographic distribution.

Clinical features are indistinguishable from those seen in actinomycosis and include cellulitis, ulcerated nodules, and abscesses that often develop draining sinuses (see Fig. 4:9 *F*). Lesions typically occur in areas of wounding, especially on the limbs and feet, and are often accompanied by lymphadenopathy. Cats often have lesions on the ventral abdomen that resemble panniculitis or opportunistic mycobacterial infection. Pyothorax may be present along with other systemic signs, such as weakness, anorexia, fever, depression, and dyspnea, and neurologic signs may be present.[1, 40, 76]

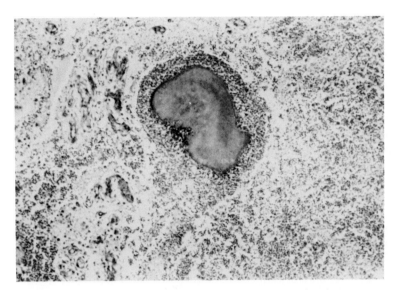

Figure 4:14. Nocardiosis. Tissue grain in pyogranulomatous dermatitis.

Diagnosis is by direct smear of fine needle aspirates, aerobic culture, and biopsy. Histopathologic study reveals nodular to diffuse dermatitis, panniculitis, or both, with or without tissue grains (Fig. 4:14). Special stains (Gram's and Brown-Brenn) are needed to demonstrate organisms. *Nocardia* spp. can be distinguished from *Actinomyces* spp. because they are partially acid fast (with modified Fite-Faraco stain) and usually branch at right angles. When branched and beaded, the organisms are similar in appearance to Chinese characters. Clinical management includes surgical drainage of infected tissues, but antibacterial therapy is mandatory. Nocardial organisms show varying sensitivity to antibiotics and the correlation between in vivo and in vitro results is variable.[1, 76] If at all possible, sensitivity data should be developed for each case. If the organism cannot be isolated, drugs that can be effective empirically include potentiated sulfa drugs, ampicillin alone or in combination with erythromycin, cephalosporins, chloramphenicol, tetracyclines, and various parenteral drugs. Treatment must be continued for at least 1 month after clinical remission. Prognosis is guarded.

■ MISCELLANEOUS BACTERIAL INFECTIONS

Brucellosis

Brucellosis is a systemic bacterial infection caused by *Brucella canis*.[1] Despite widespread dissemination in the body, systemic signs of illness are rare, as are skin lesions. Brucellosis may produce a secondary scrotal dermatitis resulting from the animal's licking the skin over painful epididymitis and orchitis.[129] Some cases may involve necrosis of the testis, with severe inflammation of the entire scrotum, and draining ulcers. *B. canis* has been isolated from the exudate.[129]

B. canis has also been isolated from a 15-month-old female laboratory beagle with chronic exudative lesions that resembled acral lick dermatitis.[41] During a period of 16 months, expanding painful lesions developed on both hocks and the dorsum of the right carpus. The lesions were hyperemic, edematous, and granulomatous, with an irregularly pitted surface. A sanguinopurulent exudate was present, and the regional lymph nodes were enlarged. Histologic examination revealed dermal, subcutaneous, and tendinous edema; pronounced lymphoid nodules; a prominent infiltration of macrophages, plasma cells, and lymphocytes; and scattered neutrophils. The enlarged lymph nodes were characterized by sinusoid histiocytosis and medullary cord plasmacytosis. These findings are typical of the tissue response to *Brucella* infection.[41] Diagnosis is supported by serologic examination findings and confirmed by culture.

Treatment of canine brucellosis should not be undertaken lightly because the infection can spread to humans and is not easily eradicated in the dog.[1] Affected dogs should be removed from breeding programs and neutered if possible. Although the organism shows in vitro sensitivity to tetracyclines, chloramphenicol, aminoglycosides, spectinomycin, rifampin, ampicillin, sulfonamides, and the quinolones, relapses are common when a specific drug is used individually for a single course of treatment. The highest rate of success has been obtained with oral minocycline combined with parenteral streptomycin.[1]

Plague

Plague is an acute, febrile, infectious disease that has a high mortality rate and is caused by the gram-negative organism *Yersinia pestis*, a bipolar coccobacillus of the family Enterobacteriaceae.[1] It is a facultative anaerobic, nonmotile, non–spore-forming organism that cannot penetrate unbroken skin but can invade mucous membranes. Plague occurs in three forms: bubonic, pneumonic, and septicemic.[53, 54] The most common is bubonic plague, in which localized abscesses form near the site of infection (especially the head and neck). The septicemic and pneumonic forms are more serious, because they may be undiagnosed until it is too late for effective treatment.

The incubation period is 1 to 3 days if the organism is ingested or inhaled, or 2 to 6 days if the organisms enter through a flea bite, a skin wound, or a mucous membrane. The course is fulminating and can lead to death. Plague exists in every continent except Australia.[1] There have been outbreaks in all states of the United States west of the Rocky Mountains, including Hawaii. Rodents and cats are highly susceptible, dogs are less susceptible, and other domestic animals are resistant. It primarily affects rodents, especially prairie dogs, rock and ground squirrels, and rats.[1, 53]

Plague typically is transmitted by fleas or by ingestion of infected animals. *Diamanus montanus* and four less common rodent-hosted fleas are the primary vectors. The common dog and cat fleas are not normally involved.[127]

An epizootic plague can develop if susceptible rodents come in contact with the *Yersinia* organisms, causing a massive die-off in the rodent colony. The sick rodents become easy prey for cats or other carnivores, and the fleas seek new hosts. Cats can spread the infection to humans by transmitting infected fleas mechanically, by bringing dead or affected rodents home (thus facilitating human contact with the rodent or its fleas), or by causing direct infection. The latter occurs by bites, contact with pus, or inhalation of droplets from a sneezing or salivating cat. Plague can be a most serious public health problem for people exposed to infected material from clinical cases.[124]

Animal health personnel handling supposed cat abscesses in endemic plague areas have contracted the disease. In endemic areas, all cats with abscesses should be handled carefully by personnel using disposable gloves and masks, and all animals with plague should be kept in isolation. Oral administration of medications should be avoided, as well as any unnecessary handling, to reduce exposure. Bedding, contaminated bandages, and animal carcasses should be placed in double plastic bags and should be incinerated.

Rodents and cats are highly susceptible to plague, whereas dogs are more resistant and often have only mild fevers. Cats experience severe systemic signs of high fever, depression, anorexia, and lymphadenopathy with abscess formation and drainage. Mortality rates in untreated cats approach 75 per cent. Approximately 50 per cent of infected cats have the bubonic form and have the systemic signs plus one or more abscesses, typically on the face, the neck, or the limbs. The systemic form is next most common, and the pneumonic form occurs in approximately 10 per cent of cases. Overlap in the three presentations occurs.[1, 53]

Diagnosis is made by culture of the exudate, by immunofluorescence of impression smears, or by serologic confirmation based on a fourfold increase in antibody titers, from acute to convalescent.[1, 53] The latter is useful only in epidemiologic investigations. It is important to be cautious about the diagnosis, because *P. multocida* is often cultured from the abscess too. Differential diagnosis should include cat abscesses, wound infections, and other pyogranulomatous diseases.

Treatment should be instituted as soon as is possible, even before the results of the diagnostic tests are available. With prompt treatment, survival rates approaching 90 per cent have been reported. Drugs of choice are streptomycin, gentamicin, chloramphenicol, and tetracycline. Some clinicians reserve tetracyclines for prophylaxis, whereas other clinicians report success with it in treatment.[1, 53] Local abscesses should be opened and drained carefully and irrigated daily with an antibacterial solution. Flea control is important to prevent further spread.

Lyme Borreliosis

Lyme borreliosis is a complex multisystemic disorder caused by the spirochete *Borrelia burgdorferi*.[1, 7, 16, 32] The organism is transmitted by hard-shelled ticks of the genus *Ixodes*. Other ticks, flies, fleas, and mosquitoes have been found to harbor the organism, but the vector status of these other arthropods and insects is uncertain.

In all species, the predominant sign of Lyme borreliosis is polyarthropathic. In humans, a characteristic expanding ringlike macule or papule (erythema chronicum migrans) develops in 1 to 2 weeks at the site of the tick bite. Although lesions of erythema chronicum migrans have been reported in dogs,[7] no histologic studies have been performed to confirm that diagnosis. No doubt such lesions do occur, but are obscured by the haircoat.

Because Lyme borreliosis is a systemic immune complex disorder, skin lesions other than erythema chronicum migrans could occur but are apparently rare. In a report of 110 seropositive dogs, 4 had skin lesion of urticaria, rash, or moist dermatitis.[32] Another investigator reported recurrent, tetracycline-responsive lesions of pyotraumatic dermatitis in seropositive dogs.[156] One author (WHM) treated a seropositive dog with small vessel cutaneous vasculitis with tetracycline. The skin lesions resolved with treatment, did not recur, and the dog seroconverted.

The diagnosis of Lyme borreliosis is corroborated by serologic study.[16] Because not all strains of *B. burgdorferi* are arthritogenic, and cross-reactivity with other spirochetes can occur, a single positive serologic finding is not diagnostic. A significant rise or fall in antibody titer is more diagnostic.

Tetracyclines and ampicillin are the drugs of choice and are typically administered for 10 to 14 days.[1] Early treatment is essential to prevent irreversible joint changes.

Trichomycosis Axillaris

Trichomycosis axillaris is a bacterial infection of the hair shafts of humans. It involves mainly axillary and pubic hair. A similar infection with *Corynebacterium* sp. has been reported in a beagle dog.[20] The animal had a diffuse, irregular, and patchy alopecia that affected the neck and flank regions. There was no dermatitis. In the involved areas, some hairs were broken off and some hair shafts displayed small, hard nodules. Masses of bacteria ensheathed the hair at those locations. Inoculated hair developed nodules that eventually involved the whole hair. Inoculation of normal hair from other dogs produced no alopecia and no bacterial growth. This is not a fungal disease, in spite of its name, and no fungal elements were seen or isolated on culturing.

This is an uncommon and inconsequential disorder that should respond readily to clipping of the hair and frequent use of antibacterial shampoos.

L-Form Infections

L-Forms are partially cell wall–deficient bacteria, which resemble *Mycoplasma*.[1, 26, 74] Retention of some cell wall, variability in size and morphologic characteristics, and the ability to revert to the parental type with in vitro passage differentiate L-forms from *Mycoplasma*. L-Forms cannot be cultured by routine techniques and may or may not be isolated with special L-form techniques. The organisms can be found by electron microscopy of fresh tissues.

Most reports of L-form infections in animals have involved cats with abscesses with or without concurrent polyarthropathy.[26, 74] The cats are febrile, are depressed, and have one or more draining abscesses, typically over joints. The draining exudate is nonodoriferous and contains numerous nontoxic neutrophils and macrophages. The neutrophils often contain ingested erythrocytes, vacuoles, and granules. Treatment with the antibiotics used to treat routine feline abscesses results in no improvement. Rapid response is seen to the administration of tetracycline.

Pseudopyodermas

There is a group of dermatoses, of variable etiology, which are not pyodermas, although they resemble them. The group includes the following:

1. Callus pyoderma (see Chap. 15)
2. Juvenile cellulitis (see Chap. 17)
3. Other pyoderma-like dermatoses
   a. Acne (see Chap. 13)
   b. Intertrigo (fold dermatitis) (see Chap. 15)
   c. Linear IgA dermatosis (see Chap. 8)
   d. Sterile panniculitis (see Chap. 17)
   e. Pemphigus erythematosus (see Chap. 8)
   f. Pemphigus foliaceus (see Chap. 8)
   g. Sterile eosinophilic pustulosis (see Chap. 17)
   h. Sterile pyogranuloma syndrome (see Chap. 17)
   i. Subcorneal pustular dermatosis (see Chap. 17)

REFERENCES

General
1. Greene, C. E.: Infectious Diseases of the Dog and Cat. W. B. Saunders Co., Philadelphia, 1990.

Specific
2. Ackerman, L.: Cutaneous bacterial granuloma (botryomycosis) in five dogs: Treatment with rifampin. Mod. Vet. Pract. 68:404, 1987.
3. Allaker, R. P., et al.: Occurrence of *Staphylococcus intermedius* on the hair and skin of normal dogs. Res. Vet. Sci. 5:174, 1992.
4. Allaker, R. P., et al.: Colonization of neonatal puppies by staphylococci. Br. Vet. J. 148:523, 1992.
5. Allaker, R. P., et al.: Population sizes and frequency of staphylococci at mucocutaneous sites in healthy dogs. Vet. Rec. 130:303, 1992.
6. Angarano, D. W., MacDonald, J. M.: Efficacy of cefadroxil in the treatment of bacterial dermatitis in dogs. J. Am. Vet. Med. Assoc. 194:57, 1989.
7. Appel, M. J. G.: Lyme disease in dogs and cats. Comp. Cont. Educ. 12:617, 1990.
8. Armstrong, J. P.: Systemic *Serratia marcescens* infections in a dog and a cat. J. Am. Vet. Med. Assoc. 184:1143, 1984.
9. Ascher, F., et al.: Controlled trial of ethyl lactate and benzoyl peroxide shampoos in the management of canine surface pyoderma and superficial pyoderma. In: von Tscharner, C., Halliwell, R. E. W. (eds.). Advances in Veterinary Dermatology, Vol. 1. Baillière-Tindall, London, 1990, p. 375.
10. Awad-Masalmeh, V. M., et al.: Bakteriologische Untersuchungen zur Pyodermie des Hundes Therapeutischen Einsatzeiner autogenen Vakzin. Wien Tierärztl Mschr. 75:232, 1986.
11. Becker, A. M., et al.: *Propionibacterium acnes* immunotherapy in chronic recurrent canine pyoderma. J. Vet. Intern. Med. 3:26, 1989.

12. Berg, J. N., et al.: The occurrence of anaerobic bacteria in diseases of the dog and cat. Am. J. Vet. Res. 40:877, 1979.
13. Berg, J. N., et al.: Clinical models for anaerobic bacterial infection in dogs and their use in testing the efficacy of clindamycin and lincomycin. Am. J. Vet. Res. 45:1299, 1984.
14. Berg, J. N., et al.: Identification of the major coagulase-positive *Staphylococcus* sp. of dogs as *Staphylococcus intermedius*. Am. J. Vet. Res. 45:1307, 1984.
15. Blum, J. R., et al.: The clinical manifestations of a genetically determined deficiency in the third component of complement in the dog. Clin. Immunol. Immunopathol. 34:304, 1985.
16. Breitschwerdt, E. B.: Laboratory diagnosis of tick-transmitted diseases in the dog. In: Kirk, R. W., Bonagura, J. D. (eds.). Kirk's Current Veterinary Therapy XI. W. B. Saunders Co., Philadelphia, 1992, p. 252.
17. Breitschwerdt, E. B., et al.: Rhinitis, pneumonia, and defective neutrophil function in the Doberman pinscher. Am. J. Vet. Res. 48:1054, 1987.
18. Buchanan, A. M., Scott, J. L.: *Actinomyces hordeovulneris,* a canine pathogen that produces L-phase variants spontaneously with coincident calcium deposition. Am. J. Vet. Res. 54:2552, 1984.
19. Buchanan, A. M., et al.: *Nocardia asteroides* recovery from a dog with steroid- and antibiotic-unresponsive idiopathic polyarthritis. J. Clin. Microbiol. 18:702, 1983.
20. Buck, G. E., et al.: Isolation of a corynebacterium from beagle dogs affected with alopecia. Am. J. Vet. Res. 35:297, 1974.
20a. Burrows, A. K.: Residual Antimicrobial action of 2% mupirocin ointment (Bactoderm). Proc. Am. Acad. Vet. Dermatol. Am. Coll. Vet. Dermatol. 10:35, 1994.
21. Campbell, K. L., et al.: Immunoglobulin A deficiency in the dog. Canine Pract. 16:7, 1991.
22. Caprile, K. A.: Maintenance antibacterial agents in recurrent pyoderma. Vet. Med. Rep. 2:297, 1990.
23. Carakostas, M. C., et al.: Subcutaneous dermatophilosis in a cat. J. Am. Vet. Med. Assoc. 185:675, 1984.
24. Carb, A. V., Liu, S. K.: *Actinobacillus lignieresii* infection in a dog. J. Am. Vet. Med. Assoc. 154:1062, 1969.
25. Carpenter, J. L., et al.: Tuberculosis in five basset hounds. J. Am. Vet. Med. Assoc. 192:1563, 1988.
26. Carro, T., et al.: Subcutaneous abscesses and arthritis caused by a probable bacterial L-form in cats. J. Am. Vet. Med. Assoc. 194:1583, 1989.
27. Chambers, E. D., Severin, G. A.: Staphylococcal bacterin for treatment of chronic staphylococcal blepharitis in the dog. J. Am. Vet. Med. Assoc. 185:422, 1984.
28. Chastain, C. B., et al.: Dermatophilosis in two dogs. J. Am. Vet. Med. Assoc. 169:1079, 1976.
29. Christensen, G. D.: Coagulase-negative staphylococci—saprophyte or parasite? Int. J. Dermatol. 22:463, 1983.
30. Chusid, M. J., et al.: Defective polymorphonuclear leukocyte metabolism and function in canine cyclic neutropenia. Blood 46:921, 1975.
31. Clerex, C., et al.: Tuberculosis in dogs: A case report and review of the literature. J. Am. Anim. Hosp. Assoc. 28:207, 1992.
32. Cohen, N. D., et al.: Clinical and epizootiologic characteristics of dogs seropositive for *Borrelia burgdorferi* in Texas: 110 cases (1988). J. Am. Vet. Med. Assoc. 197:893, 1990.
33. Cox, H. U., et al.: Antimicrobial susceptibility of coagulase positive staphylococci isolated from Louisiana dogs. Am. J. Vet. Res. 44:2039, 1984.
34. Cox, H. U., Hoskins, J. D.: Distribution of staphylococcal species on clinically healthy cats. Am. J. Vet. Res. 46:1824, 1985.
35. Cox, H. U., et al.: Species of staphylococcus isolated from animal infections. Cornell Vet. 74:124:1984.
36. Cox, H. U., Schmeer, N.: Protein A in *Staphylococcus intermedius* isolates from dogs and cats. Am. J. Vet. Res. 47:1881, 1986.
37. Couto, C. G., et al.: In vitro immunologic features of Weimaraner dogs with neutrophil abnormalities and recurrent infections. Vet. Immunol. Immunopathol. 23:103, 1989.
38. Couto, C. G.: Patterns of infection associated with immunodeficiency. In: Kirk, R. W., Bonagura, J. D. (eds.). Kirk's Current Veterinary Therapy XI. W. B. Saunders Co., Philadelphia, 1992, p. 223.
39. Crowe, D. T., Kowalski, J. J.: Clostridial cellulitis with localized gas formation in a dog. J. Am. Vet. Med. Assoc. 169:1094, 1976.
40. Davenport, D. J., Johnson, G. C.: Cutaneous nocardiosis in a cat. J. Am. Vet. Med. Assoc. 188:728, 1986.
41. Dawkins, B. G., et al.: Pyogranulomatous dermatitis associated with *Brucella canis* infection in a dog. J. Am. Vet. Med. Assoc. 181:1432, 1982.
42. Day, M. J., Penhale, W. J.: Serum immunoglobulin A concentrations in normal and diseased dogs. Res. Vet. Sci. 45:36, 1988.
43. DeBoer, D. J., et al.: Evaluation of commercial staphylococcal bacterin for management of idiopathic recurrent superficial pyoderma in dogs. Am. J. Vet. Res. 51:636, 1990.
44. DeBoer, D. J., et al.: Clinical and immunological responses of dogs with recurrent pyoderma to injection of staphylococcus phage lysate. In: von Tscharner, C., Halliwell, R. E. W. (eds.). Advances in Veterinary Dermatology, Vol. 1. Baillière-Tindall, London, 1990, p. 335.
45. DeBoer, D. J., Pukay, B. P.: Recurrent pyoderma and immunostimulants. In: Ihrke, P. J., Mason, I. S., White, S. D. (eds.). Advances in Veterinary Dermatology, Vol. 2. Pergamon Press, Oxford, 1993, p. 443.
46. deLisle, G. W., et al.: A report of tuberculosis in cats in New Zealand, and the examination of strains of *Mycobacterium bovis* by DNA restriction endonuclease analysis. N. Z. Vet. J. 38:10, 1990.
47. Devriese, L. A.: Identification and characterization of staphylococci isolated from cats. Vet. Microbiol. 9:279, 1984.
48. Devriese, L. A., DePelsmaecker, K.: The anal region as a main carrier site of *Staphylococcus intermedius* and *Streptococcus canis* in dogs. Vet. Rec. 121:302, 1987.
49. Devriese, L. A., Haesebrouch, F.: *Streptococcus suis* infection in horses and cats. Vet. Rec. 130:300, 1992.

50. Donnelly, T. M., et al.: Diffuse cutaneous granulomatous lesions associated with acid-fast bacilli in a cat. J. Small Anim. Pract. 23:99, 1982.

51. Dow, S. W., et al.: Anaerobic bacterial infections and response to treatment in dogs and cats: 36 cases (1983–1985). J. Am. Vet. Med. Assoc. 189:930, 1986.

52. Dow, S. M., Jones, R. L.: Anaerobic infections. Part I: Pathogenesis and clinical significance. Comp. Cont. Educ. 9:711, 1987.

53. Eidson, M., et al.: Clinical, clinicopathologic, and pathologic features of plague in cats: 119 cases (1979–1988). J. Am. Vet. Med. Assoc. 199:1191, 1991.

54. Emerson, J. K.: Plague. Canine Pract. 12:43, 1985.

55. Fadok, V. A.: Granulomatous dermatitis in dogs and cats. Semin. Vet. Med. Surg. (Small Anim.) 2:186, 1987.

56. Farrow, B. R. H., et al.: *Pneumocystis* pneumonia in the dog. J. Comp. Pathol. 82:447, 1972.

57. Fehrer, S. L., et al.: Identification of protein A from *Staphylococcus intermedius* isolated from canine skin. Am. J. Vet. Res. 49:697, 1988.

58. Feingold, D. S.: Gangrenous and crepitant cellulitis. J. Am. Acad. Dermatol. 6:289, 1982.

59. Feingold, D. S.: Bacterial adherence, colonization, and pathogenicity. Arch. Dermatol. 122:161, 1986.

60. Felsburg, P. J., Jezyk, P. F.: A canine model for combined immunodeficiency. Clin. Res. 30:347, 1982.

61. Felsburg, P. J.: Primary immunodeficiencies. In: Kirk, R. W., Bonagura, J. D. (eds.). Kirk's Current Veterinary Therapy XI. W. B. Saunders Co., Philadelphia, 1992, p. 448.

62. Frank, L. A., Kunkle, G. A.: Comparison of the efficacy of cefadroxil and generic and proprietary cephalexin in the treatment of pyoderma in dogs. J. Am. Vet. Med. Assoc. 203:530, 1993.

63. Giger, U., et al.: Deficiency of leukocyte surface glycoproteins mo1,LFA-1 and Leu M5 in a dog with recurrent bacterial infections: An animal model. Blood 69:1622, 1987.

64. Gross, T. L., Connelly, M. R.: Nontuberculous mycobacterial skin infections in two dogs. Vet. Pathol. 20:117, 1983.

64a. Halliwell, R. E. W., Gorman, N. T.: Veterinary Clinical Immunology. W. B. Saunders Co., Philadelphia, 1989, p. 253.

65. Hardie, E. M., Barsanti, J. A.: Treatment of canine actinomycosis. J. Am. Vet. Med. Assoc. 180:537, 1982.

66. Hart, B. L., Barrett, R. E.: Effects of castration on fighting, roaming, and urine spraying in adult male cats. J. Am. Vet. Med. Assoc. 163:290, 1973.

67. Harvey, R. G., et al.: Distribution of propionibacteria on dogs: A preliminary report of the findings on 11 dogs. J. Small Anim. Pract. 34:80, 1993.

67a. Harvey, R. G., et al: A comparison of lincomycin hydrochloride and clindamycin hydrochloride in the treatment of superficial pyoderma or in dogs. Vet. Rec. 132:351, 1993.

68. Higgins, R., Paradis, M.: Abscess caused by *Corynebacterium equi* in a cat. Can. Vet. J. 21:63, 1980.

68a. Hill, P. B., Moriello, K. A.: Canine Pyoderma. J. Am. Vet. Med. Assoc. 204:334, 1994.

69. Hinton, M., et al.: The antibiotic resistance of pathogenic staphylococci and streptococci isolated from dogs. J. Small Anim. Pract. 19:229, 1978.

70. Hirsch, D. C., et al.: Changes in prevalence and susceptibility of obligate anaerobes in clinical veterinary practice. J. Am. Vet. Med. Assoc. 186:1086, 1985.

71. Horwitz, L., Ihrke, P. J. Canine seborrheas. In: Kirk, R. W. (ed.). Current Veterinary Therapy VI. W. B. Saunders Co., Philadelphia, 1977.

71a. Ihrke, P. J.: Antibacterial therapy in dermatology. In: Kirk, R. W. (ed.). Current Veterinary Therapy IX. W. B. Saunders Co., Philadelphia, 1986, p. 566.

71b. Ihrke, P. J., Gross, T. L.: Canine mucocutaneous pyoderma. In: Bonagura J. D. (ed.): Kirk's Current Veterinary Therapy XII. W. B. Saunders Co., Philadelphia. (in press, 1995).

71c. Ihrke, P. J., Gross, T. L.: Conference in Dermatology, No. 1. Vet. Dermatol. 4:33, 1993.

72. Jezyk, P. F., et al.: Lethal acrodermatitis in bull terriers. J. Am. Vet. Med. Assoc. 118:833, 1986.

73. Jezyk, P. F., et al.: X-linked severe combined immunodeficiency in the dog. Clin. Immunol. Immunopathol. 52:173, 1989.

73a. Jordon, H. L., et al.: Disseminated *Mycobacterium avium* complex infection in three Siamese cats. J. Am. Vet. Med. Assoc. 204:90, 1994.

74. Keane, D. P.: Chronic abscesses in cats associated with an organism resembling mycoplasma. Can. Vet. J. 24:289, 1983.

75. Keane, K. A., Taylor, D. J.: Slime-producing *Staphylococcus* species in canine pyoderma. Vet. Rec. 130:75, 1992.

76. Kirpensteijn, J., Fingland, R. B.: Cutaneous actinomycosis and nocardiosis in dogs: 48 cases (1980–1990). J. Am. Vet. Med. Assoc. 201:917, 1992.

77. Krakowaka, S.: Acquired immunodeficiency diseases. In: Kirk, R. W., Bonagura, J. D. (eds.). Kirk's Current Veterinary Therapy XI. W. B. Saunders Co., Philadelphia, 1992, p. 453.

78. Kramer, T. T.: Immunity to bacterial infections. Vet. Clin. North Am. (Small Anim. Pract.) 8:683, 1978.

79. Krick, S. A., Scott, D. W.: Bacterial folliculitis, furunculosis, and cellulitis in the German shepherd: A retrospective analysis of 17 cases. J. Am. Anim. Hosp. Assoc. 25:23, 1989.

80. Kristensen, S., Krogh, H. V.: A study of skin diseases in dogs and cats. III. Microflora of the skin of dogs with chronic eczema. Nord. Vet. Med. 30:223, 1978.

81. Krogh, H. F., Kristensen, S.: A study of skin diseases in dogs and cats. Nord. Vet. Med. 28:459, 1976.

82. Kunkle, G. A., et al.: Rapidly growing mycobacteria as a cause of cutaneous granulomas: Report of five cases. J. Am. Anim. Hosp. Assoc. 19:513, 1983.

83. Kunkle, G. A. New considerations for rational antibiotic therapy of cutaneous staphylococcal infection in the dog. Semin. Vet. Med. Surg. (Small Anim.) 2:212, 1987.

84. Kwochka, K. W., Kowalski, J. J.: Prophylactic efficacy of four antibacterial shampoos against *Staphylococcus intermedius* in dogs. Am. J. Vet. Res. 52:115, 1991.
85. Kwochka, K. W.: Recurrent pyoderma. In: Griffin, C. E., Kwochka, K. W., MacDonald, J. M. (eds.). Current Veterinary Dermatology. Mosby Year Book, St. Louis, 1993, p. 3.
86. Lee, A. H., et al.: Effects of chlorhexidine diacetate, providone iodine, and polyhydroxydine on wound healing in dogs. J. Am. Anim. Hosp. Assoc. 24:77, 1988.
87. Liu, S., et al.: Canine tuberculosis. J. Am. Vet. Med. Assoc. 177:164, 1980.
88. Lloyd, D. H., Jenkinson, D. M.: The effect of climate on experimental infection of bovine skin with *Dermatophilus congolensis*. Br. Vet. J. 136:122, 1980.
89. Lloyd, D. H.: Skin surface immunity. Vet. Dermatol. News 5:10, 1980.
90. Lloyd, D. H.: The cutaneous defense mechanisms. Vet. Dermatol. News 1:9, 1976.
91. Lloyd, H., Reyss-Brion, A.: Le peroxide de benzoyle: Efficacité clinique et bacteriologique dans le traitement des pyodermites chroniques. Prat. Méd. Chirug. Anim. Cie 19:445, 1984.
92. Lloyd, D. H., et al.: Carriage of *Staphylococcus intermedius* on the ventral abdomen of clinically normal dogs and those with pyoderma. Vet. Dermatol. 2:161, 1991.
93. Lotti, T., Hartmann, G.: Atypical mycobacterial infections: A difficult and emerging group of infectious dermatoses. Int. J. Dermatol. 32:499, 1993.
94. Love, D. N., et al.: Antimicrobial susceptibility patterns of obligately anaerobic bacteria from subcutaneous abscesses and pyothorax in cats. Aust. Vet. Pract. 10:168, 1980.
95. Love, D. N., et al.: Characterization of strains of staphylococci from infections in dogs and cats. J. Small Anim. Pract. 22:195, 1981.
96. McEwan, N. A.: Bacterial adherence to canine corneocytes. In: von Tscharner, C., Halliwell, R. E. W. (eds.). Advances in Veterinary Dermatology, Vol. 1. Baillière-Tindall, London, 1990, p. 454.
97. McIntosh, D. W.: Feline leprosy: A review of forty-four cases from western Canada. Can. Vet. J. 23:291, 1982.
98. Manning, T. O.: Canine pododermatitis. Dermatol. Rep. 2:1, 1983.
99. Mason, K. V., Wilkinson, G.T.: Results of treatment of atypical mycobacteriosis. In: von Tscharner, C., Halliwell, R. E. W. (eds.). Advances in Veterinary Dermatology, Vol. 1. Baillière-Tindall, London, 1990, p. 452.
100. Mason, I. S., Lloyd, D. H.: The role of allergy in the development of canine pyoderma. J. Small Anim. Pract. 30:216, 1989.
101. Mason, I. S., Lloyd, D. H.: Scanning electron microscopic studies of the living epidermis and stratum corneum in dogs. In: Ihrke, P. J., Mason, I. S., White, S. D. (eds.). Advances in Veterinary Dermatology, Vol. 2. Pergamon Press, Oxford, 1993, p. 131.
102. Medleau, L., et al.: Frequency and antimicrobial susceptibility of *Staphylococcus* spp. isolated from canine pyodermas. Am. J. Vet. Res. 47:229, 1986.
103. Medleau, L., Blue, J. L.: Frequency and antimicrobial susceptibility of *Staphylococcus* spp. isolated from feline skin lesions. J. Am. Vet. Med. Assoc. 193:1080, 1988.
104. Medleau, L. M., et al.: Superficial pyoderma in the cat: Diagnosing an uncommon skin disorder. Vet. Med. 86:807, 1991.
105. Messinger, L. M., Beale, K. M.: A blinded comparison of the efficacy of daily and twice daily trimethoprim-sulfadiazine and daily sulfamethoxine-ormetoprim therapy in the treatment of canine pyoderma. Vet. Dermatol. 4:13, 1993.
106. Miller, R. I., Ladds, P. W.: Probable dermatophilosis in two cats. Aust. Vet. J. 60:155, 1983.
107. Miller, W. H., Jr.: Deep pyoderma in two German shepherd dogs associated with a cell-mediated immunodeficiency. J. Am. Anim. Hosp. Assoc. 27:513, 1991.
108. Monroe, W. E., Chickering, W. R.: Atypical mycobacterial infections in cats. Comp. Cont. Educ. 10:1043, 1988.
108a. Morales, C. A., et al.: Antistaphylococcal antibodies in dogs with recurrent staphylococcal pyoderma. Vet. Immunol. Immunopathol. (in press, 1994).
109. Muller, G. H., et al.: Small Animal Dermatology, 4th ed. W. B. Saunders Co., Philadelphia, 1989.
110. Mundell, A. C.: The use of clofazimine in the treatment of three cases of feline leprosy. In: von Tscharner, C., Halliwell, R. E. W. (eds.). Advances in Veterinary Dermatology, Vol. 1. Baillière-Tindall, London, 1990, p. 451.
111. Noble, W. C., Kent, L. E.: Antibiotic resistance in *Staphylococcus intermedius* isolated from cases with pyoderma in the dog. Vet. Dermatol. 3:71, 1992.
112. Paradis, M., et al.: Efficacy of enrofloxacin in the treatment of canine bacterial pyoderma. Vet. Dermatol. 1:123, 1990.
113. Paul, J. W., Gordon, M. A.: Efficacy of a chlorhexidine surgical scrub compared to that of hexachlorophene and providone-iodine. Vet. Med. 73:573, 1978.
114. Phillips, W. E., Kloos, W. E.: Identification of coagulase-positive *Staphylococcus intermedius* and *Staphylococcus hyicus* subsp. *hyicus* isolated from veterinary clinical specimens. J. Clin. Microbiol. 14:671, 1981.
115. Phillips, W. E., Williams, B. J.: Antimicrobial susceptibility patterns of canine *Staphylococcus intermedius* isolates from veterinary clinical specimens. Am. J. Vet. Res. 45:2377, 1984.
116. Pickler, M. E.: Gaseous gangrene in a dog: Successful treatment using hyperbaric oxygen and conventional treatment. J. Am. Anim. Hosp. Assoc. 18:807, 1982.
117. Plechner, A. J.: IgM deficiency in two Doberman pinchers. Mod. Vet. Pract. 60:150, 1979.
118. Price, P. M. Pyoderma caused by *Peptostreptococcus tetradius* in a pup. J. Am. Vet. Med. Assoc. 198:1649, 1991.
119. Raychaudhuri, S. P., Raychaudhuri, S. K.: Relationship between kinetics of lesional cytokines and secondary infection in inflammatory skin disorders: A hypothesis. Int. J. Dermatol. 32:409, 1993.
120. Reinke, S. I., et al.: Histopathologic features of pyotraumatic dermatitis. J. Am. Vet. Med. Assoc. 190:57, 1987.
121. Renshaw, H. W., et al.: Canine granulocytopathy syndrome. Am. J. Pathol. 95:731, 1979.

122. Richard, J. L., et al.: Experimentally induced canine dermatophilosis. Am. J. Vet. Res. 34:797, 1973.
123. Rosser, E. J. German shepherd pyoderma: A prospective study of 12 dogs. Proc. Am. Acad. Vet. Dermatol. Am. Coll. Vet. Dermatol. 9:40, 1993.
124. Rosser, W. W.: Bubonic plague. J. Am. Vet. Med. Assoc. 191:406, 1987.
125. Roth, J. A., et al.: Improvement in clinical condition and thymus morphologic features associated with growth hormone treatment of immunodeficient dwarf dogs. Am. J. Vet. Res. 45:1151, 1984.
126. Roth, R. R., James, W. D.: Microbiology of the skin. J. Am. Acad. Dermatol. 20:369, 1989.
127. Ryan, C. P.: Selected arthropod-borne diseases; plague, lyme disease, babesiosis. Vet. Clin. North Am. (Small Anim. Pract.) 17:179, 1987.
128. Schiefer, H. B., Middleton, D. B.: Experimental transmission of a feline mycobacterial skin disease (feline leprosy). Vet. Pathol. 20:460, 1983.
129. Schoeb, T. R., Morton, R.: Scrotal and testicular changes in canine brucellosis. J. Am. Vet. Med. Assoc. 172:598, 1978.
130. Schultz, R. D.: Basic veterinary immunology and a review. Vet. Clin. North Am. (Small Anim. Pract.) 8:569, 1978.
131. Scott, D. W.: Canine pododermatitis. In: Kirk, R. W. (ed.). Current Veterinary Therapy VII. W. B. Saunders Co., Philadelphia, 1980.
132. Scott, D. W.: Feline dermatology 1900–1980: A monograph. J. Am. Anim. Hosp. Assoc. 16:331, 1980.
133. Scott, D. W.: Feline dermatology 1979–1982: Introspective retrospections. J. Am. Anim. Hosp. Assoc. 20:537, 1984.
134. Scott, D. W.: Feline dermatology 1983–1985: The secret sits. J. Am. Anim. Hosp. Assoc. 23:255, 1987.
135. Scott, D. W.: Feline dermatology 1986 to 1988: Looking to the 1990s through the eyes of many counsellors. J. Am. Anim. Hosp. Assoc. 26:515, 1990.
136. Scott, D. W.: Bacteria and yeast on the surface and within non-inflamed hair follicles of skin biopsies from dogs with non-neoplastic dermatoses. Cornell Vet. 82:379, 1992.
137. Scott, D. W.: Bacteria and yeast on the surface and within non-inflamed hair follicles of skin biopsies from cats with non-neoplastic dermatoses. Cornell Vet. 82:371, 1992.
138. Scott, D. W., et al.: The combination of ormetoprim and sulfadimethoxine in the treatment of pyoderma due to *Staphylococcus intermedius* infection in dogs. Canine Pract. 10:29, 1993.
138a. Scott, D. W., et al.: Efficacy of tylosin tablets for the treatment of pyoderma due to *Staphylococcus intermedius* infection in dogs. Can. Vet. J. (in press, 1994).
139. Snider, W. R.: Tuberculosis in canine and feline populations. Review of the literature. Am. Rev. Respir. Dis. 104:877, 1971.
139a. Stewart, L. J., et al.: Cutaneous *Mycobacterium avium* Infection in a cat. Vet. Dermatol. 4:87, 1993.
140. Studdert, V. P., Hughes, K. L.: Treatment of opportunistic mycobacterial infections with enrofloxacin in cats. J. Am. Vet. Med. Assoc. 201:1300, 1992.
141. Swaim, S. F., et al.: Fusion podoplasty for the treatment of chronic fibrosing interdigital pyoderma in the dog. J. Am. Anim. Hosp. Assoc. 27:264, 1991.
142. Tredten, H. W., et al.: *Mycobacterium* bacteremia in a dog: Diagnosis of septicemia by microscopic evaluation of blood. J. Am. Anim. Hosp. Assoc. 26:359, 1990.
143. Trowald-Wigh, A., et al.: Leukocyte adhesion protein deficiency in Irish setter dogs. Vet. Immunol. Immunopathol. 32:261, 1992.
144. Walton, D. K., et al.: Cutaneous bacterial granuloma (botryomycosis) in a dog and cat. J. Am. Anim. Hosp. Assoc. 19:537, 1983.
145. Welsh, O., et al.: Amikacin alone and in combination with trimethoprim-sulfamethoxazole in the treatment of actinomycotic mycetoma. J. Am. Acad. Dermatol. 17:443, 1987.
146. White, S. D., et al.: Cutaneous atypical mycobacteriosis in cats. J. Am. Vet. Med. Assoc. 182:1218, 1983.
147. White, S. D., et al.: Occurrence of *S. aureus* on the clinically normal canine hair coat. Am. J. Vet. Res. 44:332, 1983.
148. White, S. D.: Pododermatitis. Vet. Dermatol. 1:1, 1989.
149. White, S. D.: Pyoderma in 5 cats. J. Am. Anim. Hosp. Assoc. 27:141, 1991.
150. Whitney, J. C.: Some aspects of interdigital cysts in the dog. J. Small Anim. Pract. 11:83, 1970.
151. Willemse, T., et al.: *Mycobacterium thermoresistibile*: Extrapulmonary infection in a cat. J. Clin. Microbiol. 21:854, 1985.
152. Wisselink, M. A., et al.: Immunologic aspects of German shepherd pyoderma. Vet. Immunol. Immunopathol. 19:67, 1988.
153. Wisselink, M. A., et al.: German shepherd pyoderma. A genetic disorder. Vet. Quart. 11:161, 1989.
154. Wisselink, M. A., et al.: Deep pyoderma in the German shepherd dog. J. Am. Anim. Hosp. Assoc. 21:773, 1985.
155. Woldehiwet, Z., Jones, J. J.: Species distribution of coagulase-positive staphylococci isolated from dogs. Vet. Rec. 126:485, 1990.
156. Von Tscharner, C.: Personal communication, Bad Kreuznach, Germany, 1988.
157. Yager, J. A.: The skin as an immune organ. In: Ihrke, P. J., Mason, I. S., White, S. D. (eds.). Advances in Veterinary Dermatology, Vol. 2. Pergamon Press, Oxford, 1993, p. 3.

Fungal Skin Diseases

■

Chapter Outline

■ CUTANEOUS MYCOLOGY

Fungi are omnipresent in our environment. Of the thousands of different species of fungi, only a few have the ability to cause disease in animals. The great majority of fungi are either soil organisms or plant pathogens; however, more than 300 species have been reported to be animal pathogens. A *mycosis* (pl. *mycoses*) is a disease caused by a fungus. A dermatophytosis is an infection of the keratinized tissues, claw, hair, and stratum corneum that is caused by a species of *Microsporum, Trichophyton,* or *Epidermophyton.* These organisms—dermatophytes—are unique fungi that are able to invade and maintain themselves in keratinized tissues. A dermatomycosis is a fungal infection of hair, claw, or skin that is caused by a nondermatophyte, a fungus not classified in the genera *Microsporum, Trichophyton,* or *Epidermophyton.* Dermatophytosis and dermatomycosis are different clinical entities. Fungi, however, are not nearly as common a cause of skin disease as supposed; many nonspecific, pruritic, and nonpruritic dermatoses are diagnosed as dermatomycoses on the basis of inadequate evidence. Some clinicians incorrectly use the term *grass fungus* for these problems despite the fact that contact dermatitis, atopy, or factors other than fungi are involved. On the other hand, many true fungal infections are probably not diagnosed because of the variability of clinical presentations.

General Characteristics of Fungi

The term *fungus* includes yeasts and molds. The kingdom of *Fungi* is recognized as one of the five kingdoms of organisms. The other four kingdoms are *Monera* (bacteria and blue-green algae), *Protista* (protozoa), *Plantae* (plants), and *Animalia* (animals).[1-3, 9] Fungi are eukaryotic achlorophyllous organisms that may grow in the form of a yeast (unicellular), a mold (multicellular-filamentous), or both. The cell walls of fungi consist of chitin, chitosan, glucan, and mannan and are used to distinguish the fungi from the Protista. Unlike plants, fungi do not have chlorophyll. The kingdom of Fungi contains five divisions: *Chytridomycota, Zygomycota, Basidiomycota, Ascomycota,* and *Fungi Imperfecti* or *Deuteromycota.*

Fungi have traditionally been identified and classified (1) by their method of producing conidia and spores; (2) by the size, shape, and color of the conidia; and (3) by the type of hyphae and their macroscopic appearance (e.g., by the color and texture of the colony and sometimes by physiologic characteristics). Therefore, it is important to understand the terms that describe these characteristics. A single vegetative filament of a fungus is a *hypha.* A number of vegetative filaments are called *hyphae,* and a mass of hyphae is known as a *mycelium.* Hyphae are *septate,* if they have divisions between cells, or *sparsely septate,* if they have many nuclei within a cell. This latter condition is known as *cenocytic.* The term *conidium* (pl. *conidia*) should be used only for an asexual *propagule* or unit that gives rise to genetically identical organisms. A *conidiophore* is a simple or branched mycelium bearing conidia or conidiogenous cells. A *conidiogenous cell* is any fungal cell that gives rise to a conidium. (Modern taxonomists also may use sexual reproduction characteristics and biochemical and immunologic methods for identification.) There are six major types of conidia: blastoconidia, arthroconidia, annelloconidia, phialoconidia, poroconidia, and aleuriconidia. More detailed information about fungal taxonomy can be found in other texts.[1-3, 9]

Changes in the scientific names resulting from recent taxonomic studies have caused some confusion regarding the names of pathogenic fungi. Some disease names have been based on geographic distribution or have been created by the indiscriminate lumping together of dissimilar diseases. The authors here attempt to name diseases on the basis of a single etiologic agent and common usage, tempered by contemporary knowledge of geographic distribution and current taxonomy. Mycotic diseases are divided into three categories: superficial, subcutaneous, and systemic. The first category contains the most common fungal diseases in veterinary dermatology.

Characterization of Pathogenic Fungi

Fungi that are pathogenic to plants are distributed throughout all divisions of fungi, but those that are pathogenic to animals are found primarily in the *Fungi Imperfecti* and the *Ascomycota*.[1-3, 9]

A yeast is a unicellular budding fungus that forms blastoconidia, whereas a mold is a filamentous fungus. Some pathogenic fungi, such as *Histoplasma capsulatum, Coccidioides immitis, Sporothrix schenckii,* and *Blastomyces dermatitidis,* are *dimorphic.* Dimorphic fungi are capable of existing in two different morphologic forms. For example, at 37°C (98.6°F) in enriched media or in vitro, *B. dermatitidis* exists as a yeast, but at 30°C (86°F) it grows as a mold. *C. immitis* is unique in that at 37°C (98.6°F) or in tissue, spherules containing endospores are formed. Some fungi such as *Aspergillus* form true hyphae in tissue and are a mold at either 30°C or 37°C (86°F or 98.6°F). Another manifestation of fungal growth in tissue is the presence of granules that are organized masses of hyphae in a crystalline or amorphous matrix. These granules are characteristic of the mycotic infection mycetoma and are the result of interaction between the host tissue and the fungus.

At one time, numerous fungi were thought to be pathogens. Today, with the increased use of broad-spectrum antibiotics, immunosuppressive therapy, and improved mycologic techniques, many fungi that were considered contaminants have, in fact, been found to be pathogenic. The following criteria can be helpful in differentiating pathogenic from contaminant fungi: (1) source, (2) number of colonies isolated, (3) species, (4) whether the fungus can be repeatedly isolated, and most important (5) the presence of fungal elements in the tissue. A fungus isolated from a normal sterile site, such as a biopsy specimen, warrants greater credence as a pathogen than that same fungus isolated from the surface of the skin, where it may be an airborne contaminant. The number of colonies isolated should influence the decision as to whether an organism is a contaminant or a pathogen. One isolated colony of *Aspergillus* may have resulted from an airborne conidium that floated into a plate, whereas a petri dish filled with *Aspergillus fumigatus* could represent a pathogen. Colonies that are not seen on the streak line of the agar should be considered contaminants. Certain species of fungi are definitely recognized as pathogens, however, so if even only one colony is isolated, it should be reported. Such organisms include *B. dermatitidis, H. capsulatum, C. immitis,* and *Cryptococcus neoformans.* Another indication of fungal pathogenicity is that the same fungus can be repeatedly isolated from the lesion. In order to confirm that a fungus is a cause of a mycosis, the fungal structures observed in tissue or a direct smear must correlate with the fungus identified in culture.

Although gross colonies of dermatophytes are never black, brown, or green, the proper identification of organisms in fungal cultures should be made by medical laboratory clinicians who have expertise in such matters. Detailed information on the cultural growth of three common dermatophytes *(Microsporum canis, Microsporum gypseum, Trichophyton mentagrophytes)* and commonly isolated fungal contaminants is available in other texts.[1, 2, 9]

Normal Fungal Microflora

Dogs and cats harbor many saprophytic molds and yeasts on their haircoats and skin (Table 5:1). The most common of these fungi isolated from dogs are species of *Alternaria, Aspergillus, Aureobasidium, Cladosporium, Mucor, Penicillium,* and *Rhizopus.*[15, 29, 30, 47, 58] In cats, the most commonly isolated fungi are species of *Alternaria, Aspergillus, Cladosporium, Mucor, Penicillium,* and *Rhodotorula.*[11, 15, 30a, 43] Most of these saprophytic isolates probably represent repeated transient contamination by airborne fungi or by fungi in soil.

Dermatophytes are also isolated from the haircoats and skin of normal dogs and cats.* To

---

*See references 15, 22, 29, 30a, 34, 43, 47, and 48.

Table 5:1. Saprophytic Fungi Isolated From the Haircoat and Skin of Normal Dogs and Cats

Absidia	Geotrichum
Acremonium	Gliocladium
Alternaria	Malassezia
Arthrinium	Mucor
Arthroderma	Paecilomyces
Aspergillus	Penicillium
Aureobasidium	Pestalotia
Beauveria	Phoma
Botrytis	Rhizopus
Candida	Rhodotorula
Cephalosporium	Scopulariopsis
Chaetomium	Stemphylium
Chrysosporium	Trichocladium
Cladosporium	Trichoderma
Doratomyces	Trichosporon
Epicoccum	Trichothecium
Fusarium	Ulocladium
Geomyces	Verticillium

what extent dermatophytes isolated from normal dogs and cats—such as *M. gypseum, T. mentagrophytes, Trichophyton rubrum, Trichophyton terrestre*—represent resident flora or transient flora is uncertain. For instance, it is not unheard of to isolate a geophilic dermatophyte, such as *M. gypseum*, from normal dogs or from a dog presented for a skin disease (e.g., pododermatitis) wherein these dermatophytes are playing no pathogenic role. This is particularly true in outdoor animals. *M. canis* is, however, undeniably present as a persistent infection in many asymptomatic cats.[15, 29, 30, 47, 57]

Culture and Examination of Fungi

Proper specimen collection, isolation, culture, and identification are necessary to determine the cause of a fungal infection. Detailed information on these important techniques is in Chapter 2.

■ SUPERFICIAL MYCOSES

The superficial mycoses are fungal infections that involve superficial layers of the skin, hair, and claws. The organisms may be dermatophytes such as *Microsporum* and *Trichophyton*, which are able to use keratin. However, other fungi such as *Candida (Monilia)* and *Malassezia (Pityrosporum)* may also produce superficial mycoses.

Dermatophytosis

CAUSE AND PATHOGENESIS

The dermatophytes that most frequently infect animals are *Microsporum* and *Trichophyton*. These genera can be divided into three groups on the basis of natural habitat: geophilic, zoophilic, and anthropophilic. Geophilic dermatophytes, such as *M. gypseum*, normally inhabit soil, in which they decompose keratinous debris. Zoophilic dermatophytes, such as *M. canis*, *Microsporum distortum*, and *Trichophyton equinum* have become adapted to animals and are only rarely found in soil. Anthropophilic dermatophytes, such as *Microsporum audouinii*, have become adapted to humans and do not survive in soil. Zoophilic dermatophytes often cause less inflammatory reaction in animals than geophilic or anthropophilic fungi.

Table 5:2. Dermatophytes Isolated From Dogs and Cats

Dermatophyte	Host*	Source†
Epidermophyton floccosum	B	A
Microsporum audouinii (M. langeronii, M. rivalierii)	B	A
M. canis (M. equinum, M. felineum, M. lanosum, M. obesum)	B	Z
M. cookei	B	G
M. distortum	B	Z
M. gypseum (M. fulvum, M. duboisii, Achorion gypseum)	B	G
M. nanum	B	Z
M. persicolor	B	Z
M. vanbreuseghemii	B	G
Trichophyton ajelloi (Keratinomyces ajelloi)	B	G
T. equinum	B	Z
T. erinacei (T. mentagrophytes var. *erinacei)*	B	Z
T. gallinae (M. gallinae, A. gallinae)	B	Z
T. megninii	B	A
T. mentagrophytes (T. asteroides, T. caninum, T. felineum, *T. granulosum, T. gypseum, T. quinckeanum)*	B	Z
T. rubrum (T. multicolor, T. purpureum)	B	A
T. schoenleinii (A. schoenleinii)	B	A
T. simii	D	Z, G
T. terrestre	B	G
T. tonsurans (T. accuminatum, T. cerebriforme, T. crateriforme, *T. epilans, T. fumatum, T. plicale, T. sabouraudi,* *T. sulfureum)*	B	A
T. verrucosum (T. album, T. discoides, T. faviforme, *T. ochraceum)*	B	Z
T. violaceum (T. glabrum, T. kagewaense, T. vinosum)	B	A

*B = dog and cat, D = dog.
†A = anthropophilic, G = geophilic, Z = zoophilic.

Three fungi cause the great majority of clinical cases of dermatophytosis in dogs and cats*: *M. canis, M. gypseum,* and *T. mentagrophytes.* In general, *M. canis* is the most common cause of dermatophytosis in cats and dogs.† There is, however, great variation in the proportion in which these three fungi occur in different parts of the world.[22, 34, 59] The incidence and prevalence of dermatophytosis vary with the climate and natural reservoirs. In a hot, humid climate, a higher incidence is observed than in a cold, dry climate. It has been reported that the seasonal incidence of dermatophytosis in dogs and cats in the United States varies with the species of fungus.[31b, 34] The incidence may also depend on the climate and on the amount of time the animal spends outdoors and thus more exposed to geophilic species. In general, the incidence for dogs in the northern hemisphere can be summarized as follows: (1) *M. canis* is high in the period from October to February and low from March to September; (2) *M. gypseum* is high in the period from July to November and low from December to June; (3) *T. mentagrophytes* is present all year, with a peak occurring in November and December. In general, the incidence for cats can be summarized as follows: (1) *M. canis* varies little all year; (2) *M. gypseum* and *T. mentagrophytes* are seldom reported in cats, but a slight increase may occur during the summer and fall months. Other fungi reported to cause dermatophytosis in cats and dogs are listed in Table 5:2. Rarely, dermatophytosis in dogs and cats is caused by simultaneous infection with two different fungi.[18, 19, 21]

Dermatophytes are transmitted by contact with infected hair and scale or fungal elements on animals, in the environment, or on fomites.[1, 9, 29, 30, 43a] Combs, brushes, clippers, bedding,

*See references 1, 10, 17, 22, 29, 30, 51, and 59.
†See references 1, 10, 17, 22, 29, 30, 51, and 59.

transport cages, and other paraphernalia associated with the grooming, movement, and housing of animals are all potential sources of infection and re-infection. *M. canis* can be cultured from dust, heating vents, and furnace filters.[43a] Visitors to catteries and multiple-households may introduce organisms. The source of *M. canis* infections is usually an infected cat. *Trichophyton* spp. infections are usually acquired directly or indirectly by exposure to typical reservoir hosts, which may be determined by specific identification of the fungal species or subspecies. For example, most *T. mentagrophytes* infections are associated with exposure to rodents or their immediate environment. *M. gypseum* is a geophilic dermatophyte that inhabits rich soil. Cats and dogs are usually exposed to it by digging and rooting in contaminated areas. Infections with anthropophilic species are rare; they are acquired as reverse zoonoses by contact with infected humans. Hair shafts containing infectious arthrospores may remain infectious in the environment for many months, for example, up to 18 months in the case of *M. canis.**

When an animal is exposed to a dermatophyte, an infection may be established. Mechanical disruption of the stratum corneum appears to be important in facilitating the penetration and invasion of anagen hair follicles.[1, 9, 10, 43a, 46, 54] Hair is invaded in both ectothrix and endothrix infections. The ectothrix fungi produce masses of arthrospores on the surface of hair shafts, whereas endothrix fungi do not. Fungal hyphae invade the ostium of hair follicles, proliferate on the surface of hairs, and migrate downward (proximally) to the hair bulb, during which time the fungus produces its own keratinolytic enzymes (keratinases) that allow penetration of the hair cuticle and growth within the hair shaft until the keratogenous zone (Adamson's fringe) is reached. At this point, the fungus either establishes an equilibrium between its downward growth and the production of keratin or it is expelled. Spontaneous resolution occurs when infected hairs enter the telogen phase or if an inflammatory reaction is incited. When a hair enters telogen, keratin production slows and stops; because the dermatophyte requires actively growing hairs for survival, fungal growth also slows and stops. Infectious arthrospores may remain on the hair shaft, but re-infection of that particular hair follicle does not occur until it re-enters anagen.

Cutaneous inflammation is due to toxins produced in the stratum corneum that provoke a sort of biological contact dermatitis.[5, 9, 10, 29, 30] Host factors are poorly documented, but the host's ability to mount an inflammatory response plays a critical role in determining the type of clinical lesions produced and in terminating the infection. Dermatophyte infections in healthy dogs and cats are often self-limiting. Conversely, the relatively poor inflammatory response of most typical feline dermatophyte lesions produced by *M. canis* attests to the cat's relative tolerance of this fungus, and probably accounts for the high rate of asymptomatic carriage of this species among cats.[10, 29, 30, 43a] It has been shown that *T. rubrum* and *T. mentagrophytes* produce substances (especially mannans) that diminish cell-mediated immune responses and indirectly inhibit stratum corneum turnover.[25b] These effects could predispose the animal to persistent or recurrent infections.

As with many infectious diseases, young animals are predisposed to acquiring symptomatic dermatophyte infections.† This is partly due to a delay in development of adequate host immunity. However, differences in biochemical properties of the skin and skin secretions (especially sebum), the growth and replacement of hair, and the physiologic status of the host as related to age may also play a role. Local factors, such as the mechanical barrier of intact skin and the fungistatic activity of sebum caused by its fatty acid content, are deterrents to fungal invasion.

Natural and experimental infections have been shown to incite various forms of hypersensitivity in their hosts.‡ When intradermal injections of *M. canis* glycoprotein antigens were given to normal cats and cats that had recovered from *M. canis* dermatophytosis, all previously

---

*See references 1, 9, 10, 29, 30, 40, and 43a.

†See references 1, 10, 22, 29, 30, 34, 37, and 59.

‡See references 1, 5, 9, 26b, 29, 30, 31a, 48a, and 53c.

infected cats developed immediate and delayed-type hypersensitivity reactions. By comparison, the control cats failed to develop delayed-type hypersensitivity reactions and, uncommonly (20 per cent of animals), developed immediate hypersensitivity reactions.[26] There is no correlation between circulating antibodies and protection. It is believed that the cell-mediated immune response is the mainstay of the body against fungal infection. This is corroborated by the increased incidence of fungal infections in patients with various acquired or inherited forms of immunosuppression, such as feline leukemia virus (FeLV) infection, feline immunodeficiency virus (FIV) infection, and cancer; poor nutrition and anti-inflammatory or immunosuppressive drug therapy (such as glucocorticoids) also lead to an increased incidence.* The stress of pregnancy and lactation may increase susceptibility to fungal infection.[23, 43a] The presence of ectoparasites, especially fleas and *Cheyletiella* mites, can be very important in the establishment and spread of dermatophytosis in catteries and multiple-cat households.[23, 43a]

CLINICAL FINDINGS

When clinicians rely on clinical signs alone, dermatophytosis (ringworm, tinea) is greatly overdiagnosed, especially in dogs. In studies of skin diseases in dogs and cats, the incidence of dermatophytosis is low, accounting for only 0.26 to 3.6 per cent of all cases examined.[17, 34, 37, 53a] The analysis of cultures submitted from suspected dermatophytosis cases in dogs and cats generally reveals that between 2.1 and 31 per cent (average 15 per cent) are positive.[17, 29, 34, 53b] Several other dermatoses, especially staphylococcal folliculitis and demodicosis, mimic the classic ringworm lesion. On the other hand, dermatophytosis is a diagnosis that is often missed because of the protean nature of the dermatologic findings.[10, 29, 30]

Because the infection is almost always follicular in dogs and cats, the most consistent clinical sign is one or many circular patches of alopecia with variable scaling.[29, 30] Some patients may develop the classic ring lesion with central healing and fine follicular papules and crusts at the periphery. However, signs and symptoms are highly variable and depend on the host-fungus interaction and, therefore, the degree of inflammation. Pruritus is usually minimal or absent; however, it is occasionally marked and suggests an ectoparasitism or allergy. In addition, dermatophytosis may be complicated by secondary bacterial (usually staphylococcal) infection. In vitro studies have shown that dermatophytes can produce antibiotic substances and encourage the development of penicillin-resistant staphylococci.[16, 34a]

Dog

Dogs more often exhibit the classic annular areas of peripherally expanding alopecia, scale, crust, and follicular papules and pustules (Fig. 5:1 *A, B, C,* and *D*). However, less common syndromes are frequent enough that dermatophytosis should be considered in the differential diagnosis of any annular, papular, or pustular eruption. Symmetric nasal or facial folliculitis and furunculosis, mimicking autoimmune skin disease, may be caused by a dermatophyte, especially *T. mentagrophytes*; (Fig. 5:2; also see Fig. 5:1 *E* and *F*) and *Microsporum persicolor* (Fig. 5:3). *Trichophyton* infections may also present as folliculitis and furunculosis affecting one paw or one leg (see Fig. 5:1 *G*). These infections often scar significantly; following a cure, there may be residual areas of scarring alopecia. A seborrhea-like eruption with greasy scale may be seen with generalized infections. The dermatophyte kerion is a boggy, exudative, variably well-circumscribed, nodular type of furunculosis that develops multiple draining tracts. It is often associated with *M. gypseum* or *T. mentagrophytes* infections (see Fig. 5:1 *H*). Onychomycosis is rare[13a]; it is usually associated with *T. mentagrophytes* and may present as an asymmetric (one digit, or multiple digits on one paw) paronychia or onychodystrophy.

In general, the nature of the dermatophyte cannot be determined from the clinical presenta-

---

*See references 4, 5, 9, 23, 29, 30, and 38.

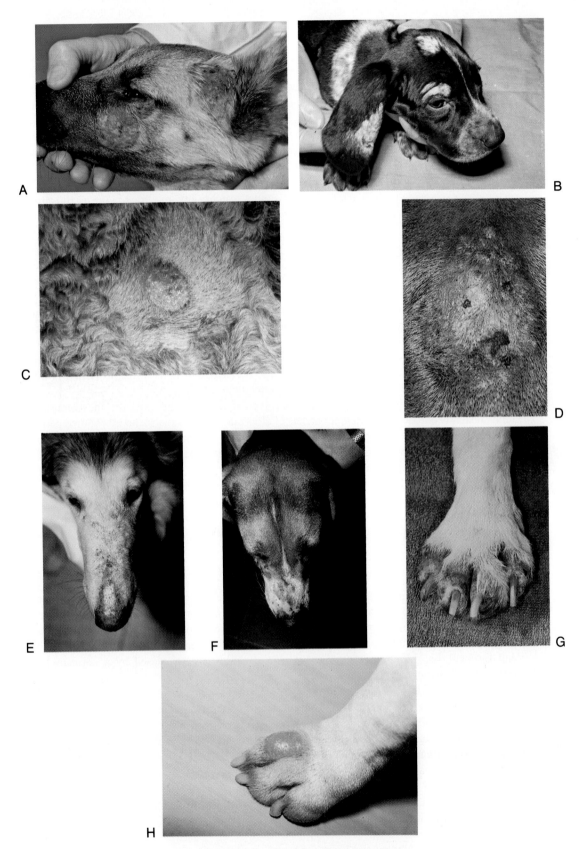

Figure 5:1 *See legend on opposite page*

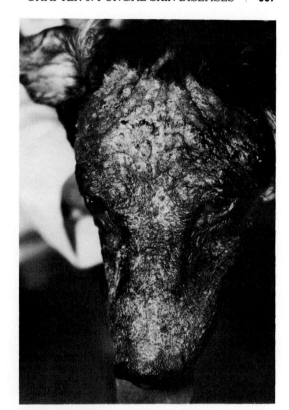

Figure 5:2. Extensive facial dermatitis in a dog caused by *T. mentagrophytes*.

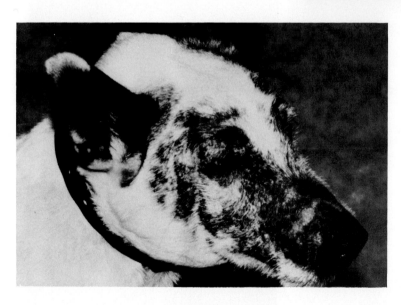

Figure 5:3. Chronic facial dermatitis with areas of hyperpigmentation and depigmentation in a dog caused by *M. persicolor*. (Courtesy D. Carlotti.)

Figure 5:1. Dermatophytosis. *A*, German shepherd puppy with annular inflammatory lesions below the eye and cranial to the pinna caused by *M. canis*. (Courtesy B. Farrow.) *B*, Pointer puppy with well-circumscribed areas of alopecia and grayish crusts above the eye and on the pinna caused by *M. canis*. *C*, Annular, erythematous, oozing, pruritic lesion resembling pyotraumatic dermatitis on a Poodle caused by *M. canis*. *D*, Crusted follicular papules and pustules on the bridge of the nose of a dog caused by *M. persicolor*. (Courtesy D. Carlotti.) *E*, Collie with a crusting, erosive, alopecic dermatitis on the bridge of the nose caused by *T. mentagrophytes*. *F*, Coonhound with a highly inflammatory nasal dermatitis caused by *T. mentagrophytes*. *G*, Severe pododermatitis in a beagle caused by *T. mentagrophytes*. *H*, Kerion on the digit of a dog caused by *M. gypseum*. Note the pinpoint draining tracts.

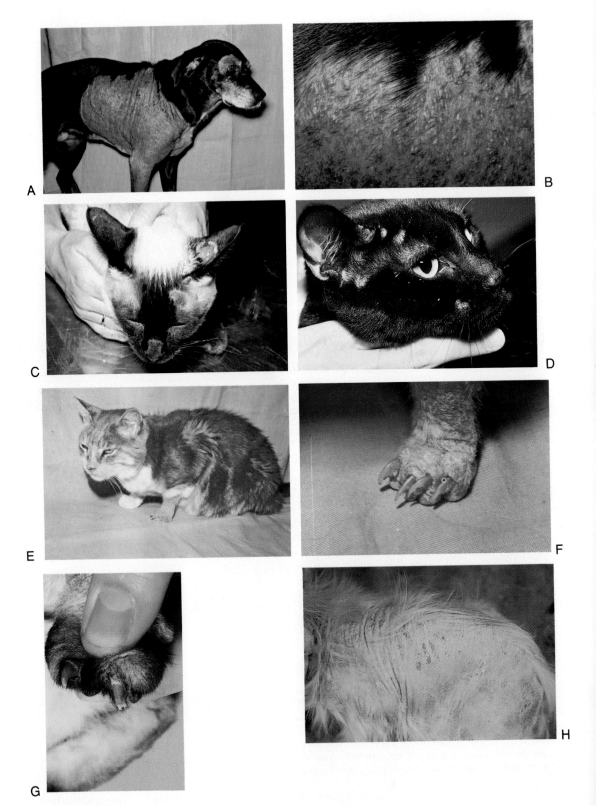

Figure 5:4 *See legend on opposite page*

tion. Dermatophyte infections are most often localized, with lesions occurring most commonly on the face, pinnae, paws, and tail.* Whereas dermatophytosis is usually a disease of young animals (less than 1 year old),[34] sylvatic ringworm (that acquired from wild mammals) occurs more commonly in adults.[59] *M. persicolor* is an increasingly recognized cause of dermatophytosis in Europe,[17a, 18, 20, 22, 59] where it typically produces facial lesions that may be predominantly scaly or papulopustular and crusty; in addition, concurrent depigmentation of the nasal planum and nostrils may occur. Extensive dermatophytosis in older dogs may be seen in association with concurrent immunosuppressive diseases (e.g., cancer, hyperadrenocorticism) or inappropriate systemic glucocorticoid therapy (Fig. 5:4 *A* and *B*). In Europe, it has been reported that dermatophytosis occurs more commonly in the Jack Russell terrier, Yorkshire terrier, and Pekinese.[48, 59]

Cat

Feline dermatophytosis most often appears as one or more irregular or annular areas of alopecia with or without scale (Fig. 5:4 *C* and *D*). Hairs in these areas often appear broken and frayed. Follicular hyperkeratosis may result in exaggerated hair follicle openings or comedo formation. The alopecia may be severe and widespread, accompanied by little evidence of inflammation. Cats occasionally have more inflammatory areas of folliculitis characterized by alopecia, erythema, scale, crust, and follicular papules (Fig. 5:4 *E* and *F*). The so-called *miliary dermatitis*, which is characterized by an often pruritic, widespread, papulocrustous dermatitis, is an uncommon manifestation of dermatophytosis that is usually caused by *M. canis*. Recurring chin folliculitis resembling feline acne may be seen.[23] Onychomycosis is rare;[13b] it is usually caused by *M. canis* and may present as an asymmetric (one digit, or multiple digits on one paw) paronychia or onychodystrophy (Fig. 5:4 *G*). Generalized seborrhea-like eruptions can be seen wherein dry or greasy scale is prominent. The condition is usually due to *M. canis*. Widespread, pruritic, exfoliative erythroderma is occasionally seen in association with *M. canis* (Fig. 5:4 *H*). Dermatophyte kerion reactions are occasionally seen in the cat, as are cases of otitis externa due to *M. canis*.[28] Dermatophytic pseudomycetoma has been reported only in Persian cats; it is characterized by one or more subcutaneous nodules that are often ulcerated and discharging. The nodules occur most commonly over the dorsal trunk or tail base (Fig. 5:5 *A* and *B*). These cats may have more typical, superficial dermatophyte lesions on other areas of the body, or they may be clinically normal except for the nodules.[8, 37, 42, 60]

In general, the nature of the dermatophyte cannot be determined from the clinical presentation. Lesions occur most commonly on the head, pinnae, and paws.† Generalized dermatophyte infection is more common in cats than in dogs.[34] As with dogs, dermatophytosis is more common in young cats (less than 1 year old),[34] but sylvatic ringworm occurs more commonly in adults.[59] Longhaired cats, especially Persians and Himalayans, are predisposed to this infection.[23, 34, 48, 53a]

---

*See references 17, 22, 24, 25, 29, 30, 33, 34, 36, 37, 45, 52, 55, 56, and 59.
†See references 12, 17, 22, 29, 30, 34, 37, 59.

Figure 5:4. Dermatophytosis. *A*, Chronic widespread dermatitis in an old dog caused by *T. mentagrophytes*. Note the strikingly well-circumscribed nature of the lesions. *B*, Close-up of the dog in *A* showing the erythematous papulovesicular dermatitis. *C*, Classic "ringworm" lesions on the left pinna and dorsal to the left eye in a Siamese cat caused by *M. canis*. *D*, Multiple annular areas of alopecia and grayish crusts on the face of a cat caused by *M. canis*. *E*, Well-circumscribed areas of alopecia and erythema on the muzzle and left front paw of a cat caused by *T. mentagrophytes*. *F*, Closer view of the paw lesion in E. *G*, Brownish paronychial exudate, leukonychia, and onychorrhexis in a cat caused by *M. canis*. *H*, Generalized exfoliative erythroderma in a Persian cat caused by *M. canis*. (Courtesy G. Wilkinson.)

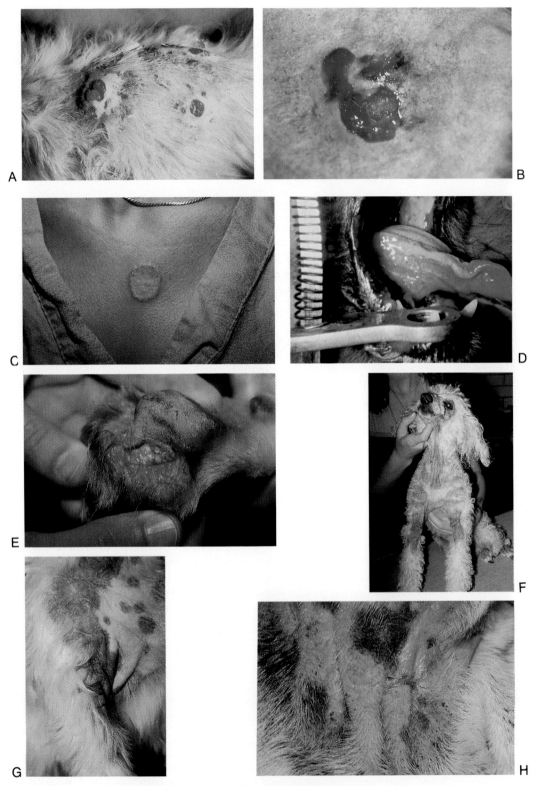

Figure 5:5 *See legend on opposite page*

Zoonotic Aspects

About 30 per cent of all cases of microsporosis and about 15 per cent of all cases of dermatophytosis (tinea) in humans are caused by *M. canis*, the vast majority of these infections being acquired from cats.[15a, 25a, 29, 53] Approximately 50 per cent of humans exposed to symptomatic or asymptomatic infected cats acquire the infection.[29, 46a, 57] In about 30 to 70 per cent of all households with infected cats, at least one person in the household becomes infected.[29, 46a, 53, 58a] The cutaneous changes with animal-origin dermatophytosis in humans are variable and most commonly occur on areas of the body that contact infected animals, such as the arms, scalp, and trunk (Fig. 5:5 *C*).[4, 53]

DIAGNOSIS

The differential diagnosis for dermatophytosis is extensive as a result of the variable clinical appearance of the disease. Because most infections are follicular, the primary differential diagnoses are staphylococcal folliculitis and demodicosis. In dogs, staphylococcal folliculitis is much more common than dermatophytosis.[29, 30, 53b] In fact, the following adage is very useful regarding dogs: "If it looks like ringworm, it is probably not! It is probably staphylococcal folliculitis!" In cats, however, dermatophytosis is more common than demodicosis and staphylococcal folliculitis. Other causes of annular areas of alopecia, crusts, and variable inflammation include pemphigus foliaceus and erythematosus, *Pelodera* dermatitis, flea bite hypersensitivity, food hypersensitivity, seborrheic dermatitis, subcorneal pustular dermatosis, and the various sterile eosinophilic folliculitides. Although alopecia areata produces annular areas of alopecia, the alopecic skin appears otherwise normal. Dermatophyte kerions may resemble other infectious or foreign-body granulomas, acral lick dermatitis, or neoplasms such as histiocytoma, mast cell tumor, and lymphoma. Dermatophytic pseudomycetoma must be differentiated from other infectious or foreign-body granulomas, sterile panniculitis, and various neoplasms.

History taking may be of limited value unless exposure is known to have occurred; this is so because clinical dermatophytosis is so variable, and the incubation period is poorly defined (in general, 4 days to 4 weeks).[10] The number, types, and sources of contact animals should be determined. The source of kittens and puppies presented for examination should be ascertained because animals from some breeding establishments, pet shops, or animal shelters may have a high incidence of infection. Evidence for contagion—in other animals or human contacts—should be sought.

Fungal tests are very useful in diagnosis. These tests are described in detail in Chapter 2.

Wood's lamp examination for fluorescence causes only certain strains of *M. canis, M. audouinii, M. distortum,* and *Trichophyton schoenleinii* to produce a positive yellow-green color on infected hairs.[1, 7, 10] Only about 50 per cent of *M. canis* infections fluoresce.* Several important pitfalls exist in the use and interpretation of the Wood's lamp (see Chap. 2).

---

*See references 7, 10, 17, 22, 29, 37, 43a, 48, 57, and 59.

Figure 5:5. Dermatophytosis and yeast infections. *A,* Ulcerated nodules (dermatophytic pseudomycetoma) over the back of a cat due to *Trichophyton* sp. *B,* Close-up of lesion in *A. C,* Annular erythema and scaling with a slightly raised papulovesicular border in a human caused by *M. canis. D,* Candidiasis in a dog. Note the whitish gray plaque on the cheek and the linear lesion on the tongue. (Courtesy N. Field.) *E,* Candidiasis in a dog. Multiple whitish gray, mucoid plaques on markedly erythematous interdigital skin. *F,* Malasseziasis. Note the symmetric, greasy, erythematous dermatitis in a poodle. (Courtesy K. Mason.) *G,* Malasseziasis secondary to atopy and glucocorticoid therapy in a Lhasa apso. Note erythema, alopecia, hyperpigmentation, lichenification, and yellowish crusts in the axilla and on the medial forearm. *H,* Malasseziasis in intertriginous areas of an English bulldog. Note moist, erythematous, alopecic dermatitis of the ventral neck.

Microscopic examination of plucked hairs and scraped scales may reveal hyphae and arthrospores in 40 to 70 per cent of the cases, and it is definitive evidence of dermatophytosis (see Chap. 2).* *M. persicolor* and *Epidermophyton floccosum* do not invade hairs, and could be called true epidermophytes.[1, 17a, 18, 20, 29]

Fungal culture of affected hair and scale is the most reliable diagnostic test and is the only way to identify the specific dermatophyte.[1, 17, 29, 30, 43a, 59] Caution is warranted here, however, because dermatophytes may be cultured from the haircoat and skin of normal cats and dogs as well as those with nonfungal skin diseases. These dermatophyte isolates may reflect a true carrier state or recent exposure to a contaminated environment (such as hunting dogs and *M. gypseum*). Although dermatophyte test medium is widely used and recommended for culturing dermatophytes,[17, 29, 30, 37, 43a] some mycologists have reported it to be unreliable and inferior to Sabouraud's dextrose agar.[48, 59] In addition, some *M. canis* isolates do not produce the initial red color change on dermatophyte test medium.[43b]

Biopsy findings are as variable as the clinical lesions, and they are not as sensitive as culture.[6, 10, 29, 30] On the other hand, when the true significance of a cultural isolation is questioned, demonstration of the organism in biopsy specimens is definitive proof of true infection. Histopathologic examination is most useful in the nodular forms of dermatophytosis—the kerion and pseudomycetoma. It may be impossible to culture the organism in such cases by collecting hair and scale. The most common histopathologic patterns observed in dermatophytosis are (1) perifolliculitis, folliculitis, and furunculosis (Figs. 5:6 and 5:7); (2) hyperplastic or spongiotic superficial perivascular or interstitial dermatitis with prominent parakeratotic or orthokeratotic hyperkeratosis of the epidermis and hair follicles; and (3) intraepidermal pustular dermatitis (suppurative, neutrophilic epidermitis). In *M. persicolor* infections, fungal hyphae are found only in the surface keratin.[17a] Dermatophytic pseudomycetoma is characterized by nodular to diffuse, granulomatous to pyogranulomatous panniculitis and dermatitis wherein the fungus is present as broad (2.5 to 4.5 μm), hyaline, septate hyphae,

---

*See references 1, 10, 17, 29, 30, 43a, 57, and 59.

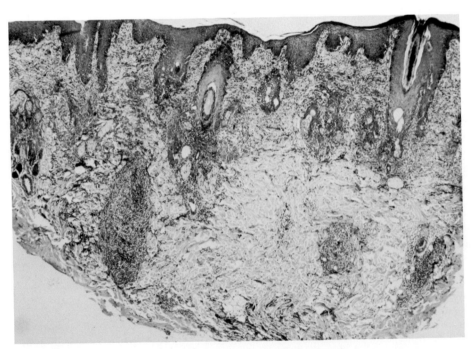

Figure 5:6. Follicularly oriented inflammation in a cat with dermatophytosis.

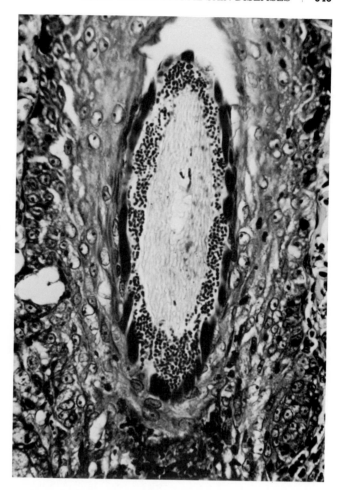

Figure 5:7. *Microsporum canis* in a cat. Note arthroconidia surrounding hair shaft. (AOG stain).

chainlike pseudohyphae, and large (12 μm) chlamydospore-like cells within grains or granules (pseudogranules) (Figs. 5:8 and 5:9). In cats with alopecia that does not appear clinically to be inflammatory, biopsy findings often reveal enormous numbers of arthrospores and hyphae associated with infected hairs, minimal lymphohistiocytic perivascular dermatitis or no apparent inflammation, and minimal orthokeratotic hyperkeratosis. Septate fungal hyphae and spherical to ovoid arthrospores may be present in and around infected hairs, in hair follicles, and within the stratum corneum of the surface epidermis. The number of fungal elements present is often inversely proportional to the severity of the inflammatory response.

Asymptomatic carriage of dermatophytes, especially of *M. canis* in cats, represents a very important and often unsuspected threat to animals and humans. In show cats, cattery cats, and cats that frequent veterinary clinics, from 6.5 to 100 per cent of the animals may be asymptomatic carriers of *M. canis*.* In one study,[43b] *M. canis* was isolated just as commonly from shorthaired cats as from longhaired cats. However, healthy pet cats and stray cats were rarely positive for *M. canis*.[40, 43a, 57] In dogs, asymptomatic carriage of *M. canis* is less common, with 0 to 10 per cent of the animals having positive fungal cultures.[22, 29, 48, 60a] Culturing asymptomatic cats and dogs requires using the brush (toothbrush, surgical scrub brush) or carpet-square method (see Chap. 2).

---

*See references 10, 15, 22, 29, 43a, 43b, 48, 50a, 57, 58c, and 60a.

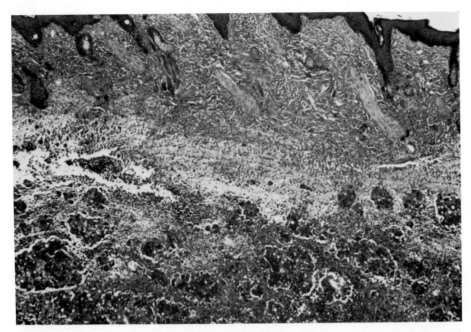

Figure 5:8. Subcutaneous dermatophytosis in a cat (*Trichophyton* sp.). Diffuse panniculitis with tissue grains.

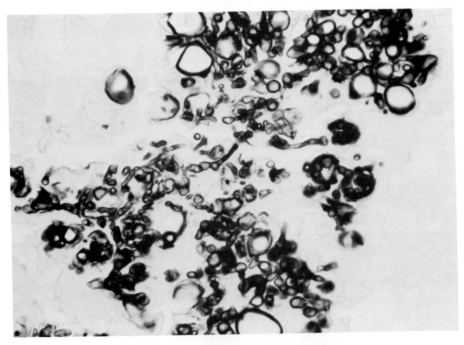

Figure 5:9. Subcutaneous dermatophytosis (*Trichophyton* sp.). Numerous hyphae with bulbous dilatations (Gomori's methanamine-silver [GMS] stain).

CLINICAL MANAGEMENT

Dermatophytosis in healthy dogs and shorthaired cats often undergoes spontaneous remission within 4 months.[10, 29, 30, 39, 59] Animals with generalized dermatophytosis, however, usually, but not always,[41a] require aggressive therapy. Even longhaired cats can undergo spontaneous resolution, but it may take 1½ to 4 years.[39, 43a] In general, sylvatic ringworm (especially *M. persicolor* and *Trichophyton* spp.) in dogs does not spontaneously resolve and requires aggressive therapy.[17a, 29, 30, 59] However, it has been reported that several cases of *T. mentagrophytes* infection in cats resolved spontaneously.[59] The goals of therapy are (1) to maximize the patient's ability to respond to the dermatophyte infection (by the correction of any nutritional imbalances and concurrent disease states, and by the termination of systemic anti-inflammatory and immunosuppressive drugs), (2) to reduce contagion (to the environment, other animals, and humans), and (3) to hasten resolution of the infection.

Topical Therapy

Every confirmed case of dermatophytosis should receive topical therapy.[29, 30, 39, 40] Hair is clipped from a wide margin (6 cm) surrounding all lesions.[29, 30, 32] Clipping should be done gently (scissors or number 10 clipper blade) so as to avoid traumatizing the skin and encouraging the spread of infection. Longhaired animals should be clipped entirely.* Clipped hair is carefully disposed of. The authors applaud and echo the warning of Carney and Moriello[23] concerning symptomatic longhaired cats: "Never anticipate a cure for dermatophytosis if the owner is unwilling to shave the cat." Creams and lotions are available for use on focal lesions, and these are typically applied every 12 hours, to include a 6-cm margin of clinically normal skin, if possible. There is a wide variety of topical antifungals available, and there is no particular advantage of one product over another (Table 5:3). For highly inflamed lesions, a product containing glucocorticoid in combination with antifungal agents may hasten resolution of clinical disease. However, because the glucocorticoid can be absorbed systemically, it is not recommended in the treatment of very young kittens and puppies or pregnant queens and bitches. Clipping and spot-treatment of dogs with focal lesions is usually curative.[22, 29, 30, 39]

For dogs and cats with multifocal or generalized skin involvement, antifungal shampoos, rinses (dips), or both are indicated. Cats that have focal lesions should also be given this treatment because they inevitably have or soon will have widespread to generalized infected hairs but are often asymptomatic.[30, 39, 40, 43a] Rinses are preferred because the entire body surface can be treated and the antifungal agent can be allowed to dry on the skin. These rinses can be applied daily—which increases the owner's time and economic commitment as well as the likelihood of excessive drying or irritation of the pet's skin—but an application every 5 to 7 days usually suffices. In a 1993 study,[58b] lime sulfur, enilconazole, chlorhexidine, and povidone-iodine were rapidly effective topical antifungal agents against *M. canis*. Ketoconazole and sodium hypochlorite were also effective, but these agents took longer to produce negative culture results. Hairs treated with captan never became culture negative. Topical medicaments are continued for 2 weeks beyond clinical cure or until fungal cultures are negative. Povidone-iodine and sodium hypochlorite are not recommended for use directly on cats because of frequent skin irritation.[10, 23]

Systemic Therapy

Dogs and cats that are not responding to topical therapy after a 2- to 4-week course of treatment should receive systemic therapy (Table 5:4).[23, 30, 39, 40] Griseofulvin is the drug of choice.†

---

*See references 22, 23, 29, 30, 39, 40, and 43a.
†See references 23, 29, 30, 39, 40, 43a, 43c, and 59.

Table 5:3. Products for Topical Treatment of Dermatophytosis

Product	Administration	Comments
Focal Lesions		
Chlorhexidine 1% ointment*	Apply q12h	Rarely irritating
Clotrimazole 1% cream†	Apply q12h	Occasionally irritating
Clotrimazole 1% and betamethasone 0.1% cream‡	Apply q12h	For highly inflamed lesions
Econazole 2% cream§	Apply q12h	Occasionally irritating
Ketoconazole 2% cream‖	Apply q12h	Occasionally irritating
Miconazole 2% cream or 1% lotion¶	Apply q12h	Occasionally irritating
Thiabendazole 4% and dexamethasone 0.1% lotion**	Apply q12h	For highly inflamed lesions
Widespread or Generalized Lesions		
Chlorhexidine 0.5% shampoo††	Bathe q1–3d	Rarely irritating
Chlorhexidine 2% solution‡‡	Rinse q1–3d	Rarely irritating, corneal ulcers
Enilconazole§§	0.2% rinse q3d	Not in United States
Ketoconazole 2% shampoo‖‖	Bathe q1–3d	Occasionally irritating
Lime sulfur¶¶	2% rinse q5–7d	Odorous, tarnishes jewelry, stains white animals and fabrics, drying, occasionally irritating
Miconazole 2% shampoo***	Bathe q1–3d	Occasionally irritating
Povidone-iodine 2% solution†††	0.4% rinse q1–3d	Irritating, sensitizing, staining
Sodium hypochlorite 0.5% solution§§§	Rinse q5–7d	Bleaches haircoat and fabrics, occasionally irritating

*Nolvasan (Fort Dodge). †Lotrimin (Schering). ‡Lotrisone (Schering). §Spectazole (Ortho). ‖Nizoral (Janssen). ¶Conofite (Pitman-Moore). **Tresaderm (Merck). ††Nolvasan (Fort Dodge). ‡‡Nolvasan (Fort Dodge). §§Imaveral (Janssen). ‖‖Nizoral (Janssen). ¶¶Lym Dyp (DVM). ***Dermazole (Allerderm). †††Weladol (Pitman-Moore). ‡‡‡Weladol (Pitman-Moore). §§§Clorox (Clorox).

Dosage and frequency protocols vary widely. Side-effects are uncommon and generally mild in dogs; they may be more common and potentially severe, however, in cats, especially Persians, Himalayans, Siamese, and Abyssinians.[23, 40, 43a] Side-effects are especially severe in cats with FIV infection, so griseofulvin probably should be avoided in these cats.[39, 43a] Griseofulvin is a teratogen and must never be used during the first two thirds of pregnancy. The reader is referred to Chapter 3 for details concerning the use of griseofulvin in dogs and cats.

Ketoconazole is very effective in the treatment of dermatophytoses in dogs and cats and has supplanted griseofulvin as the standard approach to systemic therapy in Europe.* However, ketoconazole is not labeled for use in dogs and cats in the United States, and most veterinarians reserve this drug for those cases in which griseofulvin resistance is encountered, or when the patient cannot tolerate griseofulvin.[29, 30, 39, 40, 43a] Although concern has been expressed about the

*See references 18, 19, 21, 22, 27, 29, 30, 39, 41, and 48.

Table 5:4. Products for Systemic Treatment of Dermatophytosis

Product	Dose (mg/kg)	Interval
Griseofulvin		
Microsized*	25–60	q12h
Ultramicrosized†	2.5–15	q12h
Itraconazole‡	10–20	q24–48h
Ketoconazole§	10	q12–24h

*Fulvicin U/F (Schering). †Gris-PEG (Herbert). ‡Sporanox (Janssen). §Nizoral (Janssen).

efficacy of ketoconazole against *M. canis*,[29, 30] and a report has indicated that about 50 per cent of the *M. canis* isolates from cats showed in vitro resistance to ketoconazole,[49] such concerns and in vitro findings have not been corroborated either clinically or by other in vitro studies.[30a, 31] The reader is referred to Chapter 3 for details on the use of ketoconazole in dogs and cats.

Itraconazole appears to be effective as therapy for the dermatophytoses of dogs and cats.[39, 40, 43c] However, it is not labeled for use in dogs and cats in the United States. Itraconazole may be useful when griseofulvin resistance or toxicity are encountered, or when animals cannot tolerate ketoconazole. The reader is referred to Chapter 3 for details concerning the use of itraconazole in dogs and cats.

It is important to remember that systemic antifungal therapy does not rapidly reduce contagion and is always to be used in conjunction with clipping and topical antifungal agents.* Systemic antifungal agents are administered for 2 weeks beyond clinical cure, or until fungal culture is negative, which usually requires 4 to 20 weeks. The successful treatment of infected claws always requires systemic antifungal agents (usually for 6 to 12 months) or onychectomy.[10, 29, 30, 39, 40] Dermatophytic pseudomycetoma in cats is often frustrating to treat. Lesions usually recur following wide surgical excision, and griseofulvin and ketoconazole are often ineffective or only partially effective.[29, 30, 39, 40, 42] One cat with dermatophytic pseudomycetoma was cured after 10 months of treatment with itraconazole, and another cat's disease was controlled after 18 months.[39, 40]

Fungal vaccines have been successful in Europe in the management of endemic dermatophytoses in cattle and foxes.[29, 50b] A killed *M. canis* vaccine administered to normal cats appeared to induce a similar antibody titer but less cellular immunity than those produced by clinical infection.[26a] Although there is one report[44] that has described the use of a fungal vaccine in the treatment of dermatophytosis in a cat, there have been no controlled studies published on the use of fungal vaccines to treat or prevent dermatophytosis in cats and dogs. Small companies are selling so-called *M. canis* vaccines, but their efficacy has not been demonstrated and none of them has Food and Drug Administration (FDA) approval. It is recommended that these preparations be avoided until safety and efficacy are demonstrated.[23] In the United States, a killed *M. canis* vaccine (Fort Dodge Laboratories) has recently become available for the treatment and prevention of dermatophytosis in cats. Because there is currently no published scientific information on this product, the authors cannot recommend it.

Local hyperthermia was reported to be effective therapy for focal dermatophyte lesions in dogs and cats.[35] However, such therapy is not readily accessible, it requires chemical restraint, and it is impractical for multifocal or generalized disease.

A critical feature of clinical management is the treatment of all dogs and cats in contact with the infected animal and treatment of the environment.[29, 30, 40]

Chronic and recurring cases of dermatophytosis are usually associated with (1) inappropriate therapy, including wrong drug or wrong drug dosage, inadequate duration of therapy, failure to use topicals, failure to clip the haircoat, failure to treat all other animals in the house, and failure to treat the environment; (2) underlying diseases, e.g., hyperadrenocorticism, diabetes mellitus, FeLV infection, FIV infection, or cancer; or (3) immunosuppressive drug therapy.[23, 29, 30, 38]

Management of Catteries and Multiple-Cat Households

The elimination of dermatophytosis in a cattery or other multiple-cat facility requires the separation of carriers from noncarriers, the treatment or destruction of infected animals, and the institution of measures to prevent re-infection of the premises.[23, 43a] Successful elimination of dermatophytosis requires aggressive systemic and topical therapy, interruption of breeding

---

*See references 10, 17, 29, 30, 39, 40, and 43a.

programs and show campaigns, isolation of the colony, environmental decontamination, and the testing and isolation of future cattery or household members. Such control programs are complicated by the cost of medical expenses, by the loss of revenue from the sale of cats and kittens, by the time commitment and effort required, and by the fear of permanent damage to the reputation of the cattery. This fear is often the most difficult obstacle to overcome.

M. canis is the dermatophyte involved in almost all cattery and multiple-cat household infections, especially in longhairs.[29, 30, 40, 43a] However, both *M. gypseum* and *T. mentagrophytes* have been responsible for cattery dermatophytosis in instances in which the cats were housed in screened porch buildings or outdoor runs.[23]

Control options include three general approaches.[23, 43a] The first requires total depopulation of the cattery or household, decontamination of the facility, and repopulation with only animals that test negative on three consecutive brush cultures performed at 2-week intervals. Most breeders reject this because of the loss of their gene pool. The second approach requires treatment of the entire colony and facilities with appropriate topical medications, systemic therapy, and environmental clean-up. The colony is isolated, and breeding and showing are interrupted. The third option is to treat only the kittens. This is practical only for catteries, pet shops, or kitten mills that produce kittens for the pet cat market. The following recommendations have been reprinted, with only slight modification, from Moriello's excellent article.[43a]

Specific Recommendations for the Treatment of Infected Catteries

■ *Cats*

1. Perform toothbrush fungal cultures on all cats in the cattery and all animals in the household.
2. Isolate any animals that are found to be free of *M. canis*. These animals should be quarantined in a separate facility. Reculture these animals because they will probably be found to be infected with *M. canis* when recultured.
3. Isolate the cattery. Cats should not be sold, shown, or sent on breeding loans. New members should not be added, and breeding programs should be interrupted.
4. Clip the entire haircoat of all cats, especially those of longhaired cats. Be sure that all whiskers are clipped. Clipping should be performed in a room that is easy to decontaminate. The infected hairs should be burned. The individual performing the clipping should be dressed in disposable clothing to prevent infection from animal to human. Clipping should be repeated every month until the infection is eliminated.
5. Begin aggressive topical therapy with an antifungal shampoo followed by an antifungal dip. Treatment intervals will vary, depending on the product selected and the number of cats in the cattery. Ideally, cats should be treated twice a week; this is the most cost-effective approach. The haircoat should be kept short. Topical antifungal preparations can be applied to clinical lesions.
6. If, after 4 to 8 weeks of therapy, the cats are still culture positive, initiate oral griseofulvin therapy in all **nonpregnant** queens and kittens older than 12 weeks of age. Topical therapy should be continued. Monitoring complete blood counts and platelet counts in all cats, and especially in Persians, Himalayans, Abyssinians, and Siamese cats, is highly recommended. Many clients refuse to have precautionary blood work performed because of the cost. Be sure to warn clients clearly of the potential for toxicity.
7. The duration of treatment is variable and may last from weeks to months. Continue treatment until **all** cats are culture negative, using the toothbrush technique at least twice.
8. If a griseofulvin-resistant strain is suspected, confirm that the client is administering the griseofulvin correctly. If so, submit an *M. canis* culture for griseofulvin and ketoconazole sensitivity testing. It may be necessary to contact the Center for Disease Control to locate the appropriate laboratory for performance of the testing.

■ *Environmental Decontamination*

1. *M. canis* spores remain viable in the environment for up to 18 months. All nonporous surfaces should be thoroughly vacuumed and disinfected, including all floors, walls, countertops, windowsills, and transport vehicles. Chlorhexidine or sodium hypochlorite (1:10 dilution of household bleach) is recommended. Sodium hypochlorite is the most cost-effective antifungal preparation available.
2. Destroy all bedding, rugs, brushes, combs, and the like.
3. Rugs that cannot be destroyed or removed should be washed with an antifungal disinfectant. Be sure to recommend that the client test for colorfastness. Steam cleaning of carpets has been recommended as a method of decontamination. To kill fungal spores, the temperature of the water being forced into the carpets must be at least 43.3°C (110°F). Five do-it-yourself machines were tested to determine whether this was possible. To reach a temperature of 43.3°C (110°F) at the carpet level, the water chamber had to be filled with water exceeding 76.6°C (170°F). In a household situation, achieving this required boiling water to reach this temperature. Unfortunately, the temperature of the water rapidly cooled in the clean water reservoir, and within 15 minutes of filling the chamber, the temperature of the water being forced out of the nozzle was less than 37.7°C (100°F). Steam cleaning of carpets may therefore not be a reliable method of killing *M. canis* unless an antifungal disinfectant such as chlorhexidine or sodium hypochlorite is added to the water.
4. All heating and cooling vents should be vacuumed and disinfected. Furnaces should be cleaned with high-power suction equipment by a commercial company. Furnance filters should be changed weekly.
5. The cattery should be vacuumed daily, preferably twice daily. **Do not use Fans.**
6. Cages should be disinfected daily.
7. Remind the cattery owner to disinfect all portable cages, automobiles, and so forth.
8. **Do not let the cats roam freely in the house or cattery.**

■ *Treatment of Kittens Only.*   In some situations, a cattery owner may be unable or unwilling to treat the entire cattery. If the owner is interested only in producing kittens that are not infected with *M. canis*, an alternative strategy is available. Although this strategy is not ideal, it is a reasonable alternative to depopulation and to the sale of *M. canis*–infected kittens to the public.

1. Isolate breeding and pregnant queens from the remainder of the cattery.
2. Clip the haircoat of the queens.
3. Treat the queens topically with chlorhexidine shampoos and dips twice weekly.
4. After the kittens are born, begin oral griseofulvin therapy in queens. Although griseofulvin is contraindicated in pregnant queens, some feline practitioners have routinely begun administering griseofulvin during the last week of pregnancy and have not observed any ill effects.
5. Wean the kittens as soon as possible, preferably by 4 weeks of age, and isolate them from all other cats. Some cattery owners choose to separate the kittens from the queens at birth and to raise them in isolation.
6. When the kittens are 4 weeks of age, culture all of them with a sterile toothbrush. Pending fungal culture results, begin topical therapy. Chlorhexidine and lime sulfur have been reported to be safe in young kittens. If the fungal culture indicates that the kittens are infected, begin oral griseofulvin therapy. Oral griseofulvin is not recommended for use in kittens less than 12 weeks of age; it has, however, been used in kittens as young as 6 weeks of age without any ill effects. The potential for griseofulvin toxicity should be thoroughly explained to the owner.
7. Kittens should not be sold until at least one, and preferably two, negative fungal cultures have been obtained.

■ *Monitoring Response to Therapy.* Response to therapy in both cats and kittens is best monitored via fungal culturing. The toothbrush culturing technique is recommended. It is critical that the brushing be very aggressive during this period. During treatment, the number of infective spores decreases, and if the individual sampling is not aggressive enough with combing, false-negative results could be obtained. Do not use a Wood's lamp to monitor therapy because this device is much less reliable than culturing.

■ *Preventive Measures.* The prevention of the introduction or re-introduction of *M. canis* into a cattery requires the isolation of any new cats, the isolation of cats returning from shows or breeding loans, and periodic culturing of the entire colony. Cats entering or re-entering the cattery should be cultured for *M. canis* and kept in isolation until the results are obtained. It is suggested that these cats be dipped or washed with one of the previously mentioned products during this isolation period to minimize contamination of the cattery in the event that they are infected. It is difficult to decontaminate the environment, and re-infection is possible. Ideally, there should be no visitors to the cattery so that introduction of the organism from clothing or other fomites can be prevented.

Cat shows present a tremendous threat to an *M. canis*–free cattery because it is extremely difficult to prevent re-infection from occurring and to prevent exposure to spores. The cats should be groomed in an area free of other cats, if possible, and no grooming equipment from other exhibitors should be used. The cat carriers should be covered when cats are not being examined by the judges.

Candidiasis

CAUSE AND PATHOGENESIS

Candida spp. yeasts are normal inhabitants of the alimentary, upper respiratory, and genital mucosa of mammals.[1, 61, 64] *Candida* spp., especially *Candida albicans* and *Candida parapsilosis*, are the most commonly isolated fungi from the ears, nose, oral cavity, and anus of clinically normal dogs, and dogs with candidiasis.[61–64, 67, 69] *Candida tropicalis, Candida pseudotropicalis, Candida krusei, Candida stellatoidea,* and *Candida guilliermondii* are occasionally found. *Candida* species cause opportunistic infections of skin, mucocutaneous areas, external ear canal, and claws. Factors that upset the normal endogenous microflora (prolonged antibiotic therapy) or disrupt normal cutaneous or mucosal barriers (maceration, burns, indwelling catheters) provide a pathway for *Candida* spp. to enter the body.[1, 64, 69] Once in the body, further spread of infection correlates with cell-mediated immunocompetence and neutrophil function.[63–65] Immunosuppressive disease states (diabetes mellitus, hyperadrenocorticism, viral infections, cancer, inherited immunologic defects) or immunosuppressive drug therapy predispose some animals to candidiasis.

Candidiasis has been reported under the following names in earlier literature: *candidosis, moniliasis,* and *thrush.*

CLINICAL FINDINGS

Dog

Candidiasis is a rare disease with a distinct predilection for mucous membranes (see Fig. 5:5 *D*), mucocutaneous junctions, or areas where moisture may persist and macerate the skin, such as the external ear canal and lateral pinnae, intertriginous areas, the clawbed, and interdigital areas (see Fig. 5:5 *E*).[61, 62, 64, 68] On mucous membranes, the lesions appear as foul-smelling, nonhealing ulcers covered with thick, whitish gray plaques with erythematous borders. On the skin, lesions are initially papular and pustular and evolve into oozing erythematous plaques and ulcers.[62, 67, 69] Solitary or locally grouped lesions may resemble pyotraumatic dermatitis or staphylococcal infection.[62, 69] In two dogs the lesions were more hyperkeratotic and crusted, affecting especially the nose, face, pinnae, genitalia, and footpads.[61, 67] One dog developed three nodules on the neck and lateral thighs associated with *Candida zeylanoides* following injections of calcium gluconate.[66] Candidiasis isolated to the clawbeds is rare.[13a] Candidiasis may rarely present as a mucocutaneous ulcerative disorder; however, one reported case of mucocutaneous candidiasis was probably a dog with necrolytic migratory erythema (hepatocutaneous syndrome) and secondary *C. albicans* infection.[68]

Cat

Candidiasis involving the skin is extremely rare in cats. Lesions include erythema, erosions, ulcers, crusts, and oozing in intertriginous areas, paws, and mucocutaneous junctions.[61a, 63a] One cat developed vesicles and ulcers of the mucocutaneous areas of the nose, lips, prepuce, and anus, as well as the oral cavity, following 2 weeks of tetracycline therapy for an upper respiratory infection.[7] Nystatin therapy was curative.

DIAGNOSIS

The differential diagnosis for localized forms of candidiasis includes pyotraumatic dermatitis, staphylococcal infection, and intertrigo. Mucocutaneous candidiasis must be differentiated from immunologic diseases (e.g., pemphigus vulgaris, bullous pemphigoid, systemic lupus erythematosus, erythema multiforme), drug eruptions, necrolytic migratory erythema, thallium poisoning, epitheliotropic lymphoma, and other usual infections (leishmaniasis, protothecosis, phaeohyphomycosis). Cytologic examination of direct smears reveals suppurative inflammation and numerous yeasts (2 to 6 µm in diameter) and blastoconidia (budding cells).[1, 3, 9, 64] Pseudohyphae may occasionally be seen. Biopsy findings include suppurative epidermitis, parakeratotic hyperkeratosis, and occasionally, suppurative superficial folliculitis. Numerous yeasts and blastoconidia are present in the keratin of the surface epidermis and infundibular portion of hair follicles (Fig. 5:10). Pseudohyphae and true hyphae may also be seen. *Candida* species grow on Sabouraud's dextrose agar at 25 to 30°C (77 to 86°F). The API 20C system is a convenient and reliable system for identification.

CLINICAL MANAGEMENT

Correction of predisposing causes is fundamental. Excessive moisture must be avoided. For localized lesions, clipping, drying, and topical antifungal agents are usually effective. Useful topical agents include nystatin (100,000 U/gm), 2 per cent miconazole, 1 per cent clotrimazole, 3 per cent amphotericin B, gentian violet (1:10,000 in 10 per cent alcohol), and potassium permanganate (1:3000 in water).[64] These agents should be applied 3 times daily until lesions are completely healed (1 to 4 weeks).

Oral, widespread mucocutaneous, and generalized lesions require systemic antifungal therapy.[64] Although intravenous amphotericin B is effective, ketoconazole or itraconazole administered orally are the drugs of choice (see Chap. 3).[64] Therapy should be continued for 7 to 10 days beyond clinical cure (2 to 4 weeks).

Malasseziasis

CAUSE AND PATHOGENESIS

Malassezia pachydermatis (Pityrosporum pachydermatis, Pityrosporum canis, M. canis) is a lipophilic, nonmycelial saprophytic yeast that is commonly found on normal and abnormal skin, in normal and abnormal ear canals, and in the anal sacs, rectum, and vagina of normal

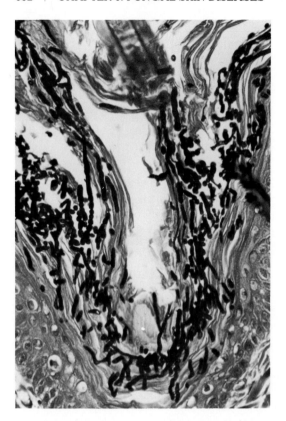

Figure 5:10. Candidiasis in a dog. Numerous yeasts and pseudohyphae in hair follicle. (Courtesy M. Pichler-Schick.)

dogs and cats.[1, 9, 76, 79, 80] Although *Malassezia* organisms can be easily isolated from the skin of normal dogs by a tape culture method, cytologic demonstration of yeasts has been difficult, with only three or fewer yeasts being observed within an entire ½-inch² (1 cm²) area of slides prepared by superficial skin scraping, clear adhesive tape, or cotton swab techniques.[69a, 72a] Alterations in skin surface microclimate or host defense may allow this normally commensal organism to become a significant pathogen. Surface microclimate factors leading to *Malassezia* proliferation include excessive sebum or cerumen production, accumulations of moisture, and subsequent disruption of the epidermal barrier.[75, 76] Allergic and bacterial skin disease may also be predisposing factors, as are the long-term glucocorticoid and antibiotic administrations rendered for these diseases.[75–77, 79] In one study,[79] the prevalence of cutaneous *Malassezia* spp. was evaluated in a semiquantitative fashion on dogs with various dermatoses (especially seborrhea, atopy, and presumptive allergy). The prevalence of higher than normal (no normal dogs studied) amounts did not correlate significantly with sample site (ventral neck, axilla, interdigital space), sex, or age. The number of *Malassezia* seen in tape strippings of skin from atopic dogs was larger than that from normal dogs, but smaller than that from dogs with *Malassezia* dermatitis.[69a] Factors associated with an increased prevalence of high *Malassezia* spp. counts were seborrheic dermatitis, recent antibiotic treatment, and breed. Genetic predisposition, possibly as a result of deficient T lymphocyte responses to the yeast, has been suggested to occur in West Highland White terriers.[72, 81] The yeast produces lipases that can liberate fatty acids, and zymogen in the yeast cell wall activates complement.[75, 76] Both of these actions could contribute to cutaneous inflammation. In addition, immediate and delayed hypersensitivity responses to *Malassezia* antigen are common in humans with atopy, suggesting that yeast hypersensitivity is important in some individuals.[73, 79]

CLINICAL FINDINGS

Dog

Malassezia dermatitis is an uncommon but increasingly recognized dermatosis in dogs.[75, 76] It occurs in adult dogs of any age and breed, but the following breeds appear to be predisposed: silky terrier, Australian terrier, Maltese terrier, Jack Russell terrier, West Highland White terrier, Basset hound, Chihuahua, Poodle, Shetland sheepdog, collie, German shepherd, dachshund, Cocker spaniel, and Springer spaniel.[70, 76–79] The dermatitis often begins in the summer or highly humid months, which also correspond to the allergy season (pollens, molds), and then persists into winter.[76] About 50 per cent of the dogs have underlying diseases, especially seborrhea, allergies, and bacterial pyodermas.[75–79]

Pruritus is a major sign and is virtually constant. Dogs with generalized skin disease (exfoliative erythroderma) are erythematous, greasy, scaly (yellow or slate gray), and crusty. They often have an offensive, greasy, seborrheic odor (Fig. 5:11 A; also see Fig. 5:5 F, G, and H).[75, 76] Regional dermatitis occurs on the ears, lips, muzzle, interdigital spaces, ventral neck, medial thighs, axillae, perianal region, intertriginous areas.[70, 71, 76, 78] Focal scaly plaques and erythematous macules and patches may coalesce into serpiginous tracts. Occasionally, the dog is presented for so-called frenzied fits of nose and lip scratching with the front paws. Otitis externa associated with *Malassezia* infection is discussed in Chapter 18.

Cat

Malassezia dermatitis is rarely reported in cats; when found, it may be associated with a black and waxy otitis externa (see Chap. 18), recalcitrant feline chin acne, and a generalized erythematous scaly dermatitis (exfoliative erythroderma).[8a, 61a, 76, 76a] Recurrent, generalized *Malassezia* dermatitis has been observed in cats with FIV infection.[79]

DIAGNOSIS

The differential diagnosis is extensive, and includes atopy, food hypersensitivity, flea bite hypersensitivity, drug eruption, superficial staphylococcal folliculitis, demodicosis, feline acne, scabies, acanthosis nigricans, contact dermatitis, seborrheic dermatitis, and epitheliotropic lymphoma.[76] The diagnosis can be even more perplexing for the clinician because *Malassezia* dermatitis is often associated with or triggered by most of the potential differentials. *Malassezia* dermatitis should be considered a factor in any scaly, erythematous, oily, pruritic dermatitis in which other differentials have been eliminated by diagnostic tests and there is a lack of response to treatment (e.g., glucocorticoids, antibiotics, antiseborrheic shampoos, insecticides, miticides).

The most useful and readily available tool for the clinician presented with a suspected case of *Malassezia* dermatitis is cytologic examination.[76, 79] Samples of surface scale or grease are gathered by making a superficial skin scraping, vigorously rubbing a cotton swab on the skin surface, pressing a piece of clear cellophane tape onto lesional skin several times, or pressing a section of a clean glass microscope slide on the skin.[76, 79] Scraping and taping appear to be more reliable than swabbing.[69a] All material is transferred to a glass slide, heat fixed (but not if cellophane tape has been used), and stained for cytologic examination. One typically sees numerous round or oval, budding, yeastlike cells (3 to 8 μm in diameter). Yeasts are often seen in clusters or adhered to keratinocytes (Fig. 5:12). Biopsy findings are characterized by a hyperplastic, superficial, perivascular to interstitial dermatitis with lymphohistiocytic cells predominating (Figs. 5:13 and 5:14).[75, 77, 78, 81] The epidermis and outer root sheath of the infundibular portion of hair follicles usually show prominent spongiosis, exocytosis of lymphoid cells, and parakeratotic hyperkeratosis. Numerous yeasts, and occasionally pseudohyphae, are present in the keratin of the surface epidermis and the infundibulum of hair follicles. Neutrophils, microabscesses, pustules, and superficial folliculitis are often present when secondary bacterial

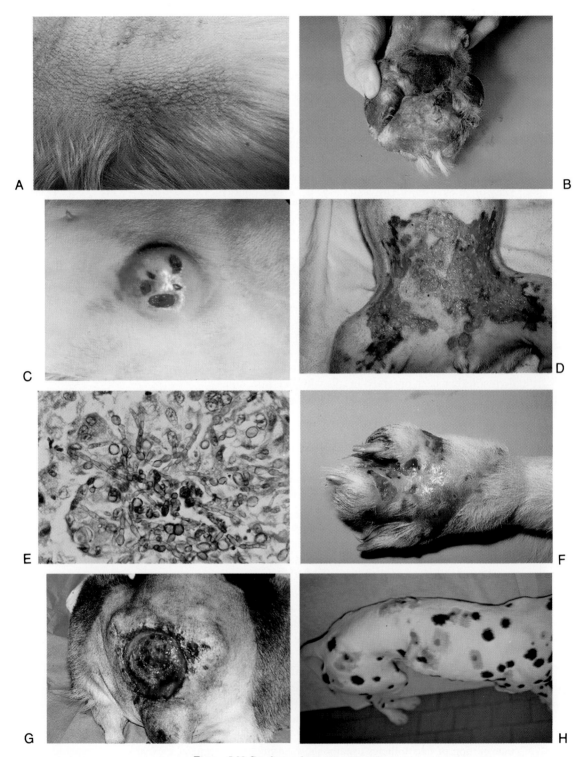

Figure 5:11 *See legend on opposite page*

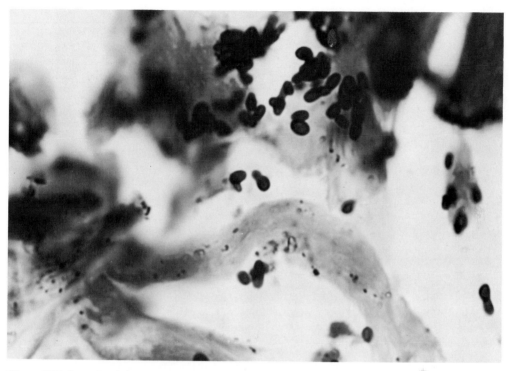

Figure 5:12. Superficial skin scraping from a dog with malasseziasis. Numerous budding yeasts among the squames.

Figure 5:11. Miscellaneous fungal infections. *A*, Malasseziasis in a dog. Alopecia, erythema, and yellowish brown, crumbly surface debris. *B*, Mycetoma in a dog. Marked swelling of footpads and multiple draining tracts. (Courtesy D. Chester.) *C*, Phaeohyphomycosis in a cat. Truncal nodule that is multifocally ulcerated. *D*, Phaeohyphomycosis in a dog. The ulcerative dermatitis on the ventral abdomen and medial thighs is more or less symmetric. (Courtesy K. Kwochka.) *E*, Phaeohyphomycosis in a cat. Numerous greenish brown fungal elements in granulomatous dermatitis. *F*, Pythiosis in a dog. Swollen paw with multiple areas of necrosis and ulceration. (Courtesy D. Chester.) *G*, Ulcerated nodules over the lumbosacral area of a dog with pythiosis. (Courtesy C. Foil.) *H*, Sporotrichosis in a Dalmatian. Widely scattered crusted plaques (hair has been clipped around each lesion).

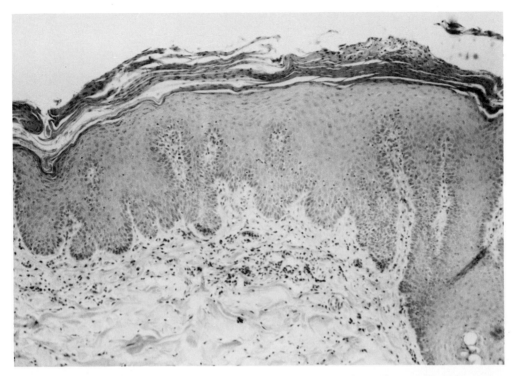

Figure 5:13. Malasseziasis in a dog. Superficial interstitial dermatitis with parakeratotic hyperkeratosis, spongiosis, and lymphocytic exocytosis.

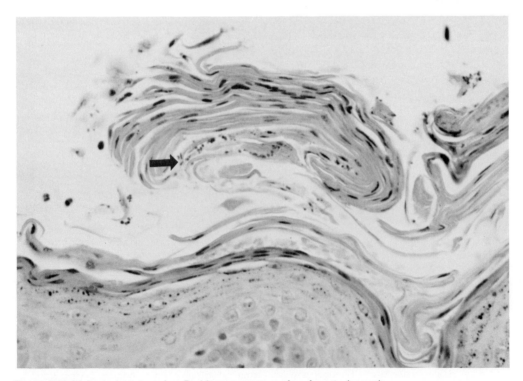

Figure 5:14. Malasseziasis in a dog. Budding yeasts in surface keratin *(arrow)*.

infection exists. It must be remembered that yeasts can occasionally be seen on the surface of biopsies from numerous canine and feline dermatoses and yet play no known role in their pathogenesis or treatment.[81a, 81b] Yeasts present in hair follicles, however, must always be assumed to be possibly pathogenic. Skin biopsy is less reliable than cytologic examination for demonstrating yeasts.[69a] Although *M. pachydermatis* grows on routine culture media, skin surface swabs often fail to isolate the yeast.[76] Ultimately, the diagnosis of *Malassezia* dermatitis rests on the response to antiyeast treatment.[69a, 76]

CLINICAL MANAGEMENT

The treatment of *Malassezia* dermatitis is best accomplished with oral ketoconazole (5 to 10 mg/kg q12h).[8a, 72, 75, 76] Pruritus is usually noticeably reduced in the first week, and cutaneous lesions resolve within 2 to 4 weeks. Therapy should be continued for 7 to 10 days beyond clinical cure. Good results have recently been achieved with itraconazole (5mg/kg q24h per os).[76a]

Selenium sulfide shampoo followed by rinses with enilconazole is reported to be very effective.[76] However, enilconazole has an offensive odor and is not licensed for use in the United States. Ketoconazole, zinc pyrithione, and chlorhexidine shampoos have also been reported to be effective.[72, 76, 78, 81] Chlorhexidine must be present at a concentration of at least 1 per cent. Shampoos are applied twice weekly until cure results. Localized *Malassezia* dermatitis may respond to the topical application of nystatin, miconazole, clotrimazole, enilconazole, ketoconazole, or chlorhexidine.[71, 74, 76] The authors have been impressed with the efficacy of daily shampoos containing selenium sulfide (Selsun Blue) for localized or regionalized lesions. In more severe or generalized cases, these shampoos can be given twice weekly and followed with 2 per cent lime sulfur dips (Lym Dyp) (see Chap. 3).

Because many cases of *Malassezia* dermatitis are associated with underlying diseases and therapeutic regimens, recognition and control of these predisposing factors is critical to prevent recurrent yeast infections.[75, 76, 77] However, when predisposing causes cannot be found or cannot be corrected, chronic maintenance therapy is necessary. This can be accomplished with weekly topical treatments or one to two times weekly oral ketoconazole administration.[72, 76, 78, 81]

Rhodotorulosis

CAUSE AND PATHOGENESIS

Rhodotorula spp. are normal inhabitants of the skin, ear canal, and alimentary tract.[1, 2, 81c] These yeastlike fungi are opportunistic pathogens of immunosuppressed individuals.

CLINICAL FINDINGS

Rhodotorulosis appears to be extremely rare. One cat had an erythematous dermatitis with adherent brown-red, doughy crusts on the nasal planum, nostrils, bridge of the nose, periocular region, and one digit.[81c] *Rhodotorula mucilaginosa* was isolated in culture. The cat was positive for FeLV and FIV.

DIAGNOSIS

Biopsy revealed an interstitial dermatitis with ovoid, yeastlike organisms in the dermis.[81c] *Rhodotorula* spp. grow on Sabouraud's dextrose agar.

CLINICAL MANAGEMENT

A cat treated with ketoconazole orally for 4 months was still in remission 18 months later.[81c]

■ SUBCUTANEOUS MYCOSES

The subcutaneous (intermediate) mycoses are fungal infections that have invaded the viable tissues of the skin.[1, 3, 4, 9] These infections are usually acquired by traumatic implantation of saprophytic organisms that normally exist in soil or vegetation. The lesions are chronic and, in most cases, remain localized. The terms used to refer to the subcutaneous mycoses have been contradictory, confusing, and frequently changing. The term *chromomycosis* includes subcutaneous and systemic diseases caused by fungi that develop in the host tissue in the form of dark-walled (pigmented, dematiaceous) fungal elements.[3, 9] Chromomycosis is separated into two forms, depending on the appearance of the fungus in tissues. In *phaeohyphomycosis*, the organism appears as septate hyphae and yeastlike cells. In *chromoblastomycosis*, the fungus is present as large (4 to 12 μm in diameter), rounded, dark-walled cells (sclerotic bodies, chromo bodies, Medlar bodies).

A *mycetoma* is a unique infection wherein the organism is present in tissues as granules or grains.[3, 9] Mycetomas may be *eumycotic* or *actinomycotic*. The etiologic agents of eumycotic mycetomas are fungi, whereas actinomycotic mycetomas are caused by members of the *Actinomycetales* order, such as *Actinomyces* and *Nocardia*, which are bacteria (see Chap. 4). Eumycotic mycetomas may be caused by dematiaceous fungi (black-grained mycetomas) or nonpigmented fungi (white-grained mycetoma). Pseudomycetomas have differences in granule formation and are caused by dermatophytes (dermatophytic pseudomycetoma) or bacteria, such as *Staphylococcus* (bacterial pseudomycetoma or botryomycosis).

The term *hyalohyphomycosis* has been proposed to encompass all opportunistic infections caused by nondematiaceous fungi (such as the *Aspergillus* spp.), the basic tissue forms of these being hyaline hyphal elements that are septate, branched, or unbranched.[3, 4, 9]

Another term that creates confusion is *phycomycosis*.[3, 4, 9] The class *Phycomycetes* no longer exists. Pythiosis (oömycosis) and zygomycosis are now the preferred terms for phycomycosis. Members of the genus *Pythium* are properly classified in the kingdom Protista and in the phylum *Oömycetes*. The phylum *Zygomycota* includes the orders *Mucorales* and *Entomophthorales*. The term zygomycosis is used to include both mucormycosis and entomophthoromycosis.

Eumycotic Mycetoma

CAUSE AND PATHOGENESIS

The fungi causing eumycotic mycetoma in dogs and cats are ubiquitous soil saprophytes that cause disease via wound contamination.[1, 9, 86, 87, 90] The condition occurs most frequently near the Tropic of Cancer between the latitudes 10°S and 30°N, including Africa, South and Central America, India, and southern Asia. The disease is rare in the United States and Europe. The most commonly reported fungus causing eumycotic mycetoma in the United States is *Pseudoallescheria boydii*.

CLINICAL FINDINGS

The three cardinal features of eumycotic mycetoma (maduromycosis) are tumefaction, draining tracts, and grains (granules) in the discharge.[84, 86–90] Lesions are usually solitary and occur most commonly on the limbs and face (see Fig. 5:11 *B*). Early papules evolve into nodules that are often painful. As lesions enlarge, they develop draining tracts that exude a serous, purulent, or hemorrhagic discharge. As some fistulas heal, scar tissue develops and forms the hard, tumor-like mass that characterizes mycetoma. Grains present in discharge vary in color, size, shape, and texture, depending on the particular fungus involved. Black- or dark-grain mycetomas are usually associated with *Curvularia geniculata*, occasionally *Madurella grisea* and *Torula* sp.[89]

White-grain mycetomas are usually caused by *Pseudoallescheria (Allescheria, Petriellidium) boydii* and, occasionally, *Acremonium hyalinum*.[82, 83, 86] Chronic infections can extend into underlying muscle, joint, or bone.

DIAGNOSIS

The differential diagnosis includes infectious and foreign-body granulomas and neoplasms. Cytologic examination of aspirates or direct smears reveals pyogranulomatous inflammation with occasional fungal elements. Fungi are easily seen by squashing and examining grains. Biopsy findings include nodular to diffuse, pyogranulomatous to granulomatous dermatitis and panniculitis. Fungal elements are present as a grain (granule, thallus) within the inflammatory reaction (Fig. 5:15). The grains (0.2 to several mm in diameter) are irregularly shaped, often taking a scalloped or scroll-like appearance, and consist of broad (2 to 6 μm in diameter), septate, branching hyphae, which often form chlamydoconidia, and a cementing substance (Fig. 5:16).[3] The fungal elements may be pigmented or nonpigmented. The fungi grow on Sabouraud's dextrose agar. Either tissue grains or punch biopsies are the preferred material for culture (see Chap. 2).

CLINICAL MANAGEMENT

Wide surgical excision is the treatment of choice.[85, 86] In some cases, amputation of an affected limb is necessary. Any attempt at antifungal chemotherapy should be based on in vitro susceptibility testing of the isolate.[86] Medical therapy is often unsuccessful. Ketoconazole and itraconazole have enjoyed erratic success.[86, 87] Treatment must be continued for 2 to 3 months past clinical cure.

Phaeohyphomycosis

CAUSE AND PATHOGENESIS

Phaeohyphomycosis (chromomycosis) is caused by a number of ubiquitous saprophytic fungi found in various soils and organic materials.[1, 94, 106] Infection occurs via wound contamination.

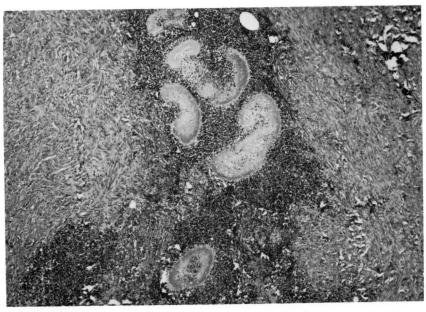

Figure 5:15. Mycetoma in a dog. Note numerous tissue grains within a pyogranuloma.

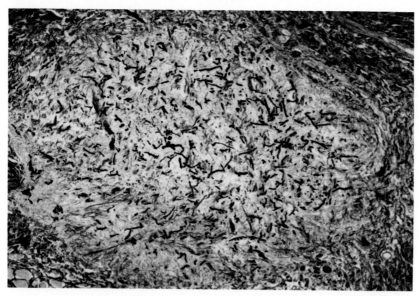

Figure 5:16. Histologic appearance (low power) of a mycetoma caused by *Curvularia geniculata* and reproduced from a section stained with Gomori's methenamine silver. It demonstrates numerous dark fungal fragments, chlamydospores, and hyphae in the center of a necrotic granulomatous reaction. (At this magnification cell types cannot be identified, but multinucleated foreign body giant cells, macrophages, neutrophils, lymphocytes, and plasma cells are present.)

These fungi have the characteristic of forming pigmented (dematiaceous) hyphal elements (but not grains) in tissues.

CLINICAL FEATURES

Dog

Phaeohyphomycosis appears to be rare in dogs. Fungi isolated include *Bipolaris spiciferum (Brachycladium spiciferum, Drechslera spiciferum), Phialemonium obovatum, Pseudomicrodochium suttonii,* and *Xylohypha bantiana (Cladosporium trichoides, C. bantianum).*[9, 91, 94, 96, 97] Solitary subcutaneous nodules, often ulcerated, may be seen especially on extremities. However, widespread nodular or necrotizing and ulcerative lesions are also seen (Fig. 5:11 *D*).[96, 106] Contiguous skeletal or disseminated infections have been reported.[94]

Cat

Phaeohyphomycosis is uncommon in cats. Fungi isolated include *Bipolaris spiciferum (Brachycladium spiciferum, D. spiciferum), X. bantiana (C. trichoides, C. bantianum), X. emmonsii, Exophiala jeanselmei (Phialophora gougerotii), Exophiala spinifera, Moniliella suaveolens, Phialophora verrucosa, Alternaria alternata, Scolecobasidium humicola,* and *Stemphylium* sp.[92–95a, 98–103, 105] In most cases, lesions are solitary and affect the paw, leg, nose, or trunk (see Fig. 5:11 *C*). Slow-growing, firm to fluctuant, subcutaneous nodules are seen. Ulceration and draining tracts may occur. Disseminated infection is rare.[94, 105a]

DIAGNOSIS

The differential diagnosis includes infectious granulomas, sterile granulomas, foreign-body granulomas, and neoplasms. In dogs with widespread mucocutaneous and footpad lesions,[96] the

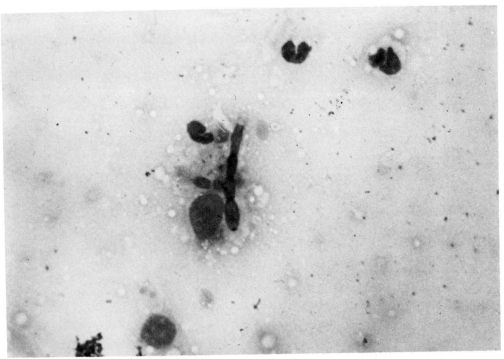

Figure 5:17. Direct smear from a cat with phaeohyphomycosis. Pigmented fungal hypha within a macrophage.

differential includes immunologic diseases (pemphigus vulgaris, bullous pemphigoid, systemic lupus erythematosus, erythema multiforme), drug eruptions, necrolytic migratory erythema, thallium poisoning, epitheliotropic lymphoma, and other unusual infections (leishmaniasis, prototheciasis, candidiasis).

Cytologic examination of aspirates or direct smears reveals granulomatous to pyogranulomatous inflammation. Pigmented fungal hyphae may be seen (Fig. 5:17). Biopsy findings include nodular to diffuse, granulomatous to pyogranulomatous dermatitis and panniculitis. Numerous fungal elements are present as broad (2 to 6 μm in diameter) pigmented, septate, branched, or unbranched hyphae with occasional chlamydoconidia and numerous round to oval, pigmented yeast forms (Medlar bodies, so-called copper pennies) (see Fig. 5:11 *E*).[3] The fungi grow on Sabouraud's dextrose agar at 25 to 35°C (77 to 95°F), and punch biopsies are the preferred material for culture.

CLINICAL MANAGEMENT

Wide surgical excision of solitary lesions may be curative, but recurrence at the same site or at new sites is common.[94, 95a, 99, 100] Chemotherapy may be curative, depending on the agent, but the response is unpredictable. This may be due to differing susceptibilities of the fungi involved, and differences in the therapeutic protocols that have been used to date. Drugs should be chosen on the basis of in vitro susceptibility testing. Ketoconazole has been used successfully and unsuccessfully, alone or in combination with flucytosine.[93, 94, 102, 104] Flucytosine has been used successfully and unsuccessfully, alone or in combination with ketoconazole or amphotericin B.[94, 95a, 98, 102, 104] Amphotericin B has been used successfully or unsuccessfully, alone or in combination with flucytosine.[94, 98, 104] In humans, itraconazole, cryosurgery, and local application of heat have also been curative in some cases.[104]

Pythiosis

CAUSE AND PATHOGENESIS

Pythium spp. are aquatic fungi that rely on aquatic plant or organic substance for their normal life cycle.[1, 2, 109] The motile zoospore stage shows chemotaxis toward damaged plant or animal tissues. Animals become infected by standing in or drinking stagnant water, and damaged skin appears to be a prerequisite for infection. Environmental conditions are probably the most influential factors governing the occurrence of pythiosis. Thus, most cases are seen during the summer and fall in tropical and subtropical areas of the world. In North America, cases are reported from the southern United States exclusively, particularly from the Gulf Coast region.

Pythium insidiosum (Pythium gracile, Hyphomyces destruens) is the species isolated from dogs, humans, and horses.[1, 106a, 109, 109b] Pythiosis has been reported under other names in the literature: phycomycosis, hyphomycosis, and oömycosis. A single case has been reported in a cat.[106b]

CLINICAL FINDINGS

Large-breed, male dogs are most commonly affected.[109] German shepherds appear to be particularly susceptible.[107, 108] Lesions may be solitary or multiple, and they are typically confined to one area of the body, especially the legs (see Fig. 5:11 *F*), face, and tail head (see Fig. 5:11 *G*). Ulcerated nodules develop, often rapidly, into large, firm to boggy masses with ulceration and draining tracts. The discharge is usually a mixture of pus and blood. The lesions are often pruritic. Early lesions on the limbs may resemble acral lick dermatitis. Some leg lesions progress to involve the entire circumference of the limb. Rarely, dogs develop locally invasive (skeletal) or disseminated infection.[109, 109a]

DIAGNOSIS

The differential diagnosis includes infectious granulomas, foreign-body granulomas, acral lick dermatitis, and neoplasms. Cytologic examination of aspirates or direct smears reveals granulomatous to pyogranulomatous inflammation wherein eosinophils are often numerous; however, fungal elements are only occasionally seen. Biopsy findings include nodular to diffuse, granulomatous to pyogranulomatous dermatitis and panniculitis. Foci of necrosis and large numbers of eosinophils are often seen. Wide (4.5 to 5.5 μm in diameter), occasionally septate, irregularly branching hyphae are numerous (Fig. 5:18) and occasinally invade blood vessel (especially arterial) walls. As a result, thrombosed blood vessels may be a prominent feature. The hyphae of zygomycetes, which are very similar to those of *Pythium* spp., are easily seen in H & E–stained sections, whereas those of *Pythium* usually require special stains. The organism often appears as clear hollow spaces in necrotic and granulomatous areas in H & E–stained sections.[109a] Pythium stains poorly with Periodic acid–Schiff, but nicely with GMS.[109a, 109b] *Pythium* spp. grow rapidly at 25 to 37°C (77 to 98.6°F) on blood agar and Sabouraud's dextrose agar, and punch biopsies are the preferred material for culture. It is advisable to submit specimens to veterinary diagnostic laboratories, where the microbiologist is more likely to be familar with *Pythium* spp.[109] *Pythium* antigen can be demonstrated in sections of paraffin-embedded tissues by an indirect immunoperoxidase technique.[109a]

CLINICAL MANAGEMENT

Wide surgical excision is the treatment of choice, but recurrence is not uncommon.[109] Amputation of an affected limb may be necessary. Because *Pythium* spp. do not share cell wall characteristics with true fungi, antifungal chemotherapy agents (amphotericin B, ketoconazole,

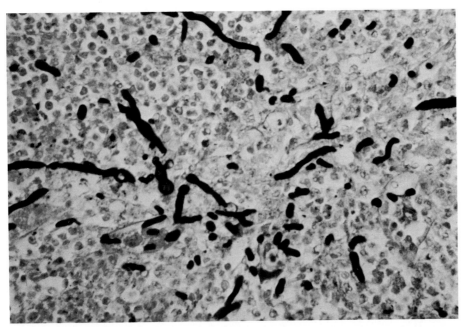

Figure 5:18. Canine pythiosis. Numerous hyphae in a pyogranulomatous dermatitis. (Courtesy C. Foil.)

flucytosine) have been disappointing in the treatment of this disease.[107–109] Autogenous *Pythium* spp. vaccines and transfer factor have been tried without success.[108, 109]

Zygomycosis

Zygomycetes are ubiquitous saprophytes of soil and decaying vegetation and a component of the normal flora of skin and haircoat.[1, 112] The portal of entry may be gastrointestinal, respiratory, or cutaneous via wound contamination. In humans, a compromised immune system is generally necessary for invasion to occur. However, in dogs and cats, such factors have not been identified in most instances.

There are two orders of *Zygomycetes* that cause disease: (1) *Mucorales*, which includes the genera *Rhizopus, Mucor, Absidia, Mortierella,* and (2) *Entomophthorales*, which includes the genera *Conidiobolus* and *Basidiobolus*. Infections caused by fungi from the order *Mucorales* were previously called *mucormycosis* and those associated with the order *Entomophthorales* were called *entomophthoromycosis*. In addition, many of the older reports of phycomycosis in dogs and cats were likely zygomycosis.[112]

CLINICAL FINDINGS

Zygomycosis appears to be rare in dogs and cats, and most infected animals have had fatal gastrointestinal disease.[110, 112, 113] Skin lesions may be solitary or multiple, are typically nodular, ulcerated, and draining, and commonly involve the extremities.[110, 114] One dog had a nonhealing bite wound in the neck caused by *Absidia corymbifera*.[111]

DIAGNOSIS

The differential diagnosis includes numerous infectious granulomas, foreign-body granulomas, and neoplasms. Cytologic examination of aspirates or direct smears reveals pyogranulomatous to granulomatous inflammation, wherein fungal elements may be visualized. Biopsy findings include nodular to diffuse, pyogranulomatous to granulomatous dermatitis and panniculitis containing numerous broad (6 to 25 μm in diameter), occasionally septate, irregular branching fungal hyphae with nonparallel sides.[3] Fungal elements are most commonly found, and are most abundant, within foci of necrosis. *Zygomycetes* grow on Sabouraud's dextrose agar, and punch biopsies are the preferred material for culture.

CLINICAL MANAGEMENT

The susceptibility of the *Zygomycetes* to antimycotic agents is quite variable and largely unknown.[112] Solitary lesions may be surgically excised. In other cases, surgical excision or debulking may be followed by chemotherapy as dictated by in vitro susceptibility tests (amphotericin B, benzimidazoles, potassium iodide).[112, 114]

Sporotrichosis

CAUSE AND PATHOGENESIS

Sporotrichosis is caused by the ubiquitous dimorphic fungus *Sporothrix schenckii*, which exists as a saprophyte in soil and organic debris.[1, 121, 122, 123a] Infection occurs as a result of wound contamination. Glucocorticoids and other immunosuppressive drugs are contraindicated in dogs or cats with sporotrichosis.[121, 122] These drugs should be avoided both during and after treatment of the disease, as immunosuppressive doses of glucocorticoids have been reported to cause a recurrence of clinical sporotrichosis as long as 4 to 6 months after apparent clinical cure.[118]

CLINICAL FINDINGS

Dog

Sporotrichosis is uncommon to rare. The disease is often related to puncture wounds from thorns or wood splinters.[121, 122] This is presumably why the disease is more commonly observed in hunting dogs.[121, 122] The *cutaneous form* of sporotrichosis is the most commonly reported.[117, 121–123] Multiple firm nodules, ulcerated plaques with raised borders, or annular crusted and alopecic areas are present, especially on the head, pinnae, and trunk (Fig. 5:19 *A*; also see Fig. 5:11). Some lesions have a verrucous appearance. Nodules may ulcerate or develop draining tracts (Fig. 5:19 *B*). Lesions are neither painful nor pruritic, and affected dogs are usually healthy otherwise. The *cutaneolymphatic form* is characterized by a nodule on the distal aspect of one limb, with subsequent ascending infection via the lymphatics.[119, 121, 122] Secondary nodules may be firm or fluctuant; they often ulcerate and discharge a brownish red exudate, and they are associated with regional lymphadenopathy. Affected dogs are usually otherwise healthy. One dog had ulcers and nodules affecting the nares, mucocutaneous junctions, scrotum, and footpads;[119] another had papulonodular otitis externa.[115] Disseminated sporotrichosis is extremely rare.[121, 122]

Figure 5:19. Miscellaneous fungal infections. *A*, Sporotrichosis. Close-up of the top of the head of the dog in 5:11 *H*. *B*, Sporotrichosis presenting as multiple papules and nodules on the bridge of the nose of a collie. *C*, Sporotrichosis presenting as multiple ulcers on the face of a cat. *D*, Multiple erythematous papules and a large, ulcerated nodule on the hand of a human with sporotrichosis. (Courtesy R. Goltz.) *E*, Large nodule with a central ulcer on the hind paw of a cat caused by *Alternaria* sp. *F*, Ulcerated nodules on the nose of a dog with blastomycosis. (Courtesy J. Brace.) *G*, Swollen digit with a focal ulceration in a dog with blastomycosis. *H*, Alopecic, erythematous nodule on the digit of a dog with coccidioidomycosis (Courtesy D. Chester).

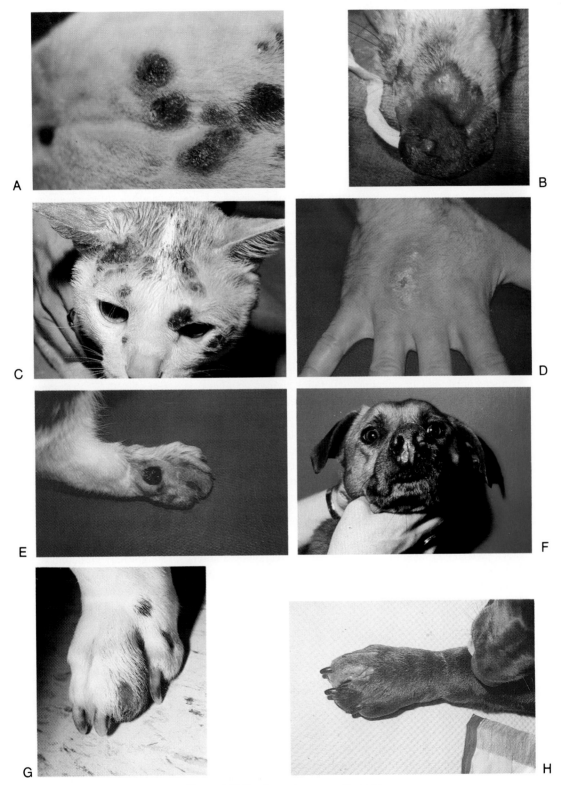

Figure 5:19 *See legend on opposite page*

Cat

Sporotrichosis is uncommon. The disease is believed to be acquired by inoculation of the organism by contaminated claws or teeth from another cat.[121, 122] This may explain why the disease is usually seen in intact male cats that roam outdoors.[121, 122] Lesions are commonly seen on the head (see Fig. 5:19 C), distal limbs, or tail base region.[13b, 121, 122] The cats may initially present with fight wound abscesses, draining tracts, or cellulitis. Affected areas ulcerate, drain a purulent exudate, and form crusted nodules. Large areas of necrosis may develop, with exposure of muscle and bone. The disease may be spread to other areas of the body (other limbs, face, pinnae) via autoinoculation during normal grooming behavior. Some cats may present with a history of lethargy, depression, anorexia, and fever, which suggest the potential for disseminated disease.[121, 122] Although affected cats frequently appear clinically to have only dermatologic disease, most have necropsy evidence of lymph node and lymphatic vessel involvement, and *S. schenckii* is commonly isolated in culture from numerous internal organs and feces.[121, 122]

Zoonotic Aspects

The zoonotic potential of sporotrichosis, especially in cats, must be seriously considered and respected.[53, 116, 121, 122, 123a, 124] There have been several reports documenting transmission of sporotrichosis to humans through contact with an ulcerated wound or the exudate from an infected cat.[53, 116, 121, 122] Human infections have occurred even though there had been no known injury or penetrating wound prior to the onset of the disease. Transmission from animals to humans has been limited to feline sporotrichosis, presumably because large numbers of organisms are found in contaminated feline tissues, exudates, and feces.[116, 121, 122] Veterinarians, veterinary technicians, veterinary students, and owners of infected cats have a higher risk of infection.[53, 116, 121, 122]

The most common form of sporotrichosis in humans is cutaneolymphatic.[4, 53] A primary lesion—which may be a papule, pustule, nodule, abscess, or verrucous growth—develops at the site of injury. This lesion may be painful. Most lesions are on an extremity (finger, hand, foot) (see Fig. 5:19 D) or the face. Secondary lesions then ascend proximally via lymphatic vessels. The cutaneous (fixed) form is less common.

DIAGNOSIS

The differential diagnosis includes other infectious granulomas, foreign-body granulomas, and neoplasms. Because of the zoonotic potential of sporotrichosis, precautions must be taken. All people handling cats suspected of having sporotrichosis should wear gloves. Gloves should also be worn when samples are taken of exudates or tissues. The gloves should then be carefully removed and disposed of. Forearms, wrists, and hands should be washed in chlorhexidine or povidone-iodine.

Cytologic examination of aspirates or direct smears reveals suppurative to pyogranulomatous to granulomatous inflammation. The organism is difficult to find in the exudates of dogs but is easily found in those of cats (Fig. 5:20). *S. schenckii* is a pleomorphic yeast that is round, oval, or cigar-shaped, 2 to 10 μm in length.[1, 3] Biopsy findings include nodular to diffuse, suppurative to granulomatous to granulomatous dermatitis (Fig. 5:21). Fungal elements are numerous and readily found in cats but rarely in dogs (Fig. 5:22). The fungi have a refractile cell wall from which the cytoplasm may shrink, giving the impression that the organism has a capsule. When this occurs, the organisms may be confused with *Cryptococcus neoformans*. *S. schenckii* grows on Sabouraud's dextrose agar at 30°C (86°F); samples submitted for culture should include both a sample of the exudate (from deep within a draining tract) and a piece of tissue (removed surgically) for a macerated tissue culture. A fluorescent antibody test is most useful in dogs because it may be positive when cultures are negative.[121, 122]

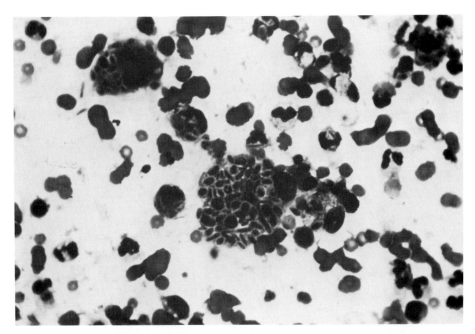

Figure 5:20. Feline sporotrichosis. Numerous yeast and cigar bodies in a macrophage. (Courtesy J.M. MacDonald.)

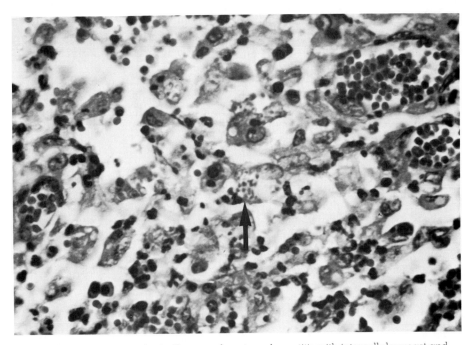

Figure 5:21. Feline sporotrichosis. Pyogranulomatous dermatitis with intracellular yeast and cigar bodies *(arrow).*

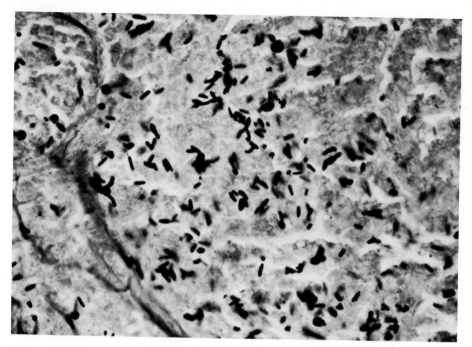

Figure 5:22. Canine sporotrichosis. Numerous yeast and cigar bodies (GMS stain).

CLINICAL MANAGEMENT

Dog

The treatment of choice is oral administration of a supersaturated solution of potassium iodide, 40 mg/kg q8 to 12h with food.[115, 117, 119, 121–123] Treatment must be continued for 30 days beyond clinical cure (4 to 8 weeks). Signs of toxicity (iodism) include ocular and nasal discharge, a dry haircoat with excessively scaling skin, vomiting, depression, and collapse.[121, 122] If iodism is observed, medication should be stopped for 1 week. The drug may then be re-instituted at the same or a lower dosage. If iodism becomes a recurrent problem or if side-effects are severe, alternative treatment should be considered.

The imidazole and triazole classes of drugs may be considered for dogs that do not tolerate iodides, are refractory to them, or relapse after apparent clinical cure.[121, 122] Ketoconazole or itraconazole may be used successfully, and are continued for 30 days beyond clinical cure. Side-effects are usually mild (see Chap. 3).

Cat

Increased sensitivity to the toxic side-effects of iodides and ketoconazole in cats poses a greater challenge for the treatment of sporotrichosis. The treatment of choice is the oral administration of a supersaturated solution of potassium iodide at 20 mg/kg q12 to 24h with food[116, 120–122, 123a] for 30 days beyond clinical cure (4 to 8 weeks). Signs of iodism include vomiting, anorexia, depression, twitching, hypothermia, and cardiovascular failure. In animals that cannot tolerate or fail to respond to iodides, ketoconazole or itraconazole should be used (see Chap. 3).[121, 122, 123a]

Rhinosporidiosis

CAUSE AND PATHOGENESIS

Rhinosporidium seeberi is a fungal organism of uncertain classification.[1, 125] Attempts to culture it using conventional fungal culture media were unsuccessful; however, the organism has been grown in tissue culture.[125] The disease is endemic in India and Argentina, but North American reports have come almost exclusively from the southern United States. It is thought that infection is acquired by mucosal contact with stagnant water or dust and that trauma is a predisposing factor.

CLINICAL FINDINGS

The disease appears to be rare, and it is reported only in dogs.[1, 125] There appears to be a predilection for large-breed, male dogs. Affected dogs typically present for wheezing, sneezing, unilateral seropurulent nasal discharge, and epistaxis. Nasal polyps may be visible in the nares or may be visualized by rhinoscopy. Single or multiple polyps varying in size from a few mm up to 3 cm are pink, red, or grayish and are covered with numerous pinpoint, white foci (fungal sporangia). Polyps may be sessile or pedunculated, and may protrude out of, or involve, the mucocutaneous area of the nostril.

DIAGNOSIS

The differential diagnosis includes numerous infectious granulomas and neoplasms. Cytologic examination of nasal exudate or histologic examination of the polyp should be diagnostic. Biopsy findings include a fibrovascular polyp containing numerous sporangia (spherules) having a thick, double outer membrane. The sporangia vary from 100 to 400 μm in diameter, and contain a variable number of sporangiospores (endospores).[1, 125] A variable number of lymphocytes, plasma cells, and neutrophils are often found where sporangiospores (2 to 10 μm in diameter) have been released into the surrounding connective tissue.

CLINICAL MANAGEMENT

Surgical excision is the treatment of choice, although recurrence 6 to 12 months following surgery has been reported.[125] Successes have been reported with dapsone or ketoconazole administered orally (see Chap. 3); however, the utility of medical therapy in canine rhinosporidiosis requires further evaluation.

Alternariosis

CAUSE AND PATHOGENESIS

Alternaria spp. are ubiquitous saprophytic fungi in soil and organic debris and a common component of the flora of the canine and feline integument.[1, 4] They cause opportunistic wound infections.

CLINICAL FINDINGS

Alternaria spp. are rarely reported to cause skin disease in dogs and cats. In the dog, dermatologic abnormalities attributed to *Alternaria* spp. infection include (1) poorly circumscribed areas of alopecia, erythema, and scaling, especially in intertriginous or traumatized areas of skin,[126, 143] and (2) nodular, ulcerated, depigmented inflammation of the nose *(Alternaria tenuissima)*.[127] In the cat, *Alternaria* spp. have been associated with phaeohyphomycosis *(Alternaria alternata)*[8, 93] and ulcerated nodule on the paw (see Fig. 5:19 *E*).

DIAGNOSIS

The differential diagnosis for superficial inflammatory disease includes staphylococcal folliculitis, demodicosis, dermatophytosis, and malasseziasis. The differential diagnosis for nodules includes infectious and foreign-body granulomas and neoplasms. Cytologic examination of aspirates or direct smears from nodular lesions reveals pyogranulomatous inflammation and numerous fungal elements. Biopsy findings include nodular to diffuse pyogranulomatous dermatitis and panniculitis with numerous broad (3 to 6 μm in diameter), septate, branched or unbranched hyphae. *Alternaria* spp. grow on Sabouraud's dextrose agar. Punch biopsies are the preferred culture material.

CLINICAL MANAGEMENT

Surgical excision of nodules may be curative. Antifungal chemotherapy should be based on in vitro susceptibility tests. One dog was cured after 8 weeks of oral ketoconazole.[127]

■ SYSTEMIC MYCOSES

Deep mycoses are fungal infections of internal organs that may secondarily disseminate by hematogenous spread to the skin. Fungi that cause deep mycoses exist as saprophytes in soil or vegetation. These infections are usually not contagious because the animal inhales conidia from a specific ecologic niche. Skin lesions that occur via primary cutaneous inoculation are very rare, and animals with skin lesions are assumed to have systemic infection until proven otherwise. The deep mycoses are discussed only briefly here. The reader is referred to texts on mycology and infectious diseases for additional information.

Blastomycosis

CAUSE AND PATHOGENESIS

Blastomyces dermatitidis is a dimorphic saprophytic fungus.[1, 3, 9, 14, 139] The reservoir is thought to be sandy, acid soil, and proximity to water. Even within endemic areas, the fungus does not seem to be widely distributed. Most people and dogs living in such areas show no serologic or skin test evidence of exposure. A point source where the exposure occurs within an enzootic area is more likely. Blastomycosis (Gilchrist's disease, Chicago disease) is principally a disease of North America, but it has been identified in Africa and Central America. In North America, blastomycosis has a well-defined endemic distribution that includes the Mississippi, Missouri, Ohio, and St. Lawrence River Valleys and the middle Atlantic states.

CLINICAL FINDINGS

Dog

Blastomycosis is an uncommon disease in endemic areas. Young (2 to 4 years old), male dogs of large breeds and sporting breeds (especially Doberman pinscher, Labrador retriever, Bluetick Coonhound, Treeing-walker Coonhound, Pointers, Weimaraners) are predisposed.[139, 140] A larger number of cases are seen in the fall.[140] Clinical signs usually include anorexia, weight loss, coughing, dyspnea, ocular disease, lameness, and skin disease.[139] Up to 40 per cent of dogs with blastomycosis have skin lesions that include firm papules, nodules, and plaques, ulcers, draining tracts, and subcutaneous abscesses.[139] Lesions are usually multiple and may be found anywhere; however, the nasal planum (see Fig. 5:19 *F*), face, and clawbeds (see Fig. 5:19 *G*) appear to be preferred sites.

Cat

Blastomycosis is very rare in cats. Dyspnea, draining skin lesions (especially the digits), and weight loss are the most prominent clinical signs.[7, 139] Siamese cats may be predisposed.

DIAGNOSIS

A history of travel to an endemic area should increase the clinician's index of suspicion. Cytologic examination of aspirates or direct smears is often diagnostic, revealing suppurative to pyogranulomatous to granulomatous inflammation containing round to oval yeastlike fungi (5 to 20 μm in diameter) that show broad-based budding and have a thick, refractile, double-contoured cell wall (Fig. 5:23). Biopsy findings include nodular to diffuse, suppurative to pyogranulomatous to granulomatous dermatitis, wherein the fungus is usually found easily (Fig. 5:24). Culture of cytologic specimens is not recommended for in-hospital laboratories because of the danger of infection from the mycelial form of the organisms. Only after an extensive search for the organisms has been made should serologic testing (agar-gel immunodiffusion, enzyme-linked immunosorbent assay) be used to help establish a diagnosis.[139]

CLINICAL MANAGEMENT

All animals with clinical blastomycosis should be treated because spontaneous remission is rare.[14, 139] Although either amphotericin B (83 per cent response rate) or ketoconazole (62 per cent rate) may be effective alone, the treatment of choice is the sequential administration of these two antifungal agents.[14, 139] Itraconazole is more effective than ketoconazole, and appears to produce cure rates comparable to those achieved with amphotericin B.[139]

PUBLIC HEALTH CONSIDERATIONS

Penetrating wounds contaminated by the organisms have produced infections in humans.[139] Care should be taken to avoid getting bitten when handling infected animals. Accidental inoculation of organisms by contaminated knives or needles should be avoided at necropsy or

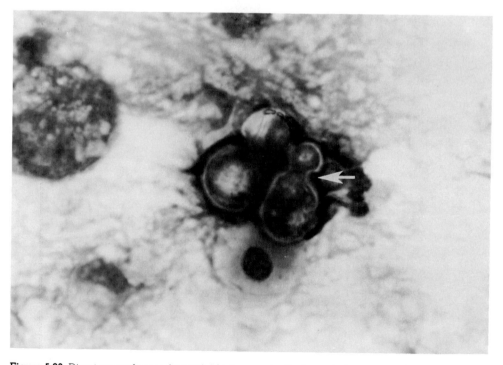

Figure 5:23. Direct smear from a dog with blastomycosis. Oval yeasts demonstrate broad-based budding *(arrow)*. (Courtesy T. French.)

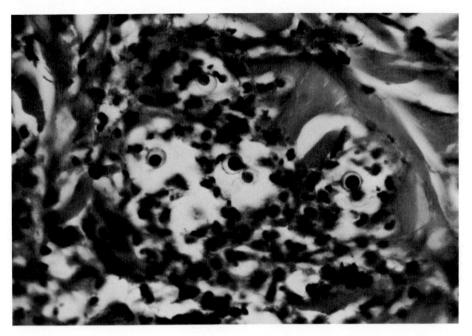

Figure 5:24. Canine blastomycosis. Large, round, thick-walled yeast bodies (H & E stain).

during fine-needle aspiration. Culturing of the organism should be limited to laboratories with proper facilities.

Coccidioidomycosis

CAUSE AND PATHOGENESIS

Coccidioides immitis is a dimorphic saprophytic soil fungus.[1, 3, 9, 14, 141] The ecologic niche of this fungus is characterized by sandy, alkaline soils, high environmental temperature, low rainfall, and low elevation. Geographically, this area is referred to as the Lower Sonoran Life Zone, and includes the southwestern United States, Mexico, and Central and South America. Serologic surveys indicate that most human and canine inhabitants of the endemic area become infected. Coccidioidomycosis has also been called *San Joaquin Valley Fever.*

CLINICAL FINDINGS

Dog

Coccidioidomycosis is an uncommon disease in endemic areas.[14, 141] Young (1 to 4 years old) male dogs are predisposed, and the boxer and Doberman pinscher are predisposed to disseminated infections. Clinical signs usually include coughing, dyspnea, persistent or fluctuating fever, anorexia, weight loss, lameness, skin disease, and ocular disease.[14, 141] Skin lesions are usually multiple and include papules, nodules, abscesses, draining tracts, and ulcers. Skin lesions almost always occur over sites of infected bone (especially the distal diaphyseal, metaphyseal, and epiphyseal areas of long bones) (see Fig. 5:19 *H*).

Cat

Coccidioidomycosis is extremely rare in cats.[14, 141] Clinical signs include anorexia, weight loss, cough, dyspnea, lameness, ocular disease, and chronic draining skin lesions.

DIAGNOSIS

A history of travel to an endemic area should increase the clinician's index of suspicion. Cytologic examination of aspirates or direct smears reveals suppurative to pyogranulomatous to granulomatous inflammation. Fungal elements are seldom found (Fig. 5:25 *B*)[141] Biopsy findings include nodular to diffuse, suppurative to pyogranulomatous to granulomatous dermatitis and panniculitis. Fungal elements are usually present but may be sparse. The organisms are present in spherule (20 to 200 μm in diameter) and endospore (2 to 5 μm in diameter) forms (Fig. 5:25).[1, 3, 141]

Attempts should not be made to culture *C. immitis* in veterinary practices because of the risk of human infection.[141] Culturing of the organism should be limited to laboratories with appropriate facilities. Serologic tests (precipitin, complement fixation) are useful for diagnosis.[141]

CLINICAL MANAGEMENT

All animals with clinical coccidioidomycosis should be treated because spontaneous remission is unlikely.[141] The current drug of choice is ketoconazole.[14, 141] Treatment of animals with disseminated disease should continue for a minimum of 1 year. Amphotericin B is used to treat animals that cannot tolerate or do not respond to ketoconazole.[14, 141]

Cryptococcosis

Cryptococcus neoformans is a ubiquitous, saprophytic, yeastlike fungus that is most frequently associated with droppings and the accumulated filth and debris of pigeon roosts.[1, 7, 9, 134] The establishment and spread of infection are highly dependent on host immunity; however, underlying diseases are often not detected in dogs and cats with cryptococcosis.[134, 137a] Both experimental and natural cases of cryptococcosis in dogs and cats are accelerated or worsened by glucocorticoid therapy.[134] In the cat, cryptococcal infection has often been seen in association with FeLV or FIV infections.[7, 14, 128, 128a, 134] Cryptococcosis has also been called *European blastomycosis* and *torulosis*.

CLINICAL FINDINGS

Dog

Cryptococcosis is a rare disease.[14, 134] Young (average age 3 years) large-breed dogs are predisposed. Clinical signs include various abnormalities of the central nervous system and eyes.[14, 134] Skin lesions are found in about 20 per cent of the cases; these lesions are characterized by papules, nodules, ulcers (Fig. 5:26 *A*), abscesses, and draining tracts. The nose, lips, and clawbeds are often affected.[13a, 134]

Cat

Cryptococcosis is an uncommon disease, but it is the most common deep mycosis of the cat.[7, 14, 134] Clinical signs occur from abnormalities of the upper respiratory, cutaneous, central nervous, and ocular systems.[7, 14, 134] In about 70 per cent of the cases with upper respiratory signs, a flesh-colored, polyp-like mass is visible in the nostril, or a firm to mushy subcutaneous swelling over the bridge of the nose is evident (Fig. 5:26 *B*). The skin or subcutaneous tissues are involved in about 40 per cent of the cases.[7, 14, 134] Lesions are usually multiple and include papules, nodules (Fig. 5:26 *C*), abscesses, ulcers, and draining tracts.[7, 128, 131, 134, 137, 138] Skin lesions can occur anywhere but most commonly involve the face, pinnae, and paws.

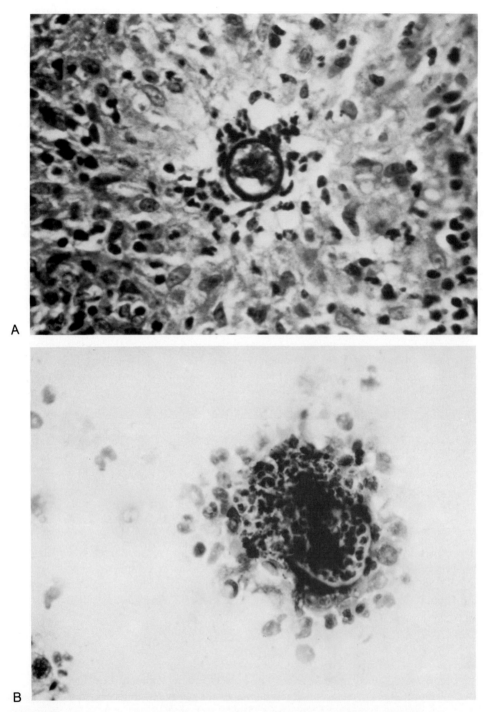

A

B

Figure 5:25. *A*, Canine coccidioidomycosis. *Coccidioides immitis* spherule in center of pyogranuloma (PAS stain). *B*, Direct smear from a dog with coccidioidomycosis. Ruptured spherule releasing endospores and surrounded by degenerate neutrophils. (Courtesy T. French.)

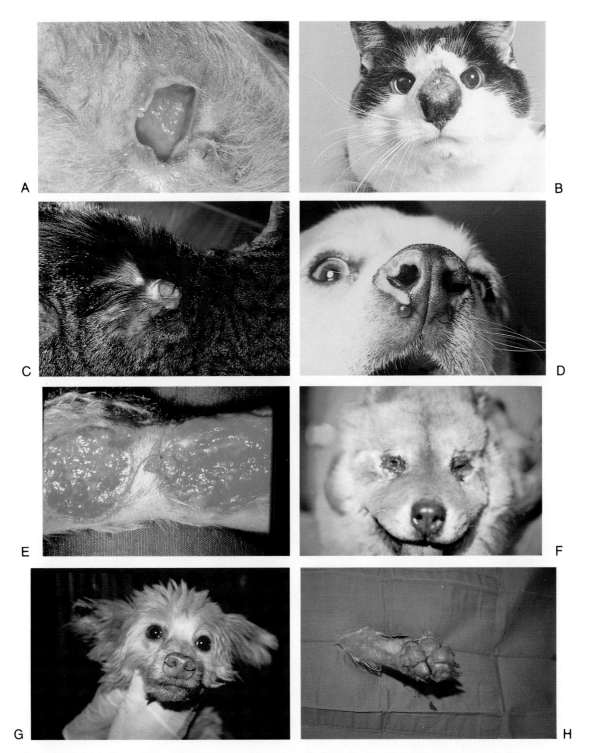

Figure 5:26. Miscellaneous fungal infections. *A,* Necrosis and ulceration in a dog with cryptococcosis. *B,* Granulomatous nasal dermatitis in a cat with cryptococcosis. *C,* Ulcerated nodule containing gelatinous exudate on the back of a cat with cryptococcosis. *D,* Multifocal areas of depigmentation and ulceration of the nostrils in a dog with nasal aspergillosis. *E,* Ulcers on the leg of a dog with aspergillosis. (Courtesy R. Halliwell.) *F,* Chronic blepharitis with sticky, black exudate in a Chow Chow caused by *Aspergillus niger. G,* Swollen, erythematous, ulcerated nose of a dog with protothecosis. (Courtesy J. Perrier.) *H,* Swollen, ulcerated footpads of a dog with protothecosis. (Courtesy J. Perrier.)

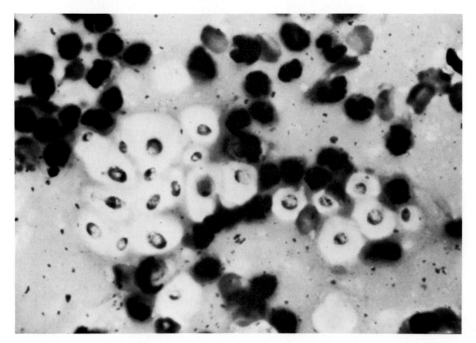

Figure 5:27. Canine cryptococcosis. Encapsulated yeast bodies in direct smear (NMB stain).

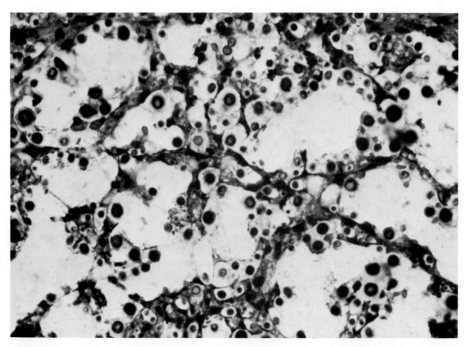

Figure 5:28. Feline cryptococcosis. Numerous encapsulated yeast bodies on a cystic background (Mucicarmine stain).

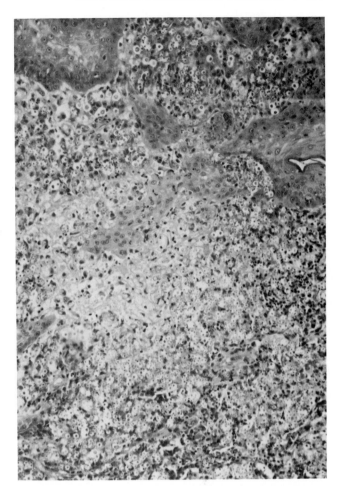

Figure 5:29. Feline cryptococcosis. Numerous encapsulated yeast bodies in pyogranuloma (H & E stain).

DIAGNOSIS

Cytologic examination of aspirates or direct smears reveals pyogranulomatous to granuloma-tous inflammation with numerous pleomorphic (round to elliptical, 2 to 20 μm in diameter) yeastlike organisms. These show narrow-based budding and are surrounded by a mucinous capsule of variable thickness, which forms a clear or refractile halo (Fig. 5:27).[1, 3, 9, 134] Biopsy findings include a cystic degeneration or vacuolation of the dermis and subcutis that is surpris-ingly acellular (sometimes likened to an infusion of soap bubbles) (Fig. 5:28) or a nodular to diffuse, pyogranulomatous to granulomatous dermatitis and panniculitis (Fig. 5:29) containing numerous organisms. Mayer's mucicarmine is a useful special stain because it stains the organism's capsule (carminophilic) a red color.[3, 134] The only clinically useful serologic test is a latex agglutination test that detects cryptococcal capsular antigen.[132, 134] It may be negative, however, in cats with disease apparently isolated to the skin.[132, 134, 137a] The test may also be used to monitor response to therapy.[132, 134, 136, 137a]

CLINICAL MANAGEMENT

The drugs of choice are ketoconazole, itraconazole, and fluconazole.[129, 130, 131, 133, 134, 136, 137] The combination of ketoconazole and flucytosine, with lower doses of both, may produce more rapid cures and a reduction in side-effects.[135, 137a] Amphotericin B, flucytosine, and the combi-nation of both drugs have also been successfully used to treat cryptococcosis.[7, 14, 128, 134, 138]

Rarely, solitary lesions in animals with primary cutaneous cryptococcosis can be surgically excised and the animals cured.[131, 134]

Histoplasmosis

Histoplasma capsulatum is a dimorphic saprophytic soil fungus.[1, 3, 9, 140, 142] The organism prefers areas with moist, humid conditions and soil containing nitrogen-rich organic matter such as bird and bat excrement. Most cases of histoplasmosis occur in the central United States in the Ohio, Missouri, and Mississippi River Valleys. Surveys indicate that most human and canine inhabitants of endemic areas become infected.

CLINICAL FINDINGS

Dog

Histoplasmosis is an uncommon disease in endemic areas.[14, 142] Young (less than 4 years old) dogs are usually affected, and Pointers, Weimaraners, and Brittany spaniels may be predisposed.[14, 142] Clinical signs include anorexia, weight loss, fever that is unresponsive to antibiotic therapy, coughing, dyspnea, gastrointestinal disease, ocular disease, and skin disease.[14, 142] Skin lesions are usually multiple, occur anywhere on the body, and are characterized by papules, nodules, ulcers, and draining tracts.

Cat

Histoplasmosis is an uncommon disease in endemic areas.[14, 142] Most affected cats are younger than 4 years old, and most have disseminated disease. Clinical signs include depression, weight loss, fever, anorexia, dyspnea, ocular disease, and skin disease.[14, 142] Skin lesions are usually multiple, occur anywhere on the body, and are characterized by papules, nodules, ulcers, and draining tracts.

DIAGNOSIS

A history of travel to an endemic area should increase the clinician's index of suspicion. Cytologic examination of aspirates or direct smears reveals pyogranulomatous to granulomatous inflammation containing numerous small (2 to 4 μm in diameter), round yeast bodies with a basophilic center and lighter halo caused by shrinkage of the yeast during staining (Fig. 5:30).[1, 3, 9, 142] Biopsy findings include nodular to diffuse, pyogranulomatous to granulomatous dermatitis with numerous intracellular organisms (Fig. 5:31). At present, no reliable serologic test exists.[14, 142] Attempts to culture *H. capsulatum* in a routine practice setting are not recommended because of the pathogenic potential of this organism.[142]

CLINICAL MANAGEMENT

All animals with clinical histoplasmosis should be treated because spontaneous remission is unlikely.[142] The current drug of choice is ketoconazole.[14, 142] For severe or fulminating cases, the combination of ketoconazole and amphotericin B is recommended.[14, 142] Itraconazole and fluconazole have shown promise in early trials.

Aspergillosis

CAUSE AND PATHOGENESIS

Aspergillus spp. are ubiquitous fungi that exist in nature as soil and vegetation saprophytes and as a component of normal skin, haircoat, and mucosal flora in humans and animals.[11, 144, 145] In

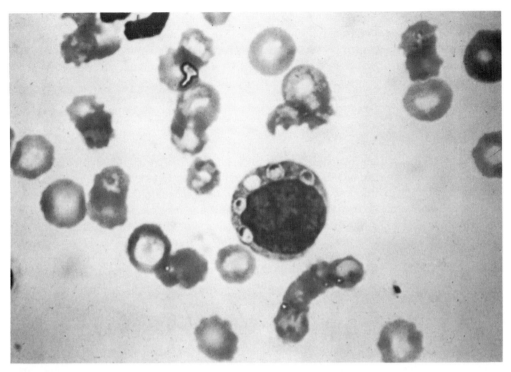

Figure 5:30. Direct smear from a dog with histoplasmosis. Multiple small, intracytoplasmic yeasts in a macrophage. (Courtesy T. French.)

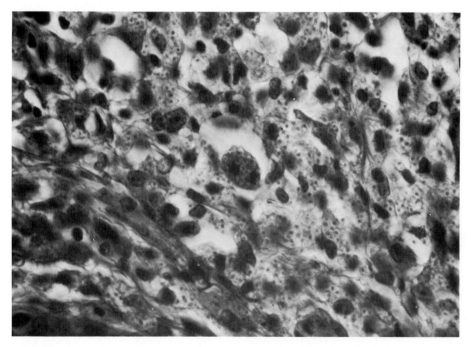

Figure 5:31. Canine histoplasmosis. Numerous small, intracellular yeast bodies in a granuloma (H & E stain).

humans, many cases of aspergillosis are associated with immunosuppression; in dogs, however, predisposing factors are not usually identified.[144] The organism is believed to produce opportunistic infections by invading mucosal or cutaneous surfaces. *A. fumigatus* is the most common species encountered in nasal aspergillosis, with *A. niger, A. nidulans,* and *A. flavus* being occasionally involved.[144, 145] In disseminated aspergillosis, infection has involved, in decreasing frequency, *A. terreus, A. deflectus, A. flavipes,* and *A. fumigatus.*[144, 145]

CLINICAL FINDINGS

To date, cutaneous and mucocutaneous aspergillosis has been reported only in dogs. Dolichocephalic and mesocephalic breeds are more susceptible to nasal aspergillosis, but there is no apparent age or sex predilection.[144, 145] Inflammation, depigmentation, ulceration, and crusting of the external nares and, occasionally, the nasal planum may be seen secondary to nasal discharge (Fig. 5:26 *D*). Most cases of disseminated aspergillosis have occurred in German shepherds and have been reported from Australia or California.[144] These dogs may develop cutaneous nodules, abscesses, and draining tracts, as well as oral ulcers. *Aspergillus* spp. have rarely been associated with cutaneous nodules and ulcers (Fig. 5:26 *E*) or blepharitis (Fig. 5:26 *F*) in otherwise healthy dogs.

DIAGNOSIS

The differential diagnosis includes other infectious diseases, neoplastic diseases, and in the case of nasal aspergillosis, various immune-mediated disorders such as discoid and systemic lupus erythematosus, pemphigus foliaceus and erythematosus, and drug eruption. Cytologic examination of aspirates or direct smears reveals suppurative to pyogranulomatous inflammation, with fungal elements occasionally visualized. Biopsy findings include nodular to diffuse suppurative or pyogranulomatous dermatitis or necrotizing dermatitis with minimal inflammation. Organisms are usually plentiful and characterized by broad (3 to 6 μm in diameter) septate, dichotomously branched hyphae (Figs. 5:32 and 5:33).[3] *Aspergillus* spp. can be grown on Sabouraud's dextrose agar.

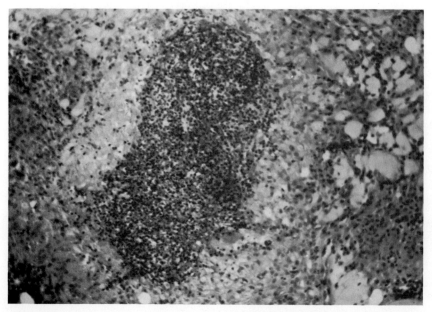

Figure 5:32. Aspergillosis in a dog. Note pyogranulomatous dermatitis. (Courtesy R. Halliwell.)

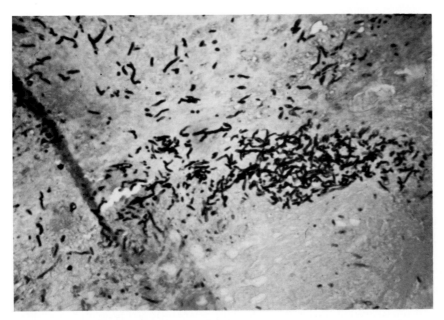

Figure 5:33. Aspergillosis in a dog. Note branching fungal hyphae within dermal pyogranuloma (GMS stain). (Courtesy R. Halliwell.)

In nasal aspergillosis, blind culture or cytologic examination of discharge is often unrewarding and can erroneously suggest that the disease is bacterial in origin.[144] Heavy growths of *Pseudomonas* spp. or other *Enterobacteriaceae* are common. In addition, up to 40 per cent of normal dogs or dogs with nasal neoplasia will have *Aspergillus* or *Penicillium* spp. cultured from nasal swabs.[144, 145] Rhinoscopy allows fungal plaques (a white, yellow, or light green mold) to be visualized and sampled directly for cytologic, histopathologic, and cultural examinations. Serologic diagnosis is possible using agar gel immunodiffusion, counter immunoelectrophoresis, or enzyme-linked immunosorbent assay techniques.[144, 145]

CLINICAL MANAGEMENT

Thiabendazole (10 to 20 mg/kg q12h) or ketoconazole (5 to 10 mg/kg q12h) administered orally eliminates the disease in about 50 per cent of the cases.[144, 145] Itraconazole (5 mg/kg q12h) or fluconazole (2.5 to 5 mg/kg q12h) may be more effective, but few clinical trials have been conducted to date.[144] These medications must be administered for 3 to 4 weeks beyond clinical cure, so a total of 6 to 8 weeks of treatment are required. For nasal aspergillosis, the most successful therapeutic regimen is enilconazole administered topically for 7 to 10 days through tubes implanted into each nasal chamber via the frontal sinuses.[144, 145] To date, no form of therapy has been successful in disseminated aspergillosis.[14]

Paecilomycosis

CAUSE AND PATHOGENESIS

Paecilomyces spp. are ubiquitous saprophytic, yeastlike fungi that exist in nature in soil and decaying vegetation.[1, 4, 9] In humans, disease occurs in individuals that are immunosuppressed. The organism is presumed to produce opportunistic infections by invading mucosal or cutaneous surfaces. Evidence for immunosuppression has not been present for most reported cases of paecilomycosis in dogs and cats.

CLINICAL FINDINGS

Dog

The disease appears to be extremely rare. Most dogs have had disseminated infections with no skin lesions.[4, 148, 149] One dog had severe, chronic, bilateral otitis externa characterized by severe hyperplasia, ulceration, pain, and a brownish black aural discharge.[149] Another dog had an ulcerated, crusted nodule in the region of the left caudal mammary gland.[148] Both dogs developed disseminated disease.

Cat

The disease appears to be extremely rare. One cat developed an ulcerated, nonhealing nodule on a paw that was caused by *Paecilomyces fumosoroseus*.[146] The cat subsequently developed other cutaneous, nasal, and disseminated lesions despite receiving ketoconazole orally at 10 to 40 mg/kg/day.

DIAGNOSIS

The differential diagnosis includes numerous infectious granulomas and neoplasms. Cytologic examination of aspirates or direct smears reveals pyogranulomatous inflammation and numerous pleomorphic fungal elements, including thick, branched, septate pseudohyphae and round to oval, often budding, yeastlike structures (3 to 7 μm in diameter).[9, 146, 148, 149] Biopsy findings include nodular to diffuse pyogranulomatous dermatitis with numerous fungal elements. *Paecilomyces* spp. grow on Sabouraud's dextrose agar, and punch biopsy is the preferred material for culture.

CLINICAL MANAGEMENT

Paecilomyces spp. are usually resistant to amphotericin B but may be susceptible to benzimidazole compounds such as ketoconazole or itraconazole (see Chap. 3).[147, 148] Ketoconazole was of no benefit in one dog[148] and one cat[146] with paecilomycosis. Too few cases have been treated to allow detailed therapeutic and prognostic recommendations.

Protothecosis

CAUSE AND PATHOGENESIS

Prototheca spp. are ubiquitous, saprophytic achlorophyllous algae that inhabit raw and treated sewage, the slime flux of trees, animal wastes, and contaminated and stagnant water.[1, 152, 154] In North America, most cases are reported from the southern United States. The organism causes opportunistic infections, and disseminated disease is often associated with dysfunction of host immunity. The portal of entry is believed to be the colon in disseminated infections and wound contamination in cutaneous lesions. The virulence of the *Prototheca* organisms may differ; only *Prototheca wickerhamii* is isolated from cutaneous infections in dogs and cats, and *Prototheca zopfii* is nearly always isolated from disseminated infections in dogs.[154]

CLINICAL FINDINGS

Dog

Protothecosis is a rare disease. Collies appear to be predisposed, and the majority of *Prototheca* spp. infections have occurred in females.[154] Dogs with disseminated protothecosis frequently have colitis and ocular and central nervous system involvement, but they rarely have skin lesions.[154] Disseminated disease is almost always associated with *P. zopfii.*

Dogs with cutaneous or mucocutaneous prototothecosis usually do not have clinical signs of systemic involvement, and infection is invariably due to *P. wickerhamii.*[151, 153–155] Dermatologic lesions may include multiple papules and nodules, often over pressure points, or nodules and ulcers involving mucocutaneous junctions (especially nostrils) and footpads (see Fig. 5:26 *G* and *H*).

Cat

Protothecosis is a rare disease. Only cutaneous involvement has been reported, and all cats were in good health otherwise. Skin lesions may be solitary to multiple; they occur as firm papular to nodular masses or fluctuant subcutaneous growths.[150, 154] Lesions have most commonly been present on the paws and legs, but they have also occurred on the nose, head, and pinnae, and on the base of the tail. Only *P. wickerhamii* has been isolated.

DIAGNOSIS

The differential diagnosis includes infectious, foreign body, and sterile granulomas, abscesses, and neoplasms. Cytologic examination of aspirates or direct smears reveals pyogranulomatous to granulomatous inflammation with numerous intracellular spherules that are round, oval, or polyhedral, and vary from 2 to 25 μm in diameter.[1, 3, 9, 154] The fungi reproduce by endosporulation, and internal cleavage planes are seen in larger spherules, which may contain 2 to 20 endospores. Biopsy findings include nodular to diffuse, pyogranulomatous to granulomatous dermatitis and panniculitis with numerous fungal elements (Figs. 5:34 and 5:35). *Protheca*

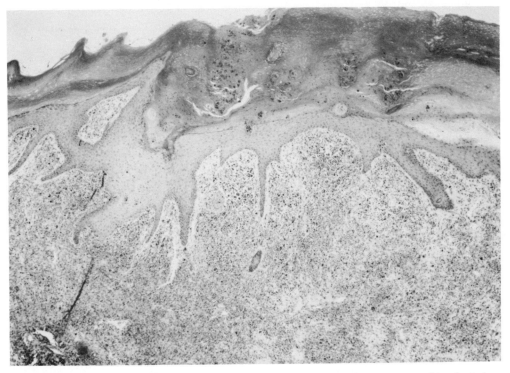

Figure 5:34. Protothecosis in a dog. Diffuse granulomatous dermatitis with numerous multinucleated histiocytic giant cells.

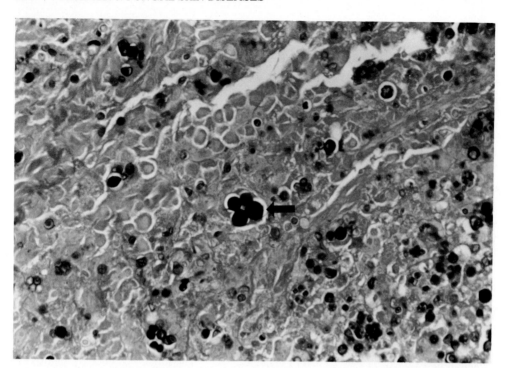

Figure 5:35. Protothecosis in a dog. Numerous organisms demonstrate internal cleavage planes *(arrow)* (GMS stain).

spp. grow on Sabouraud's dextrose agar at 25°C (77°F) and blood agar at 37°C (98.6°F), and punch biopsies are the preferred material for culture. The API 20C system can be used on cultures for species identification, as can fluorescent antibody techniques on formalin-fixed tissue.[1, 154]

CLINICAL MANAGEMENT

Solitary lesions in otherwise healthy patients, especially cats, may be surgically excised and the patient cured.[154] A variety of antimicrobials (including amphotericin B and sodium iodide) have been tried therapeutically, but treatment has failed in most instances. Amphotericin B and tetracycline act synergistically to inhibit the growth of *P. wickerhamii*; this combination has been successfully used to treat protothecosis in humans.[154] Ketoconazole (see Chap. 3) administered orally has been curative in some cases in dogs and humans.[154, 155] Therapy is usually prolonged (2 to 4 months) and should be continued for 3 to 4 weeks beyond clinical cure.

Trichosporonosis

CAUSE AND PATHOGENESIS

Trichosporon spp. are ubiquitous yeastlike fungi that exist in nature as soil saprophytes and as a minor component of normal skin, haircoat, and mucosal flora in humans and animals.[1, 4, 9] In humans, most cases of trichosporonosis have been disseminated, fatal, and reported in association with severe immunosuppression. The organism is believed to produce opportunistic infections by invading mucosal or cutaneous surfaces.[156] In cats, evidence for immunosuppression has not been present in all affected animals, but one had multicentric lymphoma.

CLINICAL FINDINGS

To date, trichosporonosis has been reported only in cats,[156, 157] and the disease appears to be extremely rare. Affected cats have presented with solitary papular or nodular lesions on the nostril, or a solitary ulcerated nodule at the site of a bite wound on a distal limb. *Trichosporon beigelii (Trichosporon cutaneum)* and *Trichosporon pullulans* have been isolated in culture.

DIAGNOSIS

The differential diagnosis includes numerous infectious granulomas, foreign-body granulomas, and neoplasms. Cytologic examination of aspirates or direct smears reveals pyogranulomatous inflammation and numerous pleomorphic fungal elements, including septate, branching hyphae, arthroconidia (2.5 $\times$ 10.4 μm), and pleomorphic blastoconidia (2.5 to 8 μm in diameter).[156, 157] Biopsy findings include nodular to diffuse pyogranulomatous dermatitis with numerous fungal elements. Mycotic invasion of blood vessels may be seen; this often results in areas of necrosis. *Trichosporon* can be grown on Sabouraud's dextrose agar, and punch biopsies are the preferred material for culture.

CLINICAL MANAGEMENT

Trichosporon spp. are generally more susceptible to benzimidazole compounds than amphotericin B or flucytosine.[156] Affected cats should be treated with oral ketoconazole or itraconazole (see Chap. 3). Not enough cases have been treated to allow detailed therapeutic and prognostic recommendations.

Geotrichosis

CAUSE AND PATHOGENESIS

Geotrichum candidum is a ubiquitous soil saprophyte and a minor component of the normal flora of the oral cavity, gastrointestinal tract, and integument.[1, 147] The organism is believed to produce opportunistic infections by invading mucosal or cutaneous surfaces.

CLINICAL FINDINGS

Geotrichosis appears to be extremely rare. *Geotrichum* was cultured from both a cat with a nonhealing wound on its back and its owner, who had a granulomatous infection of the skin and subcutis.[7] One dog had a symmetric onychodystrophy from which *Geotrichum* was repeatedly isolated.[13a]

DIAGNOSIS

Cytologic examination of aspirates or direct smears reveals suppurative to pyogranulomatous inflammation with broad (3 to 6 μm in diameter), septate, infrequently branched hyphae, spherical yeastlike cells, and rectangular or cylindrical arthroconidia (4 to 10 μm wide) with rounded or squared ends.[1, 3, 7] Biopsy findings include nodular to diffuse, suppurative to pyogranulomatous dermatitis with numerous fungal elements. *Geotrichum* grows on Sabouraud's dextrose agar, and punch biopsies are the preferred material for culture.

CLINICAL MANAGEMENT

There is little information available on the treatment of geotrichosis. One cat and its owner were cured with amphotericin B.[7]

REFERENCES

General Laboratory, Pathology, and Clinical Bibliography

1. Carter, G. R., Cole, J. R., Jr.: Diagnostic Procedures in Veterinary Bacteriology and Mycology V. Academic Press, New York, 1990.
2. Carter, G. R., Chengappa, M. M.: Essentials of Veterinary Bacteriology and Mycology IV. Lea and Febiger, Philadelphia, 1991.
2a. Kwon-Chung, K. J., Bennett, J. E.: Medical Mycology. Lea and Febiger, Philadelphia, 1992.
3. Chandler, F. W., Watts, J. C.: Pathologic Diagnosis of Fungal Infections. ASCP Press, Chicago, 1987.
4. Fitzpatrick, T. B., et al.: Dermatology in General Medicine IV. McGraw-Hill Book Co., New York, 1993.
5. Greene, C. E.: Infectious Diseases of the Dog and Cat. W. B. Saunders Co., Philadelphia, 1990.
6. Gross, T. L., et al.: Veterinary Dermatopathology. Mosby Year Book, St. Louis, 1992.
7. Holzworth, J.: Mycotic diseases. In: Holzworth, J. (ed). Diseases of the Cat. Medicine and Surgery, Vol. 1. W. B. Saunders Co., Philadelphia, 1987, p.320.
8. Mialot, M., Chermette, R.: Lésions cutanées pseudotumorales d'origine mycosique chez le chat. Proc GEDAC 7:28, 1991.
8a. Moriello, J. A.: The cutaneous mycoses of dogs and cats. Vet. Rep. 1:1, 1988.
9. Rippon, J. W.: Medical Mycology III. W. B. Saunders Co., Philadelphia, 1988.
10. Scott, D. W.: Feline dermatology 1900–1978: A monograph. J. Am. Anim. Hosp. Assoc. 16:331, 1980.
11. Scott, D. W.: Feline dermatology 1979 to 1982: Retrospective introspections. J. Am. Anim. Hosp. Assoc. 20:537, 1984.
12. Scott, D. W.: Feline dermatology 1983–1985: The Secret Sits. J. Am. Anim. Hosp. Assoc. 23:255, 1987.
13. Scott, D. W.: Feline dermatology 1986–1988: Looking to the 1990s through the eyes of many counsellors. J. Am. Anim. Hosp. Assoc. 26:515, 1990.
13a. Scott, D. W., Miller, W. H., Jr.: Disorders of the claws and clawbed in dogs. Comp. Cont. Educ. 14:1448, 1992.
13b. Scott, D. W., Miller, W. H., Jr.: Disorders of the claws and clawbed in cats. Comp. Cont. Educ. 14:449, 1992.
14. Wolf, A. M., Troy, G. C.: Deep mycotic diseases. In: Ettinger, S. J. (ed.). Textbook of Internal Medicine III. W. B. Saunders Co., Philadelphia, 1989, p.341.

Dermatophytosis

15. Aho, R. Saprophytic fungi isolated from the hair of domestic and laboratory animals with suspected dermatophytosis. Mycopathologia 83:65, 1983.
15a. Alteras, I., et al.: The increasing role of *Microsporum canis* in the variety of dermatophyte manifestations reported from Israel. Mycopathologia 94:105, 1986.
16. Bibel, D. J., Smiljanic, R. J.: Interactions of *Trichophyton mentagrophytes* and micrococci in skin culture. J. Invest. Dermatol. 72:133, 1979.
17. Blakemore, J. C.: Dermatomycosis. In: Kirk, R. W. (ed.). Current Veterinary Therapy V. W. B. Saunders Co., Philadelphia, 1974, p. 422.
17a. Bond, R., et al.: Chronic dermatophytosis due to *Microsporum persicolor* infection in three dogs. J. Small Anim. Pract. 33:571, 1992.
18. Bourdeau, P., et al.: Quelques formes rares de dermatomycoses des carnivores domestiques. 2ᵉ cas: Dermatite généralisée du chien due à une infection mixte par *Microsporum persicolor* et à *Microsporum gypseum*. Point Vét. 14:69, 1983.
19. Bourdeau, P., Chermette, R.: Formes rares de dermatomycoses des carnivores. IIIᵉ cas: Dermatite localisée du chien due à une infection mixte par *Trichophyton mentagrophytes* et *Trichophyton erinacei*. Point Vét. 19:619, 1987.
20. Bourdeau, P. Quel est votre diagnostic? Point Vét. 19:665, 1987.
21. Bussieras, J., et al.: Quelques formes rares de dermatomycoses des carnivores domestiques. 1ᵉʳ cas: Dermatite généralisée du chien, due à une infection mixte par *Microsporum canis* et par *Trichophyton mentagrophytes*. Point Vét. 13:43, 1982.
22. Carlotti, D., Couprie, B.: Dermatophyties du chien et du chat: Actualités. Prat. Méd. Chirurg. Anim. Cie. 23:449, 1988.
23. Carney, H. C., Moriello, K. A.: Dermatophytosis: Cattery management plan. In: Griffin, C. E., et al (eds.). Current Veterinary Dermatology. Mosby–Year Book, St. Louis, 1993, p. 34.
24. Chatterjee, A., et al.: Isolation of *Microsporum distortum* from ringworm lesions in a dog. Indian J. Anim. Health 19:159, 1980.
25. Connole, M. D.: Keratinophilic fungi in cats and dogs. Sabouraudia 4:45, 1965.
25a. Constable, P. J., Harrington, J. M.: Risks of zoonosis in a veterinary service. Br. Med. J. 284:246, 1982.
25b. Dahl, M. V.: Suppression of immunity and inflammation by products produced by dermatophytes. J. Am. Acad. Dermatol. 28:S19, 1993.
26. DeBoer, D. J., et al.: Immunological reactivity to intradermal dermatophyte antigens in cats with dermatophytosis. Vet. Dermatol. 2:59, 1991.
26a. DeBoer, D. J., Moriello, K. A.: Experimental feline dermatophytosis—effect of a fungal cell wall vaccine. Proc. Annu. Memb. Meet. Am. Acad. Vet. Dermatol. Am. Coll. Vet. Dermatol. 9:11, 1993.
26b. DeBoer, D. J., Moriello, K. A.: Humoral and cellular immune responses to *Microsporum canis* in naturally occurring feline dermatophytosis. Proc. Annu. Memb. Meet. Am. Acad. Vet. Dermatol. Am. Coll. Vet. Dermatol. 9:43, 1993.
27. DeKeyser, H., Van den Brande, M.: Ketoconazole in the treatment of dermatomycosis in cats and dogs. Vet. Quart. 5:142, 1983.

28. Dreisörner, H., et al.: Otitis externa durch *Microsporum canis* bei Katzen. Kleintierpraxis 9:230, 1964.
29. Foil, C. S.: Dermatophytosis. In: Greene, C. E. (ed.). Infectious Diseases of the Dog and Cat. W. B. Saunders Co., Philadelphia, 1990, p. 659.
30. Foil, C. S.: Dermatophytosis. In: Griffin, C. E., et al. (eds.). Current Veterinary Dermatology. Mosby Year Book, St. Louis, 1993, p. 22.
30a. Gambale, W., et al.: Dermatophytes and other fungi of the haircoat of cats without dermatophytosis in the city of Sao Paulo, Brazil. Feline Pract, 21:29, 1993.
31. Gabal, M. A.: Antifungal activity of ketoconazole with emphasis on zoophilic fungal pathogens. Am. J. Vet. Res. 47:1229, 1986.
31a. Jones, H. E.: Immune response and host resistance of humans to dermatophyte infection. J. Am. Acad. Dermatol. 28:S12, 1993.
31b. Kaplan, W., Ivens, M. S.: Observations on seasonal variations in incidence of ringworm in dogs and cats in the U.S.A. Sabouraudia 1:91, 1961.
32. Knudsen, E. A.: The areal extent of dermatophyte infection. Br. J. Dermatol. 92:413, 1975.
33. Kushida, T., Watanabe, S.: Canine ringworm caused by *Trichophyton rubrum*: Probable transmission from man to animal. Sabouraudia 13:30, 1975.
34. Lewis, D. T., et al.: Epidemiology and clinical features of dermatophytosis in dogs and cats at Louisiana State University: 1981–1990. Vet. Dermatol. 2:51, 1991.
34a. Leyden, J. J.: Progression of interdigital infections from simplex to complex. J. Am. Acad. Dermatol. 28:S7, 1993.
35. Lueker, D. C., Kainer, R. A.: Hyperthermia for the treatment of dermatomycosis in dogs and cats. Vet. Med. Small Anim. Clin. 76:658, 1981.
36. Mansfield, P. D., Stringfellow, J. S.: Isolation of *Microsporum vanbreuseghemii* from skin lesions of a dog. J. Am. Vet. Med. Assoc. 197:875, 1990.
37. Medleau, L., Ristic, Z.: Diagnosing dermatophytosis in dogs and cats. Vet. Med. 87:1086, 1992.
38. Medleau, L., Kuhl, K. A.: Dealing with chronic recurring dermatophytosis. Vet. Med. 87:1101, 1992.
39. Medleau, L., White-Weithers, N. E.: Treating and preventing the various forms of dermatophytosis. Vet. Med. 87:1096, 1992.
40. Medleau, L., Moriello, K. A.: Feline dermatophytosis. In: Kirk, R. W. (ed.). Current Veterinary Therapy XI. W. B. Saunders Co., Philadelphia, 1992, p. 547.
41. Medleau, L., Chalmers, S. A.: Ketoconazole for treatment of dermatophytosis in cats. J. Am. Vet. Med. Assoc. 200:77, 1992.
41a. Medleau, L., Chalmers, S. A.: Resolution of generalized dermatophytosis without treatment in dogs. J. Am. Vet. Med. Assoc. 201:1891, 1992.
42. Miller, W. H., Jr., Goldschmidt, M. H.: Mycetoma in a cat caused by a dermatophyte: A case report. J. Am. Anim. Hosp. Assoc. 22:255, 1986.
43. Moriello, K. A., DeBoer, D. J.: Fungal flora of the coat of pet cats. Am. J. Vet. Res. 52:602, 1991.
43a. Moriello, K. A.: Management of dermatophyte infections in catteries and multiple-cat households. Vet. Clin. North Am. (Small Anim. Pract.) 20:1457, 1990.
43b. Moriello, K. A., DeBoer, D. J.: Fungal flora of the haircoat of cats with and without dermatophytosis. J. Med. Vet. Mycol. 29:285, 1991.
43c. Moriello, K. A., DeBoer, D. J.: Efficacy of griseofulvin and itraconazole in the treatment of experimental feline dermatophytosis. Proc. Annu. Memb. Meet. Am. Acad. Vet. Dermatol. Am. Coll. Vet. Dermatol. 10:38, 1994.
44. Mosher, C. L., et al. Treatment of ringworm *(Microsporum canis)* with inactivated fungal vaccine (a case report). Vet. Med. (S.A.C.) 72:1343, 1977.
45. Muhammed, S. I., Mbogwa, S.: The isolation of *M. nanum* from a dog with skin lesions. Vet. Rec. 21:573, 1974.
46. Okuda, C., et al.: Fungus invasion of human hair tissue in tinea capitis caused by *Microsporum canis*: Light and electron microscopic study. Arch. Dermatol. Res. 281:238, 1989.
46a. Pepin, G. A., Oxenham, M.: Zoonotic dermatophytosis (ringworm). Vet. Rec. 118:110, 1986.
47. Philpot, C. M., Berry, A. P.: The normal fungal flora of dogs. A preliminary report. Mycopathologia 87:155, 1984.
48. Pinard, M., et al.: Diagnostic et prophylaxie des teignes des carnivores domestiques. Etude critique à partir d'une enquête à l'Ecole nationale vétérinaire d'Alfort. Rec. Méd. Vét. 163:1107, 1987.
48a. Pinter, L., et al.: The value of enzyme-linked immunosorbent assay (ELISA) in the sero-diagnosis of canine dermatophytosis due to *Microsporum canis*. Vet. Dermatol. 3:65, 1992.
49. Puccini, S., et al.: *In vitro* susceptibility to antimycotics of *Microsporum canis* isolates from cats. J. Am. Vet. Med. Assoc. 201:1375, 1992.
50. Quaife, R. A., Lutwyche, P.: *Microsporum cookei* as the suspected cause of ringworm in a dog. Vet. Rec. 110:311, 1982.
50a. Quaife, R. A., Womar, W. M.: *Microsporum canis* isolates from show cats. Vet. Rec. 110:333, 1982.
50b. Rybnikář, A., et al.: Prophylactic and therapeutic use of a vaccine against trichophytosis in a large herd of silver foxes and arctic foxes. Acta Vet., Brno. 60:285, 1991.
51. Sagmeister, H.: Diagnostic der Dermatomykosen. Wien. Tierärztl. Mschr. 76:196, 1989.
52. Scott, D. W., et al.: Dermatophytosis due to *Trichophyton terrestre* infection in a dog and cat. J. Am. Anim. Hosp. Assoc. 16:53, 1980.
53. Scott, D. W., Horn, R. T., Jr.: Zoonotic dermatoses of dogs and cats. Vet. Clin. North Am. (Small Anim. Pract.) 17:117, 1987.
53a. Scott, D. W., Paradis, M.: A survey of canine and feline skin disorders seen in a university practice: Small Animal Clinic, University of Montréal, St. Hyacinthe, Québec, (1987–1988). Can. Vet. J. 31:830, 1990.

53b. Stenwig, H.: Isolation of dermatophytes from domestic animals in Norway. Nord. Vet. Med. 37:161, 1985.

53c. Sparkes, A. H., et al.: Humoral immune responses in cats with dermatophytosis. Am. J. Vet. Res. 54:1869, 1993.

54. Takatori, K., et al.: Microscopic observation of human hairs infected with *Microsporum ferrugineum*. Mycopathologia 81:129, 1983.

55. Terreni, A. A., et al.: *Epidermophyton floccosum* infection in a dog from the United States. Sabouraudia J. Med. Vet. Mycol. 23:141, 1985.

56. Tewari, R. P.: *Trichophyton simii* infections in chickens, dogs, and man in India. Mycopathol. Mycol. Appl. 39:293, 1969.

57. Thomas, M. L. E., et al.: Inapparent carriage of *Microsporum canis* in cats. Comp. Cont. Educ. 11:563, 1989.

58. Van Cutsem, J., et al.: Survey of fungal isolates from alopecic and asymptomatic dogs. Vet. Rec. 116:568, 1985.

58a. Warner, R. D.: Occurrence and impact of zoonoses in pet dogs and cats at US Air Force bases. Am. J. Public Health 74:1239, 1984.

58b. White-Weithers, N.: Evaluation of topical therapies for the treatment of dermatophytosis in dogs and cats. Proc. Annu. Memb. Meet. Am. Acad. Vet. Dermatol. Am. Coll. Vet. Dermatol. 9:29, 1993.

58c. Woodgyer, A. J.: Asymptomatic carriage of dermatophytes by cats. N. Z. Vet. J. 25:67, 1977.

59. Wright, A. I.: Ringworm in dogs and cats. J. Small Anim. Pract. 30:242, 1989.

60. Yager, J. A., et al.: Mycetoma-like granuloma in a cat caused by *Microsporum canis*. J. Comp. Pathol. 96:171, 1986.

60a. Zaror, L., et al.: The role of cats and dogs in the epidemiological cycle of *Microsporum canis*. Mykosen 29:185, 1986.

Candidiasis

61. Bourdeau, P., et al.: Hyperkératose et candidose cutanée chez un chien. Etude d'un cas. Rec. Méd. Vét. 160:803, 1984.

61a. Carlotti, D. N., et al.: Les mycoses superficielles chez le chat. Prat. Méd. Chirurg. Anim. Cie. 28:241, 1993.

62. Dale, J. E.: Canine dermatosis caused by *Candida parapsilosis*. Vet. Med. Small Anim. Clin. 67:548, 1972.

63. Ehrensaft, D. V., et al.: Disseminated candidiasis in leukopenic dogs. Proc. Soc. Exp. Biol. Med. 160:6, 1979.

63a. Gerding, P. A., Jr., et al.: Ocular and disseminated candidiasis in an immunosuppressed cat. J. Am. Vet. Med. Assoc. 204:1635, 1994.

64. Greene, C. E., Chandler, F. W.: Candidiasis. In: Greene, C. E. (ed.). Infectious Diseases of Dogs and Cats. W. B. Saunders Co., Philadelphia, 1990, p. 723.

65. Holøoymoen, J. I., et al.: Systemisk candidiasis (moniliasis) hos hund. En kasusbeskrivelse. Nord. Vet. Med. 34:362, 1982.

66. Ichijo, S., et al.: A canine case of cutaneous phyma caused by *Candida zeylanoides*. Jpn. J. Vet. Med. Assoc. 37:773, 1984.

67. Kral, F., Uscavage, J. P.: Cutaneous candidiasis in a dog. J. Am. Vet. Med. Assoc. 136:612, 1960.

68. Pichler, M. E., et al.: Cutaneous and mucocutaneous candidiasis in a dog. Comp. Cont. Educ. 7:225, 1985.

69. Schwartzman, R. M., et al.: Experimentally induced cutaneous moniliasis *(Candida albicans)* in the dog. J. Small Anim. Pract. 6:327, 1965.

Malasseziasis

69a. Bond, R., Sant, R. E.: The recovery of *Malassezia* pachydermatis from canine skin. Vet. Dermatol. News. 15:25, 1993.

70. Dufait, R.: *Pityrosporum canis* as the cause of canine chronic dermatitis. Vet. Med. Small Anim. Clin. 78:1055, 1983.

71. Dufait, R.: Over de werkingran enkele imidazoleverbindingen op *Pityrosporum canis*. Vlaams Diergeneesk. Tijdschr. 50:99, 1981.

72. Fontaine, J., Remy, I.: Quel est votre diagnostic? Point Vét. 24:385, 1992.

72a. Kennis, R. A.: Quantitation and topographical analysis of *Malassezia* organisms on normal canine skin. Proc. Annu. Memb. Meet. Am. Acad. Vet. Dermatol. Am. Coll. Vet. Dermatol. 9:23, 1993.

73. Kieffer, M., et al.: Immunological reactions to *Pityrosporum ovale* in adult patients with atopic and seborrheic dermatitis. J. Am. Acad. Dermatol. 22:739, 1990.

74. Lorenzini, R., et al.: *In vitro* sensitivity of *Malassezia* spp. to various antimycotics. Drugs Exp. Clin. Res. 11:393, 1985.

75. Mason, K. V., Evans, A. G.: Dermatitis associated with *Malassezia pachydermatis* in 11 dogs. J. Am. Anim. Hosp. Assoc. 27:13, 1991.

76. Mason, K. V.: Cutaneous *Malassezia*. In: Griffin, C. E., et al. (eds.). Current Veterinary Dermatology. Mosby–Year Book, St. Louis, 1993, p. 44.

76a. Mason, K. V., Stewart, L. J.: Malassezia and canine dermatitis. In: Ihrke, P. J., et al. (eds). Advances in Veterinary Dermatology II. New York: Pergamon Press, 1993, p. 399.

77. McNeil, P. E.: *Pityrosporum* in canine skin biopsies. Vet. Dermatol. News. 13:17, 1991.

78. Pedersen, K.: Seboreisk dermatitis hos 10 hunde forårsaget af *Malassezia pachydermatis (Malassezia canis)*. Dansk Veterinaer. 75:513, 1992.

79. Plant, J. D., et al.: Factors associated with and prevalence of high *Malassezia pachydermatis* numbers on dog skin. J. Am. Vet. Med. Assoc. 201:879, 1992.

80. Sanguinetti, V., et al.: A survey of 120 isolates of *Malassezia (Pityrosporum) pachydermatis*. Mycopathologia 85:93, 1984.

81. Scott, D. W., Miller, W. H., Jr.: Epidermal dysplasia and *Malassezia pachydermatis* infection in West Highland white terriers. Vet. Dermatol. 1:25, 1989.

81a. Scott, D. W.: Bacteria and yeast on the surface and within noninflamed hair follicles of skin biopsies from dogs with nonneoplastic dermatoses. Cornell Vet. 82:379, 1992.
81b. Scott, D. W.: Bacteria and yeast on the surface and within noninflamed hair follicles of skin biopsies from cats with nonneoplastic dermatoses. Cornell Vet. 82:371, 1992.

Rhodotorulosis
81c. Bourdeau, P., et al.: Suspicion de dermatomycose à *Rhodotorula mucilaginosa* chez un chat infecté par le FeLV et le FIV. Rec. Méd. Vét. 168:91, 1992.

Eumycotic Mycetoma
82. Allison, N., et al.: Eumycotic mycetoma caused by *Pseudallescheria boydii* in a dog. J. Am. Vet. Med. Assoc. 194:797, 1989.
83. Baszler, T., et al.: Disseminated pseudallescheriasis in a dog. Vet. Pathol. 25:95, 1988.
84. Beale, K. M., Pinson, D.: Phaeohyphomycosis caused by two different species of *Curvularia* in two animals from the same household. J. Am. Anim. Hosp. Assoc. 26:67, 1990.
85. Coyle, V., et al.: Canine mycetoma: A case report and review of the literature. J. Small Anim. Pract. 25:261, 1984.
86. Foil, C. S.: Eumycotic mycetoma. In: Greene, C. E. (ed.). Infectious Diseases of Dogs and Cats. W. B. Saunders Co., Philadelphia, 1990, p. 738.
87. McElroy, J. A., et al.: Mycetoma: Infection with tumefaction, draining sinuses, and "grains." Cutis 49:107, 1992.
88. Mezza, L. E., Harvey, H. J.: Osteomyelitis associated with maduromycotic mycetoma in the foot of a dog. J. Am. Anim. Hosp. Assoc. 21:215, 1985.
89. van den Broek, A. H. M., Thoday, K. L.: Eumycetoma in a British cat. J. Small Anim. Pract. 28:827, 1987.
90. Welsh, O.: Mycetoma. Current concepts in treatment. Int. J. Dermatol. 30:387, 1991.

Phaeohyphomycosis
91. Ajello, L., et al.: Phaeohyphomycosis in a dog caused by *Pseudomicrodochium suttonii*. Mycotaxon 12:131, 1980.
92. Bostock, D. E., et al.: Phaeohyphomycosis caused by *Exophiala jeanselmei* in a domestic cat. J. Comp. Pathol. 92:479, 1982.
93. Dhein, C. R., et al.: Phaeohyphomycosis caused by *Alternaria alternata* in a cat. J. Am. Vet. Med. Assoc. 193:1101, 1988.
94. Foil, C. S.: Phaeohyphomycosis. In: Greene, C. E. (ed.). Infectious Diseases of Dogs and Cats. W. B. Saunders Co., Philadelphia, 1990, p. 737.
95. Jang, S. S., et al.: Feline abscesses due to *Cladosporium trichoides*. Sabouraudia 15:115, 1977.
95a. Kettlewell, P., et al.: Phaeohyphomycosis caused by *Exophiala spinifera* in two cats. J. Med. Vet. Mycol. 27:257, 1989.
96. Kwochka, K. W., et al.: Canine phaeohyphomycosis caused by *Drechslera spicifera*: A case report and literature review. J. Am. Anim. Hosp. Assoc. 20:625, 1984.
97. Lomax, L. G., et al.: Osteolytic phaeohyphomycosis in a German shepherd dog caused by *Phialemonium obovatum*. J. Clin. Microbiol. 23:987, 1986.
98. McKeever, P. J., et al.: Chromomycosis in a cat: Successful medical therapy. J. Am. Anim. Hosp. Assoc. 19:533, 1983.
99. McKenzie, R. A., et al.: Subcutaneous phaeohyphomycosis caused by *Moniliella suaveolens* in two cats. Vet. Pathol. 21:582, 1984.
100. Muller, G. H., et al.: Phaeohyphomycosis caused by *Drechslera spicifera* in a cat. J. Am. Vet. Med. Assoc. 160:150, 1975.
101. Padhye, A. A., et al.: *Xylohypha emmonsii* sp. nov., a new agent of phaeohyphomycosis. J. Clin. Microbiol. 26:702, 1988.
102. Pukay, B. P., Dion, W. W.: Feline phaeohyphomycosis: Treatment with ketoconazole and 5-FC. Can. Vet. J. 25:130, 1984.
103. Sousa, C. A., et al.: Subcutaneous phaeohyphomycosis (*Stemphyllium* sp. and *Cladosporium* sp. infections) in a cat. J. Am. Vet. Med. Assoc. 185:673, 1984.
104. Tuffanelli, L., Milburn, P. B.: Treatment of chromoblastomycosis. J. Am. Acad. Dermatol. 23:728, 1990.
105. Van Steenhouse, J. L., et al.: Subcutaneous phaeohyphomycosis caused by *Scolecobasidium humicola* in a cat. Mycopathologia 102:123, 1988.
105a. Waurzyniak, B. J., et al.: Dual systemic mycosis caused by *Bipolaris spicifera* and *Torulopsis glabrata* in a dog. Vet. Pathol. 29:566, 1992.
106. Weissenböck, H., et al.: Phäohyphomykose—2 Fallberichte bei Hund und Katze und eine Literaturübersicht. Wien. Tierärztl. Monatsschr. 77:277, 1990.

Pythiosis
106a. Bentinck-Smith, J., et al.: Canine pythiosis—isolation and identification of Pythium insidiosum. J. Vet. Diagn. Invest. 1:295, 1989.
106b. Bissonnette, K. W., et al.: Nasal and retrobulbar mass in a cat caused by Pythium insidiosum. J. Med. Vet. Mycol. 29:39, 1991.
107. English, P. B., Frost, A. J.: Phycomycosis in a dog. Aust. Vet. J. 61:291, 1984.
108. Foil, C. S. O., et al.: A report of subcutaneous pythiosis in five dogs and a review of the etiologic agent *Pythium* spp. J. Am. Anim. Hosp. Assoc. 20:959, 1984.

109. Foil, C. S.: Oömycosis (pythiosis). In: Greene, C. E. (ed.). Infectious Diseases of Dogs and Cats. W. B. Saunders Co., Philadelphia, 1990, p. 731.
109a. Howerth, E. W., et al.: Subcutaneous pythiosis in a dog. J. Vet. Diagn. Invest. 1:81, 1989.
109b. Triscott, J. A., et al.: Human subcutaneous pythiosis. J. Cut. Pathol. 20:267, 1993.

Zygomycosis
110. Ader, P. L.: Phycomycosis in fifteen dogs and two cats. J. Am. Vet. Med. Assoc. 184:1216, 1979.
111. English, M. P., Lucke, V. M.: Phycomycosis in a dog caused by unusual strains of *Absidia corymbifera*. Sabouraudia 8:126, 1970.
112. Foil, C. S.: Zygomycosis. In: Greene, C. E. (ed.). Infectious Diseases of Dogs and Cats. W. B. Saunders Co., Philadelphia, 1990, p. 734.
113. Miller, R. I., Turnwald, G. H.: Disseminated basidiobolomycosis in a dog. Vet. Pathol. 21:117, 1984.
114. Pavletic, M. M., MacIntire, D.: Phycomycosis of the axilla and inner brachium in a dog: Surgical excision and reconstruction with a thoracodorsal axial pattern flap. J. Am. Vet. Med. Assoc. 18:1197, 1982.

Sporotrichosis
115. Dion, W. M., Speckmann, G.: Canine otitis externa caused by the fungus *Sporothrix schenckii*. Can. Vet. J. 19:44, 1978.
116. Dunstan, R. W., et al.: Feline sporotrichosis: A report of five cases with transmission to humans. J. Am. Acad. Dermatol. 15:37, 1986.
117. Londero, A. T., et al.: Two cases of sporotrichosis in dogs in Brazil. Sabouraudia 3:273, 1964.
118. Macdonald, E., et al.: Reappearance of *Sporothrix schenckii* lesions after administration of Solu-Medrol to infected cats. Sabouraudia 18:295, 1980.
119. Moriello, K. A., et al.: Cutaneous-lymphatic and nasal sporotrichosis in a dog. J. Am. Anim. Hosp. Assoc. 24:621, 1988.
120. Netto, A., Wong, W. T.: Sporotrichosis in the cat. Malaysian Vet. J. 8:185, 1987.
121. Rosser, E. J., Jr.: Sporotrichosis. In: Griffin, C. E., et al. (eds.). Current Veterinary Dermatology. Mosby–Year Book, St. Louis, 1993, p. 49.
122. Rosser, E. J., Dunstan, R. W.: Sporotrichosis. In: Greene, C. E. (ed.). Infectious Diseases of Dogs and Cats. W. B. Saunders Co., Philadelphia, 1990, p. 707.
123. Scott, D. W., et al.: Sporotrichosis in three dogs. Cornell Vet. 64:416, 1974.
123a. Werner, A. H., Werner, B. E.: Feline sporotrichosis. Comp. Cont. Educ. 15:1189, 1993.
124. Zamri-Saad, M., et al.: Feline sporotrichosis: An increasingly important zoonotic disease in Malaysia. Vet. Rec. 127:480, 1990.

Rhinosporidiosis
125. Breitschwerdt, E.: Rhinosporidiosis. In: Griffin, C. E., et al. (eds.). Current Veterinary Dermatology. Mosby–Year Book, St. Louis, 1993, p. 711.

Alternariosis
126. Baumgärtner, W., Posselt, H. J.: Kutane Alternariose bei Hunden mit unspezifischen Dermatitiden. Kleintierpraxis 28:353, 1983.
127. Weiss, R., et al.: Schimmelpilzmykose beim Hund durch *Alternaria tenuissima*. Kleintierpraxis 33:293, 1988.

Cryptococcosis
128. Dye, J. A., Campbell, K. L.: Cutaneous and ocular cryptococcosis in a cat: Case report and literature review. Comp. Anim. Pract. 2:34, 1988.
128a. Ferrer, L., et al.: Cryptococcosis in two cats seropositive for feline immunodeficiency virus. Vet. Rec. 131:393, 1992.
129. Hansen, B. L.: Successful treatment of severe feline cryptococcosis with long-term high doses of ketoconazole. J. Am. Anim. Hosp. Assoc. 23:193, 1987.
130. Malik, R., et al.: Cryptococcosis in cats: Clinical and mycological assessment of 29 cases and evaluation of treatment using orally administered fluconazole. J. Med. Vet. Mycol. 30:133, 1992.
131. Medleau, L., et al.: Cutaneous cryptococcosis in three cats. J. Am. Vet. Med. Assoc. 187:169, 1985.
132. Medleau, L., et al.: Clinical evaluation of a cryptococcal antigen latex agglutination test for diagnosis of cryptococcosis in cats. J. Am. Vet. Med. Assoc. 196:1470, 1990.
133. Medleau, L., et al.: Evaluation of ketoconazole and itraconazole for treatment of disseminated cryptococcosis in cats. Am. J. Vet. Res. 51:1454, 1990.
134. Medleau, L., Barsanti, J. A.: Cryptococcosis. In: Greene, C. E. (ed.). Infectious Diseases of Dogs and Cats. W. B. Saunders Co., Philadelphia, 1990, p. 687.
135. Mikiciuk, M. G., et al.: Successful treatment of feline cryptococcosis with ketoconazole and flucytosine. J. Am. Anim. Hosp. Assoc. 26:199, 1990.
136. Noxon, J. O., et al.: Ketoconazole therapy in canine and feline cryptococcosis. J. Am. Anim. Hosp. Assoc. 22:179, 1986.
137. Pentlarge, V. W., Martin, R. A.: Treatment of cryptococcosis in three cats using ketoconazole. J. Am. Vet. Med. Assoc. 188:536, 1986.
137a. Shaw, S. E.: Successful treatment of 11 cases of feline cryptococcosis. Aust. Vet. Pract. 18:135, 1988.
138. Wilkinson, G. T., et al.: Successful treatment of four cases of feline cryptococcosis. J. Small Anim. Pract. 24:507, 1983.

Blastomycosis
139. Legendre, A. M.: Blastomycosis: In: Greene, C. E. (ed.). Infectious Diseases of Dogs and Cats. W. B. Saunders Co., Philadelphia, 1990, p. 669.
140. Rudmann, D. G., et al.: Evaluation of risk factors for blastomycosis in dogs: 857 cases (1980–1990). J. Am. Vet. Med. Assoc. 201:1754, 1992.

Coccidioidomycosis
141. Barsanti, J. A., Jeffery, K. L.: Coccidioidomycosis: In: Greene, C. E. (ed.). Infectious Diseases of Dogs and Cats. W. B. Saunders Co., Philadelphia, 1990, p. 696.

Histoplasmosis
142. Wolf, A. M.: Histoplasmosis. In: Greene, C. E. (ed.). Infectious Diseases of Dogs and Cats. W. B. Saunders Co., Philadelphia, 1990, p. 679.

Aspergillosis
143. Nooruddin, M., et al.: Cutaneous alternariosis and aspergillosis in humans, dogs, and goats in Punjab. Indian J. Vet. Med. 6:65, 1986.
144. Sharp, N. J. H.: Aspergillosis and penicilliosis. In: Greene, C. E. (ed.). Infectious Diseases of Dogs and Cats. W. B. Saunders, Philadelphia, 1990, p. 714.
145. Sharp, N. J. H., et al.: Canine nasal aspergillosis and penicilliosis. Comp. Cont. Educ. 13:41, 1991.

Paecilomycosis
146. Elliott, G. S., et al.: Antemortem diagnosis of paecilomycosis in a cat. J. Am. Vet. Med. Assoc. 184:93, 1984.
147. Foil, C. S.: Hyalohyphomycosis. In: Greene, C. E. (ed.). Infectious Diseases of Dogs and Cats. W. B. Saunders Co., Philadelphia, 1990, p. 735.
148. Littman, M. P., Goldschmidt, M. H.: Systemic paecilomycosis in a dog. J. Am. Vet. Med. Assoc. 191:445, 1987.
149. Patterson, J. M., et al.: A case of disseminated paecilomycosis in the dog. J. Am. Anim. Hosp. Assoc. 19:569, 1983.

Protothecosis
150. Dillberger, J. E., et al.: Prototothecosis in two cats. J. Am. Vet. Med. Assoc. 192:1557, 1988.
151. Macartney, L., et al.: Cutaneous prototothecosis in the dog: First confirmed case in Britain. Vet. Rec. 123:494, 1988.
152. Pore, R. S.: *Prototheca taxonomy.* Mycopathologia 90:129, 1985.
153. Sudman, M. S., et al.: Primary mucocutaneous prototothecosis in a dog. J. Am. Vet. Med. Assoc. 163:1372, 1973.
154. Tyler, D. E.: Prototothecosis. In: Greene, C. E. (ed.). Infectious Diseases of Dogs and Cats. W. B. Saunders Co., Philadelphia, 1990, p. 742.
155. Wilkinson, G. T., Leong, G.: Prototothecosis in a dog. Aust. Vet. Pract. 18:147, 1988.

Trichosporonosis
156. Greene, C. E., Chandler, F. W.: Trichosporosis. In: Greene, C. E. (ed.). Infectious Diseases of Dogs and Cats. W. B. Saunders Co., Philadelphia, 1990, p. 728.
157. Doster, A. R., et al.: Trichosporonosis in two cats. J. Am. Vet. Med. Assoc. 190:1184, 1987.

Parasitic Skin Diseases

■

Chapter Outline

Animal skin is exposed to attack by many kinds of animal parasites.[58, 69, 147, 174, 196] Each species has a particular effect on the skin; the effect can be mild, as in the case of an isolated fly or mosquito bite, or severe, as in the case of generalized demodicosis or canine scabies. Although the reaction of the skin to the infestation may be slight, the common parasitisms must be considered here because the dermatologist is the logical consultant in such cases.

When ectoparasites are vectors or intermediate hosts of bacterial, rickettsial, or parasitic diseases, they become more important than when they produce only their own effect. A severe local or systemic reaction may result when toxins are injected into the skin (e.g., tick paralysis). The larvae of some parasites live in wounds or on macerated skin and produce a condition known as myiasis. The most serious dermatologic concern occurs when the dermatosis produced by parasites living in or on the skin produces irritation and sensitization.

Some parasites (*Cheyletiella* mites and biting lice) live on the skin, subsisting on the debris and exudates that are produced on its surface. Other parasites (fleas, sucking lice, and ticks) live on the skin but periodically penetrate its surface to draw nourishment from blood and tissue fluids. Still other parasites (demodectic and sarcoptic mites) live within the skin for at least part of their life cycle, producing more severe cutaneous effects. The reaction of the skin to these insults varies from trivial to lethal but usually includes inflammation, edema, and an attempt to localize the foreign body, toxin, or excretory products of the parasite. These secretions are often allergenic and cause itching and burning sensations.

■ HELMINTH PARASITES

Ancylostomiasis and Uncinariasis (Hookworm Dermatitis)

The larvae of *Ancylostoma braziliense, A. caninum,* and *Uncinaria stenocephala* cause a characteristic skin lesion in humans that is called creeping eruption. The skin lesions that these larvae produce in dogs or cats are not as severe, because these animals are their specific hosts.[21] The skin lesions are often incidental to completion of the normal life cycle of the parasite, with the larvae quickly abandoning the skin and proceeding to other parts of the body. Although percutaneous entry can lead to completion of the life cycle, larvae penetrating by this route rarely mature.[141] The larvae are present on the grass and in the soil of runs and paddocks during the spring and summer in cool climates, and animals exposed to them become infected. Thus, the disease is essentially one of kenneled dogs on grass or earth runs that have poor sanitation.

Cutaneous lesions seem to be more prevalent in areas with predominant infection with *U. stenocephala* (Ireland, parts of England, and the United States), although animals with ancylostomiasis may also have skin lesions. *U. stenocephala* produces a marked dermatitis on skin penetration but rarely completes its life cycle by this route. It is insignificant as a blood sucker compared with *A. braziliense* or *A. caninum*.[5, 21] The latter can complete its life cycle via skin penetration.

Hookworm dermatitis has been produced by natural and experimental infestations with *U. stenocephala*.[26] With both types of infection, similar clinical and histologic lesions were produced. The third-stage larvae enter the dog's skin on areas of the body that frequently contact the ground. The larvae approach the skin up a temperature gradient to a peak at the animal's approximate body temperature. They enter primarily at an area of desquamation on the skin, although a few larvae may use hair follicles. The larvae enter the horny layer parallel to the skin surface, and there is little evidence of enzymatic activity. The larvae are thought simply to exert pressure by undulating activity, the forward movement being achieved by pushing back against rigid keratinized cells. This route follows the line of least resistance through the outer layers.[133] After they are through the epidermis, the dermis appears to cause little hindrance to the migrating larvae. After larvae pass through tissue, the cells reunite and there is little lasting evidence of their passage.[133] Some other species of hookworm larvae cause loss of integrity of the epidermis as they penetrate it.

Clinical signs of hookworm dermatitis are initially red papules on the parts of the body in frequent contact with the ground. Later, these areas become uniformly erythematous and then thickened and alopecic. The feet are especially affected (Fig. 6:1). However, the skin of the sternum, ventral abdomen, posteromedial thighs, and tail may also be involved. Skin over the bony prominences of the elbows, hocks, and ischial tuberosities may have more obvious lesions owing to the thickened skin and hair loss. The interdigital webs may be erythematous, and the feet may be swollen, painful, and hot. The footpads become spongy and soft, especially at the pad margins, where the tissue can be readily grooved and often stripped from the underlying dermis (Fig. 6:2). The chronic inflammation causes the claws to grow rapidly and to appear deformed. The claws may be friable and may break off, leaving thick, tapered stumps. Arthritis of the interphalangeal joints may be present too.[5] Pruritus is a constant finding but varies in its intensity.

Histopathologic examination reveals varying degrees of perivascular dermatitis (hyperplastic or spongiotic) with eosinophils and neutrophils. The epidermis may contain recent larval migration tracts, which may occasionally be traced into the dermis as linear tracts of neutrophils and eosinophils. Larvae are rarely found but, if present, are surrounded by clusters of neutrophils, eosinophils, and mononuclear cells. Hypersensitivity has been suggested as a cause of the lesions.[185]

Diagnosis can be made with reasonable certainty by the clinical signs, a positive fecal examination finding of hookworm eggs, and a history of poor housing and sanitation. Differential diagnosis may be complicated by a coincidental infection with hookworms. Differential diagnostic possibilities include demodectic mange, contact dermatitis, and intradermal penetration by parasites such as *Strongyloides* and schistosomal agents.

Treatment should emphasize cleaning of the premises, frequent removal of feces, and generally improved hygiene, combined with appropriate routine anthelmintic treatment and prophylaxis of all dogs in the kennel. Dry, paved runs or periodic treatment of dirt or gravel

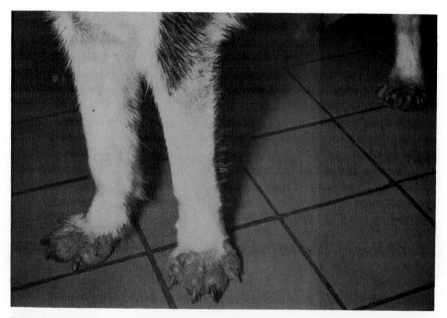

Figure 6:1. Hookworm dermatitis. A Siberian husky confined to a dirt-based run and affected with *A. caninum* shows lesions of chronic hookworm dermatitis on all four feet. There is alopecia, erythema, swelling, and crusting.

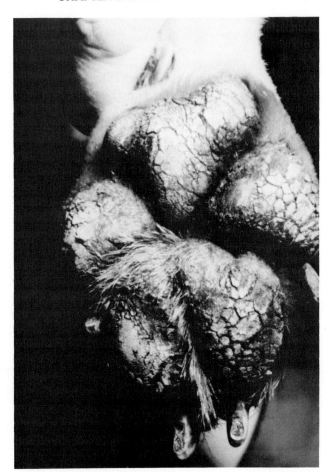

Figure 6:2. Digital hyperkeratosis due to hookworm *(Uncinaria stenocephala)* pododermatitis. (Courtesy K. Thoday.)

runs with 4.5 kg (10 lb) of borax per 30 m² (100 ft²) of run may be helpful, but borax or salt kills vegetation. Attention to measures designed to improve foot health are important. Claws should be kept trimmed short to improve foot conformation and help to alleviate joint stress. The paws should be kept clean and dry. Exercising dogs on new clean pasture is beneficial.

Pelodera Dermatitis

Pelodera dermatitis (rhabditic dermatitis) is a local erythematous, nonseasonal pruritic dermatitis caused by a cutaneous infestation with the larvae of *Pelodera strongyloides.*

Under filthy conditions, the larvae of the free-living nematode *P. strongyloides* may invade the skin of dogs. The adult parasites have a direct life cycle and live in damp soil or decaying organic material, such as rice hulls, straw, and marsh hay that has been stored in contact with the ground for many months. The larvae may invade the skin of animals that comes in contact with contaminated soil or hay.[197] The larvae are about 600 μm long (Fig. 6:3) and may be found in skin scrapings from affected skin or in the associated bedding. In histologic sections, larvae and some parthenogenetic female nematodes may be found in the hair follicles where a typical folliculitis is present.

Pasyk[168] described *Pelodera* dermatitis in an 11-year-old girl who slept with a pet dog with the condition. The larvae invaded the epidermis and hair follicles, and the inflammatory infiltrate of mononuclear and eosinophilic cells surrounded necrotic hair follicles and extended to capillaries and venules of the upper dermis. It was noted that the child might have contracted the infestation from the dog, but it seems more reasonable that both individuals were infested

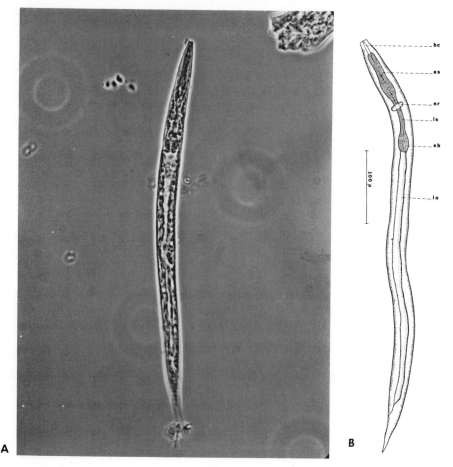

Figure 6:3. *A*, Larva of the free-living nematode, *Pelodera strongyloides*. (Courtesy J. Georgi.)
B, Larva of *P. strongyloides*: bc = buccal capsule; es = esophagus; nr = nerve ring; is = isthmus;
eb = esophageal bulb; in = intestine. (From Willers, W. B.: *Pelodera strongyloides* in
association with canine dermatitis in Wisconsin. J. Am. Vet. Med. Assoc. 156:319, 1970.)

from the same environmental source. Harmon[97] and Smith and colleagues[194] reported that human skin infections with larval nematodes can be contracted from dogs with *A. braziliense*, *A. caninum*, *U. stenocephala*, *Gnathostoma spinigerum*, and *Strongyloides stercoralis*, as well as *P. strongyloides*.

Clinical features of *Pelodera* dermatitis include a distribution of skin lesions that typically involves areas that contact the ground—feet, legs, perineum, lower abdomen and chest, and tail (see Fig. 6:4 *A*).[16, 109, 210] The affected skin is erythematous and partially to completely alopecic. Multiple papules later develop to crusts, scales, and secondary infection from the constant scratching (Fig. 6:4 *B*). Pruritus varies from mild to intense.

Diagnosis is by skin scrapings, which readily reveal small, motile nematode larvae (625 to 650 μm in length). Larvae and adults can also be identified in contaminated litter by using the Baermann technique.[16] The history of contaminated bedding and pruritus together with the skin scraping findings should be diagnostic, but the differential diagnostic possibilities include hookworm dermatitis, dirofilariasis, and strongyloidiasis (all on the basis of the larval findings). Grossly, skin lesions may suggest contact dermatitis, bacterial folliculitis, demodicosis, or scabies.

Skin biopsy reveals varying degrees of perifolliculitis, folliculitis, and furunculosis (Fig. 6:5). Nematode segments are present within hair follicles and dermal pyogranulomas. Eosinophils are numerous.

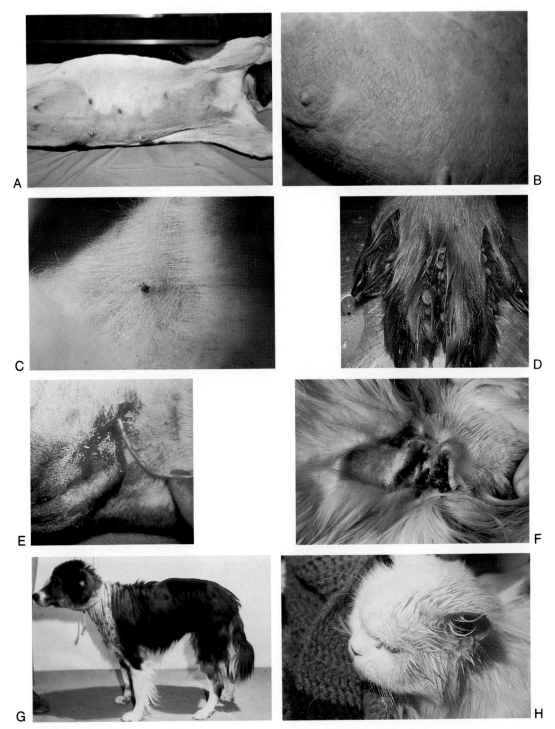

Figure 6:4. *A*, Ventral chest and abdomen of a beagle with *Pelodera* dermatitis. The involved areas are alopecic and erythematous. *B*, Close view of the skin of the patient in *A*, showing intense erythema, multiple papules, and alopecia. *C*, Tick bite. Note the erythematous nodule with a tick attached. *D*, Tick infestation. Pododermatitis in a dog associated with numerous interdigital ticks. *E*, Dracunculiasis. Ulcerated skin lesion of an English pointer's neck with a female adult emerging from a fistula. (Courtesy G. G. Doering.) *F*, Dark brown, waxy exudate and crusts in the ear of a dog with *Otodectes cynotis*. (Courtesy R. L. Collinson.) *G*, Dog with a severe case of generalized otodectic mange. *H*, Erythema and excoriation of pinna and temporal region in a cat with *O. cynotis*.

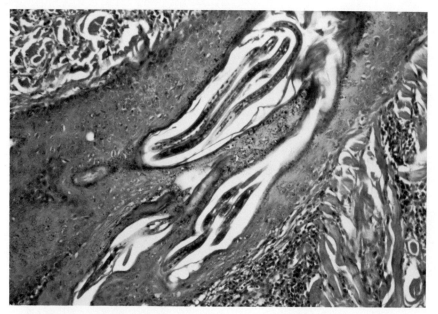

Figure 6:5. *Pelodera* dermatitis in a dog. Numerous nematodes within hair follicle.

Treatment is simple and effective. Complete removal and destruction of bedding are mandatory. Beds, kennels, or cages should be thoroughly washed and sprayed with an insecticide such as malathion and diazinon. The bedding should be replaced with cedar or other wood shavings, cloth, or shredded paper. The patient should be bathed with a warm water shampoo to soften and remove crusts and then with a parasiticidal dip, as for scabies. This procedure usually results in prompt relief of itching and rapid healing. Although repeated parasiticidal dips have been recommended in the past, it is highly unlikely that they are necessary.[16] Prednisolone may be given for a few days to help to stop the pruritus; systemic antibiotics may be indicated for any secondary pyoderma. The infestation is self-limited and resolves spontaneously after the animals are removed from the source of contamination.

Strongyloides stercoralis–like Infection

In a single report, an apparently rare cutaneous manifestation of *S. stercoralis* infection was reported in 5 of 10 Boston terriers in a kennel.[130] Three weeks after a new pup was placed in the kennel, 6-month-old puppies developed mucoid, blood-flecked feces; anemia; general lymphadenopathy; and focal dermatitis. The hair was rough, dull, and dry, and crusted lesions of 1 cm in diameter were on the tail, distal hindlegs, the ventral trunk, and other areas with ground contact. Some pups had a severe, hemorrhagic pododermatitis. The dogs were housed in outdoor pens with concrete and shaded grassy areas. Fecal samples contained large embryonated and unembryonated ova (80 by 35 μm) and first-stage larvae (200 μm). The ova were larger than those of *S. stercoralis* (normally 55 by 32 μm), and this parasite usually sheds only first-stage larvae in the feces. When feces were cultured for 18 hours, free-living adults and third-stage larvae were produced.

Treatment with thiabendazole,[130] 11.4 mg/kg once daily orally for 5 days, or ivermectin,[131] 200 to 800 μg/kg orally, can be effective, but retreatments may be necessary.

Anatrichosomiasis

Anatrichosomiasis is a type of larval migrans caused by the nematode *Anatrichosoma cutaneum*, which produces blisters on the hands and feet of monkeys and humans in Africa. A case caused by an *Anatrichosoma* sp. worm was reported in a 13-year-old South African cat.[186] The cat was presented for lameness with necrosis, sloughing, and ulceration of the footpads of all four feet. Treatment was not attempted, and the cat was euthanized. Histopathologic findings included superficial perivascular dermatitis with numerous worms and bioperculate eggs located in necrotic migratory tracts within the epidermis (Fig. 6:6). Female worms averaging 42 mm in length were identified only as *Anatrichosoma* sp.[186]

A female, 5-month-old boxer was found to be passing double-operculate eggs in its feces. Similar eggs were obtained from skin scrapings taken from a raised, flaking, erythematous nodule on the dorsal midline in the lumbar region. The nodule was removed surgically, and the eggs from the scraping and the nematode segments found in histologic sections were identified as an *Anatrichosoma* sp.[104]

Schistosomiasis

Schistosoma cercariae of ducks, shore birds, voles, mice, or muskrat (natural hosts) penetrate the skin of humans, or other warm-blooded animals that are abnormal hosts, and produce a pruritic dermatitis (*Schistosoma* dermatitis).

Schistosome eggs are shed in the feces of the natural host. The miracidia hatch within 20 minutes and must either find a mollusk (snail) host within 12 hours or die. They form sporocysts in the mollusk and hatch in 4 weeks as cercaria. These are shed into water but die in 24 hours unless they reach a warm-blooded natural host. In the natural host, they go to the liver and the intestinal wall, where eggs are laid and passed in the feces.[107] These parasites are trematodes: *Trichobilharzia ocellata*, *T. stagmicolae*, and *T. physellae* infest waterfowl of the Great Lakes area, whereas *Austrobilharzia variglandis* affects ducks and terns in Florida and Hawaii.[197] In humans, the condition has been called swimmers' itch, clam diggers' itch, and rice paddy itch. These conditions occur because the cercariae penetrate the skin of the abnormal host and produce clinical disease. Although skin exposed to infested bodies of water from spring to fall may become infected, animals are more apt to be swimming and the cercariae are

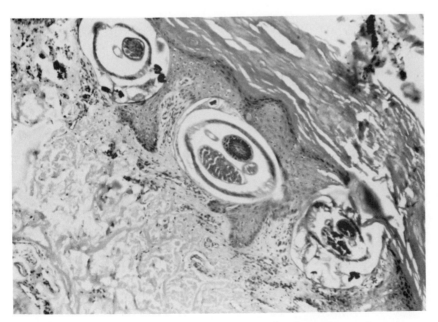

Figure 6:6. Anatrichosomiasis. Nematode segments within the epidermis of a cat's footpad.

much more numerous in the water on bright warm days of midsummer; thus, infection is most common then.

At the time of penetration, the cercariae produce macules and wheals that last 15 to 20 hours. These later develop into papules and, after 2 to 4 days, into vesicles. These stages are intensely pruritic. They are often confused with mosquito, chigger, or flea bites. Healing takes place in 5 to 7 days, as the cercariae are walled off by an acute inflammatory reaction, with infiltration of neutrophils, lymphocytes, and eosinophils. Some humans with the condition have only one strong reaction and on subsequent exposures seem immune, but most people experience increasingly severe reactions on each re-exposure.

Local treatment of the skin is not effective, except with palliative antipruritic lotions. Control measures should primarily emphasize staying out of the water. Actions such as removing water vegetation that encourages snail populations or killing the mollusks by adding dilute copper sulfate solution to small ponds are of limited value. The authors are not aware of documented cases of canine schistosomiasis in the literature but have seen dogs that had signs and a history suggestive of the problem.

Dracunculiasis

Dracunculus insignis is a parasite of dogs and wild carnivores of North America.[87, 111, 164, 173] *D. medinensis* (guinea worm) affects humans, cats, and other animals in Asia and Africa.[150, 201] *D. insignis* has been reported to affect the dog, raccoon, mink, fox, otter, and skunk.[87] The intermediate host is a *Cyclops* (a crustacean) that is ingested from contaminated water by the host. The larvae develop in the host during a period of 8 to 12 months. The adults develop in the subcutaneous tissue of the abdomen and limbs. Usually, a nodule forms, and eventually, a fistula develops (Fig. 6:7). Just before the fistula opens, the host may show urticaria, itching, and a slight fever. When the host enters cool water, the female worm is stimulated to release larvae (Fig. 6:8), which escape through the cutaneous fistula. Some larvae may enter the blood, but they can be distinguished from *Dirofilaria* and *Dipetalonema* larvae by their long tapered tails. One can also apply cold water to the fistula to stimulate the female worm and then make a smear of the exudate to identify the larvae.

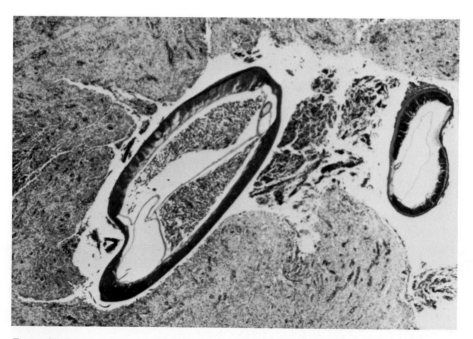

Figure 6:7. Dracunculiasis. Nematode segments in an abscess.

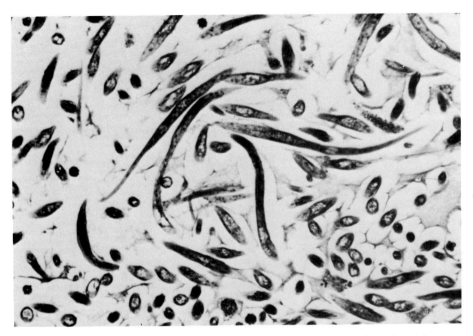

Figure 6:8. Dracunculiasis. Characteristic larvae (enlargement of section from the adult nematode segments as seen in Figure 6:7).

Clinical features are chronic, single to multiple nodules on the limbs, the head, or the abdomen that eventually ulcerate and do not heal (see Fig. 6:4 *E*). The lesions are often painful and pruritic. The adult parasites (female, 17 by 70 cm; male, 17 by 22 cm) may occasionally be seen in fistulae. Exfoliative cytologic study may reveal neutrophils, eosinophils, and macrophages as well as larvae (about 500 μm length). Histologic examination of an excised lesion reveals a pseudocyst containing adult and larval nematodes surrounded by fibrosis and eosinophilic pyogranulomatous inflammation.[164]

Treatment is to remove the worm gently by *carefully* winding it up on a stick during a period of several days. Subsequently, healing of the fistula is prompt.[197] However, the nodule may be excised surgically.[111] Soulsby[197] suggested that large doses of diethylcarbamazine or thiabendazole for 2 or 3 days kill both adults and larvae, whereas Subrahmanyam and associates[201] used metronidazole in a dog at dosages of 200 mg twice daily for 10 days with apparent success. Thiabendazole, metronidazole, and nitridazole are effective for reducing the severity of the clinical signs, encouraging spontaneous expulsion of the worms, and facilitating extraction.[164]

Control measures depend on decontaminating water supplies. With time, the incidence of disease decreases and the disease dies out. Dracunculiasis can be prevented also by drinking only water that is passed through a fine filter.

Dirofilariasis

Adults of *Dirofilaria immitis* live in the heart, and larvae are found in the blood and occasionally in the subcutaneous tissues. Adult worms can rarely be found in abscess-like lesions in the skin, especially on the legs.[38, 56, 186] The microfilaria rarely cause skin disease. Although pustular eruptions, ulcerative dermatitis, and scabies-like dermatitis have been associated with dirofilariasis,[30, 136, 143] the cause-and-effect relationship was not well established in those cases. A pruritic papulonodular dermatitis has been proved to be associated with these larvae and probably results from a hypersensitivity to the larvae.[149, 184, 189]

Dogs with cutaneous dirofilariasis (heartworm dermatitis) typically have a chronic, pruritic dermatitis with ulcerated papules, nodules, and plaques. Lesions are most commonly found on the head or the limbs but can be seen anywhere. Response to antibiotics, topical agents, sedatives, and glucocorticoids is poor.

Peripheral eosinophilia and a positive Knott's test for microfilaria are common findings but lesions can occur in dogs with occult filariasis.[189] Histopathologic examination revealed varying degrees of angiocentric pyogranulomatous dermatitis. Microfilarial segments were present intravascularly and extravascularly within the granulomatous dermal nodules. Eosinophils varied in number from few to numerous. Many of the blood vessels in the central areas of the lesions contained microfilariae, but none of the deep dermal or subcutaneous vessels outside the lesions showed cellular infiltrates or microfilariae. Immunohistochemical staining shows positive immunoreaction of the microfilaria with anti–immunoglobulin G (IgG) serum.[149]

With standard heartworm treatments, the lesions become nonpruritic within 2 weeks and heal completely within 8 weeks.

Other Filarial Infections

A large number of filarial nematodes are found worldwide. The adults reside in subcutaneous tissues, whereas microfilaria circulate in the blood. Typically, no disease is caused by either life stage, but the microfilaria can be confused with those of *D. immitis*. Ocular onchocerciasis has been reported in dogs from the western United States.[83] Adult worms and larvae were found within the pyogranulomatous mass and were either causal or coincidental. Various nonspecific skin changes (e.g., swelling and hyperpigmentation) have been associated with *Dirofilaria repens*[114] and other filarial nematodes.[30] It is not clear whether the parasites induced the dermatitis or were a coincidental finding in some pre-existing skin disease. Because the clinical findings were similar to those seen in filarial dermatitis in other species (e.g., equine onchocerciasis), the nematode is probably causal.

Miscellaneous Helminthic Infections

Parasitology textbooks[85, 197] list hundreds of trematodes, cestodes, and nematodes of domestic and feral animals. Because pets are frequently bitten by the insect vectors for the various parasites or ingest the parasite by eating the natural host or some intermediate stage (e.g., dracunculiasis), aberrant infection can occur and probably is more common than reported. In the unnatural host, the parasite may complete its life cycle if the natural and new hosts are similar (e.g., dog and fox) or may die or encyst in an abnormal site, often the skin. Internal and cutaneous infection has been reported in a dog with *Taenia crassiceps*.[36] Subcutaneous abscesses have been reported in dogs with *Habronema* spp.[181] and *Gnathostoma spinigerum*[10] and in a cat with *Lagochilascaris major*.[47] If there is systemic involvement, the parasite should be identified specifically so that an appropriate parasiticide can be selected. When the parasite has encysted in the skin or the subcutis, the wound should heal with removal of the parasite and good wound care.

■ ARTHROPOD PARASITES

Arachnids

Arachnids differ from insects in the absence of wings, the presence of four pairs of legs in adults, and fusion of the head and the thorax. With ticks and mites, the head, the thorax, and the abdomen are fused so that they have lost their external signs of segmentation. The mouthparts and their base together are called the *gnathostoma*, or *capitulum*. The rest of the parasite consists of fused elements of the head along with the thorax and abdomen, together called the *idiosoma*. There are separate sexes.

PARASITIC TICKS

Ticks differ from mites in their larger size, the hairless or short-haired leathery body, the exposed armed hypostoma, and the presence of a pair of spiracles near the coxae of the fourth pair of legs. Most ticks are not host specific. Ticks are divided into argasid or soft, ticks and ixodid, or hard, ticks. The argasid ticks are more primitive and less often parasitic, produce fewer progeny, and infest the premises occupied by their hosts. Ixodid ticks are more specialized and highly parasitic, produce more progeny, and infest the open country frequented by their hosts.[147]

Argasid (Soft) Ticks

Argasid ticks are more commonly parasites of birds and are found frequently in warmer climates. In regions where they are endemic, they may infest all types of wild and domestic animals. They have no dorsal plate, the sexes are similar, the capitulum is not visible dorsally, and the spiracles lie in front of the third pair of unspurred coxae. Ticks of this class seldom travel far from their lairs and are often nocturnal feeders. Only one species is discussed.

■ *Spinous Ear Tick.* *Otobius megnini* is found in the external ear canal of dogs and cats. Its range is limited to the southern United States, especially the Southwest. The larvae and nymphs infest the ear canal of the host, producing acute otitis externa, pain, and occasional convulsions. Often, the ear canals become packed with immature ticks, but in some cases, only a few are found. Adults are fiddle shaped with a constriction in the middle, but they are not spiny and do not feed, because they are not parasitic. Adults can live 6 to 12 months in a protected environment and lay 500 to 600 eggs. Eggs hatch in days, and larvae typically feed immediately but can survive unfed for 2 to 4 months. The larvae, engorged on lymph from the ear canal, are yellow or pink. They are about 0.3 cm and spherical, with three pairs of minute legs. After 5 to 10 days of feeding, they develop into nymphs. The nymphs, which also inhabit the ear canal, are bluish gray with four pairs of yellow legs (Fig. 6:9). They are widest in the middle, and the skin has numerous sharp spines. The nymphs feed for 1 to 7 months before molting to adults.

Damage from spinous ear ticks results from the loss of blood and lymph. In addition, severe irritation and secondary otitis cause vigorous head shaking and scratching. Treatment involves mechanically removing ticks with forceps, spraying or dipping the coat with insecticidal materials such as pyrethroids and malathion, and treating the otitis externa.

Reinfestation is a problem, so destruction of the lairs or nests of the ticks is important. Spraying the sheds, grounds, woodpiles, and other homesites with malathion or chlorpyrifos may be effective. An amitraz tick collar (Preventic [Virbac]) may prevent reinfestation.

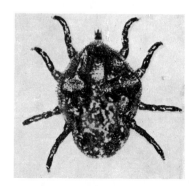

Figure 6:9. Nymph of *Otobius megnini*, the spinous ear tick. (From Lapage, G.: Monnig's Veterinary Helminthology and Entomology, 5th ed. Williams & Wilkins Co., Baltimore, 1962.)

Ixodid (Hard) Ticks

Hard ticks possess a chitinous shield, the scutum, which covers the dorsal surface of the male and the anterior dorsal part of the female tick. The capitulum is visible dorsally at the anterior end, and its base is important taxonomically. The sexes are dissimilar, although both are bloodsuckers. It is beyond the scope of this text to identify ticks specifically, but because *Rhipicephalus sanguineous* (in comparison with *Dermacentor*) can reproduce easily in buildings and thus presents special control problems, a few key features for identifying genera are described (Fig. 6:10).

Rhipicephalus is recognized by the vase-shaped base of the capitulum, by elongated spiracles, and by triangular adanal plates in the male tick. The fourth coxae are no larger than the other three. *Dermacentor* ticks are characterized by the large fourth coxae, the rectangular base of the capitulum, and the ornate scutum.

The general life cycle of ixodid ticks is similar, although each species may vary slightly in some details. Eggs hatch in 2 to 7 weeks. Larvae feed for 3 to 12 days and then drop from the host for 6 to 90 days before molting. Nymphs also feed for a short period (3 to 10 days) before an extended, off-host rest (17 to 100 days). Adults are hardy (up to a 19-month life span) and prolific, with egg lays of 2000 to 8000. Generally, completion of the life cycle necessitates three hosts, preferably animals of varied size, for the larva, nymph, and adult, although some species pass through all stages on the same mammal. If the complicated life cycle is interrupted, the tick can survive for long periods or hibernate through the winter. Although the life cycle is usually completed in a single year, it may extend for 2 or 3 years.

While off the host, these ticks infest ground that is covered with small bushes and shrubs. They resist cold but are susceptible to strong sunlight, desiccation, and excessive rainfall. They require a moist environment.

■ *Common Species of Ixodid Ticks Affecting Dogs and Cats*

■ *Rhipicephalus sanguineus.* The brown dog tick is widely distributed in North America and causes the primary tick problem in many sections of the United States. It can survive indoors, owing to its low moisture requirements, and can complete its life cycle with only one animal as host. Although its principal host is the dog, it is found on other canine and feline species,

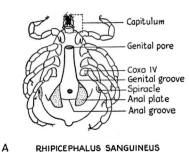

A   RHIPICEPHALUS SANGUINEUS

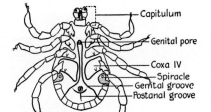

B   DERMACENTOR ANDERSONI

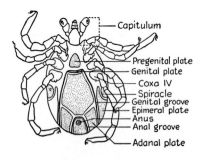

C   IXODES RICINUS

Figure 6:10. Ventral view of various species of male ixodid ticks, showing genital and anal grooves, coxae, and plates. Differential characteristics are indicated by heavy lines and dotted areas. (From Belding, D. L.: Textbook of Parasitology. Appleton-Century-Crofts, New York, 1965; redrawn from Hegner, Root, Augustine, and Huff: Parasitology. Appleton-Century Company, 1938.)

rabbits, horses, and humans. It requires three distinct hosts (but perhaps the same animal) in its life cycle. It can transmit babesiosis and anaplasmosis, *Ehrlichia canis* and *Francisella tularensis* infection, and can cause tick paralysis.

■ *Dermacentor variabilis.* The American dog tick is also widely distributed in North America but is especially common along the Atlantic coast in areas of shrub and beach grass. The principal host of the adult tick is the dog, but humans, domestic animals, and large fur-bearing mammals may be attacked. The principal host of the immature tick is the field mouse, but other small rodents, or larger mammals may be infested. It spreads Rocky Mountain spotted fever, St. Louis encephalitis, tularemia, and anaplasmosis, and causes tick paralysis.

■ *Other Ticks That May Affect Dogs and Cats.* These include *Dermacentor andersoni* (Rocky Mountain wood tick), *Dermacentor occidentalis* (Pacific or West Coast tick), *Ixodes scapularis* (black-legged tick), *Ixodes dammini* (deer tick), and *Amblyomma maculatum* (Lone Star tick).

Damage from Ticks

Ticks injure animals by causing irritation via their bites; by producing hypersensitivity reactions (Fig. 6:11) (see Chap. 8); by serving as vectors for bacterial, rickettsial, viral, and protozoal diseases; and by producing tick paralysis through their poisonous secretions (see Fig. 6:4 *C* and *D*).

Tick paralysis has been produced by 12 ixodid species, including *D. variabilis*, and is seen in many hosts including dogs and cats. The paralysis is caused by a protein toxin produced by the salivary glands of the tick. It may be elaborated by ovarian function, as it is associated with egg production. Individual ticks vary in their toxin-producing capacity, although those attached near the spine and neck seem to produce a more severe intoxication. The toxin affects the lower motor neurons of the spinal cord and cranial nerves and produces a progressive ascending flaccid paralysis.[8, 110]

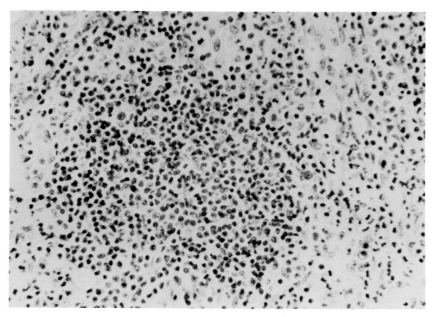

Figure 6:11. Tickbite granuloma in a dog. Central nodule of lymphoplasmacytic inflammation (pseudolymphoma) with peripheral eosinophils. (Courtesy E. Walder.)

Treatment and Control of Ticks

In cases of tick paralysis, rapid recovery follows mechanical removal of the complete tick or ticks. When animals are infested by small numbers of ticks, manual removal from the host is simple and easy. An effective method is to soak the tick in alcohol, grasp the head parts at the surface of the skin gently with a 5-inch curved Crile mosquito hemostat, and apply firm traction. Ticks are commonly found in the ears and between the toes. The collected ticks should be soaked in alcohol or an insecticide until dead.

For cases of heavy or persisting infestations, the dog may be treated topically with malathion, chlorpyrifos, or pyrethrin or pyrethroid sprays or dips. Only pesticides registered for cats should be used for that species. The amitraz tick collar for dogs is reported to be highly effective in detaching or preventing the attachment of ticks.[14]

Infestations of *R. sanguineus* in houses and kennels can often be controlled or eliminated by repeated spraying of woodwork, crawl spaces, pipe clearances, and cracks with chlorpyrifos. For severe infestations, professional exterminators should be employed.

Outdoor control measures are usually impractical but can help limit the number of ticks. Their habitat can be destroyed by cutting and burning brush and grass, by cultivating land, and by rotating pastures. In urban areas, grass and shrubbed areas can be treated with appropriately registered pesticides. Application is done in the spring and repeated once during midsummer.

PARASITIC MITES

Mites are members of the order Acarina. They are smaller than ticks and do not have a leathery covering; the hypostome may be unarmed, and some mites have spiracles on the cephalothorax. Parasitic mites are chiefly ectoparasites of the skin, mucous membranes, or feathers, but a few are endoparasites. They are distributed worldwide, are found on plants and animals, cause direct injury to animals, and spread disease. Because of their prevalence and clinical importance, four parasitic mites—*Cheyletiella* spp., *Demodex* spp., *Sarcoptes scabiei* (var. *canis*), and *Notoedres cati*—and the diseases they cause are discussed in depth.

Most disorders discussed subsequently can be effectively treated with topical pesticides or oral or parenteral avermectins (ivermectin and milbemycin). Currently, the avermectins are licensed only in dogs for monthly administration at low dosages. Their acaricidal dosages are much higher (ivermectin: 200 to 600 μg/kg; milbemycin: 1 to 2 mg/kg). Use at these doses in dogs or any use in the cat is an extralabel drug use and should not be considered unless no licensed product exists, the licensed products cannot be used because of animal idiosyncrasies, or the licensed product is not effective. Casual use could subject the veterinarian to legal action, especially if the animal had an adverse reaction.

Dermanyssus gallinae

This mite attacks poultry (poultry mite), wild and cage birds, dogs, and cats, as well as humans. It is called the red mite, but it is red only when engorged with blood. At other times, it is white, gray, or black. The engorged adult, which is the largest form, is only 1.1 mm in size (Fig. 6:12). It lives in nests and cracks in cages or houses. After a meal of blood, it lays up to seven eggs at a time. They hatch to six-legged nymphs that do not feed. After 48 hours, these molt to eight-legged protonymphs that feed and molt, 48 hours later, to deutonymphs. These also feed and molt 48 hours later to adults. The whole cycle takes only 7 days under ideal conditions, but without feeding opportunities, it may last 5 months.

This mite affects dogs and cats only rarely and almost accidentally.[46] Wild birds nesting in the eaves of houses have mites, which may enter open windows and affect people and animals living there.[24] Ramsay and Mason[171] found such large numbers of mites covering a dog's body that the small grayish white mites crawling on the hair resembled the ''walking'' dandruff of

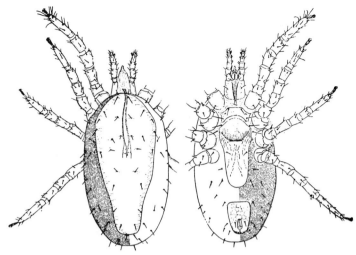

Figure 6:12. *Dermanyssus gallinae* (Degeer). Left, dorsal view of female; right, ventral view of female. (From Lapage, G.: Monnig's Veterinary Helminthology and Entomology, 5th ed. Williams & Wilkins Co., Baltimore, 1962.)

cheyletiellosis. In that case, itching was not severe. Most cases occur in pets that have access to chicken houses or live in recently converted poultry quarters. Clinical signs include erythema and papulocrustous, intensely pruritic eruptions, especially over the back and the extremities. Diagnosis is made by finding the mites in skin scrapings. Almost any insecticidal bath, dip, or spray eliminates the mites. The affected premises that initiated the infection should be treated to prevent reinfestation.

Lynxacarus radovsky

The small cat fur mites are endemic in Australia and Hawaii[23] and have been reported in Florida[70, 89] and Texas.[45] They have elongated bodies, 430 to 520 μm in length, and flaplike sternal extensions. These contain the first two legs, which grasp the hair of the host (Fig. 6:13). All the legs have terminal suckers. Because all fur mites are generally alike, a competent parasitologist is needed for accurate species identification. These mites are not highly contagious and infection typically occurs by direct contact, but fomites may be important for transmission.[45] Bowman[23] reported only 1 of 14 cats in a group to be affected. Usually, there is little itching. The mites attach to the hair and give a salt-and-pepper appearance to the dull and dirty coat. Although hair is easily epilated, the skin either is normal or has a widespread papulocrustous eruption. Mites usually congregate along the topline attached to the terminal parts of the hair. However, they may occasionally be found all over the body. Diagnosis is made by isolation of mites on skin scrapings or acetate tape impression. Treatment with insecticidal sprays or dips, lime sulfur dips weekly, or ivermectin[70] is usually adequate.

Trombiculiasis

Although 20 of about 700 species of chigger mites (harvest mites) can cause disease, only two are reported here.

■ ***Eutrombicula (Trombicula) alfreddugesi (North American Chigger) and Neotrombicula (Trombicula) autumnalis.*** The adult form is a scavenger living on decaying vegetable material. It is orange red, is about the size of the head of a pin, and lives about 10 months, producing probably one generation per year. The eggs are laid in moist ground and hatch to six-legged red larvae that are parasitic and feed on animals. They drop to the ground and become nymphs, and finally adults (Fig. 6:14). The entire cycle is complete in 50 to 70 days, but adult female

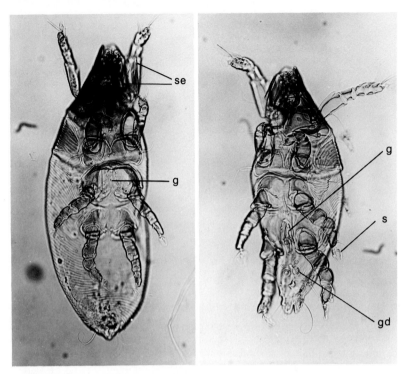

Figure 6:13. *A, Lynxacarus radovsky,* female in ventral view: se = sternal extensions; g = genitalia. Body length = 515 μm. *B, L. radovsky,* male in ventral view: g = genitalia; s = sucker; gd = genital disc. Body length = 430 μm. (From Bowman, W. L., Domrow, R.: The cat-fur mite in Australia. Austl. Vet. J. 54:403, 1978. Photographs by R. Wilson.)

mites may live longer than a year. They are usually found in areas where the skin is in contact with the ground, such as the legs, the feet, the head, the ears, and the ventrum. Signs are variable. The bite usually produces severe irritation and an intensely pruritic papulocrustous eruption (Fig. 6:15 *B*), but it may also cause nonpruritic papules, pustules, and crusts. Secondary scaling and alopecia may appear. Mites may be found in and around the ears of cats but are easily distinguished from *Otodectes* (ear mites) by their intense orange-red color (Fig.

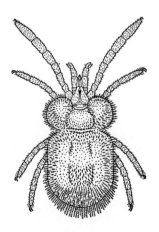

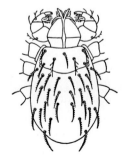

Figure 6:14. *A, Trombicula alfreddugesi* (North American chigger) adult; *B, T. alfreddugesi* larva, dorsal view (legs omitted). (From Belding, D. L.: Textbook of Parasitology. Appleton-Century-Crofts, New York, 1965.)

X 20

X 100

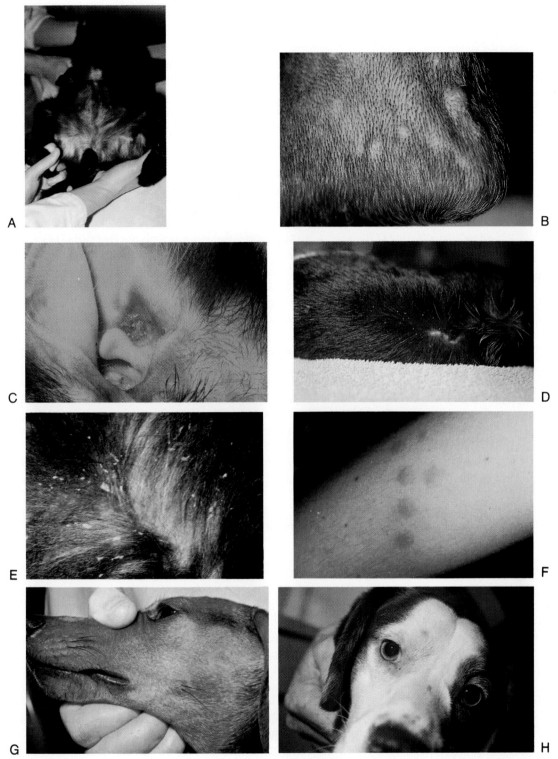

Figure 6:15. *A,* Self-induced hypotrichosis in a cat with *Otodectes cynotis. B,* Papules on the medial elbow of a dog due to chigger bites. *C,* Orange chigger mites on a crust in the temporal region of a cat. (Courtesy T. Manning.) *D,* Scaling over the dorsum of a cat with cheyletiellosis. (Cat is lying on its side on a green towel.) *E, Cheyletiella* infestation in dog. The white specks are walking dandruff. *F,* Papular urticaria of human skin due to *Cheyletiella blakei* bites. *G,* Localized demodicosis. A single alopecic patch at the commissure of the lips. *H,* Periocular alopecia and erythema in a dog with localized demodicosis.

6:15 *C*) and their tight adherence to the skin.[27, 66, 88, 96, 125] When removed from the host for microscopic examination, they should be placed in mineral oil immediately or they will escape.

Chiggers are seasonal in summer and fall and are especially common in the central United States. Affected patients have a history of environmental contact in woods and fields. Skin biopsy reveals varying degrees of superficial perivascular dermatitis (spongiotic or hyperplastic) in which eosinophils are numerous.

Treatment is successful with one or two parasiticidal dips or topical otic preparations containing a parasiticide (Tresaderm).[88] Patients must be kept from contaminated areas to prevent reinfestation. Systemic corticosteroids administered for 2 to 3 days help to relieve the itching, if present.

■ *Walchia americana.* This is a chigger mite that has been reported to be common in squirrels and small rodents in the southwestern and eastern United States and has been reported in the cat.[125] The larvae live on the surface of the skin. Their salivary secretions allow them to feed on tissue liquids of the host. A walled-off channel is formed on the skin surface as a host reaction that attempts to isolate the parasite. The larvae detach and enter decaying wood for a quiet period. Active nymphs emerge and forage, become quiet again as they pass through the imagochrysalis stage, and then emerge as adults. These feed principally on the Collembolla insect (spring tail). The adults lay many eggs, which hatch to parasitic larvae. Some chiggers have a special liking for certain body locations on the host. The mite prefers the ventrum but is also found on the ears and the back.

In the cat reported by Lowenstine and colleagues,[125] the lesions were on the ventral trunk, the medial surface of the legs, and the interdigital spaces. Lesions could be palpated, but the hair needed to be parted carefully to see them easily. There was nodular thickened skin, and the surface was cracked and scaly, with moist, serous yellow exudate. The paws were swollen, and the claws were cracked. The cat shook its feet as if it had stepped into something noxious. Close inspection revealed nonpruritic papules (0.1 to 0.3 cm) with a few wheals and flares. Skin scrapes produced few mites, but a skin biopsy specimen contained many mites.

Histopathologic examination reveals varying degrees of intraepidermal pustular to vesicular dermatitis. Hyperkeratosis is marked, and mite segments are seen within the epidermis. Eosinophils and mast cells are numerous.

Treatment with insecticidal powders for the mites and broad-spectrum antibiotics for the secondary infection produces a good response in 10 days.

Otodectes cynotis

O. cynotis (ear mite) is a psoroptid mite that does not burrow but lives on the surface of the skin. Adult mites are large and white and move freely. The anus is terminal, they have four pairs of legs, and all except the rudimentary fourth pair of the female mite extend beyond the body margin. All legs of the male mite bear short, unjointed stalks (pedicles) with suckers, which are also present on the first two pairs of legs of the females.

The life cycle lasts 3 weeks. The egg is laid with a cement that sticks it to the substrate. After a 4-day incubation, it hatches to produce the six-legged larva. At this point, the larva feeds actively for 3 to 10 days, rests for 10 to 30 hours, and hatches to the protonymph, which has eight legs, although the last pair are small. After a simple active and resting stage, the protonymph molts into the deutonymph. The deutonymph is usually approached by the male adult (Fig. 6:16), and the two become attached (end to end) by the pair of dorsal posterior suckers on the body of the nymph and those on the rear legs of the adult male mite. If a male adult is produced from the deutonymph, the attachment has no physiologic significance; however, if a female mite emerges, copulation occurs at that moment, and the female mite becomes egg bearing. Female mites that are not attached, and thereby do not permit copulation at the moment of ecdysis, do not lay eggs. Sexual dimorphism occurs only in the adult form. The

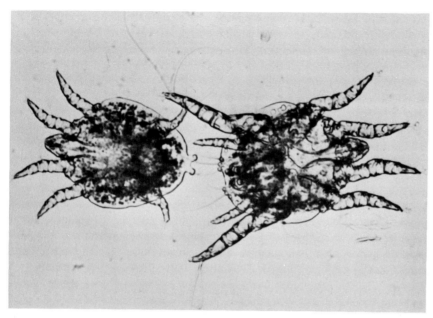

Figure 6:16. Larger male *O. cynotis* mite approaching a deutonymph.

first four legs of all stages bear unjointed, short stalks and suckers, but only the adult male mites have suckers on the rear legs. Adults have approximately a 2-month life span.

The mites feed on epidermal debris and tissue fluid from the superficial epidermis. In this way, the host is exposed to, and immunized against, mite antigen.[170, 205] There is no delayed hypersensitivity, but a reaginic antibody develops early in the disease and precipitating antibodies later in its course.

As the mites feed, the epithelium of the ear canal is irritated and the canal fills with cerumen, blood, and mite exudate. This discharge has the classic coffee grounds appearance (see Fig. 6:4 *F*). Clinical symptoms are variable, especially in cats. Some cats with massive amounts of discharge show no clinical signs, whereas other cats have intense otic pruritus with minimal discharge (see Fig. 6:4 *H*). Dogs tend to have otic pruritus with minimal discharge. Lesions may be restricted to the external ear canal, but mites are commonly found on other areas of the body, especially on the neck, rump, and tail.[13, 185] These ectopic mites often cause no disease, but some animals have a pruritic dermatitis, which can resemble flea bite hypersensitivity, atopy, or food hypersensitivity (see Figs. 6:4 *G* and 6:15 *A*).[17, 94, 119] Other conditions to be ruled out include pediculosis, *Pelodera* dermatitis, scabies, and chigger bites. Ear mites are highly contagious and especially prevalent in the young. The mites are not host specific,[196] so all contact animals should be presumed to be infected. Mites can cause a transient papular dermatitis in humans[99] or rarely become a true otic parasite.[124]

Control of mites is especially difficult in kennel or cattery situations, where multiple animals are found together. Weisbroth and colleagues[206] noted little effect from attempts at control using dichlorvos (Vapona) flea collars. Suggestions for flea control are also appropriate here. Thorough cleaning and insecticidal treatment of the premises with residual materials are desirable. These procedures should be combined with complete treatment of all parts of every animal in contact, using appropriate flea sprays, powders, or dips. This is the most important part of therapy. It should be repeated weekly for 4 weeks.

Local treatment of the ears is important. Many miticidal agents are available commercially. Some contain only parasiticides, whereas other agents contain ceruminolytic agents or antibiotics. Neomycin sulfate–thiabendazole–dexamethasone solution (Tresaderm) is also effective in treating ear mites and its thiabendazole component may have some ovicidal activity.[62] Before and during treatment with any product, the ear canals should be cleaned of all debris to allow better dispersion of the medication. Treatment at the manufacturer's suggested interval should be continued for a minimum of 30 days. Because of its probably ovicidal activity, Tresaderm can be effective with only 14 days of treatment.

Ivermectin is effective in otodectic mange in both dogs and cats when given orally or subcutaneously at dosages of 200 to 400 μg/kg.[13, 77, 195, 213] Most animals receive two doses separated by 2 weeks. Body or otic treatment with a parasiticide is unnecessary. This treatment should be reserved for intractable animals or kennel or cattery situations.

Pneumonyssoides caninum

P. caninum is a mite of unknown incidence; it inhabits the nasal passages and sinuses of dogs.[131a] Most infested dogs are asymptomatic. When signs result, they include serous to catarrhal rhinitis-sinusitis, sneezing, excessive lacrimation, and other signs that could be confused with those of respiratory allergy. Some dogs have facial pruritus.[153] Diagnosis is by mite identification at rhinoscopy or in nasal flushes. The only effective treatment is ivermectin.[153]

Environmental Mites

Many species of free-living mites can be found in grains, in hay and straw, and in the house. These mites can cause skin disease by accidental parasitism on mammals[121] or by the induction of allergic reactions when the exoskeletons, body parts, or excreta are inhaled, absorbed percutaneously, or ingested.[91, 204] The latter method is most important, especially with *Dermatophagoides pteronyssinus* and *D. farinae*, the two most common species of house dust mites. Atopic dogs (see Chap. 8) often show positive reactions to these mites, but the absolute significance of those reactions is uncertain.

Environmental mites may be susceptible to parasiticides used in flea control programs, but the natural habitat of these mites makes their eradication difficult. Hay and straw mite problems can be resolved by removing the hay and straw or by using fresh straw, which should contain the natural foodstuffs of these mites.[121] Food storage mites can be eliminated only by destroying the food. House dust mite populations can be decreased by removal of carpets and frequent and thorough vacuuming of floors, furniture, and bedding. These cleaning procedures may help but do not completely resolve the pet's problem because the basis for the dermatitis is allergy and not direct parasitism.

Cheyletiellosis

Cheyletiella dermatitis (walking dandruff) is usually a mild, nonsuppurative mite-induced dermatitis produced by *Cheyletiella* spp. living on the surface of the skin.

■ *Cause and Pathogenesis.* *Cheyletiella* mites are large mites that affect cats, dogs, rabbits, and humans.[193] The incidence of the disease is unknown because signs are so variable but it is probably less prevalent now because of the widespread use of flea control products, which also kill this mite. The three species of mites may go freely to various host species.[19, 37, 146, 148, 196] In general, *Cheyletiella yasguri* is considered the species found in dogs;[76] *Cheyletiella blakei*, the species in cats;[137, 154] and *C. parasitovorax*, the species in rabbits. Other *Cheyletiella* species also may infest dogs or cats.[135] Experimental transfer of *C. yasguri* between dogs and rabbits suggests that the various species do not have extreme host specificity.[76] All species can transiently affect contact humans.[123]

The large mites (385 μm) have four pairs of legs bearing combs instead of claws (Fig. 6:17). The most diagnostic feature of *Cheyletiella* spp. is the accessory mouthparts or palpi that terminate in prominent hooks (Fig. 6:18). The heart-shaped sensory organ on genu I is diagnos-

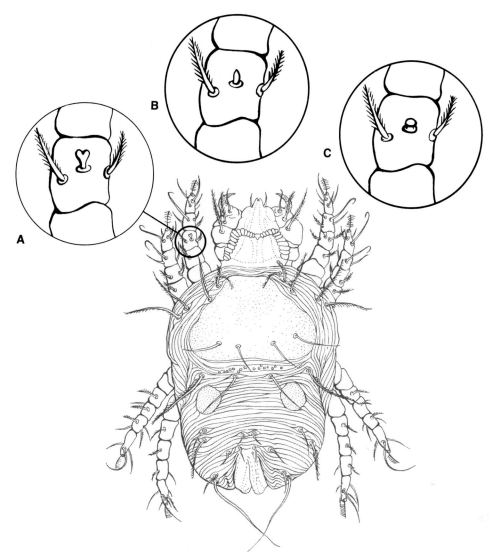

Figure 6:17. Artist's sketch of adult female *Cheyletiella yasguri* mite, showing characteristic saddle-shaped body and diagnostic hooks of the accessory mouthparts. Insert *A* shows the heart-shaped sense organ on genu I that typifies *Cheyletiella yasguri*. Insert *B* shows the conical sense organ on genu I that typifies *Cheyletiella blakei*. Insert *C* shows the global sense organ on genu I that typifies *Cheyletiella parasitovorax*.

tic of *C. yasguri*, the cone-shaped sensory organ is diagnostic of *C. blakei*, and the global sensory organ is diagnostic of *C. parasitovorax*.

The mites do not usually burrow but live in the keratin layer of the epidermis and are not associated with hair follicles. They move about rapidly in pseudotunnels in epidermal debris but periodically attach themselves firmly to the epidermis, pierce the skin with their stylet chelicerae, and become engorged with a clear colorless fluid. The ova are smaller than louse nits and are attached to hairs by fine fibrillar strands. In contrast, louse eggs are cemented firmly to the host's hairs (Fig. 6:19).

Cheyletiella mites are not predacious on other mites. The entire life cycle is completed on one host and goes through the typical egg, larval, nymphal, and adult stages. The life cycle is approximately 21 days. The mite is an obligate parasite, as larvae, nymphs, and adult male

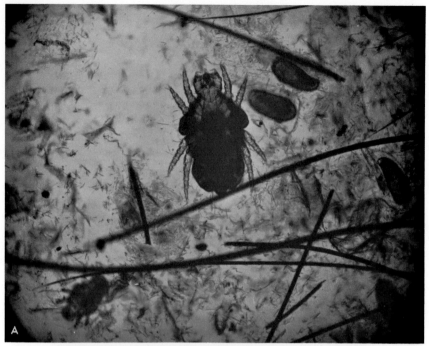

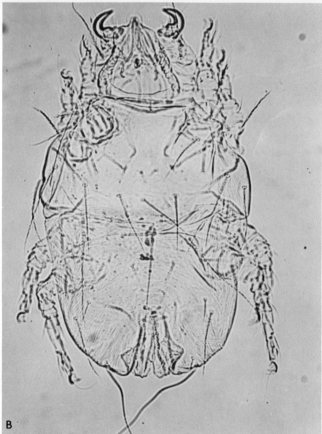

Figure 6:18. *A, C. yasguri* adult, larva, and eggs from skin scraping (low power). *B, C. yasguri* adult mite showing the diagnostic hooks of the accessory mouthparts.

Figure 6:19. Comparison of eggs attached to hair. Left, *Cheyletiella* egg. Small, attached at one end by filaments. Right, louse egg. Large, adhering closely to hair along most of its length.

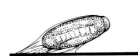
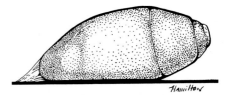

mites are thought to die soon after leaving the host. Adult female mites are more hardy and may live free of their host for up to 10 days.[37, 148] Eggs that are shed into the environment with the pet's hair may be important sources of reinfestation.[146] Stein[198] reported seeing *Cheyletiella* mites crawling in and out of the nostrils of cats and thus added a new twist to the epidemiology and therapy of the disease.

The mites are highly contagious, especially between young host animals, and humans may be affected too. Both dogs and cats may be a source of human infection.[123] In one survey, 27 of 41 catteries that had problems with a pruritic dermatitis had animals with cheyletiellosis.[161] In 20 per cent of these situations, humans cases were also found. *C. blakei* was isolated in all cases. *Cheyletiella* infestation often causes a mild feline dermatosis but probably should be of more concern as a cause of human parasitic dermatitis transmissible from cats.[154]

There is no doubt that the public health aspects of this parasite are important, because frequent contact with infected animals may produce an uncomfortable skin disease in humans. Human infestations vary in severity, but after direct contact with infested animals has occurred, grouped, erythematous macules form on the arms, the trunk, and the buttocks (see Fig. 6:15 *F*). These rapidly develop a central papule that becomes vesicular and then pustular, finally rupturing to produce a yellow crusted lesion that is frequently excoriated because of the intense pruritus. Although the lesions are severely inflamed, they are well demarcated from surrounding skin. Older lesions have an area of central necrosis, which is highly diagnostic. Constant animal contact is usually needed to maintain human infections. With no further infestation, lesions subside in 3 weeks.

Symptoms in dogs and cats are variable and range from virtually none to an intensely pruritic dermatitis. Initially, most infested animals develop a dorsally oriented dry scaling with minimal or no pruritus (see Fig. 6:15 *D*). These initial signs are probably due to inflammation caused by the mites' feeding. Because a cat's natural grooming removes both scale and mites and eggs (both can be found in feces), these initial signs tend to be less noticeable and disease progression is often slower than in the nongrooming dog. With time, the scaling becomes more severe and widespread (see Fig. 6:15 *E*), hair loss can occur, and the level of pruritus tends to increase. In some animals, the intensity of the pruritus is well out of proportion to the number of mites present, suggesting the development of a hypersensitivity to the mite.[146] Animals in this latter group can have an exfoliative erythroderma or a scabies-like condition with the same distribution of lesions and intensity of pruritus. Some cats have a widespread papulocrustous eruption (miliary dermatitis).[19, 148, 196]

■ *Diagnosis.* The diagnosis is confirmed by identifying the mite or its eggs. This can be difficult, especially in cats. Techniques used to identify the mite include direct examination of the animal with a powerful magnifying glass and examination of superficial skin scrapings obtained with a scalpel, acetate tape impressions, a large amount of hair and scale collected with a flea comb, or fecal flotations.[166] In the feces, *Cheyletiella* eggs resemble hookworm eggs but they are three to four times larger (230 by 100 μm) and are often embryonated. The success rate of each technique depends on the length of the animal's coat, the size of the area sampled, and most importantly, the number of mites present.

The most reliable method appears to be the flea combing technique, but this test can be negative in 15 per cent of dogs[165] and 58 per cent of cats.[166] Hair and scale collected in the comb can be evaluated in two ways. The first involves transferring the material to a Petri dish, covering it with mineral oil, and examining its contents with a dissecting microscope. In the second method, the hair and debris are dissolved by treating the sample with 10 per cent potassium hydroxide in a warm water bath for approximately 30 minutes. After this treatment, fecal flotation solutions are added and the solution is centrifuged at 1500 rpm for 10 minutes. The surface layer is examined microscopically at low power for mites or eggs. Each method has advantages and disadvantages, and no studies have been done to compare the two methods. In the absence of positive mite identification, a therapeutic trial may be necessary to confirm or negate the diagnosis.

The differential diagnosis depends on the clinical presentation. If just scaling is present in dogs, the differential diagnosis includes primary seborrhea, intestinal parasitism, poor nutrition, demodicosis, otodectic mange, pediculosis, and flea infestation. If intense pruritus occurs, scabies, flea bite hypersensitivity, and food hypersensitivity must also be considered. For cats, diabetes mellitus and liver disease must be included if seborrhea is present, whereas feline scabies and the other differential diagnostic possibilities for miliary dermatitis must be considered with pruritus.

Histopathologic study reveals varying degrees of superficial perivascular dermatitis (hyperplastic or spongiotic). In some cases, an interface lichenoid lymphoplasmacytic dermatitis is seen. Mite segments are occasionally found within the hyperkeratotic stratum corneum (Fig. 6:20). Eosinophils vary in number, from few to many.

■ *Treatment.*   In many instances, *Cheyletiella* infestation can be resolved by the weekly application of various pesticides to all dogs and cats in contact with the mites. Product selection and its route of administration depend on the species, the age of the animals, and the nature of the animals' coat and dermatitis. Lime sulfur dips or the various flea products are usually effective when applied weekly for 3 to 4 weeks. Conventionally, environmental treatment was not recommended.

Many veterinarians have recognized cases in which these treatments did not work or relapses occurred. These problems can result from poor pesticide application, resistance to pesticide, nasal sequestration of mites, or reinfestation from the environment. One investigator reported

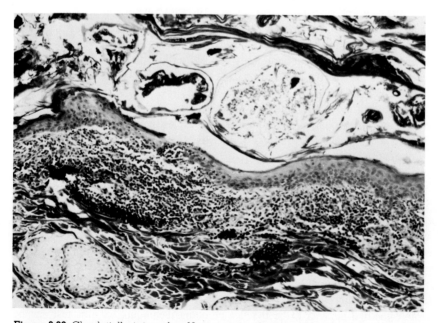

Figure 6:20. Cheyletiellosis in a dog. Note sections of mites within the stratum corneum.

the failure of some routine flea products, the need to treat some animals for long periods, and the isolation of live mites from furniture.[146] She recommended flea-type environmental treatments every second week and treatment of animals with lime sulfur, pyrethrins, or amitraz (dogs only) for 6 to 8 weeks.

If relapse occurs, nasal sequestration is known, the owners are physically disabled, or kennels or catteries are infested, satisfactory control usually necessitates the use of ivermectin at 200 to 300 μg/kg.[165, 166] Two to three treatments at 14-day intervals should be sufficient.

Canine Demodicosis

Demodicosis (demodectic mange, follicular mange, or red mange) is an inflammatory parasitic disease of dogs characterized by the presence of larger-than-normal numbers of demodectic mites. The initial proliferation of mites may be due to a genetic or immunologic disorder.

■ *Cause and Pathogenesis*

■ *Parasite.* The mite *Demodex canis* (Leydig, 1859) is part of the normal fauna of canine skin and is present in small numbers in most healthy dogs.[157–159] Another mite with different morphologic features has been recognized in some dogs with generalized demodicosis.[132a] This mite could be a mutant of *D. canis* or a second species of mite that has gone unrecognized. The skin of dogs with demodicosis is ecologically favorable to the reproduction and growth of demodectic mites. They seize this opportunity to colonize the hair follicles and to populate the skin by the thousands. The resulting alopecia and erythema are known as *demodicosis*. The entire life cycle of the mite is spent on the skin.[180] The parasite resides within the hair follicles and rarely the sebaceous glands, where it subsists by feeding on cells, sebum, and epidermal debris. The variant mite appears to inhabit only the surface keratin and not the hair follicles.[132a]

Four stages of *D. canis* may be demonstrated in skin scrapings (Fig. 6:21). Fusiform eggs hatch into small, six-legged larvae, which molt into eight-legged nymphs and then into eight-legged adults (Fig. 6:22).[159] The male adult measures 40 by 250 μm and the female adult is 40 by 300 μm. Mites (all stages) may be found in the lymph nodes, the intestinal wall, the spleen, the liver, the kidney, the urinary bladder, the lung, the thyroid gland, blood, urine, and feces. However, mites found in these extracutaneous sites are usually dead and degenerate, and represent simple drainage to these areas by blood or lymph. Sako and Yamane[178] found that 76 per cent of the dogs with generalized demodicosis that were examined had mites in their superficial and deep lymph nodes, but the numbers were small compared with those in the skin, and the percentages of adults, nymphs, larvae, and eggs were the same.

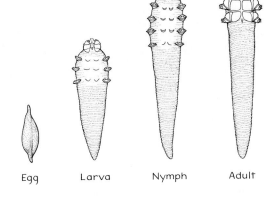

Figure 6:21. Adult and immature forms of *Demodex canis.*

Egg   Larva   Nymph   Adult

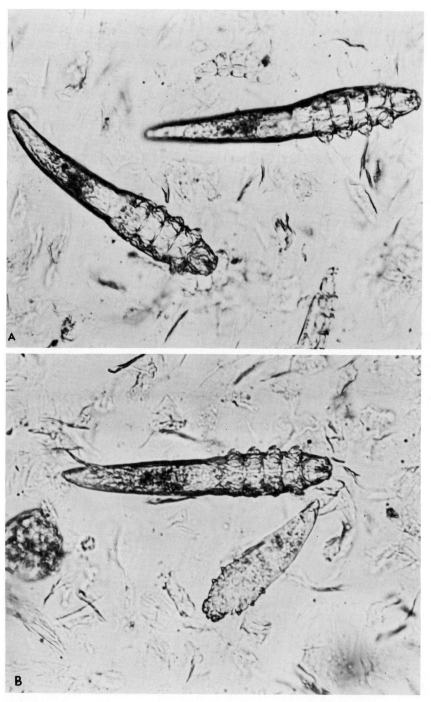

Figure 6:22. *Demodex canis* (×500). *A*, Two adults (four pairs of legs). *B*, Adult and larva (three pairs of stubby legs).

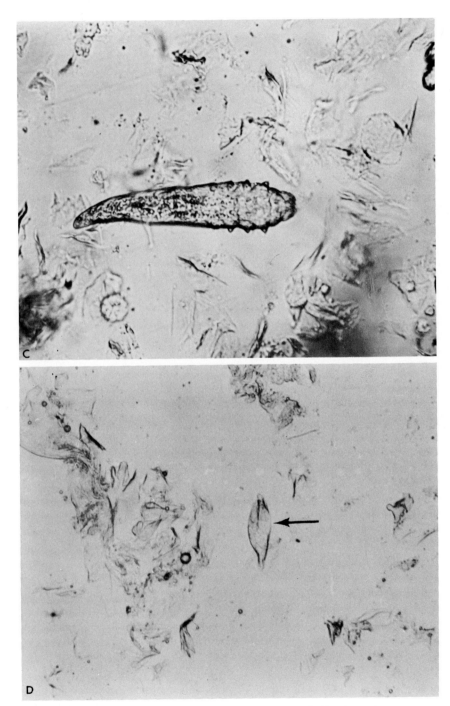

Figure 6:22 *Continued C*, Nymph (four pairs of stubby legs). *D*, Egg *(arrow)*.

■ *Transmission.* D. canis is a normal resident of canine skin. Transmission occurs from the bitch to nursing neonates by direct contact during the first 2 or 3 days of neonatal life.[80] Mites may be demonstrated in the hair follicles of puppies by the time they are 16 hours old. The mites are first observed on the muzzle of the puppies, which emphasizes the importance of direct contact and nursing. When puppies were taken by cesarean section and raised away from the infected bitch, they did not harbor mites, indicating that in utero transmission does not occur.[157, 187] Similarly, mites cannot be demonstrated in stillborn puppies.[179] Although mites can be transferred to normal adults by the application of mite-laden solutions to their skin or by close confinement with a dog with generalized demodicosis,[71, 72] progressive disease does not occur. Any lesions that occur resolve spontaneously.[179, 187]

Sako[180] found the thermotactic zone of D. canis to be between 16 and 41°C (60 to 106°F). Movement of the mites ceased at environmental temperatures below 15°C (59°F). Under various laboratory and artificial conditions, mites could live away from dogs for as long as 37 days.[180] However, these mites lost their ability to infect (invade the hair follicles of) dogs. On a more practical note, after they are on the surface of the skin, mites are rapidly killed by desiccation in 45 to 60 minutes at 20°C (68°F) and a relative humidity of 40 per cent.[158]

■ *Types of Demodicosis.* Two types of demodicosis are generally recognized: localized and generalized. The course and the prognosis of the two types are vastly different. Localized demodicosis occurs as one to several small, circumscribed, erythematous, scaly nonpruritic to pruritic areas of alopecia, most commonly on the face and the forelegs. The course is benign and most cases resolve spontaneously. Generalized demodicosis usually covers large areas of the body but can be more localized, especially when the disease first starts. A dog who has five localized lesions or more, has involvement of an entire body region (e.g., facial area), or has complete involvement of two feet or more has generalized demodicosis. The disease may stay restricted in its scope or may become more generalized. Even with localization of the lesions, the pathogenesis, prognosis, and treatment regimens remain the same.

Generalized demodicosis usually starts during puppyhood (3 to 18 months). If the lesions do not resolve spontaneously or receive adequate treatment, the patient carries the disease into adulthood. It is not uncommon to make the diagnosis of generalized demodicosis in dogs older than 2 years of age. The majority of these cases occur in dogs between 2 and 5 years of age, and most of these dogs have had a chronic skin disease. These dogs typically have had the demodicosis from puppyhood but went undiagnosed. Dogs who first experience the disease at 4 years of age or older have true adult-onset demodicosis.

True adult-onset generalized demodicosis is rare, but when it occurs, it can be as serious as the juvenile form. It has been observed to start in dogs as old as 14 years. Internal disease, malignant neoplasia, or treatment with immunosuppressive drugs is often diagnosed in adult-onset demodicosis patients within 1 to 2 years of the onset of the skin lesions.[7, 54a, 162] In these cases, the dog has tolerated and controlled the demodectic mites as part of its normal cutaneous fauna for years. If the resistance of the host decreases, the mites suddenly multiply by the thousands. One can speculate that some internal diseases may cause immunosuppression or otherwise lower the dog's capacity to control the number of mites, and adult-onset demodicosis occurs. Owners need to be warned that, even if the generalized demodicosis is cured, the dog must be observed carefully for the development of major systemic illnesses and malignant neoplasia in the future.

In pododemodicosis, the disease is confined to the paws, although some dogs have a higher-than-normal population of mites in their clinically normal skin. Pododemodicosis can occur as a result of generalized demodicosis, in which the lesions heal everywhere except on the paws. The foot can be involved, especially in Old English sheepdogs, without generalized lesions. The digital, interdigital, and plantar involvements are almost always complicated by secondary bacterial infections (see Fig. 6:23 *G* and *H*).

Demodicosis may occasionally occur as an erythematous, ceruminous otitis externa. Microscopic examination of ear wax or scrapings of the external ear canal reveals numerous demodectic mites. The ear disease may accompany more generalized lesions.

Demodicosis is more common in purebred dogs and certain breeds have far more frequent disease than other breeds. In the Cornell population, the 10 breeds with the highest statistical risk of generalized demodicosis are the Shar Pei, West Highland White terrier, Scottish terrier, English bulldog, Boston terrier, Great Dane, Weimaraner, Airedale terrier, Alaskan Malamute, and Afghan hound.[144] Demodicosis is commonly diagnosed in other breeds (e.g., Doberman pinscher), but the frequency in those breeds is not out of proportion to the number of dogs within that breed. To the authors' knowledge, any breed of dog, with the possible exception of the Mexican hairless or Chinese crested, can develop generalized demodicosis.

A hereditary predisposition has been observed regularly in breeding kennels. Certain breeders can predict which litters will have the disease. In an affected litter, all or some of the siblings experience generalized demodicosis. Elimination of affected or carrier dogs (both parents and siblings) from a breeding program greatly reduces or eliminates the incidence of demodicosis in that population of dogs. By following this strict culling program, some kennels have virtually eliminated the disease from their line. Analysis of the incidence data from one collie kennel (WHM) and one beagle kennel (DWS) conducted by the authors suggested an autosomal recessive mode of inheritance.[143]

Other predisposing factors suggested for demodicosis include age, short hair, poor nutrition, estrus, parturition, stress, endoparasites, and debilitating diseases. Most of these factors are difficult to evaluate and many are highly unlikely to be predisposing factors. Length of hair coat, size and activity of sebaceous glands, sex of the animal, and biotin deficiency have no effect on the development or progression of demodicosis.[187] In fact, the great majority of clinical cases are seen in purebred dogs that are receiving excellent diets and are otherwise in generally good condition.

■ *Pathogenesis.* If most dogs harbor the *Demodex* mite as part of their normal fauna, the question must be answered why some dogs develop demodicosis and other dogs do not. Differences in the virulence of some *Demodex* strains has been considered but seem unlikely. In litters with demodicosis, some puppies have serious disease while others remain normal. Because these normal puppies have been exposed to the same mite population as their affected littermates, demodicosis cannot be solely associated with the strain of mite. The induction of demodicosis in dogs treated with antilymphocyte serum[40] demonstrated the probable role of immunodeficiency in this disease. The development of demodicosis in adult dogs undergoing immunosuppressive treatments[162] or having cancer or serious metabolic disorders[93] supported this theory. However, broad-based immunosuppression does not explain most cases of demodicosis. If puppies with generalized demodicosis were compromised immunologically, they should develop viral disorders, pneumonias, or other systemic infections and they do not.[187, 188] Likewise, most adult dogs having cancer, especially of the lymphoreticular system, or undergoing immunosuppressive treatment for autoimmune disorders or cancer should develop demodicosis and they do not. A mite-specific immunoincompetence of varying severity helps to explain these disparities. Immunologic studies that support this theory are as follows:

■ *Nonspecific Immunity.* Nonspecific immunity in canine demodicosis has been studied in the neutrophil and complement systems. No absolute deficiencies of neutrophils or abnormalities in neutrophil morphologic features have been observed.[187, 188] Additionally, dogs with proven neutrophil dysfunction do not develop demodicosis. Limited complement studies have not shown any association of complement deficiency with demodicosis.[210a]

■ *Humoral Immunity.* Dogs with generalized demodicosis typically have normal to elevated numbers of plasma cells in their skin, bone marrow, lymph nodes, and spleen.[187, 188] When these dogs are vaccinated with Aleutian mink disease virus or canine distemper–infectious canine

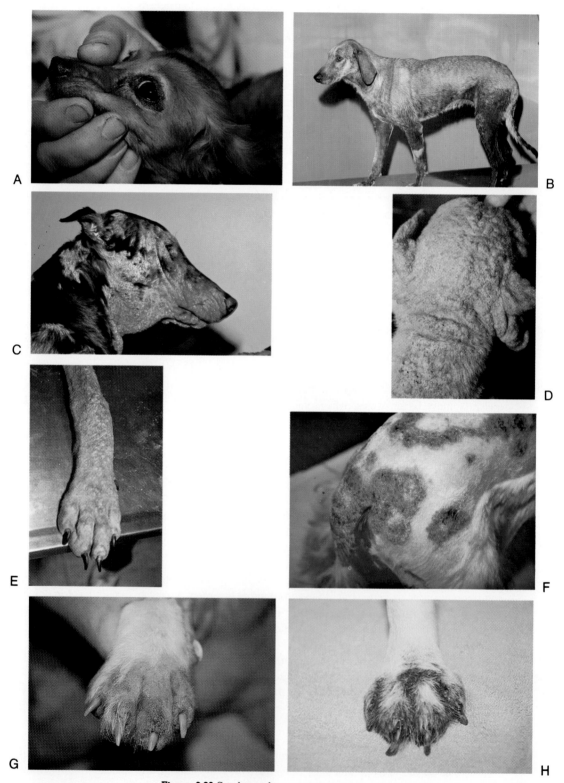

Figure 6:23 *See legend on opposite page*

hepatitis vaccine, they can mount a normal antibody response.[40] The number of IgE-bearing mast cells in the skin of dogs with demodicosis is identical to that found in specific pathogen–free dogs.[102] Most dogs with generalized demodicosis have a hyperglobulinemia and show a reactive serum protein electrophoretic pattern.[187] Dogs with IgM or IgA deficiency do not appear to be predisposed to demodicosis. All these studies demonstrate that humoral immuno-deficiency is not the cause of demodicosis and that many of these dogs have hyper-reactive B cell responses. This hyper-reactivity may be the result of T cell hyporeactivity.

■ *Cellular Immunity.* Dogs with chronic generalized demodicosis have depressed T cell function, as measured by the in vitro lymphocyte blastogenesis (IVLB) test[40, 41, 106, 187, 188] or skin testing with phytohemagglutinin, concanavalin A, or dinitrochlorobenzene.[41, 100, 103, 208] Because these dogs are rarely lymphopenic and have no hypocellularity of the T cell areas of the lymph nodes and spleen, the deficiency appears to be one of function rather than numbers.

The IVLB test can be performed by various methods, is subject to a variety of technical problems, and does not give identical results in dogs of the same breed and age.[7] Accordingly, studies using this test should be performed in a large number of dogs and the results must be evaluated by appropriate statistical analysis. Much of the work on the IVLB in dogs with demodicosis was not subject to such careful scrutiny, and the conclusions drawn may not be valid.

The original work demonstrated that the IVLB suppression seen in demodicosis was largely caused by a humoral immunosuppressive factor.[106, 188] The factor, either an immunoglobulin or an immune complex,[120] suppressed the blastogenesis of a normal dog's lymphocytes, could be made less active by dilution with fetal bovine serum or other techniques, and disappeared when the number of mites was reduced with treatment.[106, 188] These data, coupled with the normal IVLB results from dogs with localized demodicosis or early generalized disease,[7, 40, 188] resulted in the hypothesis that the immunosuppression of demodicosis was parasite induced. As the mites start to proliferate, they produced or more likely induced the humoral factor, which suppressed the immune response to the parasite and allowed the proliferation of the mites to continue unchecked.

Work by Barta and colleagues[9] seemed to refute that theory. In that study, dogs with demodicosis and no bacterial pyoderma had normal IVLB test results, whereas dogs with demodicosis and pyoderma or pyoderma alone had IVLB suppression. The degree of suppression in these latter dogs correlated with the severity of the pyoderma. The conclusion was that the immunosuppression was a consequence of the bacterial pyoderma, a common problem in demodicosis, and not the mites themselves.

More recent work refuted some of Barta's conclusions and supported the original hypothesis.[7] This study showed that dogs with either localized or generalized demodicosis of 3 weeks' duration had normal cell-mediated function when compared with that of normal dogs. When the testing was repeated 3 weeks later, 6 weeks after the appearance of clinical signs, dogs with localized demodicosis had slight depression in response to phytohemagglutinin and moderate depression in response to concanavalin A stimulation. Dogs with generalized disease had severe depression with concanavalin A, phytohemagglutinin, and lipopolysaccharide. The conclusions

Figure 6:23. *A,* Periocular alopecia and hyperpigmentation in a dog with localized demodicosis. *B,* Hound-cross with chronic generalized demodicosis. *C,* A 9-month-old Doberman pinscher whose once beautiful face is disfigured by the effects of the disease. The loose fold of skin at the throat containing numerous pustules is characteristic. *D,* Follicular papules, crusts, and alopecia over the dorsal neck and top of the head of a dog with generalized demodicosis. *E,* Follicular papules, crusts, and alopecia on the leg of a dog with generalized demodicosis. *F,* Well-demarcated, alopecic, crusted patches of generalized demodicosis with pyoderma on the rump of a West Highland White terrier. These lesions are not easily recognized unless the hair is clipped away. *G,* Canine pododemodicosis. Erythema, alopecia, hyperpigmentation of a paw. *H,* Chronic pododermatitis in a dog with pododemodicosis.

were that the immunosuppression of demodicosis is induced by the parasite and is proportional to the number of mites. Additional information in this study supported Barta's observation of the immunosuppressive nature of bacterial pyoderma. Similar results were reported from a study in which dogs with localized demodicosis, generalized demodicosis, and generalized demodicosis with secondary bacterial pyoderma were given intradermal injections of phyto-hemagglutinin.[100]

The data suggest that clinical demodicosis is a parasite-induced immunosuppressive disorder in which the immunosuppression is proportional to the number of mites present. An intercurrent pyoderma contributes to the dog's immunosuppression. This information does not answer the basic question of why mite proliferation begins or why some dogs self-cure their generalized disease.

A hereditary, *D. canis*–specific T cell defect of varying severity offers an appealing solution, which answers many questions. The hereditary component is supported by the higher preva-lence in certain breeds, and the association of demodicosis with another hereditary disease in beagles.[49] The *D. canis*–specific T cell defect is supported by studies done with *Demodex* antigen. Normal dogs and dogs that self-cure their demodicosis show an adequate delayed-type hypersensitivity skin test result, whereas dogs with chronic disease do not.[40, 41]

With a severe *D. canis*–specific defect, the dog has generalized demodicosis with its secon-dary immunosuppressive component. These dogs require vigorous treatment. With a less pro-nounced defect, the dog does not experience generalized demodicosis unless some other immunosuppressing condition occurred. If the secondary condition was resolved, the demodi-cosis could resolve spontaneously or respond rapidly and completely to fairly simple treatments. In puppies, the immunosuppressive factor could be the stress of puppyhood, whereas more serious immunosuppressive diseases would be necessary in adult dogs.

■ Clinical Features

■ *Localized Demodicosis.* A patch of skin develops mild erythema and partial alopecia. Pruritus may be present, and the area may be covered with fine silvery scales. One to several squamous patches can be present. The most common site is the face, especially the periocular area and the commissures of the mouth (see Figs. 6:15 *G* and *H* and 6:23 *A*). Next in order of occurrence are the forelegs. More rarely, one or more patches are seen on the trunk or the rear legs. Most cases occur at 3 to 6 months of age and heal spontaneously without treatment. It is rare for true localized demodicosis in a dog to progress to generalized disease. When the disease is controlled, hair begins to regrow within 30 days. Lesions can come and go over a period of several months. Recurrences are rare because the skin has apparently become a less favorable habitat for the rapid reproduction of mites or the immunocompetence of the host has returned to normal.

■ *Generalized Demodicosis.* Although localized demodicosis is a mild clinical disease, gen-eralized demodicosis is one of the most severe canine skin diseases; it can terminate fatally. The disease can be widespread from the onset (see Fig. 6:23 *B*) but usually starts with multiple poorly circumscribed areas of disease, which worsen rather than improve with time. Numerous lesions appear on the head (see Fig. 6:23 *C*), the legs, and the trunk. Each lesion gets larger, and some coalesce to form patches (see Fig. 6:23 *F*). Follicular hyperkeratosis is often marked, and close examination of lesions often reveals follicular openings accentuated and plugged with conical hyperkeratoses, while follicular casts are prominent at various levels on hair shafts. Although some dogs with demodicosis have only seborrheic changes (Fig. 6:24 *A*), mites developing in the hair follicle usually produce a folliculitis. Peripheral lymphadenopathy is marked. When secondary pyoderma complicates these lesions, edema and crusting elevate the patches into plaques. Deep folliculitis develops, and exudates are produced and form thick crusts (see Figs. 6:23 *D* to *F*).

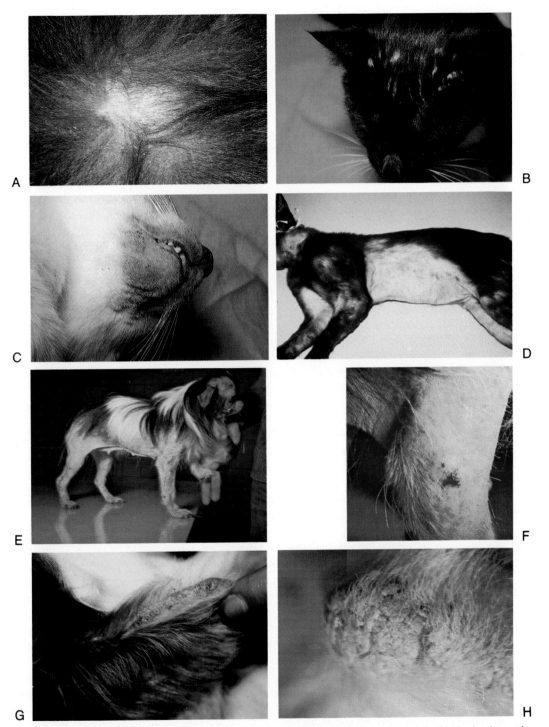

Figure 6:24. *A,* Diffuse scaling, follicular casts, and focal erythema and alopecia over the back of a dog with generalized demodicosis. *B,* Feline demodicosis. Alopecia and scaling of forehead and ears. *C,* Feline demodicosis. Alopecia and hyperpigmentation of chin and lip. *D,* Bilaterally symmetric alopecia in a cat with generalized demodicosis. (Courtesy B. Stein.) *E,* Canine scabies 4 weeks after onset in a Japanese spaniel. Fourteen dogs in a kennel were affected. This illustrates the typical distribution pattern. *F,* Closer view of same patient as in *E,* showing area on elbow where diagnostic skin scraping was made. The typical papular "rash" is well illustrated in this view. *G,* Ear margin showing characteristic grayish yellow crusts on affected skin. *H,* Crusted lesions on the elbow that are typical of a chronic case.

Bacteria thrive under these crusts and in the follicles. *Staphylococcus intermedius* is the most common bacterial organism to complicate generalized demodicosis. *Pseudomonas aeruginosa* causes severe pyogenic complications and is especially refractory when it occurs with demodectic pododermatitis. *Proteus mirabilis* is another serious secondary bacterial invader in generalized demodectic mange.

After several months, the chronically infected skin is covered with crusted, pyogenic, hemorrhagic, and follicular-furuncular lesions. The abdomen is least affected, perhaps because fewer hair follicles are in that area. Numerous lesions are concentrated on the head and neck, and involvement may be severe. Many owners elect euthanasia for their pets at this stage.

■ *Pododemodicosis.* Demodicosis can be present on the feet of dogs without generalized lesions. The case history reveals whether the dog once had generalized demodicosis that healed, except for the foot lesions, or whether the paws were the only part of the body ever affected. The digital and interdigital lesions are especially susceptible to secondary pyodermas (see Fig. 6:23 *G* and *H*). In some animals, pododemodicosis can be chronic and extremely resistant to therapy. The pain and edema is especially distressing to large dogs such as Great Danes, Newfoundlands, St. Bernards, and Old English sheepdogs.

In summary, disease in one dog can progress through the following stages: fairly localized demodicosis, generalized demodicosis, generalized pyogenic demodicosis, and chronic pyogenic pododemodicosis. Rarely, dogs may present with only demodectic otitis externa.

■ *Diagnosis.* Skin scrapings that are properly made and interpreted can establish the diagnosis of demodicosis. The affected skin should be squeezed firmly to extrude the mites from the hair follicles, and skin scrapings should be deep and extensive. Extremely fragile areas should be avoided because the resultant hemorrhage usually makes interpretation of the results difficult. Diagnosis is made either by demonstrating large numbers of adult mites or by finding an increased ratio of immature forms (ova, larvae, and nymphs) to adults. The demonstration of an occasional adult mite in skin scrapings is consistent with a diagnosis of normal skin, *not* demodicosis. However, because it is uncommon to find a *Demodex* mite in the scrapings from normal dogs, the finding of one mite should not be ignored. The dog should be scraped at several additional sites before the diagnosis of demodicosis is dismissed.

Skin scraping appears to be a straightforward, easy laboratory procedure; however, every year, the authors continue to receive cases on referral that somehow had negative findings on scraping and were misdiagnosed. Adequate skin scrapings are mandatory in all cases of canine pyoderma and seborrhea complex. When negative skin scraping findings are obtained from a Shar Pei or from a dog with fibrotic lesions, especially in the interdigital region, a skin biopsy specimen should be examined before demodicosis is ruled out.

Clinical laboratory tests in young dogs with demodicosis usually show no consistent abnormalities. Anemia of chronic disease, elevations in white blood cell numbers, hyperglobulinemia, and depressed baseline thyroid hormone levels are found in many dogs. The depressed thyroid hormone values are usually the result of the demodicosis (euthyroid sick syndrome, see Chap. 9) and not its cause. In cases of adult-onset demodicosis, these routine tests become more significant in identifying the cause of the demodicosis.[142] If baseline thyroid hormone levels are depressed, additional thyroid testing should be performed because hypothyroidism can trigger demodicosis in the adult dog.[54a, 175] Unexplained elevations in liver enzyme activity should lead to the consideration of adrenal function tests (see Chap. 9) for hyperadrenocorticism, a common cause of adult-onset demodicosis.[54a, 93]

■ *Histopathology.* Skin biopsy specimens from dogs with localized or generalized demodicosis show follicles containing mites and keratinous debris (Figs. 6:25 and 6:26) and inflammatory perifolliculitis, folliculitis, or suppurative furunculosis.[6, 32] Many cases share all three

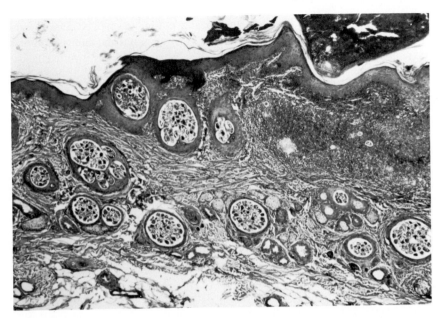

Figure 6:25. Demodicosis in a dog. Note hair follicles containing numerous mite segments and a pyogranuloma due to follicular rupture (upper right).

patterns. Mural folliculitis, in which plasma cells, lymphocytes, macrophages, mast cells, and eosinophils are found around the follicles and infiltrating the epithelium, was a consistent finding in one study of 33 dogs.[32] In the same study, 8 of 33 cases had perifollicular granulomas surrounding mite fragments and 7 of 33 had a suppurative furunculosis as the main pattern. In these 33 cases, 10 per cent of the perifollicular cells and 90 per cent of the cells infiltrating the follicular epithelium were T cells. Perifollicular melanosis is also a common finding in skin biopsy specimens from dogs with generalized demodicosis.[32a]

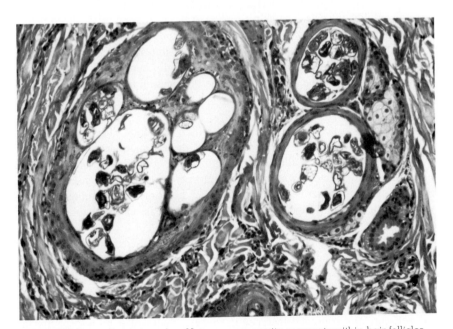

Figure 6:26. Demodicosis in a dog. Note numerous mite segments within hair follicles.

To date, skin biopsy is not reliable in differentiating localized from generalized demodicosis or in indicating whether self-cure is likely. However, if mites are numerous and there is minimal to absent cellular response or eosinophils are absent, especially when there is a furunculosis, the dog likely has severe immunosuppression.

■ ***Differential Diagnosis.*** Because skin scrapings easily reveal mites in the vast majority of cases of demodicosis, the disease should not be confused with other disorders. Generalized pyoderma may resemble demodicosis, and demodicosis should be suspected in every case of folliculitis. Dermatophytosis resembles patches of localized demodicosis. Superficial abrasions in young dogs sometimes resemble the erythematous patches of localized demodicosis. Conversely, demodicosis may be mistaken for abrasions. Muzzle folliculitis or furunculosis (acne) on the face of young dogs sometimes resembles pustular demodicosis, and certain demodectic pustules on the abdomen and inside surface of the thighs resemble canine impetigo. Differentiation can be made by examination of skin scrapings or by biopsy. Contact dermatitis exhibits erythematous papules that occasionally resemble squamous demodicosis. Pemphigus complex, lupus erythematosus, and dermatomyositis facial lesions can also mimic demodicosis.

■ ***Clinical Management***

■ ***Localized Demodicosis.*** This is a mild disease that usually heals spontaneously in 6 to 8 weeks, but may wax and wane in a localized area for months. There is no difference in healing between treated and untreated cases.[152a] There is no evidence that treatment of localized demodicosis prevents generalization in cases so destined. If the clinician believes that some form of treatment is indicated, a mild topical parasitide used to treat ear mites or benzoyl peroxide gel (OxyDex gel, Pyoben gel) can be gently massaged into the alopecic area once a day. The medication should be rubbed in the direction of the hair growth so that as few hairs as possible are pulled out. The owner should be informed that the medications and the rubbing necessary to apply them worsen the lesions for 2 to 3 weeks. This does not affect the outcome of the disease, as the lesions only appear to be getting larger. It is important to check the general health status of the dog at this time, paying special attention to diet, endoparasite problems, and vaccination needs. Amitraz is not a rational treatment for localized demodicosis.

At a return visit 4 weeks later, the veterinarian can determine whether there are any indications of generalized demodicosis. The skin scraping at the beginning of localized demodicosis often reveals numbers of live adult mites and immature forms. After 4 weeks of treatment, skin scrapings from healing cases should show fewer mites, fewer immature forms, and sometimes no live mites. If the lesions are spreading and the mite count (including the ratio of immature to adult) is high, the condition may be progressing to generalized demodicosis.

■ ***Generalized Demodicosis.*** This serious disease is difficult to treat. The owner of the affected dog must be made aware of this and informed of the estimated length and cost of treatment, as well as the prognosis for a clinical cure. Euthanasia, commonly resorted to in the past, is rarely necessary if a dedicated owner uses current treatments. With intense treatment, most cases, perhaps as many as 94 per cent, can be cured.[152a] Most of the remaining cases can be controlled with treatments. Many owners accept this regimen as an acceptable price for salvaging their pets' lives.

A discussion of euthanasia before outlining the treatment may seem strange, but it is necessary because, although the prognosis for generalized demodicosis has improved dramatically in the past 5 years, it still is not an easily treated disease. First, approximately 30 to 50 per cent of all dogs less than 1 year of age with generalized demodicosis recover spontaneously. No data are available to indicate whether treatment accelerates the dog's self-cure, and this significant rate of self-cure can confound therapeutic studies. Studies that do not specify the age of the dogs or the extent of disease cannot be evaluated critically.[78] To euthanize 6- to 12-

month-old dogs because they have severe generalized demodicosis is unwarranted, because some of them recover spontaneously if secondary pyodermas and seborrheas are controlled and the general health status is good. Dogs older than 2 years of age or dogs with adult-onset generalized demodicosis have a much less favorable prognosis. The disease can often be controlled but not always cured.

Before the institution of any treatment for the demodicosis, the dog's general health and management should be improved if necessary. This is especially true for dogs with adult-onset disease. Their disease was triggered by some systemic disorder and resolution of the underlying condition allows the dog either to self-cure its demodicosis or to respond better to treatment.

The pyoderma and seborrhea seen in dogs with demodicosis is a result of the mite infestation and cannot be cured until the mites are eradicated. However, these problems should be addressed before topical acaricidal treatment to make the skin less irritable and to allow better penetration of the dip. Antibiotic selection varies with the case, but bactericidal agents should be selected because of the probable immunosuppressed state of the dog. Because of the high frequency of deep pyodermas in these dogs, courses of treatment of 6 to 8 weeks are commonplace. Because of the expense of this long-term treatment, the temptation is to use suboptimal dosages or a shortened course of treatment. Both measures can result in more serious infections and should be avoided.

One investigator found depressed serum vitamin E levels in dogs with demodicosis and speculated that this deficiency caused suboptimal lymphocyte function and disease.[64] Supplementation with vitamin E reportedly resolved the disease in most dogs. Other investigators have not found depressed serum levels,[86] and other clinical trials have not shown vitamin E to be of significant benefit.[143] Other trials with immunomodulatory drugs (levamisole and thiabendazole) have also shown no benefit.[187, 188] Because the immunosuppression in demodicosis is parasite induced, it is not surprising that nonparasiticidal drugs are of limited benefit. Immunosuppressive drugs, especially corticosteroids, are detrimental in those dogs and should not be used. Long-term administration of corticosteroids in these dogs causes the most troublesome cases of demodicosis, which probably do not respond completely to treatment.

Amitraz is the only licensed product in the United States and Canada for the treatment of generalized demodicosis. The drug is diamide, N'-(2,4-dimethylphenyl)-N-[[(2,4-dimethyl-phenyl)imino]methyl]-N-methylmethanidamide.[71] It is marketed in the United States and Canada as Mitaban. Slightly different formulations of amitraz are marked worldwide as Ectodex Dog Wash or Taktic.[28, 29, 60]

To achieve maximal results with amitraz (Mitaban) as formulated for use in the United States and Canada, it is imperative to follow this protocol:

1. Dogs with medium-length or long coats should be clipped closely to allow the aqueous solution to contact the skin and penetrate the hair follicle better.
2. All crusts are removed. In some cases, tranquilization or anesthesia is necessary, because some crusts adhere tightly and removal without anesthesia is painful.
3. Protective ophthalmic ointment is applied to the eyes. The entire dog is washed with a medicated shampoo designed to kill bacteria and remove scales and exudates. Soaking in a whirlpool bath or a gentle stream of water is beneficial. Even though the skin may appear raw and irritated after the above procedures, the medication can have optimal contact with the affected skin. The dog is gently dried with a towel. Alternatively, the cleaning preparation can be done the day before treatment.
4. Amitraz solution is applied by wetting and sponging. The solution must be applied to the entire body—to normal as well as to affected areas of skin. Although the solution is not irritating, it is mandatory for persons applying amitraz to wear protective gloves and to work in a well-ventilated area. Amitraz causes a transitory sedative effect for 12 to 24 hours, especially after the first treatment, and some dogs become pruritic after the first few applications. Other side effects are rare and include allergic reactions (urticaria and

edema), skin irritation, and a variety of systemic signs. Severe reactions or intoxications can be treated with yohimbine and other appropriate supportive measures.[54a, 54b] The occurrence or severity of the side-effects usually diminishes with subsequent applications. Rarely, dogs have increasingly severe reactions to amitraz dips: marked weakness, ataxia, and somnolence. If amitraz therapy is still desirable, dogs can be pretreated with yohimbine, which prevents or markedly reduces the severity of these adverse effects.[143] Exposure to amitraz can cause contact dermatitis, migraine-like headaches, or asthma-like attacks in some people.

If there is pododemodicosis, the paws can be immersed in a small pan containing amitraz solution and gently massaged to facilitate penetration. One should not rinse the feet or the body. The medication should remain on the skin for 2 weeks. Although about half the drug is retained in the skin for 2 weeks, some may be lost if the dog gets wet or swims. In this case, a new application may be given before the next treatment is due.

5. Although it is not necessary to repeat clipping and shampooing before each treatment, it makes sense to remove any new crusts before each treatment.
6. Treatment is continued until multiple deep skin scraping findings are negative and then for an additional 30 to 60 days or longer. A negative scraping specimen contains no live or dead mites at any stage of their development. Adequate scraping is crucial to successful treatment. Four to six sites are a minimum. Because the face and the feet are problematic, those areas always should be scraped.
7. After treatment is stopped, the dogs should be observed carefully for the next 12 months for any signs of skin disease. If any disease occurs, scrapings should be performed immediately. One should not use recovered animals as breeders.

The preceding description outlines the protocol to be followed using the product approved by the U.S. Food and Drug Administration (FDA) for use in the United States. It is applied in a concentration of 250 ppm every 14 days. There is worldwide debate concerning the best way to use it and the prognosis for cure. Scott and Walton[190] treated 17 dogs with generalized demodicosis, and although six responded initially, all had relapses within 10 months. Kwochka and coworkers[122] reported slightly more than 50 per cent cures in a series of animals followed for 3 years. Muller[152, 152a] reported an 86 per cent recovery rate in more than 400 dogs. Kwochka[122] had much better results in a second series of patients by doubling the frequency of treatment to once weekly. Bussieras and Chermette,[29] who used the drug for 7 years, believed that it is an exceptionally effective and safe treatment of generalized demodicosis if applied weekly by sponging on the entire body at concentrations of 500 to 1000 ppm (the frequency and the levels are not approved by the FDA in the United States). Thus, it seems that the concentration of the drug and the frequency of application have much to do with successful treatment.

For daily treatment of feet or ears, amitraz in mineral oil (1:9) can be more effective than the aqueous formulation.[152] This is an extra-label formulation.

Some percentage of dogs are not cured of their generalized demodicosis with the licensed amitraz protocol. When cure is not attainable, three options are available: euthanasia, control with regularly scheduled dips every 2 to 4 weeks, or extralabel use of amitraz (Mitaban) or another U.S. Environmental Protection Agency (EPA)–registered parasiticide. It is a violation of U.S. federal law to use an EPA-registered pesticide in a manner inconsistent with its labeling, even when treating generalized demodicosis. Accordingly, the extralabel use of an EPA-registered pesticide should be the last resort.

Most investigators retreat amitraz treatment failures with that chemical but at a higher frequency (every seventh day), either at the licensed strength (250 ppm) or at higher concentrations (500, 750, or 1000 ppm). As mentioned above, these therapeutic modifications can cure some initial treatment failures. The product information on Mitaban shows an increasing frequency of side-effects as the topical concentration increases. Most side-effects are transient and of low frequency at concentrations less than 1250 ppm. It is rare for a dog who tolerated dipping at 250 ppm every 14th day to experience clinical side-effects when Mitaban is used at 500 ppm every seventh day. No published data are available on higher concentrations of Mitaban, but it can probably be used safely at 750 or 1000 ppm, as the European products are.[29]

The cure rate is increased with the extralabel use of amitraz but some dogs, perhaps as many as 20 per cent,[100a, 122] do not attain negative scraping results or experience relapse when treatment is stopped. As a therapeutic alternative for these amitraz treatment failures, ivermectin was administered on a weekly basis to dogs with chronic generalized demodicosis with disappointing results.[190] Studies with milbemycin oxime (Interceptor [Ciba-Geigy]) and daily ivermectin have given more encouraging results. When 46 dogs with chronic generalized demodicosis were given milbemycin orally on a daily basis at either 0.5 mg/kg every 24 hours or every 12 hours, 96 per cent achieved remission.[82] No clinical lesions remained, and mites could not be demonstrated by skin scraping. Forty-two per cent of the dogs in remission were cured, 29 per cent were still being followed, and 29 per cent experienced a relapse. In a similar study of 30 dogs, 25 (83 per cent) achieved remission with an overall cure rate of 54 per cent.[145] Both studies had a higher incidence of treatment failure in dogs with adult-onset demodicosis. Treatment courses were long, ranging from 60 to 300 days. Despite the high doses used and the length of administration, adverse reactions occurred in only three dogs. One dog vomited the medication when given on an empty stomach,[82] and two small dogs who received dosages of 3.4 mg/kg had transient neurologic signs (stupor, trembling, and ataxia).[145] In an ongoing study of dosages of 2 mg/kg, time to remission is quicker.[143] However, it is unclear whether this more rapid response results in higher cure rates. All of the dogs in the above studies have received the medication until skin scraping findings were negative and then for an additional 30 days. This probably was too conservative in many cases and resulted in relapses.

Other investigators have studied the efficacy of ivermectin (Ivomec [MSD Agvet]) in 17 dogs.[167, 176] Collies, Shetland sheepdogs (shelties), other herding dogs, and their crosses were excluded. The drug was administered orally once daily at 0.6 mg/kg for as long as 210 days with no adverse reactions reported. Nine dogs have finished treatment and are presumed cured, and the remainder still are under study. The authors (WHM and DWS) have treated a small number of dogs with 0.3 mg/kg/day, and the results seem comparable.

Administration of the avermectins is continued after negative scraping results are noted. Because most of the dogs receiving these drugs are amitraz treatment failures, the course of treatment after negative scraping results should probably be longer than 30 days. The specifics of each case dictate the appropriate duration, but 60 to 90 days might be sufficient. No studies have been performed using both topical amitraz and an oral avermectin, but the combination has been recommended.[122a] Because of differences in their pharmacology, no drug interactions should occur and none was reported.[122a] It is unknown whether the concurrent use of the topical product decreases the length of treatment.

If any or all of the above treatments fail, the owner has the option of using several EPA-registered pesticides not licensed for the treatment of dogs. The oldest and most labor-intensive protocol utilized a 3 per cent aqueous solution of trichlorfon (Neguvon [Miles]).[142] The solution is applied to one third of the animal's body on a rotating basis every other day until negative scraping results are achieved. The course of treatment varies, but 24 weeks of treatment is not uncommon. A newer protocol uses the farm animal formulation of amitraz (Taktic [Hoechst-Roussel]).[139] A 1250 ppm aqueous solution of the amitraz is applied to one half of the animal's body on a rotating basis. If the feet are involved, they are treated daily. When this protocol was used on 71 dogs, 56 (79 per cent) were cured with a mean course of treatment of 3.7 months. No serious side effects were noted. One report suggested that a collar containing 9 per cent amitraz was effective for the treatment of canine demodicosis,[78] but other investigators were unable to confirm this.[100a]

Dogs who achieve negative skin scraping results cannot be declared cured of their disease until 12 months after treatment is stopped. Most dogs destined to experience relapse do so during the first 6 months, but some do not have relapse until the 11th month. During this waiting period, any skin lesions that develop should be scraped and the administration of immunosuppressive drugs should be avoided. To the authors' knowledge, no dog free from disease for 12 months has had a relapse later in life unless it received immunosuppressive treatments for some other condition.

Generalized demodicosis is hereditary in young dogs. Until the mode of inheritance is established, preventive measures are impossible if affected dogs and their littermates are used for breeding. If the disease has a recessive mode of inheritance, some normal puppies in the litter will be truly normal, whereas other puppies will be carriers and will pass on the trait. Because no test is available to separate normal animals from carriers, all puppies from litters in which one or more pups is clinically affected should be culled from breeding programs. Dermatologists do not treat dogs for generalized demodicosis if they are to be used for breeding. General acceptance of this policy will eventually eradicate the disease.

Feline Demodicosis

Feline demodicosis is caused by (1) *Demodex cati*[48] and (2) a species of *Demodex* that has not yet been named.[39, 86a, 135, 209]

D. cati is much like *D. canis,* with minor taxonomic differences (Fig. 6:27 *A*). The ova are slim and oval (Fig. 6:27 *B*) rather than spindle shaped, and all immature life stages are narrower in *D. cati* than in *D. canis.* It is a rare disease that usually affects the eyelids, the periocular area, the head, and the neck (see Fig. 6:24 *B* and *C*).[81] Lesions are variably pruritic and consist of patchy erythema, scaling, crusting, and alopecia. It is the localized type of demodicosis and is usually self-limited. Feline demodicosis may also occur as a ceruminous otitis externa.[86a, 185] Lime sulfur solution or mild parasiticides used for ear mites can be used to treat the lesions. Amitraz in mineral oil (1:9) is an effective otic miticide[86a]; it has not, however, been approved for use in cats.

Generalized feline demodicosis is rare and not usually as severe as the canine form.[44, 138, 199] Cases may be more common in purebred Siamese and Burmese cats.[199] Lesions are found primarily on the head but may be on the neck, the trunk, and the limbs. The lesions consist of circumscribed macules and patches with alopecia, scaling, erythema, hyperpigmentation, and crusting. Some cats develop generalized lesions. Pruritus is variable. In two cases, large numbers of mites were found in scrapings of the ear canal of healthy cats.[48] Generalized demodicosis due to *D. cati* is usually associated with underlying disease: diabetes mellitus,[44, 158, 207] feline leukemia virus infection,[86a] systemic lupus erythematosus,[138, 185] hyperadrenocorticism, or feline immunodeficiency virus infection.[33] One case had raised exudative lesions on the lips and chin.[3] Mites and a *Staphylococcus* organism were obtained, and the cat had a marked lymphopenia associated with long-term therapy for a respiratory tract infection. *D. cati* was isolated from nose lesions in a litter of snow leopards.[67] Clinicians should be aware of its possible association with serious systemic disease. Histologic examination reveals varying degrees of perifolliculitis and folliculitis, with mites in hair follicles, or mild superficial perivascular dermatitis, with mites found in surface keratin.

Some cats respond in a short time spontaneously with mild remedies such as topical lime sulfur dips, carbaryl shampoos, malathion dips, and rotenone.[44, 138] The apparent ease with which generalized demodicosis can be treated in some cats may be explained by the often superficial location of mites in the skin of cats as compared with that in the skin of dogs. Treatment with amitraz dips at 125 ppm or 250 ppm on a weekly basis also can be beneficial.[43, 86a]

The other species of mite causing feline demodicosis is unnamed, but it bears a close taxonomic resemblance to *Demodex criceti,* which is found in the epidermal pits in the stratum corneum of hamsters.[134, 160] The mites affecting cats are shorter and have broad, blunted abdomens (see Fig. 6:27 *C* and *D*), unlike the slim, elongated abdomens of *D. cati.*[39, 134, 209]

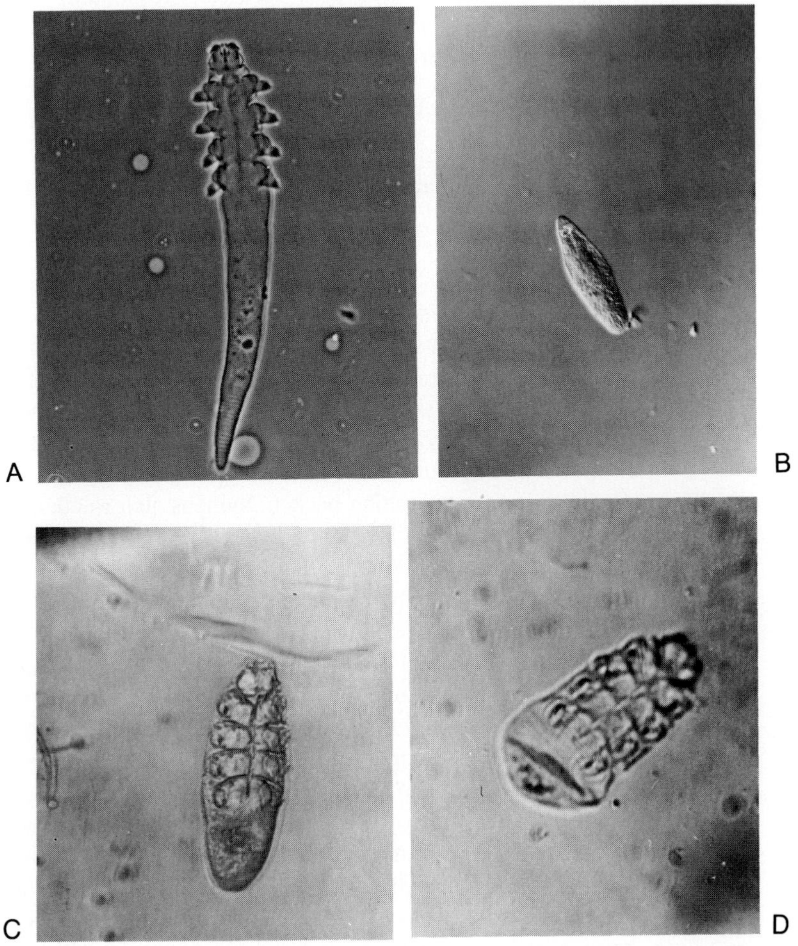

Figure 6:27. *A,* Adult *Demodex cati* in skin scraping. It is similar to *D. canis,* except for a somewhat slimmer abdomen. (Courtesy J. Georgi.) *B, D. cati* ovum in skin scraping. It is slim and oval rather than spindle shaped. (Courtesy J. Georgi.) *C, D,* Unnamed adult demodicid and ovum in skin scraping from a cat. This mite is morphologically similar to *Demodex criceti,* which is found on hamsters. Note blunt, rounded abdomen.

They are superficially located and inhabit only the stratum corneum. Skin scrapings of affected skin usually reveal numerous mites, but they can be overlooked if the slide is scanned rapidly with the four-power objective. The occurrence of two cases in the same household suggests that this mite may be transferable from adult to adult.[138]

The clinical signs of disease due to the unnamed *Demodex* sp. may be suggestive of feline scabies or allergic skin disease, with severe pruritus; alopecic, scaly, excoriated, and crusted lesions are seen, often concentrated on the head, the neck, and the elbows. Other cases have multifocal erythema and hyperpigmentation with broken, stubby hairs located on the proximal rear legs, the flanks, and the ventral abdomen. Some are cases of symmetric alopecia with or without scaling (see Fig. 6:24 *D*), which mimics feline symmetric alopecia, psychogenic alopecia, or hypersensitivity reactions.

Histologically, minimal inflammation is observed. The epidermis may be irregularly acanthotic and hyperkeratotic, with mites in the stratum corneum. No mites are found in the hair follicles.

Differential diagnosis of the second type of feline demodicosis must include all feline dermatoses that are associated with excessive grooming such as psychogenic alopecia, atopy, food hypersensitivity, feline scabies, contact dermatitis, flea bite hypersensitivity, and the demodicosis caused by *D. cati.* Careful skin scrapings are paramount in the work-up for each of these conditions to make a proper diagnosis.

The prognosis is favorable, as cases usually respond to simple treatments such as three dips with a solution of malathion or lime sulfur at weekly intervals. Cats with demodicosis caused by the unnamed mite are usually otherwise healthy.

Canine Scabies

Canine scabies (sarcoptic mange) (Fig. 6:28 A) is a nonseasonal, intensely pruritic, transmissible infestation of the skin of dogs caused by the mite *Sarcoptes scabiei* var. *canis* (Fig. 6:29). The mite is transferable to other species.[2]

■ *Cause and Pathogenesis.* The causative mite belongs to the family Sarcoptidae, as does *Notoedres cati*, the cause of feline scabies. Because these mites have much in common, their 17- to 21-day life cycles are presented together. Copulation of adults occurs in a molting pocket on the surface of the skin. The fertilized female mite excavates a burrow through the horny layer of the skin at a rate of 2 to 3 mm/d and lays eggs in the tunnel behind her. The eggs hatch as larvae and burrow to the surface of the skin, where they travel about feeding and eventually resting in a molting pocket. Nymphs also wander about the skin, but they may stay in the molting pocket until they are mature. Mites prefer skin with little hair, so they are most common on the ears, the elbows, the abdomen, and the hocks. As the disease spreads and hair is lost, they may eventually colonize large areas of the host's body. The entire life cycle may be complete in only 3 weeks.

Adult mites are small (200 to 400 μm), oval, and white with two pairs of short legs anteriorly that bear long unjoined stalks with suckers (Figs. 6:29 and 6:30). The stalks are of medium length in *N. cati* (see Fig. 6:35). Two pairs of posterior legs are rudimentary and do not extend beyond the border of the body. The posterior legs carry long bristles, not suckers, although the fourth pair of legs of the male mite have suckers. The anus of *S. scabiei* var. *canis* is terminal, whereas that of *N. cati* has a dorsal location—an important point of differentiation.

Scabies mites have hosts of preference but can cause disease in other species. *S. scabiei* var. *canis* is known to cause disease in cats, fox, and humans.[34, 59, 101, 116, 129, 155] Likewise, dogs can be infected by mites from fox and possibly even humans.[15] Reactions in humans occur within 24 hours after brief direct exposure and are characterized by pruritic papules on the trunk and arms (see Fig. 6:28 D). Pruritus is severe, especially when the skin is warm—as it is in bed at night or after a warm shower. Mites burrow but usually remain on the aberrant host for only a few days. The lesions regress spontaneously in 12 to 14 days, if only a few mites were transmitted and contact with affected dogs is terminated. However, with many mites and prolonged repeated contact, the human lesions persist for long periods.

Variations in the above syndrome have been reported in which human patients did not develop lesions until 3 to 4 days after exposure.[155] This may represent a hypersensitivity reaction, and patients reacting more quickly may have been sensitized previously. In one case, lesions continued to spread for several weeks after animal contacts were removed.[155] Skin scrapings revealed mites and mite eggs, one of which later hatched. In this case, the skin lesions were typical of canine scabies in humans, and the mites came from a positively identified case of canine scabies; thus, it appears that the mite was able to propagate in the human host. (One can speculate, in view of the unusual course, about whether this might have been a case in which human scabies in the dog was returned to its natural host.) There is one report, however, of a child with Norwegian scabies caused by *S. scabiei* var. *canis*.[129] Similar mites were found on three dogs in the household and on all other members of the family.

Canine *Sarcoptes* mites can live on human beings for at least 6 days and produce ova during that time.[57] Itching started within 2 hours of experimental implantation of mites, so it was concluded that hypersensitivity was not a factor.[57] In general, human infestations clear spontaneously when the affected dog is removed from contact.

The off-host survival time of scabies mites depends on the relative humidity and tempera-

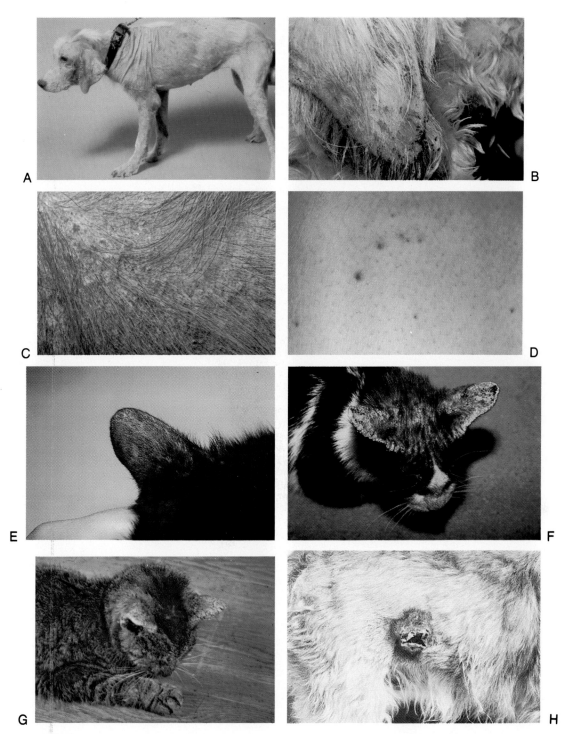

Figure 6:28. *A*, Generalized erythema and alopecia of dog with extensive scabies. *B*, Margin of the ear (pinna) is a characteristic site. *C*, Grayish crusts on the body mimic seborrheic dermatitis. Hemorrhagic area is from skin scraping (positive). *D*, Crusted papules on human skin (forearm), the typical lesion of canine scabies in humans. *E*, Pinnal alopecia, scale, and crust in an early case of feline scabies. *F*, Chronic feline scabies. Note marked crusting and excoriation on pinnae and head. *G*, Dry, crusted lesions on the edges of the ears and face are typical of feline scabies. *H*, Spider bite. Focal area of necrosis and slough in the flank of a dog.

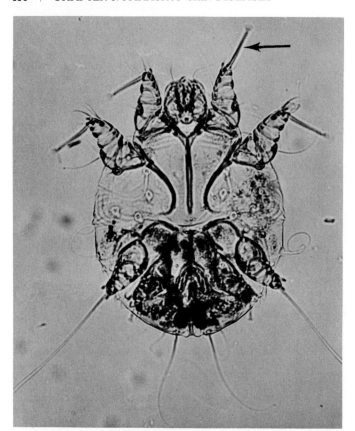

Figure 6:29. Adult *Sarcoptes scabiei* var. *canis*. Note the long unjointed stalks and suckers.

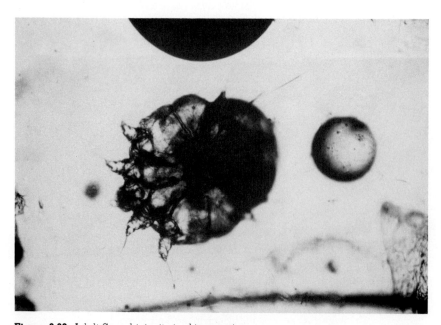

Figure 6:30. Adult *S. scabiei* mite in skin scraping.

ture. Female mites and nymphs generally survive longer than do male mites or larvae, and low temperature and high humidity prolong survival.[1] At 10 to 15°C (50 to 59°F), female mites and nymphs could survive for 4 to 21 days, depending on the humidity. At room temperature (20 to 25°C, 68 to 77°F) all stages can survive for 2 to 6 days. These mites can be point sources of infection for other animals.[146, 148]

■ *Clinical Features.* The distribution pattern of canine scabies typically involves the ventral portions of the abdomen, the chest, and the legs.[73] The ears and the elbows, favorite habitats of mites, are almost always affected and are premiere places for obtaining diagnostic scrapings (see Fig. 6:24 *E* to *H*). However, some animals have no ear lesions. The disease spreads rapidly and can involve the entire body (see Fig. 6:28 *A*), but the dorsum is usually spared. Alopecia is present, and early skin lesions are characteristic. These are pruritic, reddish papulocrustous eruptions (see Fig. 6:24 *F*). Typically, they have thick yellowish crusts, and the intense and constant itching soon produces extensive excoriation (see Fig. 6:28 *B* and *C*). These patients are miserable because they are constantly scratching themselves. Itching is thought to be more severe in warm environments (e.g., indoors or by the stove).

The incubation period for scabies is unknown. When fox mites were transferred to dogs, there was a lag period of 6 to 11 days before signs developed and those were mild.[15] In the natural situation, infested dogs should start to itch a few days after infection. The pruritus is at a low level and is proportional to the number of mites. As the number of mites increases, the pruritus becomes more severe, but there is some point at which the pruritus explodes in severity. This is usually 21 to 30 days after exposure and probably signifies the development of hypersensitivity to the mite.[90, 202] After the mite is established, the course may last weeks or years. Unfortunately, it is often misdiagnosed as an allergy and treated with only corticosteroids. In long-term cases, hyperpigmentation of the affected skin is common. Most patients also have a generalized lymphadenopathy.

Some dogs never have the classic lesions of scabies. They scratch incessantly and have few, if any, real lesions other than mild erythema and occasional excoriations. They are often treated for an allergy with systemic corticosteroids but without benefit. These dogs have had scabies ever since they came in contact with an infected dog or environment, but mites are not found in skin scrapings. Thorough grooming may have removed superficial mites and crusts, so only a few mites remain—enough to cause pruritus, but too few to find. These dogs respond rapidly and dramatically to proper antiscabies therapy.

In cats, *S. scabiei* infestation is rare and variable in clinical presentation. There are pruritic pinnal and facial papules; generalized crusts, scale, and pruritus; and self-induced hair loss with no skin lesions.[63a] Temporary transmission from cats to humans has been reported.[63a] Affected cats are often immunosuppressed prior to infestation.

■ *Diagnosis.* Scabies mites can be difficult to demonstrate, especially when the patient is intensely pruritic, has had the disease for a long time, or has received multiple baths or dips. Scabies should be considered in any dog with nonseasonal, intense pruritus, especially when the pruritus does not stop with the administration of 1.1 mg/kg of prednisone. When scabies is a differential diagnostic possibility, it can be excluded only by the animal's failure to respond to adequate treatment.

A helpful, although nonspecific, test for scabies is the pinnal-pedal reflex. The edge of the dog's pinna is rubbed or scratched and the test is positive if the dog's hindleg attempts to scratch the ear region. Between 75 and 90 per cent of dogs with scabies have a positive pinnal-pedal reflex.[90, 143] The test may be negative if no ear lesions are present. Because hypersensitivity to the mite appears to be important in the pruritus of scabies and mites of various species may share some cuticular or fecal antigens, anecdotal reports on the diagnostic accuracy of skin testing with house dust mite antigen have arisen. The authors have not been able to substantiate this finding, with positive results seen in only 22 per cent[143] or 36 per cent[90] of proven scabies cases.

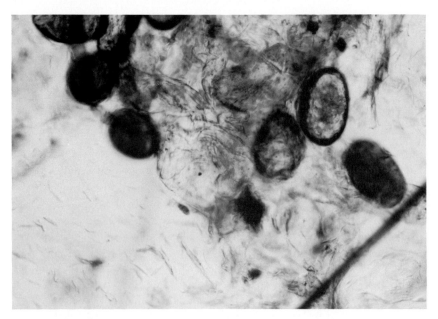

Figure 6:31. Multiple S. *scabiei* ova in skin scraping.

The absolute confirmation of the diagnosis necessitates that some stage of the mite or its feces be seen via skin scrapings. Multiple scrapings are necessary. For scraping, one should choose skin sites that have not been excoriated. In these areas, one should look for red, raised papules with yellowish crusts on top (Fig. 6:28 *C*). The ear margins, the elbows, or the hocks are primary scraping sites because the mites seem to prefer these areas. Large amounts of material are collected and spread on slides with mineral oil, and every field should be examined carefully. One mite (see Fig. 6:30), egg (Fig. 6:31), or dark brown oval fecal pellets (Fig. 6:32)

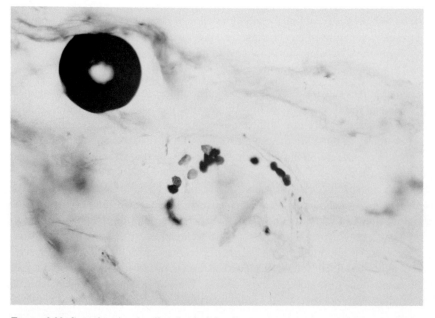

Figure 6:32. S. *scabiei* fecal pellets (scybala) in linear arrangement in skin scraping.

are diagnostic. Depending on the number of scrapings taken, mites may be seen in only 20 per cent of cases.[90]

If the clinical features are suggestive, a presumptive diagnosis of canine scabies should be made and the dog treated for the disease. One of the best diagnostic aids is the prompt response to therapy. Other laboratory aids are of less significance, but a few patients have mites in the feces, and a few cases are diagnosed on the basis of skin biopsies. A hemogram may reveal eosinophilia or nonregenerative anemia. Thoday[202] reported that dogs with scabies had serum levels of IgA and IgM that were lower, and those of IgG that were higher, than levels in normal dogs. IgA and IgM levels in the scabietic dogs returned to normal with scabicidal therapy.

Histologic examination may be useful but is rarely conclusive, unless actual mites are seen in the biopsy specimen. One should always select an active papule, undisturbed by excoriation, as the biopsy specimen. Mites may rarely be found in the superficial epidermis and the stratum corneum (Fig. 6:33). Histopathologic study reveals varying degrees of superficial perivascular or superficial interstitial dermatitis (hyperplastic or spongiotic). A suggestive histopathologic clue is the presence of focal areas of epidermal edema, exocytosis, degeneration, and necrosis (epidermal "nibbles") (Fig. 6:34). Eosinophils vary in number, from few to many, probably relative to recent glucocorticoid therapy. Focal parakeratotic hyperkeratosis is often pronounced.

Differential diagnosis should include contact dermatitis, atopy, food hypersensitivity, *Malassezia* dermatitis, *Pelodera* dermatitis, cheyletiellosis, otodectic dermatitis, and dirofilariasis. Any one of these dermatoses at a particular stage might resemble scabies. Failure to find mites should not eliminate the diagnosis of scabies and doing so is a common mistake. Many such cases are erroneously treated as an allergy. Careful history, physical examination, or appropriate cultures, biopsy, and examination of scrapings, and especially response to acaricidal medicaments, usually satisfactorily resolve the diagnostic problem.

■ *Treatment.* The mites must be eradicated. Treatment should be started as soon as the diagnosis is made or suspected. This disease is highly contagious in a kennel or a hospital. The only licensed method of treatment for canine scabies is the repeated application of a topical parasiticide. If the dog has a dense coat, the hair should be clipped. All patients should be

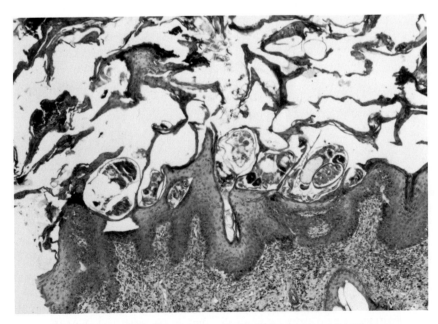

Figure 6:33. Canine scabies. Note mite segments within stratum corneum.

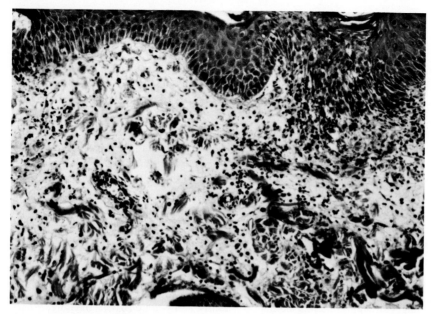

Figure 6:34. Canine scabies. Hyperplastic perivascular dermatitis with focal epidermal necrosis and exocytosis ("nibbles").

bathed with an antiseborrheic shampoo to remove crusts and other debris, and then an acaricidal dip should be applied thoroughly and allowed to soak every inch of the skin surface. Spot treatment is ineffective. Particular care should be taken around the ears and the eyes; the skin in those regions is often severely infected, yet delicate and easily irritated by parasiticidal dips. Administration of systemic corticosteroids in full antiallergic dosages (1.1 mg/kg of prednisone or prednisolone daily) for 2 to 3 days is useful to provide relief from scratching and to stop self-mutilation until the mites are eliminated.

Many of the proven scabicides (e.g., lindane and chlordane) are no longer available for veterinary use and mite resistance to some pesticides, especially the organophosphates, has been suggested. These problems limit the number of dips available, and no topical treatment can be considered 100 per cent effective. A 2 to 3 per cent lime sulfur dip is widely used. The solution can be made from orchard spray concentrates or from LymDyp (Dermatologics for Veterinary Medicine). The solution is miticidal, antifungal, antibacterial, and antipruritic with little or no potential for toxicity. It has an unpleasant odor, stains light-colored coats, and can irritate the skin. It has little residual activity so it must be applied weekly. Amitraz is reported to be an effective agent when used at 250 ppm once to three times at 2-week intervals.[74, 212] This is an extralabel use of this pesticide. Other products may be effective and should be used in accord with the label directions. Regardless of which dip is used, treatment should be continued until all active lesions are resolved. Typically, a 4- to 6-week course of treatment is necessary. The dog's pruritus starts to decrease with the first treatment and lessens with each subsequent treatment. At the end of the dips, any residual pruritus should be minimal.

Ivermectin is so effective in the treatment of scabies[90, 146, 182, 213] that response to it is used as a diagnostic test when scrapings are negative. The drug is given orally or subcutaneously at dosages of 0.2 to 0.4 mg/kg every 14 days until the condition is resolved. This is an extralabel use of this drug, and these exaggerated dosages should not be administered to collies, Shetland sheepdogs, Old English sheepdogs, other herding dogs, or their crosses. In dogs with proven scabies, one treatment can be curative,[182] but most dogs are given a second dose. Rarely is a third dose necessary. Typically, the dog's pruritus is reduced by 50 per cent or more 7 to 10 days after the first treatment and disappears gradually during the next 3 to 4 weeks. This residual pruritus is probably a result of the animal's hypersensitivity to the parasite. Before treatment, the pruritus often responds poorly to corticosteroid administration but is steroid responsive after the mites are killed. If ivermectin is given to a dog with suspected scabies and its pruritus is not significantly reduced during the second week, the dog probably does not have scabies. Interestingly, some owners report that improvement was seen for the first few days after treatment but it was not sustained. This transient response may be due to some anti-inflammatory actions of the product.[167]

Preliminary studies with milbemycin oxime (Interceptor [Ciba-Geigy]) suggest that this avermectin may be as effective as ivermectin.[143] To date, all dogs given 2 mg/kg orally on days 0, 7, and 14 have been cured. Because this drug has a low incidence of side effects in collies,[82, 145] it may be a useful systemic treatment for scabies in dogs in which ivermectin is contraindicated.

Most cases of scabies in a single-pet household can be resolved by treatment of the animal alone. In multiple-dog households, all contact dogs should be treated, even if they exhibit no signs, because asymptomatic carriers have been identified. Because the parasite can live in the environment for up to 21 days, cleaning and applying an environmental pesticide may be indicated.[146] This is most important when numerous mites are found on scraping, especially when multiple dogs are involved.

Humans who do not have lesions at the onset of treatment of the dog should not develop any. If lesions were present, they may persist for 7 to 14 days but new lesions should not develop. Development of new lesions indicates inadequate treatment of the dogs, environmental infestation, or true human scabies, which could have been transferred to the dogs. The owners should be referred to a human dermatologist.

Feline Scabies

Feline scabies (notoedric mange) is a contagious parasitic disease of cats caused by *N. cati.*

■ ***Cause and Pathogenesis.*** *N. cati* (Fig. 6:35) primarily attacks cats but may also infect foxes, dogs, and rabbits.[68, 69] It causes transient lesions in humans.[203] The mites are obligate parasites that probably survive off the host for only a few days. The disease is highly contagious by direct contact and characteristically affects whole litters and both sexes of adult cats. Affected animals have large numbers of mites, which are easily found on skin scrapings.[68] Notoedric mange appears in epizootics; it is rarely diagnosed in some parts of the country but is endemic and common in others.

The mite belongs to the family Sarcoptidae, and because its basic life cycle and structure

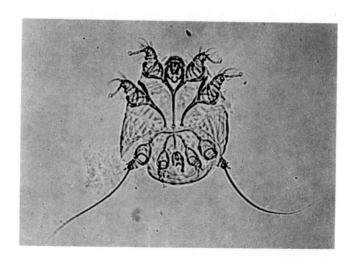

Figure 6:35. Adult *Notoedres cati.* Note the medium-length stalks, the striated integument, and the lack of a terminally located anus. The mite is smaller than *S. scabiei* var. *canis.*

are similar to those of canine scabies, the two are discussed together on page 434. The main features of taxonomic differentiation for the clinician are that *N. cati* mites are smaller than *Sarcoptes canis* and have medium-length unjointed sucker-bearing stalks on their legs. They also have more body striations and, most importantly, have a dorsal anus as compared with the terminal anus of *Sarcoptes*.[85] The abundant mites are much easier to find on skin scrapings than they are in cases of *S. canis*.

■ *Clinical Features.* The distribution is typical. Lesions first appear at the medial proximal edge of the pinna of the ear (see Fig. 6:28 *E*). They spread rapidly to the upper ear, the face, the eyelids, and the neck (see Fig. 6:28 *F* and *G*). They also extend to the feet and the perineum. This probably results from the cat's habits of washing and of sleeping in a curled position.

Female mites burrow into the horny layer of the epidermis between hair follicles. These burrows appear on the skin surface in the center of minute papules. The skin soon becomes thickened, wrinkled, and folded and later is covered with dense, tightly adhering, yellow to gray crusts (see Fig. 6:24 *G*). There is partial alopecia in affected areas. Intense pruritus develops, and the excoriations produced by scratching may become secondarily infected. As the disease progresses, the hair loss and skin lesions spread until large areas of the body are involved. Peripheral lymphadenopathy is usually present.

■ *Diagnosis.* The distribution of lesions and the intensity of the pruritus are highly suggestive. Identification of the mites is diagnostic. Scrapings should be examined with the 10-power objective with reduced light because the mites are small and become less visible with intense

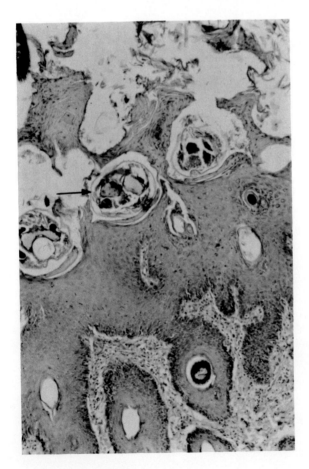

Figure 6:36. Histopathologic section of cat skin with three *N. cati* mites in the stratum corneum. The arrow points to the central mite. Note extensive acanthosis, hyperkeratosis, parakeratosis, prominent rete ridges, and infiltration of inflammatory cells in the superficial dermis. (Courtesy B. Bagnall.)

light. The differential diagnosis should rule out *Otodectes* infection, cheyletiellosis, atopy, food hypersensitivity, pemphigus foliaceous or erythematosus, and systemic lupus erythematosus.

Histopathologic study reveals varying degrees of superficial perivascular or superficial interstitial dermatitis (hyperplastic or spongiotic). Mite segments may be found within the superficial epidermis (Fig. 6:36). Eosinophils vary in number from few to many, probably reflecting recent glucocorticoid administration. Focal parakeratotic hyperkeratosis is usually pronounced.

■ *Treatment.* Many parasiticidal agents are contraindicated because of extreme toxic effects in cats. Sulfur in various forms is usually safe. With the cat under sedation, the hair is clipped, if necessary, and the cat is bathed in warm water and soap to loosen scales and debris. A 2 to 3 per cent warm water solution of lime sulfur should be applied and allowed to dry on the skin. The dip is repeated every seventh day until the condition is resolved. Six to eight treatments may be necessary. All cats on the premises must be treated, because cats in preclinical stages of the disease might be carriers. The response to treatment is usually rapid and complete if all cats are thoroughly treated and re-exposure is prevented. Amitraz as used in demodicosis can be effective. Ivermectin given subcutaneously at 0.3 mg/kg is effective.[12, 195] Amitraz and ivermectin are *not* approved for use on cats in the United States.

SPIDERS

The numbers of spiders are arachnids that inhabit woodpiles, old buildings, and refuse areas. The four species of spiders that are medically important in the United States are the black widow *(Latrodectus mactans)*, the red-legged widow *(Latrodectus bishopi)*, the brown recluse *(Loxosceles reclusa)*, and the common brown spider *(Loxosceles unicolor)*.[117, 211]

Spider bites occur most commonly on the forelegs and the face. Bites of spiders of the genus *Latrodectus* (the widows) initially consist of two small puncture marks with local erythema. The local reaction may develop into granulomatous nodules within a few days. Bites of spiders of the genus *Loxosceles* (the brown spiders) initially appear as puncture marks surrounded by local erythema.[11] Within a few hours, they become vesicular and painful. The next day the lesions turn black and become necrotic, and a large indolent ulcer develops (see Fig. 6:28 *H*). Skin biopsy reveals a nodular to diffuse necrotizing dermatitis and panniculitis (Fig. 6:37).

Systemic reactions to spider bites may be severe. They may be manifested by salivation, nausea and diarrhea, ataxia and convulsions, or paralysis, any of which occur within 6 to 48 hours. Generalized urticaria can result from the ingestion or bites of less venomous spiders.

Although spider bites are rarely recognized and reported, they are probably underdiagnosed in veterinary medicine.[140] Diagnosis should be based on history and the physical examination findings. Recommended early bite wound therapy includes local infusion with 2 per cent lidocaine and triamcinolone acetonide.[156] Systemic support with the administration of analgesics, calcium gluconate, and epinephrine and glucocorticosteroids may be needed. In the case of bites of *Latrodectus* spp., the local infusion of 1 ml of antivenin is recommended.[156] Chronic ulcers may take months to heal and may be best treated by surgical excision.

The numbers of spiders can be controlled by cleaning up woodpiles and outdoor sites; by eliminating scattered debris; and by spraying insecticides under appliances, in cupboards, in cracks in basement and attic floors, and outdoors under eaves and in window wells and woodpiles.

Insects

The numerous species of insects play important roles in the health of animals as vectors of disease and as irritants to the skin. Insect's heads bear appendages and sensory organs, such as antennae and simple or compound eyes. The structure of the masticatory mouthparts varies, depending on the feeding habits. The thorax typically carries two pairs of wings and three pairs

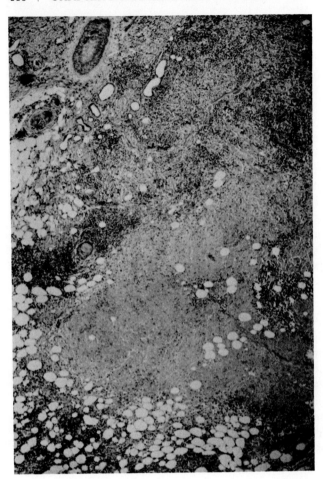

Figure 6:37. Spider bite histologic view. Nodular area of necrotizing dermatitis and panniculitis.

of legs. The abdomen is segmented and terminates in the male hypopygium or the female ovipositor. The body is encased in hard chitinous plates connected by flexible membranes.

The life cycles of insects are of three types: direct development, incomplete metamorphosis, and complete metamorphosis. In the first type, the newly hatched insect is a small replica of the adult. Incomplete metamorphosis occurs in primitive insects, and the larvae differ from adults in size, proportion, and lack of wings. Complete metamorphosis is found in more specialized species. The wormlike larva differ from the adult in regard to feeding habits. After several molts, the larva pupates and emerges as an adult. The larva and the pupa possess characteristic hairs, bristles, and appendages, which are of taxonomic importance. The duration of adult pupal and larval stages varies with the species and the environment.

Insects have medical importance because of the damage they can do to the skin and because their stings, bites, or body parts can be allergens. Insect hypersensitivity, aside from flea bite hypersensitivity, has received much attention and helps to explain the severe skin reactions to seemingly trivial bites.[91] Equally as important, insects seem to be a source of inhaled allergen for some dogs or cats with atopy-like conditions. These animals have the classic signs of atopy but either show no intradermal or serologic reactions to common inhaled allergens or do not respond to immunotherapy. Ants, moths, houseflies, butterflies, and cockroaches are probably important as strictly inhaled allergens. Mosquitos, biting flies, and honeybees can cause disease through both their bites and the inhalation of their body parts. Hypersensitivity to these insects can be documented by intradermal tests.[91] It remains to be seen how effective immunotherapy can be.

PEDICULOSIS

Pediculosis is infestation with lice (Fig. 6:38 *A*).

■ *Cause and Pathogenesis.* Lice are small, degenerate, dorsoventrally flattened, wingless insects that do not undergo true metamorphosis. The eyes are reduced or absent, and each leg bears one or two claws. There is one pair of spiracles on the mesothorax and usually six pairs on the abdomen. Lice are host specific and spend their entire life on their host. They survive only a few days if separated from the host. Lice are spread by direct contact or by contaminated brushes, combs, and bedding. The operculated white eggs (nits) are cemented firmly to the hairs of the host. In contrast, *Cheyletiella* ova are smaller and loosely attached to the hair shafts (see Fig. 6:19). The nymph hatches from the egg, undergoes three ecdyses (molting), and becomes the adult. The entire cycle lasts 14 to 21 days.

Lice are divided into two suborders: Anoplura, or sucking lice, and Mallophaga, or biting lice.

■ *Anoplura.* These have mouthparts adapted for sucking the blood of the host. With heavy infestations, they produce sufficient anemia to cause weakness, and some animals become distraught and ill-tempered because of the chronic irritation. The only species found commonly on dogs is *Linognathus setosus* (Figs. 6:39 *A* and 6:40 *C*).

■ *Mallophaga.* These so-called biting lice feed on epithelial debris and hair, but some species also have mouthparts adapted for drawing blood from their hosts. Because they are active, they may cause more irritation than do sucking lice, and rubbing by their host may cause alopecia. *Trichodectes canis* (Fig. 6:40 *A*) is the common biting louse of dogs. It may act as the intermediate host of the dog tapeworm, *D. caninum. Felicola subrostratus* infests cats (Fig. 6:41; also see Fig. 6:39 *B*) and may either be asymptomatic or cause severe pruritus with dermatitis and hair loss on the back. *Heterodoxus spiniger* may be found on dogs in warm climates only (see Fig. 6:40 *B*). A single case of *Phthirus pubis* (human pubic louse) infesting a dog has been reported. The dog, which had no clinical signs, slept in the bed of its owner, who was infested with the louse.[79]

■ *Clinical Features.* Lice can be highly irritating to the host and can cause intense itching. They accumulate under mats of hair and around the ears and body openings. Sucking lice produce anemia and severe debilitation, especially in young animals. Sucking lice do not move rapidly and are easily seen and caught (see Fig. 6:38 *A*). Biting lice, however, move rapidly and may be difficult to find and capture.

Lice produce a few direct lesions, but excoriations and secondary dermatitis from scratching may be severe. Pediculosis may look like miliary dermatitis in cats and like flea bite hypersensitivity in dogs. Papules and crusts may be found (see Fig. 6:38 *B*). Debilitated, anemic, and frustrated patients are often ill-tempered and difficult to handle. The patient's coat is often dirty, matted, and ill-kept, as this is a disease of neglect often associated with overcrowding and poor sanitation. The animal has a mousy odor, especially when wet.

In some cases, animals are asymptomatic carriers or have only seborrhea sicca with variable pruritus. Pediculosis is often more prevalent in the winter months, perhaps owing to the growth of longer, heavier haircoats and closer contact among animals. In addition, the high ambient and skin surface temperature during summer can be lethal to lice.

Pediculosis is a rare diagnosis in most veterinary practices. Lice are easily killed by common flea shampoos, sprays, or powders; consequently, owners usually eliminate these parasites with routine grooming care. More insecticidal shampoos are used today than were used many years ago, and louse infestation has decreased proportionately.

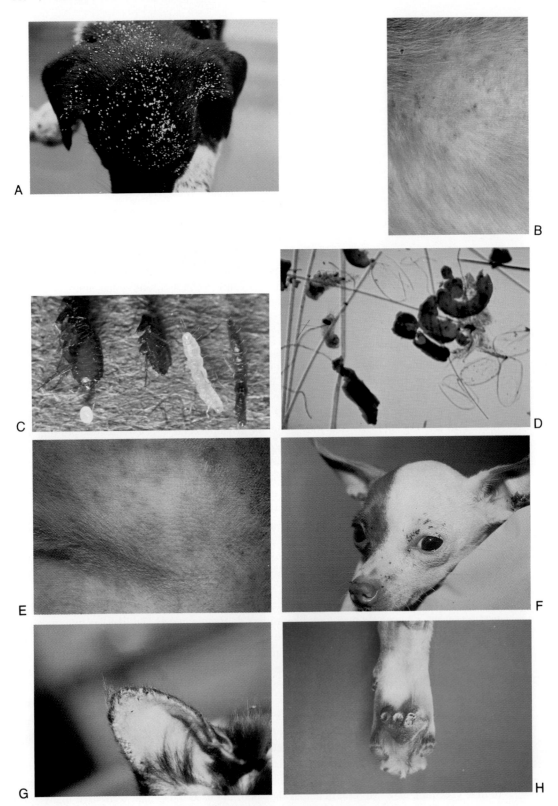

Figure 6:38 *See legend on opposite page*

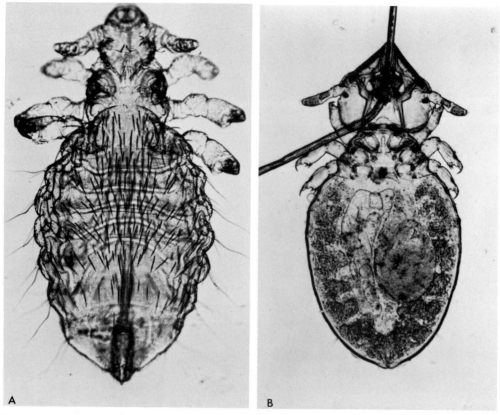

Figure 6:39. *A, L. setosus,* adult male. *B, F. subrostrata,* egg-bearing female.

■ *Diagnosis.* Diagnosis is made by physical examination to find and identify the lice. The acetate tape impression method of immobilizing lice for identification is described in Chapter 2.

Differential diagnosis of pediculosis should include seborrhea, scabies, flea bite hypersensitivity, cheyletiellosis, and *Dermanyssus, Lynxacarus,* or *Trombicula* infestations. Skin scrapings and acetate tape examinations should resolve any diagnostic questions. Histopathologic examination reveals varying degrees of superficial perivascular dermatitis (hyperplastic or spongiotic). Eosinophils are usually prominent.

■ *Treatment.* All affected animals and other animals in close association with them should be treated. Thick mats and hair tags should be clipped away. After a regular soap and water shampoo, the animal should be soaked or sprayed thoroughly with a good insecticide. Lice are susceptible to almost all parasiticidal agents. Ivermectin was reported to be effective when given at 0.2 mg/kg subcutaneously once.[192]

Figure 6:38. *A,* Multiple louse nits on the head of a dog. (Courtesy J. King.) *B,* Multiple erythematous, crusted papules on the back of a dog with pediculosis. *C,* Stages of life cycle of the flea (from left to right): Adult female with egg, adult male, mature larva ready to pupate (white), young larvae after first blood meal (red). The pupa is not illustrated. *D,* Empty flea egg cases (lower right), young yellow-white larvae (upper left) and blood fecal crusts from adult fleas to be used as larval food. *E,* Erythematous papules on the abdomen of a dog with flea bite hypersensitivity. *F,* Sticktight fleas *(Echidnophaga gallinacea)* on the face of a dog. (Courtesy G. Kunkle.) *G,* Multiple crusted papules on the margin of the pinna of a cat with European rabbit flea infestation. (Courtesy R. Harvey.) *H,* Multiple ulcers due to *Tunga penetrans* on the metacarpal pad of a dog. (Courtesy J. King.)

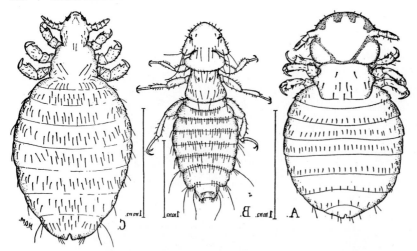

Figure 6:40. Dog lice. *A, Trichodectes canis. B, Heterodoxus spiniger. C, Linognathus setosus.* (From Lapage, G.: Monnig's Veterinary Helminthology and Entomology, 5th ed. Williams & Wilkins Co., Baltimore, 1962.)

■ *Cats.* Cats can be treated with pyrethrin or carbamate shampoos. After being dried, cats can be sprayed or dusted with products containing pyrethrins. Treatment should be repeated within 10 to 14 days, because not all the nits may be killed and any that remain will have hatched by that time. Two per cent lime sulfur dips are also effective.

■ *Dogs.* Stronger medications with residual action can be used on dogs, although lice are easily killed with the preparations noted above. Bathing the dog with a shampoo containing synergized pyrethrin or a pyrethroid is effective. Dogs can then be dipped with any residual flea dip. A second or third treatment in 10 to 14 days is recommended. These treatments are usually highly effective.

Severely anemic and depressed patients with extreme parasite infestation may go into shock and die after vigorous treatment. It is best to transfuse blood, provide a high-protein diet, and reduce the number of parasites with pyrethrin sprays first. More complete treatment as outlined can be given several days later.

It is advisable to clean thoroughly bedding, the premises, and grooming implements at least once, even though lice do not live long when they are off the host.

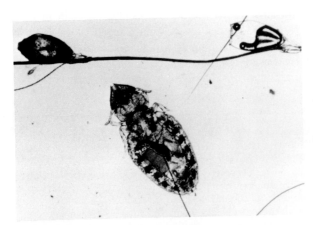

Figure 6:41. *Felicola subrostrata,* egg-bearing female. On the left is an intact egg; on the right, an empty case.

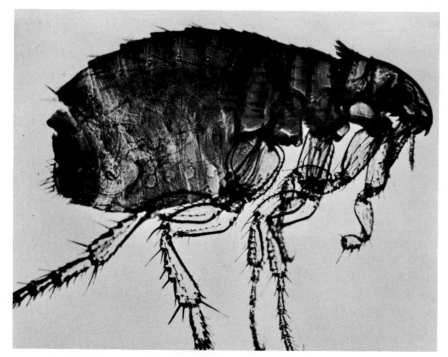

Figure 6:42. *Ctenocephalides felis felis* adult.

FLEAS

Fleas are small, brown, wingless insects with laterally compressed bodies (Fig. 6:42). Male fleas are smaller than female fleas, and the chitinous head bears antennae, eyes, combs, and suctorial mouthparts (Fig. 6:43). The prothoracic and genal combs are useful taxonomically. Each segment of the three-sectioned thorax bears a pair of powerful legs terminating in two curved claws. The structure adapts fleas for powerful jumping, which enables them to transfer

Figure 6:43. *A, Ctenocephalides canis,* female. Head and pronotum showing one of the antennae and the genal and pronotal combs. *B, C. felis felis,* female. Head and pronotum showing one of the antennae and the genal and pronotal combs. (From Lapage, G.: Veterinary Parasitology, 2nd ed. Charles C Thomas, Springfield, IL, 1967.)

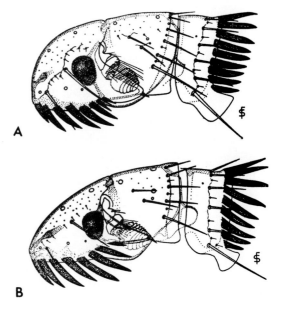

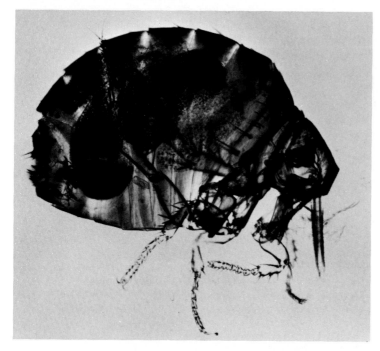

Figure 6:44. *E. gallinacea* (sticktight flea) adult.

from host to host. Because of their dependence on the host for protection and food, fleas spend their entire adult life on the host or other contact animals.[54]

There are more than 2000 species and subspecies of fleas worldwide.[53] Although dogs and cats could be transient hosts for virtually any species of flea, only *Ctenocephalides felis, C. canis, Pulex* spp., and *Echidnophaga gallinacea* are of medical concern in most pets. The rabbit flea, *Spilopsyllus cuniculi,* is problematic in some parts of Europe and Australia.[98, 200]

Worldwide, *Ctenocephalides* spp. are of greatest medical concern. Surveys on flea-infested dogs and cats have shown that *C. felis felis* is the most common species, with prevalence figures of greater than 92 per cent in dogs and 97 per cent in cats.[53, 127] *C. canis* is far less common and is not found on most dogs or cats. *E. gallinacea* (Fig. 6:44), the sticktight poultry flea, can occasionally infest pets, especially in warm climates.[113] For transfer to occur, the pet's environment must be or have been occupied by birds. *Pulex irritans,* the human flea (Fig. 6:45), is an uncommon finding on most dogs, although one study found high rates of infestation in some dogs.[112] Given the choice between infesting humans or dogs, *P. irritans* appears to prefer the dog but transfers from the dog to contact humans. Because *P. irritans* may be important as a plague vector, the infestation of pets may have some public health significance.

Fleas develop by complete metamorphosis from the egg to the adult through three larval stages and one pupal stage. Details of the life cycle are illustrated in Figure 6:38 C. The biology of only *C. felis felis* has been well described, and developmental data may not apply to other species. The female flea lays her eggs on the host. These eggs are ovoid, white, and 0.5 mm in

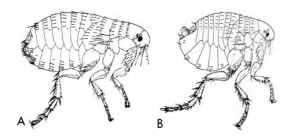

Figure 6:45. *Pulex irritans*, the human flea (×17). *A,* female; *B,* male. (From Herns, W. B., James, M. T.: Medical Entomology, 5th ed. The Macmillan Co., New York, 1961.)

A   B

length. Because they are not sticky, the eggs fall from the host into the environment, where the life cycle is completed. Development is independent of the host's presence but is dependent on the macroenvironmental and microenvironmental conditions. Ambient temperature and relative humidity are critical for the flea's development and its timing. Because of their negative phototactism and positive geotropism, flea larvae move deep into carpets, down cracks in wood floors, and under the soil surface or organic debris outside. In these protected environments, the local temperature and humidity can be different from those of the gross environment and the life cycle can be completed more rapidly than expected.

Flea eggs typically hatch in 1 to 10 days. At 70 per cent relative humidity, the hatching rate increases fourfold when the temperature is increased from 13 to 35°C (55 to 95°F).[53] Newly hatched larvae move to dark protected areas, where they feed on organic debris and, most importantly, adult flea feces (Fig. 6:38 *D*). Two molts are completed before the third larval instar enters the pupal phase. The larval phase is completed in 5 to 11 days if sufficient food is available and the climate is ideal. Dryness, high heat, and extreme cold are deleterious to the larvae.

At the end of the larval phase, the third instar produces a silklike cocoon in which pupation occurs. At 80 per cent humidity and 27°C, adult cat fleas can start to emerge in 5 days. Peak emergence occurs at day 8 to 9. Emergence is not automatic but depends on the presence of appropriate stimuli, especially temperature and physical pressure. Without the proper stimulus, the adult flea can remain in the cocoon for as long as 140 days.[53] These pre-emerged adults can emerge rapidly when the proper stimulus occurs, leading to a massive explosion in the number of fleas.

In most households, *C. felis felis* takes 3 to 4 weeks to complete its life cycle, with extremes of 12 to 174 days recorded.[53, 126, 127] The newly emerged adults require a host for long-term survival. Under standard households conditions, most nonhosted, nonfed adult fleas do not survive after 12 days. If the fleas have fed for a few days before separation from the host, they die much more rapidly in the environment. If fleas are not removed from the host, they can survive for more than 100 days.

The female flea starts egg production 3 to 4 days after her first blood meal. Production varies, with peaks of 40 to 50 eggs per day recorded. Under environmental conditions that allow a 21-day life cycle, one mating female flea who lays 20 eggs per day, 50 per cent of which hatch to females, can be responsible for an infestation of more than 20,000 adults and more than 160,000 preadult forms in 60 days.

The biology of *E. gallinacea* is slightly different. After copulation, the female flea burrows into the skin, where the eggs are laid. The eggs hatch on the host, but the larvae fall into the environment, where the remainder of the life cycle is completed.[113]

Ctenocephalides canis is the most common flea isolated from dogs in Ireland.[6a] The ideal temperature and relative humidity for the development of *C. canis* are 25°C (77°F) and 75 per cent, respectively. When reared on cats, *C. canis* did not develop beyond the first larval stages.

Most species of fleas move freely around their host's body and can be found virtually anywhere. *E. gallinacea* has a preference for the facial region (see Fig. 6:38 *F*). During feeding, the flea releases material into the dermis to prevent blood clotting. *S. cuniculi*, the rabbit flea, has a preference for the pinna and periauricular areas (see Fig. 6:38 *G*). *Tunga penetrans* burrows into the skin and produces significant damage at the site of attachment (see Fig. 6:38 *H*).

The flea's saliva contains a variety of substances that can be irritating or allergenic (see Fig. 6:38 *E*). Signs associated with flea feeding are variable and depend on the number of fleas present, the tolerance of the host for skin irritation, and most importantly, the presence or absence of hypersensitivity to the flea saliva (Chap. 8). Nonallergic individuals can harbor variable numbers of fleas with little or no clinical response to them. These animals are at risk for a blood loss anemia. Seventy-two female fleas can consume a total of 1 ml of blood per day.[53] All animals, but especially those of small size, can lose a considerable amount of blood per day when they are heavily infested. However, the irritant nature of the flea's bite is usually somewhat protective for the animal. As the flea population increases, the animal's grooming behavior or scratching increases, which dislodges the flea and decreases the population feeding at any one time. Aside from the blood loss and skin damage they cause, fleas are intermediate hosts for the tapeworm *Dipylidium caninum* and could be vectors for various infectious agents.

FLEA CONTROL

Fleas are ubiquitous and, depending on the climate, can cause a seasonal or nonseasonal problem for pets and their owners. Any animal that contacts other dogs or cats, frequents grooming parlors or kennels, or is exercised in areas open to other pets or wildlife should be considered exposed. Preventive environmental and animal treatments can minimize or abort more serious problems. Measures discussed below can be both prophylactic and therapeutic but need to be used much more vigorously when the pet and its local environment are heavily infested. Prevention is the key to good flea control.

Control necessitates routine regular treatment of all pets in the house, the house, and the yard. Poor treatment in any one area, especially the house, can make the whole program unsatisfactory. Most programs employ the use of pesticides on the animals and in their environment. Pesticide use is strictly controlled in the United States and most other countries. Use of a product in a manner inconsistent with its labeling is a violation of U.S. federal law. Veterinarians who encourage extralabel use (e.g., more frequent application, use on an species of animal not cited on the label, and outdoor use of an indoor product) of a pesticide are in violation of federal law, even if commonly accepted practice indicates that use in such a manner is appropriate.

Most pesticides have some residual activity,[118] and levels can build up in the animal and its environment with repeated use. It is paramount that the veterinarian be aware of all pesticides used on the animal and its environment.[126, 127] If the same type of insecticide (e.g., organophosphate) is used on both the pet and the environment, intoxication can result from absorption from both sites.

External Environment

Because flea eggs fall to the ground, the infested pet's yard is seeded with fleas when the pet goes out or when stray dogs, cats, or feral animals visit the area. Fleas may develop from these eggs, depending on where they fall and what the climate is. Flea larvae are sensitive to heat and desiccation. Relative humidities below 50 per cent and temperature above 35°C (95°F) are lethal to flea larvae.[53] Accordingly, adults should not develop on paved areas, on deck surfaces, or in short-cut, sun-exposed lawn. Eggs that fall in protected areas (e.g., under decks, in crawl spaces, and in tall vegetation) can develop. All woodlands and uncultivated fields should be considered infested.

The first and most environmentally sound step in outdoor flea control involves restriction of the pet from the trouble spots. Crawl spaces, areas under decks, and garden areas should be fenced off and pets should not be allowed to roam in woods or fields. Exercise in short-cut, sun-exposed fields is allowed. Areas that cannot be avoided by the pet should be cleaned of organic debris frequently and treated with a pesticide registered for outside use. Powder, liquid, and granular formulations of carbamates or organophosphates are available.[126, 127] Nonmicroencapsulated liquids have a shorter residual action than do the powder or granular formulations. Recently, a novel biopesticide system for outdoor flea control has been marketed (Interrupt-Veterinary Product Laboratories). This product contains harmless nematodes, *Steinernema carpocapsae*, which kill flea larvae and pupae in the grass and soil.[192a] The efficacy of this system is not known yet.

A commonly overlooked outdoor point source of infestation is the family vehicle. If the pet travels with the family, the vehicle can be seeded with eggs. It is ill-advised to apply a residual pesticide inside the vehicle. Fumes that could develop when the vehicle sits in the sun with the windows closed could make the passengers ill. The vehicle should be vacuumed thoroughly and frequently. If a pesticide is necessary, only short-acting, low-toxicity agents (e.g., pyrethrin) should be applied. The vehicle should be well ventilated before use.

Internal Environment

The house is usually most difficult in the flea control process, especially if the household has multiple pets. Although the infestation is heaviest in areas where the pets rest, any area that is traversed or casually visited must also be treated. If cats are present, virtually every square foot of the house can be infested.

Thorough cleaning is mandatory. Vacuuming with a powerful machine can reduce the flea burden by removing some of the pre-emerged stages. All areas should be vacuumed, but special attention should be paid to the furniture, the floor beneath the furniture, the baseboard areas, and all carpets, especially those with a long nap. The vacuum should be emptied after the cleaning. Carpet cleaning can be beneficial. Steam kills larval stages, but most nonprofessional steam cleaners do not produce true steam. Carpet temperatures from these machines may be too low to kill larvae. Even if the cleaning is not larvicidal, it removes organic debris and flea feces, the foodstuff of the larvae. One drawback to carpet cleaning is that the local humidity in the carpet can be increased to the ideal flea level for days to weeks. Any newly deposited eggs or missed pre-emerged stages may accelerate their development because of this environmental improvement. Accordingly, cleaned carpets should be treated with a pesticide. During the cleaning phase, the pet's bedding should be washed or replaced. Preliminary information suggests that flea traps may be of some benefit, but environmental ultrasonic devices are of no use.[25]

Unless the household is devoid of carpets and upholstered furniture, pesticides are necessary. Owners have the choice of applying the agents themselves or hiring a professional. The latter probably costs more. However, when owners put a dollar value on their time and realize that most professional services use products not available to the general public and usually include retreatment visits in the initial price quote, professional treatment becomes cost competitive. If professional services are employed, the owner should provide the clinician with the names of the products used to ensure that they are compatible with the animal products being administered.

Health and environmental concerns have led to the use of various nontraditional pesticides, especially sodium borate. The borate compounds have rapid ovicidal and larvicidal activity, probably through a dehydrating mechanism. Owner-applied and professionally applied products are available. The professionally applied product (Rx for Fleas, Inc.) is guaranteed for 1 year, provided the carpets are not cleaned, and has a reported efficacy of greater than 99 per cent.[127]

Most homeowners want to attack the flea problem themselves, and a wide variety of pesticides and methods of delivery are available. Whatever plan is developed, it must address the displaced adult flea, the pre-emerged adults, and all the immature forms. Insecticides with little residual action, so-called quick kill products, have no place in a flea control program as the sole agent, except for spot treatment of trouble areas such as the pet's sleeping area. Products selected should be either residual insecticides or quick kill products coupled with an insect growth regulator. Because many owners are concerned about their own health as well as that of their pet, the most widely used residual insecticides are those that are microencapsulated (Sectrol and Duratrol [3M Animal Care Products]). The microencapsulation stabilizes the insecticide and allows small amounts of the compound to be released on almost a continual basis. Enough insecticide is present to kill fleas but not enough to produce intoxication. Sectrol (microencapsulated pyrethrins) should be reapplied every 30 days, whereas Duratrol (microencapsulated chlorpyrifos) is claimed to have 90-day activity. Both products allow more frequent application.

Insect growth regulators (e.g., methoprene and fenoxycarb) prevent the pupation of flea larvae.[84, 191] At the licensed concentration in products for the animal's premises, they have no effect on eggs, pre-emerged adults, or adults. At higher concentrations, methoprene may have ovicidal activity.[163] If these products are applied in the house before fleas are introduced, infestation should be aborted. Methoprene is degraded by sunlight and should be reapplied at least every 30 weeks. Fenoxycarb is sunlight stable and lasts 12 months. When the household is already infested, growth regulators alone are not sufficient.

A wide variety of insecticide plus growth regulator products are available through veterinarians, pet stores, and other outlets. The insecticide kills displaced adult fleas and some pre-emerged adults, whereas the growth regulator prevents larval development. However, because neither component affects larvae that have just pupated and some pre-emerged adults probably do not emerge during the period of activity of the insecticide, fleas may be seen in the house. If the house was massively infested, fleas can be expected in 5 to 14 days[53, 126, 127] and retreatment with a quick kill insecticide is necessary. If the infestation was mild, this retreatment may not be necessary.

The most common complaint heard when owners treat their house is that the product did not work because they continue to see fleas. Although this apparent failure may be a result of insect resistance to the parasiticide,[55, 118, 183] the continued infestation most likely results from poor application and not inferior product. Thorough treatment of a house takes a great deal of time and effort, and most uneducated owners apply the products incorrectly.

Perhaps the biggest setback in good flea control was the development of the fogger. The advertisements for these products have stressed their ease of use but not their drawbacks. These room aerosols treat unnecessary areas (e.g., tabletops) and miss vital spots (e.g., under furniture, in room corners, and in closets). These problems are magnified when the owner uses only the number of foggers necessary to cover the number of square feet of the house with no regard to intervening walls and passageways, which interrupt aerosol dispersion.

The most effective methods of indoor flea control involve hand-directed spraying of the pesticide. Products are available in aerosol form in cans, hand-operated sprays, and concentrates for dilution and application via hand-pressurized spray tanks. If large areas are to be treated, hand-operated sprays are the poorest method of delivery because hand fatigue occurs. The spraying should start in the center of the room and work toward the walls. All trouble spots (e.g., under furniture) should be sprayed carefully. Foggers can be used to decrease the amount of spraying necessary in large rooms. After the corners of the rooms and trouble spots are hand-sprayed, a well-designed fogger can be discharged to cover unobstructed areas.

Owners should be instructed to follow the manufacturer's directions carefully. Specific schedules for retreatment should be developed and followed. This is often the weak link in the program. Many clients postpone retreatment until new fleas are seen. At this point, the fleas are established, and retreatment is much more labor intensive and expensive.

Animal

None of the currently available flea eradication products for animal use is 100 per cent effective in killing or repelling fleas. Hence, good environmental control to limit the number of fleas reaching the animal is needed. Another problem with these products is that their residual efficacy under field conditions is usually far shorter than that found in the laboratory. In dogs who swim frequently, most topical products have no residual effect. Accordingly, the best pesticide to use in any particular situation is one that satisfies safety concerns and has limited restrictions on its use. Products that indicate some frequency of application but allow use as necessary give the veterinarian maximal flexibility.

Ideally, all dogs and cats in the household should be treated with the same vigor, even if only one animal has problems. Failure to treat the other animals, especially if they are allowed to roam outside, is a point source of infestation for the troubled pet via environmental seeding of eggs. In households with a large number of pets, most owners do not treat the apparently unaffected animals with the same vigor as they do the allergic ones. The owners should be encouraged to use the most effective method of control on the normal animals that their situation allows.

All animal flea control programs should be designed to prevent all flea bites. The number of fleas in the environment plus the owner's willingness and ability to do the treatments determine whether the goal is achievable. The key is regular use of the product. Haphazard use of an excellent product gives poor results. Before the specifics of a program are designed, the owner should be questioned about what he or she can do on a regular basis. Product selection is based on the owner's constraints. The following discussion demonstrates strengths and weaknesses of various tools in the control program.

■ *Flea Collars.*   Flea collars are available to kill fleas (e.g., insecticidal collars), repel fleas (e.g., ultrasonic devices), or kill flea eggs laid on the animal (Ovitrol Flea Egg Collar [Vet-Kem]). Ultrasonic collars are of no value, and insecticidal collars have limited indications.[52, 61, 172] Under ideal situations, insecticidal collars can reduce the flea burden but do not eliminate it. For the pet that is allergic to fleas, reduction is not sufficient and the insecticide in the collar can preclude the use of other similar products. Insecticidal collars should be reserved for contact animals, especially free-roaming cats, when the owner does not routinely use other methods of control. As mentioned above, methoprene, depending on its concentration, is reported to kill flea eggs and is the basis for the Ovitrol Flea Egg Collar. Use of the collar is restricted to dogs, and the stated efficacy is 4 months. The collar contains no adulticide, so it is aimed at keeping the environment and not the dog flea free. No published studies on its efficacy are available.

■ *Flea Shampoos or Cream Rinses.*   Insecticidal shampoos are excellent grooming products but have a limited place in a serious flea control program. Correct use of the shampoos, which many owners do not achieve, can kill the fleas on the animal's body, but rinsing removes any residual protection. Because the bathing must be followed by the application of some other insecticide, one must question their routine use. Flea shampoos often cost more than grooming products and have been known to cause reactions, so they cannot be considered an innocuous part of the program.

Insecticidal cream rinses (Defend Cream Rinse [Pitman-Moore]) claim residual activity against fleas for up to 7 days. The true efficacy is unknown, because it depends on how well the product was applied and how much remained after the light rinsing suggested by the manufacturer.

■ *Flea Powders.*   Flea powders contain talc and various insecticides and repellents. Effective application puts the product on the skin, where it can have prolonged residual activity if it is not removed. Powders have limited applicability in animals with dense undercoats, short coats, or significant areas of hair loss. Because the talc absorbs sebum, repeated application of powder dulls the coat and dries the skin. Many powders have been reformulated with higher concentrations of active ingredients. Caution should be exercised when using these stronger products, because too frequent application can lead to a high residual concentration of insecticides.

■ *Systemic Flea Products.*   Systemic products are designed to kill adult fleas or interrupt their life cycle when the flea feeds on treated blood. The product is either given orally (Proban [Miles]; Program [Ciba-Geigy]) or applied to the skin (Pro-Spot [Miles]), where it is transdermally absorbed. Proban[22, 51, 65] and Pro-Spot[31] contain organophosphates, cythioate and fenthion, respectively. Program contains the insect growth regulator lufenuron. The product can be used in dogs and cats but is not yet available in the United States.

Proban is administered twice weekly, whereas Pro-Spot is applied every 14th day. Fleas feeding on the animal near the administration point should receive a lethal dose of the insecticide. With time to the next administration, the organophosphate levels in the animal's blood decline and can reach an ineffective level. Fleas feeding during this window are not killed, and females can lay fertile eggs.

Problems with these insecticidal products include the potential for intoxication, the need for careful use of other cholinesterase inhibitors on the animal or in its environment, the introduction of irritants or allergens into the animal's skin while the flea is feeding, and their variable efficacy. These problems make the use of these products as licensed unsatisfactory as the sole means of flea treatment in a heavily infested environment, especially when the pet is allergic to fleas. These products may have some place in a flea control program if they are used before the environment is infested. Because the licensed administration gives a window of inefficacy, some topical products must be used in the control program. Some investigators question the use of the systemic product if topical agents are needed, whereas other researchers suggest that the systemic therapy makes topical treatment less rigorous and more effective because fewer fleas are present. Obviously, the merit of these products depends on the household situation and how willing or capable the owners are to use other products.

As discussed above, environmental infestation is the major problem in a flea control program. The use of a systemic insect growth regulator (e.g., lufenuron) may minimize this problem. Eggs laid by the female feeding on treated blood do not hatch and pre-existing larvae feeding on flea feces containing the regulator also do not mature.[105a, 163] Because adults are not affected, other flea control products have to be used.

Over the years, various lay products containing garlic, thiamine, brewers' yeast, sulfur, and other natural ingredients have been touted as systemic flea repellents. There is no clinical evidence that these products are effective.[95, 185]

■ **Liquid Products.** Various proprietary, nonproprietary, and homemade liquid flea control products are used. Although home remedies (e.g., Skin-So-Soft [Avon]) can have some efficacy,[63] data on other commonly used products (e.g., pennyroyal oil) are not available. The proprietary products rarely contain a single active ingredient and usually are mixtures of insecticides, repellents, and potentiators. Each product is labeled for species and age range use and directions for its application. Intoxication can occur if the animal is sensitive to one ingredient or if the label directions are not followed.[50, 126] These products come in aerosol sprays, hand-pumped sprays, foams, dips, and special vehicles. As with any other product, its efficacy is influenced by its formulation and how well it is applied.

Aerosol sprays are of no real use; the other modes of application have use in different situations. Dips, or more appropriately rinses, are the most effective, in that a uniform concentration of the product can easily be applied to the skin, regardless of the nature of the haircoat. Drawbacks include the smell of the product, the tendency for dips to dry the coat and the skin, the long drying time, and the limited number of products licensed for cats. Because most cats hate repeated dippings, the latter is of minimal concern.

Hand-pumped sprays are basically prediluted dips that are usually more cosmetically pleasing and expensive. Most animals can be dipped just as effectively with these sprays as they can with traditional dips, but application time increases significantly. This method is ineffective in animals with dense undercoats, and many cats resent the use of sprays. If an owner likes the spray method but finds the prepackaged products too expensive to use regularly, the owner can be instructed to make his or her own spray from a dip concentrate, provided the label instructions do not exclude this use. The owner purchases a misting spray bottle and marks it clearly with a permanent marker. The dip's dilution instructions are followed, but only that amount necessary to treat the animal or fill the reservoir bottle is made. Some dips allow reuse of diluted emulsions, whereas other dips make no reference to it or specifically prohibit it. In these latter situations, only that volume necessary to treat the animals should be made. These homemade sprays have the odor and coat-drying problems of the dip, but their relatively low cost may offset the disadvantages.

Flea foams (mousse) are special liquids that leave the can as a foam, which is applied to the hair. As the foam is massaged into the coat, the bubbles burst and the liquid reaches the skin. If the foam is applied correctly, the coat is left damp. This formulation is of most value in small animals, especially cats, who resent the application of traditional liquids.

Various special vehicle flea products are available through veterinarians or pet supply houses. Some lay products supposedly contain agents that bind the insecticide to the hair shaft for a prolonged residual effect. Similar products were marketed through veterinarians but are no longer available, suggesting poor performance of the product.

One special vehicle veterinary product is Defend Exspot Insecticide for Dogs (Coopers) (65 per cent permethrin). The owner applies one or two packages of the product to the dorsum of the dog, and supposedly the special vehicle allows the product to spread to all skin surfaces. It is difficult to believe that a product applied between the shoulder blades spreads in a uniform fashion to all areas of the body, especially the distal extremities. If spread was incomplete or attained nonlethal concentrations in some areas, resistance might develop. In fact, initial clinical experiences with this product have shown that treated dogs rarely have fleas over the dorsolateral aspects of their bodies, but numerous fleas are found on the face and the distal limbs.

DIPTERA (FLIES)

Medically, flies form a most important order of arthropods, as they transmit, or are intermediate hosts for, many bacterial, viral, protozoal, and helminthic disease agents. However, their effects on skin are minor and are limited to bites (mosquitoes, stable flies, black flies, and deer flies) and to myiasis.

The reaction to insect bites varies, because some animals are less attractive or less susceptible to certain flies. The local lesion is an irritant reaction that may become less severe with repeated exposures. The systemic reaction to injected antigen, however, often increases with repeated exposures (e.g., to bee and mosquito antigens), and severe local edema or anaphylaxis may develop.

The primary lesion is a wheal or papule around a bleeding point (Fig. 6:46 D). The reaction may be transient or may persist for weeks. In the latter case, a pseudocarcinomatous hyperplasia develops, with scaling and alopecia. A superficial and deep perivascular or diffuse dermal infiltrate of eosinophils, plasma cells, and lymphocytes may be present.

■ *Fly Dermatitis.* Adult male and female stable flies *(Stomoxys calcitrans)* are peculiarly adapted for attacking the skin of the host and sucking blood. The rasping teeth and blades of the labella tear open the skin, and the labella and whole proboscis are plunged into the wound to suck blood. The entire action is highly irritating to the host and conducive to spreading disease.

The flies usually attack the face or the ears of dogs. The multiple bites are commonly found on the tips of the ears (Fig. 6:46 A) or at the folded edge of the skin in dogs whose ears are tipped over (such as Shetland sheepdogs and collies) (Fig. 6:46 B). Erythema and hemorrhagic crusts, caused by oozing serum and blood, are typical lesions. Pruritus varies from mild to severe, presumably reflecting the absence or presence of sensitization. Affected dogs are always housed outdoors and are often confined so that they cannot escape the fly attacks.

Ordinary fly repellents, fly or flea spray, or pastes made of flea powder applied to the affected skin help to prevent repeated bites. Many flea sprays and powders contain complex organic compounds as repellents. The patient should be housed indoors during the day, if possible, until the lesions heal. Topical medications such as antibiotic-corticosteroid ointment (Panalog) may be beneficial. The affected skin should be kept clean and dry. The source of the

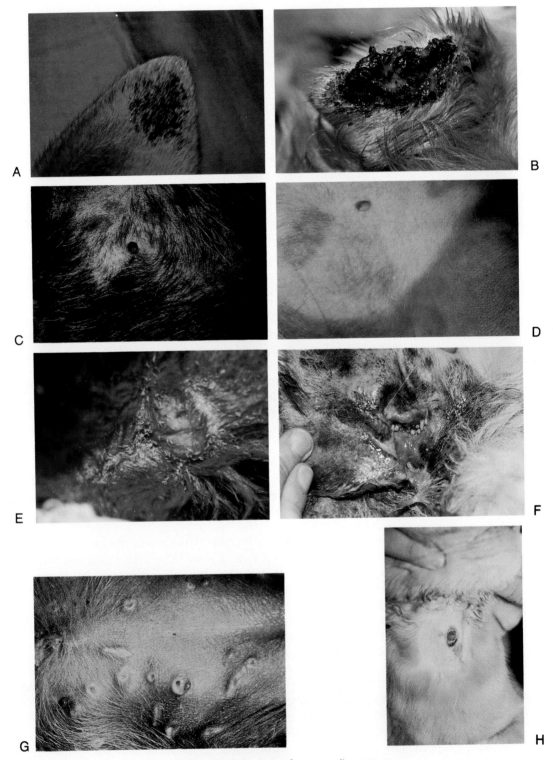

Figure 6:46 See legend on opposite page

flies should be investigated, and straw piles, manure pits, and other likely areas can be sprayed with an insecticide.

Black flies (*Simuliidae* spp.) are tiny biting flies that reproduce in shaded areas with running water. They are seasonal in early spring and summer and, during that time, cause severe reactions in people and animals. Their bites are concentrated on hairless areas such as the abdomen (Fig. 6:46 *C*), the head, the ears, and the legs (Fig. 6:46 *D*). The lesions are intensely pruritic papules, crusts, and ulcers, with hemorrhage and severe excoriation that result in circumscribed areas of necrosis. Some animals have highly diagnostic annular, macular lesions characterized by a small, pinpoint, puncture, surrounded by a larger blanched zone of edema, with a highly erythematous rim. Pruritus is variable. Horsefly (*Tabanus*), deer fly (*Chrysops*), and mosquito bites tend to be less reactive than are black fly bites, but they are all diagnosed, managed, and prevented in the same way as described for stable flies.

■ ***Mosquito Dermatitis.*** Most animals develop a pruritic papule only at the site of the mosquito's bite. Some cats apparently are hypersensitive to some mosquito salivary antigen (see Chap. 8) and develop a pruritic, erosive, crusting dermatitis of the bridge of the nose; papular to nodular lesions on the pinnae; or hyperkeratosis and swelling of the pads.[133] Lesions resolve with or without treatment when the cat is isolated from mosquitos and recur within 24 hours of new bites.

Histologically, the lesions are characterized by an eosinophilic interstitial to diffuse dermatitis with or without intraepidermal eosinophilic microabscesses or a nodular eosinophilic granulomas with collagen degeneration. Some cats show positive intradermal test reactions to mosquito extracts.

Lesional resolution is hastened by the administration of glucocorticoids but may be incomplete with continued mosquito feeding. Unless the cat tolerates repeated applications of insect repellents, management changes are necessary. Because mosquitos feed primarily from dusk to dawn, the cat should be kept in a screened cage or room during those hours.

■ ***Myiasis.*** Although maggots can have medical use,[151] natural infection is detrimental to the patient's health. The adult forms of many dipterous flies place eggs on the wet, warm skin of debilitated, weakened animals with draining wounds or urine-soaked coats (Fig. 6:46 *E* and *F*).[105] Animals that are attractive are not equally so at all stages to all flies. As the skin breaks down and liquefies, it becomes a more ideal habitat to further attract a second or third species of fly. Calliphorids (blowflies) feed on only dead tissue, whereas sarcophagids (flesh flies) attack living tissue.[105] True screwworms, *Cochliomyia hominovorax*, have been eliminated from large areas of North America but exist in other areas. They are obligate parasites of living tissue and are never common in dogs and cats.[35] *Habronema* larvae can rarely cause disease in animals housed near horses.[181] Specific identification is not important in the treatment of most myiasis cases. If necessary, larvae can be kept until adult flies develop, or the posterior aspect of the larvae can be examined for posterior spiracles and stigmal plates that are taxonomically significant.

The larvae found in cutaneous myiasis are highly destructive and produce lesions over extensive areas with punched-out round holes (Fig. 6:46 *G*) in the skin.[18, 105, 169] These may

---

Figure 6:46. *A*, Fly dermatitis on a German shepherd's pinna. Hemorrhagic crusts form from the oozing blood and serum that result from the rasping mouthparts of stable flies *(Stomoxys calcitrans)*. *B*, Collie with folded ear shows extensive fly bite lesions at the fold of the ear with secondary pyoderma. *C*, Multiple erythematous fly bites on a dog's abdomen. *D*, Multiple ecchymotic black fly bites on the glabrous skin of a canine abdomen. *E*, Myiasis. Moist exudative skin lesions attract flies. Note many white fly larvae on the surface of skin and hair. *F*, Myiasis *(Sarcophaga* sp.) complicating otitis externa in a dog. *G*, Multiple crateriform ulcers due to *Cordylobia anthropophaga* on the abdomen of a dog (Courtesy J. Van Heerden.) *H*, *Cuterebra* sp. larva protruding from a fistula in the ventral neck region of a cat (area has been clipped).

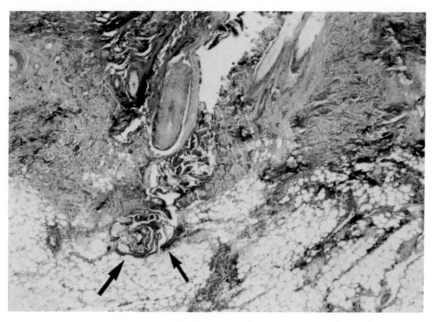

Figure 6:47. *Sarcophaga* sp. larva *(arrow)* surrounded by necrotizing dermatitis.

coalesce to form broad defects with scalloped margins. The larvae may be found under the skin and in the tissues (Figs. 6:47 and 6:48). Favorite locations are around the nose, eyes, mouth, anus, and genitalia, or adjacent to neglected wounds (Figs. 6:46 *E* and *F*). Severely infested animals may die of shock, intoxication, or infection.[105] Myiasis is always a disease of neglect.

Treatment necessitates clipping hair away from the lesions and cleaning them with an antibacterial shampoo or wound flush. The larvae must be meticulously removed from deep crevices and from under the skin. If the patient is stable, the diseased tissue should be surgically

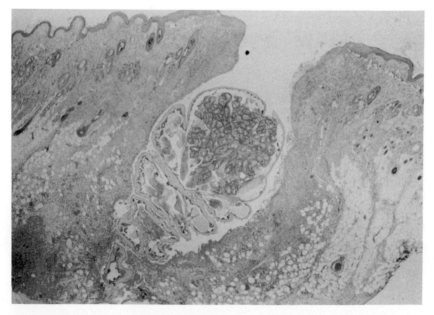

Figure 6:48. *C. anthropophaga* larva surrounded by necrotizing dermatitis and panniculitis. (Courtesy J. Van Heerden.)

debrided. Pyrethrin or pyrethroid sprays or dips should be applied to the area to kill any maggots that were missed.[105] Daily routine wound care is necessary, and the patient should be housed in screened, fly-free quarters. Usually, healing is rapid and complete, but one should also be concerned about the original cause. Fecal or urinary incontinence, a continually wet coat, fold dermatoses, or constant salivation or lacrimation, together with poor hygiene, can predispose the animal to myiasis. These underlying factors must be corrected as a primary part of therapy.

Some larvae, especially those of *Cordylobia anthropophaga* (Fig. 6:46 *G*), *Dermatobia hominis,* several species of *Cuterebra* (see below) and *Wohlfahrtia,* and possibly *Habronema* spp. can penetrate normal skin and produce single to multiple nodular to necrotic lesions.[20, 75, 177, 181] Dogs and cats can act as transport for flies via their encysted larvae and introduce them to new countries.[75] Treatment of individual lesions is as above, but repeated application of insect repellents and management changes are important to prevent new lesions.

■ *Cuterebra Species Infestation.* Adult *Cuterebra* flies are large and beelike with vestigial mouthparts, but they neither bite nor feed. They are not directly attracted to a host species but deposit eggs on stones or vegetation near the entrance to the burrows or nests of animals to which they are probably attracted at night. Animals become infested as they pass through areas contaminated with the eggs of *Cuterebra* spp. Larvae enter the body via natural body openings, by skin penetration, or by ingestion as the animal grooms contaminated fur.[4, 85] The natural hosts are usually rabbits and other rodents, and in these animals, the parasites exhibit host and site specificity.[115] Rabbit *Cuterebra* are less host specific and usually affect cats and dogs.

Because cats and dogs are abnormal hosts, the larvae undergo aberrant migrations and have been reported in the brain, the pharynx, the nostrils, and the eyelids. Typical cases involving the skin are usually localized to the regions of the head, the neck, or the trunk. Cases usually occur in late summer or fall, when the larvae enlarge and produce a swelling of 1 cm in diameter, which develops a fistula (see Fig. 6:46 *H*).

Treatment involves incising or spreading the fistulous opening and extracting the grub with a mosquito forceps. Care should be taken to avoid crushing the larva, as retained parts may produce allergic or irritant reactions. The infected wound should be treated, but healing is slow.

Identification is usually possible, because the second instar larvae are 5 to 10 mm in length and cream to gray in color, with 10 to 12 visible body segments, the first 8 to 10 of which are encircled by 3 to 4 rows of scattered dark spines and spinules. They have well-developed cranial mouth hooks but no head capsule or legs. Molting occurs, and the third instar is the dark, thick, heavily spined larva that the clinician sees in the subcutaneous or submucosal pocket.

HYMENOPTERA (BEES, WASPS, AND HORNETS)

These venomous insects are not parasitic. They possess membranous wings and mouthparts for chewing, sucking, and licking. The ovipositor of the female insect is adapted for stinging. The female insect has paired venom glands that express a toxin during the sting. When bees and certain wasps sting, the tip of the abdomen and the whole poison apparatus break off and remain in the wound. The gland may continue to express poison, so the stinger should be removed from the skin as soon as possible. Other wasps and hornets may sting repeatedly, because they remain intact. Local redness, edema, and inflammation soon develop (Fig. 6:49), and in some animals, angioedema or anaphylaxis can occur. Intoxication is possible with a large number of stings.[42] If cardiac and respiratory impairment result, the patient may die.

Facial eosinophilic folliculitis and furunculosis has been described in dogs (see Chap. 8) and is thought to be due to the sting of a venomous insect, especially the wasp.[91, 92] Dogs have an acute onset of a pruritic papular to nodular facial dermatitis.[108] Lesions may be single or multiple, are crusted, and may be ulcerated if the patient traumatizes them. Grossly, the lesions

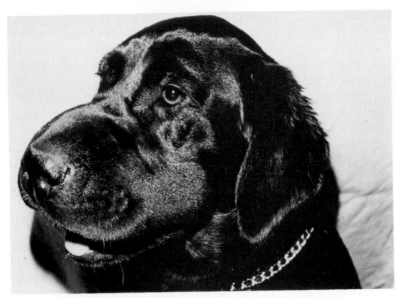

Figure 6:49. Bee sting. The local edema, pain, and redness on the nose of this Labrador retriever disappeared within 3 hours after systemic corticosteroid therapy.

cannot be differentiated from those of other causes of folliculitis or furunculosis, but cytologic evaluation of the exudate shows numerous eosinophils and no signs of infection. Histologically, an eosinophilic folliculitis or furunculosis is seen, often accompanied by areas of collagen degeneration and mucinosis.[92] Lesions resolve slowly without treatment. If the patient is pruritic, the administration of topical or oral corticosteroids hastens the resolution of the lesions. The stinger should be removed, if it can be located. In severe cases with anaphylaxis, epinephrine should be given intramuscularly and glucocorticoids should be administered intravenously. If urticaria is present, epinephrine or large doses of prednisolone followed by a rapid-acting antihistamine should be administered systemically. The application of hot compresses may relieve local pain. Subsequent bites or multiple bites make the reaction more severe.

ANTS

The fire ant (*Solenopsis invicta*) is found in South America and the southeastern United States.[170a] These ants inhabit urban and rural settings. When their nest is disturbed, they swarm out, cover nearby objects, and deliver numerous stings. Fire ants attach themselves by pinching skin with their mandibles; they then arch their bodies and inject venom through an abdominal stinger. The venom is primarily composed of a unique alkaloid (solenopsin A) that is cytotoxic and hemolytic.

In dogs, the initial fire ant sting is painless, but it is followed within 15 minutes by erythematous, pruritic swellings less than 1 cm in diameter.[170a] These swellings enlarge to be up to 2 cm in diameter in about 6 hours; they then regress and disappear within 48 hours.

Histopathologic findings include vertically oriented, linear bands of full-thickness dermal necrosis with surrounding edema and numerous eosinophils.[170a]

CATERPILLARS

The caterpillar larvae of certain Lepidoptera (butterflies and moths) can cause skin reactions.[36a, 169a] Such reactions are recognized commonly in dogs, rarely in cats, in the Mediterranean region of Europe. Pine and oak caterpillars (*Thaumetopoea* spp.) are most frequently involved. Bristles from these caterpillars contain thaumatopine, which causes mast cell degranulation and histamine release.

Animals (and humans) may be envenomated upon direct contact with the caterpillars or their nests, or by contact with airborne bristles. Most cases of skin reactions are seen in the spring in young, curious dogs. Clinical signs include the sudden onset of facial pruritus, urticaria, or angioedema. The lips and muzzle are most severely affected. In addition, the tongue is swollen and ptyalism is pronounced. In severe cases, necrotic areas may develop in the skin and on the lateral and distal portions of the tongue.

Therapy includes the use of glucocorticoids, antihistamines, and in severe cases, epinephrine.

REFERENCES

1. Arlian, L. G., et al.: Survival of adults and developmental stages of *Sarcoptes scabiei* var. *canis* when off the host. Exp. Appl. Acarol. 6:181, 1989.
2. Arlian, L. G., et al.: Cross infestivity of *Sarcoptes scabiei*. J. Am. Acad. Dermatol. 10:979, 1984.
3. Bailey, R. G., Thompson, R. C.: Demodectic mange in a cat. Aust. Vet. J. 57:49, 1981.
4. Baird, C. R.: Development of *Cuterebra ruficrus* (Diptera: Cuterebridae) in six species of rabbits and rodents with a morphological comparison of *C. ruficrus* and *C. jellisoni* third instars. J. Med. Entomol. 9:81, 1972.
5. Baker, K. P.: Clinical aspects of hookworm dermatitis. Vet. Dermatol. Newsl. 4:16, 1979.
6. Baker, K. P.: Studies on the tissue response to the genus *Demodex*. Vet. Dermatol. Newsl. 4:16, 1979.
6a. Baker, K. P., Elharam, S.: The biology of *Ctenocephalides canis* in Ireland. Vet. Parasitol. 45:141, 1992.
7. Barriga, O. O., et al.: Evidence of immunosuppression by *Demodex canis*. Vet. Immunol. Immunopathol. 32:37, 1992.
8. Barsanti, J. A.: Botulism, tick paralysis and acute polyradiculoneuritis. In: Kirk, R. W. (ed.). Current Veterinary Therapy VII. W. B. Saunders Co., Philadelphia, 1980.
9. Barta, O., et al.: Lymphocyte transformation suppression caused by pyoderma—Failure to demonstrate it in uncomplicated demodectic mange. Comp. Immunol. Microbiol. Infect. Dis. 6:9, 1983.
10. Bate, M., et al.: *Gnathostoma spinigerum* in a dog's leg. Aust. Vet. J. 60:285, 1983.
11. Berger, R. S.: The unremarkable brown recluse spider bite. J. Am. Med. Assoc. 225:1109, 1973.
12. Bigler, B., et al.: Este erfolgversprechende Ergebnisse in der Behandlung von *Notoedres cati* mit Ivermectin. Schweiz. Arch. Tierheilkd. 126:365, 1984.
13. Bilger, D., Drion, M.: Dermatite à *Otodectes cynotis*. Point Vét. 16:92, 1984.
14. Blagburn, B. L., et al.: Efficacy of the preventic (9% amitraz) collar for control of *Rhipicephalus sanguineus* and *Dermacentor variabilis* infestations on dogs. In: Proceedings of the 1993 North American Veterinary Conference, Vol. 7, 1993, p. 387.
15. Bornstein, S.: Experimental infection of dogs with *Sarcoptes scabiei* derived from naturally infected wild red foxes *(Vulpes vulpes)*: Clinical observations. Vet. Dermatol. 2:151, 1991.
16. Bourdeau, P.: Cas de dermatite à rhabitides *(Pelodera strongyloides)* chez un chien. Point Vét. 16:5, 1984.
17. Bourdeau, P.: Quel est votre diagnostic? Point Vét. 16:102, 1984.
18. Bourdeau, P.: Quel est votre diagnostic? Point Vét. 17:456, 1985.
19. Bourdeau, P.: Les cheyletielloses des carnivores domestiques. Rec. Méd. Vét. 164:979, 1988.
20. Bourdeau, P., et al.: Myiase à *Dermatobia hominis*. Rec. Méd. Vét. 164:901, 1988.
21. Bowman, D. D.: Hookworm parasites of dogs and cats. Comp. Cont. Educ. 14:585, 1992.
22. Bowen, P. M., Caldwell, N. J.: Use of cythioate to control external parasites on cats and dogs. Vet. Med. (S.A.C.) 77:79, 1982.
23. Bowman, W. L.: The cat fur mite *(Lynxacarus rhadovsky)* in Australia. Aust. Vet. J. 54:403, 1978.
24. Brockis, D. C.: Mite infestations (letter). Vet. Rec. 107:315, 1980.
25. Brown, C. R., et al.: The efficacy of ultrasonic pest controllers for fleas and ticks. J. S. Afr. Vet. Assoc. 62:110, 1991.
26. Buelke, D. L.: Hookworm dermatitis. J. Am. Vet. Med. Assoc. 148:735, 1971.
27. Bullmore, C. C., et al.: Feline trombiculosis. Feline Pract. 6:36, 1976.
28. Bussieras, J.: Le traitement de la démodécie du chien par l'amitraz. Rec. Méd. Vét. 155:685, 1979.
29. Bussieras, J., Chermette, R.: Amitraz and canine demodicosis. J. Am. Anim. Hosp. Assoc. 22:779, 1986.
30. Carmichael, J., Bell, F. R.: Filariasis in dogs in Uganda. J. S. Afr. Vet. Assoc. 14:12, 1943.
31. Carr, S. H.: Clinical observations on the topical use of fenthion. Canine Pract. 7:69, 1980.
32. Caswell, J. L., et al.: Canine demodicosis: A retrospective histopathologic study. Proc. Am. Acad. Vet. Dermatol. 9:93, 1993.
32a. Cayatte, S. M., et al.: Perifollicular melanosis in the dog. Vet. Dermatol. 3:165, 1992.
33. Chalmers, S., et al.: Demodicosis in two cats seropositive for feline immunodeficiency virus. J. Am. Vet. Med. Assoc. 194:256, 1989.
34. Charlesworth, E. N., Johnson, J. L.: An epidemic of canine scabies in man. Arch. Dermatol. 110:574, 1974.
35. Chermette, R.: A case of canine otitis due to screwworm, *Cochliomyia hominivorax*, in France. Vet. Rec. 124:641, 1989.
36. Chermette, R., et al.: Subcutaneous *Taenia crassiceps* cysticercosis in a dog. J. Am. Vet. Med. Assoc. 203:263, 1993.

36a. Chermette, R., Chareyre, G.: A propos des chenilles processionnaires. Point Vét. 26:9:1993.
37. Cohen, S. R.: *Cheyletiella* dermatitis (in rabbit, cat, dog, man). Arch. Dermatol. 116:435, 1980.
38. Coles, L. D., et al.: Adult *Dirofilaria immitis* in hind leg abscesses of a dog. J. Am. Anim. Hosp. Assoc. 24:363, 1988.
39. Conroy, J. D., et al.: New *Demodex* sp. infesting a cat: A case report. J. Am. Anim. Hosp. Assoc. 18:405, 1982.
40. Corbett, R., et al.: Cellular immune responsiveness in dogs with demodectic mange. Transplant. Proc. 7:557, 1975.
41. Corbett, R. B., et al.: The cell-mediated immune response: Its inhibition and in vitro reversal in dogs with demodectic mange. Fed. Proc. 35:589, 1976.
42. Cowell, A. K., et al.: Severe systemic reactions to *Hymenoptera* stings in three dogs. J. Am. Vet. Med. Assoc. 198:1014, 1991.
43. Cowman, L. A., et al.: Generalized demodicosis in a cat responsive to amitraz. J. Am. Vet. Med. Assoc. 192:1442, 1988.
44. Chesney, C. J.: Demodicosis in the cat. J. Small Anim. Pract. 30:689, 1989.
45. Craig, T. M., et al.: *Lynxacarus rhadovsky* infestation in a cat. J. Am. Vet. Med. Assoc. 202:613, 1993.
46. DeClerg, J., Nachtegaele, L.: *Dermanyssus gallinae* infestation in a dog. Canine Pract. 18:34, 1993.
47. Dell'Porto, A., et al.: Ocorrencia de *Lagochilascaris major* Leiper, 1910 em Gato (*Felis catus domesticus* L) no estado de Sao Paulo, Brasil. Rev. Fac. Med. Vet. Zootec. 25:173, 1988.
48. Desch, C., Nutting, W. B.: *Demodex cati*, Hirst, 1919: A redescription. Cornell Vet. 69:280, 1989.
49. Dodds, J.: Bleeding disorders: Their importance in everyday practice. Proc. Am. Anim. Hosp. Assoc. 44:147, 1977.
50. Dorman, D. C., et al.: Fenvalerate/*N,N*-diethyl-*m*-toluamide (Deet) toxicosis in two cats. J. Am. Vet. Med. Assoc. 196:100, 1990.
51. Dryden, M. W.: Differential activity of cythioate against female and male *Ctenocephalides felis* in cats. Am. J. Vet. Res. 53:801, 1992.
52. Dryden, M. W., et al.: Effects of ultrasonic flea collars on *Ctenocephalides felis* on cats. J. Am. Vet. Med. Assoc. 195:1717, 1989.
53. Dryden, M. W.: Biology of fleas of dogs and cats. Comp. Cont. Educ. 15:569, 1993.
54. Dryden, M. W.: Host association, on-host longevity and egg production of *Ctenocephalides felis felis*. Vet. Parasitol. 34:117, 1989.
54a. Duclos, D. D., et al.: Prognosis for treatment of adult-onset demodicosis in dogs: 34 cases (1979–1990). J. Am. Vet. Med. Assoc. 204:616, 1994.
54b. Duncan, K. L.: Treatment of amitraz toxicosis. J. Am. Vet. Med. Assoc. 203:1115, 1993.
55. El-Gassar, L. M., et al.: Insecticide resistance in the cat flea. J. Econ. Entomol. 79:132, 1986.
56. Elkins, A. D., et al.: Interdigital cyst in the dog caused by an adult *Dirofilaria immitis*. J. Am. Anim. Hosp. Assoc. 26:71, 1990.
57. Estes, S. A., et al.: Experimental canine scabies in humans. J. Am. Acad. Dermatol. 9:397, 1983.
58. Fadok, V. A.: Miscellaneous parasites of the skin (part I). Comp. Cont. Educ. 2:707, 782, 1980.
59. Fain, A.: Epidemiological problems of scabies. Int. J. Dermatol. 17:20, 1978.
60. Farmer, H., Seawright, A. A.: The use of amitraz (*N'*-(2,4-dimethylphenyl)-*N*-[[(2,4-dimethylphenyl)imino]-methyl]-*N*-methylmethanimidamide) in demodicosis in dogs. Aust. Vet. J. 56:537, 1980.
61. Farrell, R. K., et al.: Toxicity of flea collars. J. Am. Vet. Med. Assoc. 166:1054, 1975.
62. Faulk, R. H., et al.: Effect of Tresaderm against otoacariasis: A clinical trial. Vet. Med. (S.A.C.) 73:307, 1978.
63. Fehrer, S. L., Halliwell, R. E.: Effectiveness of Avon's Skin-So-Soft as a flea repellent on dogs. J. Am. Anim. Hosp. Assoc. 23:217, 1987.
63a. Ferguson, E. A.: Four cases of acariasis in the cat caused by Sarcoptes scabiei. Proc. Br. Vet. Dermatol. Study Grp. 16:9, 1994.
64. Figueiredo, C., et al.: Clinical evaluation of the effect of vitamin E in the treatment of generalized canine demodicosis. In: Ihrke, P. J., et al. (eds.). Advances in Veterinary Dermatology, Vol. 2. Pergamon Press, Oxford, 1993, p. 247.
65. Fisher, M. A., et al.: Efficacy of cythioate against fleas on dogs and cats. Vet. Dermatol. 1:46, 1989.
66. Fleming, E. J., et al.: Miliary dermatitis associated with *Eutrombicula* infestation in a cat. J. Am. Anim. Hosp. Assoc. 27:529, 1991.
67. Fletcher, K. C.: Demodicosis in a group of juvenile snow leopards. J. Am. Vet. Med. Assoc. 177:896, 1980.
68. Foley, R. H.: A notoedric manage epizootic in an island's cat population. Feline Pract. 19:8, 1991.
69. Foley, R. H.: Parasitic mites of dogs and cats. Comp. Cont. Educ. 13:783, 1991.
70. Foley, R. H.: An epizootic of a rare fur mite in an island's cat population. Feline Pract. 19:17, 1991.
71. Folz, S. D., et al.: Evaluation of a new treatment for canine scabies and demodicosis. J. Vet. Pharmacol. Ther. 1:199, 1978.
72. Folz, S. D.: Demodicosis (*Demodex canis*). Comp. Cont. Educ. 5:116, 1983.
73. Folz, S. D.: Canine scabies (*Sarcoptes scabiei* infestation). Comp. Cont. Educ. 6:176, 1984.
74. Folz, S. D., et al.: Evaluation of a sponge-on therapy for canine scabies. J. Vet. Pharmacol. Ther. 7:29, 1984.
75. Fox, M. T., et al.: *Timber* fly (*Cordylobia anthropophaga*) myiasis in a quarantined dog in England. Vet. Rec. 130:100, 1992.
76. Foxx, T. S., Ewing, S. A.: Morphologic features, behavior, and life history of *Cheyletiella yasguri*. Am. J. Vet. Res. 30:269, 1969.
77. Franc, M., et al.: Essai de traitement de l'otacriase du chat par les ivermectines. Rev. Méd. Vét. 136:683, 1985.
78. Franc, M., Soubeyroux, H.: Le traitement de la démodécie du chien par un collier à 9 per cent amitraz. Rev. Méd. Vét. 137:583, 1986.

79. Frye, F. L., Furman, D. P.: Phthiriasis in a dog. J. Am. Vet. Med. Assoc. 152:1113, 1968.
80. Gaafer, S. M., Greeve, J.: Natural transmission of *Demodex canis* in dogs. J. Am. Vet. Med. Assoc. 148:1043, 1966.
81. Gabbert, N., Feldman, B. F.: A case report—Feline *Demodex*. Feline Pract. 6:32, 1976.
82. Garfield, R. A., Reedy, L. M.: The use of oral milbemycin oxime (Interceptor) in the treatment of chronic generalized demodicosis. Vet. Dermatol. 3:231, 1992.
83. Gardiner, C. H., et al.: Onchocerciasis in two dogs. J. Am. Vet. Med. Assoc. 203:828, 1993.
84. Garg, R. C., et al.: Pharmacologic profile of methoprene, an insect growth regulator, in cattle, dogs, and cats. J. Am. Vet. Med. Assoc. 194:410, 1989.
85. Georgi, J., Georgi, M.: Parasitology for Veterinarians, 5th ed. W. B. Saunders Co., Philadelphia, 1990.
86. Gilbert, P. A., et al.: Serum vitamin E levels in dogs with pyoderma and generalized demodicosis. J. Am. Anim. Hosp. Assoc. 28:407, 1992.
86a. Gisseliere, Y.: Five cases of feline demodicosis. Proc. Br. Vet. Dermatol. Study Grp. 16:16, 1994.
87. Giovengo, S. L.: Canine dracunculiasis. Comp. Cont. Educ. 15:726, 1993.
88. Greene, R. T., et al.: Trombiculiasis in a cat. J. Am. Vet. Med. Assoc. 188:1054, 1986.
89. Greve, J. H., Gerrish, R. R.: Fur mites *(Lynxacarus)* from cats in Florida. Feline Pract. 11:28, 1981.
90. Griffin, C. E.: Scabies. In: Griffin, C. E., et al. (eds.). Current Veterinary Dermatology. Mosby–Year Book, St. Louis, 1993, p. 85.
91. Griffin, C. E.: Insect and arachnid hypersensitivity. In: Kwochka, K. W., MacDonald, J. M. (eds.). Current Veterinary Dermatology. Mosby Year Book, St. Louis, 1993, p. 133.
92. Gross, T. L.: Canine eosinophilic furunculosis of the face. In: Ihrke, P. J., Mason, I. S., White, S. D. (eds.). Advances in Veterinary Dermatology, Vol. 2. Pergamon Press, Oxford, 1993, p. 211.
93. Guaguère, E.: La démodécie du chien adulte. A propos de 22 cas. Prat. Méd. Chirurg. Anim. Cie 26:411, 1991.
94. Guaguère, E.: Dermatite miliare à *Otodectes cynotis* chez un chat. Prat. Méd. Chirurg. Anim. Cie 5:705, 1992.
95. Halliwell, R. E. W.: Ineffectiveness of thiamine (vitamin B_1) as a flea-repellent in dogs. J. Am. Anim. Hosp. Assoc. 18:423, 1982.
96. Hardison, J. L.: A case of *Eutrombicula alfreddugesi* (chiggers) in a cat. Vet. Med. (S.A.C.) 72:47, 1977.
97. Harmon, R. R. M.: Parasites, worms, and protozoa. In: Rook, A., et al. (eds.) Textbook of Dermatology. Blackwell Scientific Publications, Oxford, 1979.
98. Harvey, R. G.: Dermatitis in a cat associated with *Spilopsyllus cuniculi*. Vet. Rec. 126:89, 1990.
99. Harwick, R. P.: Lesions caused by canine ear mites. Arch. Dermatol. 114:130, 1978.
100. Havrileck, B., et al.: Suivi immunitaire individuel de chiens démodéciques par intradermoréactions à la phyto-hemagglutinin. Applications au prognostic. Rev. Méd. Vét. 140:599, 1989.
100a. Havrileck, B., Ducos de Lahitte, J.: Traitement et pronostic de la démodécie canine. L'Action Vét. 1150:34, 1990.
101. Hawkins, J. A., et al.: *Sarcoptes scabiei* infestation in a cat. J. Am. Vet. Med. Assoc. 190:1572, 1987.
102. Healy, M. C., Gaafar, S. M.: Demonstration of reaginic antibody (IgE) in canine demodectic mange: An immunofluorescent study. Vet. Parasitol. 3:107, 1977.
103. Healy, M. C., Gaafar, S. M.: Immunodeficiency in canine demodectic mange. II. Skin reactions to phytohemagglutinin and concanavalin A. Vet. Parasitol. 3:133, 1977.
104. Hendrix, C. M., et al.: *Anatrichosoma* sp. infection in a dog. J. Am. Vet. Med. Assoc. 191:984, 1987.
105. Hendrix, C. M.: Facultative myiasis in dogs and cats. Comp. Cont. Educ. 13:86, 1991.
105a. Hink, W. F., et al.: Evaluation of a single oral dose of lufenuron to control flea infestations in dogs. Am. J. Vet. Res. 55:822, 1994.
106. Hirsch, D. C., et al.: Suppression of in vitro lymphocyte transformation by serum from dogs with generalized demodicosis. Am. J. Vet. Res. 36:195, 1975.
107. Hoeffler, D. F.: Swimmer's itch. Cutis 19:461, 1977.
108. Holtz, C. S.: Eosinophilic dermatitis in a Siberian husky cross. Calif. Vet. 44:11, 1990.
109. Horton, M. L.: Rhabditic dermatitis in dogs. Mod. Vet. Pract. 61:158, 1980.
110. Ilkiw, J. E.: Tick paralysis in Australia. In: Kirk, R. W. (ed.). Current Veterinary Therapy VII. W. B. Saunders Co., Philadelphia, 1980.
111. Johnson, G. C.: *Dracunculus insignis* in the dog. J. Am. Vet. Med. Assoc. 165:553, 1974.
112. Kalkofen, U. P., Greenberg, J.: Public health aspects of *Pulex irritans* infestations in dogs. J. Am. Vet. Med. Assoc. 165:903, 1974.
113. Kalkofen, U. P., Greenberg, J.: *Echidnophaga gallinacea* infestations in dogs. J. Am. Vet. Med. Assoc. 165:447, 1974.
114. Kamalu, B. P.: Canine filariasis caused by *Dirofilaria repens* in southeastern Nigeria. Vet. Parasitol. 40:335, 1991.
115. Kazocos, K. R., et al.: *Cuterebra* species as a cause of pharyngeal myiasis in cats. J. Am. Anim. Hosp. Assoc. 16:773, 1980.
116. Kershaw, A.: *Sarcoptes scabiei* infestation in a cat. Vet. Rec. 124:537, 1989.
117. King, K. E.: Spider bites. Arch. Dermatol. 123:41, 1987.
118. Koehler, P. G., et al.: Residual efficacy of insecticides applied to carpet for control of cat fleas. J. Econ. Entomol. 79:1036, 1986.
119. Kraft, W., et al.: Die *Otodectes cynotis* Infestation von Hund und Katze. Tierarztl. Prax. 16:409, 1988.
120. Krawiec, D. R., Gaafar, S. M.: Studies on immunology of demodicosis. J. Am. Anim. Hosp. Assoc. 16:669, 1980.
121. Kunkle, G. A., et al.: Dermatitis in horses and man caused by the straw itch mite. J. Am. Vet. Med. Assoc. 181:467, 1982.

122. Kwochka, K. W., et al.: The efficacy of amitraz for generalized demodicosis in dogs: A study of two concentrations and frequencies of application., Comp. Cont. Educ. 2:234, 1980.

122a. Kwochka, K. W.: Demodicosis. In: Griffin, C. E., et al. (eds.). Current Veterinary Dermatology. Mosby–Year Book, St. Louis, 1993, p. 72.

123. Lee, B. W.: *Cheyletiella* dermatitis: A report of 14 cases. Cutis 47:111, 1991.

124. Lopez, R. A.: Of mites and man. J. Am. Vet. Med. Assoc. 203:606, 1993.

125. Lowenstine, L. J., et al.: Trombiculosis in a cat. J. Am. Vet. Med. Assoc. 175:289, 1979.

126. MacDonald, J. M., Miller, T. A.: Parasiticide therapy in small animal dermatology. In: Kirk, R. W. (ed.). Current Veterinary Therapy 9. W. B. Saunders Co., Philadelphia, 1986.

127. MacDonald, J. M.: Flea allergy dermatitis and flea control. In: Griffin, C. E., et al. (eds.). Current Veterinary Dermatology. Mosby Year Book, St. Louis, 1993, p. 57.

128. Maillard, R.: Quel est votre diagnostic? Point Vét. 19:569, 1987.

129. Maldonado, R. R., et al.: Norwegian scabies due to *Sarcoptes scabiei* var. *canis*. Arch. Dermatol. 113:1733, 1977.

130. Malone, J. B., et al.: *Strongyloides stercoralis*–like infection in a dog. J. Am. Vet. Med. Assoc. 176:130, 1980.

131. Mansfield, L. S., et al.: Ivermectin treatment of naturally acquired and experimentally induced *Strongyloides stercoralis* infections in dogs. J. Am. Vet. Med. Assoc. 20:726, 1992.

131a. Marks, S. I., et al.: Pneumonyssoides caninum: the canine nasal mite. Compend. Cont. Educ. 16:577, 1994.

132. Mason, K. V., et al.: Mosquito bite–caused eosinophilic dermatitis in cats. J. Am. Vet. Med. Assoc. 198:2086, 1991.

132a. Mason, K. V.: A new species of *Demodex* mite with *D. canis* causing canine demodicosis: A case report. Proc. Am. Acad. Vet. Dermatol. Am. Coll. Vet. Dermatol. 9:92, 1993.

133. Matthews, B. E.: Mechanics of skin penetration by hookworm larvae. Vet. Dermatol. Newsl. 6:75, 1981.

134. McDougal, B. J., Novak, C. P.: Feline demodicosis caused by an unnamed *Demodex* mite. Comp. Cont. Educ. (S.A.C.) 8:820, 1986.

135. McGarry, J. W.: Recurrent infestation of a cat by *Cheyletiella eruditus* (Shrank 1781). Vet. Rec. 125:18, 1989.

136. McKee, A. J.: Microfilaria found in the skin. Vet. Med. 33:115, 1938.

137. McKeever, P. J., Allen, S. K.: Dermatitis associated with *Cheyletiella* infestation in cats. J. Am. Vet. Med. Assoc. 174:718, 1979.

138. Medleau, L., et al.: Demodicosis in cats. J. Am. Anim. Hosp. Assoc. 24:85, 1988.

139. Medleau, L. M., et al.: Efficacy of daily amitraz therapy for generalized demodicosis in dogs: Two independent studies. Proc. Am. Acad. Vet. Dermatol. Am. Coll. Vet. Dermatol. 7:41, 1991.

140. Meerdink, G. L.: Bites and stings of venomous animals. In: Kirk, R. W. (ed.). Current Veterinary Therapy VIII. W. B. Saunders Co., Philadelphia, 1983.

141. Miller, T. A.: Vaccination against hookworm diseases. Adv. Parasitol. 9:153, 1971.

142. Miller, W. H.: Canine demodicosis. Comp. Cont. Educ. 4:334, 1980.

143. Miller, W. H., Jr., Scott, D. W.: Unpublished observations.

144. Miller, W. H., Jr., et al.: Dermatologic disorders of the Chinese Shar Peis: 58 cases (1981–1989). J. Am. Vet. Med. Assoc. 200:986, 1992.

145. Miller, W. H., Jr., et al.: Efficacy of milbemycin oxime in the treatment of generalized demodicosis in adult dogs. J. Am. Vet. Med. Assoc. 203:1426, 1993.

146. Moriello, K. A.: Treatment of *Sarcoptes* and *Cheyletiella* infestations. In: Kirk, R. W., Bonagura, J. D. (eds.). Kirk's Current Veterinary Therapy XI: Small Animal Practice. W. B. Saunders Co., Philadelphia, 1992, p. 558.

147. Moriello, K. A.: Common ectoparasites of the dog. Part I, Fleas and ticks. Canine Pract. 14:7, 1987.

148. Moriello, K. A.: Cheyletiellosis. In: Griffin, C. E., et al. (eds.). Current Veterinary Dermatology. Mosby–Year Book, St. Louis, 1993, p. 90.

149. Mozos, E., et al.: Cutaneous lesions associated with canine heartworm infection. Vet. Dermatol. 3:191, 1992.

150. Muhammad, G.: *Dracunculus medinensis* in a bull terrier (a case report). Indian Vet. J. 67:967, 1990.

151. Mulder, J. B.: The medical marvels of maggots. J. Am. Vet. Med. Assoc. 195:1497, 1989.

152. Muller, G. H.: Demodicosis treatment with Mitaban liquid concentrate (amitraz). J. Am. Anim. Hosp. Assoc. 19:435, 1983.

152a. Muller, G. H., et al.: Small Animal Dermatology, 4th ed. W. B. Saunders Co., Philadelphia, 1989, p. 376.

153. Mundell, A. C., et al.: Ivermectin in the treatment of *Pneumonyssoides caninum*. A case report. J. Am. Anim. Hosp. Assoc. 26:393, 1990.

154. Niyama, M., Ohbayashi, M.: *Cheyletiella blakei* in a cat. Jpn. J. Vet. Sci. 41:395, 1979.

155. Norins, A. L.: Canine scabies in children. Am. J. Dis. Child. 117:239, 1969.

156. Northway, R. B.: A therapeutic approach to venomous spider bites. Vet. Med. (S.A.C.) 80:38, 1985.

157. Nutting, W. B.: Hair follicle mites (Acari: Demodicidae) of man. Int. J. Dermatol. 15:79, 1976.

158. Nutting, W. B.: Hair follicle mites (*Demodex* spp.) of medical and veterinary concern. Cornell Vet. 66:214, 1976.

159. Nutting, W. B., Desch, C. E.: *Demodex canis*: Redescription and reevaluation. Cornell Vet. 68:139, 1978.

160. Nutting, W. B.: *Demodex crecti*, notes on its biology. J. Parasitol. 44:328, 1958.

161. Ottenshot, T. R. F., Gil, D.: Cheyletiellosis in long-haired cats. Tijdschr. Diergeneeskd. 103:1104, 1978.

162. Owen, L. N.: Transplantation of canine osteosarcoma. Eur. J. Cancer 5:615, 1969.

163. Palma, K. G., et al.: Mode of action of pyriproxyfen and methoprene on eggs of *Ctenocephalides felis* (Siphonaptera: Pulicidae). J. Med. Entomol. 30:421, 1993.

164. Panciera, D. L., Stockham, S. L.: *Dracunulus insignis* infection in a dog. J. Am. Vet. Med. Assoc. 192:78, 1988.

165. Paradis, M., Vileneuve, A.: Efficacy of ivermectin against *Cheyletiella yasguri* infestation in dogs. Can. Vet. J. 29:633, 1988.

166. Paradis, M., et al.: Efficacy of ivermectin against *Cheyletiella blakei* infestation in cats. J. Am. Anim. Hosp. Assoc. 26:125, 1990.

167. Paradis, M., et al.: Efficacy of daily ivermectin treatment in a dog with amitraz-resistant, generalized demodicosis. Vet. Dermatol. 3:85, 1992.

168. Pasyk, K.: Dermatitis rhabditidosa in an 11-year-old girl. Br. J. Dermatol. 98:107, 1978.

169. Penny, D. S.: Fly strike in a dog. Vet. Rec. 125:79, 1989.

169a. Poisson, L., et al.: Quatre cas d'envenimation par les chenilles processionnaires du pin chez le chien. Point Vét. 25:992, 1994.

170. Powell, M. B., et al.: Reaginic hypersensitivity in *Otodectes cynotis* infestation of cats and mode of mite feeding. Am. J. Vet. Res. 41:877, 1980.

170a. Rakich, P. M., et al.: Clinical and histologic characterization of cutaneous reactions to stings of the imported fire ant (*Solenopsis invicta*) in dogs. Vet. Pathol. 30:555, 1993.

171. Ramsay, G. W., Mason, P. C.: Chicken mite *(D. gallinae)* infesting a dog. N. Z. Vet. J. 23:155, 1975.

172. Randall, W. F., et al.: Field evaluation of antiflea collars for initial and residual efficacy in dogs. Vet. Med. (S.A.C.) 75:606, 1980.

173. Rash, D. M., Benzon, S. P.: Dracunculosis in a dog. Mod. Vet. Pract. 62:701, 1981.

174. Reedy, L. M.: Common parasitic problems in small animal dermatology. J. Am. Vet. Med. Assoc. 188:362, 1986.

175. Reedy, N. R., et al.: Serum thyroxine levels in canine demodicosis. Indian J. Anim. Sci. 61:1300, 1991.

176. Ristic, Z.: Ivermectin in the treatment of generalized demodicosis in the dog. Proc. Am. Acad. Vet. Dermatol. Am. Coll. Vet. Dermatol. 9:31, 1993.

177. Roosje, P. J., et al.: A case of *Dermatobia hominis* in a dog in the Netherlands. Vet. Dermatol. 3:183, 1992.

178. Sako, S., Yamane, O.: Studies on the canine demodicosis. II. The significance of presence of the parasite in lymphatic glands of affected dogs. Jpn. J. Parasitol. 11:93, 1962.

179. Sako, S., Yamane, O.: Studies on the canine demodicosis. III. Examination of the oral-internal infection, intrauterine infection, and infection through respiratory tract. Jpn. J. Parasitol. 11:499, 1962.

180. Sako, S.: Studies on the canine demodicosis. IV. Experimental infection of *Demodex folliculorum* var. *canis* to dogs. Trans. Tottori Soc. Agri. Sci. 17:45, 1964.

181. Sanderson, T. P., et al.: Cutaneous habronemiasis in a dog. Vet. Pathol. 27:208, 1991.

182. Scheidt, V. J., et al.: An evaluation of ivermectin in the treatment of sarcoptic mange in dogs. Am. J. Vet. Res. 45:1201, 1984.

183. Schwinghammer, K. A., et al.: Comparative toxicity of ten insecticides against the cat flea, *Ctenocephalides felis*. J. Med. Entomol. 22:512, 1985.

184. Scott, D. W.: Nodular skin disease associated with *Dirofilaria immitis* infection in the dog. Cornell Vet. 59:233, 1979.

185. Scott, D. W.: Feline dermatology 1900–1978: A monograph. J. Am. Anim. Hosp. Assoc. 16:331, 1980.

186. Scott, D. W.: Feline dermatology 1972–1982: Introspective retrospections. J. Am. Anim. Hosp. Assoc. 20:537, 1984.

187. Scott, D. W., et al.: Studies on the therapeutic and immunologic aspects of generalized demodectic mange in the dog. J. Am. Anim. Hosp. Assoc. 10:233, 1974.

188. Scott, D. W., et al.: Further studies on the therapeutic and immunologic aspects of generalized demodectic mange in the dog. J. Am. Anim. Hosp. Assoc. 12:203, 1976.

189. Scott, D. W., Vaughn, T. C.: Papulonodular dermatitis in a dog with occult filariasis. Comp. Anim. Pract. 1:31, 1987.

190. Scott, D. W., Walton, D. K.: Experiences with the use of amitraz and ivermectin for the treatments of generalized demodicosis in dogs. J. Am. Anim. Hosp. Assoc. 21:535, 1985.

191. Shaaya, E.: Interference of the insect growth regulator methoprene in the process of larval-pupal differentiation. Arch. Insect. Biochem. Physiol. 22:233, 1993.

192. Shastri, U. V.: Efficacy of ivermectin against lice infestation in cattle, buffaloes, goats, and dogs. Indian Vet. J. 68:191, 1991.

192a. Silverman, J., et al.: Infection of cat flea, *Ctenocephalides felis* (Bouche) by *Neoaplectana carpocapsai* Weiser. J. Nematol. 14:394, 1982.

193. Smiley, R. L.: A review of the family Cheyletiellidae (Acarina). Ann. Entomol. Soc. Am. 63:1056, 1970.

194. Smith, J. D., et al.: Larva currens; cutaneous strongyloides. Arch. Dermatol. 112:1161, 1976.

195. Song, M. D.: Using ivermectin to treat feline dermatoses caused by external parasites. Vet. Med. 86:498, 1991.

196. Sosna, C. B., Medleau, L.: Symposium on external parasites. Vet. Med. 87:537, 1992.

197. Soulsby, E. J. L.: Helminths, Arthropods, and Protozoa of Domesticated Animals, 7th ed. Lea & Febiger, Philadelphia, 1982.

198. Stein, B.: Personal communication, 1982.

199. Stogdale, L., Moore, D. J.: Feline demodicosis. J. Am. Anim. Hosp. Assoc. 18:427, 1982.

200. Studdert, V. P., et al.: Dermatitis of the pinnae of cats in Australia associated with European rabbit flea. Vet. Rec. 123:624, 1988.

201. Subrahmanyam, B., et al.: *Dracunculus medinesis* (guinea worm) infestation in a dog and its therapy with Flagyl. Indian Vet. J. 63:637, 1976.

202. Thoday, K. L.: Serum immunoglobulin concentrations in canine scabies. In: Ihrke, P. J., et al. (eds.). Advances in Veterinary Dermatology, Vol. 2. Pergamon Press, Oxford, 1993, p. 211.

203. Thomsett, L. R.: Mite infestations of man contracted from dogs and cats. Br. Med. J. 3:93, 1968.

204. Vollset, I.: Immediate type hypersensitivity in dogs induced by storage mites. Res. Vet. Sci. 40:123, 1986.

205. Weisbroth, S. H., et al.: Immunopathology of naturally-occurring otodectic otoacariasis in the domestic cat. J. Am. Vet. Med. Assoc. 165:1088, 1974.
206. Weisbroth, S. H., et al.: Efficacy of Vapona-containing flea collars for control of *Otodectes* mites. Cornell Vet. 64:549, 1979.
207. White, S. D., et al.: Generalized demodicosis associated with diabetes mellitus in two cats. J. Am. Vet. Med. Assoc. 191:448, 1987.
208. Wilkie, B. N., et al.: Deficient cutaneous response to PHA-P in healthy puppies from a kennel with a high prevalence of demodicosis. Can. J. Comp. Med. 43:415, 1979.
209. Wilkinson, G. T.: Demodicosis in a cat due to a new mite species. Feline Pract. 13:32, 1983.
210. Willers, W. B.: *Pelodera strongyloides* in association with canine dermatitis in Wisconsin. J. Am. Vet. Med. Assoc. 156:319, 1970.
210a. Wolfe, J. H., Halliwell, R. E. W.: Total hemolytic complement values in normal and diseased dog populations. Vet. Immunol. Immunopathol. 1:287, 1980.
211. Wong, R. C., et al.: Spider bites (in depth review). Arch. Dermatol. 123:98, 1987.
212. Yathiraji, S., et al.: Treatment of scabies in canines with amitraz. Indian Vet. J. 67:867, 1990.
213. Yazwinski, T. A., et al.: Efficacy of ivermectin against *Sarcoptes scabiei* and *Otodectes cynotis* infestation of dogs. Vet. Med. (S.A.C.) 76:1749, 1981.

Viral, Rickettsial, and Protozoal Skin Diseases

■

Chapter Outline

These dermatoses are apparently rare in dogs and cats. Additionally, many of those that have been reported are associative or circumstantial in nature. This chapter is a brief overview of proven and suspected skin diseases of viral, rickettsial, and protozoal origin in dogs and cats.

■ VIRAL DISEASES

Feline Leukemia Virus Infection

The feline leukemia virus (FeLV) is an oncogenic immunosuppressive retrovirus.[1, 12] Although it can induce skin tumors (lymphoma, fibrosarcoma), FeLV most commonly affects the skin by its cytosuppressive actions. Clinical signs include chronic or recurrent gingivitis or pyoderma (folliculitis, abscess, paronychia), poor wound healing, seborrhea, exfoliative dermatitis, generalized pruritus, and cutaneous horns.[18] Diagnosis is supported by positive immunofluorescent antibody or serologic tests. Recent immunohistochemical tests with anti–glycoprotein 70 antisera have been able to detect viral antigen in the skin.[6] This testing should clarify whether the noninfectious manifestations are caused by or coincidental with FeLV infection.

Feline Immunodeficiency Virus Infection

Feline immunodeficiency virus (FIV) is another retrovirus that causes a variety of cytosuppressive disorders in the cat.[1, 24] The most common clinical sign is chronic or recurrent oral disease (gingivitis, periodontal disease, stomatitis). Dermatologic signs include chronic or recurrent abscesses, chronic infections of the skin and ears, and demodicosis.[5, 24]

The clinical signs of FIV and FeLV overlap; therefore, the two conditions cannot be differentiated on the basis of signs alone. Co-infection with both viruses can occur, with marked synergism of immunosuppression.[24] Diagnosis of FIV infection is supported by serologic testing.

Feline Cowpox Virus Infection

Cowpox virus is a member of the *Orthopoxvirus* genus that has sporadically caused infections of domestic and exotic cats in various European countries.[1, 2, 15, 20–22] The natural reservoir is unknown but probably is small wild mammals. Cats typically become infected through wounding while hunting these wild mammals. Cat to cat, cat to human, or cat to dog transmission can also occur.[22]

There appears to be no age, breed, or sex predisposition to infection, and many cases are recognized in the fall of the year.[2] The primary lesion in the disease is an infected bite wound, typically on the head, neck, or forelimb. Local viral replication worsens the primary lesions and is the point source for the subsequent viremia. During the viremic phase, some cats develop mild pyrexia, inappetence, and depression. Ten to 14 days after the primary lesion, multiple secondary lesions develop over the body. The secondary or pox lesions are initially macular but progress to ulcerated, papular to nodular lesions that crust rapidly (Fig. 7:1 *A* and *B*).

Figure 7:1. *A*, Footpad ulceration in feline poxvirus infection. (Courtesy R. Gaskell.) *B*, Focal oozing and crust in the temporal area of a cat with feline poxvirus infection. (Courtesy R. Gaskell.) *C*, Ballooning degeneration and eosinophilic intracytoplasmic inclusion bodies in feline poxvirus infection. *D*, Exfoliative dermatitis on the head and pinnae of a dog with leishmaniasis. (Courtesy Z. Alhaidari.) *E*, Mucocutaneous ulceration in a dog with visceral leishmaniasis. (Courtesy A. Koutinas.) *F*, Purpura, ulceration, and crusting on the paw of a dog with leishmaniasis. (Courtesy Z. Alhaidari.) *G*, Multifocal ulceration of the scrotum in a dog with Rocky Mountain spotted fever. *H*, Edema, purpura, and scaling on the scrotum of a dog with babesiosis. (Courtesy D. Carlotti.)

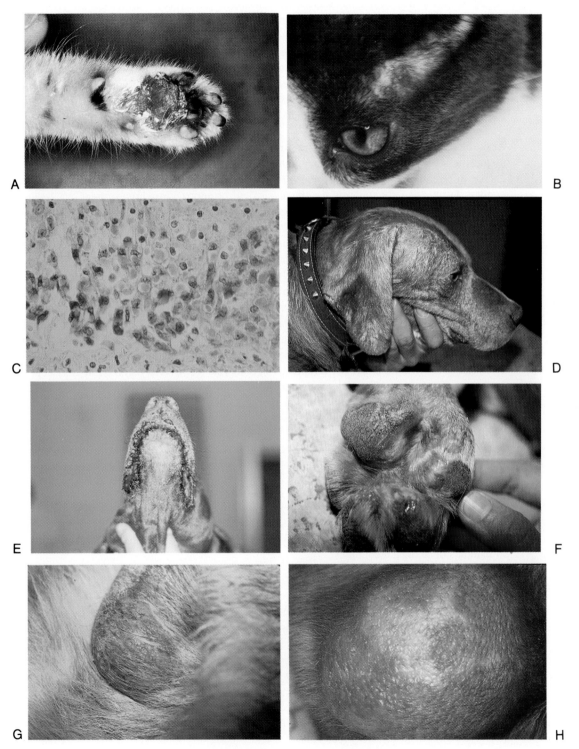

Figure 7:1 *See legend on opposite page*

Pruritus is variable, and approximately 20 per cent of infected cats develop oral vesiculation or ulceration.[1, 2] Lesions heal slowly over 3 to 4 weeks and may be permanently scarred. During the development and course of the secondary lesions, systemic signs of illness are uncommon unless the cat has some intercurrent immunosuppressive disease.

The differential diagnosis includes bacterial and fungal infections, eosinophilic granuloma, and neoplasia (especially mast cell tumor and lymphoma). Definitive diagnosis is made by skin biopsy, serologic testing, and virus isolation.[3] Dermatohistopathologic findings include hyperplasia, ballooning degeneration, reticular degeneration, microvesicle formation, and necrosis of the affected epidermis and the outer root sheath of the hair follicle (Fig. 7:1 C). Eosinophilic intracytoplasmic inclusion bodies are found within keratinocytes.

The diagnosis of cowpox is based on the results of diagnostic tests. Serum samples and fresh biopsy or scab material in viral transport medium are submitted to an appropriate diagnostic laboratory for serologic examination and viral isolation, respectively. Serologic tests cannot differentiate cowpox from other orthopox viruses. Histopathologic examination of secondary lesions usually supports the diagnosis, and orthopox virus involvement can be demonstrated by immunohistochemical techniques[2] or electron microscopy. Virus isolation is currently the only method of making a precise diagnosis.

There is no specific therapy for cowpox infection. If secondary bacterial infections of the skin or other organs occur, appropriate antibacterial therapy should be instituted. Severely ill animals, which typically have an underlying immunosuppressive disorder, require intense supportive care and may have to be euthanized. Glucocorticoids are contraindicated.

Feline cowpox has zoonotic potential for contact cats, dogs, and humans.[8, 21, 22] These contact infections are uncommon; they can be serious, however, especially if the individual is immunologically compromised. A fatality in a human receiving corticosteroids has been documented.[21] Accordingly, all infected cats should be isolated and handled carefully. The cowpox virus can remain viable under dry temperature conditions for several years, but it is susceptible to various disinfectants, especially to hypochlorite solutions.[2]

No data are available to indicate whether infection confers long-lasting immunity. To prevent possible re-infection, hunting should be prohibited.

Feline Infectious Peritonitis

Feline infectious peritonitis is a systemic viral disease caused by strains of coronaviruses. Effusive and noneffusive forms are most common.[1] Skin lesions other than those associated with debility have not been reported. Several cats experimentally infected have developed ulcerative lesions around the head and neck (Fig. 7:2).[16a] Histopathologic tests showed changes typical of a superficial vasculitis, and viral antigen was demonstrated in blood vessel walls by immunohistochemical techniques.

Canine Distemper

Canine distemper is caused by a paramyxovirus.[1] In addition to severe respiratory, gastrointestinal, and neurologic disorders, the virus may produce skin lesions in some animals. Because of their general debility, some dogs, and especially very young puppies, develop widespread impetigo. The classic skin manifestation of distemper is the so-called hard pad disease, in which the dog develops nasal (Fig. 7:3) and footpad (Fig. 7:4) hyperkeratosis of varying severity. Although a variety of diseases (e.g., pemphigus foliaceus, lupus erythematosus, drug eruption) induce nasodigital hyperkeratosis, animals with those disorders are often not as systemically ill as dogs with distemper and have more widespread skin lesions. Distemper, necrolytic migratory erythema (see Chap. 9), and generic dog food skin disease (see Chap. 16) all can produce the nasodigital lesions and similar systemic signs of illness. The index of suspicion for distemper should be high when the pads are much harder to the touch than the degree of hyperkeratosis would suggest and the dog's vaccination history is poor.

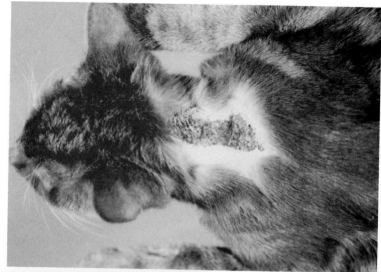

Figure 7:2. Well-demarcated necrosis and ulceration over the dorsal neck of a cat with feline infectious peritonitis.

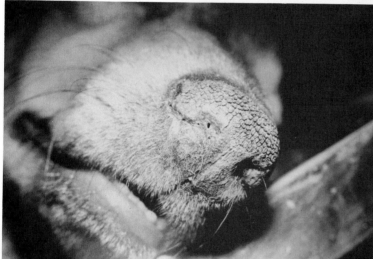

Figure 7:3. Nasal hyperkeratosis in a dog with canine distemper.

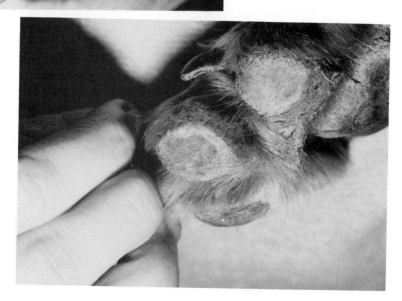

Figure 7:4. Digital hyperkeratosis in a dog with canine distemper.

Contagious Viral Pustular Dermatitis

Contagious viral pustular dermatitis (orf, contagious ecthyma) is a disease that is found primarily in sheep and goats and is caused by a parapoxvirus.[19] Contagious viral pustular dermatitis was reported in a pack of hounds allowed to feed on sheep carcasses.[23] Lesions consisted of circular areas of acute moist dermatitis, ulceration, and crusts. The predilection site was around the head. Skin biopsy revealed epidermal hyperplasia, ballooning degeneration, acantholysis within the stratum spinosum, and marked infiltration of neutrophils. Saline suspensions of skin biopsies were applied to the scarified skin of a normal sheep. Crusts removed from the inoculation sites were processed for electron microscopy, and parapoxvirus virus particles were readily seen.

Therapy for contagious viral pustular dermatitis is topical and according to symptoms. The usual course of the disease in animals is 1 to 4 weeks. The disease may be transmitted to humans if broken skin is exposed to lesion material or contaminated objects. Generally, contagious viral pustular dermatitis is a benign disease in humans and results in the formation of a solitary lesion, especially on the hands. Lesions in humans are characterized by maculae that progress through a papular, nodular, and papillomatous stage. The lesions are usually centrally umbilicated and occasionally are bullous. Complications of contagious viral pustular dermatitis in humans include regional lymphadenopathy, lymphangitis, secondary bacterial infection, and, rarely, generalized or systemic disease.

Pseudorabies

Pseudorabies is an acute, fatal viral disease caused by an α-herpesvirus.[1] Pigs are the main reservoir of infection. Dogs and cats can be infected by contact with an infected animal or, more typically, by eating raw pork products or offal. Incubation periods range from 2 to 10 days,[13] and death typically occurs within 48 hours of the onset of clinical signs.[17]

Early work suggested that intense, maniacal upper body pruritus was the cardinal feature of the disease in dogs.[13] More recent work, however, showed that this sign occurred in only 52 per cent of affected dogs.[17] Ptyalism was a universal finding, followed by restlessness, anorexia, ataxia, and a variety of other neurologic abnormalities. When present, the pruritus is intense and leads to self-mutilation, typically of the head and ears. In cats, the neurologic signs seem to predominate.[1]

The diagnosis can be confirmed by virus isolation. Treatment is usually not attempted; when it is, the result is unrewarding. Prevention by means of strict hygienic procedures is of paramount importance.

Feline Rhinotracheitis Infection

Feline rhinotracheitis infection occasionally causes oral and cutaneous ulcers.[1,9] The cutaneous ulcers are usually superficial and multiple and can occur anywhere on the body, including the footpads. Stress or trauma to the skin might precipitate the development of the ulcers. Skin biopsies reveal epidermal ulceration with subjacent dermal necrosis and a mixed inflammatory infiltrate. Basophilic intranuclear inclusion bodies may be visualized in the keratinocytes or dermal histiocytes. Herpesvirus can be cultured from the skin; more diagnostically, it can be seen in the keratinocytes via electron microscopy.[6]

Feline Calicivirus Infection

Oral ulceration is reported to be more common with calicivirus infection than with rhinotracheitis.[1] Sporadic reports associate infection with skin lesions of the feet or perineum.[7,14] The tissues are swollen, tender, and ulcerated. Although calicivirus was isolated from the skin in one case, no histopathologic tests were performed to demonstrate whether the virus was causal or a contaminant. Because some infected cats can develop a presumed immune-mediated arthropathy,[14] it is reasonable to assume that the virus can induce primary skin lesions.

Canine Papillomavirus Infection

Papillomaviruses belong to the papovavirus family and are either known to cause or suspected to cause oral papillomatosis, cutaneous papillomas, and cutaneous inverted papillomas in dogs (see Chap. 19). Two new syndromes have been recognized that are probably associated with papillomavirus infection in dogs.

The first syndrome involves the development of multiple "warts" on the footpads of young dogs.[16a] Affected dogs are 1 to 2 years of age at the onset of symptoms. They develop discrete, firm, hyperkeratotic, often hornlike lesions on multiple pads of two or more paws. In the dogs studied, lesions were not detected elsewhere. If the lesions are large or involve the weightbearing surface of the pad, lameness can occur. The lesions wax and wane in severity, and individual lesions may spontaneously resolve but new ones develop. Histologically, the lesions have the characteristics of viral papillomas; to date, however, efforts to demonstrate the virus have been unrewarding. Treatment with topical keratolytic or softening (e.g., water and petrolatum) agents removes the hyperkeratotic debris, softens the lesions, and decreases the dog's discomfort, but it does not appear to alter the course of infection. Spontaneous resolution of all lesions has not been recognized.

The second syndrome involves the development of multiple discrete and pigmented papules, plaques, or nodules. The cases recognized have occurred in young adult dogs (3 to 5 years) with no prior history of skin disease.[10, 16a, 17a] Lesions could be singular but typically were multiple from the onset, involved any skin surface, and became more numerous with time. Histologically, the lesions were sharply demarcated and characterized by surface and infundibular follicular epithelial pseudocarcinomatous hyperplasia and dysplasia. No koilocytosis or inclusion bodies were seen. Immunohistochemical staining with rabbit antibovine papillomavirus antisera (DAKO) demonstrated papillomavirus antigen.[16a, 17a] The lesions can persist unchanged for over 18 months, but singular or multiple intraepidermal carcinomas may develop.[10, 17a] No effective treatment is known.

Feline Papillomavirus Infection

Although papillomas are occasionally recognized in cats, there was no evidence for their viral induction in cats until 1990.[4a] Two aged Persian cats were described with multiple hyperkeratotic plaques.[4] The lesions were of variable size, predominately truncal in location, and hyperpigmented in one case. Histopathologic studies showed surface and follicular infundibular epithelial hyperplasia and dysplasia with koilocytosis. Intracytoplasmic inclusion bodies were seen and papillomavirus-like particles were demonstrated on electron microscopy. Immunohistochemical staining demonstrated papillomavirus antigen that had characteristics of a novel feline papillomavirus. Other cases with similar features were subsequently reported.[6, 8a] The cats were assumed to be immunocompromised.

Many cases of multicentric squamous cell carcinoma in situ have been recognized in the cat since 1990[1a, 11, 16] (see Chap. 19). The lesions from these cats also showed surface and follicular hyperplasia and dysplasia, but there was far more cellular atypia and koilocytosis was absent. Immunohistochemical staining with rabbit antibovine papillomavirus antisera has demonstrated inconsistent results, but staining has been seen in some cats.[16a] These data would suggest that the feline papillomavirus induces long-lasting dysplastic lesions that eventually become neoplastic.

Therapeutic options are limited. Surgical removal is usually impractical because of the numbers of lesions, their location, or both, and because new lesions appear after surgery. Topical treatment with 5-fluorouracil, which can be effective in humans and dogs,[16] is contraindicated in cats because of its neurotoxicity. Preliminary work suggests that beta radiation therapy (strontium-90 plesiotherapy) is an effective treatment for early lesions;[16] as with surgery, however, it does not prevent new lesions.

Neoplasia

Papovaviruses cause cutaneous and mucosal papillomas (warts) in the dog (see Chap. 19). Feline sarcoma virus produces cutaneous fibrosarcomas in young cats (see Chap. 19). FeLV and feline sarcoma virus have been associated with the development of lymphosarcoma, liposarcoma, melanoma, hemangioma, and multiple cutaneous horns in cats (see Chap. 19).

For as yet unknown reasons, postvaccination alopecia and panniculitis appear to have increased in frequency. Of greatest concern is the possible development of cutaneous neoplasms at the injection sites. Investigators have noted an increased frequency of fibrosarcomas at common sites of vaccination in cats,[19a] and rabies vaccines have been incriminated most commonly (see Chap. 19). It is unknown whether the neoplasm is induced solely by the virus or is modulated by adjuvants in the vaccines. Until further data are available, it is advisable to monitor any postvaccination reactions carefully and to perform wide surgical excision at the first sign of changing clinical appearance.

■ RICKETTSIAL DISEASES

Canine Rocky Mountain Spotted Fever

Rocky Mountain spotted fever is caused by the rickettsial agent, *Rickettsia rickettsii*, and is transmitted by ticks.[1, 25, 27–28] It is a seasonal disease in the United States, with cases occurring between April and September. Infected dogs develop fever, anorexia, lethargy, peripheral lymphadenopathy, and signs of neurologic dysfunction, which may be accompanied by erythema, petechiation, edema, and occasionally necrosis and ulceration of the oral, ocular, and genital mucous membranes and the skin of the nose, pinnae, ventrum, scrotum (see Fig. 7:1 *G*), and distal limbs and feet. Edema of the extremities is frequently seen. The epididymis of male dogs may be painful and swollen. Hematologic changes may include anemia, leukopenia, or leukocytosis and thrombocytopenia. Skin biopsy reveals necrotizing vasculitis (Fig. 7:5).

Dogs with Rocky Mountain spotted fever have a fourfold rise in serum antibody titer to *R*.

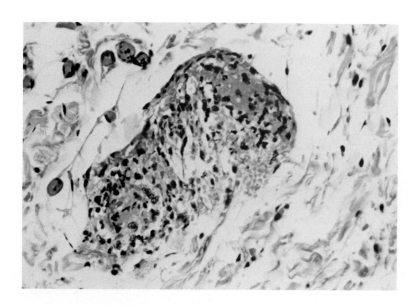

Figure 7:5. Leukocytoclastic vasculitis in a dog with Rocky Mountain spotted fever.

rickettsii. Direct immunofluorescence testing for *R. rickettsii* antigen in formalin-fixed skin biopsy specimens is often positive (antigen seen within vascular endothelium).[1]

Therapy includes tetracycline (22 mg/kg q8h orally) or chloramphenicol (20 mg/kg q8h orally) for 1 to 2 weeks and supportive care. Doxycycline (10 to 20 mg/kg q12h orally) can be effective when used for 1 week.[1, 28] The dog presents a potential public health danger when infested with *R. rickettsii*–infected ticks; there is also a danger when blood or tissues from rickettsemic dogs are handled without suitable protection.

Feline Haemobartonellosis

Feline haemobartonellosis (feline infectious anemia) is an acute or chronic disease of domestic cats characterized by fever, depression, anorexia, and macrocytic hemolytic anemia.[1] It is caused by the rickettsial agent *Haemobartonella felis.* Cutaneous hyperesthesia and alopecia areata have been reported to occur in cats with acute and chronic haemobartonellosis[26]; however, no pictures, photomicrographs, or details of any kind were provided to substantiate these cutaneous diagnoses.

■ PROTOZOAL DISEASES

Feline Toxoplasmosis

Toxoplasmosis is a multisystemic disease caused by the coccidian *Toxoplasma gondii.*[1] Toxoplasmosis has been rarely reported to cause various cutaneous lesions in humans[30] and firm nodules in the skin of the legs in cats.[38a, 42] Histopathologic findings in cats were reported to be necrotizing dermatitis and vasculitis with *Toxoplasma* (Fig. 7:6).

Canine Caryosporosis

Coccidia of the genus *Caryospora* have a complicated life cycle involving rodents, reptiles, and raptors.[1, 37] Infection occurs by ingestion of an infected host and results primarily in diarrhea. These organisms have been suspected[51, 54] or identified[37] in puppies that developed pustules, plaques, or nodules on the skin of the trunk. The tissue reaction was pyogranulomatous with eosinophils, and numerous organisms in various stages were identified in macrophages and connective tissue cells (Fig. 7:7).

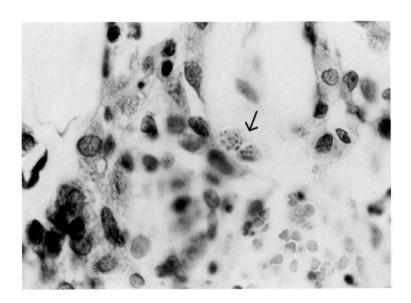

Figure 7:6. *Toxoplasma gondii* tachyzoites *(arrow)* in endothelial cells of a cat with cutaneous toxoplasmosis.

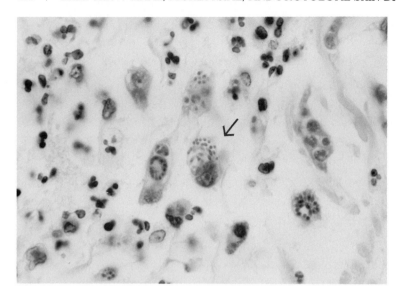

Figure 7:7. Tachyzoites *(arrow)* of *Caryospora* in pyogranulomatous dermatitis of a dog. (Courtesy J. Dubey.)

Canine Neosporosis

Neosporosis is caused by *Neospora caninum*, a newly described protozoan.[1, 35, 36, 49a] Because its tachyzoites and tissue cysts resemble those of *Toxoplasma gondii*, the organism has doubtless existed unrecognized for years. Its complete life cycle is unknown.

Dogs of any age can be infected, but clinical signs are more severe in young dogs. Neurologic and muscular signs predominate, but skin lesions were described in 1 of 23 dogs.[35] The dog had a rapidly spreading, pruritic, ulcerative dermatitis of the perineal region, eyelid, neck, and thorax. Histologically, the involved areas showed a pyogranulomatous and eosinophilic necrotizing dermatitis with severe congestion, thrombosis, and infarction. Tachyzoites were seen within macrophages, neutrophils, and, rarely, in endothelial cells.

Information on treatment is sparse, but that used for toxoplasmosis might be of benefit.

Canine Sarcocystosis

Sarcocystis organisms are widespread in nature, especially in cattle and sheep.[1] Dogs and cats become infected by ingesting tissue cysts (sarcocysts). *Sarcocystis* species are typically not pathogenic for dogs and cats, although there has been one report of a dog with chronic diarrhea who developed multiple cutaneous abscesses over the whole body and especially on the hind limbs.[38] Biopsy showed severe necrotizing, fibrinosuppurative dermatitis with numerous neutrophils and fewer eosinophils and macrophages. Vessels were congested and plugged, and numerous protozoal organisms were seen within macrophages and, occasionally, in endothelial cells of vessels.

Canine Babesiosis

Canine babesiosis is a tick-borne hematozoan disease caused by three species of *Babesia*[1]: *Babesia canis*, which is worldwide in its distribution, and *Babesia gibsoni* and *Babesia vogeli*, which are more restricted. Infection induces a parasitemia that results in varying clinical signs. Asymptomatic carriers exist.

Aside from the oral or cutaneous petechial and ecchymotic hemorrhages associated with thrombocytopenia or disseminated intravascular coagulation, skin lesions are rare. Reported lesions include ulcerative stomatitis, urticaria, angioedema, and necrosis of the distal extremities (see Fig. 7:1 *H*).[31] No histopathologic studies have been reported; therefore; it is not known whether lesions are the result of vascular insufficiency or damage from specific parasite-induced changes.

Leishmaniasis

Leishmaniasis is a serious protozoal infection caused by a variety of *Leishmania* spp.* Disease is most common in humans and dogs but can be seen in cats and other domestic animals. The disease is worldwide in distribution. In the Old World, most cases in dogs occur in the Mediterranean basin and Portugal, but reports have originated in France, Germany, Switzerland, the Netherlands, and other countries. In the New World, the disease is endemic in South and Central America; endemic foci have been reported in Texas, Oklahoma, Ohio, Michigan, and Alabama.[30a, 40] Dogs imported from endemic areas may develop the disease months or years later, so cases could be recognized anywhere. The disease is transmitted to humans and animals by bloodsucking sandflies of the genus *Lutzomyia* in the New World and *Phlebotomus* in the Old World. Domestic and wild dogs, rodents, and other wild mammals are the reservoir. Because of the occurrence of open lesions, some investigators have expressed concern regarding the possibility of direct or mechanical transmission from dog to dog or from dog to humans.[48, 52]

The incubation period varies from weeks to several years. The disease primarily affects dogs less than 5 years old. Skin lesions occur in approximately 90 per cent of dogs with visceral involvement.[1, 49] The most common finding is an exfoliative dermatitis with silvery white, asbestos-like scaling. The exfoliation can be generalized but usually is most pronounced on the head, pinnae, and extremities (see Fig. 7:1 *D*). Nasodigital hyperkeratosis may accompany the scaling, and the involved skin can be hypotrichotic to alopecic. Periocular alopecia (lunettes) is common. The next most common presentation is an ulcerative dermatitis (see Fig. 7:1 *E* and *F*). Other findings include onychogryposis, paronychia, sterile pustular dermatitis, nasal depigmentation with erosion and ulceration, and nodular dermatitis.

Systemic signs of illness are many and varied. Over 50 per cent of involved dogs show decreased endurance, weight loss, and somnolence.[1, 49] Because of the parasitemia and the host's immunologic response to the organism, physical abnormalities are varied. Generalized lymphadenopathy and hepatosplenomegaly are nearly universal findings. Other common abnormalities include muscle wasting, cachexia, intermittent fever, keratoconjunctivitis, and lameness.

Leishmaniasis is rarely reported in cats,[29, 42, 52] and they are quite resistant to experimental infection.[47] Reported cutaneous lesions include nodules or crusted ulcers on the lips, nose, eyelids, and pinnae.

The differential diagnosis includes pemphigus foliaceus, systemic lupus erythematosus, zinc-responsive dermatosis, necrolytic migratory erythema, sebaceous adenitis, and lymphoma. Laboratory findings usually include nonregenerative anemia, hyperglobulinemia, hypoalbuminemia, and proteinuria.

Tests for immune-mediated diseases (Coombs tests, antinuclear antibody, lupus erythematosus preparation, rheumatoid factor) can be positive in dogs with leishmaniasis.[30a] In one study, over 80 per cent of infected dogs had a positive antinuclear antibody titer.[49] Because many of the clinical signs of leishmaniasis overlap with those of systemic lupus erythematosus, immunodiagnostic test results must be interpreted carefully when a dog comes from an endemic area.

Demonstration of anti-Leishmania antibodies or the organism itself confirms the diagnosis. Although dogs can have positive serologic test results in the absence of clinical disease, spontaneous elimination of the parasite is rare; therefore, positive test results indicate infection.[1] However, the indirect immunofluorescence test, which is the test most commonly used, can

---

*See references 1, 39–41, 43–49, 52, and 53.

give false negative results in 10 to 20 per cent of infected dogs.[49] Amastigotes are most easily seen with Giemsa stain and are found most often in smears from lymph nodes or bone marrow (Fig. 7:8). Identification in other tissues is more difficult and often unrewarding.

Skin biopsy findings vary considerably. Orthokeratotic and parakeratotic hyperkeratosis are usually prominent; the inflammatory infiltrate typically consists of macrophages with fewer numbers of lymphocytes and plasma cells. Granulomatous perifolliculitis, interstitial dermatitis, superficial and deep perivascular dermatitis, lichenoid interface dermatitis, nodular dermatitis, lobular panniculitis, suppurative folliculitis, and intraepidermal pustular dermatitis are the nine inflammatory patterns that have been recognized in leishmaniasis; this large number reflects the clinical variability of the disease.[49] The three most common patterns are granulomatous perifolliculitis (Fig. 7:9), superficial and deep perivascular dermatitis, and interstitial dermatitis. It is common for a dog to have more than one pattern of inflammation present. In the perifollicular pattern, total obliteration of the sebaceous glands occurs in approximately 45 per cent of the cases. This sebaceous destruction no doubt contributes to the high frequency of clinical exfoliation. The *Leishmania* organisms are found intracellularly and extracellularly in approximately 50 per cent of cases. They are round to oval, 2 to 4 μm in size, and contain a round, basophilic nucleus and a small, rodlike kinetoplast (Fig. 7:10). Although visible in routine stains, Leishmania organisms are best seen when Giemsa stain is used. Immunohistochemical techniques facilitate the identification of the organism.

At this writing, canine leishmaniasis is considered an incurable disease. Relapses months to years after treatment are to be expected. These relapses are probably due to incomplete eradication of the parasite but could also represent re-infection. Accordingly, with the poor prognosis for cure and the possible reservoir status of the dog for human infection, euthanasia may be indicated.

When treatment is indicated, the most widely used treatment is meglumine antimonate (Glucantime).[1, 39, 40] Doses of 100 mg/kg are administered intravenously or subcutaneously every day for 3 to 4 weeks. In France, Glucantime is often given intravenously at 200 to 300 mg/kg every other day for 15 to 20 treatments.[7] Studies in humans and dogs have suggested that the antileishmanial activity of liposome-encapsulated meglumine antimonate is vastly superior to that of the unencapsulated drug.[32, 33] Other drugs that have been used in canine leishmaniasis include (1) sodium stibogluconate (Pentostam) administered intravenously or subcutaneously, 30 to 50 mg/kg daily for 3 to 4 weeks; (2) pentamidine (Lomidine) administered intramuscularly, 4 mg/kg every other day for at least 15 days; (3) metronidazole admin-

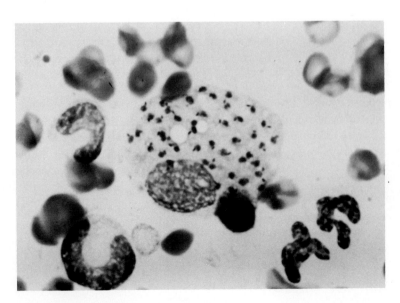

Figure 7:8. Macrophage containing numerous Leishman-Donovan bodies. (Courtesy T. French.)

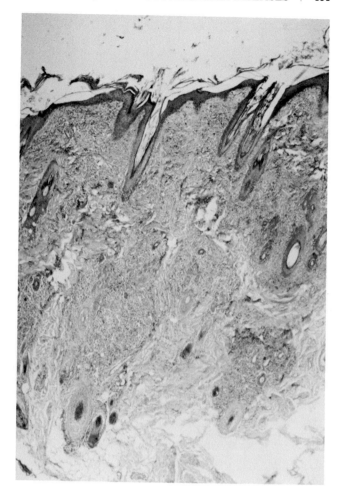

Figure 7:9. Perifollicular granulomatous dermatitis in a dog with visceral leishmaniasis.

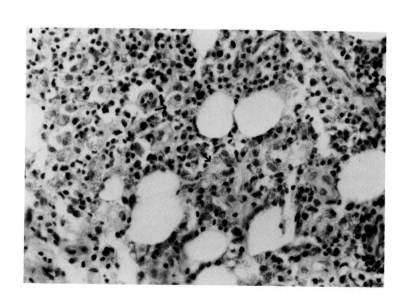

Figure 7:10. Leishman-Donovan bodies *(arrows)* in pyogranulomatous panniculitis of a dog with visceral leishmaniasis.

istered orally, 10 to 15 mg/kg q12h for 15 days; and (4) ketoconazole (Nizoral) administered orally, 15 to 30 mg/kg/day for 2 months or longer.[1, 40]

Successful treatment of feline leishmaniasis has not been reported.

In humans, many other drugs have occasionally been advocated for the treatment of leishmaniasis, including rifampicin, 8-aminoquinolines, levamisole, allopurinol, amphotericin B, and dapsone.[33, 34, 40]

REFERENCES

General Textbook Sources
1. Greene, C. E.: Infectious Diseases of the Dog and Cat. W. B. Saunders Co., Philadelphia, 1990.

Viral Diseases
1a. Baer, K. E., et al.: Feline epidermal squamous cell carcinoma *in situ*. Proc. Am. Acad. Vet. Dermatol. and Am. Coll. Vet. Dermatol., 9, 1993, p. 100.
2. Bennett, M., et al.: Feline cowpox virus infection. J. Small Anim. Pract. 31:167, 1990.
3. Bennett, M., et al: The laboratory diagnosis of orthopox virus infection in the domestic cat. J. Small Anim. Pract. 26:653, 1985.
4. Carney, H. C., et al.: Papillomavirus infection of aged Persian cats. J. Vet. Diagn. Invest. 2:294, 1990.
4a. Carpenter, J. L., et al. Cutaneous xanthogranuloma and viral papilloma on an eyelid of a cat. Vet. Dermatol. 3:187, 1992.
5. Chalmers, S., et al.: Demodicosis in two cats seropositive for feline immunodeficiency virus. J. Am. Vet. Med. Assoc. 194:256, 1989.
6. Clark, E. G., et al.: Primary viral skin disease in three cats caused by three different viruses and confirmed by immunohistochemical and/or electron microscopic techniques on formalin-fixed tissue. Proc. Am. Acad. Vet. Dermatol. and Am. Coll. Vet. Dermatol., 9, 1993, p. 56.
7. Cooper, L. M., Sabine, M.: Paw and mouth disease in a cat. Aust. Vet. J. 48:644, 1972.
8. Egberink, H. F., et al.: Isolation and identification of a poxvirus from a domestic cat and a human contact case. J. Vet. Med. B 33:237, 1986.
8a. Egberink, H. E., et al.: Papillomavirus associated skin lesions in a cat seropositive for feline immunodeficiency virus. Vet. Microbiol. 31:117, 1992.
9. Flecknell, P.A., et al.: Skin ulceration associated with herpesvirus infection in cats. Vet. Rec. 104:313, 1979.
10. Gross, T. L., et al.: Multifocal intraepidermal carcinoma in a dog histologically resembling Bowen's disease. Am. J. Dermatopathol. 8:509, 1986.
11. Gross, T. L., et al.: Veterinary Dermatopathology. Mosby–Year Book, Inc., St. Louis, p. 340, 1992.
12. Hoover, E. A., Mullins, J. I.: Feline leukemia virus infection and diseases. J. Am. Vet. Med. Assoc. 199:1287, 1991.
13. Howard, D. R.: Pseudorabies in dogs and cats. In: Kirk, R. W. (ed.). Current Veterinary Therapy IX. W. B. Saunders Co., Philadelphia, 1986, p. 1071.
14. Love, D. N., et al.: Feline calicivirus associated with pyrexia, profound anorexia, and oral and perineal ulceration in a cat. Aust. Vet. Pract. 17:136, 1987.
15. Maenhout, T., et al.: Drie Gevallen Van Koepokkeninfektie bij de Kat in Belgie. Vlaams. Diergenerskd. Tijdschr. 60:66, 1991.
16. Miller, W. H. Jr., et al.: Multicentric squamous cell carcinomas *in situ* resembling Bowen's disease in five cats. Vet. Dermatol. 3:177, 1992.
16a. Miller, W. H. Jr., Scott, D. W.: Unpublished observations, 1994.
17. Monroe, W. E.: Clinical signs associated with pseudorabies in dogs. J. Am. Vet. Med. Assoc. 195:599, 1989.
17a. Nagata, M., et al: Pigmented plaques associated with papillomavirus infections in dogs. Proc. Annu. Memb. Meet. Am. Acad. Vet. Dermatol. and Am. Coll. Vet. Dermatol. 10:14, 1994.
18. Scott, D. W.: Feline dermatology 1900–1978: A monograph. J. Am. Anim. Hosp. Assoc. 6:331, 1980.
19. Scott, D. W.: Large Animal Dermatology. W. B. Saunders Co., Philadelphia, 1988.
19a. Shanely, K. J.: Acquired nonendocrine alopecias of the dog and cat. In: Bonagura, J. D. (ed.). Kirk's Current Veterinary Therapy XII. W. B. Saunders Co., Philadelphia (in press, 1994).
20. Thomsett, L. R.: Feline poxvirus infection. In: Kirk, R. W. (ed.). Current Veterinary Therapy IX. W. B. Saunders Co., Philadelphia, 1986, p. 605.
21. Vestey, J. P., et al.: What is human catpox/cowpox infection? Int. J. Dermatol. 30:696, 1991.
22. von Bomhard, D., et al.: Zur Epidemiologie, Klink, Pathologie und Virologie der Katzen-Pocken-Infektion. Kleintierpraxis 37:219, 1992.
23. Wilkinson, G. T., et al.: Possible "orf" (contagious pustular dermatitis, contagious ecthyma of sheep) infection in the dog. Vet. Rec. 87:766, 1970.
24. Yamamoto, J. K., et al.: Epidemiologic and clinical aspects of feline immunodeficiency virus infection in cats from the continental United States and Canada and possible mode of transmission. J. Am. Vet. Med. Assoc. 194:213, 1989.

Rickettsial Diseases
25. Greene, C. E., et al.: Rocky Mountain spotted fever in dogs and its differentiation from canine ehrlichiosis. J. Am. Vet. Med. Assoc. 186:465, 1985.

26. Gretillati, S.: Feline haemobartonellosis. Feline Pract. 14:22, 1984.
27. Rutgers, C., et al.: Severe Rocky Mountain spotted fever in five dogs. J. Am. Anim. Hosp. Assoc. 21:361, 1985.
28. Weiser, I. D., et al.: Dermal necrosis associated with Rocky Mountain spotted fever in four dogs. J. Am. Vet. Med. Assoc. 195:1756, 1989.

Protozoal Diseases

29. Barnes, J. C., et al.: Diffuse cutaneous leishmaniasis in a cat. J. Am. Vet. Med. Assoc. 202:416, 1993.
30. Binazzi, M.: Profile of cutaneous toxoplasmosis. Int. J. Dermatol. 25:357, 1986.
30a. Bravo, L., et al. Canine leishmaniasis in the United States. Comp. Cont. Educ. 15:699, 1993.
31. Carlotti, D. N., et al.: Skin lesions in canine babesiosis. In: Ihrke, P. J., et al. (eds.). Advances in Veterinary Dermatology. Vol. 2. Pergamon Press, Oxford, 1993, p. 229.
32. Chapman, W. L., et al.: Antileishmanial activity of liposome-encapsulated meglumine antimonate in the dog. Am. J. Vet. Res. 45:1028, 1984.
33. Chong, H.: Oriental sore. A look at trends in and approaches to the treatment of leishmaniasis. Int. J. Dermatol. 25:615, 1986.
34. Dogra, J., et al.: Dapsone in the treatment of cutaneous leishmaniasis. Int. J. Dermatol. 25:398, 1986.
35. Dubey, J. P., et al.: Newly recognized fatal protozoan disease of dogs. J. Am. Vet. Med. Assoc. 192:1296, 1989.
36. Dubey, J. P., et al.: Neosporosis in dogs. Vet. Parasitol. 36:147, 1990.
37. Dubey, J. P., et al.: *Caryospora*-associated dermatitis in dogs. J. Parasitol. 76:552, 1990.
38. Dubey, J. P., et al.: Fatal cutaneous and visceral infection in a Rottweiler dog associated with a sarcocystis-like protozoan. J. Vet. Diagn. Invest. 3:72, 1991.
38a. Dubey, J. P., Carpenter, J. L.: Histologically confirmed clinical toxoplasmosis in cats: 100 cases (1952–1990). J. Am. Vet. Med. Assoc. 203:1556, 1993.
39. Ferrer, L.: Leishmaniasis. In: Kirk, R. W., Bonagura, J. D. (eds.). Kirk's Current Veterinary Therapy XI. W. B. Saunders Co., Philadelphia, 1992, p. 266.
40. Frank, L. A.: Leishmaniasis: In the USA too? Proc. Am. Acad. Vet. Dermatol. and Am. Coll. Vet. Dermatol., 9:51, 1993.
41. Gothe, R.: Leismaniosen des Hundes in Deutschland: Erregerfauna und Biologie, Epidemiologie, Klinik, Patho-genesis, Diagnose, Therapie und Prophylaxie. Kleintierpraxie 36:69, 1991.
42. Holzworth, J.: Diseases of the Cat: Medicine and Surgery. W. B. Saunders Co., Philadelphia, 1987.
43. Keenan, C. M., et al.: Visceral leishmaniasis in the German Shepherd dog. I. Infection, clinical disease, and clinical pathology. Vet. Pathol. 21:74, 1984.
44. Keenan, C. M., et al.: Visceral leishmaniasis in the German Shepherd dog II. Pathology. Vet. Pathol. 21:80, 1984.
45. Kerdel-Vegas, F.: American leishmaniasis. Int. J. Dermatol. 21:291, 1982.
46. Nelson, D. A., et al.: Clinical aspects of cutaneous leishmaniasis acquired in Texas. J. Am. Acad. Dermatol. 12:985, 1985.
47. Kirkpatrick, C. E., et al.: *Leishmania chagasi* and *L. donovani*: Experimental infections in domestic cats. Exp. Parasitol. 58:125, 1984.
48. Longstaffe, J. A., et al.: Leishmaniasis in imported dogs in the United Kingdom: A potential human health hazard. J. Small Anim. Pract. 24:23, 1983.
49. Koutinas, A. F., et al.: Skin lesions in canine Leishmaniasis (Kala-Azar): A clinical and histopathologic study on 22 spontaneous cases in Greece. Vet. Dermatol. 3:121, 1993.
49a. Odin, M., Dubey, J. P.: Sudden death associated with *Neospora caninum* myocarditis in a dog. J. Am. Vet. Med. Assoc. 203:831, 1993.
50. Pumarola, M., et al.: Canine leishmaniasis associated with systemic vasculitis in two dogs. J. Comp. Pathol. 105:279, 1991.
51. Sangster, L. T., et al.: Coccidia associated with cutaneous nodules in a dog. Vet. Pathol. 22:186, 1985.
52. Schawalder, P.: Leishmaniose bei Hund und Katze. Kleinter-Praxis 22:237, 1977.
53. Sellon, R.: Leishmaniasis in the United States. In: Kirk, G. W., Bonagura, J. D. (eds.). Current Veterinary Therapy XI. W. B. Saunders Co., Philadelphia, 1992, p. 271.
54. Shelton, G. C., et al.: A coccidia-like organism associated with subcutaneous granulomata in a dog. J. Am. Vet. Med. Assoc. 152:263, 1968.

Immunologic Skin Diseases

■

Chapter Outline

Because of the incredible expansion of knowledge in basic and clinical immunology, it has become difficult to keep up with new information related to clinical immunology. Even the narrower subject of immunodermatology has seen a tremendous emergence of new discoveries, findings, and laboratory techniques. An adequate review of this information is decidedly beyond the scope of this chapter. For the practitioner, student, and academician interested in details, numerous texts on immunology and immunodermatology are available.* In this section, we confine ourselves to a brief overview of new concepts regarding immunology of the skin.

The immune system and its inflammatory component are complex models of biological activity and interaction. There is a tendency to dissect the immune response into its individual components and to discuss them as autonomous functional units. Immune responses are interwoven and interdependent, however, and manipulation of one component influences others. The newer studies have shown that the skin itself is a very integral and active component of the immune system. These observations led to the hypothesis that the skin, like the gastrointestinal tract, may be a functioning lymphoid organ; as such, it has been referred to as skin-associated lymphoid tissue (SALT).[40] Even prior to the development of the SALT concept, it was suggested that the skin functions as a primary immunologic organ. The term skin immune system (SIS) has also been proposed to describe the components of the skin, excluding the regional lymph nodes, that constitute SALT.[5] In the following sections, we attempt to briefly review the specifics of the skin immune system so that the reader is familiar with the tremendous gains in knowledge and future avenues for work that will lead to further discoveries.

■ SKIN IMMUNE SYSTEM

The skin immune system (SIS) contains two major components, the cellular and humoral. The cellular component comprises keratinocytes, epidermal dendritic cells (Langerhans' cells), lymphocytes, tissue macrophages, mast cells, endothelial cells, and granulocytes. The humoral components include immunoglobulins, complement components, fibrinolysins, cytokines, eicosanoids, neuropeptides, and antimicrobial peptides. Virtually all inflammatory and some noninflammatory skin diseases involve alterations of or an interaction between one or both parts of the SIS. As a result, it becomes inappropriate to consider immunologic disease as a category if one is to include all skin diseases that involve the immune system. Therefore, this chapter presents those diseases classically described as allergic (hypersensitive) or autoimmune (primary immune-mediated).

The epidermis is often considered the producer of the effective barrier between the outside world and the body's inside environment. In this role, the epidermis acts as a mechanical barrier, because it is often the first component of the body exposed to environmental agents

*See references 4, 5, 9, 12, 13, 20, 27, 31, 37, 41, 43, 44, 51, 53, 56, 57, and 59.

such as viruses, bacteria, toxins, insects, arachnids, and allergens. The epidermis also plays an active role in the body's immunologic response to these external factors. Before the immune system can respond to these external factors, however, their presence has to be recognized. Recognition may occur at one of two levels: on the surface of the epidermis or in the dermis. If an intact epidermis is present, it would seem most likely that recognition of an environmental agent occurs in the epidermis. For many immunologic responses, including helper T cell induction, antigens must first be processed for presentation to lymphocytes. Classically, this occurs by macrophages, which express class II major histocompatibility complex (MHC) antigens, but other cells with class II MHC antigens may be involved. Because macrophages are present in the dermis and do not normally reside in the epidermis, this function is served by other cells. The epidermis contains two very important cells of the SIS that probably contribute to this function: the Langerhans' cell and keratinocyte.

Keratinocytes

Keratinocytes do much more than produce keratin, surface lipids, and intercellular substances. They play a major role in the SIS. It is now clear that keratinocytes produce a wide variety of cytokines that have important roles in mediating cutaneous immune responses, inflammation, wound healing, and the growth and development of certain neoplasms.[3] Keratinocytes, especially when perturbed by exposure to interferon gamma (IFN-γ), express MHC II antigens.[5] This expression is required for cells to be antigen-presenting cells for T cell responses. Though keratinocytes are capable of phagocytosis, their role as antigen-processing cells is controversial. The primary requisites for antigen processing, MHC II expression and phagocytosis, are present, however. Keratinocytes may also be stimulated to produce the leukocyte adhesion molecule, ICAM-1. Besides production of these immunologically important cell-surface markers, keratinocytes have been shown to be very capable producers of a variety of cytokines. They are the primary epidermal source for cytokines.[5] Probably the most immunologically important is interleukin-1 (IL-1). Keratinocytes store IL-1, which is readily released following damage to the cells. In fact, release of IL-1 from keratinocytes is essentially a primary event in skin disease.[36] Interleukin-1 stimulates further release of IL-1 from neighboring keratinocytes as well as the production and release of interleukins IL-3, IL-6, and IL-8, tumor necrosis factor alpha (TNF-α), and a variety of granulocyte-monocyte-macrophage stimulating and activating factors.[5, 33, 36, 37] Keratinocytes may also play a role in tissue repair by production of multiple growth factors. Another important role is the down-regulation of immune responses, to which keratinocytes contribute by the production of immunosuppressive mediators such as prostaglandin E_2 and transforming growth factors. Considering the diverse functions, activities, and mediators produced by keratinocytes, it has become obvious that the epidermis plays a major role in the immune response and that keratinocytes do not function only as a mechanical barrier to environmental substances.[5, 62]

Langerhans' Cells

Langerhans' cells, which appear as suprabasilar clear cells on skin sections stained routinely with hematoxylin and eosin (H & E), are the major antigen-presenting cells of the epidermis. They are bone marrow–derived monocyte/macrophage–type cells. The Langerhans' cell is characteristically identified in the epidermis by the electron-microscopic presence of Birbeck granules. These granules are often absent in the dog (see Chap. 1), however. In the dog, CD1a is considered the best marker for Langerhans' cells and has been shown to label canine epidermal dendritic cells. Langerhans' cells express class II MHC antigens as well as receptors for C3b, Fc-IgG, and Fc-IgE. The main function of Langerhans' cells is antigen-specific T cell activation.[5, 37, 41] They bind epidermal antigens and then present the antigens to the lymphoid tissues (regional lymph node), where helper T cell lymphocytes in particular are activated.

Langerhans' cells may bind some antigens, such as certain haptens, directly on their cell surface with MHC II receptors. In other situations, such as with globular proteins, the antigens may require processing, which involves phagocytosis, internalization, and intracellular proteolysis. In addition, they produce other cytokines such as IL-1.

Lymphocytes

Lymphocytes are bone marrow–derived cells that may be divided into three main types: B (bursa- or bone marrow–derived) cells, T (thymus-dependent) cells, and null cells. *B cells* are characterized by possessing surface immunoglobulins, Fc receptors, and C3b receptors. B cells differentiate into *plasma cells,* which produce the immunoglobulins IgG, IgM, IgA, and IgE, and they are responsible for antibody immunity. The growth and development of B cells occurs in two phases. The first is antigen-independent and yields B cells that express IgM and IgD. The second phase is the differentiation into Ig-secreting or memory B cells and requires a specific antigen.[37, 41] The second phase is partly controlled by cytokines released by T cells, with interleukins IL-1, IL-2, IL-4, IL-5, and IL-10 all being shown to play roles in growth or differentiation. Interleukin-4 in particular is essential for B cells to switch into IgE-producing plasma cells.[37] In human beings, B lymphocytes are rarely found in normal skin and, even in dermatologic disease, are much less common than T cells.[5] Considering the relative increase in the frequency of plasma cells in canine compared with human cutaneous disease, however, the importance of B lymphocytes in the dog may be relatively greater. Humoral immunity is described as providing primary defense against invading bacteria and neutralization activity against circulating viruses.

T cells are formed in the thymus and may be divided into two major types on the basis of the T cell receptors present. Classically, T cells are considered responsible for cell-mediated immunity. We now know, however, that certain subpopulations of T cells are involved in contact hypersensitivity, whereas others serve completely different functions. As T cells mature in the thymus, they develop surface receptor molecules, some of which are referred to by the cluster differentiation nomenclature (CD). The receptor molecules expressed on a T cell are critical in determining the future function of the cell. At least seven different CD molecules have been recognized, as well as other functionally important receptors. The major division of T cells is to classify them as helper (CD4 +) or suppressor (CD8 +) T cells. In general, helper T cells may stimulate B cell responses and other T cells, and may function in recognition of antigens presented with MHC II receptors.

More recently, two types of helper T cells have been recognized in mice and humans. These two subtypes, Th1 and Th2, differ in the cytokines and, therefore, the effects they produce; Th2 cells produce IL-4, IL-5, and IL-10, whereas Th1 cells produce IL-2, IFN-γ, and TNF-α.[5, 37, 41]

Suppressor T cells recognize antigens displayed with MHC I molecules. Typically, these cells are cytotoxic or down-regulating and suppress the B and T cell responses. Exceptions to these generalizations occur, however, and the exact function of a T cell depends on the overall presence of the many different receptor-ligand interactions that occur on its surface. T cells play a central role in directing and modifying the immune response. Functions of T cells include: (1) helping B cells make antibody (helper T cells), (2) suppressing B cell antibody production (suppressor T cells), (3) directly damaging "target" cells, (4) mediating delayed hypersensitivity reactions, (5) suppressing delayed hypersensitivity reactions mediated by other T cells, (6) modulating the inflammatory response with lymphokines, (7) inducing graft rejection, and (8) producing graft-versus-host reactions. T cell lymphokines may amplify or dampen phagocytic activity, collagen production, vascular permeability, and coagulation phenomena. T cells can kill microorganisms and other cells, or they can recruit effector cells to perform this function. T cell function is known to be suppressed by numerous infections (staphylococcal pyoderma, demodicosis, blastomycosis, canine distemper, feline leukemia virus infection, feline immunodeficiency virus infection), cancers, and drugs.[20, 40, 57]

Tissue Macrophages

The end stage of the mononuclear phagocyte system (MPS) is the tissue macrophage, which in the dermis has also been considered the precursor cell to the dermal dendrocyte.[5, 41] In lymph nodes and other tissues, there are dendritic macrophage type cells that are also believed to be part of the MPS. These cells are all bone marrow–derived and pass through the blood circulation as monocytes. These cells have a wide variety of activities and morphologically may appear differently, especially in inflammation. Tissue macrophages, epithelioid cells, and multinucleated histiocytic giant cells are all MPS cells found in a variety of inflammatory diseases. They serve the critical function of processing and presenting antigens, especially for T cell activation. The MPS also plays major roles in wound healing, granulopoiesis, erythropoiesis, and antimicrobial defense (especially against intracellular pathogens). Monocytes and macrophages may secrete numerous enzymes, cytokines, inflammatory mediators, histamine-releasing factors, and inhibitors when stimulated. Some mediators upgrade inflammation, whereas others inhibit inflammatory activity in order to prevent too much tissue destruction from inflammation.

Mast Cells

Mast cells are believed to be of monocytogenous origin.[5, 37, 40, 41] They have been recognized for many years, and their importance in immediate hypersensitivity diseases is well documented. Their role in other skin diseases, however, such as contact dermatitis and bullous pemphigoid, and in the process of fibrosis has only recently been recognized.[37] This relates to the diverse effects and interactions mast cells have with other cells and structures of the skin (Fig. 8:1). Mast cells serve as repositories for or synthesizers of numerous inflammatory mediator substances. The mediators present vary by species studied and, in some situations, according to the type and tissue location of the mast cells.[37] Some mediators are universally present, such as histamine, leukotrienes, eosinophil chemotactic factor of anaphylaxis (ECF-A), and proteolytic enzymes. There are two main categories of mediators. Preformed mediators are produced and stored in mast cell granules, which are modified lysosomes that develop from the Golgi apparatus (Table 8:1).[37] Mast cells also produce mediators that are newly synthesized at the time of activation and degranulation (Table 8:2). The major roles of mast cells probably consist of the recruitment of eosinophils and neutrophils, immunoglobulins, and complement from the circulation and the regulation of the immunologic response (Tables 8:1 and 8:2). Mast cells may be divided morphologically and functionally into type I (atypical, mucosal) and type II (typical, connective tissue) cells.[5, 37, 40, 41] *Mucosal* and *connective tissue* are misleading terms, because both types of mast cells occur in mucosa and connective tissue. This heterogeneity of mast cells has been demonstrated in dog skin.[40] The skin of atopic dogs contains at least two subsets of mast cells that are distinguished in the following ways: (1) histologically, by metachromatic staining properties in different fixatives, and (2) functionally, by response to antigen in vivo (see discussion of canine atopy).

Mast cell degranulation may be initiated by a variety of substances, including allergens cross-linking two surface IgE molecules (or IgGd), complement components C3a and C5a, eosinophil major basic protein, some hormones (estrogen, gastrin, somatostatin), substance P, and a group of cytokines referred to as histamine-releasing factors.[20, 37, 41] Other exogenous compounds known to cause mast cell degranulation include anti-IgE, compound 48/80, opiates, concanavalin A, and calcium ionophores. The different types of mast cells may be affected differently, depending on the compound that causes degranulation. Variability in degranulation, the mediators released, quantity, and time course may occur. Another secretory mechanism for

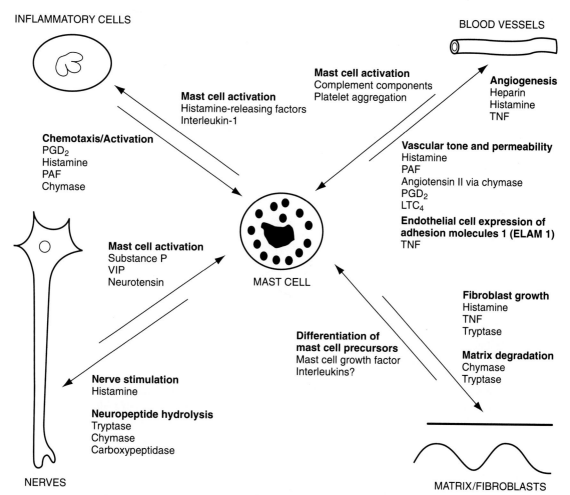

Figure 8:1. Schematic representation of the documented interactions of human mast cells with other cells and structures in skin. Factors identified in rodent species only are not shown. (From Goldstein, S.M., Wintroub, B.V.: The cellular and molecular biology of the human mast cell. In: Fitzpatrick, T.B., et al.: Dermatology in General Medicine, Vol. V, 4th ed. McGraw-Hill, New York, 1993, p. 365.)

Table 8:1. Preformed Mediators of Human Mast Cells

Mediator	Functions
Histamine	H_1 and H_2 receptor-mediated effects on smooth muscle, endothelial cells, and nerve endings
Tryptase	Cleaves C3 and C3a
	Degrades VIP and CGRP kallikrein-like activity
	Activates fibroblasts
Chymases	Function unclear
	Cleave neuropeptides, including substance P
Carboxypeptidase	Acts in concert with other neutral proteases
Acid hydrolases	Break down complex carbohydrates
Arylsulfatase	Hydrolyses aromatic sulfate esters
ECF-A	Eosinophil chemotaxis and ''activation''
Neutrophil chemotactic factor	Neutrophil chemotaxis and ''activation''
Heparin	Anticoagulant, anticomplementary
	Modifies activities of other preformed mediators
Chondroitin sulfate	Function unknown
Cytokines (eg, TNF-α, IL-4, IL-3, IL-5, and IL-6)	See Table 8:6

Table 8:2. Pharmacologic Activities of Newly Generated Mast Cell Mediators

Mediator	Abbreviation	Pharmacologic Actions
Prostaglandin D_2	PGD_2	Bronchoconstriction; peripheral vasodilation; coronary and pulmonary vasoconstriction; inhibition of platelet aggregation; neutrophil chemoattraction; augmentation of basophil histamine release
Prostaglandin F_2	9-α, 11-β- PGF_2	Bronchoconstriction; peripheral vasodilation; coronary vasoconstriction; inhibition of platelet aggregation
Thromboxane A_2	TXA_2	Vasoconstriction; platelet aggregation; bronchoconstriction
Leukotriene B_4	LTB_4	Neutrophil chemotaxis, adherence and degranulation; augmentation of vascular permeability
Leukotriene C_4	LTC_4	Bronchoconstriction; increase in vascular permeability; arteriolar constriction
Leukotriene D_4	LTD_4	Bronchoconstriction; increase in vascular permeability
Leukotriene E_4	LTE_4	Weak bronchoconstriction; enhancement of bronchial responsiveness; increase in vascular permeability
Platelet-activating factor	PAF	Platelet aggregation; chemotaxis and degranulation of eosinophils and neutrophils; increase in vascular permeability; bronchoconstriction; engenders hypotension

histamine release has been described.[37] It has been referred to as piecemeal secretion and transfer to the cell surface by microvesicles.

Interestingly, histamine has two types of effects on hypersensitivity reactions, pro-inflammatory and anti-inflammatory. The pro-inflammatory effects of histamine (see Table 8:1) are mediated through histamine$_1$ (H_1) receptors and resultant decreases in intracellular cyclic adenosine monophosphate (cAMP). Also, H_1 receptors mediate pruritus, and the trauma associated with pruritus may lead to further tissue and keratinocyte damage. The anti-inflammatory effects of histamine (inhibition of the release of inflammatory mediator substances from mast cells, neutrophils, lymphocytes, and monocyte-macrophages) are mediated through H_2 receptors and resultant increases in cAMP. Canine and feline blood vessels have been reported to possess both H_1 and H_2 receptors.[40]

Endothelial Cells

The vascular endothelium is now known to be a very active cell type that is important in inflammation, immune responses, and tissue repair.[11, 37, 41, 52] In response to various cytokines, endothelial cells express adhesion molecules (integrin, selectin, and immunoglobulin gene families) on their surfaces. These molecules allow for the homing of the activated lymphocytes, monocytes, and granulocytes into the site of inflammation. Without this ability to home, the circulating effector cells could not respond to an immunologic or inflammatory event. In addition, activated endothelial cells can synthesize and secrete numerous substances such as cytokines (including IL-1, IL-6, and IL-8), fibronectin, collagen IV, proteoglycans, blood clotting factors, growth factors, and granulocyte-macrophage colony-stimulating factor (CSF). Defects in endothelial cell adhesion molecule expression may result in disorders that mimic immunodeficiencies owing to defective migration of lymphocytes, monocytes, or granulocytes (see Chap. 4).

Granulocytes

Neutrophils have, as their major roles, the function of phagocytosis and subsequent destruction and elimination of phagocytized material. In a sense, they are the scavengers of immunologically identified debris. They are considered most important in containing infection. Owing, however, to their numerous chemoattractants (Table 8:3) and intracellular products (Table 8:4),

Table 8:3. Chemoattractants for Neutrophils

Bacterial products	Lipid chemotactic factors (HETE, etc.) from
C5a (derived from complement activation; tissue, virus, and	mast cells
bacterial enzymes cleave C5)	Lysosomal proteases
C3a	Collagen breakdown products
C567	Fibrin breakdown products
Kallikrein	Plasminogen activator
Denatured protein	Prostaglandins
Lymphokines	Leukotrienes (especially LTB_4)
Monokines	Immune complexes
Neutrophil chemotactic factor (NCF) from mast cells	
ECF-A from mast cells	

neutrophils are omnipresent participants in most immune and virtually all inflammatory reactions.[20, 37, 41, 55]

Neutrophil dysfunctions have been described in dogs with pyoderma and generalized demodicosis (see Chap. 4), but are likely secondary to the skin disease. In addition, primary (hereditary) neutrophil dysfunctions are described (see Chap. 4).

Eosinophils, effector cells in hypersensitivity reactions, also participate in the downgrading of inflammation and defense of the host against extracellular parasites.[5, 37, 41] They are also phagocytic (immune complexes, mast cell granules, aggregated immunoglobulins, and certain bacteria and fungi). Though, in the past, numerous eosinophil chemoattractants have been described, their true role has been questioned, and other, previously unrecognized factors (LTB_4) may have been responsible.[35, 37, 41] Eosinophils are noteworthy for their preformed mediators stored within the eosinophilic granules but like other inflammatory cells, they also newly synthesize leukotrienes and a variety of cytokines when activated (Table 8:5).

Major basic protein (also found in basophils), eosinophil cationic protein, and eosinophil peroxidase are potent toxic mediators. Additionally, eosinophil degranulation results in the production of membrane-derived mediators such as leukotrienes and platelet-activating factor.

Basophils and mast cells are the major effector cells in hypersensitivity reactions. In skin diseases, basophils are particularly important in cutaneous basophil hypersensitivity, a T cell–controlled reaction important in host responses to various ectoparasites. Basophils are some-

Table 8:4. Neutrophil Products

ANTIMICROBIAL ENZYMES	HYDROLASES
Lysozyme	Cathepsin B
Myeloperoxidase	Cathepsin D
	N-Acetyl-β-
PROTEASES	glucosaminidase
Collagenolytic proteinase	β-Glucuronidase
Collagenase	β-Glycerophosphatase
Elastase	
Cathepsin G	OTHERS
Leukotrienes	Lactoferrin
Gelatinase	Eosinophil chemotactic
	factor
	Leukotrienes
	Pyrogen
	Prostaglandins
	Thromboxanes
	Platelet-activating factor

Table 8:5. Granule-Associated Eosinophil Products and Their Functions

Product	Function
Lysophospholipase	Formation of crystalline structure
Major basic protein	Helminthotoxin; cytotoxin; neutralizes heparin; bactericidal
Eosinophil cationic protein	Neutralization of heparin; decrease in coagulation time; alters fibrinolysis; helminthotoxin; neurotoxin
Eosinophil-derived neurotoxin	Neurotoxin
Eosinophil peroxidase	Inactivation of leukotrienes; oxidative killing of microorganisms and parasites; stimulation of mast cell secretion
Collagenase	Denaturing of type I and type III collagen
Arylsulfatase B	Inactivates leukotrienes

what similar to mast cells, in that they have high-affinity receptors for IgE and contain high levels of histamine.

Humoral Components

The humoral components as described in the SIS include immunoglobulins, complement components, fibrinolysins, cytokines, eicosanoids, neuropeptides, and antimicrobial peptides. The changes observed in inflammation are mediated, however, by numerous substances derived from the plasma, from cells of the damaged tissue, and from infiltrating monocytes, macrophages, lymphocytes, and granulocytes. The interactions among cells, neurons, expression of cell receptors, cytokines, and other soluble mediators determine the inflammatory response. Some mediators augment inflammation, and others suppress it. Some mediators antagonize or destroy other mediators, and others amplify or generate other mediators. All mediators and cells normally act together in a harmonious fashion to maintain homeostasis and to protect the host against infectious agents and other noxious substances. Many mediators may be preformed and stored with the effector cells; others mediators are produced only in response to damage or appropriate receptor activation. A complete summary of all inflammatory mediator substances is beyond the scope of this chapter; the interested reader is referred to the various references cited on the first page of the chapter.

COMPLEMENT SYSTEM

Complement is a group of plasma and cell membrane proteins that induce and influence immunologic and inflammatory events.[20, 37, 41, 57] The critical step in the generation of biological activities from the complement proteins is the cleavage of C3. There are two pathways for the cleavage of C3. The classic pathway requires the presence of immunoglobulin and immune complexes. The alternative (properdin) pathway does not require immunoglobulin and may be directly activated by bacteria, viruses, and some abnormal cells. There is also a pathway to amplify C3 cleavage, and an effector sequence. The final effect of this sequence is the production of a membrane attack complex, which causes cell lysis. As the effector sequence progresses, a variety of complement components are formed that have other effects. These other components play a role in neutralization of viruses, solubilization of immune complexes, and interaction with receptors on other cells. Many inflammatory cells have receptors for degradation products of C3 and C5. These activated receptors are important in phagocytosis, immune regulation, and mast cell and basophil degranulation. Hemolytic complement levels in dogs are reported to be decreased with enteropathies, hepatopathies, systemic lupus erythematosus, and systemic glucocorticoid therapy.[20, 40, 61] A genetically determined (autosomal recessive) deficiency of C3 has been reported in Brittany spaniels that have recurrent bacterial skin infections and sepsis (see Chap. 4).

IMMUNE COMPLEXES

Immune complexes are a heterogeneous group of immunoreactants formed by the noncovalent union of antigen and antibody.[5, 10, 20, 37, 40, 41] Many factors influence the formation, immunochemistry, biology, and clearance of these reactants. Circulating immune complexes influence both the afferent and efferent limbs of the immune response and can mediate tissue damage in certain pathologic states. Circulating immune complexes can be measured by a number of generally unavailable techniques, including C1q-binding, solid-phase C1q, conglutinin, and Raji cell assays. Circulating immune complexes have been detected in numerous human dermatoses and probably play an important role in the pathogenesis of systemic lupus erythematosus and vasculitis. Circulating immune complexes have been demonstrated in 6 per cent of a normal dog population, in contrast to 25 per cent of a population of sick dogs,[40] as well as in numerous conditions such as diabetes mellitus, hypothyroidism, arthropathies, nephropathies, neuropathies, mycotic and parasitic infections, systemic and discoid lupus erythematosus, cutaneous vasculitis, generalized demodicosis, and bacterial pyoderma.[10, 40]

CYTOKINES

A variety of cells, including all the cells of the SIS, synthesize and secrete low-molecular-weight glycoprotein, hormone-like molecules now referred to as *cytokines.* Cytokines are transiently produced and exert their biological activities via specific cell-surface receptors of target cells, which may be expressed only after activation of the cell.[5, 21, 37, 41, 62] Each mediator usually has multiple overlapping activities. Cytokines are substances that were found to regulate the growth and differentiation of cells of the immune or hematopoietic system. Initially, they were discovered in association with lymphocytes and termed *lymphokines,* which is no longer as appropriate. Cytokines were also formerly called *monokines, secretory regulins,* and *peptide regulatory factors.*

Numerous cytokines have been described, and typically, they may perform several different functions, depending on the tissue they interact with and what other cytokines are present.[5, 37, 41] These other cytokines may affect the same cell in a permissive, inhibitor, additive or suppressive manner. In any case, cytokines play a key role in inducing and modulating inflammatory reactions, especially in cell-mediated immune reactions and delayed-type hypersensitivity reactions (Table 8:6).

EICOSANOIDS

The metabolites of the oxidation of arachidonic acid are potent biological mediators or modulators termed *eicosanoids.*[5, 13, 37, 41] The eicosanoids include two main types of molecules, the prostanoids and leukotrienes. Prostanoids (prostaglandins and thromboxanes) are derived by the metabolism of arachidonic acid by cyclooxygenase. Leukotrienes and their precursors—hydroperoxyeicosatetraenoic acids (HPETEs) and hydroxyeicosatetraenoic acids (HETEs)—are derived by the metabolism of arachidonic acid by the three enzymes of lipoxygenation, 5-, 12-, and 15-lipoxygenase.

Arachidonic acid is normally found as a constituent of cell membranes and is released following specific receptor stimulation and membrane dissolution after cellular injury. Its release is produced by the action of phospholipases, especially phospholipase A, with the free arachidonic acid being immediately metabolized. Glucocorticoids inhibit the action of phospholipases, possibly by the induction of lipocortin, at pharmacologically achieved levels. This is thought to be a major anti-inflammatory mechanism of glucocorticoid therapy. The effects of arachidonic acid formation are quite variable according to the species, tissue, and cellular source, the presence of stereospecific receptors, and the generation of secondary mediators.[37, 54] Different tissues express variable levels of the cytosolic lipoxygenases. The 5-lipoxygenase

Table 8:6. Immunologic Properties of Cytokines

Cytokine	Properties
INTERLEUKINS	
IL-1	Immunoaugmentation (promotes IL-2, IFN-γ, CSF production by T cells); promotes B cell activation (promotes IL-4, IL-5, IL-6, IL-7 production); stimulates macrophages and fibroblasts
IL-2	Activates T and natural killer (NK) cells; promotes cell growth and immunoglobulin production
IL-3	Promotes growth of early myeloprogenitor cells, eosinophils, mast cells, and basophils
IL-4	Promotes B cell activation and IgE switch; promotes T cell growth; synergistic with IL-3 for mast cell growth
IL-5	Eosinophil growth; B cell growth; T cell growth
IL-6	Terminal differentiation factor for cells and polyclonal immunoglobulin production; enhances IL-4–induced IgE production; promotes T cell proliferation and cytotoxicity; promotes NK cell activity
IL-7	Lymphoprotein
IL-8	Chemoattractant for neutrophils, T lymphocytes, basophils; increases histamine release from basophils
IL-9	Maturation of erythroid progenitor cell tumor growth; synergistic with IL-3 for mast cell growth
IL-10	Thymocyte proliferation; cytotoxic T lymphocyte differentiation; B cell growth and differentiation
IL-11	Megakaryocyte and plasma cell growth
IL-12	Cytotoxic lymphocyte maturation
COLONY-STIMULATING FACTORS	
Granulocyte CSF	Neutrophil growth
Monocyte CSF	Monocyte growth
Granulocyte-monocyte CSF	Monomyelocytic growth
INTERFERONS	
IFN-α	Antiviral; antiproliferative; immunomodulating (activation of macrophages; proliferation of B cells; stimulation of NK cells); inhibit fibroblasts
IFN-β	Antiviral; antiproliferative; immunomodulating (activation of macrophages; proliferation of B cells; stimulation of NK cells); inhibit fibroblasts
IFN-γ	Immunomodulating (activation of macrophages; proliferation of B cells; stimulation of NK cells); antiproliferative; antiviral; inhibit fibroblasts
TUMOR NECROSIS FACTORS	
TNF-α	Inflammatory, immunoenhancing, and tumoricidal
TNF-β	Inflammatory, immunoenhancing, and tumoricidal
TNF-$\beta_{1,2,3}$	Fibroplasia and immunosuppression

pathway predominates in neutrophils, monocytes, macrophages, and mast cells, whereas the 15-lipoxygenase pathway predominates in eosinophils and in endothelial and epithelial cells. Typically, eicosanoids have autocrine and paracrine functions that are important locally for host defense, and then they are inactivated or degraded. Abnormalities in production or control mechanisms may occur, however, leading to local or systemic tissue damage and disease.

The actions of eicosanoids are quite diverse. The understanding of how they function in disease is further complicated by the complex interactions that occur but that are not included in many laboratory studies. Table 8:7 summarizes some of the activities that eicosanoids may have in skin disease.[5, 37, 41]

Phospholipase A activity also results in the production of platelet-activating factor (PAF) when it removes arachidonic acid from cell membranes. PAF is not an eicosanoid but a phospholipid that also acts as an inflammatory mediator. It is produced from a variety of cells, although in humans, neutrophils and eosinophils produce the largest amounts.[5, 37, 41] Platelet-

Table 8:7. Effects of Eicosanoids in Skin Disease

Eicosanoid	Effect
$LTC_4/D_4/E_4$	Vascular dilation and increased permeability
LTB_4	Leukocyte chemotaxis and activation; increased endothelial adherence of leukocytes; stimulates keratinocyte proliferation; enhances NK cell activity; hyperalgesia
12-HETE	Stimulates smooth muscle contraction
15-HETE	Hyperalgesia; inhibits cyclooxygenase; inhibits mixed lymphocyte reaction; stimulates suppressor T cells; inhibits NK cell activity
15-HPETE	Suppresses T lymphocyte function and Fc receptors
PGE_2	Plasma exudation; hyperalgesia; stimulates cell proliferation; suppresses lymphocyte and neutrophil function
PGF_2	Vasoconstriction; synergy with histamine and bradykinin on vascular permeability; stimulates cell proliferation
PGD_2	Smooth muscle relaxation
PGD_2/PGI_2	Suppression of leukocyte function; vasodilation and increased permeability

activating factor primes cells to have augmented responses to other stimuli and has its greatest effects on eosinophils and monocytes. It is an extremely potent eosinophilic chemoattractant and stimulates their degranulation and release of leukotrienes. A chemoattractant for mononuclear cells, PAF stimulates their release of IL-1, IL-4, and TNF-α.

Adhesion Molecules

Glycoproteins critical for cell-to-cell contact and communication, adhesion molecules play an integral role in cutaneous inflammation and immunology.[21, 60, 62] The *integrin family* includes membrane glycoproteins with α and β subunits, such as vascular cell adhesion molecule–1 (VCAM-1) on endothelial cells, which binds T lymphocytes and monocytes via vascular leukocyte adherin–4 (VLA-4), and fibronectin and laminin, which bind keratinocytes and mast cells. The *immunoglobulin gene superfamily* contains intercellular adhesion molecule–1 (ICAM-1), found on keratinocytes, Langerhans' cells, and endothelial cells, which binds leukocytes via leukocyte function–associated antigen–1 (LFA-1) or CD11a/CD18. The *selectin family* includes lectin adhesion molecule–1 (LECAM-1 or L-selectin) on lymphocytes, which binds endothelial leukocyte adhesion molecule–1 (ELAM-1 or E-selectin), and Gmp-140 (P-selectin) as a "homing" mechanism.

■ TYPES OF HYPERSENSITIVE REACTIONS

Clinical hypersensitivity disorders were divided on an immunopathologic basis, by Gell and Coombs, into four types:[5, 20, 31, 57]

> Type I: immediate (anaphylactic)
> Type II: cytotoxic
> Type III: immune complex
> Type IV: cell mediated (delayed)

Subsequently, two other types of hypersensitivity reactions have been described: late-phase reactions and cutaneous basophil hypersensitivity. Clearly, these six reactions are oversimplified because of the complex interrelationships that exist among the effector cells and the numerous components of the inflammatory response. In most pathologic events, immunologically initiated responses almost certainly involve multiple components of the inflammatory process. In reality, many diseases may involve a combination of reactions, and their separation into distinct pathologic mechanisms rarely occurs. For example, IgE (classically involved in type I hypersensitivity reactions) and Langerhans' cells (classically involved in type IV hypersensitivity reactions) may interact in a previously unrecognized fashion in the development of human atopic dermatitis. Even the classic type IV reaction is not as straightforward as we used to think, as evidence suggests that mast cells and eosinophils may play a role.

Realization that this scheme has become a simplistic approach to immunopathology has provoked other investigators to modify the original scheme of Gell and Coombs, often to a seemingly hopeless degree of hairsplitting.[40] In this section, we briefly examine the classic Gell and Coombs classification of hypersensitivity disorders, because (1) it is still somewhat applicable to discussions of cutaneous hypersensitivity diseases and (2) it is still the immunopathologic scheme used by most authors and by major immunologic and dermatologic texts.

Type I (anaphylactic, immediate) hypersensitivity reactions are classically described as those involving genetic predilection, reaginic antibody (IgE) production, and mast cell degranulation. A genetically programmed individual absorbing a complete antigen (e.g., ragweed pollen) responds by producing a unique antibody (reagin, IgE). IgE is homocytotropic and avidly binds membrane receptors on tissue mast cells and blood basophils. When the eliciting antigen comes in contact with the specific reaginic antibody, a number of inflammatory mediator substances are released and cause tissue damage. This reaction occurs within minutes and gradually disappears within an hour. It is important to note that older terms such as *reaginic antibody, homocytotropic antibody,* or *skin-sensitizing antibody* are *not* strictly synonymous with *IgE,* because subclasses of IgG may also mediate type I hypersensitivity reactions. The classic examples of diseases that involve type I hypersensitivity reactions in dogs and cats are urticaria, angioedema, anaphylaxis, atopy, food hypersensitivity, flea bite hypersensitivity, and some drug eruptions.

Late-phase immediate hypersensitivity reactions (LPRs) have been recognized and studied.[5, 20, 37, 41, 54] The onset of these mast cell–dependent reactions occurs 4 to 8 hours after challenge (neutrophils and eosinophils found histologically). They persist up to 24 hours, in contrast to classic type I reactions, which abate within 60 minutes. The initial reaction is histologically characterized by an infiltrate of neutrophils and eosinophils, which changes to a predominance of mononuclear cells. These late-phase reactions can be reproduced with intradermal injections of leukotrienes, kallikrein, or platelet-activating factor (PAF). Although LPRs to the intradermal injection of allergens have been recorded in dogs,[54] the clinical importance of late-phase reactions remains to be defined in dogs and cats. These reactions, however, are suspected to play a role in flea bite hypersensitivity.

Type II (cytotoxic) hypersensitivity reactions are characterized by the binding of antibody (IgG or IgM), with or without complement, to complete antigens on body tissues. This binding of antibody, with or without complement, results in cytotoxicity or cytolysis. Examples of type II hypersensitivity reactions in dogs and cats are pemphigus, pemphigoid, cold agglutinin disease, and some drug eruptions.

Type III (immune complex) hypersensitivity reactions are characterized by the deposition of circulating antigen-antibody complexes (in slight antigen excess) in blood vessel walls. These immune complexes (usually containing IgG or IgM) then fix complement, which attracts neutrophils. Proteolytic and hydrolytic enzymes released from the infiltrating neutrophils produce tissue damage. Type I hypersensitivity reactions and histamine release may be important in the initiation of immune complex deposition. Examples of type III hypersensitivity reactions in dogs and cats are systemic lupus erythematosus, leukocytoclastic vasculitis, some drug eruptions, and bacterial hypersensitivity.

Type IV (cell-mediated, delayed) hypersensitivity reactions classically do not involve antibody-mediated injury. An antigen (classically, an incomplete antigen referred to as a *hapten*) interacts with an antigen-presenting cell (APC). In the skin, the APC is the Langerhans' cell. The APC usually internalizes the antigen and digests it, then presents a peptide fragment bound to MHC class II immune response antigens on the cell surface. The processed antigen is then presented to T cells, leading to the production of "sensitized" T lymphocytes. These sensitized

T lymphocytes respond to further antigenic challenge by releasing lymphokines that produce tissue damage. In mouse models, there is evidence that the development of type IV hypersensitivity may involve mast cells and, in some situations, small amounts of IgE.[37] It has been suggested that the term *cell-mediated* is an unfortunate misnomer for this type of immunologic reaction, which is no more or less cell mediated than antibody-dependent reactions, which themselves are ultimately due to the participation of a lymphocyte or plasma cell.[40] Classic examples of type IV hypersensitivity reactions in dogs and cats are contact hypersensitivity, flea bite hypersensitivity, and some drug eruptions.

Cutaneous basophil hypersensitivity (CBH) may be mediated by T cells or homocytotropic antibody (IgE or IgG). It is characterized by a marked basophil infiltrate and fibrin deposition. These reactions occur about 12 hours after intradermal allergen injections and may peak in intensity from 24 to 72 hours.[5, 37, 41] CBH is considered important in the development of immunity to ticks and in the pathogenesis of flea bite hypersensitivity.[20]

Type I, type II, and type III hypersensitivity reactions together form the ''immediate'' hypersensitivity reactions. They are all antibody-mediated; thus, there is only a short delay (from minutes to a few hours) before their tissue-damaging effects become apparent. Type IV hypersensitivity is the ''delayed'' hypersensitivity reaction. It is *not* antibody mediated, and it classically requires 24 to 72 hours before becoming detectable. This concept has also been further evaluated so that type III, type IV, CBH, and late-phase reactions are all regarded as having delayed in time manifestations varying from 4 to 48 hours.[37]

■ SPECIALIZED TESTS FOR IMMUNOLOGIC DISEASES

Combining the sciences of genetics, molecular biology, and immunology has led to the development of vast numbers of immunologic tests and methodologies. A multitude of tests and assays are available at the research level, but the veterinary practitioner, by practicality, is still quite limited. The various tests used clinically are described with the disease(s) they are most commonly used for.

■ HYPERSENSITIVITY DISORDERS

Urticaria and Angioedema

Urticaria (hives) and angioedema are variably pruritic, edematous skin disorders, that are immunologic or nonimmunologic in nature. They are uncommon in the dog and rare in the cat.

Cause and Pathogenesis

Urticaria and angioedema result from mast cell or basophil degranulation. They may result from many stimuli, both immunologic and nonimmunologic.[13, 37, 40, 65] Immunologic mechanisms include type I and III hypersensitivity reactions. Nonimmunologic factors that may precipitate or intensify urticaria and angioedema include physical forces (pressure, sunlight, heat, exercise), psychologic stresses, genetic abnormalities, and various drugs and chemicals (aspirin, narcotics, foods, food additives). Atopic humans have a higher incidence of urticaria and angioedema, but no such predilection has been reported in dogs and cats. Factors reported to have caused urticaria and angioedema in dogs and cats are listed in Table 8:8.[40, 44, 65]

Clinical Features

No age, breed, or sex predilections have been reported for urticaria and angioedema in dogs and cats. Clinical signs may be acute (most common) or chronic. In humans, acute urticaria and angioedema are empirically defined as episodes lasting less than 6 weeks, whereas chronic

Table 8:8. Factors Reported to Have Caused Urticaria and Angioedema in Dogs and Cats

Foods
Drugs (penicillin, ampicillin, tetracycline, vitamin K, propylthiouracil, amitraz, doxorubicin, radiocontrast agents)
Antisera, bacterins, and vaccines (panleukopenia, leptospirosis, distemper-hepatitis, rabies, feline leukemia)
Stinging and biting insects (bee, hornet, mosquito, black fly, spider, ant)
Allergenic extracts*
Blood transfusions
Plants (nettle, buttercup)
Intestinal parasites (ascarids, hookworms, tapeworms)
Infections (staphylococcal pyoderma, canine distemper)*
Sunlight*
Excessive heat or cold*
Estrus*
Dermatographism*
Atopy*
Psychogenic factors*

*Reported in dogs only.

episodes last longer. Urticarial reactions are characterized by localized or generalized wheals, which may or may not be pruritic and usually do not exhibit serum leakage or hemorrhage (Figs. 8:2 and 8:3). Characteristically, the wheals are evanescent lesions, with each lesion persisting less than 24 hours. Urticarial lesions may occasionally assume bizarre patterns (serpiginous, linear, arciform, annular, papular). Hair may appear raised in these areas. Angioedematous reactions are characterized by localized or generalized large, edematous swellings, which may or may not be pruritic and exhibit serum leakage or hemorrhage (Fig. 8:4).

Diagnosis

The differential diagnosis for urticaria includes folliculitis, vasculitis, erythema multiforme, lymphoreticular neoplasia, and mast cell tumor. Staphylococcal folliculitis often manifests as slightly raised tufts of hair (tufted papules) and is the most common cause of misdiagnosed ''urticaria'' in dogs with short haircoats. Juvenile cellulitis, infectious cellulitis, mast cell tumor, and lymphoreticular neoplasia are the most common considerations in the differential diagnosis for angioedema. Definitive diagnosis is based on history, physical examination, and pursuit of the etiologic factors listed in Table 8:8. A specific etiologic diagnosis can usually be made in acute cases, but chronic urticaria and angioedema are extremely frustrating diagnostic challenges, with 75 to 80 per cent of such cases in human patients defying specific etiologic diagnosis.

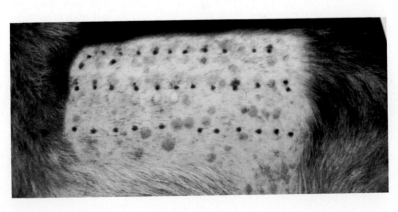

Figure 8:2. Numerous wheals in a dog with urticaria that occurred following clipping, marking with ink, and giving intradermal injections of allergens.

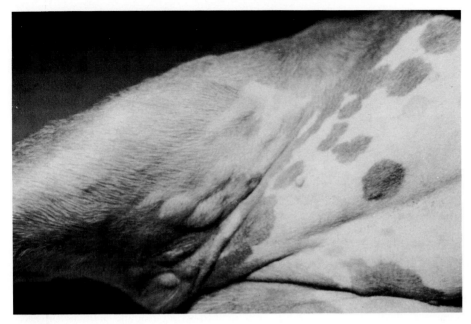

Figure 8:3. Urticaria in groin following amitraz dip.

■ *Histopathology.* Skin biopsy shows a variable, nondiagnostic pattern, from simple vascular dilatation and edema in the superficial and middle dermis to pure superficial perivascular to interstitial dermatitis with varying numbers of mononuclear cells, neutrophils, mast cells, and eosinophils (uncommon).[17, 63] Leukocytoclastic vasculitis is rarely seen. Direct immunofluorescence testing of urticarial lesions in humans is usually negative but occasionally reveals immunoglobulin, complement, or both in blood vessel walls (especially when the histologic reaction is vasculitis).

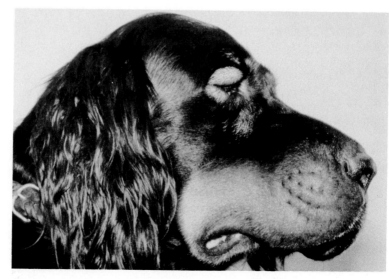

Figure 8:4. Angioedema due to phenamidine administration. Note swollen lips and eyelids. (Courtesy D. N. Carlotti)

Clinical Management

The prognosis for urticarial reactions is favorable, because general health is not usually affected. The prognosis for angioedema varies with severity and location. Angioedematous reactions involving the nasal passages, pharynx, and larynx may be fatal.

Therapy consists of (1) elimination and avoidance of known etiologic factors and (2) treatment of symptoms with epinephrine (epinephrine 1:1000 at 0.1 to 0.5 ml subcutaneously or intramuscularly) or glucocorticoids (prednisolone or prednisone at 2 mg/kg, given orally, intramuscularly, or intravenously), or both. Antihistamines have not been adequately evaluated for efficacy in treating chronic urticaria. They are ineffective for the treatment of acute reactions but may be useful for the prevention of future reactions or in the management of chronic cases. Some cases of chronic urticaria in dogs respond quite well to antihistamine therapy, although several agents may have to be tried to find the one that works best for a given patient (see Chap. 3).

Canine Atopy

Atopy (atopic disease, allergic inhalant dermatitis) is a genetically programmed disease of dogs in which the patient becomes sensitized to environmental antigens that in nonatopic animals create no disease. Additionally, *atopy* has been defined as an reaginic antibody-mediated disease.[19] Though allergen-specific IgE has been classically associated with the disease, a large body of literature also supports the importance of allergen-specific IgG.[43, 96, 132, 165–167]

Cause and Pathogenesis

Strong breed predilections, familial involvement, and limited breeding trials have demonstrated that canine atopy is genetically programmed.[20, 40, 44, 142] The exact mode of inheritance is unknown, and a pilot study failed to demonstrate any clear-cut relationship between dog leukocyte-antigen typing and canine atopy.[40] In addition to genetics, other factors may be important in the development of clinical atopy. One study has shown an association between the month of birth and the incidence of canine atopy.[155] Dogs studied that were born during the onset of pollen seasons more commonly developed atopy than control dogs. This finding would suggest that dogs may be particularly susceptible to primary sensitization during the first 4 months of life. Birth during nonpollen seasons would tend to disfavor the development of sensitization, whereas birth during pollen seasons would tend to increase the incidence of sensitization. Parasitic diseases may augment the production of IgE to other environmental allergens.[19] Viral infections, or at least vaccination with modified live viral vaccines, have been shown to augment production of IgE specific for environmental allergens.[16, 98, 99] It is important to note, however, that most of these dogs do not develop clinical signs while housed in a laboratory environment (OL Frick, personal communication, 1991). At least in humans, the amount of allergen exposure and size of allergen may also contribute to the development of atopy as well as the type of symptoms manifested.[149]

Canine atopy has been classified as a type I hypersensitivity reaction. Genetically predisposed dogs absorb percutaneously, inhale, and possibly ingest various allergens that provoke allergen-specific IgE or IgG production. In the United States, it has been traditional to espouse the primary importance of allergen-specific IgE.[19, 20, 40, 44] The European view, however, is that allergen-specific IgG (IgGd subclass) is key[43] and that allergen-specific IgE cannot even be detected in many atopic dogs and normal dogs experimentally sensitized to allergens.[43, 165, 166]

IgE (and IgGd) fixes to tissue mast cells, especially in the skin, the primary target organ of canine atopy. When mast cell–fixed IgE reacts with its specific allergen or allergens, mast cell degranulation and release or production of many pharmacologically active compounds ensue. Canine IgE is (1) not precipitated in the presence of antigen, (2) inactivated at 56°C, (3) not complement fixing, (4) antigenically similar to human IgE, and (5) capable of passively transferring atopic sensitivities to normal dogs by Prausnitz-Küstner (P-K) testing.[20, 40, 44] Atopic dogs are also known to develop late-phase reactions (at 6 hours) to intradermally injected allergens,[74] although the clinical or therapeutical significance of these reactions is unknown.

The exact role of IgE in the pathogenesis of atopy remains unclear. The following observations can be made in human atopy: (1) 20 per cent of the patients have normal or low serum IgE levels; (2) atopy has been recognized in patients with agammaglobulinemia; and (3) abnormally increased serum IgE levels generally do not fluctuate consistently during exacerbations, remissions, or treatment.[13, 37] Additionally, in neither humans nor dogs does the positive skin test result that detects the presence of allergen-specific IgE or IgGd produce the type of skin lesion seen with the clinical disease. In fact, many dogs are not even pruritic at the skin test site. Work in human atopic dermatitis has revealed a much more complex pathogenesis. A more complex pathogenesis is likely to be involved in the dog as well.

In humans, the genetic abnormality in atopic dermatitis appears to be an immunologic skin dysfunction that may be altered by bone marrow transplantation.[91] Abnormalities of the SIS in atopic humans include: (1) endothelial cells that abnormally express adhesion molecules, (2) an increase in T cells that are predominantly T helper cells, particularly the Th2 subclass, (3) hyperstimulatory epidermal Langerhans' cells and increased dermal Langerhans' cells, (4) B cell overproduction of IgE, (5) IgE on Langerhans' cells, and (6) increased dermal levels of eosinophil-derived major basic and cationic proteins without obvious tissue eosinophils.* It is obvious that the pathogenesis is much more complex than genetically programmed alterations in IgE production.

In dogs, there also are other interesting findings. Some investigators were unable to detect allergen-specific IgE in the serum of dogs with naturally occurring atopy or in dogs experimentally sensitized to dinitrochlorophenol and *Toxocara canis* eggs.[165, 166] Willemse and associates,[165, 166] however, demonstrated a reaginic antibody, confirmed by passive cutaneous anaphylaxis (PCA) and P-K testing, in the IgGd subclass. Unfortunately, determining that the results became negative following IgG absorption, which would have proved that the reaginic antibody was an IgG, was not done. Total IgE levels are not elevated in atopic dogs.[19, 20, 106, 124] Even allergen-specific IgE, as measured by commercial laboratories, may not be elevated in atopic dogs.[89] This finding, however, was in contrast to the research laboratory findings of Halliwell,[19, 20] which showed that allergen-specific IgE is associated with atopic disease. These findings would suggest that (1) immunoglobulins other than the classic IgE may be involved in the pathogenesis of atopy or (2) elevated IgE and IgGd levels are simply an epiphenomenon, a coincident feature of disordered cell regulation in atopy, rather than an essential pathogenic factor.[5, 37, 40, 43, 44, 167] Serum IgA levels may be low in atopic dogs.[81, 106] The significance of this is unknown, though the lowering of local immune responses or an increase in antigen absorption and presentation could potentially result.

The advent of in vitro tests that measure serum allergen-specific IgE levels has offered another tool to assess IgE production. These tests have shown in a number of studies that normal dogs also produce allergen-specific IgE and that the titers do not correlate with clinical disease. These observations in dogs and other work in humans have led to the hypothesis that heterogeneity of IgE may exist, with only one or some select types being involved in atopic disease.[5, 19, 37, 78] In this hypothesis, two basic types of IgE would exist: IgE− and IgE+. Individuals with serum and tissue-bound IgE− would have minimal or no skin disease, whereas those with IgE+ would have atopic skin disease. Another possibility is that the sensitivity to IgE and the ability of target cells to degranulate may constitute the underlying abnormality in atopic disease.

A newer concept also questions the initial site of immunologic stimulation. In human atopic patients, IgE has been found on epidermal Langerhans' cells.[37, 41, 78, 118, 119] This finding has

---

*See references 5, 37, 41, 76, 78, 91, and 109.

raised the question whether immune dysfunction occurs following percutaneous absorption of allergen and its processing by abnormal Langerhans' cells as the initial step in the induction and development of atopic disease.[118, 119] These allergen-processing Langerhans' cells then normally migrate to regional lymph nodes, where they stimulate a helper T cell response. In humans with atopic dermatitis, however, Langerhans' cells may be able to stimulate T cells locally. This ability could lead, in the atopic patient, to an exaggerated T lymphocyte response. Special stains of skin samples from humans with atopic dermatitis have revealed that lesional skin contains increased numbers of activated helper T cells of the subclass Th2.[118, 119] These helper T cells may preferentially induce IgE-producing B cells by themselves producing IL-4, IL-5, and IL-10.[37, 41, 118, 119] These interleukins stimulate mast cell and eosinophil activation and proliferation. Though eosinophils are not seen in lesional skin from human atopic dermatitis patients, the presence of eosinophil major basic and cationic proteins indicates that eosinophils were present.[5, 37, 41, 108]

In humans, similar changes to naturally occurring lesions can be induced at allergen patch test sites in patients with atopic dermatitis but not normal patients or patients with rhinitis or asthma.[13, 37] The patch test–induced lesions produced are also grossly similar to naturally occurring atopic dermatitis lesions, in contrast to intradermal test reactions. These observations imply that percutaneous absorption is important and that the pathogenesis involves helper T cells and eosinophils. Similar patch test studies have not been done in the dog. Intradermal test reactions do not, however, mimic the clinical lesions seen in the atopic dog, and in many cases, they are not pruritic, suggesting that intradermally deposited antigen does not reproduce the natural disease. In addition, the predominance of skin lesions in canine atopy occurring in contact areas would support the importance of percutaneous penetration of allergen.[16, 19, 20] Therefore, the percutaneous absorption of antigen may better explain the clinical disease, and future studies in dogs may yield a new understanding of the pathogenesis of canine atopy.

A summary of current thought as to the possible pathogenesis of atopic skin disease might go as follows:

Percutaneously absorbed allergens (allergen penetration probably enhanced by inherent defect of epidermal barrier function) encounter allergen-specific IgE on Langerhans' cells, whereupon the allergens are trapped, processed, and presented to allergen-specific T lymphocytes. There is a subsequent preferential expansion of allergen-specific Th2 cells, which produce IL-3, IL-4, IL-5, IL-6, and IL-10. The imbalance in allergen-specific Th2 cells (with a resultant increase in IL-4–stimulated production of allergen-specific IgE) and allergen-specific Th1 cells (with a resultant decrease in interferon alpha inhibition of allergen-specific IgE production) culminates in enhanced production of allergen-specific IgE by B lymphocytes.[22, 76, 78, 79, 138, 151]

An older theory focused on β-adrenergic blockade as the underlying abnormality of atopy.[40, 44] Though it is not accepted as the major pathologic abnormality, it may play a role in the pathogenesis. Szentivanyi proposed the β-adrenergic theory of atopic disease in 1968.[40] He suggested that the heightened sensitivity of atopic human beings to various pharmacologic agents could be due to a blockage of β-adrenergic receptors in the tissues. Since that time, there has been an explosion of investigative effort in the field of the cyclic nucleotides.[5, 37, 40, 41] In brief, the cyclic nucleotides cyclic adenosine monophosphate (cAMP) and cyclic guanosine monophosphate (cGMP) appear to serve as the intracellular effectors of a variety of cellular events. They are viewed as exerting opposing influences in a number of systems.

A number of pharmacologic agents are known to act via various cell receptors to influence intracellular levels of cAMP and cGMP. In general, substances that elevate intracellular cAMP levels (β-adrenergic drugs, prostaglandin E, methylxanthines, histamine, and other mediator substances) or reduce intracellular cGMP levels (anticholinergic drugs) tend to stabilize the cells (lymphocytes, monocyte-macrophages, neutrophils, mast cells) and inhibit the release of various inflammatory mediators. On the other hand, substances that reduce cAMP levels (α-adrenergic drugs) or elevate cGMP levels (cholinergic drugs, ascorbic acid, estrogen, levamisole) tend to labilize the cells and promote the release of inflammatory mediators. Further studies in the area of cyclic nucleotides and biological regulation may produce significant advances in the areas of disease pathomechanism and control of immunologic inflammation.

Studies in a Basenji-Greyhound model of atopy have revealed the following findings: (1) airway hypersensitivity to methacholine, citric acid, and leukotrienes, (2) elevated blood histamine and leukotriene levels after antigen challenge, (3) blunted cAMP response to β-adrenergic agents, (4) adenylate cyclase activities and β-adrenergic receptor numbers and affinities similar to those in normal dogs, and (5) elevated levels of phosphodiesterase.[40, 44, 85, 86] These studies suggest that the blunted cAMP responses in atopic dogs are due to increased phosphodiesterase activity, rather than to defects in the β-adrenergic receptor–adenylate cyclase system.

Katz introduced the concept of *allergic breakthrough*.[20, 40, 44] Normally, according to this concept, IgE antibody production is maintained at a low magnitude following sensitization because of the existence of a normal suppressive or ''damping'' mechanism that exists specifically to limit the quantity of IgE antibodies produced during any particular response. If any one of a number of possible perturbations (respiratory viral infections, endoparasites, hormonal fluctuations) disturbs this damping mechanism in such a way as to diminish the overall damping capabilities to a sufficiently low level, and if, when the damping threshold is lowered, the individual becomes exposed to sufficient levels of allergen, sensitization resulting in allergic breakthrough occurs. This may explain why some atopic dogs have a temporary worsening of their disease following their annual vaccinations.

Atopic dogs are known to be prone to secondary bacterial pyoderma and, possibly, *Malassezia* infections. A variety of abnormalities are present in atopic dogs that may explain these infections. Atopic dog corneocytes have greater adherence for *Staphylococcus intermedius*.[113a] Intradermal injection of histamine causes increased percutaneous penetration of staphylococcal antigens in normal dogs, suggesting that the inflamed skin of atopic dogs would also be more accessible to staphylococcal antigens and, perhaps, staphylococcal pyoderma.[113] Cell-mediated immunity is also depressed.[122] A similar situation occurs in human atopic dermatitis patients. It has been shown that, however, in dogs, many of these abnormalities are the result of the allergic reaction and not a primary abnormality.[120–123] Atopic humans often have exaggerated responses to patch or intradermal testing with *Malassezia* antigens, and flares of their dermatitis may respond to antiyeast therapy.[138] A similar phenomenon is likely to occur in atopic dogs.

The average serum histamine concentration in atopic dogs was reported to be equal to that of normal dogs (15.3 ± 7.75 ng/ml)[124] or *lower* (1.46 ng/ml) than that of normal dogs (3.66 ng/ml).[137] The average response of the serum histamine concentration of atopic dogs to nasal aerosols of antigens that had given positive results on intradermal skin testing was 0.98 ng/ml (before antigenic exposure) to 2.70 ng/ml (10 to 20 minutes after exposure).[137] Nasal exposure to antigens that did *not* give positive reactions on intradermal skin testing resulted in average values of 0.76 ng/ml pre-exposure and 1.48 ng/ml postexposure.[137] Cutaneous histamine concentrations were always greater in atopic dogs than in normal dogs but did not correlate with plasma histamine concentrations.[124]

Atopic dogs have lower levels of plasma triglycerides than normal dogs after being fed corn oil.[153] It is unknown whether this finding represents impaired fat absorption or increased plasma clearance.

Clinical Features

Atopy is universally recognized and, in areas with fleas, is the second most common hypersensitivity skin disorder of dogs, probably affecting around 10 per cent of the canine population.*

Certain breeds are known to have a predilection for canine atopy, including Chinese Shar Peis, Cairn terriers, West Highland White terriers, Scottish terriers, Lhasa apsos, Shih tzus,

---

*See references 19, 32, 40, 43, 44, 83, 84, 125, 143, and 144.

wirehaired fox terriers, Dalmatians, Pugs, Irish setters, Boston terriers, golden retrievers, boxers, English setters, Labrador retrievers, miniature Schnauzers, Belgian Tervurens, and Beaucerons.[40, 43, 44, 83, 125, 143, 144] Canine atopy is reportedly seen more commonly in females than in males, though some studies show no sex predilections.

The age of onset of clinical signs in atopic dogs varies from 6 months to 7 years, with about 70 per cent of the dogs first manifesting clinical signs between 1 and 3 years of age. An exception to this general rule would be the Shar Pei breed, wherein the signs of atopy may begin as early as 3 months of age. Other cases, and certain breeds (Akita, Golden retriever) may occasionally be seen that develop signs prior to 6 months of age. This may partly reflect the environment (allergen load) that the puppies are raised in and is more commonly seen when both parents are atopic.[16, 44] Clinical signs may initially be seasonal or nonseasonal, depending on the allergens involved. About 80 per cent of all atopic dogs eventually have nonseasonal clinical signs.[16, 40, 43, 44, 143] About 80 per cent of the atopic dogs initially manifest clinical signs in the period from spring to fall, and about 20 per cent begin in winter.[44, 143]

The initial lesion is pruritus of areas with either no visible lesion or slightly erythematous macules. An exception to the rule is the atopic English bulldog, which often presents with erythema, edema, and other secondary skin lesions but little or no history of pruritus. The presence of a primary papular rash should suggest another or coexistent disease. The skin lesions seen in atopic dogs are usually those associated with self-trauma, secondary bacterial pyoderma, and secondary seborrheic skin disease.[16, 40, 43, 44, 143] The self-trauma, chronic inflammation, and secondary bacterial pyoderma or *Malassezia* dermatitis may result in complete or partial alopecia, salivary staining, papules, pustules, circular crusted papules, hyperpigmentation, and lichenification (Fig. 8:5 *A*). In general, the presence of lichenified, crusty, or greasy plaques is associated with secondary bacterial pyoderma or *Malassezia* dermatitis (Fig. 8:5 *B*). Pruritus usually involves the face (Fig. 8:5 *C*), paws (Fig. 8:5 *D* and *E*), distal extremities, anterior elbows, and ventrum, or some combination thereof (Fig. 8:5 *F* and *G*). Generalized cutaneous involvement may eventually be present in about 40 per cent of the dogs. Atopic otitis externa (Fig. 8:5 *H*) and conjunctivitis may be present in about 50 per cent of the dogs.[16, 40, 43, 44, 143] Secondary bacterial pyoderma (folliculitis, furunculosis), pyotraumatic dermatitis, or acral lick dermatitis may be present in as many as 68 per cent of atopic dogs.[16, 40, 43, 44, 144] Marked seborrhea is seen in 12 per cent of atopic dogs.[16, 40, 144] Close inspection reveals, however, that most atopic dogs have mild scaling in most pruritic areas. The haircoat is often dryer in these areas as well, though in some dog breeds (especially German shepherd, Chinese Shar Pei, Lhasa apso, Shih tzu), it may be greasy.[16] Hyperhidrosis may be present in 10 to 20 per cent of atopic dogs.[40, 44, 143] Seborrheic skin disease, hyperhidrosis, secondary bacterial infections, and secondary *Malassezia* infections may all contribute to the objectionable odor of atopic dogs.

Some atopic dogs have a seasonally recurrent pruritic bacterial folliculitis or furunculosis. Antibiotic therapy resolves the skin lesions and the pruritus. Whether these atopic dogs are truly nonpruritic and asymptomatic without their infections, or whether their owners tolerate or ignore low levels of licking, chewing, and scratching (perhaps believing them to be normal for their dogs), is unclear. In any case, these dogs are skin test positive, and successful hyposensitization or anti-inflammatory drug therapy prevents recurrence of the bacterial skin disease.

Noncutaneous clinical signs reported to occur occasionally in atopic dogs include rhinitis, asthma, cataracts, urinary and gastrointestinal disorders, and hormonal hypersensitivity.[16, 40, 43, 44, 143] Atopic female dogs may exhibit irregular estrus cycles, low conception rates, and high

---

Figure 8:5. Canine atopy. *A*, Marked inflammation and secondary bacterial infection of ventrum. *B*, Secondary bacterial pyoderma or *Malassezia* dermatitis is usually present in these ventral thoracic and abdominal lichenified lesions. *C*, Severe periocular excoriation and secondary bacterial infection. *D*, Paw licking results in rust-colored digital hairs. *E*, Severe pedal excoriation and secondary bacterial infection. *F*, Erythema, edema, and alopecia involving muzzle and perioral, periocular, and pinnal areas is a commonly seen pattern. *G*, Classic presentation of face, axillae, and paws. *H*, Pinnal erythema with secondary accumulations of excessive cerumen.

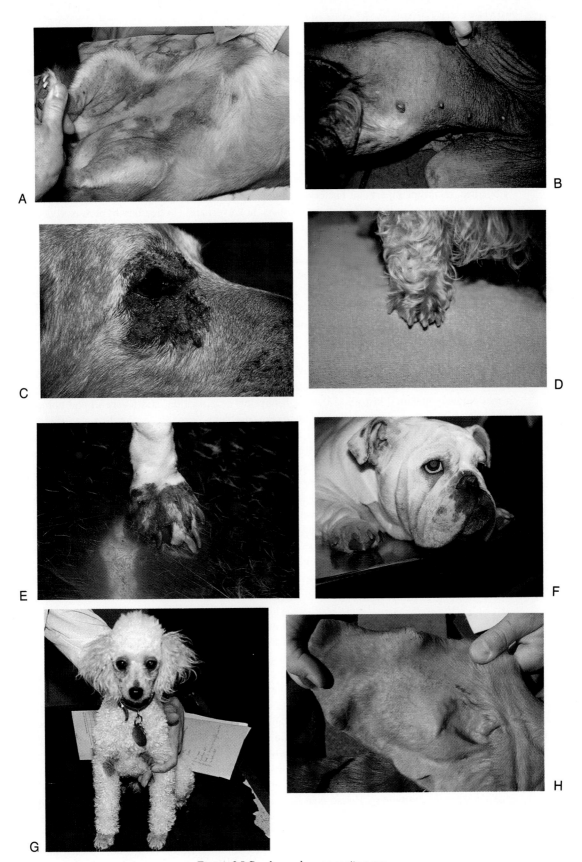

Figure 8:5 See legend on opposite page

incidence of pseudopregnancy.[40, 44] It has not been determined what proportion of the secondary infections, cases of seborrhea, and noncutaneous signs are induced or influenced by previous therapies used.

Diagnosis

The differential diagnosis is lengthy, considering the wide variation of presenting signs and secondary complications that may occur—for example, pruritic facial dermatitis, pruritic podo-dermatitis, pruritic otitis externa, pruritic ventral dermatitis, pruritic generalized dermatitis, seborrhea, recurrent superficial bacterial pyoderma, and *Malassezia* dermatitis. The more common considerations in the differential diagnosis, however, are: (1) flea bite hypersensitivity, (2) food hypersensitivity, (3) scabies, (4) insect hypersensitivity, (5) contact dermatitis (primary irritant or hypersensitivity), (6) intestinal parasite hypersensitivity, (7) bacterial folliculitis, and (8) *Malassezia* dermatitis. In dogs under 12 months of age, endoparasitic hypersensitivity, insect hypersensitivity, scabies, and food hypersensitivity are the major possibilities to pursue. Flea bite hypersensitivity only rarely causes facial dermatitis, conjunctivitis, or otitis externa, but many atopic dogs (as many as 75 per cent) have concurrent flea bite hypersensitivity.[20, 40, 43, 44, 82] Therefore, when these other cutaneous reaction patterns are present in a flea-hypersensitive dog, atopy may also be present and is most rapidly ruled out by intradermal skin testing. In addition, atopic dogs may have concurrent food hypersensitivity.[82, 228]

The diagnosis is based on history, physical examination, ruling out other possible diagnoses, and intradermal testing. It cannot be overemphasized that allergy tests are *never* a substitute for a meticulously gathered history, a thorough physical examination, and a careful and complete elimination of other diagnoses and concurrent problems. Owing to the low specificity of commercial in vitro tests, they should not be used to make a diagnosis of atopic disease.[16] Peripheral and tissue eosinophilias are rare in atopic dogs, unless the dogs have concurrent ectoparasitisms, insect hypersensitivities, or endoparasitisms.[40, 44]

A tentative diagnosis of canine atopy can be made on the basis of history, clinical signs, and laboratory tests to rule out other possibilities. A definitive diagnosis of atopy and revelation of the allergens involved may be made with intradermal (skin) testing and, to some extent, in vitro (serologic) allergy tests. The intradermal test is thought to be superior to the scratch, prick, and in vitro allergy tests.[40, 43, 44, 71] Because of the very common occurrence of ''false-positive'' (clinically insignificant) reactions obtained, in vitro allergy testing should not be used alone to diagnose atopy, but it may be helpful in determining which allergens to include in a hyposensitization formula.

■ *Intradermal Allergy Testing.* A limited number of studies have been conducted to document optimum intradermal testing procedures. Unfortunately, different commercial allergen sources were sometimes used, making comparisons impossible, and the studies have not directly compared different commercial sources of allergens. Studies with aqueous allergens made by Greer Laboratories have shown that, for most allergens, 0.05 ml of 1000 protein nitrogen units (PNU) per ml is not reactive in most normal dogs and cats. Exceptions are mold mix 2, which probably should not be used, and house dust. If house dust is used, it should be used at 125 PNU/ml or less. House dust mite is currently preferred by many authors.[43] House dust is a heterogenous mixture of animal and human danders, molds, house dust mites, insect debris, bacteria, food particles, breakdown products of clothing, and inorganic substances, and each lot can vary in its antigenicity and irritability.[158, 159] House dust mites are thought to be the major allergenic component. House dust has been used for years to test and hyposensitize dogs and cats,[40, 44] however, and a 1991 study showed that the reactivities of house dust and house dust mite allergens in atopic dogs were very comparable.[159] This same study indicated that there was a strong positive correlation between reactions to house dust mite and flea antigen but not between house dust and kapok or mixed feathers. Other allergens that have given controversial results are cattle hair, wool, feathers, tobacco, and cat dander as causes of false-positive (irritant) skin test reactions.[16, 40, 43, 44] Cattle hair, wool, feathers, and mold mixes should be used at 250 to 500 PNU/ml. In general, the recommended aqueous test allergen concentration is 1000 PNU/ml or 1:1000 weight/volume (w/v).

■ *Allergen Selection.* Skin test allergen selection is an important subject. Consultations with allergen firms and national pollen charts reviewing prevalence of pollens in the practice area help the clinician decide what to test for. It is important to select allergens from a reputable allergen supply house and then not to switch, because experience with one source becomes important. Tremendous unresolved problems surround the standardization of allergenic extracts, including standards for raw material collection, methods of measuring the purity of raw materials, techniques for identifying many substances, a variety of methods of manufacturing, and determination of allergen stability and potency.[16, 40, 43, 44] Bioactivity of commercial products varies from 10-fold to 1000-fold, and no relationship was found between bioactivity and concentrations declared in PNU or w/v.[43, 44]

Testing with allergen *mixes* is not recommended.[16, 40, 43, 44] Such mixes frequently result in false-negative reactions because individual allergens within the mix may be in a concentration too dilute for detection. More important, the patient may be allergic to only one of the allergens within the mix, making hyposensitization based on the mix result less specific. In fact, one most likely ends up hyposensitizing with allergens that the pet is not allergic to and, potentially, inducing new allergies. One report has indicated, however, that treating normal dogs with irrelevant antigens administered according to a common hyposensitization protocol induced neither skin test positivity nor clinical signs of allergy.[88] Skin testing with commercial ''regional'' allergen kits that use mixes is unsatisfactory. Instead, discussions with the supply house regarding the most important allergens for the practice area may be the most appropriate way to perform cost-effective and accurate tests for the client's budget.

Allergens commonly reported to be important in dogs are house dust mites, house dust, human dander, feathers, kapok, molds, weeds, grasses, and trees.* In the United States, most animals are multisensitive,[40, 44, 140, 143] but polysensitization is reportedly rare in Europe.[43, 130] In fact, European dogs are often sensitive only to house dust mite, and even when other allergens give positive reactions, hyposensitization is frequently undertaken using only house dust mite and re-evaluated in 1 year.[43, 130] The most important allergens in Europe are reported to be house dust, house dust mite, and human dander.[43, 82, 125, 126] *Acarus siro* (a storage mite found in poorly dried and stored cereals) antigen has been reported to cause positive skin test reactions in 75 per cent of the atopic dogs tested.[157] In addition, other insect antigens (moth, black fly, housefly, deer fly, mosquito, black ant) have been reported to cause positive reactions in many atopic dogs as well as in atopic suspects that were skin test negative to all other commonly tested allergens.[16, 168, 258, 259] One case of canine atopy was related to marijuana exposure.[93]

It is essential to remember that a positive skin test reaction means *only* that the patient has skin-sensitizing antibody, mast cells that degranulate on antigen exposure, and target tissue that responds to the released mediators. A positive reaction does not necessarily mean that the patient has clinical allergy to the allergen(s) injected. Thus, it is essential that positive skin test reactions be interpreted in light of the patient's history. By the same token, a negative skin test reaction does not necessarily mean that the patient is not atopic. Ten to 30 per cent of the otherwise classically atopic dogs may have negative skin test reactions.[16, 40, 43, 44] This group probably reflects either failure (by limiting the number of test allergens used) to challenge dogs with the appropriate allergens or the intervention of various factors known to produce false-negative reactions, as listed in Table 8:9.

Many factors may lead to false-positive or false-negative skin test reactions in dogs (see Tables 8:9 and 8:10).[40, 43, 44] These factors must be carefully considered when skin testing is

---

*See references 16, 40, 43, 44, 82, 126, 140, and 143.

Table 8:9. Reasons for False-Negative Intradermal Skin Test Reactions

Subcutaneous injections
Too little allergen:
    Testing with mixes
    Outdated allergens
    Allergens too dilute (1000 PNU/ml recommended)
    Too small volume of allergen injected
Drug interference:
    Glucocorticoids
    Antihistamines
    Tranquilizers
    Progestational compounds
    Any drugs that lower blood pressure significantly
Anergy (testing during peak of hypersensitivity reaction)
Inherent host factors
    Estrus, pseudopregnancy
    Severe stress (systemic diseases, fright, struggling)
Endoparasitism or ectoparasitism? (''blocking'' of mast cells with antiparasitic IgE?)
Off-season testing (testing more than 1 to 2 months after clinical signs have disappeared)
Histamine ''hyporeactivity''

performed. False-positive reactions to house dust mite have been reported in 60 per cent of dogs with scabies.[130] The most common cause of negative skin test reactions is the recent administration of certain drugs: glucocorticoids, antihistamines, progestagens. There are no reliable withdrawal times for these drugs. Guidelines have been arbitrarily determined by clinicians, with rare studies conducted to confirm them. One study that evaluated hydroxyzine therapy inhibition of intradermal test results for flea allergen demonstrated suppression up to 10 days.[72] Even this study has to be interpreted carefully, because some authorities believe that different allergens may be more easily suppressed and that flea antigen in particular is less inhibited by drugs.[247] General rules of thumb for drug withdrawal times prior to skin testing are: 3 weeks for oral and topical glucocorticoids, 8 weeks for injectable glucocorticoids, 10 days for antihistamines, and 10 days for products containing omega-3/omega-6 fatty acids.

Studies of intradermal test reactions in normal dogs have generally yielded the following findings: (1) no breed differences, (2) either no age differences or decreased reactivity with increasing age, (3) either no sex differences or increased reactivity of females to some allergens, (4) decreased reactivity to some allergens with increasing haircoat pigmentation, (5) decreased reactivity to histamine in hospitalized dogs compared with normal household dogs (stress related?), (6) weekly intradermal injections of allergens resulting in multiple positive reactions to allergens that originally tested negative (usually after weekly injections for 8 weeks), and

Table 8:10. Reasons for False-Positive Intradermal Skin Test Reactions

Irritant test allergens (especially those containing glycerin; also some house dust, feather, wool, mold, and all food preparations)
Contaminated test allergens (bacteria, fungi)
Skin-sensitizing antibody only (prior clinical or present subclinical sensitivity)*
Poor technique (traumatic placement of needle; dull or burred needle; too large a volume injected; air injected)
Substances that cause nonimmunologic histamine release (narcotics)
''Irritable'' skin (large reactions seen to all injected substances, including saline control)
Dermatographism
Mitogenic allergen

*These reactions would be more appropriately termed ''clinically insignificant.''

(7) previous treatment with allergens not inducing positive reactions.[40, 43, 44, 69, 70, 88, 141] Although many commercial skin test antigens contain measurable amounts of histamine, the quantity is not sufficient to cause false-positive skin test reactions.[128]

Clearly, intradermal testing is not a procedure to be taken lightly. It requires keen attention to details and possible pitfalls, together with experience and lots of practice. Intradermal testing is, however, the preferred method of diagnosing canine atopy and determining appropriate immunotherapy.[16, 40, 44, 84, 89, 94, 115, 133] Clinicians who cannot conduct skin tests on dogs on a weekly or biweekly basis will probably be unhappy with the results. In experienced hands, however, the intradermal test is a powerful tool in the diagnosis and management of canine atopy. When possible, cases should be referred to clinicians who specialize in this subject.

■ *Procedure for Intradermal Allergy Testing*

A commonly used procedure for intradermal testing is as follows:
1. Make sure the patient at least reacts to histamine. One-twentieth (0.05) ml of 1:100,000 histamine phosphate is injected intradermally. A wheal 10 to 20 mm in diameter should be present at 15 to 30 minutes after injection. If the histamine wheal is small (less than 10 mm) to absent, postpone intradermal skin testing, and test the animal with histamine on a weekly basis until the expected reaction is seen. *A positive reaction does not invariably indicate that testing will be unaffected by previous drugs.* Rarely, cutaneous reactivity to histamine returns prior to cutaneous reactivity to allergen.
2. Chemical restraint is helpful and may decrease the endogenous release of glucocorticoids. One study has indicated that intradermal skin testing performed in nonsedated dogs provoked hypercortisolemia, which was inhibited by prior sedation.[97] The hypercortisolemia produced in nonsedated dogs did not change intradermal skin test reactions, however. The combination of xylazine hydrochloride (Rompun, 0.25 to 0.5 mg/kg IV) and atropine sulfate is usually satisfactory for skin testing and is probably the most common form of chemical restraint employed.[40, 69, 73] Other acceptable chemical restraint protocols include: thiamylal (17.5 mg/kg IV) with or without maintenance with halothane, isoflurane, or methoxyflurane; and tiletamine-zolazepam (4 mg/kg IV).[73, 86, 87, 117] Place the animal in lateral recumbency for testing.
3. The skin over the lateral thorax is the preferred test site. Because different areas of skin vary in responsiveness, the site used should be consistent from patient to patient. Gently clip the hair with a No. 40 blade, using *no* chemical preparation to clean the test site. Use a felt-tipped pen to mark each injection site. Place injection sites at least 1.5 cm apart, avoiding dermatitic areas.
4. Using a 26- to 27-gauge, ⅜-inch (0.9 cm) needle attached to a 1-ml disposable syringe, carefully inject, intradermally, 0.05 ml of saline or diluent control (negative control) and 0.05 ml of 1:100,000 histamine phosphate (positive control) and all the appropriately mixed test allergens. Skin testing–strength antigens should have been made fresh from concentrate within 12 weeks of use. Read the test sites at 15 and 30 minutes. Prevent the animal from traumatizing the test area.
5. By convention, a 2-plus (2+) or greater reaction is considered to be potentially significant and must be carefully correlated with the patient's history. With experience, positive reactions may be "guesstimated" by visual inspection. It is strongly recommended, however, that the novice *measure* the diameter of each wheal in millimeters. A positive skin test reaction may then be objectively defined as a wheal having a diameter that is equal to or larger than that halfway between the diameters of the wheals produced by the saline and histamine controls. In addition to the objective assessment of size, a subjective assessment of erythema and turgidity of the wheals is also utilized in determining a positive reaction. The size of positive skin test reactions does *not* necessarily correlate with their clinical importance. Late-phase immediate reactions (6 hours) and delayed skin test site reactions (24 to 48 hours after injection) are occasionally seen and are of

unknown significance. Pruritus at some positive reaction sites occasionally occurs and can be managed with cold compresses or topical steroids. Systemic reactions (anaphylaxis) to intradermal skin testing are extremely rare in dogs.

■ *In Vitro Testing*

■ *Serologic Allergy Tests.* The radioallergosorbent test (RAST), enzyme-linked immunosorbent assay (ELISA), and liquid-phase immunoenzymatic assay are three tests that detect relative levels of allergen-specific IgE in the serum. The RAST and ELISA attach the allergens to be tested to a solid substrate such as a paper disk or polystyrene well. The liquid-phase immunoenzymatic assay does not use a solid phase initially but mixes a labeled allergen with the patient's serum. The combined labeled allergen-antibody complex is subsequently bound by the label to the plastic well. This method in humans has been shown to decrease the incidence of false-positive results due to background, nonspecific IgE.[16] In general, these tests are not to be used alone for the diagnosis of atopy.[16, 84, 89, 115]

Total serum IgE levels are very much higher in dogs than in human beings, with the mean level in normal dogs reported to be about 190 μg/ml, which is similar to that found in atopic dogs.[19, 20, 40, 44, 124] The highest serum IgE levels are found in dogs with endoparasitism. It has also been shown in the dog that the higher levels of total IgE contribute to an increased incidence of false-positive or irrelevant serologic reactions.[16, 102, 112]

Serologic allergy tests have numerous advantages over intradermal testing, including: (1) no patient risk (no need to sedate; no risk of anaphylactic reactions); (2) convenience (no need to clip patient's haircoat, chemically restrain patient, or keep patient at clinic while preparing for, performing, and evaluating test); (3) lower likelihood that result will be influenced by prior or current drug therapy; and (4) the ability to be used in patients with widespread dermatitis or dermatographism.[43, 147, 148] The disadvantages of serologic tests are that they are more expensive, so that group testing (mixes of allergens) are used and that "false-positive" (clinically insignificant) results are exceedingly common.[16, 89, 101, 148] Perhaps the most frustrating and irritating aspect of the proliferation of companies offering serologic allergy testing in dogs is that, with few exceptions, there is absolutely no scientific information available that would confirm (or deny) the reliability and usefulness of the service(s) being provided. Information is now becoming available on some of these tests, and some very important points must be made about them.

Technologically, the ELISA appears to be more reproducible than the RAST[66, 101] and the liquid-phase immunoenzymatic assay (VARL).[129] Although these tests are purported to be species specific, one study revealed that the canine RAST, but not the ELISA, indicated that all horses, goats, cats, and humans tested were also allergic![66] With all of the technologies involving the determination of allergen-specific IgE, virtually all normal dogs, all dogs with any kind of skin disease, and all atopic dogs have at least one, and usually multiple, positive reactions.[66, 89, 101, 110, 115] According to the European literature, false-positive results are rarely obtained with the ELISA for allergen-specific IgG in nonatopic dogs.[96, 132] Investigators in the United States reported, however, that allergen-specific IgG was detectable in the majority of nonatopic as well as all atopic dogs.[107] In addition, factors that produce high levels of serum IgE in dogs (ectoparasitism, endoparasitism) can provoke false-positive reactions with serologic allergy testing.[102, 112] The point, here, is that false-positive reactions are to be *expected* with serologic allergy testing. Hence, it is absolutely critical (1) that the candidates for testing undergo meticulous work-up, so that atopy is the only possible remaining diagnosis and (2) that the test results obtained be very carefully evaluated in light of the patient's dermatologic history.

The results of serologic allergy testing correlate poorly with those of intradermal allergy testing.* Short-term treatment with anti-inflammatory doses of glucocorticoids probably does not influence the results of serologic allergy testing,[116] but long-term treatment may cause false-

---

*See references 66, 89, 101, 103, 110, 115, and 165.

negative reactions.[16, 101, 148] Attempts to create in-office allergy screening tests have, to date, been unsuccessful.[114, 127]

In spite of the inherent pitfalls of serologic allergy testing, the results are not without value. When hyposensitization is rendered on the basis of carefully interpreted serologic allergy tests performed on meticulously selected patients, about 60 per cent of the dogs have good to excellent responses.* This overall response rate is similar to that reported for hyposensitization based on the results of intradermal testing.[44] The percentage of dogs with excellent responses appears to be higher, however, when hyposensitization is based on intradermal testing.[16, 115] Some reports indicate that occasional dogs who had negative intradermal tests, or who had failed to respond to hyposensitization based on intradermal allergy testing, responded well to hyposensitization based on serologic allergy testing.[16, 67]

In part, the discrepancies between serologic and intradermal testing may be explained by numerous difficulties in technique, sensitivity, and so forth. It is also important, however, to realize that they test for two different things, so correlations are not expected (Table 8:11). The differences may also indicate that two types of IgE are present, that tissue-bound IgE does not correlate with circulating levels, or that immediate skin test reactivity and the presence of allergen-specific antibodies are no more than secondary features (epiphenomena) of atopy.[16, 19, 20, 40, 44]

Considering all the current available information, the authors and others suggest that intradermal testing is the preferred method for diagnosis of canine atopy.[40, 44, 73, 89, 133] When intradermal testing is not available, when intradermal testing gives negative results in an otherwise classic atopic dog, or when hyposensitization based on intradermal testing is unsuccessful, however, serologic allergy testing may be used.

■ *Basophil Degranulation Test.* The in vitro basophil degranulation test has been reported to show promise in the diagnosis of canine atopy.[42, 43] The test, however, requires fresh blood, must be run within 24 hours, is very time consuming and labor intensive, and is unlikely to become anything more than a research tool.

---

*See references 16, 67, 115, 133, 134, 146, 148, and 160.

Table 8:11. Comparison of Intradermal and In Vitro Allergy Tests in Dogs

Feature	Intradermal	In Vitro
Detects reaginic antibody	Yes	Yes
Detects presence of reaginic antibody in serum	No	Yes
Detects presence of cutaneous mast cells with reaginic antibody present on them	Yes	No
Determines capability of inducing a cutaneous type I hypersensitivity reaction on exposure to antigen	Yes	No
Test results are inhibited by antihistamines and glucocorticoids	Yes	No
Sensitivity (%)	70 to 90	100
Specificity (%)	>90	0 to 50
Risk to patient	Rare but possible anaphylaxis or sedative reaction	Only serum sample required
Availability	Limited to certain practices; often requires referral	Excellent
Cost per antigen tested	Inexpensive	Relatively expensive
Clinic overhead	Relatively high	Little to none

■ *Major and Minor Diagnostic Criteria.*   Because of the difficulties associated with the in vivo and in vitro diagnosis of atopy, the concept of major and minor diagnostic features has been introduced in an attempt to provide consistency in the diagnosis of atopy in dogs and humans.[167] For dogs, the following criteria have been proposed:

At least three of the following *major* features should be present:

Pruritus
Facial and/or digital involvement
Lichenification of the flexor surface of the tarsus or the extensor surface of the carpus
Chronic or chronically relapsing dermatitis
An individual or familial history of atopy
A breed predilection

At least three of the following *minor* features should also be present:

Onset of signs before 3 years of age
Facial erythema and cheilitis
Bacterial conjunctivitis
A superficial staphylococcal pyoderma
Hyperhidrosis
Immediate skin test reactivity to inhalant allergens
Elevated allergen-specific IgGd
Elevated allergen-specific IgE

To date, no reported studies have documented the validity and reliability of using these criteria to diagnose canine atopy. Additionally, it has been suggested that a tentative diagnosis of atopic disease requires ruling out other major possibilities, because the criteria just listed determine what patients may have atopy but do not exclude the possibility of some other diagnoses.[16]

■ *Histopathology.*   Skin biopsy of atopic dogs reveals variable degrees of superficial perivascular dermatitis (pure, spongiotic, hyperplastic) with lymphocytes and histiocytes usually predominating (Figs. 8:6 and 8:7).[17, 63, 143] Though statistically there is a very mild tissue eosinophilia,[124] it will not be noted during routine histopathologic examination. The presence of a significant tissue eosinophilia suggests another or concurrent disease. The presence of numerous neutrophils or plasma cells or both indicates infection, usually secondary bacterial pyoderma. Therefore, histopathology is more helpful in suggesting that further diagnostics are indicated and does not make a diagnosis of atopy. Similar dermal changes of a milder degree may be seen in clinically normal skin from atopic dogs. Histopathologic findings consistent with secondary bacterial pyoderma (suppurative folliculitis, perifolliculitis, intraepidermal pustular dermatitis) are commonly seen in specimens of skin from atopic dogs.

Clinical Management

Prognostically, atopic dogs have about an 80 per cent chance of developing nonseasonal disease. Natural desensitization is uncommon. One placebo-controlled study revealed, however, that about 20 per cent of atopic dogs improve by greater than 50 per cent after receiving placebo for 9 months.[164] In general, over 90 per cent of atopic dogs can be satisfactorily controlled. The client must be made aware, however, that treatment is usually required for life and that therapeutic modifications over the life of the dog are to be expected. Before the clinician discusses the details of therapy with the client, it is imperative to mention that some allergens may be tolerated by an individual without any disease manifestations, but a small increase in that load (one or more allergens) may push the individual over the pruritic threshold and initiate clinical signs.[40, 44] Equally important when considering the cause of dermatologic

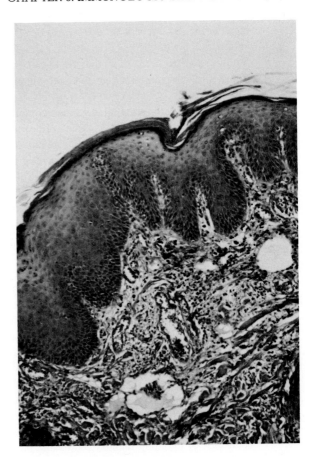

Figure 8:6. Canine atopy. Hyperplastic perivascular dermatitis. (From Scott, D.W.: Observations on canine atopy. J. Am. Anim. Hosp. Assoc. 17:91, 1981.)

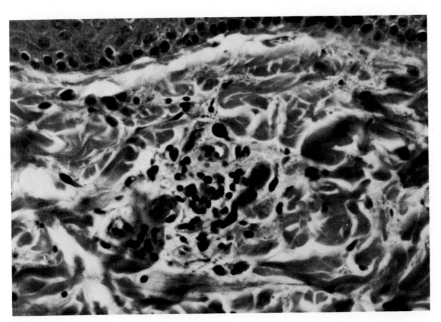

Figure 8:7. Canine atopy. Perivascular accumulation of mononuclear cells. (From Scott, D.W.: Observations on canine atopy. J. Am. Anim. Hosp. Assoc. 17:91, 1981.)

disorders is the concept of *summation of effect;* for example, a subclinical hypersensitivity in combination with a flea infestation, a mild bacterial pyoderma, or a dry environment may produce marked discomfort that could be absent if any one of the disorders existed alone.[40, 44] Thus, it is very important to evaluate all possible contributions to the clinical signs in "allergic" dogs.

Therapy for atopy includes various combinations of avoidance, topical therapies (see Chap. 3), hyposensitization, and systemic antipruritic drugs (see Chap. 3).[16, 40, 43, 44] In most cases, a single drug does not give the safest and most efficacious results, and the clinician should approach the management of the atopic dog with a complete treatment plan.[16, 100] Development of a treatment plan needs to consider multiple variables, including seasonality, distribution and amount of involved skin, cost, willingness of client to administer the treatment, acceptability to the patient, and risk to the patient. Optimally, the clinician incorporates avoidance, topical therapy (especially shampooing), and fatty acids into the treatment plan.

■ *Avoidance.* Avoidance of allergens is not always possible or practical. Such manipulations and their benefits are not generally possible without accurate identification of the offending allergen(s) by allergy testing. Because many patients have multiple reactivities and most allergens cannot be avoided, the effective use of this approach is rarely possible as a sole therapy. It is still an important aspect of the management, however, because it will often decrease the allergen load. Additionally, some patients may greatly benefit from avoidance of confirmed allergens such as feathers (pillows, birds), cats (dander), newsprint (newspaper), and tobacco smoke.[16, 40, 44, 143] With other allergens, complete elimination may be impossible but a decrease in exposure may be achievable (Table 8:12).[75] For example, house dust mite exposure can be decreased by keeping the pet outdoors more, or at least out of bedrooms and off fabric furniture; mold exposure can be decreased by removing or cleaning mildewed items, houseplants, and carpeting in bathrooms and by keeping bread refrigerated; cotton exposure can be decreased by avoiding laundry rooms and closets and by making sure that the dog's bedding is made from synthetic material. In atopic humans involved in a controlled trial wherein vacuuming and miticide were used in an attempt to eradicate house dust mites, the number of mites decreased, but the patients derived no clinical benefit.[90]

■ *Topical Therapy.* Topical therapy is utilized in two main ways. The first is through shampoos and rinses, which remove allergens from the skin and help to eliminate dry skin.[16, 100] The second is through topical antipruritic agents, which are usually most effective for treating localized areas of pruritus. These therapies are covered in Chapter 3. In general, most atopic dogs should be bathed at least every 1 or 2 weeks. It should be remembered that atopic dogs often have sensitive, easily irritated skin. Hypoallergenic and colloidal oatmeal–containing shampoos are preferred.

■ *Hyposensitization.* Hyposensitization (immunotherapy), which has been described as the mainstay of therapy in canine atopy, is indicated in animals in which avoidance of antigens is impossible, signs are present for more than 4 to 6 months of the year, and antipruritic drugs are unsatisfactory.* Virtually no attempts have been made to standardize hyposensitization regimens in the dog or to scientifically compare their merits. Thus, published regimens vary in the form of allergen used (aqueous, alum precipitated, propylene glycol suspended, glycerinated), the number and frequency of injections given in the induction phase, the dose of allergen administered, the potency of allergenic extract, and the route of administration (subcutaneous, intramuscular, intradermal). The vast majority of clinicians use only the subcutaneous route when hyposensitizing for atopy. Numerous authors have written about the benefits of hyposensitization, with most reporting a 50 to 80 per cent rate of good to excellent

---

*See references 16, 40, 43, 44, 68, 75, and 95.

Table 8:12. Practical Environmental Management for the Atopic Canine

Allergen	Avoidance Suggestions
House dust	Keep dog out of room when cleaning/vacuuming for several hours
House dust mite	Use plastic zippered cover over dog bed
	Wash bedding in hot water (> 70° C)
	Avoid letting dog sleep on overstuffed furniture (if dog sleeps on human's bed, use plastic mattress/pillow covers)
	Avoid stuffed toys
	Keep dog overnight or during working hours in uncarpeted rooms
	Frequently damp-mop the dog's "holding" room
	Run air conditioner during hot and humid weather
Molds	Keep dog out of damp basements
	Keep dog away from barns
	Keep dog away while lawn is mowed
	Avoid dusty dog foods
	Clean and disinfect humidifiers
	Avoid having large numbers of houseplants
	Avoid using as the dog's "holding" room any room with a high moisture level (bathroom, laundry room)
	Keep dog out of crawl spaces under house
	Use dehumidifiers
	Clean with chlorine bleach solutions
Pollens	Keep dog out of fields
	Keep grass cut short
	Rinse dog off after periods in high grasses/weeds
	Keep dog indoors at dusk and early morning during heavy pollen season
	Use air conditioners
	Keep dog away while mowing lawn

Modified from Bevier DE: Long-term management of atopic disease in the dog. Vet. Clin. North Am. [Small Anim. Prac.] 20:1491, 1990.

responses.* A double-blind study of hyposensitization in atopic dogs (alum-precipitated allergens versus an alum-based placebo) found a 59 per cent improvement with the vaccine and a 21 per cent improvement with a placebo.[164] It is well accepted that hyposensitization is an effective, valuable, and relatively safe treatment for atopic dogs.

The mechanism of action of hyposensitization is unclear. Various hypotheses are (1) humoral desensitization (reduced levels of IgE), (2) cellular desensitization (reduced reactivity of mast cells and basophils), (3) immunization (induction of "blocking antibody"), (4) tolerization (generation of allergen-specific suppressor cells), and (5) some combination thereof.[37, 40, 44]

Three forms of allergens have been used for hyposensitization of atopic dogs.[40, 43, 44] *Aqueous allergens,* which are rapidly absorbed, necessitate smaller doses and require multiple, frequent injections, constitute by far the most commonly used type today. A variety of hyposensitization dose protocols are utilized, but most of the aqueous regimens are modifications of the schedule shown in Table 8:13. Some specialists, including the authors, utilize just the two more potent concentrations and keep the intervals at no more than 14 days for the first 4 months of therapy. *Alum-precipitated allergens* are intermediate in action between the aqueous allergens and emulsion allergens. They are more slowly absorbed than the aqueous allergens; as a result, larger doses, fewer and less frequent injections, and more rapid hyposensitization are possible. Concern has been expressed about the possible carcinogenicity of alum precipitates, which are increasingly less available today. In the United States, alum-precipitated formulations for immunotherapy are available for only a small number of allergens. In Europe, however, they are the allergens most commonly used and recommended.[43, 160, 164] *Emulsion allergens* (aqueous

*See references 16, 40, 43, 44, 92, 95, 115, 126, 146, 148, and 160.

Table 8:13. Hyposensitization Schedule for Aqueous Allergens*

Injection No.	Day No.	Vial 1 (100 to 200 PNU/ml)†	Vial 2 (1000 to 2000 PNU/ml)	Vial 3 (10,000 to 20,000 PNU/ml)
1	1	0.1 ml		
2	2	0.2 ml		
3	4	0.4 ml		
4	6	0.8 ml		
5	8	1.0 ml		
6	10		0.1 ml	
7	12		0.2 ml	
8	14		0.4 ml	
9	16		0.8 ml	
10	18		1.0 ml	
11	20			0.1 ml
12	22			0.2 ml
13	24			0.4 ml
14	26			0.8 ml
15	28			1.0 ml
16	38			1.0 ml
17	48‡			1.0 ml

*Injections are given subcutaneously.

†Protein nitrogen unit (PNU) value of each vial represents the total of *all* allergens used.

‡Thereafter, repeat injections (1.0 ml) every 20 to 40 days, as needed.

allergens in propylene glycol, glycerin, or mineral oil) are the most slowly absorbed, allowing the largest doses, the least number of injections, and the most rapid hyposensitization.

By convention, no more than 10 allergens have been used at once for hyposensitization.[40, 44] Evidence suggests, however, that larger numbers may be utilized. Success has safely been achieved with the inclusion of up to 30 or more allergens in aqueous vaccines for atopic dogs.[68] In fact, larger numbers may increase the success rate. In one report,[68] dogs were treated with up to 40 allergens, and the response rate was 72 per cent in dogs treated with 1 to 10 allergens, 86 per cent in dogs treated with 11 to 20 allergens, and 78 per cent in dogs treated with 21 or more allergens. In animals with multiple sensitivities (e.g., 20 to 30 or more), the allergens should be selected on the basis of history, the probable presence of that allergen in the environment, the frequency at which the allergen is known to react in that region, and the duration of the allergen's presence. Cross-reactivity may also be utilized in the decision. In general, most grasses cross-react and may be represented by one of two major groups. Weeds are the group next most cross-reactive, and trees are the least.

Depending on which form of the allergen is being utilized, a beneficial response may be seen as early as 1 month or as late as 1 year after hyposensitization is begun.* "Booster" injections of allergens are administered as needed (when clinical signs first begin to reappear), and depending on the form of allergens involved and the vaccine protocol being used, boosters may be needed every week to every 6 months. When aqueous allergens are used, animals that require injections more frequently than every 10 days are usually given smaller volume of allergen.[16] In general, 0.1 ml per day is utilized by the authors for these short intervals. Experience with the patient allows the owner and the veterinarian to predict how long the patient will be asymptomatic following booster injections. Boosters are then administered shortly before clinical signs would be expected to flare up. Intervals between boosters may vary at different times of the year.

In general, atopic dogs require lifetime administration of vaccine. There is no strong indication that breed, age, sex, or duration of clinical signs affects the success of hyposensitization.

*See references 16, 40, 43, 44, 95, 126, 146, and 160.

There is some evidence, however, that long-term disease (clinical signs for 5 years or more) and older age at the onset of clinical signs (over 5 years old) indicate a poorer response to hyposensitization.[146] Most authors report that the likelihood of successful hyposensitization is greater in animals with few positive reactions; others disagree.[68, 146, 160] However, one of the authors of this book (CEG) believes that animals with numerous reactions, but primarily limited to pollens, do better. Regional variations may also occur. One author (CEG) with practices in Las Vegas and Southern California has a better success rate in Las Vegas (80 per cent) than in Southern California (60 per cent) with the same protocols. Boxers and West Highland White terriers have been reported to show a poorer response to hyposensitization.[160]

Response to immunotherapy is allergen specific.[95, 115] Thus, response to hyposensitization was much better in atopic dogs when it was based upon allergy testing (70 per cent good to excellent responses) than when it was administered with standard regional allergens with no regard to allergy testing (18 per cent, identical to placebo response).[67]

Adverse reactions to hyposensitization are uncommon but may occur in up to 5 per cent of patients.[68, 92] They include (1) intensification of clinical signs for a few hours to a few days, (2) local reactions (edema with or without pain or pruritus) at injection sites, and (3) anaphylaxis. Serious reactions have been reported to occur in less than 1 per cent to 1.25 per cent.[19, 68] Adverse reactions are treated according to symptom. Intensification of clinical signs is the most common side effect seen. It may indicate that the animal's maximum tolerance dose of allergens has been exceeded and that the final hyposensitizing dose achieved needs to be lowered. In humans, most studies on the possible long-term adverse effects of hyposensitization have failed to demonstrate any clinical or immunologic abnormalities. One study of 20 consecutive human patients with polyarteritis nodosa, however, revealed that in six patients, the onset of vasculitis symptoms coincided with hyposensitization for atopy.[40]

In the severely affected, nonseasonally atopic dog, it may be necessary to control the symptoms with systemic glucocorticoids during hyposensitization. As long as prednisolone or prednisone doses are kept as low as possible and administered on an alternate-day basis (see Chap. 3), hyposensitization can still be successful.[40, 44]

■ *Systemic Antipruritic Agents*

■ *Nonsteroidal Drugs.* A number of nonsteroidal drugs have been used to treat canine atopy. Little or no work has been done to document the effect of some; they include: orgotein (metalloprotein, nonsteroidal anti-inflammatory), phenothiazine tranquilizers, barbiturates, and levamisole.[40, 44] Studies of nonsteroidal antipruritic agents in dogs with hypersensitivity skin disease indicated that aspirin (25 mg/kg orally q8h), vitamin E (400 IU orally q12h), zinc methionine (Zinpro, 1 tablet/9.1 kg orally q24h), and vitamin C (25 mg/kg orally q12h) are rarely effective.[40, 145]

Multiple studies have shown, however, that several antihistamines, products containing omega-3/omega-6 fatty acids, and combinations thereof are effective (see Chap. 3). Of the numerous antihistamines that have been evaluated in atopic dogs, the following have been the most useful: clemastine (0.05 to 0.1 mg/kg orally q12h), amitriptyline (1 mg/kg orally q12h), hydroxyzine (2.2 mg/kg orally q8h), chlorpheniramine (0.4 mg/kg orally q8h), and diphenhydramine (2.2 mg/kg orally q8h).[145] It is essential to remember that response to antihistamines is quite individualized, and the clinician may need to try several before the one that is best for any given patient is found. Additionally, antihistamines are most effective when used as *preventive* antipruritic drugs; they are usually ineffective for bringing severe pruritus rapidly under control. Lastly, any one antihistamine has only a 10 to 30 per cent chance of being effective in any given patient. Products containing omega-3/omega-6 fatty acids (e.g., DVM Derm Caps) are effective for the control of pruritus in about 15 per cent of atopic dogs. These agents should be given for at least 3 weeks before their efficacy is assessed.

Judicious use of these agents may allow up to 60 per cent of cases of canine atopy to be satisfactorily managed without glucocorticoids. In addition, the use of these nonsteroidal agents often permits a significant reduction in required glucocorticoid doses.[77, 105, 127a, 145]

■ *Systemic Glucocorticoids.* Systemic glucocorticoids are usually very effective for the management of atopy. They are, however, the most dangerous of the treatments commonly utilized to treat atopy. As such, their use should be limited to cases with active seasons lasting less than 4 to 6 months or for which safer options are not effective. Prednisolone or prednisone is administered orally (1 mg/kg q24h) in the morning until pruritus is controlled (3 to 10 days), and then on an alternate-day (morning) regimen (see Chap. 3) as needed. This schedule is relatively safe compared with long-acting corticosteroids. Some cases become less and less responsive to glucocorticoids with the passage of time. It must be remembered that the response to systemic glucocorticoids is not an all-or-none phenomenon (see Chap. 3) and that one glucocorticoid may be very effective when another was unsatisfactory. Also, the combination of other treatments may allow for a reduction in the glucocorticoid dose required.[145]

■ *Other Agents.* In humans with atopic dermatitis, recent studies have demonstrated the therapeutic benefits of cyclosporine,[154] INF-γ,[104, 135] injectable allergen-antibody complexes,[111] and thymopentin.[150] To the authors' knowledge, there are no similar reports in dogs.

Feline Atopy

Feline atopy (feline atopic disease) was first described in 1982, yet the documentation of feline IgE is still awaited.[188] *Feline atopy* is a pruritic disease in cats that have positive intradermal test reactions to environmental allergens. It is considered the second most common hypersensitivity in the cat. An inherited predisposition has not been documented, though reports of cases with familial involvement suggest a genetic component.[189, 193]

Cause and Pathogenesis

Feline atopy is caused by an exaggerated or inappropriate response of the affected cat to environmental allergens. The most common environmental allergens are nonseasonal (positive reactions in over 90 per cent of cats tested).[173, 186, 189] In a study of 28 atopic cats, 50 per cent were mainly positive to nonseasonal allergens, and 48 per cent were reactive to both nonseasonal and seasonal allergens.[186] This study also showed immediate reactivity to flea allergen in 40 per cent of the cats. Another study of 10 atopic cats reported 100 per cent reactivity to the house dust mite, *Dermatophagoides farinae.*[173]

The pathogenesis of the inappropriate response is unknown, though it is believed that a reaginic antibody is present in the skin. The reaginic antibody causes an immediate reaction to the intradermal injection of antigens.[40, 44, 173, 186, 193] The determination of the antibody class responsible and its localization to cutaneous mast cells have not been documented but the response is believed to occur as in the dog. That a reaginic antibody exists and resembles IgE is supported not just by the positive intradermal test but also by other studies, which showed that: (1) cats infested with ear mites develop cutaneous hypersensitivity that is eliminated by exposing the serum to heat and mercaptoethanol, (2) positive skin test reactions in normal and atopic cats may be passively transferred to normal cats, and this reaction is heat labile, (3) the reaginic antibody sensitizes bladder smooth muscle and cross-reacts with canine IgE, and (4) hyposensitization is effective in the management of atopic cats.[40, 44, 171, 177, 178, 193] Recent studies with a monoclonal antibody against a putative feline IgE showed reactivity against feline IgA and IgM, as well.[178]

Clinical Features

No breed or sex predilections have been demonstrated. Young cats appear to be predisposed; 75 per cent of the atopic cats with miliary dermatitis in one study developed clinical signs between 6 and 24 months of age.[189] The most consistent feature of atopy is pruritus, which 100 per cent of the cats demonstrate.[173, 176, 193] The pruritus may not, however, be obvious to the owner, particularly of cats presenting with noninflammatory alopecia. In these cases, other indirect evidence of pruritus may be found, such as vomiting from hair balls, hair in feces, tufts of hair in the cat's hiding areas, hair in the cat's teeth, and trichograms revealing broken and chopped-off distal ends of hairs, suggesting licking and chewing as the cause of the hair loss.

The clinical lesions of feline atopy are quite variable. The four most commonly reported cutaneous reaction patterns are self-induced alopecia (fur mowing) (Fig. 8:8 *B*), eosinophilic granuloma complex lesions (Fig. 8:8 *C*), miliary dermatitis, and initially nonlesional pruritus of the face, neck, and pinnae (Fig. 8:8 *A*).[170, 173, 174, 176, 189, 193] Some cats manifest various combinations of these four patterns.[176, 193] Erythematous macules, papules, and excoriations may also be seen, usually in association with one or more of the more common lesions. Recurrent swelling of the chin or lower lip (eosinophilic granuloma) may be seen. The pruritus and lesions may be localized or generalized. Localized involvement often includes the abdomen, groin, lateral thorax, and caudal thighs. The head, neck, and forelegs are also commonly involved. Although the pinna is commonly affected, the ear canal is usually spared. Some cats manifest a recurrent, pruritic, ceruminous otitis externa that is typically misdiagnosed as ear mite infestation. Rarely, cats manifest an erythematous papulopustular eruption characterized clinicopathologically as a sterile eosinophilic folliculitis and furunculosis.[190] Noncutaneous signs may also be observed. Sneezing was reported in 50 per cent of the cases in one study, and conjunctivitis may also be present.[173] Chronic coughing and feline asthma may rarely occur from atopy, with or without concurrent skin disease.[20] Lymphadenopathy is frequently seen in chronic cases that have miliary dermatitis, excoriations, or eosinophilic plaques.[189] Though secondary bacterial pyoderma is rarely reported as a complication of feline atopy, one author (CEG) frequently encounters it in chronic cases with lymphadenopathy. Up to 25 per cent of atopic cats may have concurrent food hypersensitivity, or flea bite hypersensitivity, or both.[236] This presentation can greatly complicate the diagnostic work-up as well as the therapeutic regimen.

Diagnosis

The wide variation of clinical lesions reported in atopic cats requires the consideration of a lengthy differential diagnosis for feline atopy. It is more practical to consider the presenting lesion and history and then to develop a differential diagnosis. The most common presentations are clinically noninflammatory alopecia, eosinophilic granuloma complex lesions (see Chap. 17), miliary dermatitis, and pruritus of the face or pinnae. The common differential diagnosis for these presentations include flea bite hypersensitivity, food hypersensitivity, cheyletiellosis, otodectic mange, dermatophytosis, and psychogenic alopecia.

The diagnosis of feline atopy is based on a compatible history and physical findings along with ruling out the two major alternatives, flea bite hypersensitivity and food hypersensitivity. A definitive diagnosis requires a positive intradermal allergy test reaction. Good flea control and a poor response to a 9- to 13-week course of a hypoallergenic diet, respectively, are required to rule out the two alternatives. In some cases, this approach may not be practical, because it requires keeping the cat indoors. Cytologic examination of skin lesions usually reveals eosinophils, and occasionally basophils, though this picture is not specific for atopy but may also be seen with food and flea bite hypersensitivity (Fig. 8:9). The presence of degenerate neutrophils with intracellular bacteria indicates secondary bacterial pyoderma. A peripheral eosinophilia is usually present, unless the patient has recently received glucocorticoids.[193]

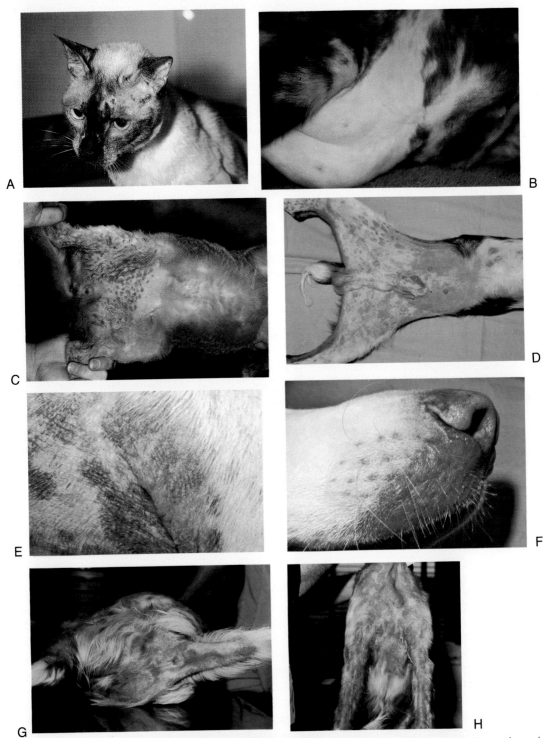

Figure 8:8. *A*, Feline atopy. Facial excoriations. *B*, Feline atopy. Self-induced symmetric alopecia. Note enlarged mammary glands, as this cat was receiving but not responding to megestrol acetate. *C*, Feline atopy. Eosinophilic plaques and alopecia. Note the linearity to the lesions that occur from licking. *D*, Contact hypersensitivity affecting the glabrous skin with papules and patches of erythema. *E*, Contact hypersensitivity. Axilla of affected dog shows erythema and papules—the primary lesions. *F*, Plastic dish dermatitis. The erythematous patch on the lip and alopecia are caused by contact with a plastic dish during eating. Note partial depigmentation of the tip of the nose. *G*, Erythema and alopecia over the perineum, ventral tail, and caudal thighs of a dog with food hypersensitivity. *H*, Severe erythema and alopecia over the ventral neck and chest and the front legs of a dog with food hypersensitivity.

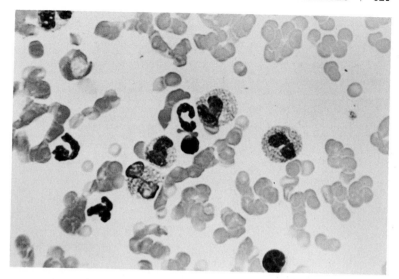

Figure 8:9. Feline atopy. Cytologic examination reveals numerous eosinophils and lesser numbers of nondegenerate neutrophils.

■ *Allergy Testing.* As with canine atopy, an intradermal allergy test is the only test currently known to aid in the diagnosis of feline atopy.[40, 44, 176] Commercially available serologic allergy tests (RAST, ELISA) that claim to diagnose feline atopy by detecting allergen-specific IgE are available. These commercial tests have not been adequately evaluated, and to date, the companies offering them have been reluctant, unwilling, or unable even to document that they are truly detecting allergen-specific IgE, which has yet to be completely characterized and purified. Additionally, these companies have not yet shown that their serologic tests are specific or sensitive. A recent study[178a] compared the results of intradermal allergy tests and a commercially available serologic allergy test (ELISA) in atopic cats, and concluded that the ELISA was *not* a useful diagnostic test. Though anecdotal reports of successful hyposensitization based on serologic allergy testing exist,[169] there are no published reports. For these reasons, the authors cannot currently recommend the serologic allergy tests for feline atopy.

Experience with intradermal allergy testing is limited in the cat compared with the dog. One study evaluated testing solutions in normal cats, and overall, the same protocol for aqueous allergens as that used in the dog was considered effective for the cat.[171, 173, 188, 189] Age, allergen, coat color, and sex have a minor effect on skin test reactivity.[171] Some normal cats reacted to low concentrations of allergen, particularly house dust, firebush, and flea. It was shown, however, that at least some of the reactions in normal cats are not irritant but most likely are mediated by reaginic antibodies, because they could be passively transferred.[171]

■ *Procedure.* The technique for feline intradermal allergy testing is similar to that described in the dog, with the following exceptions:

1. Sedation with ketamine, ketamine and diazepam, tiletamine-zolazepam, or a general gas anesthetic is usually utilized for restraint.[40, 176, 185, 189]
2. Extra care should be taken to make sure that all the injections are intradermal.
3. The test site should be examined at 5 and 20 minutes post injection, because feline reactions sometimes occur and fade rapidly, within 10 minutes.
4. Reactions, including those to histamine, are often much subtler than those seen in dogs.

A study has shown that intradermal allergy testing in cats, with and without prior sedation, produced marked increases in the concentrations of plasma cortisol, corticotropin, and α-melanocyte–stimulating hormone.[194] This may explain the typically weak responses to skin testing seen in cats compared with dogs. It is also interesting that some atopic cats are as reactive as any dog. Whether this reflects a different group of atopic cats or has any prognostic significance has yet to be determined. Immediate skin test reactivity in cats was reported to return 2 weeks after stopping oral prednisone administration and 4 weeks after the administration by injection of methylprednisolone acetate.[172]

■ *Histopathology.*   Skin biopsies of atopic cats are not diagnostic but are valuable for looking for evidence of some of the alternative diagnoses.[17, 63, 191] Additionally, the histopathologic findings may vary according to the clinical lesion sampled. Biopsy specimens from clinically noninflammatory alopecic areas typically have a normal to slightly hyperplastic epidermis with a mild superficial perivascular dermatitis wherein lymphocytes or mast cells are predominant. Inflammatory lesions (facial and pinnal pruritus; miliary dermatitis) reveal moderate to marked epidermal hyperplasia, spongiosis, serocellular crusts, erosions or ulcerations, and variable degrees of superficial or deep perivascular dermatitis, wherein eosinophils are usually the dominant inflammatory cell (Fig. 8:10).[191] Intraepidermal mast cells have also been seen in skin specimens from atopic cats, primarily those with eosinophilic plaques.[45] This finding is not specific for feline atopy. Specimens from atopic cats with eosinophilic granuloma complex lesions reveal changes typical of those lesions (see Chap. 17). In some cats, eosinophilic folliculitis and furunculosis are prominent.[191] To date, atopy, food hypersensitivity, and flea bite hypersensitivity cannot be differentiated histologically.

Clinical Management

The prognosis for feline atopy is good, although some cases are extremely difficult to manage. Concurrent flea bite hypersensitivity, food hypersensitivity, and bacterial pyoderma greatly interfere with achieving a favorable therapeutic response, and care should be taken to alleviate these complications. Treatment is usually required for life, during which multiple different therapies may be utilized. The treatment plan may involve the use of avoidance,[187] glucocorticoids, antihistamines, fatty acids, and hyposensitization (see discussion of canine atopy). The treatment selected will vary according to many client and patient factors. Generally, the differences in risks of therapy among the different treatments is not gravely important, because cats appear relatively resistant to the acute and chronic side effects of glucocorticoids.[40, 44, 193] In addition, glucocorticoid regimens tend to be less expensive and more convenient than the alternative forms of therapy. As a result, most atopic cats are managed with some form of glucocorticoid therapy.[193] Topical therapy is uncommonly utilized in the cat owing to the actual

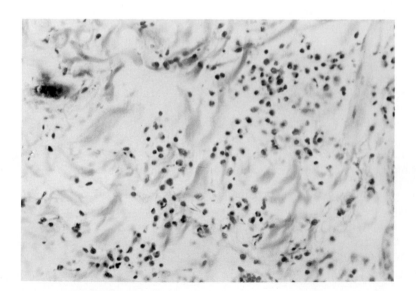

Figure 8:10. Feline atopy. Perivascular and interstitial infiltrations of predominantly eosinophils.

or perceived difficulty in bathing cats. In cats that tolerate bathing, however, and whose owners are willing, this practice can have a very beneficial effect.

Glucocorticoids are the mainstay of therapy in atopic cats.[193] The most common reason they are not used is that owners are concerned about the risks of glucocorticoids (inappropriately extrapolated from experience in humans or dogs) and the occasional objectionable side-effects. Other contraindications to their use in the cat are concurrent infections (viral, bacterial, fungal), diabetes mellitus, pancreatitis, renal failure, and perhaps, pregnancy.[193] The simplest glucocorticoid treatment is with repositol methylprednisolone acetate (Depo-Medrol) given subcutaneously or intramuscularly at 20 mg per cat or 5 mg/kg.[40, 170, 193] It may be given as needed but not more frequently than every 8 weeks and preferably every 12 weeks. Alternatively, or if methylprednisolone acetate is ineffective, triamcinolone acetonide (Vetalog), 5 mg per cat every 8 to 12 weeks as needed, may be utilized. In cases that do not respond adequately or in which injectable glucocorticoids produce adverse side-effects, or when clients prefer, oral glucocorticoids may be utilized (see Chap. 3). Most commonly, prednisone or prednisolone (2.2 mg/kg q24h) is given until the patient is in remission (5 to 10 days), followed by an alternate-day regimen.

Antihistamines are also effective in cats.[193] In contrast to dogs, cats are relatively sensitive to these drugs, and those other than chlorpheniramine and clemastine should be used cautiously until further studies are reported. One study demonstrated an excellent response in 73 per cent of atopic cats to chlorpheniramine at 2 mg/cat q12h.[182] Many other investigators have also reported favorable, though not as good, results with chlorpheniramine; therefore, it is considered the antihistamine of choice in the atopic cat. Clemastine, 0.67 mg per cat orally q12h, was shown to adequately control pruritus in 50 per cent of the cases treated.[184] For a complete discussion of antihistamines, see Chapter 3.

Fatty acid supplements (see Chap. 3) have also been reported to be effective in the management of feline atopy.[193] Although fewer studies have been reported in cats than in dogs, current information would indicate that from 50 to 75 per cent of treated cats have a good response to products containing omega-3/omega-6 fatty acids.[179, 180, 183] In addition, it has been reported that cats also benefit from the synergistic effects of combining fatty acids (DVM Derm Caps Liquid) with either chlorpheniramine or glucocorticoids.[192, 193] As a result of these good therapeutic results, the possible synergistic effects achievable, and the safety of these products, any cat that will readily ingest a liquid fatty acid supplement in its daily diet should initially be treated with it. If the supplement alone fails to control the pruritus adequately, antihistamines or glucocorticoids can be added.

It has been reported that oxatomide, a mast cell stabilizer, is effective in many atopic cats.[186] The drug is administered orally, 15 to 30 mg per cat q12h, with a good response seen in about 50 per cent of treated cats. The major reported side-effect is polyphagia.

Hyposensitization is an option available in cases for which intradermal allergy testing has determined what the cats are specifically allergic to. In some cats, hyposensitization is the best option other than repositol glucocorticoids, because it is given by injection and relatively infrequently once the maintenance dose is reached. The same protocol as for the dog is most commonly utilized (see discussion of canine atopy). One author (CEG) has found that many of the cases that respond to hyposensitization stay improved, even with a lower volume (0.5 ml) of maintenance injections. Hyposensitization utilizing either aqueous or alum-precipitated allergens is reported to give favorable responses in 70 per cent of cases.[173, 176, 181, 186, 188, 189]

Contact Hypersensitivity

Contact hypersensitivity (allergic contact dermatitis) is a rare, variably pruritic, maculopapular dermatitis usually affecting sparsely haired skin in contact areas.

Cause and Pathogenesis

Very few reports of naturally occurring contact hypersensitivity in dogs and cats have been documented by patch testing. Thus, most of the literature and data on naturally occurring *allergic contact dermatitis* in dogs and cats are of dubious validity and value. In reality, there is often a huge overlap between what has been called contact hypersensitivity and primary irritant contact dermatitis in the veterinary literature.[19, 20, 40, 44] Classically, contact hypersensitivity represents a type IV hypersensitivity reaction wherein lymphocytes are the dominant cell type.* Langerhans' cell numbers are decreased in contact hypersensitivity but not in primary irritant contact dermatitis.[195] TNF-α has been reputed to be a critical mediator in classic contact hypersensitivity reactions.[209] In dogs, however, histopathologic examination has given conflicting and confusing results.[40] In a Danish study wherein positive patch test reactions underwent biopsy and histopathologic examination, the neutrophil was the dominant inflammatory cell.[210] Limited case studies in the dog have also implicated eosinophils as a cellular component of contact hypersensitivity in the dog.[196, 197, 199, 202a, 206] These contrasting findings indicate that contact hypersensitivity in the dog may have a different pathogenesis from that in other species, and from one dog to another, depending on the allergen(s) involved. Further work in this area is needed.

It has been noted that atopy is present in about 20 per cent of the dogs with contact hypersensitivity.[205] Whether this reflects similar breed predispositions, similarities in basic immunologic pathogenesis between contact hypersensitivity and atopic disease, or abnormalities in the epidermal barrier of atopic dogs that predispose to penetration of haptens that cause contact hypersensitivity remains to be determined. In fact, canine atopy itself may be a type of contact hypersensitivity, a type I (immediate) contact hypersensitivity (see discussion of atopy).

Experimental attempts to induce contact hypersensitivity in dogs and cats have given inconsistent results. Nobreus and colleagues,[204] using a modified "maximization technique" of intradermal and topical sensitization, successfully sensitized dogs to dinitrochlorobenzene. They showed that the sensitization could be transferred to normal dogs with thoracic duct lymphocytes and that sensitization could be suppressed with antilymphocyte serum. Krawiec and Gaafar[200] successfully sensitized dogs to dinitrochlorobenzene with intradermal and topical challenge. Schultz and Adams[208] reported that helminth antigens, tissue antigens, viral antigens, bacterial antigens, fungal antigens, protein antigens, dinitrochlorobenzene, and mitogens had been used experimentally and clinically in dogs and cats to elicit delayed-type hypersensitivity responses in the skin, with limited reproducibility or irreproducible results. Schultz and Maguire[207] induced delayed-type hypersensitivity in normal cats with dinitrochlorobenzene.

Spontaneous, well-documented cases of contact hypersensitivity are found rarely in the veterinary literature. Though poison ivy and poison oak may be transferred to humans from dogs carrying the oleoresins in their haircoats, only rare cases occur in the dog, and documentation of these by patch testing has not been published. Other plants, however, have rarely been documented as a cause of contact hypersensitivity. Kunkle and Gross[201] reported a beautifully documented case of naturally occurring contact hypersensitivity to *Tradescantia fluminensis* (wandering Jew plant) in a dog. Sensitivity to *Hippeastrum* (Amaryllidaceae) leaves and bulbs was documented in a dog in the Netherlands.[212] Asian jasmine was also shown to be a cause in a case documented with patch testing and resolution upon avoidance.[202a] Interestingly in this last case, multiple intraepidermal eosinophilic pustules were revealed on histopathologic examination of the patch test site. Dandelion leaves were well documented as a cause in one dog.[199] Cedar wood was also reported as a cause of contact hypersensitivity, although patch testing was not performed to document the case.[197] Indoor or synthetic products that contain allergens are a major cause of disease in humans but, again, are rarely documented to cause

---

*See references 5, 13, 37, 40, 43, 44, 195, and 211.

disease in dogs. In a Danish study, confirmed contact hypersensitivity to the following substances was documented: thiuram mix, cobalt chloride, nickel sulfate, quinoline mix, colophony, black rubber mix, wood alcohols, epoxy resin, balsam of Peru, carba mix, formaldehyde, fragrance mix, ethylenediamine, primin, wood tar, and naphthyl mix.[209a, 210] Well-documented cases were also reported in three dogs to synthetic textiles, though the allergenic component was not identified.[199] Carpet deodorizer and a plastic shopping bag were suspected but not proven to be contact allergens in a dog[198] and cat,[203] respectively. Neomycin is a commonly mentioned, but rarely documented contact allergen in dogs and cats.[211] Because it is often present in otic preparations, neomycin is most frequently incriminated as a cause of "allergic contact otitis externa."

It can be concluded from the preceding summary of investigations that contact hypersensitivity *can* be induced in dogs and cats, but only with difficulty and with inconsistent results in comparison with tests on humans and guinea pigs. The incidence of naturally occurring disease is much lower than in humans and rarely as well documented as in humans. Additionally, the pathogenesis of the lesions needs to be studied, because there may be species differences or even multiple pathogenic mechanisms in the dog, as evidenced by the strikingly different histopathologic findings reported from clinical lesions or in positive patch tests.

Clinical Features

Naturally occurring contact hypersensitivity is reported to account for about 1 to 5 per cent of all canine dermatoses[40, 44, 202, 205, 210, 211] and to be rare in cats. The authors consider it a very rare disease. A 1993 symposium on contact hypersensitivity in the dog had very small numbers of cases presented, and most case reports were very old.[196, 197, 199, 202a, 206] Walton[40] reported that over 20 per cent of his cases of canine contact hypersensitivity occurred in yellow Labrador retrievers. In a study of 22 cases (confirmed by closed patch testing) of contact hypersensitivity in dogs in Denmark,[209a] 50 per cent of the dogs were German shepherds, whereas this breed accounted for only 16 per cent of the purebred registered dogs. Other breeds described but not documented to be at increased risk are: wirehaired fox terriers, Scottish terriers, West Highland White terriers, and Golden retrievers.[205] These are breeds also at risk for atopy. French Poodles are also reported to be at risk.[205, 210] No age or sex predilection has been documented.

Although contact hypersensitivity can be produced in dogs after a 3- to 5-week sensitization period, the sensitization period for dogs and cats with naturally occurring disease exceeds 2 years in over 70 per cent of cases.[40, 44, 205, 209a, 210] Substances reported to cause naturally occurring "allergic contact dermatitis" in dogs and cats are listed in Table 8:14. Again, virtually none of these substances, other than those previously listed, has been well documented with patch testing.

Clinical signs of contact hypersensitivity include varying degrees of dermatitis, which tend to be confined to hairless or sparsely haired areas of skin in contact regions: ventral aspect of paws (*not* pads); ventral abdomen (Fig. 8:8 *D*), thorax (Fig. 8:8 *E*), and neck; scrotum; point of chin; perineum; and lateral aspect of pinnae. If the allergen is in a topical medicament in liquid, aerosol, or powder form, cutaneous reactions may also be seen in haired areas as well (Fig. 8:11). Reactions to rubber or plastic dishes and rawhide chew toys are usually confined to the lips and nose (Fig. 8:8 *F*). Acute skin lesions consist of various combinations of erythema, macules, papules, and, rarely, vesicles. Although vesicles are the classic lesions seen in most species, they are rare in dogs and cats and often manifest themselves only at the microscopic level in acute lesions. Chronic lesions are often alopecic plaques that may be hyperpigmented or hypopigmented, excoriated, and lichenified. Secondary bacterial pyoderma or seborrheic skin disease, or both, may be present.[205, 209a, 210, 211] Pruritus varies, from mild to intense. Contact hypersensitivities may be seasonal or nonseasonal, depending on the allergens involved. In households with several dogs or cats, involvement of a single animal would

Table 8:14. Substances Reported to Cause Naturally Occurring "Allergic Contact Dermatitis" in Dogs and Cats

Substance Category	Examples
Plants	Pollens and resins (grasses, trees, weeds), jasmine blooms, poison ivy, poison oak, wandering Jew, dandelion leaves, Asian jasmine, cedar wood, *Hippeastrum*
Medications	Topicals, neomycin, tetracaine and other "caines," soaps, shampoos (especially those containing tars and creosols), petrolatum, lanolin, disinfectants, insecticides (shampoos, dips, sprays, flea and tick collars and medallions)
Highly chlorinated water	
Home furnishings	Fibers (wool, nylon, synthetics), dyes, mordants, finishes, polishes, cleansers, rubber and plastic products, detergents, cat litter, collars (leather, metal), deodorants, cement, nickel, dichromate

suggest hypersensitivity, whereas clinical signs in several animals would point to irritant reactions or contagious disease.

Diagnosis

The differential diagnosis includes primary irritant contact dermatitis, atopy, food hypersensitivity, canine scabies, insect hypersensitivity, *Pelodera* dermatitis, hookworm dermatitis, staphylococcal folliculitis, and *Malassezia* dermatitis.

Definitive diagnosis is based on history, physical findings, and results of provocative exposure and patch testing.

Provocative exposure involves avoiding contact with suspected allergenic substances for up to 14 days.[40, 44, 202, 205, 209a, 211] The animal is first bathed with a nonirritating, hypoallergenic shampoo to remove all possible allergenic substances from the skin and haircoat, then placed in a "nonallergenic" environment for up to 14 days. The animal is then re-exposed to its

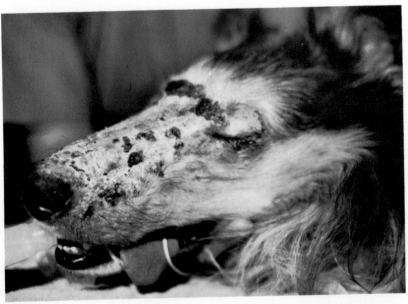

Figure 8:11. Contact dermatitis due to neomycin (Panolog) on the bridge of the nose of a dog.

normal environment or to suspect substances, one at a time, and is observed for an exacerbation of the dermatosis over 7 to 10 days. Provocative exposure is time consuming, requires a patient and dedicated owner, and is frequently impossible to undertake. Additionally, without biopsy or patch testing, provocative exposure does *not* reliably distinguish between hypersensitivity and irritant skin reactions. To better define the reactions, skin biopsy specimens taken from acute lesions induced by the exposure should be studied.

The patch test is the method for documenting contact hypersensitivity.* In the classic closed patch test, the test substance is applied to a piece of cloth or soft paper that is then placed directly on intact skin, covered with an impermeable substance, and affixed to the skin with tape. After 48 hours the patch is removed, and the condition of the underlying skin examined.

Owing to the logistical problems of applying and securing patch test substances to dogs and cats, patch testing is rarely done. The sliding of the material and irritation from tape leads to much misinterpretation of results. The use of ether to remove the tape and the adhesive (Scanpar) tends to minimize but not eliminate these problems.[205] Walton[210a] recommended open patch testing in the dog and listed suggested allergen concentrations and vehicles for canine patch testing. In open patch testing, the allergen is merely rubbed into a suitable marked test site of normal skin, and the test site is then examined daily over 5 days. Walton[210a] reported that positive patch test reactions in dogs are much less inflammatory than those seen in human beings and guinea pigs, usually consisting of mild erythema and edema and variable degrees of pruritus. In a Danish study, 63 per cent of the affected dogs were monosensitive and 23 per cent were sensitive to two allergens.[210]

For now, performing closed patch tests with suspected allergens in their natural state is probably the most sensible way to proceed. The dorsolateral thorax is gently clipped, and suspected allergens are applied to the skin (preferably with Scanpar), taped in place, and secured under a body bandage. The test materials are removed in 48 hours, and the test sites are observed for the following 3 to 5 days. Optimally, marginally suspect test sites should undergo biopsy, but more fulminant reactions can be considered positive. Substances eliciting positive reactions should be tested on normal animals to make sure that they are not irritants. A standardized patch test has been recommended for dogs.[205, 210] Limited testing in control dogs has been done, and further work is warranted before this test is fully endorsed. Additionally, many of the documented causes of contact hypersensitivity in dogs would have been missed by the test, because they are local plants or materials not included in this standard battery. Therefore, a complete work-up still requires that materials from the dog's local environment be tested in addition to the standardized battery. These natural materials can be chopped up, mixed with petrolatum, and applied with the Finn Chambers or placed in the center of a 2 × 2-inch gauze pad.

■ *Histopathology.* In experimentally induced contact hypersensitivity in dogs and cats, skin biopsy revealed varying degrees of superficial perivascular dermatitis, with mononuclear cells predominating.[200, 207] In other attempts to induce type IV hypersensitivity reactions in dog and cat skin, however, biopsies revealed varying degrees of superficial perivascular dermatitis in which neutrophils prevailed.[208] In naturally occurring contact hypersensitivity of dogs, cats, and human beings, skin biopsy is nondiagnostic, showing varying degrees of superficial perivascular dermatitis (spongiotic, hyperplastic) wherein neutrophils or mononuclear cells may predominate.[13, 17, 40, 63] Specimens taken from positive patch test reaction sites in dogs with spontaneous contact hypersensitivity revealed that neutrophils were the dominant dermal inflammatory and were commonly associated with neutrophilic exocytosis and even focal epidermal necrosis.[210] No significant differences are found in the number of mononuclear inflammatory cells or in their subclasses in skin from humans with allergic or primary irritant contact dermatitis.[5, 37]

---

*See references 5, 37, 40, 44, 205, 209a, 210, 210a, and 211.

Histopathologic findings consistent with secondary bacterial pyoderma or seborrheic skin disease, or both, may be present.

Clinical Management

The prognosis for contact hypersensitivity depends on the offending allergen. Therapy of contact hypersensitivity in dogs and cats may include avoidance of allergens or the use of glucocorticoids. Avoidance of allergens is preferable but may be impossible, either because of the nature of the substances or because they cannot be identified. In such instances, glucocorticoids are usually very effective but will often be needed for life. Some animals can be managed with topical glucocorticoids alone (see Chap. 3). Other animals require systemic glucocorticoids. Prednisolone or prednisone may be administered orally at 1 mg/kg (dog) or 2 mg/kg (cat) daily for 5 to 7 days, and then on an alternate-day regimen as needed (see Chap. 3).

Hyposensitization to certain contactants has been shown to be possible in humans.[13, 37] Such hyposensitization, however, is usually limited and temporary. In general, attempts to hyposensitize human beings, dogs, and cats to contactants have been totally unsuccessful.[13, 37, 40, 44, 209a, 210, 210a]

It has been reported that pentoxifylline (a methylxanthine derivative) suppresses the production of TNF-α by leukocytes and keratinocytes and also down-regulates adhesion molecule expression.[209] This drug may, thus, have unique application to the treatment of contact hypersensitivity.

Canine Food Hypersensitivity

Food hypersensitivity (food allergy, food intolerance) is a nonseasonal, pruritic skin disorder of dogs that is associated with the ingestion of a substance found in the dog's diet. Presumably it is a hypersensitivity reaction to an antigenic ingredient. This may not always be the case, however, and food intolerance may also be occurring and be incorrectly called food hypersensitivity.[218, 219] The term *food hypersensitivity* is still accepted, however, because of its common usage and because of the difficulty differentiating between hypersensitivity and intolerance in practice.[219]

Cause and Pathogenesis

Diet has long been recognized as a cause of hypersensitivity-like skin reactions in dogs, cats, and human beings. Although the pathomechanism of food hypersensitivity is unclear, type I hypersensitivity reactions are well documented and the most common type of hypersensitivity reactions in humans, although type III and IV reactions have been suspected.[37, 40, 44, 219] *Immediate* (within minutes to hours) and *delayed* (within several hours to days) reactions to foods have also been seen in the dog and cat.[40, 44, 214, 228, 236] Most commonly, the allergen is a glycoprotein present within the food, and this glycoprotein may become recognizable only after digestion or heating and preparation of the food. Whether sensitization occurs in the intestinal mucosa or to absorbed allergen is unknown. Typically, initial presentation of antigen to the gut mucosa results in a local, predominantly IgA immune response that reduces the amount of antigenic material absorbed across the mucosa.[218, 219] There is also a backup mechanism by which antigenic material that is absorbed is cleared via formation of IgA-containing immune complexes. Despite these defenses, an immunologic response to a variety of food antigens often occurs in both normal individuals and those with proven food hypersensitivity.[218, 219] Possibly a damaged intestinal tract, such as from internal parasites or a viral enteritis, allows the bypassing of the normal defense mechanism. Additionally, the predisposition to develop IgE antibody may be enhanced by a concurrent parasitic infection.[19] Because these conditions occur in young dogs, and food hypersensitivity often develops in young dogs, it becomes a tempting hypothesis that needs to be studied.

The documentation of an allergic mechanism is rarely confirmed in the dog. Food intolerance is also likely to occur in the dog and may mimic food hypersensitivity reactions. Intolerance is an adverse food reaction that does not have an immunologic basis.[218] One type of intolerance, the anaphylactoid reaction, mimics food hypersensitivity because it causes an anaphylaxis-type reaction, owing to the presence of histamine or substances that cause endogenous release of histamine in a nonimmunologic fashion.[37, 218, 219] Attention has also been focused on a heterogenous group of cytokines called histamine-releasing factors.[37, 218, 219] After being initially generated by antigenic exposures, these cytokines can cause histamine release in the absence of the provoking antigen, and this release can continue for some time after the antigen is removed. Such a mechanism could explain the long delay (10 to 13 weeks) reported between the initiation of a hypoallergenic diet and clinical improvement in some food-hypersensitive dogs.

Little information is available on the dietary items responsible for food hypersensitivity, because few owners are willing to separate a diet into its components and to feed each item individually to identify the responsible allergen. In vitro (serologic) tests cannot be relied on to detect allergens that cause hypersensitivity because they are positive in most normal dogs and in most dogs with other skin diseases.[231] These tests are also positive in most dogs with proven hypersensitivity to food but, in most cases, not to the important allergens determined by test meal investigations.[231] Evidence to date suggests that most dogs are sensitive to a single or a few dietary substances and that beef, dairy products, chicken, wheat, chicken eggs, corn, and soy are the most common offenders.[213, 214, 220, 223, 230] In one study, beef was by far the most common allergen, eliciting reactions in 70 per cent of the dogs.[214] Interestingly, 9 per cent of the dogs in the same study reacted to a rice product. Table 8:15 lists dietary items reported to have caused food hypersensitivity in dogs. Though food additives (including preservatives) are often blamed by the public (particularly by naturalists), these substances are rarely documented to cause food hypersensitivity in dogs.

Clinical Features

It has been estimated that food hypersensitivity accounts for (1) as many as 1 per cent of all canine and feline dermatoses in a general practice and (2) about 10 per cent of all canine allergic skin diseases (excluding parasitic allergy).[40, 44, 213, 215] Studies have indicated that food hypersensitivity in dogs and cats accounted for about 5 per cent of all skin diseases and 15 per cent of the allergic dermatoses.[214, 216] Food hypersensitivity is the third most common hypersensitivity skin disease in dogs after flea bite hypersensitivity and atopy.

Table 8:15. Dietary Items that Have Caused Food Hypersensitivity in the Dog

Artificial food additives (Gum carrageenan)	Horse meat
Beef	Kidney beans
Canned foods	Lamb and mutton
Chicken	Oatmeal
Corn	Pasta
Cow's milk	Pork
Dairy products (whey)	Potatoes
Dog biscuits	Rabbit
Dog foods (including prescription canned and dry d/d®)	Rice flour and rice
Eggs	Soy
Fish (variety)	Turkey
Food preservatives	Wheat

No age or sex predilections have been documented for canine food hypersensitivity. Though there is no age predilection, it is important to note that many cases occur in young dogs and may raise the index of suspicion above that of atopic disease when pruritus occurs in dogs under 6 months of age.[216, 220, 228] Most investigators have not found a breed predilection.[40, 44, 214, 232] Other investigators, however, found that Cocker and Springer spaniels, Labrador retrievers, collies, Miniature Schnauzers, Chinese Shar Peis, West Highland White terriers, Wheaton terriers, boxers, dachshunds, Dalmatians, Lhasa apsos, German shepherds, and Golden retrievers were at increased risk.[216, 220, 228] Food hypersensitivity can cause a wide variety of lesions and can be considered in any pruritic dog.[40, 214, 215, 226] Pruritus, with or without a primary eruption, is the only consistent finding. There is no classic set of cutaneous signs pathognomonic for food hypersensitivity in the dog. A variety of primary and secondary skin lesions are seen. These include papules, plaques, pustules, wheals, angioedema, erythema, ulcers, excoriation, lichenification, pigment changes, alopecia, scales, crusts, and moist erosions that appear as areas of pyotraumatic dermatitis (Fig. 8:12 *A;* also see Fig. 8:8 *G* and *H*). In general, the major complaint is pruritus, and the pruritus is nonseasonal and often poorly responsive to glucocorticoids. If the offending food is a snack or table food, the signs can be episodic, depending on how often the dog eats it. Any distribution of skin involvement may be seen, but the ears, distal limbs, axillae, and groin appear commonly affected.[216, 220, 226, 228] In some dogs, disease is limited to the ears or flea allergy area.[220, 228]

Pruritic, bilateral otitis externa (frequently with secondary bacterial or *Malassezia* infections) along with secondary seborrheic skin disease, bacterial pyoderma, or both are commonly seen in conjunction with food hypersensitivity.[214, 216, 220, 228] Secondary bacterial pyodermas most commonly present as superficial folliculitis, though folliculitis and furunculosis as well as bacterial pododermatitis may occur. Some dogs present with only a recurrent bacterial pyoderma, with or without pruritus, wherein all clinical signs resolve with antibiotic therapy.[220] Concurrent gastrointestinal disturbances (vomiting, diarrhea, colic) have been reported in 10 to 15 per cent of the dogs. In experimentally induced food hypersensitivity, the most common abnormality seen was an increase in the number of bowel movements. When food-hypersensitive dogs were fed diets containing the offending allergen, they averaged about 3 bowel movements per day, versus 1.5 bowel movements per day when fed an allergen-free diet. One author (CEG) has observed that pruritic dogs with more than three bowel movements per day are more likely to have food hypersensitivities as part of the reason for their pruritus. In humans, the noncutaneous symptoms associated with food hypersensitivity are numerous (''tension-fatigue syndrome''), and malaise and dullness have been observed in dogs. Seizures have been rarely described as being responsive to hypoallergenic diets.[40] Rosser had two dogs with a seizure history in his 51 food-hypersensitive dogs.[228]

Diagnosis

The differential diagnosis of canine food hypersensitivity consists of atopy, drug reaction, flea bite hypersensitivity, pediculosis, intestinal parasite hypersensitivity, scabies, *Malassezia* dermatitis, seborrheic skin disease, and bacterial folliculitis. At present, the definitive diagnosis of food hypersensitivity in dogs is reliably made only on the basis of elimination diets and test meal investigations. In the past it was (incorrectly) recommended that dogs suspected to have food-hypersensitivity be fed a ''hypoallergenic'' diet for 21 days. A 21-day protocol would have diagnosed only 26 per cent of the food-hypersensitive dogs in Rosser's prospective study.[228] This observation suggests that the incidence of food hypersensitivity may be much higher than previously thought. Studies have indicated that complete resolution or maximal improvement of clinical signs may require use of a hypoallergenic diet for 10 to 13 weeks.[216, 228]

Hypoallergenic diets must be individualized for each patient, on the basis of careful dietary history. The objectives of the diet are (1) to feed the animals dietary substances that they are not commonly exposed to and (2) to feed the animals a diet that is free of additives (colorings,

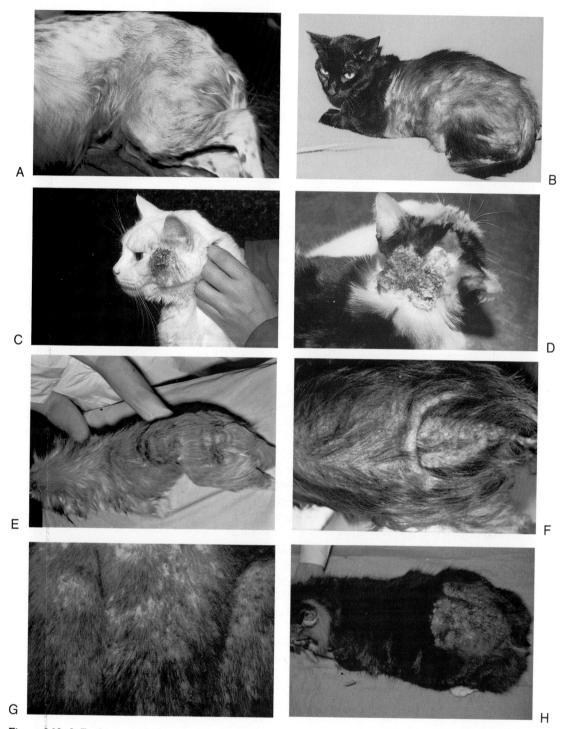

Figure 8:12. *A,* Erythema and alopecia over the lateral thighs of a dog with food hypersensitivity. *B,* Hypotrichosis of trunk and rump due to hair pulling in a cat with food hypersensitivity. *C,* Feline food hypersensitivity due to milk. Severe excoriation of the preauricular area. *D,* Feline food hypersensitivity due to fish. Severe excoriation of the neck. *E,* Chronic flea bite hypersensitivity in a Pekingese, showing alopecia, hyperpigmentation, and lichenification on the lower back and tail base. *F,* Canine flea bite hypersensitivity. After many seasons of affliction, area of the lower back and tail becomes hairless, thickened, gray, and folded. *G,* Feline flea bite hypersensitivity. The individual miliary lesions are shallow excoriations covered with a small brown crust. Some crusts have been removed to show the lesion's base. *H,* Feline flea bite hypersensitivity. Numerous miliary lesions clustered on the back of a cat. Area has been clipped to expose lesions.

flavorings, preservatives). Switching from one commercial diet to another or using commercially prepared ''hypoallergenic'' diets is not satisfactory. Frequently used components of a hypoallergenic diet include lamb, fileted whitefish, tuna fish canned in water, rabbit, venison, turkey, rice, and potatoes, depending on the dietary history.[40, 213, 232] These diets are usually not adequately balanced and, in young growing dogs, should not be fed without supplements.[229] Because the calcium content of such diets is particularly low, a nondairy calcium source as well as vitamins and essential fatty acids, at the minimum, should be added to the diet. An alternative protocol, though not as accurate as feeding a carefully selected home-prepared diet, is to feed a commercially prepared limited protein source diet. A variety of limited and different protein diets are now being manufactured by several companies, and they are very attractive because they are convenient and nutritionally complete.[215] It is critical to understand, however, that the reliability of virtually none of these commercially prepared diets has been confirmed in known food-hypersensitive dogs. To the authors' knowledge, only two commercial diets have undergone this kind of scrutiny: canned d/d and dry d/d manufactured by Hill's Pet Products. When known food-hypersensitive dogs were fed these two diets, 15 to 25 per cent became pruritic again.[222, 232]

Feeding a strict diet is critical, and the dog's owner must be counseled to allow nothing but water and the limited diet to enter the dog's mouth. The authors see many referred dogs whose owners have become frustrated because they believe that food hypersensitivity has been ruled out; on closer questioning, it is often determined that the dog is still eating the offending foods. The dogs may still be receiving treats such as rawhide chewies, flavored dietary supplements or medicines, or be receiving medication in food such as cheese or a piece of hot dog. The major clinical sign being evaluated during the elimination diet is the pruritus. The level of pruritus should markedly decrease, but this may be gradual and may take 4 to 8 weeks to become evident. Because up to 30 per cent of food-hypersensitive dogs have other concurrent hypersensitivities (especially atopy or flea bite hypersensitivity), the response to a hypoallergenic diet may be partial (for instance, 50 per cent reduction in pruritus).[214, 216, 220, 226, 228, 232] The diagnosis is then *confirmed* by feeding the animal its normal diet and seeing the dermatosis exacerbate in 10 to 14 days.[217, 220, 228]

Routine laboratory tests are not useful in diagnosing canine food hypersensitivity. Blood or tissue eosinophilia is rare in the dog.[40, 44, 213] Prick, scratch, intradermal, and serologic (RAST, ELISA) tests with food allergens in dogs with food hypersensitivity are worthless.[217, 222, 224, 231] One group of investigators was unable to demonstrate antigen-specific IgE antibodies in the serum of proven food-hypersensitive dogs using the P-K and oral P-K tests.[221] Numerous factors may influence the applicability of whole food extracts for skin testing and serologic testing, including the effects of cooking, processing, digestion, metabolism, additives, and contaminants on the original whole food substance. Gastroscopic food sensitivity testing has been described.[216a, 227] This modality would be inconvenient for routine clinical use, and further studies need to be done to determine its usefulness. The basophil degranulation test has also shown some promise for the diagnosis of food hypersensitivity, but larger, controlled studies are needed.[42, 43] This test is not currently available in the United States, requires rapid and special handling of blood, is very labor intensive, and is unlikely ever to be more than a research tool.

■ *Histopathology.* Skin biopsy reflects the variability of the gross morphology of skin lesions. It is usually characterized by varying degrees of superficial perivascular dermatitis (pure, spongiotic, hyperplastic), with mononuclear cells or neutrophils usually predominating.[17, 40, 63] Histopathologic changes consistent with secondary bacterial pyoderma are commonly present.

Clinical Management

The prognosis for food hypersensitivity is usually good. Therapy consists of avoiding offending foods or using systemic antipruritic agents. *Hypoallergenic* diets are formulated by adding single foodstuffs to the diet, one at a time, and evaluating each item for 10 to 14 days. In this way, a tolerable, varied diet can usually be achieved over the course of 4 to 6 months. Such diets need to be balanced with vitamin, mineral, and fatty acid supplements. As a compromise, animals can be ''provoked'' daily, for 10 to 14 days at a time, by being fed each of the major food items reported to cause food hypersensitivity in dogs (beef, dairy products, wheat, soy) to determine whether one of these items exacerbates the condition.[213, 220] On the basis of information obtained from this provocation, a commercial food that does not contain the offending substance can usually be selected. About 20 per cent of food-hypersensitive dogs, however, cannot consume *any* commercial diet and must be maintained on a home-prepared diet.[216, 226, 228, 232] Rarely, animals develop further dietary hypersensitivities and require re-evaluation by elimination diets and test meal investigations.

When hypoallergenic diets are not feasible, systemic glucocorticoids and/or antihistamines may be used to suppress clinical signs. Food hypersensitivity may, however, be difficult to control with these drugs. A complete response to systemic glucocorticoids is seen in only 50 per cent of food-hypersensitive dogs.[214, 216, 220, 228]

Feline Food Hypersensitivity

Feline food hypersensitivity (food allergy, food intolerance) is a nonseasonal pruritic skin disorder of cats that has been described for many years. This condition is described as both uncommon and the third most common hypersensitivity in the cat. The reported incidence ranges from 1 to 6 per cent of all feline dermatoses.[40, 214, 216] It has also been described as being relatively more common in cats than in dogs.[225] A report of 34 cats with the cutaneous reaction patterns of miliary dermatitis, eosinophilic granuloma complex, and self-induced alopecia indicated that food hypersensitivity was the second most common cause, accounting for 17 per cent of the cases.[176] Flea bite hypersensitivity was diagnosed in 70 per cent and atopy in 13 per cent of the cases, respectively. Further studies are warranted to determine the prevalence of these diseases. Little research, either clinical or experimental, has been done on food hypersensitivity in cats.

Cause and Pathogenesis

A type I hypersensitivity has been documented to occur in the cat.[230] The same report also showed, however, that IgG may also have been involved in the pathogenesis. The presence of concurrent flea bite hypersensitivity, atopy, contact hypersensitivity, or a combination of them suggests that a predisposition to allergies of any type may be a factor.[214, 225, 228] It additionally suggests that the mechanism may involve more than a type I hypersensitivity, because the associated diseases vary in their allergic mechanism. In most clinical cases, the pathomechanism is not determined, and in fact, only the association between diet and pruritus or dermatitis is established. Food intolerance, as discussed in the dog, may also play a role in the pathogenesis. Very little controlled work has been done regarding the offending allergens or materials in the diets that result in the dermatitis. In two studies, provocative exposure testing showed fish, beef, and dairy products to be the most common allergens.[234, 238] In two studies, about 30 per cent of the food-hypersensitive cats were unable to eat any commercially prepared diet without developing pruritus and dermatitis.[236, 238] Other studies have strongly implicated even such things as clam juice and lamb baby food.[214, 230, 235, 236] The frequent use and ready availability of commercial diets that contain lamb or other unusual protein sources is likely to induce some allergic reactions and make selecting a test diet more difficult. The authors and others[235] have seen cats present with or develop food hypersensitivity to lamb, both that found in commercial products and home-cooked. Table 8:16 lists all the foods currently reported to have caused food hypersensitivity in the cat.

Table 8:16. Substances Reported to Have Caused Food Hypersensitivity in the Cat

Dairy products (milk, cheese)	Lamb and mutton
Fish	Eggs
Beef	All commercial foods (various proteins, as well as preservatives
Pork	and dyes)
Chicken	Clam juice
Rabbit	Cod liver oil
Horse meat	Benzoic acid

Clinical Features

The mean age of onset of feline food hypersensitivity is 4 to 5 years, with no age predilection documented. In one study, however, 46 per cent of the cats developed the disease by 2 years of age.[236] Siamese or Siamese cross cats may be at risk, because they accounted for 30 per cent of the cases in two studies,[214, 236] and in one study had a relative risk factor of 5.0.[236] No sex predilection has been documented.

The most consistent clinical finding is pruritus, which is present in 100 per cent of the cases. The pruritus is typically nonseasonal. Some cats' owners like to rotate the commercial diets fed to their cats so as to provide variety, however. This practice can result in an irregularly recurrent pruritic dermatosis. Pruritus most commonly involves the face (Fig. 8:12 *C*), head, pinnae, and neck (Fig. 8:12 *D*), or combinations of these.* Generalized pruritus may also be seen.[20, 40, 225] The other common cutaneous reaction patterns are self-induced alopecia (Fig. 8:12 *B*), miliary dermatitis, and eosinophilic granuloma complex lesions. Rarely, cats manifest an erythematous papulopustular eruption characterized clinicopathologically as a sterile eosinophilic folliculitis and furunculosis.[190, 191] Other reported nonpruritic signs are angioedema, urticaria, and conjunctivitis.[20, 236] Gastrointestinal (usually diarrhea but also vomiting) disease is present in 10 to 15 per cent of the cases.[40, 44, 234] Lymphocytic-plasmocytic colitis may be a manifestation of food hypersensitivity in cats.[233] Sneezing, malaise, and dullness have been reported.[40, 214] Peripheral lymphadenopathy, which can be quite marked, may be present.[189]

Up to 25 per cent of food-hypersensitive cats have other concurrent hypersensitivities, especially atopy or flea bite hypersensitivity.[214, 236] These multiple hypersensitivities can greatly complicate the diagnostic work-up. About 50 per cent of food-hypersensitive cats do not completely respond to systemic glucocorticoids.[214, 216, 236]

Diagnosis

The differential diagnosis varies according to the clinical presentation. The most common alternatives are atopy, flea bite hypersensitivity, psychogenic alopecia and dermatitis, dermatophytosis, otodectic mange, cheyletiellosis, and notoedric mange. The diagnosis is suggested by utilizing an elimination diet trial that results in a significant reduction in the clinical signs. The diagnosis is confirmed if clinical signs recur when the cat is fed its previous diet.

Hypoallergenic diets must be individualized for each cat according to previous dietary history. Some common favorites are lamb or ham baby food, ground rabbit, and venison. One of these may be fed alone or mixed in a blender with potato or rice. Studies have shown that these diets are not nutritionally balanced and feeding them to young growing animals could lead to a deficiency disease.[229] Therefore, it may be prudent to recommend that the diet be at least supplemented with taurine tablets, calcium tablets (dicalcium phosphate), safflower oil, and a multiple vitamin that does not contain additives. Commercially prepared ''hypoallergenic'' diets are not reliable. In some cases, however, such a diet is all the client will agree to

---

*See references 214, 216, 226, 234, 236, 238, and 239.

try. In these instances, the client should be told that negative results do not rule out the possibility of food hypersensitivity and that a diet with totally different ingredients from the cat's previous diet should be utilized. The number of commercially prepared ''hypoallergenic'' diets is increasing daily, or so it seems.[215] It is essential to remember that, with very few exceptions, none of these diets has been scientifically evaluated in confirmed food-hypersensitive cats. To the authors' knowledge, only two commercial diets have been evaluated in cats—canned d/d for dogs, and feline d/d, manufactured by Hill's Pet Products—and about 20 per cent of the cats became pruritic and dermatitic while consuming these products.[237, 238] In many cases, to adequately perform the dietary trial, the cat may have to remain completely indoors.[225] Studies have shown that the previously recommended 3-week dietary trial is not adequate.[214, 216, 236] Improvement may occur rapidly, gradually, or late, but the diet should be continued for 9 to 13 weeks so that maximum response is achieved. Cats that have concurrent atopy or flea bite hypersensitivity show a partial response. To confirm the diagnosis, the cat is then fed its former diet for 10 to 14 days to see whether the pruritus or dermatitis is reproduced.[216, 236]

Intradermal allergy testing and serologic tests are believed to suffer from the same problems as discussed for canine food hypersensitivity—that is to say, they are *worthless*!

■ *Histopathology.* Skin biopsy is not diagnostic but is especially useful for ruling out other diagnostic possibilities.[17, 63, 191] The histopathologic findings are quite variable, as are the clinical lesions (see discussion of feline atopy). The most common reaction pattern is a superficial or deep perivascular dermatitis wherein eosinophils are the dominant inflammatory cell.[191] Some cases are seen that lack eosinophils, whereas others are primarily composed of a dense infiltrate of mast cells that may be misinterpreted as mast cell neoplasia.[17] Eosinophilic folliculitis and furunculosis may occasionally be a feature of feline food hypersensitivity.[17, 191] Biopsy specimens from eosinophilic granuloma complex lesions show the typical histopathologic findings for those lesions (see Chap. 17).

Clinical Management

The optimum treatment for feline food hypersensitivity is the avoidance of the offending allergen(s). This is best accomplished by feeding a limited protein source commercial diet, alleviating the problem of having to balance a home-prepared diet. Examples of limited-protein diets are Feline d/d (Hill's Pet Products), Rabbit and Rice (Nature's Recipe), and Chicken formula cat food (Iams). Fortunately, the pet food industry has been responding to this problem by developing new diets with atypical protein sources in them. About 30 per cent of food-hypersensitive cats, however, cannot be successfully managed with *any* commercially prepared diet. It is especially important that a home-prepared diet to be fed long-term be balanced and, at the minimum, supplemented with calcium, taurine, essential fatty acids, vitamins, and minerals. The supplements required depend on the diet, and consultation with a nutrition text or nutritionist may be necessary. The development of a hypersensitivity to a component of the new diet may occur,[235] and it has been suggested that this development is more common in cats than dogs.[225] One author (CEG) has seen a cat that developed new allergies to three consecutive diets over 2 years, at which point the client elected to treat with glucocorticoids long-term. In other situations, avoidance is impossible because the cat is outdoors and finds other sources of allergenic substances to eat. In these cases, systemic glucocorticoids, antihistamines, or fatty acids may be utilized (see Chap. 3). The efficacy of antihistamines and fatty acids for the management of food-hypersensitive cats has not been reported. In cases, however, that require high levels of systemic glucocorticoids or that do not respond to them, antihistamines and fatty acids may have a beneficial effect.

Parasitic Hypersensitivity

Parasites are known to be potent inducers of IgE and often elicit an eosinophilic response.[19, 20] Therefore, it is not surprising that they commonly induce hypersensitivity reactions in dogs and cats.

CANINE FLEA BITE HYPERSENSITIVITY

Flea bite hypersensitivity (flea allergy dermatitis) is a pruritic, papular dermatitis in dogs that become sensitized to allergens produced by fleas. It is the most common hypersensitivity skin disorder in dogs.

Cause and Pathogenesis

Flea saliva and whole flea extracts contain several potentially antigenic substances, including polypeptides, amino acids, aromatic compounds, and fluorescent materials. These substances are complete antigens, and not haptens as was previously described for the guinea pig. Multiple studies have shown that at least 15 different antigens are present. Gel filtration of flea saliva revealed that allergens were present in a high-molecular-weight fraction (about 4000 to 1,500,000 daltons) and in a highly fluorescent aromatic fraction (less than 1000 daltons). Individual dogs may react to completely different groups of allergens, though the most consistently reacting allergens appear in the range of 25 to 58 kD.[19, 20, 40, 244, 249] It was also demonstrated that *Ctenocephalides felis felis, Pulex irritans,* and *Pulex simulans* shared one or more antigens and that guinea pigs and human beings sensitized to one type of flea reacted to all species.

Most dogs that are hypersensitive to flea saliva have immediate skin test reactions to the intradermal injection of flea antigen, indicating a type I hypersensitivity reaction and an antigen with a molecular weight of 5 to 100 kD (nonhaptenic).[20, 40, 44] The orderly sequence of flea hypersensitivity that develops in guinea pigs does not occur in dogs and cats,[19, 20, 40] and dogs and cats rarely, if ever, achieve natural desensitization.[40, 44] Many flea-hypersensitive dogs also have delayed skin test reactions, and up to 30 per cent have only a delayed reaction.[130, 240] Biopsy specimens taken from skin lesions that are 4 to 18 hours old show changes compatible with cutaneous basophil hypersensitivity, and specimens from lesions that are 24 to 48 hours old, changes compatible with a delayed-type hypersensitivity reaction.[20, 241, 244] It has been suggested that late-phase IgE-mediated reactions are also involved in canine flea bite hypersensitivity.[19] It is likely that animals do *not* develop skin lesions as a result of flea infestation unless they are flea hypersensitive.

Studies on intradermal allergy test reactions to flea antigen and on the serum levels of antiflea IgE and IgG in flea-naive dogs, experimentally maintained dogs, as well as dogs kept as pets or in animal shelters with and without flea bite hypersensitivity have indicated that dogs continually exposed to fleas and flea-naive dogs have low antibody levels and negative intradermal tests reactions compared with flea-hypersensitive dogs. These observations suggest that continually exposed dogs may become partially or completely immunologically tolerant.[19, 20, 243] Experimentally, intermittent flea exposure was shown to induce both immediate and delayed intradermal reactions, and converting from intermittent to continuous exposure did not eliminate these reactions.[19, 20, 243] It has been suggested that, if a dog has an abundance of fleas and no evidence of a hypersensitivity reaction, it might be prudent to refrain from introducing a diligent flea-control program.[20, 40]

Whereas up to 40 per cent of the normal dog population in flea-endemic areas may have positive intradermal allergy test reactions to flea antigen, up to 80 per cent of the atopic dogs in the same area may be positive.[19, 20, 40] This finding suggests that the atopic state may predispose dogs to developing flea bite hypersensitivity. Another study, however, indicated that only 36 per cent of atopic dogs were also flea hypersensitive.[82]

Clinical Features

Most authors indicate that no breed or sex predilections are apparent.[40, 44] In a French study, however, setters, Fox terriers, Pekingese, spaniels, and Chow Chows were predisposed.[82] Although dogs may develop flea bite hypersensitivity at any age, it is rare for clinical signs to develop in animals less than 6 months of age. The most common age of onset is 3 to 5 years.

Canine flea bite hypersensitivity is characterized by a pruritic, papular dermatitis.[40, 44, 240, 247] The flea bite induces a wheal or papule that persists for up to 72 hours. Crusts may develop on the surface of the papules. Chronic pruritus may lead to alopecia, lichenification, crusting, and hyperpigmentation. Lesions are typically confined to the dorsal lumbosacral area, caudomedial thighs, ventral abdomen, and flanks (Fig. 8:12 *E* and *F*). Crusted papules in the umbilical area may be particularly suggestive of flea bite hypersensitivity. Generalized cutaneous signs may be present in severely hypersensitive animals. Pyotraumatic dermatitis ("hot spots"), secondary bacterial pyoderma, and secondary seborrhea are common in chronic cases. Owing to the constant, excessive chewing, some dogs wear down their incisors. Fibropruritic nodules are occasionally seen in chronic cases and are usually present in the dorsal lumbar area (see Chap. 19).

The presence of otitis externa, severe pedal pruritus, or facial pruritus strongly suggests the presence of another concurrent hypersensitivity, such as atopy or food hypersensitivity. Flea bite hypersensitivity is usually distinctly seasonal (summer and fall) in areas of the world with cold winters. In warm climates, or where household infestation persists, flea bite hypersensitivity may be nonseasonal, although clinical signs are still usually more severe in summer and fall.

Diagnosis

The differential diagnosis includes food hypersensitivity, atopy, drug reaction, pediculosis, cheyletiellosis, intestinal parasite hypersensitivity, *Malassezia* dermatitis, and bacterial folliculitis.

Definitive diagnosis is based on history, physical examination, intradermal skin testing with flea antigen, and response to therapy. The morphology and distribution of the skin lesions are very suggestive. The presence of fleas or flea dirt is also a helpful finding and optimally is found. It has also been suggested that a diagnosis cannot be made without evidence of fleas.[19] A recent bath or dip or vigorous grooming, however, may eliminate the fleas and flea dirt. In fact, 15 per cent of the dogs with flea bite hypersensitivity do not have evidence of flea infestation (fleas, flea excrement) at the time of examination.[82] In the authors' opinion, not finding evidence of fleas does not rule out the diagnosis, but it does cause one to question the diagnosis. More importantly, the mere presence of fleas on a pruritic dog does not mean the animal has flea bite hypersensitivity. In fact, the diagnosis of flea hypersensitivity does not preclude the presence of another disease. When fleas consistently are not seen on flea-hypersensitive dogs, and the client has performed adequate flea control, the persistence of pruritus should prompt the clinician to look for a concurrent hypersensitivity such as atopy or food hypersensitivity. Eosinophilia is often present.[40]

■ *Histopathology.* Skin biopsy is nondiagnostic, revealing varying degrees of superficial perivascular (pure, spongiotic, hyperplastic) to interstitial dermatitis, with eosinophils often being a predominant cell type.[17, 40, 63, 241] In addition, eosinophilic intra-epidermal microabscesses in association with epidermal edema and necrosis (epidermal nibbles) may be seen (Fig. 8:13). Histopathologic findings consistent with secondary bacterial pyoderma (suppurative folliculitis, intraepidermal pustular dermatitis) are common.

Intradermal testing is an excellent method to help confirm the diagnosis of flea bite hypersensitivity. In the United States, one commercial aqueous flea antigen (Flea Antigen, Greer Laboratories) has emerged as a very reliable product.[20, 40, 44] This product is injected intradermally (0.05 ml of 1:1000 w/v aqueous solution), along with positive (histamine) and negative

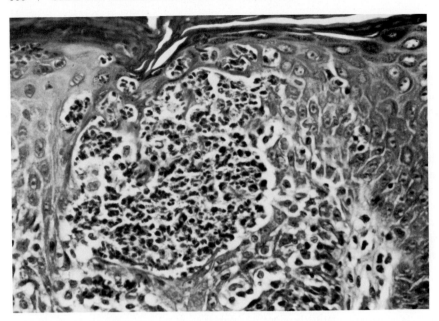

Figure 8:13. Canine flea bite hypersensitivity. Epidermal eosinophilic microabscess.

(saline) controls, and skin reactions are read at 15 and 30 minutes and at 12, 24, and 48 hours. The majority of flea-hypersensitive dogs have both immediate and delayed reactions. About 30 per cent have only delayed reactions. The delayed reactions are often very mild compared with the typical immediate reaction. The only change may be mild erythema or increased dermal thickness. It is essential to remember that a positive test reaction *only* means that the patient has skin-sensitizing antibody or a cellular response to flea antigen. It does *not* necessarily mean that the patient has clinical hypersensitivity. Thus, although virtually all flea-hypersensitive dogs and cats have positive skin test reactions to flea antigen, so does a portion of the normal dog population, and so do some dogs with other dermatoses. Current or recent administration of drugs, especially glucocorticoids and progestogens, can cause false-negative intradermal test reactions. In some cases, a positive reaction in a dog on glucocorticoid therapy is reliable.[246, 247] With negative reactions, however, testing should be repeated after a longer period of steroid withdrawal. It is also recommended to test for house dust or house dust mites at the same time.[32, 130] This limited intradermal test with saline, histamine, flea, and house dust mite antigens allows for the recognition of many dogs that have concurrent atopy. A positive house dust mite reaction occurs in about 50 per cent of the atopic dogs.

In vitro (serologic) tests are offered for diagnosis of flea bite hypersensitivity. In an experimental laboratory evaluation, the in vitro tests were valuable if the flea antigen was optimized by partial purification.[19] The current available commercial tests are of questionable value, however. First, they detect only IgE-mediated disease, and up to 30 per cent of flea-hypersensitive dogs primarily have delayed intradermal reactions. Second, in contrast to results with other allergen tests, one of the authors (CEG) has seen many negative results in flea-hypersensitive dogs that had positive immediate intradermal skin test reactions. Lastly, some normal dogs had positive serologic test results, suggesting that both sensitivity and specificity need to be further evaluated.

Clinical Management

In general, it has been classically thought that flea bite hypersensitivity in dogs tends to worsen as the animals age. Clinical signs begin a little earlier in the season, persist a little longer, and tend to become progressively more severe. Naturally occurring desensitization is apparently rare. This concept has come into question, however, with some evidence that occasional dogs improve as they age.[19]

Therapy of flea bite hypersensitivity may include flea control (see Chap. 6), systemic glucocorticoids, and hyposensitization.[247] Flea control and glucocorticoids are usually quite effective for the management of short-term or long-term flea bite hypersensitivity in colder climates but are less so in subtropical to tropical climates. Prednisolone or prednisone is given orally at 1 mg/kg daily for 5 to 7 days and then in an alternate-day regimen (see Chap. 3), as needed. Dogs with severe flea bite hypersensitivity and heavy flea exposure may require 2.2 mg/kg daily to achieve remission, and then need much higher alternate-day dosages. If gluco-corticoids are undesirable or unsatisfactory, some flea-hypersensitive dogs may respond to antihistamines (chlorpheniramine, 0.4 mg/kg q8h orally; diphenhydramine, 2.2 mg/kg q8h orally; or hydroxyzine, 2.2 mg/kg q8h orally) or omega-3/omega-6 fatty acid–containing products.[145] Of course, the single most effective therapy would be separating the fleas from the pet or eliminating the fleas. This involves concentrating extermination efforts on the indoor and outdoor premises. Aggressive flea control programs are necessary (see Chap. 6). Repellents need to be applied frequently to dogs that visit outdoor areas that cannot be adequately treated for fleas. Employing a skillful commercial exterminator, often the most effective way of controlling fleas, is highly recommended.

The efficacy of hyposensitization in canine flea bite hypersensitivity is still controversial. Enthusiastic proponents and outspoken critics abound.[40, 44] Double-blind controlled studies in dogs showed that hyposensitization with aqueous[242] and alum-precipitated[245, 248] whole flea antigens is rarely effective as well as being expensive and time consuming. Hyposensitization was used for only 3 to 4 months in these studies, however, a much shorter time than that used for atopy (see discussion of canine atopy). Longer-term hyposensitization should be assessed in flea-hypersensitive dogs as well. On the basis of current information, treatment of canine flea bite hypersensitivity with commercially available whole flea extracts should be viewed as a last-ditch therapeutic effort that has a slim chance of success. In such instances, one could try any of the commercially available whole flea extracts: Flea Antigen (Hollister-Stier Laboratories, Haver-Lockhart Laboratories, Center Laboratories, or Greer Laboratories) or Whole Flea Extract (Nelco Laboratories). Injections are given intradermally, 0.5 to 1.0 ml once weekly, to effect (9 to 12 months?). If results are successful, booster injections can then be administered as needed (every 1 to 3 months).

FELINE FLEA BITE HYPERSENSITIVITY

Feline flea bite hypersensitivity (flea allergy dermatitis) is the most common feline hypersensitivity disease in areas where fleas are present, causing a variety of clinical syndromes all characterized by pruritus.

Cause and Pathogenesis

Though much research has been done on flea bite hypersensitivity in the dog and guinea pig, very little has been done in the cat.[19, 40] This is particularly interesting, because cats are used to maintain both research and commercial populations of the cat flea, *Ctenocephalides felis felis.* The guinea pig and dog have very different immunopathogenic responses to flea antigen; therefore, it may be inappropriate to assume that cats will react like either species. Most flea-hypersensitive cats have immediate positive intradermal test reactions to flea antigen. Delayed skin test reactions have *not* been reported in flea-hypersensitive cats.[40, 44, 251] The lack of delayed reactions suggests that the pathogenesis is different or that delayed reactions in the cat are very mild and easily missed.

Clinical Features

No age, breed, or sex predilections have been reported. Papulocrustous eruptions are the most typical lesions of flea bite hypersensitivity in the cat (Fig. 8:12 *G*). Alopecia, excoriations, crusts, and scales may also be found. Pigment changes may occur, and multifocal small melanotic macules are evidence of previous inflammatory sites (Fig. 8:14). Lesions are typically confined to the dorsal lumbosacral area (Fig. 8:12 *H*), caudomedial thighs, ventral abdomen, flanks, and neck. This cutaneous reaction pattern, referred to as *miliary dermatitis,* is particularly common in cats and may be caused by a number of specific diseases (Table 8:17). Generalized cutaneous signs may be present in severely hypersensitive animals. Flea-hypersensitive cats may also present with (1) self-induced symmetric alopecia (little or no dermatitis) or (2) eosinophilic granuloma complex lesions (indolent ulcer, eosinophilic plaque, eosinophilic granuloma, or some combination of these three lesions) (see Chap. 17).[40, 44, 193, 252] In addition, any given cat may manifest various combinations of these reaction patterns. Secondary bacterial pyoderma is occasionally seen. Cats with flea bite hypersensitivity may develop moderate to marked peripheral lymphadenopathy.[189] Rarely, cats manifest an erythematous papulopustular eruption characterized clinicopathologically as a sterile eosonophilic folliculitis and furunculosis.[190] Disease often becomes more severe as the cats age. Cats with flea bite hypersensitivity may have concurrent atopy and/or food hypersensitivity, which can greatly complicate the diagnostic work-up as well as the therapeutic regimen.

Diagnosis

The differential diagnosis depends on which clinical syndrome is being examined. Most commonly, the differential for miliary dermatitis (see Table 8:17) must be considered, with atopy, food hypersensitivity, cheyletiellosis, and dermatophytosis being the primary alternatives in most cases. The diagnosis is based on the history and physical findings. The presence of fleas, flea dirt, flea eggs, or infestation with the tapeworm *Dipylidium caninum* all provide circumstantial evidence. Recent bathing or grooming may, however, remove all evidence of fleas. Neither does the mere presence of fleas on a cat with one of the typical cutaneous reaction patterns confirm that the fleas are causing the dermatosis. Cytologic examination of papulocrustous lesions and eosinophilic granuloma complex lesions usually demonstrates numerous eosin-

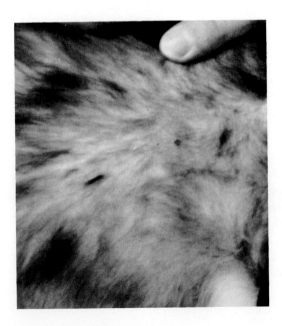

Figure 8:14. Feline flea bite hypersensitivity. Multiple foci of melanoderma/melanotrichia are evidence of previous dermatitis.

Table 8:17. Differential Diagnosis of Widespread Papulocrustous Dermatitis ("Miliary Dermatitis") in the Cat

Hypersensitivity reactions	Flea bite hypersensitivity
	Atopy
	Food hypersensitivity
	Drug reaction
	Intestinal parasite hypersensitivity
	Pemphigus foliaceus
	Feline hypereosinophilic syndrome
Ectoparasitisms	Cheyletiellosis
	Otodectic mange
	Trombiculiasis
	Cat fur mite
	Pediculosis
Infections	Dermatophytosis
	Staphylococcal folliculitis
Dietary imbalances	Biotin deficiency
	Fatty acid deficiency

ophils and occasional basophils (Fig. 8:15). Eosinophilia, occasionally with basophilia, is often present.

■ *Histopathology.* Skin biopsy is not diagnostic but typically shows varying degrees of superficial or deep perivascular to interstitial dermatitis with numerous eosinophils and mast cells.[17, 40, 63, 191] Cats presenting with clinical lesions of indolent ulcer, eosinophilic plaque, and eosinophilic granuloma have dermatohistopathologic findings consistent with those entities (see Chap. 17).

Intradermal allergy testing with flea antigen, as described for the dog, produces a positive immediate reaction.[40, 251, 252] One should remember that a positive intradermal reaction to flea antigen *only* means that the cat is sensitized to the antigens; it does *not* prove that the cat has clinical flea bite hypersensitivity. In one study, 36 per cent of the clinically normal cats that had exposure to fleas had positive immediate skin test reaction to flea antigen.[251] It is also useful to test at the same time with house dust mite to investigate the possibility of concurrent atopy.[32]

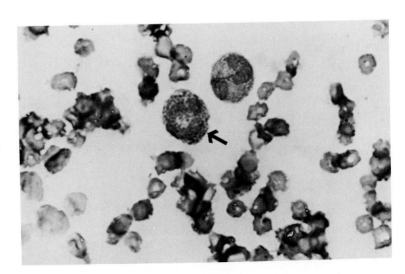

Figure 8:15. Feline flea bite hypersensitivity. Cytologic examination reveals numerous eosinophils and smaller numbers of basophils (*arrow*).

Clinical Management

Therapy of flea bite hypersensitivity includes vigorous flea control and is most successful in cats kept predominantly indoors or in a controlled environment (see Chap. 6).[247] For roaming outdoor cats, flea repellents are helpful, but they must be applied daily and are not tolerated by many cats. Repositol methylprednisolone acetate (5 mg/kg or 20 mg per cat subcutaneously every 12 weeks) or oral prednisone or prednisolone (2.2 mg/kg q24h orally for 5 to 7 days then on an alternate-day basis) are most commonly utilized for short-term relief of the hypersensitivity, or when flea control is ineffective (see Chap. 3). With severe flea infestations, the dosages of these glucocorticoids may have to be doubled or a different glucocorticoid may be needed (see Chap. 3) to achieve an adequate response. Chlorpheniramine (2 to 4 mg per cat q12h orally) or hydroxyzine (2 mg/kg q12h orally) may also be effective.[193, 252] Hyposensitization in cats has been shown to be ineffective for most cases, though an occasional cat may have a dramatic response.[250]

FELINE MOSQUITO BITE HYPERSENSITIVITY

Feline mosquito bite hypersensitivity has been described as a clinical entity in cats.[253, 254] The original descriptions of this syndrome came from Australia,[255] but not until 1988 was the etiology confirmed.[254] This is an uncommon, seasonal, predominantly facial dermatitis of cats.

Cause and Pathogenesis

An excellent study by Mason and Evans[254] documented the mosquito as the cause of this syndrome. Lesions were shown to resolve without treatment when affected cats were confined to a mosquito-free environment. Following challenge with mosquito bites, lesions developed at the sites of the bites. In addition, previously normal-haired skin was shaved and challenged with mosquito bites. Again, these sites developed the typical lesions. Intradermal allergy testing with mosquito antigen indicates that one component of the pathogenesis may involve a type I hypersensitivity. Histopathologic findings, however, include an initially perivascular, then diffuse to nodular dermatitis with an intense eosinophilic infiltrate and foci of collagen degeneration. These latter findings are not seen in typical type I reactions, suggesting that more is involved in the pathogenesis of this disorder.

Clinical Features

To date, no age, breed, or sex predilections have been recognized. The disease is seasonal, coinciding with the mosquito season. Affected cats are kept outdoors or allowed access to the outdoors. Pruritus is usually present, but the severity is variable. The earlier lesions consist of erythematous papules to plaques that often have an erosive or ulcerated, necrotic or crusted appearance (see Fig. 8:16 E). Chronic lesions include nodules, pigment changes (melanoderma or leukoderma), alopecia, and scaling (see Fig. 8:16 F). The development of multiple lesions often results in a polycyclic plaque or patch of alopecia interspersed with areas of acute lesions, scale, or crust. These lesions are usually found on the bridge of the nose and the medial aspects of the pinnae. The nasal planum and nasal philtrum may be involved and have small punctate crusted depressions. Footpads may also be affected with swelling, hyperkeratosis, fissures, and pigment changes.[254] Less commonly, the chin and lips may be affected.[253] Lymphadenopathy and, in acute cases, pyrexia may be seen.

Diagnosis

The major components of the differential diagnosis are pemphigus foliaceus or erythematosus, atopy, food hypersensitivity, and dermatophytosis. In endemic areas, feline poxvirus infection is also an alternative. The clinical presentation is fairly distinctive, and the tentative diagnosis is relatively well confirmed by keeping the cat indoors or hospitalized for 5 days, at which point the lesions are much improved. If confinement is not possible, the use of repellents on the affected areas may help establish the diagnosis. In other cases, this may be impossible or ineffective, and ruling out other possible diagnoses by biopsy and other laboratory tests helps establish a diagnosis.

■ *Histopathology.*   Skin biopsy reveals severe superficial and deep eosinophilic inflammation which is initially perivascular, then interstitial, and finally diffuse.[17, 254] Collagen degeneration, dermal mucinosis, and eosinophilic folliculitis and furunculosis are often present. Similar histopathologic changes can occur in cats with atopy, food hypersensitivity, and flea bite hypersensitivity.[191]

Clinical Management

Confinement indoors during the mosquito season, or at least during the peak mosquito feeding time, is beneficial. If this is not possible, reposital methylprednisolone acetate (20 mg per cat or 5 mg/kg subcutaneously) is usually effective and relatively safe, because this entity is a seasonal problem. Alternatively, oral glucocorticoids may be utilized (see Chap. 3). In all cases, but especially those in which glucocorticoids cannot be used, mosquito repellents in the form of pyrethrins with MGK 264, dimethyl metatolulimide (DEET), or butoxypolypropylene are helpful. Repellents do not need to be applied to the whole body, only to the short-haired and sparsely-haired areas.

INSECT AND ARACHNID HYPERSENSITIVITY

Numerous insects and arachnids exist in the normal dog and cat environment that may stimulate an immune response.[261] These hypersensitivity reactions induce a pruritic disease that involves short or sparsely haired areas.

Cause and Pathogenesis

Insects and arachnids are known to produce a number of potentially allergenic substances that may be present in their saliva, feces, or exoskeletons.[256, 258–260] Dogs have been shown to develop IgE antibodies to a variety of these allergens.[258, 259] In humans, the insect allergens may be injected (by bite or sting), inhaled, or absorbed percutaneously and induce the allergic reaction.[37] How allergen access occurs in dogs and cats has not been documented but is believed to be similar to what occurs in humans. These hypersensitivities are commonly seen in atopic animals and may even be considered a subcategory of atopy. In about 50 per cent of suspected atopic dogs that have negative intradermal test reactions to routine allergens (pollens, molds, epithelia, flea, and housedust mites), however, positive intradermal reactions to one or more insects or arachnids are present.[259]

Clinical Features

No age, breed, or sex predilections have been described. The onset may be sudden and occasionally is historically correlated with an increase in insect or arachnid numbers in the animal's environment. The primary symptom is pruritus, though an erythematous maculopapular dermatitis may be present. Depending on the offending allergen, these cases may be seasonal, with clinical signs being worst in warm weather. Chronic pruritus can lead to secondary alopecia, crusting, lichenification, and secondary bacterial pyoderma. Occasionally in chronic cases, nodules or firm plaques are present. Glabrous skin or short-haired areas are more commonly affected. As a result, the abdomen, groin, axillae, face, distal extremities, and pinnae are most commonly affected.

Diagnosis

The differential diagnosis consists of atopy, scabies, food hypersensitivity, bacterial folliculitis and furunculosis, and contact hypersensitivity. A helpful feature differentiating this type of hypersensitivity from atopy that may be seen in some cases is the presence of a papular dermatitis not associated with bacterial folliculitis.

The diagnosis is suggested by a compatible history and physical findings and is confirmed by positive intradermal test reactions to insect or arachnid antigens. Intradermal allergy testing, as described for atopy, is performed with the antigens listed in Table 8:18. Cytologic examination of a specimen taken from a papule may reveal a mixture of neutrophils and eosinophils.

■ **Histopathology.** Histopathology has not been reported for a large group of cases, but in limited numbers of animals, a hyperplastic superficial perivascular dermatitis with mononuclear cells, mast cells, and some eosinophils was found. Nodular and plaque-like lesions, additionally, show a multinodular lymphocytic to granulomatous dermatitis with numerous eosinophils.

Clinical Management

Avoidance, if possible, is the treatment of choice, but some insect and arachnid allergens are significantly aerosolized during peak seasons, making their avoidance impossible.[260] Avoidance is best accomplished by keeping the animals indoors as much as possible and utilizing an aggressive insect control regimen such as described for flea control (see Chap. 6). Medical management with glucocorticoids is usually effective. Prednisone, 1 mg/kg q24h until the condition is controlled (3 to 7 days), then on an alternate-day regimen, is most commonly utilized. Antihistamines and fatty acids (see Chap. 3) may also be tried, though their efficacy is not as good.

CANINE EOSINOPHILIC FURUNCULOSIS OF THE FACE

Canine eosinophilic furunculosis of the face is an acute, predominantly nasal and muzzle disease that seems very severe but is generally self-limiting or exquisitely responsive to glucocorticoids.

Table 8:18. Results of Intradermal Tests to Insects and Arachnids in 193 Suspect Atopic Dogs*

Antigen	% of Dogs with 3+ or 4+ Reactions	PNU
Black fly	11.4	1000
Mosquito	7.8	1000
Deer fly	9.3	1000
Horsefly	17.1	1000
Red ant	5.7	1000
Black ant	4.2	1000
Housefly	Not done	1000
Cockroach	Not done	1000

*Southern California.

Cause and Pathogenesis

This syndrome has been described in nine dogs in which the common potential inciting feature was exposure to bees or wasps.[265] The authors (DWS, WHM) have seen identical cases in winter (no flying insects present), wherein the dogs had been seen playing with or following spiders. A similar-looking, but chronic case was seen by one of the authors (CEG) in which intradermal allergy test reactions to blackfly and horsefly were positive. Eosinophils were numerous on cytologic evaluation of this dog. Because of the chronic history of the case and the lack of histopathologic evaluation, however, it may represent a different syndrome. Eosinophilic furunculosis of the face has been proposed to be some type of hypersensitivity reaction to an attack by some insect or arthropod.[265, 266] The exact pathomechanism is unknown, and further studies are needed regarding both pathomechanism and etiology.

Clinical Features

Age of onset was under 2 years in about 50 per cent of the affected dogs. Specific breed predilections are not yet determined, but typically, large or midsize breeds are affected. Toy and miniature breeds have not been described with this syndrome. No sex predilection has been determined. Onset is very acute; often the dog is normal when it goes outside but returns home within hours with fully developed lesions present. The severity of the reaction often peaks within 24 hours, and the course with just antibiotics or without treatment is 14 to 21 days. The dogs present with papules, nodules, and varying degrees of ulceration, hemorrhage, and crusts. Pruritus is usually absent or mild, but the lesions may be painful. Early lesions were described as erythematous or hemorrhagic blisters or papules. Lesions are present on the bridge of the nose, on the muzzle, and often periocularly (Fig. 8:16 *A* and *B*). Occasionally, lesions may be seen on the trunk (especially the relatively glabrous ventral abdomen and thorax) or pinnae.

Diagnosis

The differential diagnosis is staphylococcal nasal folliculitis and furunculosis. If lesions persist, then dermatophytosis may also be considered. Eosinophilic furunculosis of the face has a striking history and appearance, however, making a clinical diagnosis rather simple. Cytologic examination reveals numerous eosinophils. Occasionally, degenerate neutrophils with intracellular bacteria are seen, but they probably reflect a secondary bacterial pyoderma.

■ *Histopathology.* Skin biopsy and examination reveals eosinophilic folliculitis, perifolliculitis, and furunculosis (Figs. 8:17 and 8:18).[17, 265] Neutrophils, lymphocytes, and macrophages are also present in smaller numbers. Marked dermal and subcutaneous mucinosis and ulceration are commonly seen. Focal or multifocal areas of dermal hemorrhage or collagen degeneration (flame figures) are also often found.

Clinical Management

The prognosis is excellent. Systemic glucocorticoid therapy is very effective, with the majority of dogs responding within 36 hours and lesions being completely resolved with 10 to 14 days. Oral prednisone, 1 to 2 mg/kg q24h until lesions have greatly resolved, then on an alternate-day basis for 10 more days, is usually effective, although repositol glucocorticoids could potentially be utilized because long-term therapy is not required.

CANINE SCABIES

Hypersensitivity appears to play a considerable role in canine, porcine, and human scabies.[13, 40, 261] In humans and dogs, dermatologic changes are often completely out of proportion to the

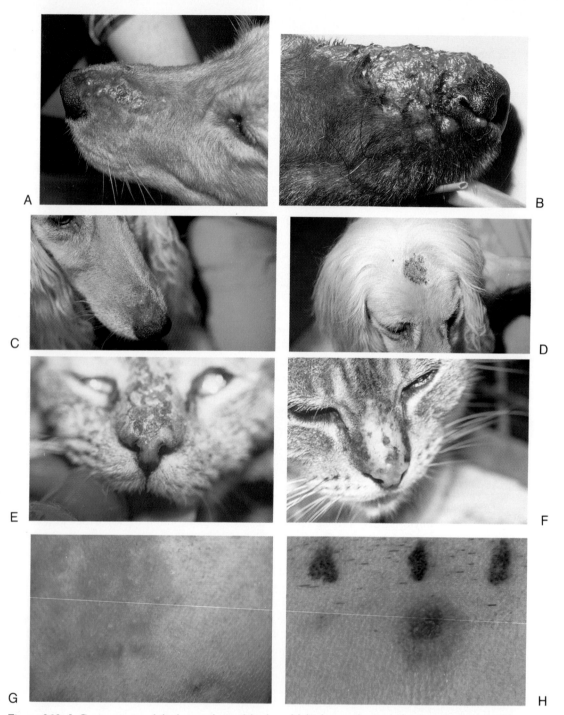

Figure 8:16. *A,* Canine eosinophilic furunculosis of the face. Multiple papules and ulcers on the bridge of the nose and upper eyelid associated with exposure to wasps. *B,* Canine eosinophilic furunculosis of the face. Erythematous papules and ulcerated, oozing nasal plaque. (Courtesy K. V. Mason) *C,* Erythematous papules on bridge of nose of a dog with cutaneous dirofilariasis. *D,* Ulcerated, crusted nodule on head of a dog with cutaneous dirofilariasis. *E,* Feline mosquito bite hypersensitivity. Plaquelike swelling, ulceration, and depigmentation of bridge of nose and nasal planum. *F,* Feline mosquito bite hypersensitivity. Note presence of mosquito on depigmented, alopecic bridge of nose and nasal planum. (Courtesy K. V. Mason) *G,* Multiple erythematous pustules on the abdomen of a dog with bacterial hypersensitivity. (From Scott, D.W., et al.: Staphylococcal hypersensitivity in the dog. J. Am. Anim. Hosp. Assoc. 14:766, 1978.) *H,* Hemorrhagic bulla skin test reaction 48 hours after the intradermal injection of *Staphylococcus aureus* bacterin-toxoid (Staphoid A–B) in a dog with bacterial hypersensitivity. (From Scott, D.W., et al.: Staphylococcal hypersensitivity in the dog. J. Am. Anim. Hosp. Assoc. 14:766, 1978.)

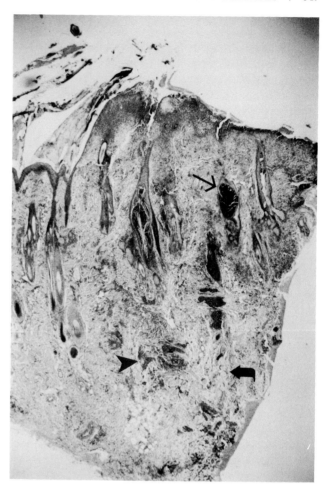

Figure 8:17. Canine eosinophilic furunculosis of the face. Note marked accumulation of eosinophils in follicles (*upper thin arrow*), numerous collagen flame figures (*notched arrow*), and prominent mucinosis of the middle and deep dermis (*curved arrow*).

number of mites present, and pruritus and dermatitis can continue for days to weeks after the mites are destroyed with miticidal agents. In the dog, other evidence suggesting the importance of hypersensitivity includes (1) presence of asymptomatic carriers, (2) rare concurrent proteinuria, and (3) rare concurrent immune complex glomerulonephritis.[40] A study evaluating immunoglobulin levels showed that scabietic dogs have low IgA and IgM and elevated IgG compared with normal dogs. Following therapy for scabies, the levels tended to go back toward normal by 9 weeks and were significantly higher for IgA.[264] Another study found specific antibodies against *Sarcoptes scabiei* var *canis* in dogs with scabies.[257]

Additional evidence for immunologic participation in the pathogenesis of human scabies includes (1) accelerated clinical response to fewer mites upon re-infestation, (2) partial immunity if cured after sensitization has occurred, (3) lower serum IgA levels in scabietic patients than in noninfested controls, (4) positive skin test reactions to scabies antigen in scabietic patients but not in noninfested controls, (5) higher incidence of circulating immune complexes in scabietic patients, (6) positive result of testing with serum from scabietic patients and scabies mite antigen in normal individuals, and (7) deposition of IgG, IgM, and C3 at the basement membrane zone and within dermal blood vessel walls on direct immunofluorescence testing of scabietic skin.[13, 40]

For further details on canine scabies, see Chapter 6.

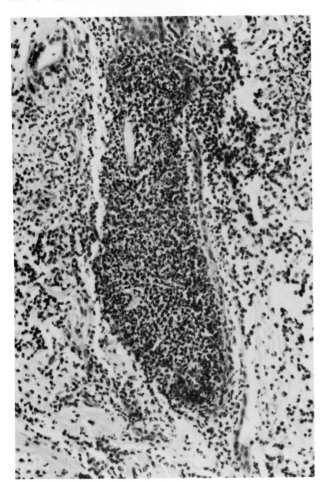

Figure 8:18. Canine eosinophilic furunculosis of the face. Hair follicle has been literally replaced by eosinophils.

TICK BITE HYPERSENSITIVITY

Cutaneous hypersensitivity reactions to tick bites have been recognized in dogs and humans.[13, 40, 261] The proposed pathomechanism of these reactions involves cutaneous basophil hypersensitivity, type III and type IV hypersensitivity responses. No age, breed, or sex predilections have been reported.

Cutaneous hypersensitivity reactions to tick bites in dogs and cats may be characterized by (1) focal areas of necrosis and ulceration, (2) nodules that may or may not be erythematous, pruritic, and ulcerated, and (3) pruritic pododermatitis. Diagnosis is based on history and physical examination.

Skin biopsy may reveal leukocytoclastic vasculitis with hemorrhage, necrosis, and ulceration (type III reaction), or nodular to diffuse dermatitis due to granulomatous or pyogranulomatous inflammation (type IV reaction), often with numerous eosinophils and lymphoid hyperplasia. Tick mouth parts are seldom found in biopsy specimens.

Therapy includes tick removal and control. Surgical excision or glucocorticoids are effective for severe or persistent reactions.

INTESTINAL PARASITE HYPERSENSITIVITY

Various intestinal parasites (ascarids, *Coccidia,* hookworms, tapeworms, whipworms) of dogs, cats, and humans may rarely be associated with pruritic dermatoses.[13, 40, 261] The pathomechanism of these dermatoses is unknown, but a type I hypersensitivity reaction is likely. Although the pathomechanism is unknown, a clear relationship between the parasite and the dermatosis is established, because (1) eliminating the parasites cures the dermatosis and (2) re-infestation with the parasite reproduces it.

Clinical signs may consist of (1) generalized or multifocal pruritic, papulocrustous dermatitis, (2) pruritic seborrheic skin disease, (3) pruritic urticaria, or (4) pruritus without skin lesions. Other signs referable to intestinal parasitism may or may not be present. No age, breed, or sex predilections have been reported.

Diagnosis is made by history, physical examination, fecal examinations, and response to therapy. Skin biopsy is nondiagnostic, revealing varying degrees of superficial perivascular dermatitis (pure, spongiotic, hyperplastic), often with small to large numbers of eosinophils.

Therapy includes elimination of the parasites and treatment of symptoms with topical (shampoos, soaks) and systemic medicaments (glucocorticoids), as indicated.

DIROFILARIASIS

Numerous rare skin disorders associated with *Dirofilaria immitis* infection (heartworm disease) have been described in dogs (see Chap. 6).[40, 261, 262] The pathomechanism of these skin disorders is unknown, although a hypersensitivity to *D. immitis* microfilaria has been suggested. No age, breed, or sex predilections have been reported.

Cutaneous syndromes reported in association with dirofilariasis in dogs include (1) a pruritic, ulcerative nodular dermatitis of the head, trunk, and limbs (see Figs. 8:16 *C* and *D*), (2) a pruritic papulocrustous dermatitis resembling canine scabies, (3) a pruritic ulcerative dermatitis of the head and limbs, (4) an erythematous, alopecic dermatitis of the chest and limbs, (5) interdigital cyst, and (6) seborrheic skin disease.

Diagnosis is based on history, physical examination, demonstration of *D. immitis* microfilaria in peripheral blood and in skin specimens, ruling out of other possible causes of the dermatosis, and response to therapy for dirofilariasis. Most dogs with dirofilariasis have peripheral eosinophilia and serum hypergammaglobulinemia.[12] About 50 per cent of affected dogs also have peripheral basophilia. In about 20 per cent of the dogs with dirofilariasis, microfilaria cannot be demonstrated in peripheral blood (occult dirofilariasis), owing to an immune-mediated reaction against microfilarial antigen. Various enzyme-linked immunosorbent assay (ELISA) methodologies for the detection of adult *D. immitis*–associated antigens (Filarochek, Mallinckrodt; Dirochek, Synbiotics; ClinEase-CH, Norden; CITE, Agri Tech Systems) are very useful for the detection of occult dirofilariasis.[12]

Histologic examination of the nodular form of cutaneous dirofilariasis reveals superficial and deep perivascular to nodular dermatitis.[17, 40, 63] Eosinophils are numerous. Pyogranulomas may be situated perivascularly, with microfilaria present intravascularly (Fig. 8:19) or interstitially surrounding extravascular microfilaria (Fig. 8:20).

Therapy consists of the administration of adulticidal and microfilaricidal drugs. Cutaneous lesions heal within 5 to 8 weeks after the completion of microfilaricidal therapy.

OTODECTIC ACARIASIS

Hypersensitivity appears to play a role in some cases of otodectic acariasis (otodectic mange, ear mites) in cats.[40, 261] Clinically, cats occasionally develop a widespread, pruritic, papulocrustous dermatitis associated with *Otodectes cynotis* infestation.[40] Immunologically, passive cutaneous anaphylaxis reactions to *O. cynotis* antigen were reported in cats with experimentally induced ear mite infestations, demonstrating the existence of reaginic antibody.[263] In addition, cats may be seen with facial or generalized pruritic dermatitis that responds to ivermectin. *Otodectes* mites may be difficult to find in some cases.

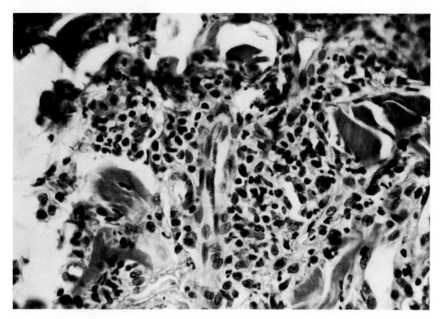

Figure 8:19. Canine cutaneous dirofilariasis. Perivascular pyogranuloma with microfilarial segment within blood vessel.

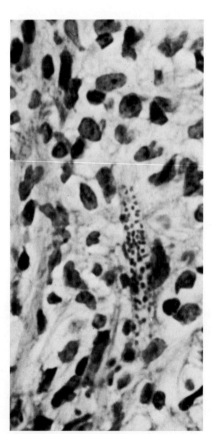

Figure 8:20. Canine cutaneous dirofilariasis. Extravascular microfilaria within a granuloma.

Hormonal Hypersensitivity

Hormonal hypersensitivity is a very rare, pruritic, papulocrustous dermatitis of dogs and humans associated with hypersensitivity reactions to sex hormones.[13, 40, 270]

Cause and Pathogenesis

Although the pathomechanism of the dermatitis is unknown, results of intradermal allergy testing in dogs and humans suggest that type I and type IV hypersensitivity reactions to endogenous progesterone, estrogen, or testosterone are involved.[270, 271] Further evidence of the immunologic nature of this disorder are: (1) in vitro basophil degranulation with histamine release in response to progesterone and (2) passive cutaneous transfer of skin test reactivity (positive P-K test result) to normal humans.[42, 271]

Clinical Features

No age or breed predilections have been reported, but over 90 per cent of the reported cases have occurred in intact females. Affected females often have a history of repeated pseudopregnancy or irregular estrual cycles or both. Dermatologic signs include a pruritic, erythematous, often papulocrustous eruption that usually begins in the dorsal rump, perineal, genital, and caudomedial thigh regions, is bilaterally symmetric, and progresses cranially (Figs. 8:21 and 8:22). The feet, face, and ears are commonly affected in chronic cases. Enlargement of the vulva and nipples is often seen (Fig. 8:23). In female dogs, the dermatologic signs usually coincide initially with estrus or pseudopregnancy or both but tend to become more severe and protracted with each episode until the dog may have some degree of pruritic dermatitis at all times. In male dogs, dermatologic signs are nonseasonal.[271]

Diagnosis

The differential diagnosis includes flea bite hypersensitivity, food hypersensitivity, atopy, drug eruption, and staphylococcal folliculitis. Definitive diagnosis is made on the basis of history,

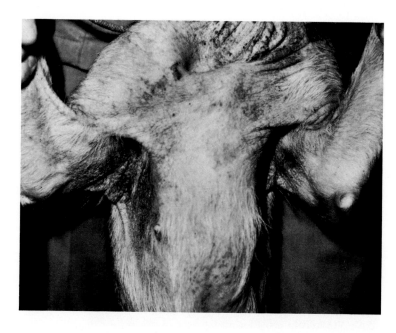

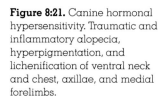

Figure 8:21. Canine hormonal hypersensitivity. Traumatic and inflammatory alopecia, hyperpigmentation, and lichenification of ventral neck and chest, axillae, and medial forelimbs.

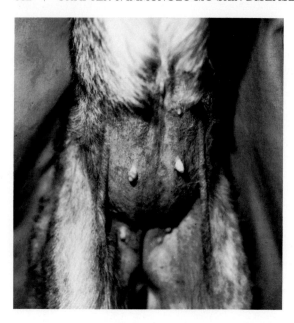

Figure 8:22. Canine hormonal hypersensitivity. Traumatic and inflammatory alopecia with gynecomastia.

physical findings, intradermal allergy test results, and response to therapy. Intradermal allergy testing has been performed with aqueous progesterone (0.025 mg), estrogen (0.0125 mg), and testosterone (0.05 mg), and the skin is observed for immediate and delayed hypersensitivity reactions.[40, 271] These hormones, however, are currently unavailable in aqueous form. The basophil degranulation test was useful in establishing the diagnosis in four bitches[42]; however, this test is currently only a research tool (see discussion of canine atopy).

■ *Histopathology.* Histopathology is nondiagnostic, revealing varying degrees of superficial perivascular dermatitis (pure, spongiotic, hyperplastic) with neutrophils or mononuclear cells predominating.

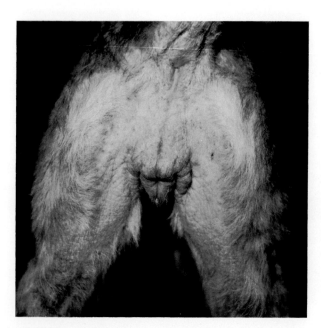

Figure 8:23. Canine hormonal hypersensitivity. Inflammatory and traumatic alopecia with lichenification and vulvar enlargement.

Clinical Management

The prognosis for hormonal hypersensitivity is favorable if neutering can be performed.[42, 270, 271] Therapy consists of ovariohysterectomy or castration and treatment of symptoms with topical and systemic medicaments, as indicated. Response to neutering is dramatic; marked improvement occurs within 5 to 10 days. Response to systemic glucocorticoids is often unsatisfactory. In females, response to repositol testosterone (1.0 mg/kg intramuscularly) is a useful presurgical diagnostic aid, with dramatic relief of pruritus occurring within 7 days. A similar response can be produced in males with the oral administration of estrogen.[271]

Bacterial Hypersensitivity

Bacterial hypersensitivity (staphylococcal hypersensitivity) is a rare, severely pruritic, pustular dermatitis in dogs associated with a presumed hypersensitivity reaction to staphylococcal antigen.

Cause and Pathogenesis

In humans, bacterial antigens are thought to elicit types I, II, III, and IV hypersensitivity reactions in the skin.[13, 40] The pathomechanism of bacterial hypersensitivity in dogs is unclear, although evidence supporting the existence of a type III, and perhaps a type I, hypersensitivity reaction has been reported.[20, 269]

Clinical Features

Clinical signs associated with canine bacterial hypersensitivity are intense pruritus in conjunction with a superficial or deep pustular and seborrheic dermatitis.[268, 269] Erythematous pustules and hemorrhagic bullae are seen with bacterial hypersensitivity (Fig. 8:16 *G* and *H*). Target or bull's eye lesions (annular or arciform areas of central erythema or hyperpigmentation, alopecia, and scaling) that spread peripherally and often coalesce are very common but nondiagnostic (see Fig. 8:12 *H*). Rarely, a dog manifests only an antibiotic-responsive, generalized, nonlesional pruritus.[267] Helpful historical clues are prior pyogenic infection, poor or incomplete response to systemic glucocorticoids, and rapid response to appropriate systemic antibiotics. Relapse after cessation of short-term antibiotic therapy is common.

Approximately 50 to 80 per cent of the dogs have concurrent diseases that appear to predispose them to, or to intensify, the bacterial hypersensitivity.[268, 269] Examples of such diseases include seborrheic skin disease, hypothyroidism, other hypersensitivities (atopy, food hypersensitivity, flea bite hypersensitivity), and foci of chronic infection (anal sacculitis, gingivitis, tonsillitis, otitis externa).

Diagnosis

The differential diagnosis consists of bacterial folliculitis, demodicosis, dermatophytosis, seborrheic skin disease, subcorneal pustular dermatosis, sterile eosinophilic pustulosis, pemphigus foliaceus, atopy, food hypersensitivity, scabies, and flea bite hypersensitivity. Definitive diagnosis is based on history, physical examination, and results of bacterial culture, skin biopsy, and intradermal allergy testing. All reported cases of canine bacterial hypersensitivity have had pure cultures of either coagulase-positive *Staphylococcus* sp. (most cases) or coagulase-negative *Staphylococcus* sp. (rare cases).

■ ***Histopathology.*** Skin biopsy reveals varying degrees of vasculitis and intraepidermal pustular dermatitis or folliculitis and furunculosis (Figs. 8:24 and 8:25).[269] The vasculitis is usually

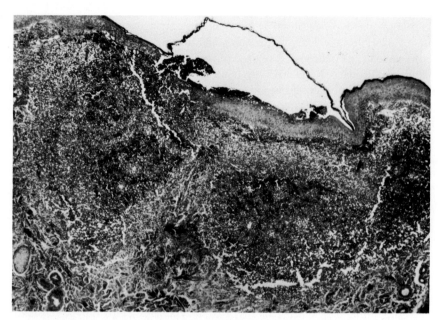

Figure 8:24. Bacterial hypersensitivity in a dog. Subepidermal hemorrhagic bulla. (From Scott, D.W., et al.: Staphylococcal hypersensitivity in the dog. J. Am. Anim. Hosp. Assoc. 14:766, 1978.)

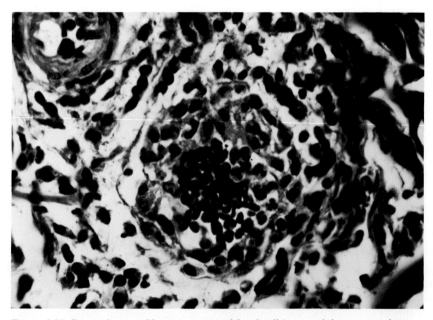

Figure 8:25. Canine bacterial hypersensitivity. Mixed-cell (neutrophils, mononuclear cells) vasculitis with endothelial swelling and degeneration and vacuolization of vessel wall. (From Scott, D.W., et al.: Staphylococcal hypersensitivity in the dog. J. Am. Anim. Hosp. Assoc. 14:766, 1978.)

mixed (neutrophils and mononuclear cells), and significant leukocytoclasis and fibrinoid degeneration are uncommon.

■ *Intradermal Allergy Testing.* Intradermal allergy testing with a staphylococcal cell wall toxoid product (Staphoid A-B) has been useful for diagnosing canine bacterial hypersensitivity.[268, 269] The product is diluted with an equal volume of sterile saline, and 0.1 ml of the mixture is injected intradermally. Virtually all dogs, normal or dermatitic from *any* cause, develop an immediate wheal and flare reaction that persists for 12 to 18 hours and appears to be irritant in nature. At 24 to 72 hours after injection, however, dogs with bacterial hypersensitivity develop erythematous, indurated oozing, pruritic reactions that may turn redpurple, become necrotic, and ulcerate (Arthus reaction) (see Fig. 8:16 *H*). Diagnostic skin testing with bacterial antigens presents problems resulting from a lack of uniformity of staphylococcal antigens, the complex antigenic structure of staphylococci and their metabolites, and various nonimmunologic cutaneous reactions.[20, 40]

Clinical Management

Treatment of canine bacterial hypersensitivity may vary, depending on the existence of concurrent diseases and the age of the dog. In those cases in which an underlying disease can be detected and successfully managed, a 3- to 8-week course of appropriate systemic antibiotics is often curative. In cases in which no underlying disease can be detected but the dog is less than 1 year of age, such a course of antibiotic therapy may still be curative.

When no underlying disease can be detected, however, and the dog is over 1 year of age, the idiopathic bacterial hypersensitivity will probably have to be managed for life with repeated antibiotic or biologic therapy. Biologic therapy is preferred, because repeated antibiotic therapy can lead to increasing bacterial drug resistance, rising drug expense, and euthanasia. Biological therapy with Staphoid A-B has been reported to be successful in 67 to 88 per cent of mature dogs with idiopathic bacterial hypersensitivity.[40, 268, 269] The product is diluted with an equal volume of sterile saline and injected intradermally and subcutaneously, as indicated in Table 8:19. Initially, the cutaneous reaction to the intradermal portion of the therapy is pronounced and resembles that seen with diagnostic testing. This intradermal reaction abates as the dog responds. Uncommonly, dogs develop severe reactions to the subcutaneous portion of the therapy—localized angioedema to generalized pruritus with or without urticaria for a few hours or up to 1 to 2 days. At this point, the subcutaneous portion of the therapy is permanently discontinued. If the dog responds well to biologic therapy, booster injections are administered as needed, usually every 1 to 3 months. Other bacterial vaccines that may be tried include Staphage Lysate and Lysigin (see Chap. 3). When biological therapy is unsuccessful, the therapy of choice for recurrent bacterial hypersensitivity is chronic antibiotic administration (see Chap. 3).

Table 8:19. Schedule for the Biologic Therapy of Canine Bacterial Hypersensitivity, Using Staphoid A-B 50:50 with Saline

Day	Intradermal Dose in ml	Subcutaneous Dose in ml
1	0.10	0.15
2	0.10	0.40
3	0.10	0.65
4	0.10	0.90
5	0.10	1.15
12	0.10	1.40
19	0.10	1.65
26	0.10	1.90

Fungal Hypersensitivity

Cutaneous hypersensitivity reactions to fungi are thought to be important in humans, but the importance of such reactions in dogs and cats is unknown.[13, 40] Hypersensitivity to *Candida albicans* infections has been suspected in some cases of paronychia and gingivitis in dogs and cats, in which the tissue response was out of proportion to the degree of infection found.[40] Fungal kerions are thought to represent hypersensitivity reactions to dermatophytes. Hypersensitivity reactions have been suspected in the pruritic widespread papulocrustous eruptions (miliary dermatitis) in cats associated with *Microsporum canis* infections.[40] *Malassezia* dermatitis may also be, in part, a hypersensitivity reaction (see Chap. 5).

■ IMMUNE-MEDIATED DISORDERS

Immune-mediated dermatoses are well recognized* but uncommon skin diseases in dogs and cats. These dermatoses have been reported to account for 1.4 and 1.3 per cent, respectively, of all canine and feline dermatoses examined by the dermatology service at a university small animal practice.[49] They have been subdivided into primary or autoimmune, and secondary or immune-mediated, the latter believed to be primarily diseases wherein tissue destruction results from an immunologic event that is not directed against self antigens.[20, 57] In autoimmune disease, antibodies or activated lymphocytes develop against normal body constituents. A major level of control of the autoreactive clones of lymphocytes is suppression by suppressor T cells that are specific for those clones.[20, 57] The development of autoimmune diseases is a reflection of a lack of control or a bypass of the normal control mechanisms. Over the years, a variety of possible defects have been described, but the exact abnormal mechanism and what induces these diseases still remains unknown. Some of the possibilities include (1) suppressor T-cell bypass, (2) suppressor T-cell dysfunction, (3) abnormal MHC II expression or interaction, (4) cytokine and receptor ligand abnormalities, (5) autoantigen modification, (6) cross-reacting antigens, (7) inappropriate interleukin-2 production, and (8) idiotype–anti-idiotype imbalance.† In addition, there is sexual dimorphism in the immune response, with female sex hormones tending to accelerate immune responses and male sex hormones tending to suppress responses.[2] In secondary immune-mediated diseases, the antigen is foreign to the body. Most commonly, the inciting antigens are drugs, bacteria, and viruses that stimulate an immunologic reaction that results in host tissue damage.[5, 20, 40, 57] Superantigens are gene products that are recognized by a large fraction of T cells and have the potential to interfere with the recognition and elimination of conventional antigens.[23] These gene products may play a role in the genesis of immune-mediated diseases.

As a group, all of these immune-mediated dermatoses are characterized by an inappropriate immune response that, to be adequately controlled, requires the use of potent immunosuppressive drugs. In the past, this primarily meant high levels of glucocorticoids and, occasionally, cyclophosphamide or azathioprine. These initial attempts at treatment, although often successful, led to many side effects (see Chap. 3). In the last 5 to 10 years, however, a variety of different treatment approaches have been evaluated, and now there are more therapeutic options available to the clinician for the management of some of these diseases. The diseases are not all optimally treated in the same way, however, nor do they have the same prognosis. Therefore, it is important that the clinician make as specific a diagnosis as possible. Although much work is occurring in human medicine regarding new approaches to the management of these diseases, very little of this information is being applied in veterinary medicine.

---

*See references 17, 20, 24, 25, 29, 32, 40, 48, 49, and 58.
†See references 1, 5, 13, 20, 30, 31, 53, and 57.

Diagnosis of Immune-Mediated Skin Disease

The diagnosis of the these dermatoses requires demonstration of characteristic dermatopathologic changes and, optimally, the autoantibodies, immune complexes, or mediators (e.g., cytotoxic T cells) of the immunologic injury. Establishing these criteria requires cutaneous biopsy (see Chap. 2). In general, the following guidelines should be observed:[15]

1. Multiple biopsies should always be taken.
2. Samples should be selected from the most representative lesions of the suspected immune-mediated diseases.
3. Punch biopsy samples should be taken in as gentle a fashion as possible; wedge biopsy by scalpel excision may be necessary.
4. Biopsy specimens for direct antibody testing should be selected from areas not secondarily infected and generally representing the earliest lesion typical for that disease; a possible exception is discoid lupus erythematosus, wherein older lesions may be preferred.
5. Sites wherein immunoglobulins are often present in normal tissue (e.g., nasal planum of dogs and cats, footpads of dogs) should not be sampled or should be interpreted appropriately (see Chap. 1).[28, 40]
7. Whenever possible, biopsy specimens should be taken when the animal is not under the effects of any glucocorticoid or immunosuppressive therapy.[15, 40, 49]
8. Samples for direct antibody detection should be sent to a veterinary immunopathology laboratory.
9. Dermatopathologic examination should be performed by a veterinary pathologist who has a special interest in dermatopathology or by a veterinary dermatologist trained in dermatopathology.

Tests used to detect the presence of autoantibodies or various immunoreactants (e.g., immunoglobulins, complement components, microbial antigens) in skin lesions include immunofluorescence and immunohistochemical (immunoperoxidase) testing (Fig. 8:26).[6, 64] Samples for direct immunofluorescent testing need to be fixed and mailed in Michel's fixative. Samples for direct immunoperoxidase testing may be formalin fixed. The results of studies of tissues processed by quick-freezing and of those kept in Michel's fixative for up to 2 weeks are comparable.[8, 40] Studies in dogs and cats suggest that specimens may reliably be preserved in Michel's fixative for at least 7 to 14 days,[40] and in some instances, specimens have successfully been preserved for 4 to 8 years.[26] The pH of Michel's fixative must be carefully maintained at 7.0 to 7.2 to ensure accurate results.[48, 49]

Testing for abnormal antibody or immune complex deposition is considered highly valuable in human medicine for many of the immune-mediated dermatoses. For the similar canine and feline diseases, however, their value is considerably less. These tests are fraught with numerous procedural and interpretational pitfalls, including method of specimen handling, choice of substrates used, method of substrate handling, specificity of conjugates, fluorescein-protein-antibody concentrations, and unitage of conjugates. An in-depth discussion of these factors is beyond the scope of this chapter; the reader is referred to Beutner and colleagues[4] for details. The incidence of positive results in the canine disorders typically varies from about 25 to 90 per cent for direct immunofluorescence testing.[14, 40, 48, 49] Positive results are much more commonly achieved with the immunoperoxidase technique. With this technique, however, the incidence of false-positive results is also much higher.[18, 38] In fact, the intercellular and basement membrane zone deposition of immunogloublins or complement can be detected from time to time in a wide variety of inflammatory dermatoses.[38, 40, 48, 49, 64] The authors and others[39] do not believe that these tests need to be routinely done in the work-up of a suspected case of immune-mediated skin disease in a dog or cat. Results of immunopathologic testing can never be appropriately interpreted in the absence of histopathologic findings.[39, 40] On the other hand, histopathologic findings are sufficiently characteristic to be diagnostic in the majority of cases.[17, 40, 63] The clinician's time and the owner's money are better spent in the careful selection and procuring of representative skin specimens and their forwarding to a knowledgeable dermatopathologist.

Indirect immunofluorescence testing (testing serum for the presence of circulating autoantibody) is rarely positive in dogs and cats and is not recommended.[40, 48, 49]

Pemphigus Complex

The pemphigus complex is a group of uncommon autoimmune diseases described in dogs and cats that is comparable to the human disease. Although there are similarities, many significant differences exist. They are vesiculobullous to pustular disorders of the skin or mucous membranes.

CAUSE AND PATHOGENESIS

In humans, the pemphigus complex is characterized histologically by intraepidermal acantholysis leading to vesicle formation, and immunologically by the presence of an autoantibody (pemphigus antibody), both bound in the skin and circulating in the serum, to the cell surface of keratinocytes.[4, 13] In dogs, only pemphigus vulgaris causes an intraepidermal vesicle. The other forms of pemphigus are typically intraepidermal pustules, a major distinction between the human and canine diseases.[17, 278] Additionally, pemphigus antibody cannot be demonstrated in the skin or serum of many dogs and cats. In humans, negative immunologic findings raise serious doubts about the diagnosis. These two differences raise questions about the pathologic similarities between the human and animal diseases. There are many animal cases with classical pathologic findings, however, and it is highly likely that a very similar disease exists. Further studies comparing cases with and without appropriate immunologic findings need to be done.

Pemphigus antigens are heterogeneous (85 to 260 kD), present in all mammalian and avian skin, and associated with desmosomal and nondesmosomal cell membrane areas.[5, 13, 275] In humans, regional variation exists in the expression of both pemphigus foliaceus and pemphigus vulgaris antigens, which also differ from each other.[284] This regional difference correlates with, and helps to explain, the distribution of lesions seen in clinical disease. Canine skin has been shown to have similar antigens.[300, 301] The pemphigus vulgaris and pemphigus foliaceus antibodies from human patients reproduce their respective clinical, histopathologic, and immunopathologic syndromes when injected into neonatal mice. Antibodies to some of these antigens are not, however, associated with pathology.

The proposed pathomechanism of blister formation in pemphigus is as follows: (1) the binding of pemphigus antibody on the antigen, (2) internalization of the pemphigus antibody and fusion of the antibody with intracellular lysomes, and (3) resultant activation and release of a keratinocyte proteolytic enzyme (plasminogen activator or another factor), which diffuses into the extracellular space and converts plasminogen into plasmin, which hydrolyzes the adhesion molecules.[13, 274, 301] The resultant loss of intercellular cohesion leads to acantholysis and blister formation within the epidermis. The pemphigus antibody–induced acantholysis is *not* dependent on complement or inflammatory cells. Experimentally, however, complement potentiates the acantholysis. What initiates the autoantibody formation is still unknown, though a virus spread by an insect vector is suspected in an endemic form of pemphigus foliaceus seen in South America.[13] It has been suggested that the black fly may play the role. This hypothesis has been supported by an epidemiologic study correlating exposure to black flies as a risk factor for the development of endemic pemphigus foliaceus.[286]

Genetic factors in humans and dogs also appear to be important. In humans, both pemphigus foliaceus and pemphigus vulgaris have HLA associations.[13] Although this has not been demonstrated in dogs, breed predispositions and familial cases have been shown.[40, 289] Other factors thought to be involved in the pathogenesis of some cases of pemphigus are drug provocation (especially penicillamine and phenylbutazone), ultraviolet light, and emotional upset.[4, 13, 40, 293, 297, 298] Drugs and chronic skin disease both seem to be important in the pathogenesis of some cases of canine and feline pemphigus.[278, 279] Interestingly, drug-induced disease in humans is less commonly associated with classic immunopathologic findings.[302] Possibly, the human drug-induced form is more similar to animal pemphigus.

Owing to the thinness, or other characteristics, of canine and feline epidermis, intraepidermal vesicles and bullae are fragile and transient. Thus, clinical lesions usually include erosions and ulcers bordered by epidermal collarettes.

DIAGNOSIS OF PEMPHIGUS: GENERAL COMMENTS

The pemphigus complex is uncommon in dogs and cats, accounting for about 0.6 per cent of all canine and feline skin disorders seen at one university small animal clinic.[49] In general, the various forms of pemphigus have relatively distinct clinical differences. Certain diagnostic features, however, can be applied to the whole group. The most important diagnostic aspects are the history, physical examination, and histopathologic findings. Detection of pemphigus antibody by direct immunofluorescence or immunohistochemical testing may also be helpful, but owing to costs, technical problems, and relatively poor diagnostic sensitivity and specificity, those tests are no longer routinely recommended. If they are performed, however, all the pemphigus variants should show an intercellular deposition of IgG or complement components (Fig. 8:26 A).[40, 297, 298] Occasionally, immunoglobulins of other classes may be found. Indirect immunofluorescence testing is rarely positive. Pemphigus erythematosus may show deposition of immunoreactants along the basement membrane zone, in addition to the intercellular findings (Fig. 8:26 B). Microscopic examination of direct smears from intact vesicles or pustules or from recent erosions often reveals numerous nondegenerate neutrophils, occasionally numerous eosinophils, and numerous acantholytic keratinocytes.[48, 298] One or two acantholytic keratinocytes may be seen in an occasional high-power microscopic field during microscopic examination in any suppurative condition, but when these cells are present in clusters or large numbers in several microscopic fields, they are strongly suggestive of pemphigus.

Skin biopsy may be diagnostic or strongly supportive in pemphigus.[17, 40, 48, 298] Intact vesicles, bullae, or pustules are essential. Because these lesions are so fragile and transient, it may be necessary to hospitalize the animal so that it can be carefully scrutinized every 2 to 4 hours for the presence of primary lesions. When a bullous lesion is observed, biopsy must be performed immediately. Multiple biopsies and serial sections will greatly increase the chances of demonstrating diagnostic histologic changes.

Electron-microscopic examination of pemphigus lesions has suggested that dissolution of the intercellular cement substance is the initial pathologic change, followed by the retraction of tonofilaments, disappearance of desmosomes, and acantholysis.[297, 298]

Results of routine laboratory determinations (hemogram, serum chemistries, urinalysis, serum protein electrophoresis) are nondiagnostic, often revealing mild to moderate leukocytosis and neutrophilia, mild nonregenerative anemia, mild hypoalbuminemia, and mild to moderate elevations of α_2, β, and γ globulins.[297, 298]

CLINICAL MANAGEMENT OF PEMPHIGUS: GENERAL COMMENTS

The prognosis for canine pemphigus appears to vary with the form and severity of the disease.[48, 297, 298] The natural course of untreated cases is unclear. Veterinarians have long recognized refractory mucocutaneous erosive or ulcerative disorders and severe exfoliative dermatoses that have resulted in the death or euthanasia of affected dogs and cats. Retrospectively, many of those dogs and cats may have had pemphigus vulgaris or pemphigus foliaceus. On the basis of the small numbers of cases documented in the veterinary literature, (1) pemphigus vulgaris

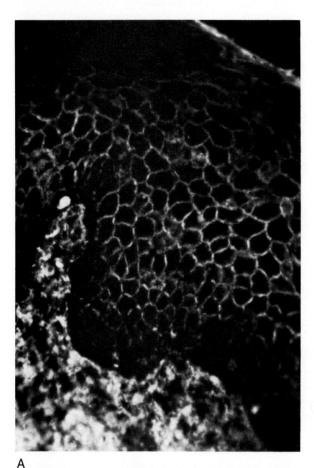

A

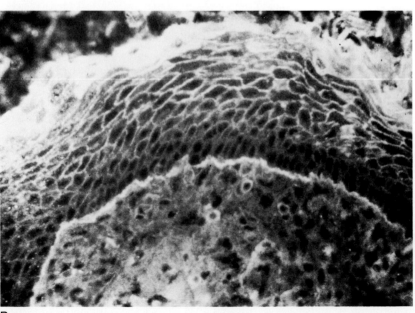

B

Figure 8:26. *A*, Canine pemphigus vulgaris. Direct immunofluorescence testing reveals host IgG within the intercellular spaces of epidermis. (From Scott, D.W., Lewis, R.M.: Pemphigus and pemphigoid in a dog and man: Comparative aspects. J. Am. Acad. Dermatol. 5:148, 1981.) *B*, Canine pemphigus erythematosus. Direct immunofluorescence testing reveals host IgG within the intercellular spaces of epidermis and along the basement membrane zone. (From Scott, D.W., Lewis, R.M.: Pemphigus and pemphigoid in a dog and man: Comparative aspects. J. Am. Acad. Dermatol. 5:148, 1981.) *C*, Canine bullous pemphigoid. Direct immunofluorescence testing reveals host IgG deposited at the basement membrane zone. (From Scott, D.W., et al.: Observations on the immunopathology and therapy of canine pemphigus and pemphigoid. J. Am. Vet. Med. Assoc. 180:48, 1982.) *D*, Canine cutaneous vasculitis. Direct immunofluorescence testing reveals host IgG within blood vessel walls.

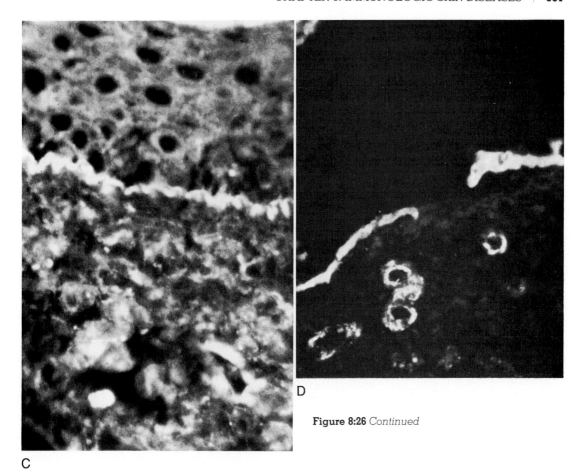

D

C

Figure 8:26 *Continued*

appears to be a severe disease that is often fatal unless treated, (2) pemphigus foliaceus is less severe but without therapy may be fatal, and (3) pemphigus erythematosus and pemphigus vegetans are usually benign disorders that rarely produce systemic signs.

Therapy of canine and feline pemphigus is often difficult, requiring large doses of systemic glucocorticoids with or without other potent immunomodulating drugs.[40, 48, 297, 298] Side-effects of these drugs are common, varying from mild to severe, and close physical and hematologic monitoring of the patient is critical. Additionally, therapy must usually be maintained for prolonged periods, if not for life. Thus, the therapeutic regimen must be individualized for each patient, and owner education is essential.

Large doses of glucocorticoids (2 to 6 mg/kg prednisone orally q24h in *dogs;* 4 to 8 mg/kg prednisone q 24 h in *cats*) will induce remission in most patients. Severe glucocorticoid side-effects, however, and the inability to achieve safe alternate-day maintenance regimens render these drugs unacceptable in about 50 per cent of cases. Glucocorticoid pulse therapy (11 mg/kg methylprednisolone sodium succinate given intravenously during a 1-hour period for 3 consecutive days) was used to induce remissions in cases of canine pemphigus that had not responded to oral glucocorticoids (see Chap. 3).

When glucocorticoids are ineffective or undesirable, other immunomodulating drugs can be used in an attempt to reduce the dosage, or eliminate the need for the former. Azathioprine is often the drug of choice in this situation in dogs (see Chap. 3). Azathioprine should be used either not at all or very cautiously in cats, because even small doses (1 mg/kg orally q48h) may produce fatal leukopenia or thrombocytopenia.[273] Chlorambucil is effective in dogs and cats, and is the preferred treatment in the cat (see Chap. 3).[291] Chrysotherapy (gold salts) is also useful, especially in cats (see Chap. 3).[29, 40, 280, 292] In animals in which significant nasal depigmentation has occurred, and photodermatitis has become an aggravating factor, photoprotection is an important therapeutic adjunct.[48, 297, 298] Avoidance of sunlight between 8:00 AM and 5:00 PM is helpful. The use of sunscreens containing para-aminobenzoic acid with high sun-protective factor values (15 or greater) is mandatory. Sunscreens should be applied 1 to 2 hours before sun exposure is anticipated and re-applied every 3 to 4 hours.

Other drugs that may be useful in individual cases include dapsone (*not* in cats), vitamin E, and omega-3/omega-6 fatty acid–containing products (see Chap. 3).

PEMPHIGUS VULGARIS

Pemphigus vulgaris has been reported in dogs and cats and appears to be the second rarest form of pemphigus.[48, 287, 298, 299] The major pemphigus vulgaris antigen is a 130-kD glycoprotein from the cadherin group of adhesion molecules.[13, 275, 285, 301] No age, breed, or sex predilections have been reported. Pemphigus vulgaris is a vesiculobullous, erosive to ulcerative disorder that may affect the oral cavity, mucocutaneous junctions (lips, nostrils, eyelids, prepuce, vulva, anus), skin, or any combination thereof (Fig. 8:27 *A* to *D*). About 90 per cent of the animals have oral cavity lesions at the time of diagnosis, and oral cavity involvement is the initial sign in about 50 per cent. Such animals often present for halitosis or excessive salivation. Cutaneous lesions occur most commonly in the axillae and groin. The Nikolsky sign may be present. The claw bed may be involved, resulting in ulcerative paronychia and onychomadesis. Pemphigus vulgaris limited to the skin is rare.[290, 296] Pruritus and pain are variable, and secondary bacterial pyoderma and lymphadenopathy may be present. Severely affected animals may be anorectic, depressed, or febrile.

Diagnosis

The differential diagnosis of pemphigus vulgaris includes bullous pemphigoid, systemic lupus erythematosus, erythema multiforme, toxic epidermal necrolysis, drug reaction, candidiasis, idiopathic ulcerative dermatitis of collies and Shetland sheepdogs, epitheliotropic lymphoma, and the numerous causes of canine and feline ulcerative stomatitis.

Pemphigus vulgaris is characterized histologically by suprabasilar acantholysis with resultant cleft and vesicle formation (Fig. 8:28).[17, 63, 297] Basal epidermal cells remain attached to the basement membrane zone like a row of ''tombstones'' (Fig. 8:29). The dermal inflammatory reaction may be scant and perivascular (cell poor) or prominent and interstitial to lichenoid (cell rich).

Management

Pemphigus vulgaris appears to have the poorest prognosis of this group. Very few cases have been diagnosed and treated, however, so these comments may not reflect what we will find

Figure 8:27. *A*, Canine pemphigus vulgaris. Annular erosions and ulcers bordered by epidermal collarettes in the inguinal region. *B*, Canine pemphigus vulgaris. Annular ulcers with collarettes near anus. *C*, Ulceration of the lips, chin, and nasal philtrum of a cat with pemphigus vulgaris. (From Manning, T.O., et al.: Pemphigus diseases in the feline: Seven case reports and discussion. J. Am. Anim. Hosp. Assoc. 18:432, 1982.) *D*, Ulceration of the hard and soft palate of a cat with pemphigus vulgaris. (From Manning, T.O., et al.: Pemphigus diseases in the feline: Seven case reports and discussion. J. Am. Anim. Hosp. Assoc. 18:432, 1982.) *E*, Multiple crusted erythematous plaques over the dorsum of a dog with pemphigus vegetans. (From Scott, D.W.: Pemphigus vegetans in a dog. Cornell Vet. 67:374, 1977.) *F*, Multiple crusted, erythematous plaques over the dorsum and side of a dog with pemphigus vegetans. (From Scott, D.W.: Pemphigus vegetans in a dog. Cornell Vet. 67:374, 1977.) *G*, Pemphigus foliaceus. Numerous pustules over thorax. *H*, Lateral surface of pinna of a dog with pemphigus foliaceus. Note pustules (early lesions) and yellow crusts (older lesions).

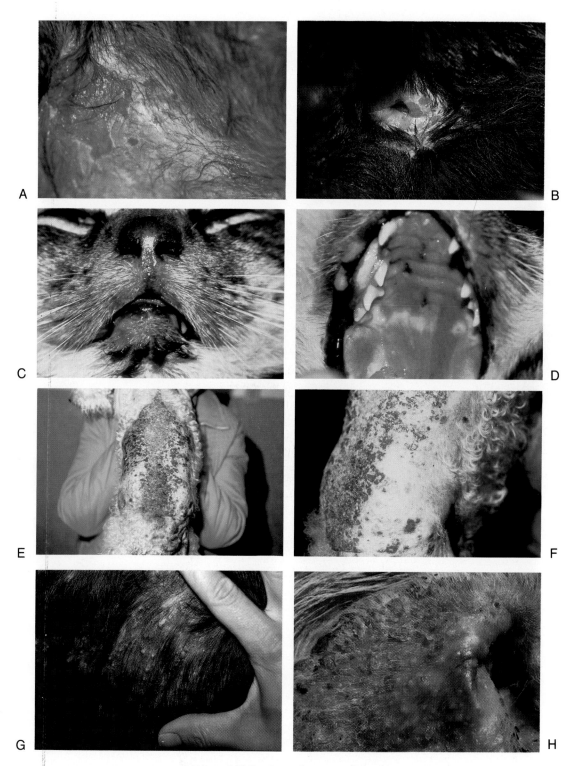

Figure 8:27 *See legend on opposite page*

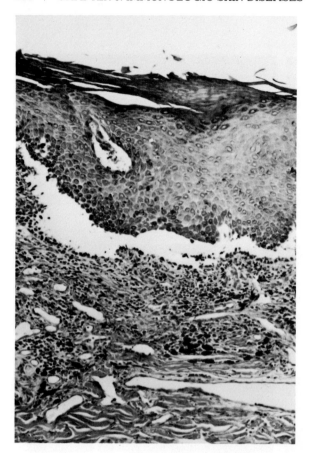

Figure 8:28. Canine pemphigus vulgaris. Suprabasilar acantholysis and cleft formation. (From Scott, D.W., et al.: Pemphigus vulgaris without mucosal or mucocutaneous involvement in two dogs. J. Am. Anim. Hosp. Assoc. 18:401, 1982.)

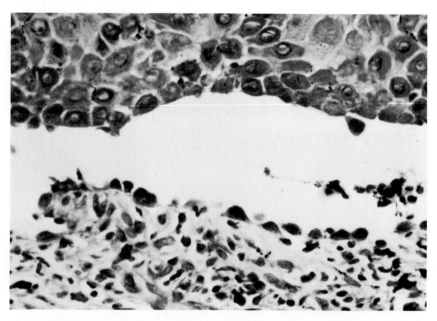

Figure 8:29. Canine pemphigus vulgaris. Suprabasilar cleft with basilar epidermal cells remaining attached to the dermis like a row of "tombstones." (From Scott, D.W., et al.: Pemphigus vulgaris without mucosal or mucocutaneous involvement in two dogs. J. Am. Anim. Hosp. Assoc. 18:401, 1982.)

with long-term experience. Without treatment, this disorder may be fatal,[297, 298] and it tends to be the most difficult form to put and retain in remission. Systemic glucocorticoids alone or in combination with azathioprine are the initial treatments of choice in *dogs,* whereas systemic glucocorticoids alone or in combination with chlorambucil would be preferred in *cats.* Combination therapy is usually required (see Chap. 3). Heparin (100 IU/kg q12h subcutaneously) was shown to have at least a temporary beneficial effect in one medically resistant case of pemphigus vulgaris.[290]

PEMPHIGUS VEGETANS

Pemphigus vegetans has been reported in the dog but is considered to be extremely rare.[294, 298] No age, breed, or sex predilections are apparent. Pemphigus vegetans is a vesiculopustular disorder that evolves into verrucous vegetations and papillomatous proliferations, which ooze and are studded with pustules (Fig. 8:27 *E* and *F*). The Nikolsky sign may be present. Pruritus and pain are variable, and the dogs are usually otherwise healthy. Pemphigus vegetans is thought to represent a more benign or abortive form of pemphigus vulgaris in an animal that has more resistance to the disease.

In a 1991 report, 16 cases of putative pemphigus vegetans were described.[288] To the authors, however, many of the dogs in these cases appeared to have "deep" pemphigus erythematosus or pemphigus foliaceus. The diagnosis of pemphigus vegetans was made on a histopathologic basis because of the presence of pustules in the epidermis and follicular infundibula. Dunstan[276] has referred to this group as having pemphigus vegetans/erythematosus and considers this entity more similar to human pemphigus vegetans, Hallopeau type. He and others[303] have proposed the name *panepidermal pustular pemphigus.*

Diagnosis

The differential diagnosis of pemphigus vegetans includes bacterial and fungal granulomas, benign familial chronic pemphigus, and cutaneous neoplasia (especially lymphoreticular neoplasia and mast cell tumor).

Pemphigus vegetans is characterized histopathologically by papillated epidermal hyperplasia, papillomatosis, and intraepidermal microabscesses that contain predominantly eosinophils and acantholytic keratinocytes (Figs. 8:30 to 8:32).[63, 297]

Management

Too few cases of pemphigus vegetans have been described, but initially, systemic glucocorticoids would be recommended. If they are not effective, azathioprine would be added.

PEMPHIGUS FOLIACEUS AND PEMPHIGUS ERYTHEMATOSUS

Pemphigus Foliaceus

Pemphigus foliaceus is the most common form of pemphigus, and perhaps the most common immune-mediated dermatosis in dogs and cats.* The major pemphigus foliaceus antigen is a 150-kD glycoprotein (desmoglein I) from the cadherin group of adhesion molecules.[275, 285, 301] No age or sex predilections have been reported. In *dogs,* Akitas, Chow Chows, dachshunds, bearded collies, Newfoundlands, Doberman pinschers, the Finnish Spitz, and Schipperkes may be predisposed.[48, 283] The mean age of onset is about 4 years, with 65 per cent of the affected

---

*See references 48, 273, 277, 281, 283, 287, 292.

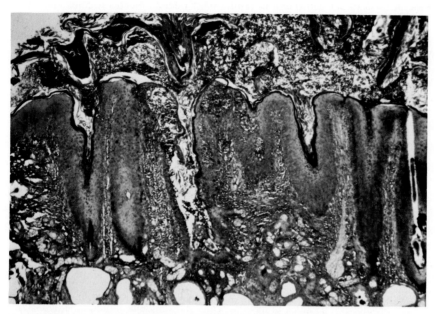

Figure 8:30. Canine pemphigus vegetans. Papillated epidermal hyperplasia, hyperkeratosis, papillomatosis, and several intraepidermal microabscesses. (From Scott, D.W.: Pemphigus vegetans in a dog. Cornell Vet., 67:374, 1977.)

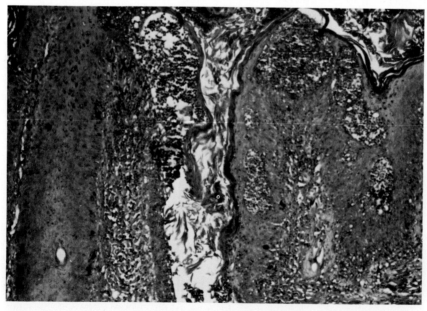

Figure 8:31. Canine pemphigus vegetans. Seven intraepidermal eosinophilic microabscesses. (From Scott, D.W., Lewis, R.M.: Pemphigus and pemphigoid in dog and man: Comparative aspects. J. Am. Acad. Dermatol. 5:148, 1981.)

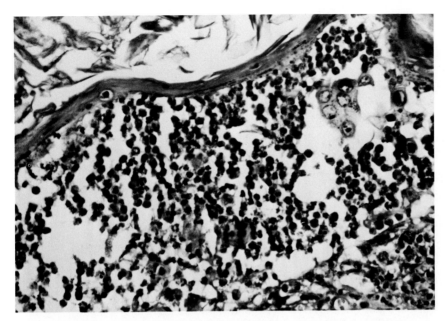

Figure 8:32. Canine pemphigus vegetans. Intraepidermal microabscess containing predominantly eosinophils and a few acantholytic keratinocytes. (From Scott, D.W.: Pemphigus vegetans in a dog. Cornell Vet. 67:374, 1977.)

dogs developing disease at 5 years or less.[283] Pemphigus foliaceus is an uncommon disease, one study showing it to account for 0.04 per cent of the hospital canine population.[283]

Pemphigus foliaceus is characterized by a pustular dermatitis (Fig. 8:27 *G*). This is an important differentiation from human pemphigus foliaceus, which starts with erythema and vesicles and may progress to pustules. Canine and feline pemphigus foliaceus does not have a vesicular phase; it is a pustular, crusting disease. Three forms of pemphigus foliaceus appear to exist in the canine.[279] The first is spontaneous canine pemphigus foliaceus. Akitas and Chow Chows may be prone to this form. The disease develops in dogs with no previous history of skin disease or drug exposure. The second form, drug-induced pemphigus foliaceus, may be more common in Labrador retrievers and Doberman pinschers. The third form is seen in dogs with a history of chronic skin disease. These dogs often have had one or more years of usually pruritic or allergic skin disease. They suddenly develop "more severe disease with new features" that ends up being diagnosed as pemphigus foliaceus. These dogs with chronic, disease-associated pemphigus foliaceus often have had multiple drug therapies, so their disease may occasionally be drug-induced.

Pemphigus foliaceus usually begins on the face and ears (Fig. 8:33 *B*); it commonly involves the feet, footpads (villous hyperkeratosis or "hard pad") (Fig. 8:33 *C* to *E*), and groin, and becomes multifocal or generalized (Fig. 8:33 *A*) within 6 months in many animals. Very early lesions consist of erythematous macules that rapidly progress through a pustular phase and end up as dry, yellow or honey-colored to brown crusts (see Fig. 8:27 *H*). There are usually scales, alopecia, and erosions bordered by epidermal collarettes. The Nikolsky sign may be present. Mucocutaneous orientation is uncommon, and oral cavity involvement is very rare. Some dogs and cats with pemphigus foliaceus present with only footpad lesions and may be lame.[272, 282] Paronychia and involvement of the nipples are commonly seen in cats (Fig. 8:33 *G*).[280] Various claw abnormalities (onychodystrophy, onychorrhexis, onychogryphosis) are occasionally seen in dogs. Nasal depigmentation is common and may result in photodermatitis (see following discussion of pemphigus erythematosus). Pruritus and pain are variable, and secondary bacterial pyoderma and peripheral lymphadenopathy may be present. Severely affected animals may be

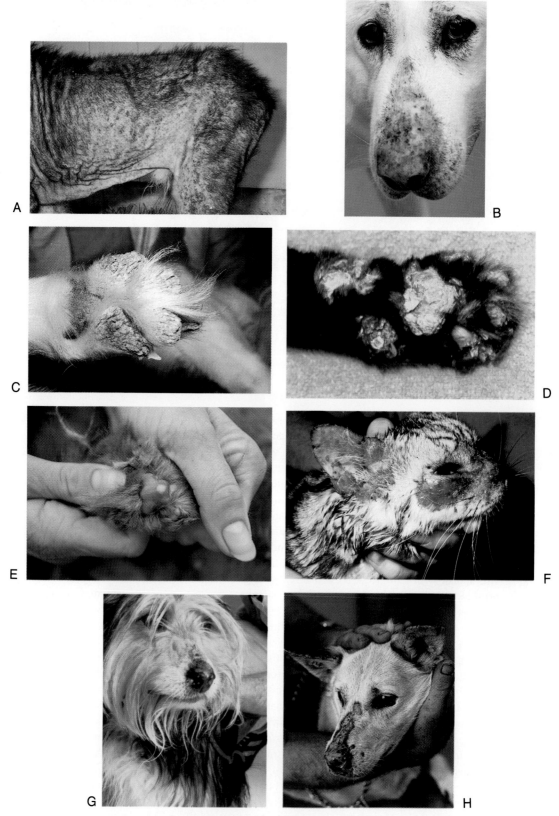

Figure 8:33 *See legend on opposite page*

anorectic, depressed, or febrile. The disease commonly has a waxing, waning course. There may be hours to days when numerous new pustules form, followed by days to weeks of crusting during which few new lesions are found.

Pemphigus Erythematosus

Pemphigus erythematosus is thought to represent a more benign form of pemphigus foliaceus.[13, 298] Some workers have also suggested it may represent a crossover syndrome between pemphigus and lupus erythematosus because of histopathologic and immunopathologic findings. Pemphigus erythematosus has been reported in dogs and cats.[48, 295, 298] No age or sex predilections are known. In dogs, collies and German shepherds may be predisposed.[48]

Pemphigus erythematosus is characterized by an erythematous, pustular dermatitis of the face and ears (Fig. 8:33 *F*). Because the primary lesions are transient, dogs and cats typically present with oozing crusts, scales, alopecia, and erosions bordered by epidermal collarettes. The Nikolsky sign may be present. Pruritus and pain are variable. The nose frequently becomes depigmented, whereupon photodermatitis becomes an aggravating factor (Fig. 8:33 *G* and *H*). If the nasal region is primarily involved, the condition is often worse in sunny weather, and the dog may be misdiagnosed as having nasal solar dermatitis (''collie nose''). Oral cavity involvement has not been reported, and affected animals are usually otherwise healthy. Occasional animals have isolated skin lesions distant from the face and ears, such as on the paws or genitalia.

Diagnosis

The differential diagnosis of pemphigus foliaceus and pemphigus erythematosus includes bacterial folliculitis, dermatophytosis, demodicosis, dermatophilosis, seborrheic skin disease, benign familial chronic pemphigus, discoid and systemic lupus erythematosus, dermatomyositis, and drug reaction. In addition, pemphigus foliaceus could be confused with subcorneal pustular dermatosis, sterile eosinophilic pustulosis, linear IgA dermatosis, necrolytic migratory erythema, leishmaniasis, and zinc-responsive dermatitis.

The definitive diagnosis of pemphigus foliaceus and pemphigus erythematosus is based on history, physical examination, direct smears, skin biopsy, and immunofluorescence or immunohistochemical testing. Pemphigus foliaceus and pemphigus erythematosus are characterized histologically by intragranular or subcorneal acantholysis with resultant cleft and vesicle or pustule formation (Figs. 8:34 and 8:35).[17, 63, 298] Within the vesicle or pustule, cells from the stratum granulosum may be seen attached to the overlying stratum corneum (granular cell ''cling-ons'') (Fig. 8:36). Either neutrophils or eosinophils may predominate within the vesicle or pustule. Pemphigus erythematosus often has a lichenoid cellular infiltrate of mononuclear cells, plasma cells, and neutrophils or eosinophils or both (Fig. 8:37). Other helpful histopathologic findings that may be seen in canine and feline pemphigus foliaceus and pemphigus erythematosus are (1) eosinophilic exocytosis and microabscess formation within the epidermis or follicular outer root sheath or both, (2) frequent involvement of the follicular outer root

---

Figure 8:33. *A,* Pemphigus foliaceus. Generalized papules, pustules, erosions, and crusts. *B,* Pemphigus foliaceus. Note symmetric dermatitis involving bridge of the nose and periocular regions. *C,* Hyperkeratosis of the footpads in a dog with pemphigus foliaceus. *D,* Hyperkeratosis of the footpads in a cat with pemphigus foliaceus. *E,* Pustule on footpad of a cat with pemphigus foliaceus. *F,* Erythema, alopecia, erosion, and crusting of the face and ear of a cat with pemphigus erythematosus. (From Scott, D.W., et al.: Pemphigus erythematosus in the dog and cat. J. Am. Anim. Hosp. Assoc. 16:815, 1980. *G,* Nasal erythema, ulceration, crusting, and depigmentation in a dog with pemphigus erythematosus. *H,* Pemphigus erythematosus demonstrating nasal depigmentation without crusting—typical of discoid lupus erythematosus—and crusted areas on nasal planum and pinna—suggestive of pemphigus foliaceus.

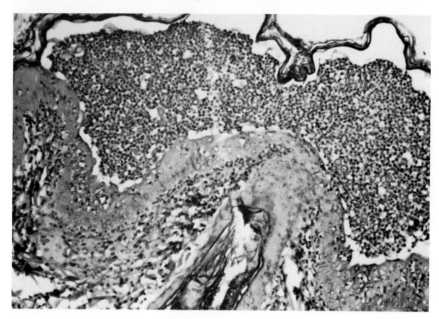

Figure 8:34. Canine pemphigus foliaceus. Numerous neutrophils and acantholytic keratinocytes within a subcorneal pustule. (From Scott, D.W., Lewis, R.M.: Pemphigus and pemphigoid in dog and man: Comparative aspects. J. Am. Acad. Dermatol. 5:148, 1981.)

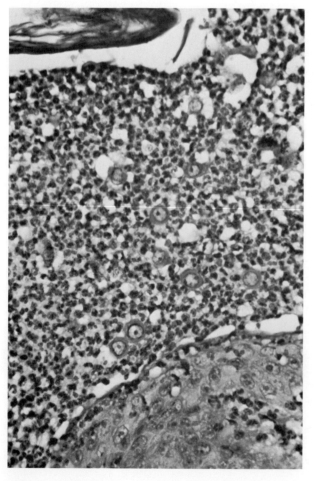

Figure 8:35. Canine pemphigus foliaceus. Numerous acanthocytes within subcorneal pustule.

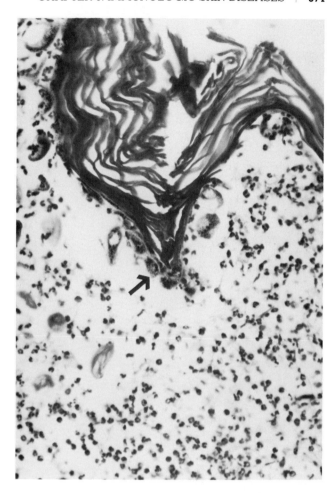

Figure 8:36. Canine pemphigus foliaceus. Intragranular acantholysis produces a "subcorneal" pustule with numerous keratinocytes from the stratum granulosum still adherent (granular "cling-ons") to the overlying stratum corneum (arrow).

sheath in the acantholytic and pustular process, and (3) acantholytic, dyskeratotic granular epidermal cells ("grains") at the surface of erosions (Fig. 8:38).

Management

The initial therapies and therapeutic options for pemphigus foliaceus and pemphigus erythematosus are different. This is an important reason to try to establish a definitive diagnosis rather than just a diagnosis of "pemphigus."

The initial treatment of choice for pemphigus foliaceus depends on the clinical presentation. Milder localized cases may be treated with topical steroids, whereas more extensive disease is usually treated with oral prednisone.[292, 298] The induction dose should be maintained until the disease is inactive, though alopecia and residual crusts may be present. Following induction, the dosage is tapered to an alternate-day regimen (see Chap. 3). In cats, patients failing to respond to prednisone may respond to dexamethasone (0.2 to 0.4 mg/kg q24h) or triamcinolone (0.4 to 0.8 mg/kg q24h), and can be safely maintained by administration of either product every second or third day. It has been suggested that oral triamcinolone may be superior to prednisone and prednisolone; however, this needs to be evaluated.[279] Oral glucocorticoids are ineffective or unsatisfactory in about 50 per cent of cases. In the dog, the next most common treatment is the addition of azathioprine for combination immunosuppressive therapy. In the cat, chlorambucil or chrysotherapy is utilized. Generally, the authors prefer chrysotherapy as the next option

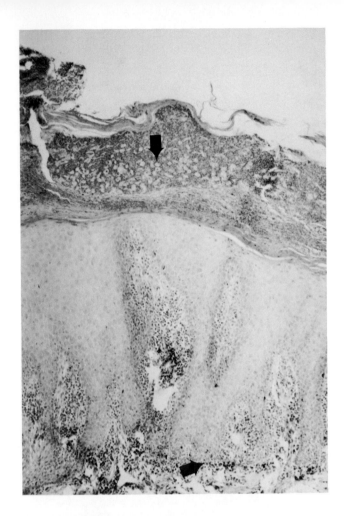

Figure 8:37. Canine pemphigus erythematosus. Note the combination of histopathologic patterns: intraepidermal pustular dermatitis with numerous acanthocytes (*upper arrow*), and interface dermatitis (*lower arrow*).

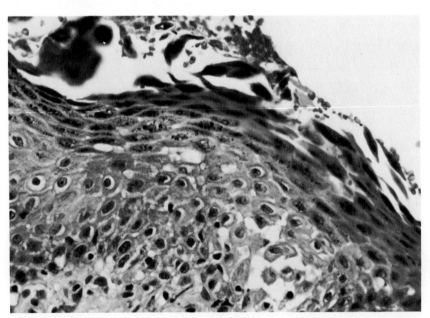

Figure 8:38. Canine pemphigus erythematosus. Acantholytic keratinocytes ("grains") within stratum granulosum at the surface of an erosion. (From Scott, D.W., Lewis, R.M.: Pemphigus and pemphigoid in dog and man: Comparative aspects. J. Am. Acad. Dermatol. 5:148, 1981.)

in the cat, because about 25 per cent of cases may be cured.[280, 292] Chrysotherapy is also an option for the dog.

Pemphigus erythematosus may initially be treated with sun avoidance and topical glucocorticoids. In dogs, the combination of tetracycline and niacinamide is effective in up to 25 per cent of cases (see Chap. 3). If this combination is not effective, systemic glucocorticoids may be added to the regimen or used alone.

Bullous Pemphigoid

Bullous pemphigoid is a rare autoimmune, vesiculobullous, ulcerative disorder of skin or oral mucosa or both that has been reported in dogs and humans.

Cause and Pathogenesis

Bullous pemphigoid is characterized histologically by subepidermal vesicle formation and immunologically by the presence of an autoantibody (pemphigoid antibody) against an antigen at the basement membrane zone of skin and mucosa.[4, 13] The cause of antibody production is still unknown. The bullous pemphigoid antigens (170 to 230 kD) are present in all mammalian and avian skin and are associated with hemidesmosomes of epidermal basal cells, both intracellularly and extracellularly, and the lamina lucida of the basement membrane.[4, 305] This protein is a homolog to desmoplakin I.[13] It has been shown that canine bullous pemphigoid antibody recognizes both the canine and human 180-kD bullous pemphigoid antigen.[306] The proposed pathomechanism of blister formation in bullous pemphigoid is as follows: (1) the binding of complement-fixing pemphigoid antibody to the antigen of the hemidesmosomes, (2) complement fixation and activation, (3) chemoattraction of neutrophils and eosinophils, and (4) release of proteolytic enzymes from the infiltrating leukocytes as well as mast cells, which disrupt dermoepidermal cohesion, resulting in dermoepidermal separation and vesicle formation.[4, 13, 40] In humans, elevated concentrations of eosinophil cationic protein, major basic protein, and neutrophil-derived myeloperoxidase were detected in blister fluid and serum of patients with bullous pemphigoid, suggesting that the release of these substances from activated granulocytes may be important in the pathogenesis of blister formation.[304] Human pemphigoid antibodies, when injected into rabbit cornea or guinea pig skin, produce locally the clinical, histologic, and immunopathologic features of bullous pemphigoid.[4, 13]

Other factors thought to be involved in the pathogenesis of some cases of bullous pemphigoid are drug provocation (especially sulfonamides, penicillins, and furosemide) and ultraviolet light.[4, 13, 293, 308] Bullous pemphigoid–like drug eruptions have been reported in dogs.[360, 372]

Clinical Features

Bullous pemphigoid is very rare in the dog, accounting for about 0.1 per cent of all canine skin disorders seen at one university small animal clinic.[49] Canine bullous pemphigoid has no reported age or sex predilections, although collies and, perhaps, Doberman pinschers appear to be predisposed to its development.[40, 307, 308] Bullous pemphigoid is a vesiculobullous, ulcerative disorder that may affect the oral cavity, mucocutaneous junctions, skin, or any combination thereof (Fig. 8:39 A and B). About 80 per cent of the dogs have oral cavity lesions at the time of diagnosis. Oral cavity involvement has been recognized either after or at the same time as the cutaneous signs and rarely as the initial event. Cutaneous lesions occur most commonly in the axillae and groin. Ulcerative paronychia, onychomadesis, or footpad ulceration may be seen. An insidious, chronic, clinically benign form of cutaneous bullous pemphigoid has been recognized in dogs, with lesions confined to the axillae, groin, or isolated mucocutaneous areas such as the anus and prepuce.[40, 308] Most cases are more severe and widespread, and they are often clinically indistinguishable from pemphigus vulgaris. The presence of intact vesicles or

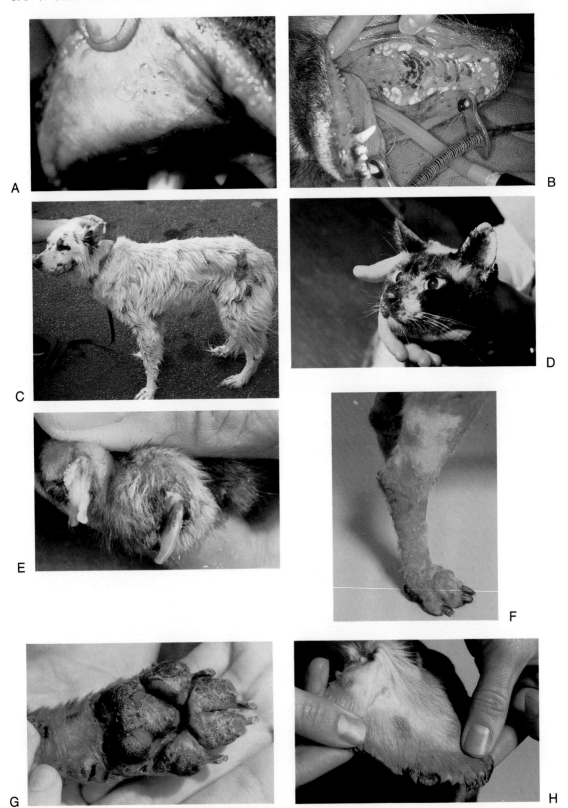

Figure 8:39 See legend on opposite page

bullae, however, is more suggestive of bullous pemphigoid. Clinical variants seen in humans—cicatricial pemphigoid (mucosal and Brunsting-Perry types), vesicular pemphigoid (pemphigoid herpetiformis), pemphigoid vegetans, pemphigoid nodularis, and erythrodermic pemphigoid—have not been recognized in dogs.[13, 308]

Vesicles and bullae are often fragile and transient. Thus, clinical lesions usually include ulcers bordered by epidermal collarettes. The pseudo–Nikolsky sign may be present. Pruritus and pain are variable, and secondary bacterial pyoderma is common. Severely affected dogs may be anorectic, depressed, or febrile, and may die because of fluid, electrolyte, and protein imbalances and septicemia.

Results of routine laboratory determinations (hemogram, serum chemistries, urinalysis, serum protein electrophoresis) are nonspecific, often revealing mild to moderate leukocytosis and neutrophilia, mild nonregenerative anemia, mild hypoalbuminemia, and mild to moderate elevations of α_2, β, and γ globulins.[48, 308] Peripheral eosinophilia is rare.[48, 308]

Diagnosis

The differential diagnosis includes pemphigus vulgaris, systemic lupus erythematosus, erythema multiforme, toxic epidermal necrolysis, idiopathic ulcerative dermatosis of collies and Shetland sheepdogs, drug reaction, epitheliotropic lymphoma, candidiasis, and the numerous causes of canine ulcerative stomatitis. Definitive diagnosis of bullous pemphigoid is based on history, physical examination, skin (or mucosal) biopsy, and immunofluorescence or immunoperoxidase testing. Microscopic examination of direct smears from intact vesicles, bullae, or recent ulcers does not reveal acantholytic keratinocytes.

Bullous pemphigoid is characterized histologically by subepidermal cleft and vesicle formation (Fig. 8:40).[13, 17, 40, 308] Acantholysis is not seen. Inflammatory infiltrates vary from mild and perivascular to marked and lichenoid (Fig. 8:41). Neutrophils and mononuclear cells usually predominate. Tissue eosinophilia is uncommon. Subepidermal vacuolar alteration appears to be the earliest prevesicle histopathologic finding (Fig. 8:42).

Electron-microscopic examination of pemphigoid lesions has revealed the following features: smudging, thickening, and interruption of the basement membrane zone; fragmentation and disappearance of anchoring fibrils, anchoring filaments, and hemidesmosomes; basal cell degeneration; and separation occurring within the lamina lucida.[40, 308]

Direct immunofluorescence or immunohistochemical testing reveals a linear deposition of immunoglobulin, and usually complement, at the basement membrane zone of skin or mucosa in 50 to 90 per cent of patients (Fig. 8:26 C).[4, 13, 48, 308] Complement component C3 is the most commonly demonstrated immunoreactant. It would appear to be important to test with all classes of immunoglobulins, because in some dogs, results are positive for only IgM or IgA. It is also important to sample intact vesicles and bullae as well as perilesional tissue. Indirect immunofluorescence testing is usually negative in canine bullous pemphigoid.[308]

Figure 8:39. *A,* Bullae on the labial mucosa of a dog with bullous pemphigoid. (From Scott, D.W., Lewis, R.M.: Pemphigus and pemphigoid in dog and man: Comparative aspects. Am. Acad. Dermatol. 5:148, 1981.) *B,* Canine bullous pemphigoid. Severe ulcerative stomatitis and cheilitis. *C,* Systemic lupus erythematosus in a dog with arthritis and generalized erythematous, alopecic, and focally ulcerative skin lesions. *D,* Alopecia, erythema, crusting, and depigmentation of the face and ear of a cat with systemic lupus erythematosus. (From Scott, D.W., et al.: A glucocorticoid-responsive dermatitis in cats, resembling systemic lupus erythematosus in man. J. Am. Anim. Hosp. Assoc. 15:157, 1979.) *E,* Bacterial paronychia in a cat with systemic lupus erythematosus. (From Scott, D.W., et al.: A glucocorticoid-responsive dermatitis in cats, resembling systemic lupus erythematosus in man. J. Am. Anim. Hosp. Assoc. 15:157, 1979.) *F,* Erythema, alopecia, and ulceration of the hind leg of a dog with systemic lupus erythematosus. *G,* Ulcerated footpads of a dog with systemic lupus erythematosus. *H,* Necrosis of the margin of the pinna in a dog with systemic lupus erythematosus.

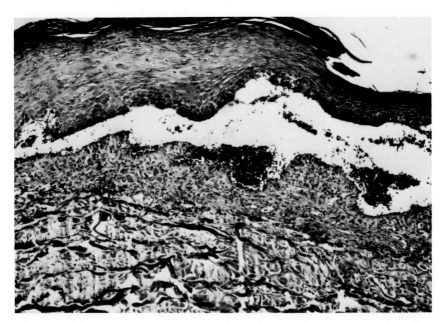

Figure 8:40. Canine bullous pemphigoid. Subepidermal vesicle and lichenoid band of inflammatory cells. (From Scott, D.W., Lewis, R.M.: Pemphigus and pemphigoid in dog and man: Comparative aspects. J. Am. Acad. Dermatol. 5:148, 1981.)

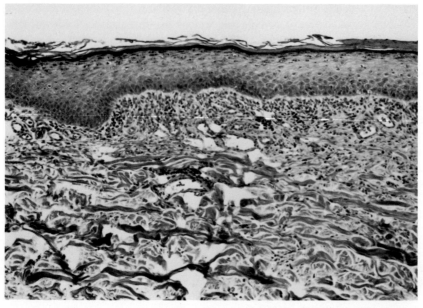

Figure 8:41. Canine bullous pemphigoid. Subepidermal vacuolar alteration and lichenoid band of inflammatory cells.

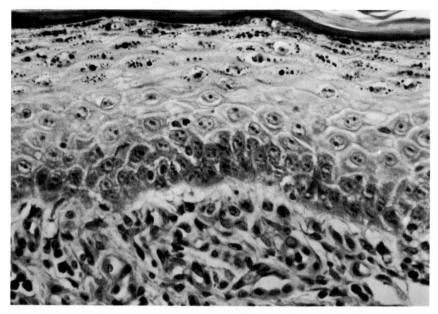

Figure 8:42. Canine bullous pemphigoid. Subepidermal vacuolar alteration.

Clinical Management

The prognosis varies according to how extensive the lesions are. The natural course of untreated cases is unclear. Veterinarians have long recognized refractory mucocutaneous ulcerative disorders that resulted in the death or euthanasia of affected dogs. Retrospectively, some of these dogs may have had bullous pemphigoid. On the basis of the small number of cases documented in the veterinary literature, canine bullous pemphigoid is usually a severe disease. Extensive cases may be fatal unless treated, although it may occasionally be a relatively benign, localized cutaneous disorder.[48, 308] Therapy of canine bullous pemphigoid is often difficult, requiring large doses of systemic glucocorticoids with or without other potent immunomodulating drugs. In one study of nine dogs with bullous pemphigoid,[308] the following observations were made: 1 mg/kg prednisolone, given orally q12h, was ineffective for controlling the disease, and 3 mg/kg prednisolone, given orally q12h, was effective for controlling the disease. Two of the nine dogs requiring the larger dose were euthanized, however, because of unacceptable side-effects, and another two died after 7 to 10 days of therapy (of acute pancreatitis). Thus, systemic glucocorticoids were unsatisfactory for treatment in four of nine dogs (44 per cent).

Bullous pemphigoid cases have, in the authors' experience, usually required combinations of immunosuppressive agents (see Chap. 3). One case (CEG) even required glucocorticoids, azathioprine, and chlorambucil to be kept in remission. Therapy usually must be maintained for prolonged periods if not for life. Thus, the therapeutic regimen must be individualized for each patient, and owner education is essential. Mild cases of canine bullous pemphigoid may be successfully managed with topical glucocorticoids or relatively low doses of systemic glucocorticoids (2.2 mg/kg/day of prednisolone or prednisone orally for induction), and therapy may occasionally even be terminated.[48, 308]

Tetracycline and erythromycin have been reported to be beneficial in the treatment of bullous pemphigoid in humans.[13, 309] It is thought that the benefit derived from these drugs is related to their abilities to inhibit neutrophil chemotaxis and random migration and to increase dermoepidermal cohesion.

Because (1) cutaneous lesions of bullous pemphigoid in humans can be induced by exposure to ultraviolet light and (2) canine bullous pemphigoid may worsen with exposure to ultraviolet light, it may be prudent to avoid direct exposure to sunlight between 8:00 AM and 5:00 PM.[13, 40, 308]

Systemic Lupus Erythematosus

Systemic lupus erythematosus is an uncommon multisystemic autoimmune disorder of dogs, cats, and humans.

Cause and Pathogenesis

The etiology of systemic lupus erythematosus appears to be multifactorial, with genetic predilection, immunologic disorder (suppressor T cell deficiency; B cell hyperactivity; deficiencies of complement components), viral infection, and hormonal and ultraviolet light modulation all playing a role.[4, 13, 40, 310] B cell hyperactivity results in a plethora of autoantibodies formed against numerous body constituents. In humans, a number of drugs (especially procainamide, hydralazine, isoniazid, penicillamine, several anticonvulsants, and contraceptives) are known to precipitate or exacerbate systemic lupus erythematosus.[4, 13] Vaccination with a modified live virus product containing distemper, hepatitis, parainfluenza, and parvovirus antigens was suspected to have precipitated systemic lupus erythematosus in a dog.[40] Tissue damage in systemic lupus erythematosus appears to be due to a type III hypersensitivity reaction. The New Zealand black mouse, the F_1 hybrid of the New Zealand black mouse, and the New Zealand white mouse develop a lupus-like disease that has many similarities to systemic lupus erythematosus in humans.[4, 13, 40, 318]

In the dog, the serologic abnormalities associated with spontaneous canine systemic lupus erythematosus can be transmitted both to normal dogs and to mice by means of cell-free extracts, thus suggesting an infective agent.[20, 40] As yet, however, none of these dogs, has developed overt systemic lupus erythematosus, indicating that other factors are involved in the pathogenesis of the clinical entity. It has been reported that dogs with systemic lupus erythematosus have lower levels of circulating thymic factors than do normal dogs, analogous to the situation in humans.[13, 40]

In a colony of dogs obtained by the mating of a male and female, each having systemic lupus erythematosus, the F_1 generation had no clinical signs; with subsequent breeding, a few dogs in the F_2 generation were affected; and clinical signs were common and marked in the F_3 generation.[311] Affected dogs had depressed suppressor T cell activity, decreased levels of serum thymulin, and decreased percentage of circulating T cells.[311]

The pathogenesis of skin lesions in systemic lupus erythematosus is unclear. Five characteristics of cutaneous lupus erythematosus are (1) photosensitivity (lesions may be produced by sunlight in both the UVB and UVA spectra), (2) keratinocyte damage (associated with contiguous T lymphocytes and macrophages), (3) lymphohistiocytic infiltration, (4) autoantibody production, and (5) immune complex deposition.[13, 313, 316, 318, 321] Skin lesions may be induced with ultraviolet light exposure. Infusion of antinuclear antibodies does not produce skin lesions, however, and immune complexes appear at the basement membrane zone *after* dermatohistopathologic changes appear.

A current hypothesis for the pathogenesis of skin lesions is as follows in genetically susceptible individuals:

1. Ultraviolet light (both UVB and UVA) penetrating to the level of epidermal basal cells induces, on the keratinocyte surface, the enhanced expression of ICAM-1 and of autoantigens previously found only in the nucleus or cytoplasm (e.g., native and denatured DNA).
2. Specific autoantibodies to these antigens that are present in plasma and in tissue fluid bathing the epidermis attach to keratinocytes and induce antibody-dependent cytotoxicity of keratinocytes.

3. Injured keratinocytes release IL-2 and other lymphocyte attractants, accounting for the resultant lymphohistiocytic infiltrate.
4. Injured keratinocytes release increased amounts of TNF-α, IL-1, and IL-6, which are associated with elevations of antinuclear antibodies (ANA), increased B cell activity, and higher production of IgM.[13, 316, 318]

Immunopathologic studies of cutaneous and oral mucosal lupus erythematosus lesions in humans have revealed a predominance of helper T cells and macrophages and a near absence of B cells and Langerhans' cells.[13] In humans, retroviral antigen has been demonstrated at the basement membrane zone of skin lesions, and evidence has been presented suggesting that the immune deposits are complement activating and may be functional and involved in the inflammatory response.[4, 13] Fibronectin, type IV collagen, and type VII collagen are all altered at the basement membrane zone of lesional skin.[315]

Clinical Features

The clinical signs associated with systemic lupus erythematosus (SLE) are varied and changeable. Because of this phenomenal clinical variability and ability to mimic numerous diseases, systemic lupus erythematosus has been called the ''great imitator.''

■ *SLE in the Dog.* Systemic lupus erythematosus is an uncommon disease in dogs.[20, 40, 49, 319] The incidence has been estimated at 0.03 per cent of the canine population.[319] There are no age or sex predilections, but collies, Shetland sheepdogs, and German shepherds are predisposed. Polyarthritis, fever, proteinuria, anemia, skin disease, and oral ulcers are the most common abnormalities in dogs. Other syndromes reported in association with canine systemic lupus erythematosus are pericarditis, polymyositis, myocarditis, pneumonitis, peripheral lymphadenopathy, splenomegaly, pleuritis, neurologic disorders (seizures, meningitis, myelitis, psychoses, polyneuropathy), and lymphedema.

The cutaneous manifestations of canine systemic lupus erythematosus are extremely diverse. They include seborrheic skin disease, cutaneous or mucocutaneous vesiculobullous disorders, footpad ulcers and hyperkeratosis, discoid lupus erythematosus, refractory secondary bacterial pyodermas, panniculitis (lupus profundus), and nasal dermatitis (see Fig. 8:34 *C* and *F* to *H*). Skin lesions may be multifocal or generalized and commonly involve the face, ears, and distal limbs. They may be exacerbated by exposure to sunlight. Pruritus is variable, and scarring is common.

■ *SLE in the Cat.* Systemic lupus erythematosus is rarely reported in cats.[49, 317] The incidence has been estimated to be 0.06 per cent of all feline hospital visits.[317] There is no apparent sex predilection, and affected cats range from 1 to 12 years old. Siamese, Persian, and Himalayan cats may be predisposed. Syndromes reported include hematologic abnormalities, neurologic or behavioral abnormalities, fever, lymphadenopathy, polyarthritis, myopathy, oral ulceration, conjunctivitis, renal failure, and subclinical pulmonary disease.

About 20 per cent of affected cats have cutaneous lesions.[49, 317] Dermatologic abnormalities include seborrheic skin disease, exfoliative erythroderma, and erythematous, scaling, crusting, alopecic, scarring dermatitis most commonly involving the face (see Fig. 8:39 *D*), pinnae, and paws (see Fig. 8:39 *E*).

Diagnosis

The differential diagnosis of cutaneous systemic lupus erythematosus is lengthy, owing to the varied and changeable cutaneous manifestations of the disorder. Typical alternative diagnoses are seborrheic skin disease, dermatophytosis, bacterial folliculitis, demodicosis, food hypersensitivity, scabies, pemphigus vulgaris, bullous pemphigoid, discoid lupus erythematosus, erythema multiforme, necrolytic migratory erythema, leishmaniasis, toxic epidermal necrolysis, candidiasis, and epitheliotropic lymphoma.

The definitive diagnosis of systemic lupus erythematosus is often one of the most challenging tasks in medicine. The disease is so variable in its clinicopathologic presentations that any dogmatic diagnostic categorization is impossible. The clinicopathologic abnormalities that are demonstrated depend on the organ systems involved and may include anemia (nonregenerative or hemolytic) with or without a positive direct Coombs' test result, thrombocytopenia with or without a positive platelet factor–3 test result, leukopenia or leukocytosis, proteinuria, hypergammaglobulinemia (polyclonal), and sterile synovial exudate obtained by arthrocentesis. The lupus erythematosus (LE) cell test may have a positive result in up to 60 per cent of the patients, but it is variable from day to day, is steroid labile, and lacks sensitivity and specificity. The assay has been discontinued in many of the leading laboratories in human medicine.[40]

The antinuclear antibody (ANA) test is currently considered the most specific and sensitive serologic test for systemic lupus erythematosus.[20, 40] It has a positive result in up to 90 per cent of cases of active systemic lupus erythematosus. In general, results from different laboratories cannot be compared. It is important to record the titer (and compare it with normals for the *same* laboratory) and the pattern of nuclear fluorescence. The rim (ring, peripheral) pattern is the one most commonly seen in systemic lupus erythematosus, but titers and patterns appear to have little or no specificity in dogs and cats. There is no clear, constant correlation between clinical disease activity and positive ANA titer.[40, 312, 314, 319, 320] It must be remembered that ANA can be detected from time to time with probably *any* disease as well as in healthy animals.[40, 317] Thus, a positive ANA titer must always be interpreted in light of other critical historical, physical, and laboratory data.

Preparations of the protozoan *Crithidia luciliae* have become commercially available for assaying patient sera for antibodies against native DNA. Large surveys employing this substrate in dogs and cats have not been reported, although preliminary reports indicate that the assay is rarely positive in dogs with systemic lupus erythematosus and in those with positive ANA titers,[40] suggesting that dogs rarely form antibodies against native DNA. The standard Farr test (radioimmunoassay) for the measurement of anti–native DNA antibodies in humans is unsatisfactory in dogs, resulting in numerous false-positive results.[40]

About 10 per cent of human patients with systemic lupus erythematosus are ANA negative.[13, 40] These patients have unique anticytoplasmic antibodies (anti-Ro), which are not detected when traditional ANA test substrates (mouse or rat liver) are employed; as a result, special substrates (calf thymus, normal human lymphocytes, human epithelial tissue culture line) are needed for such patients. The importance of this autoantibody system in dogs and cats is unknown. It could, however, explain the negative ANA results occasionally obtained in dogs with systemic lupus erythematosus.[48, 319] In one study, sera from 131 dogs were evaluated for ANA and extractable nuclear antigens (ENA), including the Ro ribonuclear protein antigen.[322] The ENA was only positive in 46 per cent of the dogs with systemic lupus erythematosus. ENA were not specific for systemic lupus erythematosus, however, because 5 per cent of healthy dogs and 11 per cent of dogs with other diseases had positive results. No dogs with systemic lupus erythematosus were Ro positive.

Investigators have attempted to better understand lupus erythematosus in humans by studying subsets of patients on the basis of one clinical characteristic (or set of them), histopathologic or immunopathologic findings, or serologic studies.[4, 13] The use of this subset approach may allow the clinician to gain insight into prognosis, improved therapy, or presumed pathogenesis. Currently, three subsets of cutaneous lupus erythematosus are recognized: chronic cutaneous (discoid) lupus erythematosus, subacute cutaneous lupus erythematosus, and acute cutaneous lupus erythematosus. The applicability of such subsets to the canine and feline diseases is currently unknown.

The dermatohistopathologic changes in systemic lupus erythematosus vary with the type of gross morphologic lesions and may be nondiagnostic.[13, 17, 63, 319] The most characteristic finding is interface dermatitis (hydropic or lichenoid or both), which may involve hair follicle outer root sheaths (Figs. 8:43 to 8:45). Other common findings are subepidermal vacuolar alteration (subepidermal bubblies), focal thickening of the basement membrane zone (Fig. 8:46), and dermal mucinosis. Uncommon findings are intrabasal to subepidermal vesicles, leukocytoclastic vasculitis, and lupus erythematosus panniculitis (see Chap. 17). In humans, these changes are often not present until the skin lesions are at least 6 weeks old.

Direct immunofluorescence or immunohistochemical testing reveals the deposition of immunoglobulin or complement or both at the basement membrane zone, often known as a positive lupus band, in 50 to 90 per cent of patients.[4, 13, 40, 48, 319] The variability in positive results reflects differences in laboratory techniques, lesion selection (age and activity of lesion), previous or current glucocorticoid therapy, and possibly other factors. In addition, immunoreactants may be found at the basement membrane zone of skin in *many* other conditions. In dogs, C3 is the most commonly detected immunoreactant, with IgA and IgM being the most commonly detected immunoglobulins.[48, 319] In humans, it is often possible to distinguish between systemic lupus erythematosus and discoid lupus erythematosus on the basis of direct immunofluorescence testing of lesional and sun-exposed normal skin. In human patients with systemic lupus erythematosus, sun-exposed normal skin may have positive lupus band in up to 60 per cent of the cases, whereas this rarely occurs in discoid lupus erythematosus.[4, 13] This criterion is of no value in the hairy dog and cat, wherein normal skin is usually negative.[48, 319] In humans, it is recommended that (1) biopsies not be taken from edematous lesions (only about 47 per cent of such lesions are positive), (2) biopsies be taken from lesions over 1 month old (only about 30 per cent are positive if less than 1 month old), (3) skin with telangiectases not be sampled (17 per cent of such lesions are positive, regardless of their etiology), and (4) all glucocorticoid and immunomodulating therapy be terminated, if possible, 3 weeks prior to biopsy.[4, 13, 40] Because no single laboratory test is diagnostic for systemic lupus erythematosus, a number of groups have produced sets of classification criteria for making the diagnosis.[20, 40] Although such criteria have acknowledged validity in humans, there is no such validation of criteria for dogs and cats. The veterinarian must rely on the recognition of multisystemic disease (especially joint, skin, kidney, oral mucosa, and hematopoietic system), positive ANA

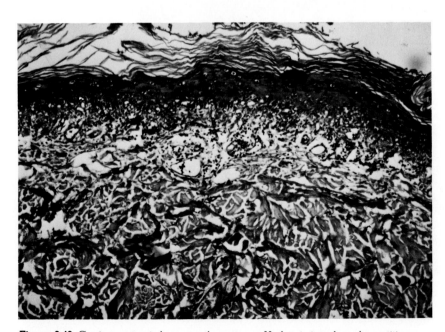

Figure 8:43. Canine systemic lupus erythematosus. Hydropic interface dermatitis.

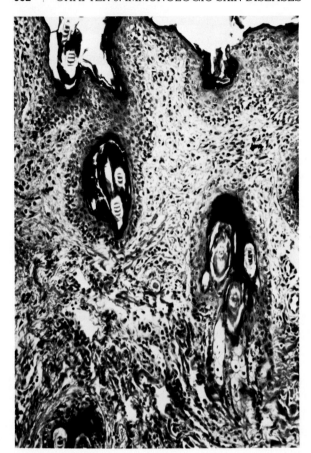

Figure 8:44. Feline systemic lupus erythematosus. Hydropic interface dermatitis. (From Scott, D.W., et al.: A glucocorticoid-responsive dermatitis in cats, resembling systemic lupus erythematosus in man. J. Am. Anim. Hosp. Assoc. 15:157, 1979.)

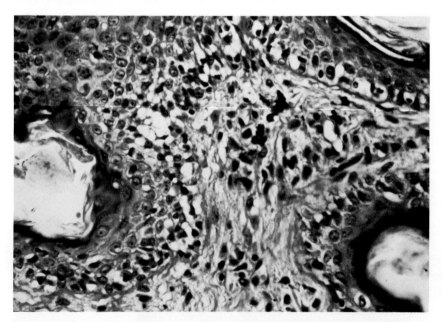

Figure 8:45. Feline systemic lupus erythematosus. Hydropic degeneration of epidermal basal cells. (From Scott, D.W., et al.: A glucocorticoid-responsive dermatitis in cats, resembling systemic lupus erythematosus in man. J. Am. Anim. Hosp. Assoc. 15:157, 1979.)

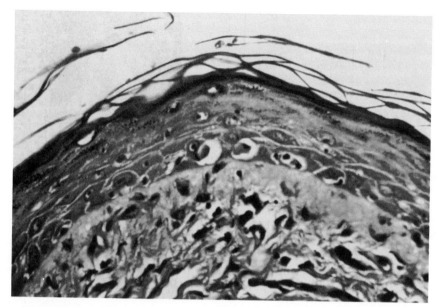

Figure 8:46. Canine systemic lupus erythematosus. Two large, round, apoptotic keratinocytes in stratum basale of epidermis can be seen in the center of the photograph. In addition, the basement membrane zone is thickened.

results, and confirmatory histopathologic and immunopathologic findings in involved skin and oral mucosa or both.[48, 319] Indirect immunofluorescence testing is negative in lupus erythematosus.

Clinical Management

The prognosis in systemic lupus erythematosus is generally unpredictable.[40, 48, 319] In the dog, it appears that patients with joint, skin, or muscle disease respond more reliably to medication and are maintained in relatively long periods of clinical remission. On the other hand, dogs with severe hemolytic anemia or thrombocytopenia or both often do not respond satisfactorily to systemic glucocorticoids and require other immunomodulating drugs or splenectomy or both. Animals with glomerulonephritis regularly develop progressive renal failure in spite of therapy.

Therapy of systemic lupus erythematosus must be individualized. The initial agent of choice is probably large doses of systemic glucocorticoids.[40, 48, 319] When systemic glucocorticoids are unsatisfactory, other immunomodulating drugs may be useful: azathioprine (Imuran) given orally at 2.2 mg/kg q24h, then q48h (*dog only*), or chlorambucil (Leukeran) given orally at 0.2 mg/kg q24h, then q48h.[40, 48, 319] Splenectomy may be needed for patients with severe hemolytic anemia or thrombocytopenia or both.

Levamisole (Levasole), given orally at 2.5 mg/kg q48h, has occasionally been beneficial in dogs and humans with systemic lupus erythematosus.[40] Chrysotherapy (injectable aurothioglucose, oral auranofin) has occasionally been used to reduce glucocorticoid requirements in dogs but would be contraindicated in patients with renal disease.[13, 29, 40] Aspirin has occasionally been effective in the management of dogs and humans.[13, 40] Other drugs used in human patients— dapsone, antiandrogens, antimalarials, colchicine, and omega-3/omega-6 fatty acids—are of undetermined benefit in dogs and cats.[13, 40] Plasmapheresis has been used to enhance initial response to chemotherapy in dogs and humans with severe systemic lupus erythematosus.[13, 34] This technique, currently used as a research tool, is hazardous and expensive.

The following statements can be made about prognosis. Over 40 per cent of the dogs with systemic lupus erythematosus are dead within 1 year after the diagnosis is made, either as a result of natural (renal disease, septicemia) or drug-induced causes, or owing to euthanasia. Dogs that respond well to therapy often do so with glucocorticoids alone and often have long-term remission on alternate-day therapy. Some dogs, in whom disease was controlled well with therapy for several months, remain in prolonged drug-free remission.[40, 319]

Several reports have indicated that people in close contact with dogs having systemic lupus erythematosus or high-titer ANA do not have greater clinical or serologic evidence of systemic lupus erythematosus compared with nonexposed human beings.[20, 40]

Discoid Lupus Erythematosus

Discoid lupus erythematosus (cutaneous lupus erythematosus) is the second most common immune-mediated dermatitis of the dog, although it remains uncommonly seen. It has been described in the cat but appears to be very rare.

Cause and Pathogenesis

Canine discoid lupus erythematosus (DLE) is a relatively benign cutaneous disease with no systemic involvement.[48, 326, 327] A relationship or progression to canine systemic lupus erythematosus has not been seen, nor has the disease been shown to be a good model for the human disorder. Sun exposure aggravates the disease in about 50 per cent of cases, suggesting that photosensitivity plays a role in the pathogenesis. In humans, it has been demonstrated that the lymphocytes infiltrating skin lesions of discoid and systemic lupus erythematosus are predominantly T cells, and that helper T cells predominate in discoid lupus, whereas suppressor T cells predominate in the systemic variety.[4, 13] In the dog, plasma cells are prominent, a feature not shared with humans, suggesting that B lymphocytes may be important and that a different pathogenesis may be occurring. A current hypothesis concerning the pathogenesis of lesion formation is presented in the discussion on systemic lupus erythematosus.

Clinical Features

■ *DLE in the Dog.*   There is probably no strong sex predilection, because both females[327] and males[325] have been reported to be predisposed. No age predilection has been reported. Collies, German shepherds, Shetland sheepdogs, Siberian huskies, Brittany spaniels, and German short-haired pointers demonstrate predilection.[48, 325, 327] Discoid lupus erythematosus has been reported to account for 0.3 per cent of the canine dermatoses examined at one university small animal practice.[49]

Clinical signs of canine discoid lupus erythematosus initially include depigmentation, erythema, and scaling of the nose (Fig. 8:47 A). Early depigmentation manifests as a slate blue or gray color change (Fig. 8:47 B). A helpful early change is the conversion of the normally rough, cobblestone-like architecture of the nasal planum into a smooth surface (Fig. 8:47 C and

Figure 8:47. *A,* Early erythema, alopecia, scaling, and depigmentation in a borzoi with discoid lupus erythematosus. (From Griffin CE, et al.: Canine discoid lupus erythematosus. Vet. Immunol. Immunopathol. 1:79, 1979.) *B,* Discoid lupus erythematosus. Note gray-blue discoloration of skin around nostrils. *C,* Nasal erythema, ulceration, and depigmentation in a dog with discoid lupus erythematosus. (From Walton, D.K., et al.: Canine discoid lupus erythematosus. J. Am. Anim. Hosp. Assoc. 17:851, 1981.) *D,* Frontal view of nose of dog in *C. E,* Depigmentation of the lip in a dog with discoid lupus erythematosus. (From Walton, D.K., et al.: Canine discoid lupus erythematosus. J. Am. Anim. Hosp. Assoc. 17:851, 1981.) *F,* Discoid lupus erythematosus. Patchy alopecia, erythema, scale, and crust of pinna. *G,* Palatine ulcers in a dog with discoid lupus erythematosus. *H,* Cold agglutinin disease in a cat. Necrosis of pinnal margin.

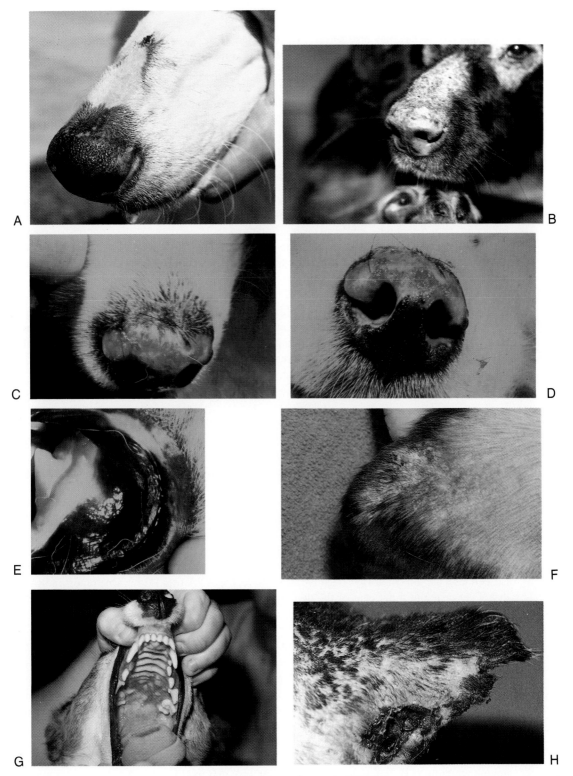

Figure 8:47 *See legend on opposite page*

D). Later lesions commonly include erosion, ulceration, and crusting. Initially, lesions tend to occur dorsally at the junction between the nasal planum and haired skin or along the ventral or medial aspects of the alar folds. Typically, with time, more extensive nasal involvement is seen, and the lesions may also spread up the bridge of the nose. Less commonly, lesions may be seen periocularly, on the pinnae (Fig. 8:47 *F*), on the distal limbs, and on the genitals. The lips may also be involved (Fig. 8:47 *E*), and small punctate ulcers may be seen in the oral cavity (Fig. 8:47 *G*), most commonly involving the tongue or palate (Fig. 8:47 *E*). Occasional dogs present only with lesions of both pinnae or with nasodigital hyperkeratosis.[323, 327, 327a] Pruritus and pain are variable. Scarring and variable degrees of permanent leukoderma are common. Rarely, deeply ulcerated nasal lesions damage arterioles, resulting in episodic, pulsatile hemorrhage. Affected dogs are otherwise healthy.

Discoid lupus erythematosus in dogs is commonly exacerbated or precipitated by exposure to ultraviolet light. Thus, the disease often is more severe in the summer and in parts of the world with sunny climates. It is very likely that many dogs previously referred to as having nasal solar dermatitis, or ''collie nose,'' actually had discoid lupus erythematosus, pemphigus foliaceus, and pemphigus erythematosus. Squamous cell carcinomas are reported to rarely develop in chronic discoid lupus erythematosus skin lesions. The authors believe, however, that this is extremely rare and would suggest that the cancer may also arise in lesions of chronic ultraviolet light damage (solar dermatitis).

■ *DLE in the Cat.*   Discoid lupus erythematosus appears to be very rare in cats.[324, 330] No age, breed, or sex predilections are reported. Lesions are most commonly seen on the pinnae and face. They are erythema, scaling, crusting, and alopecia. Pruritus is variable. Nasal dermatitis and depigmentation are less commonly seen. Lesions may be more severe when exposure to sunlight is increased. Affected cats are otherwise healthy.

Diagnosis

The most common differential diagnosis includes nasal solar dermatitis, nasal depigmentation, vitiligo-like disease, pemphigus erythematosus or pemphigus foliaceus, trauma, dermatomyositis, epitheliotropic lymphoma, drug reaction, uveodermatologic syndrome, contact dermatitis, and systemic lupus erythematosus.

Definitive diagnosis of canine discoid lupus erythematosus is based on history, physical examination, and skin biopsy. Immunopathology may be an aid to diagnosis, but in the dog, it is not believed to be required for a definitive diagnosis, because both false-positive and false-negative results occur.[15, 326] Results of routine laboratory determinations (hemogram, serum chemistries, urinalysis, serum protein electrophoresis) are usually unremarkable. The ANA and LE cell tests are almost always negative; if positive, the ANA titer is low. One report indicated that 9 per cent and 4 per cent of the dogs with discoid lupus erythematosus were positive for ENA and anti-Ro, respectively.[322]

■ *Histopathology.*   Skin biopsy reveals an interface dermatitis (hydropic, lichenoid, or both) (Figs. 8:48 and 8:49).[17, 63, 327] Focal hydropic degeneration of basal epidermal cells, pigmentary incontinence, focal thickening of the basement membrane zone, apoptotic keratinocytes, and marked accumulations of mononuclear cells and plasma cells around dermal vessels and appendages are important histopathologic features of discoid lupus erythematosus. Dermal mucinosis of variable degrees is also a common feature of canine discoid lupus erythematosus.

Immunopathologic testing reveals deposition of immunoglobulin or complement or both at the basement membrane zone.[49, 325, 327] It would appear to be important to test for individual immunoglobulin classes, as either IgG, IgM, or IgA may be the only demonstrable immunoglobulin. In humans, it is recommended that (1) edematous lesions not be biopsied (only about 47 per cent of such lesions are positive), (2) telangiectatic areas *not* be biopsied (about 17 per

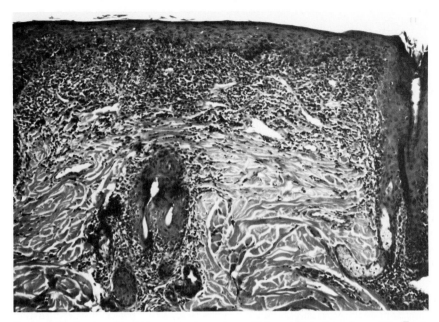

Figure 8:48. Canine discoid lupus erythematosus. Lichenoid interface dermatitis. (From Scott, D.W., et al.: Linear IgA dermatoses in the dog. Cornell Vet. 72:394, 1982.)

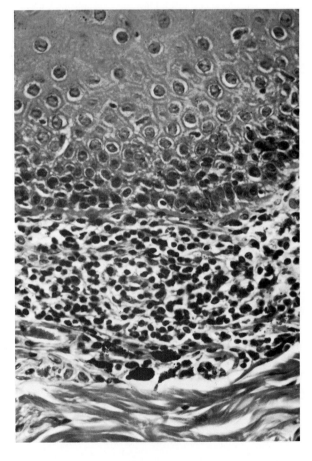

Figure 8:49. Canine discoid lupus erythematosus. Lichenoid interface dermatitis with thickening of the basement membrane zone. (From Walton, D.K., et al.: Canine discoid lupus erythematosus. J. Am. Anim. Hosp. Assoc. 17:851, 1981.)

cent of the telangiectatic skin lesions of *any* dermatosis are positive), and (3) lesions less than 1 month old *not* be biopsied (only about 30 per cent of such lesions are positive). In addition, topical or systemic glucocorticoid therapy may lead to false-negative immunopathologic findings.[15, 40, 49] The authors do not believe that immunopathologic testing is required for the diagnosis of discoid lupus erythematosus in most instances. Immunopathologic tests are also considered to be inferior to, and only supportive of, a diagnosis based on histopathologic criteria.[329, 331] Indirect immunofluorescence testing is negative in discoid lupus erythematosus.

Clinical Management

The prognosis for discoid lupus erythematosus is usually good.[49, 325, 327] Therapy will probably need to be continued for life, and marked depigmentation predisposes to sunburn.

Therapy of discoid lupus erythematosus must be appropriate to the individual.[40, 49, 325–327] Mild cases may be controlled by, and *all* cases benefit from, avoidance of exposure to intense sunlight (from 8:00 AM to 5:00 PM), the use of topical sunscreens, and the use of topical glucocorticoids (see Chap. 3). Initially, topical glucocorticoid therapy is most successful when potent agents, such as betamethasone or fluocinolone in DMSO (Synotic), are applied every 12 hours. After the dermatosis is in remission, topical glucocorticoids are applied as needed (once daily, every 48 hours, and so forth), and less potent agents (e.g., 1 to 2 per cent hydrocortisone) may be sufficient for maintenance. In some cases, a 1-month course of systemic prednisone (2.2 mg/kg orally q24h until remission is achieved, then q48h) is helpful. The topical agents may then be sufficient to maintain the remission. Though not frequently effective as the sole therapy, systemic vitamin E (400 to 800 IU daily) is recommended, because it may have a beneficial effect.[327] Vitamin E appears to have a 1- to 2-month lag phase before its benefit is recognized clinically, and systemic glucocorticoids may be used concurrently during this period. Vitamin E should be administered 2 hours before or after feeding. Two of the authors (DWS, WHM) have had good success in some cases with the oral administration of products containing omega-3/omega-6 fatty acids (DVM Derm Caps), and now use these products instead of vitamin E.

If these benign treatments are not effective in dogs, tetracycline and niacinamide in combination may be effective in up to 70 per cent of the cases (see Chap. 3).[326] In dogs under 10 kg, the dosage is 250 mg of each drug q8h, and in dogs over 10 kg, the dosage is 500 mg of each q8h. The tetracycline-niacinamide combination produces its effects within 8 weeks.

In refractory cases in dogs and cats in which the owners believe that better control is absolutely required, systemic glucocorticoids (2.2 to 4.4 mg/kg prednisolone or prednisone, given orally q24h) are often effective. For more severe or refractory cases, other systemic drugs may be added to the treatment regimen: azathioprine (2.2 mg/kg orally q24h, then q48h in *dogs only*) or chlorambucil (0.2 mg/kg orally q24h, then q48h) (see Chap. 3). Owners should understand that discoid lupus erythematosus is rarely a life-threatening disease but that some of the potent immunomodulating drugs could cause severe side-effects. In humans, discoid lupus erythematosus is often responsive to antimalarial drugs—chloroquine (Aralen), hydroxychloroquine (Plaquenil), and quinacrine (Atabrine).[13] These drugs may be useful in the dog as well, but dosage, efficacy, and toxicity need to be carefully evaluated. Other drugs occasionally found to be beneficial in humans are retinoids, dapsone, and gold (oral or injectable).[13] The usefulness of these latter compounds in dogs is currently unknown.

Cold Agglutinin Disease

Cause and Pathogenesis

Cryoglobulins and *cryofibrinogens* are proteins that can be precipitated from serum and plasma, respectively, by cooling.[13, 40, 332] Cryoglobulins have been classified into three types according to their characteristics. Type I cryoglobulins are composed solely of monoclonal immunoglobulins or free light chains (Bence Jones proteins) and are most commonly associated with lymphoproliferative disorders. Type II cryoglobulins are composed of monoclonal and polyclonal immunoglobulins and are most commonly associated with autoimmune and connective tissue disease. Type III cryoglobulins are composed of polyclonal immunoglobulins and are seen with infections, autoimmune disorders, and connective tissue diseases. Cutaneous signs associated with cryoglobulins and cryofibrinogens are due to vascular insufficiency (obstruction, stasis, spasm, thrombosis) that occur from microthrombi and vasculitis.

Clinical Features

Cold agglutinin disease (cold hemagglutinin disease, cryopathic hemolytic anemia) has been rarely reported to cause skin disease in dogs and cats.[40, 333, 333a, 334] It is an autoimmune disorder associated with cold-reacting (usually IgM) erythrocyte autoantibodies. The cryopathic autoantibody is most active at colder temperatures (0 to 4°C) but has a wide range of thermal activity (0 to 37°C). Two forms are recognized in dogs.[20] The first is associated with cold agglutinins that are IgM antibody. The second form is a nonagglutinating type, usually associated with IgG. The latter form is rarer and is not known to cause skin disease. Cold agglutinin disease represents a type II hypersensitivity reaction and has been associated with idiopathy and lead poisoning in dogs and with upper respiratory infection, lead poisoning, and idiopathy in cats.

Clinical signs of cold agglutinin disease are variable and relate to either anemia or intracapillary cold hemagglutination or both. Skin lesions include erythema, purpura, acrocyanosis, necrosis, and ulceration. Skin lesions generally involve the extremities (paws, ears, nose, tip of tail) (see Fig. 8:47 *H*) and are precipitated or exacerbated by exposure to cold (see Fig. 8:47 *H*). Hemoglobinemia may also be present.

Diagnosis

The differential diagnosis includes vasculitis, systemic lupus erythematosus, dermatomyositis, disseminated intravascular coagulation, and frostbite.

Definitive diagnosis of cold agglutinin disease is made by history, physical examination, and demonstration of significant titers of cold agglutinins. In vitro autohemagglutination of blood at room temperature can be diagnostic for cold-reacting autoantibodies. Blood in heparin or ethylenediaminetetra-acetic acid (EDTA) is allowed to cool on a slide, thus permitting the autoagglutination to be readily visible macroscopically. The reaction can be accentuated by cooling the blood to 0°C, or reversed by warming the blood to 37°C. Doubtful cases can be confirmed via Coombs' test if the complete test is performed at 4°C and the Coombs reagent has activity against IgM. Caution in interpretation of the cold Coombs' test is warranted, because normal dogs and cats may have titers up to 1:100.[40, 335]

Histopathology

Skin biopsy usually reveals necrosis, ulceration, and often secondary suppurative changes. Fortuitously sampled sections may show vasculitis, thrombotic to necrotic blood vessels, or blood vessels containing an amorphous eosinophilic substance consisting largely of precipitated cryoglobulin.[13, 332]

Clinical Management

The prognosis for cold agglutinin disease varies with the underlying cause. Therapy of cold agglutinin disease includes (1) correction of the underlying cause, if possible, (2) avoidance of cold, and (3) immunosuppressive drug regimens (e.g., glucocorticoids, azathioprine) (see Chap. 3).

Graft-Versus-Host Disease

Graft-versus-host disease is a well-recognized result of bone marrow transplantation in dogs and humans.[13, 40] The disease occurs whenever lymphoid cells from an immunocompetent donor are introduced into a histoincompatible recipient that is incapable of rejecting them. It is generally accepted that the disease results from donor T-cell responses to recipient transplantation antigens.

In dogs and humans, a bone marrow graft from a donor genetically identical for major histocompatibility complex is followed by significant graft-versus-host disease in about 50 per cent of recipients, despite post-graft immunosuppressive therapy. The principal target organs are the skin, liver, and intestinal tract. In dogs, acute graft-versus-host disease develops about 2 weeks after grafting and is characterized by erythroderma, jaundice, diarrhea, and gram-negative infections. Chronic graft-versus-host disease develops about 3 to 4 months after grafting and is characterized by exfoliative erythroderma, ulcerative dermatitis, ascites, and gram-positive infections.

Diagnosis is based on history, physical examination, and skin biopsy. Histopathologic findings in acute graft-versus-host disease include varying degrees of interface dermatitis (hydropic or lichenoid) with satellitosis.[13, 40] In chronic graft-versus-host disease, one finds variable sclerodermoid or poikilodermatous changes.

Therapy of graft-versus-host disease with various combinations of systemic glucocorticoids, azathioprine, cyclosporine, methotrexate, and antithymocyte serum have been only partially and unpredictably effective.

Cutaneous Drug Reaction

Cutaneous drug reactions (drug eruption, drug allergy, dermatitis medicamentosa) in dogs and cats are uncommon, variably pruritic, and pleomorphic cutaneous or mucocutaneous reactions to a drug.[350, 353, 360, 361]

Cause and Pathogenesis

Adverse reactions to drugs are common, and in humans, cutaneous reactions are one of the most common.[13] Drugs responsible for skin eruptions may be administered orally, topically, or by injection or inhalation. The incidence of cutaneous drug reactions in dogs and cats is unknown but is reported to be 2.2 per cent of all hospitalized human patients and 3 per 1000 courses of drug therapy.[13]

Adverse drug reactions may be divided into two major groups: (1) predictable, which are usually dose dependent and are related to the pharmacologic actions of the drugs, and (2) unpredictable, which are often dose independent and are related to the individual's immunologic response or to genetic differences in susceptibility of patients (idiosyncracy or intolerance), which are often related to metabolic or enzymatic deficiencies. Many cutaneous effects of certain drugs are predictable. For instance, many of the anticancer or immunosuppressive drugs can cause alopecia, purpura, poor wound healing, and increased susceptibility to infection through their effects on cellular biology.[13, 40, 351, 352] Doxorubicin typically causes an alopecia that begins on the head and extends to the ventral neck, thorax, and abdomen.[355, 365, 368] Hyperpigmentation and pruritus may also be seen. Immunologic reactions involved in cutaneous drug reactions include types I, II, III, and IV hypersensitivity reactions. Additionally, other immunologic reactions may occur, as evidenced by the drug-induced development of erythema multiforme, toxic epidermal necrolysis, and superficial suppurative necrolytic dermatitis of Miniature Schnauzers. Though the mechanism for these reactions is unknown, it is believed that immunologic mechanisms may play a role. Human patients with systemic lupus erythematosus and atopy are thought to be predisposed to cutaneous drug reactions,[13] but no such observations have been made for the dog and cat.

Any drug may cause an eruption (Table 8:20), though certain drugs are more frequently associated with the development of cutaneous drug eruption. The most common drugs recognized to produce hypersensitivity-like reactions in dogs and cats are sulfonamides (especially those that are trimethoprim potentiated, such as Tribrissen), penicillins, and cephalosporins.[40, 353, 360, 361, 364]

Clinical Features

Cutaneous drug reactions can mimic virtually any dermatosis (Table 8:20 and Fig. 8:50 *A* to *H*).* No age or sex predilections have been reported for canine and feline cutaneous drug

*See references 40, 357, 360, 364, 367, 372, 374, and 375.

Table 8:20. Drug Reactions Reported in Dogs and Cats

Reaction Pattern	Drugs
Urticaria-angioedema	Vaccinations, antisera, bacterins, blood transfusions, antibiotics (especially sulfonamides, penicillins, cephalosporins, tetracyclines), amitraz, propylthiouracil, levamisole, barbiturates, radiographic contrast media, etoposide, ivermectin
Fixed drug eruption	Diethylcarbamazine, 5-fluorocytosine, aurothioglucose, thiacetarsamide
Erythema multiforme	Sulfonamides, levamisole, cephalosporins, aurothioglucose, chloramphenicol, diethylcarbamazine, penicillins, L-thyroxine, gentamicin, tetracycline
Toxic epidermal necrolysis	Sulfonamides, cephalosporins, levamisole, penicillins, 5-fluorocytosine, aurothioglucose, antisera, griseofulvin, D-limonene
Bullous pemphigoid	Triamcinolone
Pemphigus	Ampicillin, cimetidine, diethylcarbamazine, sulfonamides, procainamide, thiabendazole
Lupus erythematosus	Primidone, vaccines
Mucocutaneous erythema/crust	Retinoids
Vasculitis	Penicillins, sulfonamides
Exfoliative erythroderma	Sulfonamides, lincomycin, levamisole
Pruritus (allergy-like)	Numerous (oral, injectable, topical)
Ulceration at pressure points and onychomadesis	Bleomycin
Epitheliotropic lymphoma	Ketoconazole
Patchy alopecia/pustules (follicular necrosis/inflammation and atrophy)	Levamisole, sulfonamides
Postinjection panniculitis	Subcutaneous rabies vaccine, other injectables
Postinjection vasculitis	Rabies vaccine, other vaccines and injections
Postinjection atrophy	Glucocorticoids, progestationals
Alopecia with increased susceptibility to infection	Azathioprine, chlorambucil, cyclophosphamide, doxorubicin (also flushing and pruritus), glucocorticoids, hydroxyurea, mechlorethamine
Atrophy and fragility	Diphenhydantoin
Hirsutism, papillomatosis, and lymphoplasmacytoid dermatosis	Cyclosporine
Superficial suppurative necrolytic dermatitis of miniature schnauzer	Shampoos (especially insecticidal)

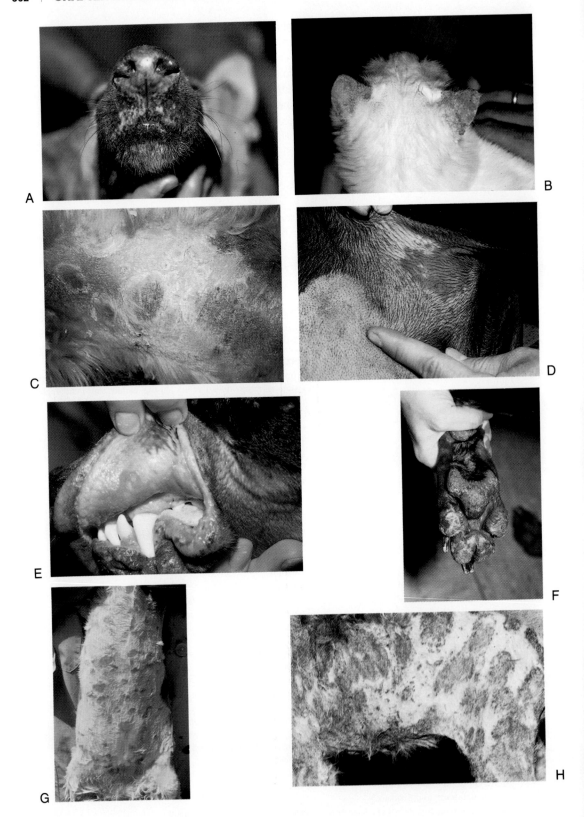

reactions. In general, no breed predilections are seen, though Poodles and certain terriers (Yorkshire, Silky) may be predisposed to rabies vaccine reactions,[361] Doberman pinschers to sulfadiazine reactions,[354] and Miniature Schnauzers to sulfonamide, gold, and shampoo (superficial suppurative necrolytic dermatitis) reactions.[378]

Although no specific type of reaction is related to only one drug, certain reactions are more commonly seen with certain drugs. The syndrome of *superficial suppurative necrolytic dermatitis of Miniature Schnauzers* has been associated only with shampoos (Fig. 8:50 *H*).[378] Adult Miniature Schnauzers of either sex develop cutaneous and systemic signs within 48 to 72 hours after shampooing (usually insecticidal). Lesions, which may be widespread or primarily ventral, include erythematous papules and plaques that develop pustulosis, becoming painful, necrotic, and ulcerative. Lesions regress spontaneously within 1 to 2 weeks with symptomatic therapy. Systemic signs include pyrexia, depression, and neutrophilia.

Erythema multiforme and toxic epidermal necrolysis have been most commonly seen with administration of sulfonamides, cephalosporins, and levamisole (Fig. 8:50 *E* to *G*).[49, 350, 360, 364, 377] Diethylcarbamazine and 5-fluorocytosine have been associated with fixed drug eruptions, especially on the scrotum of male dogs.[40, 362, 371] A hypersensitivity reaction (probably type III) associated with trimethoprim-sulfadiazine (Tribrissen) administration (probably sulfadiazine related) has been recognized in Doberman pinschers (genetically programmed?).[354] Cyclosporine has been reported to cause a lymphoplasmacytoid dermatitis with malignant features (usually a solitary plaque or nodule) in dogs and humans.[354a, 373] Methimazole may produce severe pruritus and excoriations of the face and neck of cats that are only partially responsive to glucocorticoid treatment and mimic food hypersensitivity.[358] Drugs have also been reported to produce reactions that clinically, pathologically, and immunologically resemble pemphigus (see Fig. 8:50 *C*) and pemphigoid.[349, 359, 363, 364, 366] One of the authors (DWS) has seen drug reactions (associated with ketoconazole in one case, multiple drugs in others) in dogs that were clinically and histologically indistinguishable from epitheliotropic lymphoma, as has been reported in humans.[370]

Unusual reactions to local injections are also well recognized. One such reaction is the focal vasculitis and alopecia that follows the subcutaneous administration of rabies vaccine, especially in Poodles and Yorkshire and Silky terriers (see discussion of vasculitis).[361] Another local reaction is the panniculitis associated with the subcutaneous administration of rabies vaccine in cats and dogs and of a combined rhinotracheitis-calicivirus vaccine in cats (see discussion of panniculitis, Chap. 17).[356, 376]

Because drug reaction can mimic so many different dermatoses, it is imperative to have an accurate knowledge of the medications given to any patient with an obscure dermatosis. Drug eruption may occur after a drug has been given for days or years, or a few days after drug therapy is stopped. In humans, eruptions most commonly occur within 1 week.[13] Though it has been reported in dogs that erythema multiforme usually occurs within 2 weeks, other reactions (vasculitis, atrophic dermatosis, nodules, rabies vaccine reactions) may occur months after the drug is administered.[360, 361, 367] At present, the only reliable test for the diagnosis of drug eruption is to withdraw the drug and watch for disappearance of the eruption (usually in 10 to 14 days). Occasionally, however, drug eruptions may persist for weeks to months after the offending drug is stopped.[360, 361] Purposeful re-administration of the offending drug to determine whether the eruption will be reproduced is undesirable and may be dangerous.

Figure 8:50. Drug reaction. *A*, Mucocutaneous depigmentation and ulcers due to triple sulfa. *B*, Pinnal erythema, crusting, and alopecia due to Tresaderm. *C*, Exfoliative erythroderma due to Tribrissen. *D*, Vasculitic purpura due to chloramphenicol. *E*, Ulcerative stomatitis and cheilitis associated with erythema multiforme major in a dog with *Klebsiella* otitis externa who had received numerous topical and systemic medicaments. *F*, Same dog as in *E*. Note ulcers on footpads. *G*, Multifocal ulcers on the ventral thorax and abdomen of a cat with erythema multiforme major due to cephalexin. (Courtesy E. Guaguère) *H*, Superficial suppurative necrolytic dermatitis in a miniature Schnauzer following administration of an antiseborrheic shampoo.

Diagnosis

The differential diagnosis is complex, because drug eruption may mimic virtually any dermatosis. In general, no specific or characteristic laboratory findings indicate drug eruption. Results of in vivo and in vitro immunologic tests have usually been disappointing. The basophil degranulation test has been reported to be a valuable test for detecting some hypersensitivity-induced cutaneous drug reactions.[42]

Helpful criteria for distinguishing drug hypersensitivity are as follows:

1. Hypersensitivity occurs in a minority of patients receiving the drug.
2. Observed manifestations do not resemble known pharmacologic actions for the drugs.
3. Prior exposure to drug may have been tolerated without adverse effects.
4. Reaction conforms to manifestations generally acknowledged as demonstrating hypersensitivity.
5. Reaction is reproduced by administration of small doses of the drugs or of cross-reacting drugs.
6. Resolution occurs within several days after drug is discontinued.

Identifying the specific cause of a cutaneous drug eruption can be difficult, because many patients are receiving several drugs at the same time.[13, 349]

Just as the clinical morphology of drug reactions varies greatly, so do the histologic findings. Histologic patterns recognized with cutaneous drug reactions include perivascular dermatitis (pure, spongiotic, hyperplastic), interface dermatitis (hydropic, lichenoid), intraepidermal vesiculopustular dermatitis, and subepidermal vesicular dermatitis. Eosinophils may be absent or numerous.[360, 361] In humans, eosinophils may be more prominent with drug-induced than with non–drug-induced pemphigus foliaceus.[293] Some syndromes—such as erythema multiforme, toxic epidermal necrolysis, and superficial suppurative necrolytic dermatitis—have their own characteristic histopathology. Superficial suppurative necrolytic dermatitis of Miniature Schnauzers is characterized by parakeratosis, superficial epidermal suppuration and necrosis, epidermal edema, and suppurative perivascular and perifollicular dermatitis (Figs. 8:51 and 8:52).[378] Similar changes may be seen in the follicular epithelium.

Direct immunofluorescence and immunohistochemical testing in drug reactions may reveal immunoreactants deposited in a variety of nondiagnostic patterns, especially in the walls of blood vessels and at the basement membrane zone.[40, 360, 361]

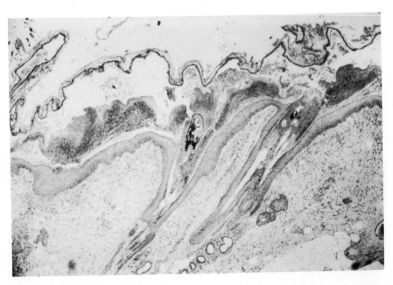

Figure 8:51. Superficial suppurative necrolytic dermatitis of miniature Schnauzers. Superficial suppuration and necrosis affecting the epidermis and hair follicle infundibulum.

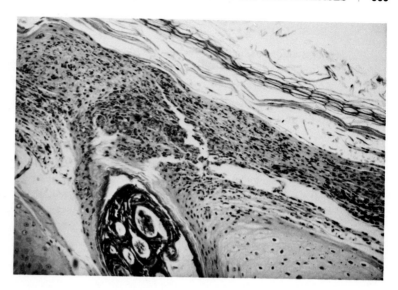

Figure 8:52. Close-up of Figure 8:51. Superficial necrosis and suppuration of the epidermis and hair follicle.

Clinical Management

The prognosis for drug reaction is usually good, unless other organ systems are involved or there is extensive epidermal necrosis. Therapy of drug reaction consists of (1) discontinuing the offending drug, (2) treating symptoms with topical and systemic medications, as indicated, and (3) avoiding chemically related drugs. Drug reactions may be poorly responsive to glucocorticoids, though some immunologically mediated reactions respond to glucocorticoids or immune-suppressive regimens (see Chap. 3).[350, 361]

Erythema Multiforme

Erythema multiforme is an uncommon, acute, usually self-limited eruption of the skin, mucous membranes, or both, characterized by distinctive gross lesions and a diagnostic sequence of pathologic changes.

Cause and Pathogenesis

Despite recognition of multiple etiologic and triggering causes, the pathogenesis of erythema multiforme is not fully understood. It is commonly considered a hypersensitivity reaction and has been associated with infections, drugs, neoplasia, and connective tissue diseases.[13, 49, 377, 383] Fadok has speculated that at least some forms of erythema multiforme, toxic epidermal necrolysis, and fixed drug eruption may reflect a drug-induced apoptosis.[350] In humans, direct immunofluorescence testing reveals immunoreactants (especially C3 and IgM) at the basement membrane zone and, in about 50 per cent of cases, in the walls of superficial dermal blood vessels.[4, 13] In addition, circulating immune complexes are often present. Erythema multiforme has been recognized in dogs in association with infections (staphylococcal folliculitis, anal sacculitis), drug therapy (aurothioglucose, cephalexin, chloramphenicol, diethylcarbamazine, gentamicin, levamisole, L-thyroxine, environmental insecticides, and trimethoprim-sulfonamide), and idiopathy.[48, 360, 377, 379, 383] A subgroup of idiopathic erythema multiforme has been described in old dogs.[17] In cats, erythema multiforme has been reported in association with drug therapy (cephalexin, penicillin, aurothioglucose).

Clinical Signs

Prodromal or concurrent clinical signs may reflect the underlying cause. As the term *multiforme* implies, the skin lesions are variable, but they are usually characterized by an acute, rather symmetric onset of (1) erythematous macules (Fig. 8:53 *B*) or slightly elevated papules that spread peripherally and clear centrally, producing annular (target) or arciform patterns (Fig. 8:53 *A*), (2) urticarial plaques, (3) vesicles and bullae, or (4) some combination thereof. The lesions and patients with maculopapular eruptions are usually asymptomatic (erythema multiforme minor). Occasionally, animals become systemically ill (fever, depression, anorexia) and have rather extensive vesiculobullous and ulcerative lesions of the mucocutaneous areas, oral mucosa, conjunctiva, pinnae, axillae, and groin (erythema multiforme major, Stevens-Johnson syndrome) (Fig. 8:50 *E* to *G*).[364, 380] The maculopapular form of erythema multiforme is characterized by *lack* of surface pathology (lack of scale, crust, oozing, hair loss). The urticarial form of erythema multiforme is characterized by a normal overlying skin and haircoat and the *persistence* of urticarial lesions, as opposed to the evanescent nature of the wheals in true urticaria.

Diagnosis

The differential diagnosis includes bacterial folliculitis, dermatophytosis, demodicosis, urticaria, and other vesicular and pustular disorders. Definitive diagnosis is made on the basis of history, physical examination, ruling out of alternatives with laboratory testing, and skin biopsy. Skin biopsy findings vary with the gross morphology of the lesions.[13, 40, 63] *Maculopapular* lesions are characterized histologically by hydropic interface dermatitis with prominent single-cell necrosis of keratinocytes and satellitosis of lymphocytes and macrophages (Figs. 8:54 and 8:55). The infundibular region of hair follicle outer root sheath epithelium is often similarly affected. A superficial interstitial or, rarely, a dense lichenoid inflammatory infiltrate is seen. *Urticarial* lesions are characterized by hydropic interface dermatitis and striking dermal edema (Fig. 8:56). Dermal collagen fibers become vertically oriented and attenuated, presenting a weblike appearance (''gossamer'' collagen). *Vesiculobullous* lesions are characterized by segmental full-thickness coagulation necrosis of epithelium (Fig. 8:57). A superficial perivascular accumulation of predominantly lymphohistiocytic cells is typical, and subepidermal cleft and vesicle formation may occur owing to separation of the necrotic epithelium from the underlying connective tissue at the basement membrane zone.

Clinical Management

Erythema multiforme may run a mild course, spontaneously regressing within a few weeks. An underlying cause should be sought and corrected, whenever possible, a procedure that will also result in spontaneous resolution of the erythema multiforme.[13, 40] Severe vesiculobullous cases of erythema multiforme require supportive care and an exhaustive search for underlying causes. The usefulness of systemic glucocorticoids and other immunomodulating drugs in erythema multiforme is controversial, and severe vesiculobullous eruptions are usually poorly responsive to these drugs.[13] They may be beneficial, however, if given in high, immunosuppressive doses in severe erythema multiforme major that is drug-induced.[13, 350, 380, 381] Anecdotal reports suggest that cyclosporine[350] or etretinate[382] may be useful in idiopathic erythema multiforme in dogs.

Toxic Epidermal Necrolysis

Toxic epidermal necrolysis is a rare, variably painful, vesiculobullous and ulcerative disorder of skin and oral mucosa in dogs, cats, and human beings. It is often considered to be closely related to or part of a spectrum that includes erythema multiforme major.

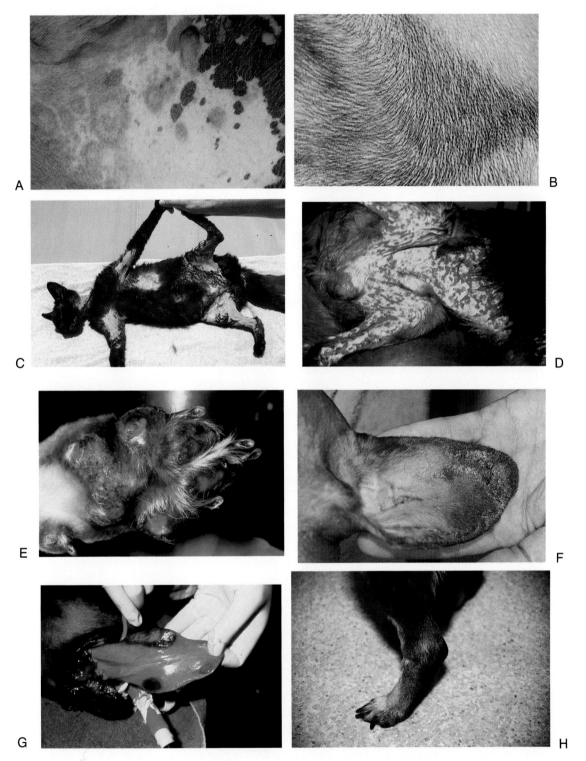

Figure 8:53. *A*, Erythema multiforme minor in a dog caused by Tribrissen. Annular, erythematous, bull's eye lesions in flank. *B*, Canine erythema multiforme due to cephalexin. Serpiginous erythema. *C*, Toxic epidermal necrolysis in a cat. (From Rosenkrantz W.S.: Cutaneous drug reactions. In: Griffin CE, et al. (eds.): Current Veterinary Dermatology. St. Louis, Mosby Year Book, 1993.) *D*, Severe ulceration of the ventrum, medial thighs, and scrotum of a dog with toxic epidermal necrolysis due to levamisole. (Courtesy G. T. Wilkinson) *E*, Ulcerated footpads in a dog with idiopathic leukocytoclastic vasculitis. *F*, Cutaneous idiopathic vasculitis in a dog. Necrosis and ulceration tracing pinnal vasculature. *G*, Punctate ulcers on the tongue of a dog with idiopathic leukocytoclastic vasculitis. *H*, Pitting edema of the hock in a dog with vasculitis.

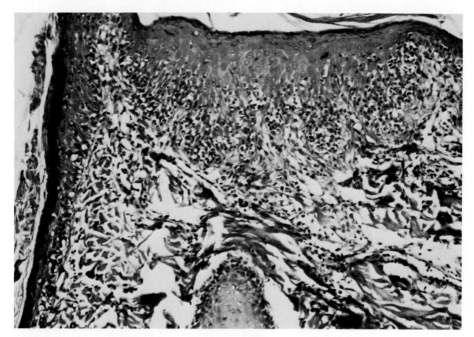

Figure 8:54. Canine erythema multiforme. Hydropic interface dermatitis.

Cause and Pathogenesis

Toxic epidermal necrolysis has been temporally associated with drugs (50 per cent of cases; especially penicillins, cephalosporins, levamisole, 5-fluorocytosine), toxins, infections, malignancies, and other systemic disorders (Table 8:21).[13, 49, 372, 377, 385, 386] A 1992 report implicated topical flea dips in both a dog and cat that developed toxic epidermal necrolysis.[384] Some cases are idiopathic. Although the pathomechanism of toxic epidermal necrolysis is unknown, immunopathologic mechanisms are most often suggested.[13] It has been suggested that drug-induced erythema multiforme major and toxic epidermal necrolysis may relate to defective epidermal detoxification of drug-induced byproducts. Fadok proposed that apoptosis may be

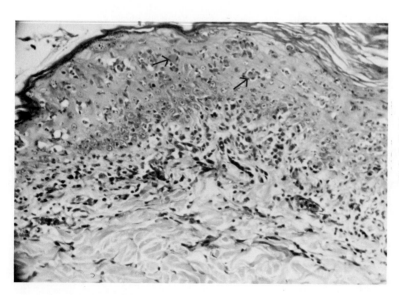

Figure 8:55. Canine erythema multiforme minor. Note interface dermatitis and marked single-cell necrosis of keratinocytes (arrows).

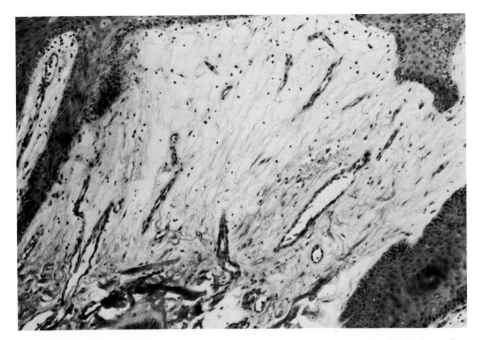

Figure 8:56. Canine erythema multiforme. Marked dermal edema with vertical stretching of collagen fibers ("gossamer collagen").

induced and that it is massive and sudden in toxic epidermal necrolysis but is localized and more gradual in erythema multiforme.[350]

Clinical Features

There are no apparent age, breed, or sex predilections. Clinically, toxic epidermal necrolysis is usually characterized by an acute onset of constitutional signs (pyrexia, anorexia, lethargy, depression) and a multifocal or generalized vesiculobullous disease (Fig. 8:53 *C* and *D*). Vesicles and bullae, necrosis, and resultant ulcers with epidermal collarettes may be found

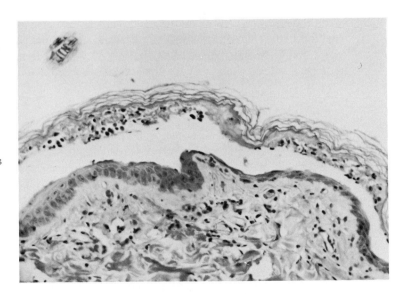

Figure 8:57. Canine erythema multiforme major. The upper half of the epidermis has undergone coagulation necrosis and has separated from the viable epidermis below.

Table 8:21. Etiologic Factors Associated with Toxic Epidermal Necrolysis in Dogs and Cats

Dog	Cat
Bacterial endocarditis	FeLV antiserum (caprine)
Myeloproliferative disease	Cephaloridine
Cholangiohepatitis	Ampicillin
Hepatic necrosis	Hetacillin
Splenic fibrosarcoma	Phomset dip
Levamisole	D-Limonene
Cephalexin	Griseofulvin
5-Fluorocytosine	Idiopathic
D-Limonene	
Aurothioglucose	
Sulfonamides (especially trimethoprim-potentiated)	
Idiopathic	

anywhere in the skin and often involve the oral mucosa, mucocutaneous junctions, and footpads. Nikolsky's sign is usually present. Cutaneous pain is usually moderate to marked.

Diagnosis

The differential diagnosis is relatively limited in severe cases with constitutional signs and the acute history and includes burns, systemic lupus erythematosus, erythema multiforme major, and epitheliotropic lymphoma.

Definitive diagnosis is based on history, physical examination, and skin biopsy. A hemogram usually reveals neutropenia or neutrophilia.[49] In humans, persistent neutropenia portends a fatal outcome.[13]

■ *Histopathology.* Histopathologic findings in toxic epidermal necrolysis are identical, regardless of underlying cause. They consist of hydropic degeneration of basal epidermal cells, full-thickness coagulation necrosis of the epidermis, and minimal dermal inflammation (silent dermis or cell-poor inflammation) (Fig. 8:58).[17, 40, 63] Dermoepidermal separation results in subepidermal vesicles (Fig. 8:59). The periodic acid–Schiff (PAS) positive basement membrane zone, when present, is usually located at the floor of the vesicles. The infundibular region of hair follicle outer root sheath epithelium may be similarly affected. It must be emphasized that toxic epidermal necrolysis is not usually the definitive diagnosis. It is imperative to remember that toxic epidermal necrolysis is only a cutaneous reaction pattern, and every attempt must be made to find the underlying cause.

Results of direct and indirect immunofluorescence testing are usually negative.[13, 49, 360, 364]

Clinical Management

The prognosis for toxic epidermal necrolysis is guarded to poor, pending identification of the underlying cause, with a 20 to 50 per cent mortality rate in humans. The mortality is greatest in idiopathic cases, wherein a precipitating factor cannot be recognized and specifically corrected. The sequelae and prognosis are similar to those of a massive second-degree burn, owing to fluid, electrolyte, and colloid losses and to secondary infections that compound the loss of epidermal barrier function.

Treatment is (1) correction of the underlying cause and (2) symptomatic and supportive measures (fluids, antibiotics, topicals, and so on). The use of systemic glucocorticoids is controversial, some investigators believing that these drugs are at best not helpful and at worst detrimental.[13] The administration of systemic glucocorticoids may be indicated, however, in

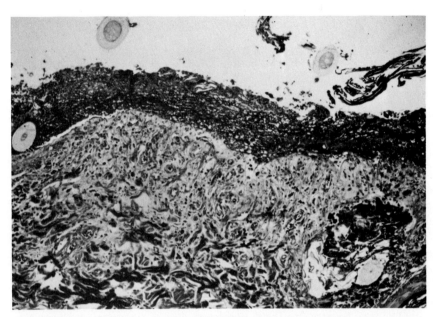

Figure 8:58. Canine toxic epidermal necrolysis (associated with staphylococcal endocarditis). Full-thickness epidermal coagulation necrosis with minimal inflammation. (From Scott, D.W., et al.: Toxic epidermal necrolysis in two dogs and a cat. J. Am. Anim. Hosp. Assoc. 15:271, 1979.)

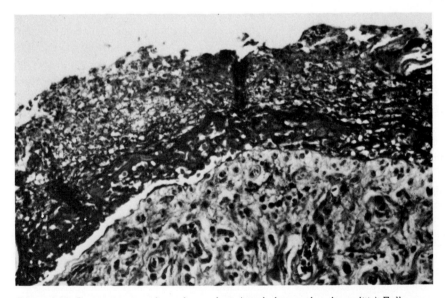

Figure 8:59. Canine toxic epidermal necrolysis (staphylococcal endocarditis). Full-thickness epidermal coagulation necrosis with subepidermal cleft formation. (From Scott, D.W., et al.: Toxic epidermal necrolysis in two dogs and a cat. J. Am. Anim. Hosp. Assoc. 15:271, 1979.)

drug-induced cases.[13] Recovery (depending on the identification and correction of the underlying cause) usually occurs in 2 to 3 weeks.

Vasculitis

Cutaneous vasculitis is an uncommon disorder in dogs that is characterized by purpura, necrosis, and ulceration often involving the extremities. It is rare in cats.

Cause and Pathogenesis

Vasculitides are classified histologically into neutrophilic, lymphocytic, granulomatous, and mixed forms. The neutrophilic forms may be leukocytoclastic (neutrophil nuclei undergo karyorrhexis, resulting in "nuclear dust") or nonleukocytoclastic.[9, 13, 49] Vasculitis can occur via immune and nonimmune mechanisms.[20, 344] As a cause of cutaneous disease, vasculitis most commonly is believed to be immunologically mediated and the result of a drug reaction.[20] It has been postulated that differences in membrane receptors (probably, adhesion molecules and cytokines) for immunoglobulin and complement on leukocytes may account for the different histologic appearances of neutrophilic and lymphocytic vasculitides.[4] The pathomechanism of most cutaneous vasculitides is assumed to involve type III hypersensitivity reactions. Type I hypersensitivity reactions may be important in the initiation of immune complex deposition in blood vessel walls.

Cutaneous vasculitis may be associated with coexisting disease (infections, malignancies, connective tissue disorders such as lupus erythematosus) or precipitating factors (drugs) or it may be idiopathic (about 50 per cent of all cases).[9, 13, 49, 344, 346] Infections may induce immune complex or septic vasculitis.[17] Focal cutaneous vasculitis reactions at the site of rabies vaccination have been described in dogs, and rabies viral antigen was detected in blood vessel walls.[348]

Clinical Features

Cutaneous signs of vasculitis usually include palpable purpura, hemorrhagic bullae or pustules, necrosis, punched-out ulcers, and occasionally acrocyanosis, especially involving the extremities (paws, pinnae, lips, tail, scrotum, and oral mucosa), and may clearly be associated with vascular pathways (Fig. 8:53 E to G). Hemorrhages may be seen within the claw. The lesions may or may not be painful. In some animals, widespread erythema that may be purplish or cyanotic is seen. The erythematous skin does *not* blanch with diascopy, confirming its purpuric nature.[344] Rarely, subcutaneous nodules may be noted, which represent a panniculitis caused by septal vasculitis.[344, 347] Constitutional signs may be present, including anorexia, depression, and pyrexia. Pitting edema of extremities, polyarthropathy, and myopathy have been reported in some dogs (Fig. 8:53 H).[344] Any age, breed, or sex may be affected, but dachshunds and Rottweilers may be predisposed.[49]

A *proliferative thrombovascular necrosis of the pinnae* has been recognized in dogs.[345] The

---

Figure 8:60. *A,* Pinnal thrombovascular necrosis with erythema of pinnal apex and linear crust on lateral surface and margin of pinna. *B,* Wedge-shaped hyperpigmented to erythematous plaque with ulceration of pinnal margin in a dog with pinnal thrombovascular necrosis. *C,* Canine linear IgA dermatosis. Annular, coalescing areas of alopecia, scaling, crusting, and hyperpigmentation. *D,* Canine uveodermatologic syndrome. Depigmentation of nose, muzzle, and periocular skin. *E,* Canine uveodermatologic syndrome. Depigmentation of lips. *F,* Uveodermatologic syndrome in an Akita. (From MacDonald JM: Uveodermatologic syndrome in the dog. In: Griffin CE, et al. (eds.): Current Veterinary Dermatology. Mosby Year Book, St. Louis, 1993.) *G,* Feline relapsing polychondritis. Swollen, curled, misshapen pinnae. (Courtesy E. Guaguère) *H,* Feline relapsing polychondritis. Swollen, violaceous pinna. (Courtesy E. Guaguère)

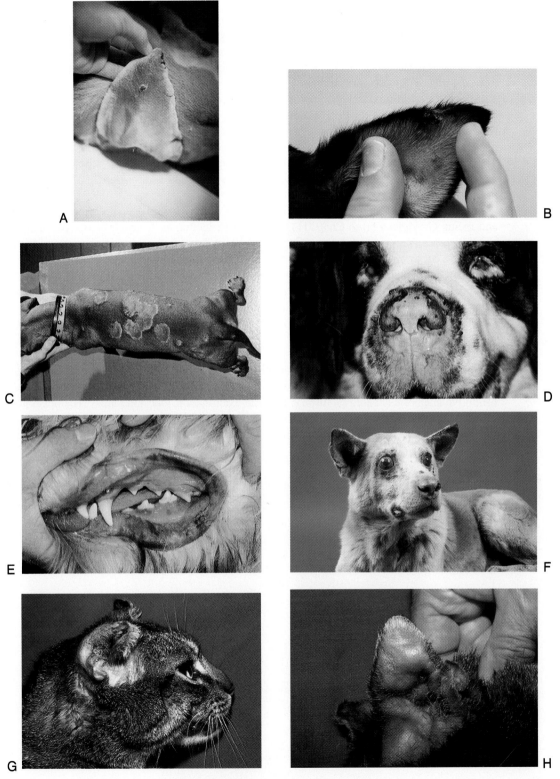

Figure 8:60 *See legend on opposite page*

etiology is unknown, and there are no apparent age, breed, or sex predilections. Lesions begin on the apical margins of the pinnae and spread along the concave surface. An elongated necrotic ulcer is at the center of the lesions. There is often a thickened, scaly, hyperpigmented zone surrounding the ulcers (Fig. 8:60 *A* and *B*). The lesions are wedge shaped, with the wide base at the pinnal apex. As the ulcer enlarges, the older areas undergo complete necrosis, resulting in a deformed pinnal margin.

A *focal cutaneous vasculitis and alopecia at the sites of rabies vaccination* has been described in dogs.[17, 348, 361] Poodles and Yorkshire and Silky terriers appeared predisposed. Reactions were characterized by roughly annular areas of variable alopecia, hyperpigmentation, and, less commonly, scaling or erythema overlying a variably indurated dermis and subcutis. The caudal or lateral thigh, or the withers are typically affected (Fig. 8:61). The lesions generally appear 3 to 6 months following the subcutaneous administration of vaccine and persist for months to years.

An *idiopathic cutaneous and renal glomerular vasculopathy* has been described in kenneled and racing Greyhounds (see Chap. 11).[343] No age (6 months to 6 years) or sex predilections exist. Palpable purpura, with lesions pinpoint to 10 cm in diameter, is most commonly seen on the tarsus, stifle, or inner thigh. Within 1 to 2 days, the lesions ulcerate and discharge a serosanguineous fluid. The ulcers are well-demarcated and usually extend into the subcutis. Healing is slow, resulting in scar formation within 1 to 2 months. Some dogs develop pyrexia, lethargy, polydipsia, polyuria, vomiting, dark or tarry stools, and acute renal failure.

Diagnosis

The differential diagnosis includes a coagulopathy, systemic lupus erythematosus, cold agglutinin disease, frostbite, disseminated intravascular coagulation, and lymphoreticular neoplasia. Definitive diagnosis is based on history, physical examination, and skin biopsy. Histopathology reveals varying degrees of neutrophilic or lymphocytic vasculitis (Fig. 8:62), possibly reflecting the age of the lesions and the types of immunoreactants.[17, 63] Fibrinoid necrosis is not usually

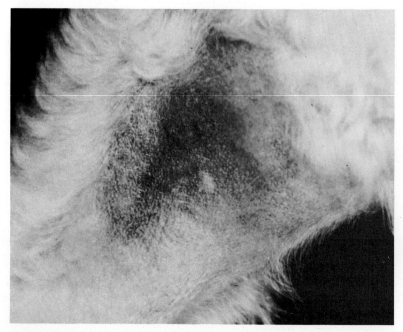

Figure 8:61. Alopecic, hyperpigmented plaque on caudomedial thigh of a Poodle due to postvaccinal vasculitis.

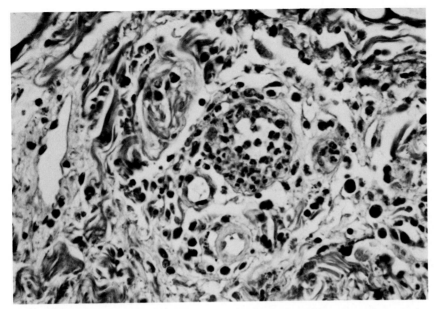

Figure 8:62. Canine cutaneous idiopathic leukocytoclastic vasculitis. Degeneration of blood vessel wall with leukocytoclasis and "nuclear dust" formation. (From Manning, T.O., Scott, D.W.: Cutaneous vasculitis in a dog. J. Am. Anim. Hosp. Assoc. 16:61, 1980.)

present. Involvement of deep dermal vessels may suggest systemic disease. When the deep vasculature is affected, necrosis of appendages and subcutaneous fat may be seen. The lesions most likely to show diagnostic changes are those from 8 to 24 hours old. In some biopsies the diagnosis of vasculitis vasculopathy is suspected on the basis of a cell-poor hydropic interface dermatitis and the loss of definition and staining intensity of hair follicles ("fading follicles"). Once the diagnosis of cutaneous vasculitis has been established, it is imperative that underlying etiologic factors be sought and eliminated (Table 8:22). Cutaneous vasculitis has been reported in dogs with bacteremia, systemic lupus erythematosus, rheumatoid arthritis, polyarteritis no-

Table 8:22. Etiologic Factors in Cutaneous Vasculitis

Infections	Bacterial
	Mycobacterial
	Fungal
	Viral
	Protozoal
	Rickettsial
Injection of foreign proteins	Sera
	Vaccines
	Hyposensitization
Drugs	Antibiotics
Other diseases	Systemic lupus erythematosus
	Discoid lupus erythematosus
	Dermatomyositis
	Plasma cell pododermatitis
	Hereditary pyogranuloma and vasculitis of Scottish terriers
	Idiopathic vasculopathy of Greyhounds
	Familial vasculopathy of German Shepherds
	Rheumatoid arthritis
	Ulcerative colitis
	Malignancies

dosa, Rocky Mountain spotted fever, ehrlichiosis, drug reactions, and staphylococcal hypersensitivity, and as an idiopathic occurrence.[40, 49, 344] In addition, lymphocytic or eosinophilic vasculitis has been recognized in dogs with drug reaction and in dogs with severe scabies and flea bite hypersensitivity.[40]

Proliferative thrombovascular necrosis of the pinnae is characterized by arteriolar proliferation, sclerosis, hyalin degeneration, and eventually thrombosis.[345] No inflammatory vasculitis is present. *Focal vasculitis and alopecia subsequent to rabies vaccination* is characterized by vasculitis affecting the arterioles of the deep dermis and subcutis, septal panniculitis, fat necrosis, focal lymphoid nodules, and marked atrophy of the overlying adnexa.[348] *Idiopathic cutaneous and renal glomerular vasculopathy* is characterized by mild to severe changes in the arterioles and arteries of the deep dermis and subcutis.[343] These changes range from increased eosinophilia of the tunica media to pyknosis and karyorrhexis and, occasionally, fibrinoid necrosis. Vascular thrombosis and ischemia result in purpura and cutaneous infarcts.

Direct immunofluorescence or immunohistochemical testing may demonstrate immunoglobulin or complement, or both, in vessel walls and occasionally at the basement membrane zone in both the neutrophilic and lymphocytic forms of cutaneous vasculitis (Fig. 8:26 *D*).[4, 13, 49] These tests are usually not needed, however, and are not particularly useful for diagnosis; if they are performed, they must be done within the first 4 hours after lesion formation. Studies in humans have shown that the intradermal injection of 0.02 ml of a histamine phosphate solution into the skin of patients with active cutaneous vasculitis was a reliable method for demonstrating the deposition of immunoreactants, with direct immunofluorescence testing of the injection site performed 4 hours after injection.[4]

Dogs with active vasculitis may have increased levels of circulating immune complexes, decreased levels of serum complement, and hypergammaglobulinemia.[40]

Clinical Management

It is difficult to predict the course of the disease in any individual case. A single episode lasting a few weeks may occur, or the disorder may be chronic or recurrent. The outcome depends on the extent of internal organ involvement (especially renal and neurologic) and the underlying or precipitating factor(s).

Treatment of vasculitis consists of correction of the underling cause and immunomodulatory drug treatment.[13, 49] In some cases, systemic prednisone or prednisolone (2 to 4 mg/kg orally q24h) is effective.[344] For other cases that are refractory to glucocorticoids, sulfones such as dapsone (1 mg/kg orally q8h, *not* cats) or sulfasalazine (20 to 40 mg/kg orally q8h) may be effective (see Chap. 3).[40, 344, 346] Cyclophosphamide has been useful in some patients,[40] and colchicine is often beneficial in humans.[13] Azathioprine has been effective in some dogs. In some cases, therapy can be stopped after 4 to 6 months of treatment. Other patients require long-term maintenance therapy with lower drug doses and reduced frequency of administration (see Chap. 3).

Proliferative thrombovascular necrosis of the pinnae is slowly progressive and unresponsive to all medical therapies that have been tried.[345] Possibly, pentoxifylline would be helpful in thrombotic pinnal diseases through its effect of increasing peripheral perfusion (see Chap. 3). The current treatment of choice is partial surgical removal of the pinna. Relapses have occurred only when attempts were made to save as much tissue as possible. *Focal cutaneous vasculitis and alopecia subsequent to injections* are best treated by complete surgical excision.

Canine Linear IgA Dermatosis

Linear IgA dermatosis is a very rare idiopathic, sterile superficial pustular dermatosis of dachshunds, characterized histologically by subcorneal pustules and immunologically by the deposition of IgA at the basement membrane zone of affected skin.[49, 387] It is not analogous to a similarly named dermatosis of humans.[4, 13]

Clinically, linear IgA dermatosis is characterized by a multifocal to generalized pustular dermatitis. The trunk is typically involved. Secondary skin lesions include annular areas of alopecia, erosion, epidermal collarettes, hyperpigmentation, scaling, and crusting (see Fig. 8:62 C). Pruritus is minimal to absent, and the dogs are otherwise healthy. All cases to date have been recognized in adult dachshunds of either sex.

The differential diagnosis includes bacterial folliculitis, dermatophytosis, demodicosis, pemphigus foliaceus, and subcorneal pustular dermatosis. Cytologic examination of pus reveals nondegenerate neutrophils, no microorganisms, and an occasional or no acanthocytes. Diagnosis is based on culture (negative), skin biopsy (intraepidermal pustular dermatitis, with numerous nondegenerate neutrophils and minimal acantholysis) (Fig. 8:63), and direct immunofluorescence or immunohistochemical testing (IgA deposited at the basement membrane zone).

Therapy consists of large doses of prednisolone or prednisone (2.2 to 4.4 mg/kg orally q24h, then an alternate-day regimen) or dapsone (1 mg/kg orally q8h, then as needed) (see Chap. 3). Interestingly, glucocorticoids may work in one case and not another. The same is true of dapsone.

Canine Uveodermatologic Syndrome

The uveodermatologic syndrome (Vogt-Koyanagi-Harada–like syndrome) is a rare, idiopathic syndrome of concurrent granulomatous uveitis and depigmenting dermatitis in dogs.

Cause and Pathogenesis

The cause of this syndrome is unknown. The syndrome has many similarities to the Vogt-Koyanagi-Harada syndrome in humans, which is currently thought to represent an autoimmune disorder.[13, 336, 338–340] In humans, cell-mediated hypersensitivity to melanin and melanocytes has been demonstrated. Antiretinal antibodies were demonstrated in a dog.[341]

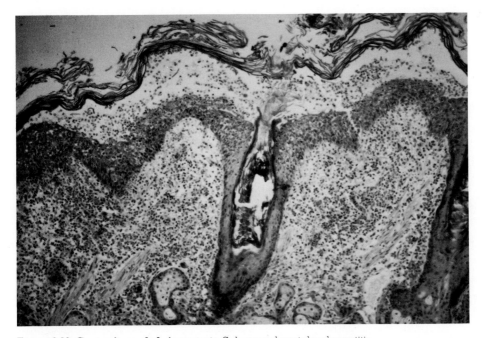

Figure 8:63. Canine linear IgA dermatosis. Subcorneal pustular dermatitis.

Clinical Features

In humans, the Vogt-Koyanagi-Harada syndrome has three phases: (1) a *meningoencephalitic* phase with prodromata of fever, malaise, headache, tinnitus, nausea, and vomiting, (2) an *ophthalmic* phase with photophobia, uveitis, decreased visual acuity, and potential blindness, and (3) a *dermatologic* phase with poliosis (90 per cent of cases), alopecia (73 per cent), and vitiligo (63 per cent).[13] The dermatologic signs are usually symmetric, especially involving the head, neck, and eyelids, and they usually mark the convalescent stage when the uveitis begins to abate. The pigmentary changes tend to be permanent.

In dogs, there are no apparent age or sex predilections, but Akitas, Samoyeds, and Siberian huskies appear predisposed.[338–340, 342] The syndrome is usually characterized by the acute onset of uveitis and concurrent or subsequent depigmentation of the nose, lips, eyelids, and occasionally the footpads, scrotum, anus, and hard palate (Fig. 8:60 *D* to *F*). Oral ulcerations may rarely be seen (Fig. 8:60 *F*).[339, 342] In most cases, skin lesions are mild, consisting of well-demarcated depigmentation with or without mild erythema and scale. Some cases, however, progress or even rapidly develop more marked dermatitis, with depigmented areas developing varying degrees of erosion, ulceration, and crusting. Perhaps some of the dermatitis may be associated with exposure to sunlight (photodermatitis).[40] Patchy leukotrichia may be present in the areas surrounding the cutaneous depigmentation. Rarely, leukoderma and leukotrichia may be widespread.[337] Clinicopathologic evidence of a meningoencephalitic phase is rarely seen in dogs.

Diagnosis

The definitive diagnosis is based on history, physical examination, and skin biopsy. Histopathologic findings in specimens taken from early skin lesions are characterized by lichenoid interface dermatitis, wherein large histiocytes are a major cellular component (Figs. 8:64 and 8:65).[17, 49, 63] Pigmentary incontinence is pronounced, but hydropic degeneration of epidermal basal cells is rarely seen. Histopathologic findings in the eye include granulomatous panuveitis and retinitis. Results of direct and indirect immunofluorescence testing are usually negative.[49]

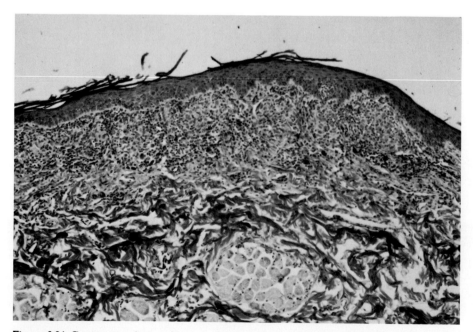

Figure 8:64. Canine uveodermatologic syndrome. Lichenoid interface dermatitis.

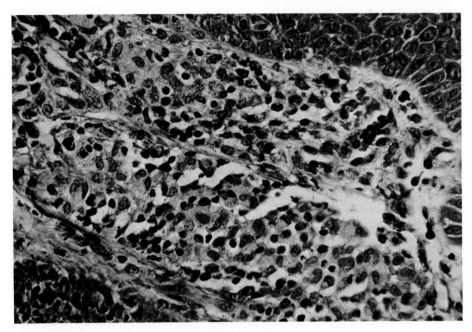

Figure 8:65. Close-up of Figure 8:64. Numerous histiocytes in lichenoid band.

Clinical Management

Patients with poorly controlled uveitis often develop posterior synechiae with secondary glaucoma, cataracts, and vision loss. Thus, aggressive early treatment is essential. Topical or subconjunctival glucocorticoids and topical cycloplegics (e.g., atropine) are beneficial in patients with anterior uveitis. Systemic glucocorticoids and azathioprine are needed to combat posterior uveitis and dermatologic signs.[340, 342] If the disease is treated early, variable degrees of cutaneous repigmentation (sometimes complete) usually occur. Occasionally, these cases may respond to systemic glucocorticoids alone, but because blindness may result from delaying an effective therapy and because more aggressive therapy is often required, the authors recommend combination immunosuppressive therapy. Dogs usually require long-term alternate-morning oral glucocorticoid therapy (e.g., 0.25 to 1.1 mg/kg prednisone or prednisolone) to prevent recurrence.[49] The response of the skin lesions should not be utilized to assess response to therapy, because uveitis may be active while the skin is improving.[339] Ophthalmic examinations should be periodically performed even when the cutaneous changes are in remission.

Feline Relapsing Polychondritis

Relapsing polychondritis is a rare disease of cats and humans characterized by inflammation and destruction involving both articular and nonarticular cartilaginous structures.[13, 389]

Cause and Pathogenesis

Relapsing polychondritis is often classified among the immune-mediated diseases because of similarities to rheumatoid arthritis and lupus erythematosus as well as its favorable response to immunomodulatory therapy. In humans, antibodies against type II collagen are demonstrated.[13] In cats, all patients tested have been either feline leukemia virus (FeLV)–or feline immunodeficiency virus (FIV)–positive.[388, 389]

Clinical Features

Affected cats present with a history of swollen, erythematous, painful ears.[47, 388, 389] When examined, the pinnae are swollen and meaty, erythematous to violaceous, and curled and deformed (Figs. 8:60 *G* and *H*). Cats may be otherwise healthy or may show signs of pyrexia, lethargy, and anorexia.

Diagnosis

Biopsies reveal lymphoplasmacytic inflammation, loss of cartilage basophilia, and cartilage necrosis (Figs. 8:66 and 8:67). Hematologic examinations may demonstrate variable degrees of neutrophilia, lymphocytosis, and hyperglobulinemia.

Clinical Management

Cats that are in no pain and show no systemic signs may do fine without therapy. In one cat, systemic glucocorticoids were ineffective, but dapsone (1 mg/kg q24h) induced a remission within 2 weeks.[389] Permanent deformity of the pinnae is to be expected, whether or not the cat is treated.

Immunoproliferative Enteropathy of Basenji Dogs

Immunoproliferative enteropathy of Basenjis is characterized by chronic intractable diarrhea, progressive emaciation, and gastropathy.[40, 390] An autosomal recessive inheritance of the condition has been hypothesized. A similar disease exists in humans.

Basenjis of either sex and a wide age range are affected. Skin lesions are variable and may consist of either alopecia, hyperpigmentation, hyperkeratosis, and marginal necrosis and ulceration of the pinnae or a symmetric alopecia of the ventrum. The haircoat is often dry and dull.

Diagnosis is based on history, physical examination, and laboratory testing. Most affected

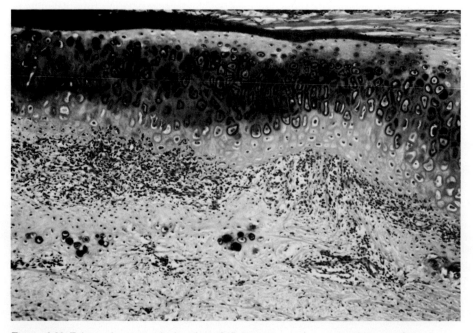

Figure 8:66. Feline relapsing polychondritis. Inflammation and necrosis of ear cartilage.

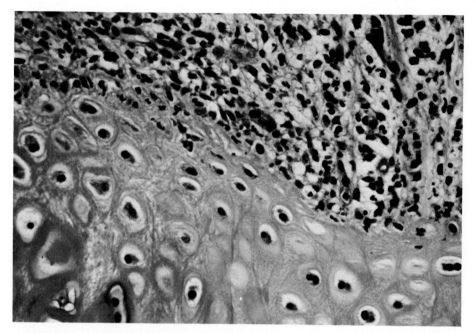

Figure 8:67. Close-up of Figure 8:66.

dogs have hypergammaglobulinemia. Some dogs are hypothyroid. Intestinal biopsy reveals lymphoplasmacytic enteritis.

Dermatohistopathologic findings are nondiagnostic. Alopecic skin is characterized by endocrinopathic changes, probably reflecting hypothyroidism. Dermatitic pinnae are characterized by ulcerative perivascular dermatitis, necrosis, and changes consistent with secondary bacterial infection. Although the clinical appearance of the pinnae is suggestive of a vasculopathy, histologic evidence of vessel disease has not been reported.

Therapy is provided according to symptoms and is often disappointing. Genetic counseling, avoidance of stress, and high-quality commercial diets are indicated. Systemic glucocorticoids may be beneficial.

Alopecia Areata

Alopecia areata is a rare disorder of dogs and cats characterized by patches of noninflammatory hair loss.

Cause and Pathogenesis

Alopecia areata is of unknown pathogenesis.[13] Genetic, endocrine, and psychological factors have been thought to play a role in humans with alopecia areata. In addition, the following observations in humans with alopecia areata have suggested that this disorder may have an immune basis: (1) accumulations of lymphoid cells (helper T cells) around hair bulbs during the active phase of the disease, (2) occasional association of alopecia areata with other immune-mediated diseases, (3) increased incidence of various autoantibodies in alopecia areata, (4) decreased numbers of circulating T cells, (5) abnormal presence of Langerhans' cells in the follicular bulb, (6) the deposition of C3 or IgG and IgM or both at the basement membrane zone of the hair follicles in lesional and normal scalp as revealed by direct immunofluorescence testing, and (7) the therapeutic benefit of inducing delayed-type hypersensitivity. Morphologic

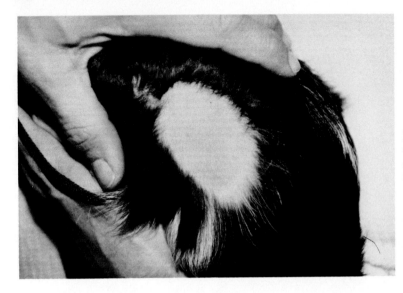

Figure 8:68. Canine alopecia areata. Well-circumscribed annular alopecia over hip region.

abnormalities of melanocytes in follicular bulbs have been described in humans with alopecia areata.

Clinical Features

In dogs and cats, alopecia areata is characterized by focal or multifocal patches of asymptomatic, noninflammatory alopecia.[17, 40] There are no apparent age, breed, or sex predilections. The alopecic areas are well circumscribed, and the exposed skin appears normal (Fig. 8:68). Chronically alopecic areas may become variably hyperpigmented. Lesions may occur anywhere, especially the head, neck, and trunk, and are usually asymmetric. Microscopic examination of hairs plucked from the margin of enlarging lesions reveals a mixture of normal telogen, dysplastic, and ''exclamation point'' hairs—short, stubby hairs with frayed, fractured, pigmented distal ends whose shafts undulate or taper toward the proximal end (Fig. 8:69).

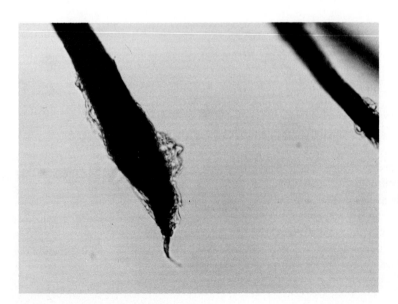

Figure 8:69. Canine alopecia areata. Trichogram may reveal hair shafts with suddenly tapered ends (''exclamation points'').

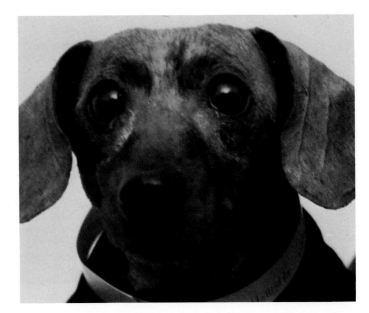

Figure 8:70. Alopecia areata in a dachshund. Alopecia of pinnae and around eyes.

Occasionally, alopecia areata may be confined to the dark-haired areas of multicolored haircoats (Fig. 8:70).

Diagnosis

The differential diagnosis includes traction alopecia, injection reactions, acquired pattern alopecia, topical steroid reaction, follicular dysplasia, dermatophytosis, demodicosis, staphylococcal folliculitis, psychogenic alopecia, and endocrinopathies. Definitive diagnosis is based on the insidious onset of asymptomatic, well-circumscribed areas of noninflammatory alopecia and on skin biopsy.

■ *Histopathology.* The characteristic early histopathologic findings include a peribulbar accumulation of lymphocytes, histiocytes, and plasma cells.[17, 63] This has been described as looking like a swarm of bees (Fig. 8:71). This early change may be difficult to demonstrate, however, requiring multiple biopsies from the advancing edges of early lesions. Later, the histopathologic findings consist of a predominance of catagen and telogen hair follicles as well as follicular atrophy. Hair follicles may be distorted in contour. Chronic lesions may show complete absence of hair follicles and a fibrous tract associated with orphaned apocrine and sebaceous glands and arrector pili muscles.

Clinical Management

The prognosis for alopecia areata in humans is usually good; most patients make a complete recovery within 3 to 5 years with or without therapy. Although topical, intralesional, or systemic glucocorticoids are often recommended for the treatment of alopecia areata in humans, dogs, and cats, there is no evidence that they are beneficial.[13, 40] The biological behavior of alopecia areata in dogs and cats is unclear. Most dogs spontaneously recover after a course of 6 months to 2 years.[40] Initial hair regrowth is often a color lighter than normal (leukotrichia).

Amyloidosis

Amyloidosis is a generic term that signifies the abnormal extracellular deposition of one of a family of unrelated proteins that share certain characteristic staining properties and ultrastruc-

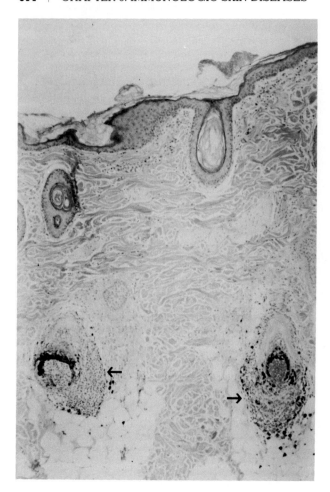

Figure 8:71. Canine alopecia areata. Peribulbar accumulations of lymphocytes ("swarm of bees") and pigmentary incontinence (*arrows*).

tural features.[9, 13] Amyloidosis is not a single disease entity, and amyloid may accumulate as a result of a variety of different pathogenetic mechanisms. In the dog and cat, most cases of amyloidosis are related to deposition of immunoglobulin light chains.[17, 20]

Although the pathogenesis of amyloidosis is unclear, it is morphologically related to cells of the mononuclear phagocytic system, plasma cells, and keratinocytes. Functional studies suggest that such cells play at least a partial role in the genesis of amyloidosis. In dogs and cats, amyloidosis is usually associated with chronic inflammatory disease and accumulations of plasma cells.[17, 20]

Most commonly, amyloidosis is an internal disease, usually affecting the kidneys.[20] Cutaneous lesions are described in dogs with systemic amyloidosis and primary cutaneous disease.[17] Cutaneous lesions with systemic amyloidosis associated with a monoclonal gammopathy was reported in an adult female Cocker spaniel.[392] Cutaneous hemorrhage could be induced by flicking the abdominal skin briskly with a finger or by removing hair (Fig. 8:72). If the skin was traumatized severely, blood oozed through the skin within seconds and clotted immediately. Skin biopsy revealed an amorphous, homogeneous, eosinophilic superficial dermis. The walls of the blood vessels in the involved area were thickened by deposition of the homogeneous eosinophilic material (Fig. 8:73). The material was Congo red–positive (congophilia), and a green birefringence of the material was seen in Congo red–stained sections examined with polarized light (dichroism). A monoclonal serum IgG paraprotein was found. No treatment was given, and the dog remained unchanged for 14 months.

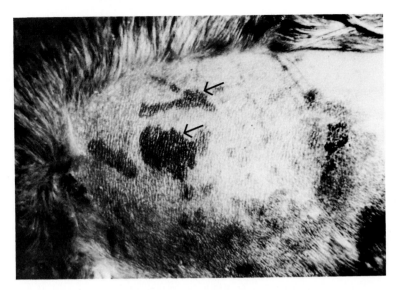

Figure 8:72. Canine cutaneous amyloidosis. Ecchymoses produced by traumatizing the skin (pinch purpura) (*arrows*). (Courtesy R.M. Schwartzman)

Mucocutaneous amyloidosis unassociated with monoclonal gammopathy, was reported in a 3-year-old Brittany spaniel.[391] The dog had multiple, whitish to ulcerated papular and plaquelike lesions on the tongue and gingiva, and oozing ulcers on the footpads, ventral surface of the interdigital spaces, and multiple pressure points (elbows, stifles).

Primary nodular cutaneous amyloidosis has been described as the most common type of cutaneous amyloidosis in dogs and cats.[17] Solitary or grouped dermal or subcutaneous nodules may occur anywhere but more commonly involve the ear. Some nodules may ulcerate secondary to necrosis. The differential diagnosis for these lesions would be neoplasia, cysts, and infectious or sterile nodular granulomas. Diagnosis is made by histopathologic examination, which shows multiple dermal accumulations of amorphous eosinophilic material. Small numbers of plasma cells are found, as well as macrophages and small numbers of lymphocytes.

The diagnosis of amyloidosis is confirmed by biopsy.[17] Solitary nodules unassociated with systemic disease can be successfully excised. Successful treatment of multiple lesions is not reported.

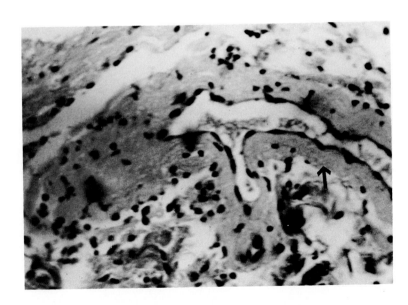

Figure 8:73. Canine cutaneous amyloidosis. Dermal blood vessel wall is markedly thickened by amyloid deposition (*arrow*). (Courtesy R.M. Schwartzman)

REFERENCES

General

1. Abdou, N.I.: The idiotype-antiidiotype network in human autoimmunity. J. Clin. Immunol. 5:365, 1985.
2. Ahmed, S.A., et al.: Sex hormones, immune responses, and autoimmune diseases. Am. J. Pathol. 121:531, 1985.
3. Ansel, J., et al.: Cytokine modulation of keratinocyte cytokines. J. Invest. Dermatol. 94:101S, 1990.
4. Beutner, E.H., et al.: Immunopathology of the Skin III. Churchill Livingstone, New York, 1987.
5. Bos, J.D.: Skin Immune System. CRC Press, Boca Raton, FL, 1989.
6. Bradley, G.A., Calderwood Mays, M.B.: Immunoperoxidase staining for the detection of autoantibodies in canine autoimmune skin disease; comparison to immunofluorescence results. Vet. Immunol. Immunopathol. 26:105, 1990.
7. Braquet, P., et al.: Perspectives in platelet-activating factor research. Pharmacol. Rev. 39:97, 1987.
8. Caciolo, P.L., et al.: Michel's medium as a preservative for immunofluorescent staining of cutaneous biopsy specimens in dogs and cats. Am. J. Vet. Res. 45:128, 1984.
9. Dahl, M.V.: Immunodermatology II. Year Book Medical Publishers, Chicago, 1988.
10. DeBoer, D.J., et al.: Circulating immune complex concentrations in selected cases of skin disease in dogs. Am. J. Vet. Res. 49:143, 1988.
11. Doré, M., et al.: Production of a monoclonal antibody against canine GMP-140 (P-selectin) and studies of its vascular distribution in canine tissues. Vet. Pathol. 30:213, 1993.
12. Ettinger, S.J.: Textbook of Veterinary Internal Medicine, III. W.B. Saunders Co., Philadelphia, 1989.
13. Fitzpatrick, T.B., et al.: Dermatology in General Medicine III. McGraw-Hill, New York, 1993.
14. Griffin, C.E., Rosenkrantz, W.S.: Direct immunofluorescence testing: A comparison of two laboratories in the diagnosis of canine immune-mediated skin disease. Semin. Vet. Med. Surg. 2:202, 1987.
15. Griffin, C.E.: Diagnosis and management of primary autoimmune skin disease: A review. Semin. Vet. Med. Surg. 2:173, 1987.
16. Griffin, C.E., et al.: Current Veterinary Dermatology. Mosby Year Book, Inc., St. Louis, 1993.
17. Gross, T.L., et al.: Veterinary Dermatopathology: A Macroscopic and Microscopic Evaluation of Canine and Feline Skin Disease. Mosby Year Book, Inc., St. Louis, 1992.
18. Haines, D.M., et al.: Avidin-biotin peroxidase complex immunohistochemistry to detect immunoglobulin in formalin fixed skin biopsies in canine autoimmune skin disease. Can. J. Vet. Res. 51:104, 1987.
19. Halliwell, R.E.W.: Clinical and immunological aspects of allergic skin diseases in domestic animals: In: von Tscharner, C., Halliwell, R.E.W. (eds): Advances in Veterinary Dermatology I. Ballière-Tindall, Philadelphia, 1990, p. 91.
20. Halliwell, R.E.W., Gorman, N.T.: Veterinary Clinical Immunology. W.B. Saunders Co., Philadelphia, 1989.
21. Hargis, A.M., Liggit, H.D.: Cytokines and their role in cutaneous injury. In: Ihrke, P.J., et al. (eds): Advances in Veterinary Dermatology II. Pergamon Press, New York, 1993, p. 325.
22. Hauser, C., et al.: T helper cells grown with hapten-modified cultured Langerhans' cells produce interleukin 4 and stimulate IgE production by B cells. Eur. J. Immunol. 19:245, 1989.
23. Hauser, C., Orbea, H.A.: Superantigens and their role in immune-mediated diseases. J. Invest. Dermatol. 101:503, 1993.
24. Henfry, J.I.: Autoimmune skin disease in dogs. In Pract. 13:131, 1991.
25. Hewicker-Trautwein, M., et al.: Zur Diagnostic bullöser und nicht-bullöser autoimmuner Hautkrankheiten bei Hund und Katze. Kleintierpraxis 37:135, 1992.
26. Ihrke, P.J., et al.: The longevity of immunoglobulin preservation in canine skin utilizing Michel's fixative. Vet. Immunol. Immunopathol. 9:161, 1985.
27. Ihrke, P.J., et al. (eds): Advances in Veterinary Dermatology II. Pergamon Press, New York, 1993.
28. Kalaher, K.M.: The value of immunofluorescence testing. In: Kirk, R.W. (ed): Current Veterinary Therapy XI. W.B. Saunders Co., Philadelphia, 1992, p. 503.
29. Kristensen, F., Mehl, N.B.: Autoimmune lidelser hos hund og kat. Behandling med guldsalte. Dansk Vet. Tidsskr. 72:883, 1989.
30. Kromer, G., et al.: Is autoimmunity a side-effect of interleukin 2 production? Immunol. Today 7:199, 1986.
31. Lewis, R.M., Picut, C.A.: Veterinary Clinical Immunology. Lea & Febiger, Philadelphia, 1989.
32. Locke, P.H., et al.: Manual of Small Animal Dermatology. British Small Animal Veterinary Association, Shurdington, 1993.
33. Luger, T.A., Schwartz, T.: Evidence for an epidermal cytokine network. J. Invest. Dermatol. 95:100S, 1990.
34. Matus, R.W., et al.: Plasmapheresis in five dogs with systemic immune-mediated disease. J. Am. Vet. Med. Assoc. 187:595, 1985.
35. McEwan, B.J., et al.: The response of the eosinophil in acute inflammation in the horse. In: von Tscharner, C., Halliwell, R.E.W. (eds): Advances in Veterinary Dermatology I. Baillière-Tindall, Philadelphia, 1990, p. 176.
36. McKenzie, R.C., Sauder, D.N.: The role of keratinocyte cytokines in inflammation and immunity. J. Invest. Dermatol. 95:105S, 1990.
37. Middleton, E., et al.: Allergy Principles and Practice IV. Mosby Year Book, Inc., St. Louis, 1993.
38. Moore, F.M., et al.: Localization of immunoglobulins and complement by the peroxidase antiperoxidase method in autoimmune and nonautoimmune canine dermatopathies. Vet. Immunol. Immunopathol. 14:1, 1987.
39. Mottier, S., von Tscharner, C.: Immunohistochemistry in skin disease: Diagnostic value? In: von Tscharner, C., Halliwell, R.E.W. (eds): Advances in Veterinary Dermatology I. Baillière-Tindall, 1990, p. 479.
40. Muller, G.H., et al.: Small Animal Dermatology, IV. W.B. Saunders Co., Philadelphia, 1989.
41. Nickoloff, B.J.: Dermal Immune System. CRC Press, Boca Raton, FL, 1993.

42. Prélaud, P.: The basophil degranulation test in the diagnosis of canine allergic skin disease. In: von Tscharner, Halliwell, R.E.W. (eds): Advances in Veterinary Dermatology I. Baillière-Tindall, Philadelphia, 1990, p. 117.
43. Prélaud, P.: Les Dermites Allergiques du Chien et du Chat. Masson, Paris, 1991.
44. Reedy, L.M., Miller, W.H., Jr.: Allergic Skin Diseases of Dogs and Cats. W.B. Saunders Co., Philadelphia, 1989.
45. Scott, D.W.: Epidermal mast cells in the cat. Vet. Dermatol. 1:65, 1990.
46. Scott, D.W.: Feline dermatology, 1979–1982: Introspective retrospections. J. Am. Anim. Hosp. Assoc. 20:537, 1984.
47. Scott, D.W.: Feline dermatology, 1983–1985: "The secret sits." J. Am. Anim. Hosp. Assoc. 23:255, 1987.
48. Scott, D.W., et al.: Immune-mediated dermatoses in domestic animals: Ten years after—part I. Comp. Cont. Educ. 9:423, 1987.
49. Scott, D.W., et al.: Immune-mediated dermatoses in domestic animals: Ten years after—part II. Comp. Cont. Educ. 9:539, 1987.
50. Scott, D.W., et al.: Miliary dermatitis: A feline cutaneous reaction pattern. Proc. Annu. Kal Kan Semin. 2:11, 1986.
51. Stone, J.: Dermatology, Immunology and Allergy. Mosby Year Book, Inc., St. Louis, 1985.
52. Swerlick, R.A., Lawley, T.J.: Role of microvascular endothelial cells in inflammation. J. Invest. Dermatol. 100:111S, 1993.
53. Thiers, B.H., Dobson, R.L.: Pathogenesis of Skin Disease. Churchill Livingstone, New York, 1986.
54. Thomsen, M.K.: Species specificity in the generation of eicosanoids: Emphasis on leukocyte-activating factors in the skin of allergic dogs and humans. In: Ihrke, P.J., et al. (eds): Advances in Veterinary Dermatology II. Pergamon Press, New York, 1993, p. 63.
55. Thomsen, M.K.: The Role of Neutrophil-Activating Mediators in Canine Health and Disease. Ballerup, Copenhagen, 1991.
56. Thompson, J.P.: Basic immunologic principles of allergic disease. Semin. Vet. Med. Surg. 6:247, 1991.
57. Tizard, I.R.: Veterinary Immunology: An Introduction, IV. W.B. Saunders Co., Philadelphia, 1992.
58. van den Broek, A.: Autoimmune skin diseases in cats. In Pract. 13:175, 1991.
59. von Tscharner, C., Halliwell, R.E.W.: Advances in Veterinary Dermatology I. Ballière-Tindall, Philadelphia, 1990.
60. Walsh, L.J., Murphy, G.F.: Role of adhesion molecules in cutaneous inflammation and neoplasia. J. Cutan. Pathol. 19:161, 1992.
61. Wolfe, J.H., Halliwell, R.E.W.: Total hemolytic complement values in normal and diseased dog populations. Vet. Immunol. Immunopathol. 1:287, 1980.
62. Yager, J.A.: The skin as an immune organ. In: Ihrke, P.J., et al. (eds): Advances in Veterinary Dermatology II. Pergamon Press, New York, 1993, p. 3.
63. Yager, J.A., Scott, D.W.: The skin and appendages. In: Jubb, K.V.F., et al. (eds): Pathology of Domestic Animals IV. Academic Press, New York, 1993, p. 531.
64. Zipfel, W., et al.: Demonstration of immunoglobulins and complement in canine and feline autoimmune and nonautoimmune skin diseases with the direct immunofluorescence and indirect immunoperoxidase method. J. Vet. Med. A. 32:494, 1992.

Urticaria and Angioedema
65. Noxon, J.O.: Anaphylaxis, urticaria, and angioedema. Semin. Vet. Med. Surg. 6:265, 1991.

Canine Atopy
66. Ackerman, L.: Diagnosing inhalant allergies: Intradermal or *in vitro* testing. Vet. Med. 83:779, 1988.
67. Anderson, R.K., Sousa, C.A.: *In vitro* versus *in vivo* testing for canine atopy: In: Ihrke, P.J., et al. (eds): Advances in Veterinary Dermatology II. Pergamon Press, New York, 1993, p. 425.
68. Angarano, D.W., MacDonald, J.M.: Immunotherapy in canine atopy. In: Kirk, R.W., Bonagura, J.D. (eds). Current Veterinary Therapy XI. W.B. Saunders Co., Philadelphia, 1991, p. 505.
69. August, J.R.: The intradermal test as a diagnostic aid for canine atopic disease. J. Am. Anim. Hosp. Assoc. 18:164, 1982.
70. August, J.R.: The reaction of canine skin to the intradermal injection of allergenic extracts. J. Am. Anim. Hosp. Assoc. 18:157, 1982.
71. Ballauf, B.: Vergleich von Intrakutan—und Pricktest in der Allergiediagnostik beim Hund. Tierarztl. Prax. 19:428, 1991.
72. Barbet, J.L., Halliwell, R.E.W.: Duration of inhibition of the immediate skin test reactivity by hydroxyzine hydrochloride in dogs. J. Am. Vet. Med. Assoc. 194:1565, 1989.
73. Beale, K.M., et al.: Effects of sedation on intradermal skin testing in flea-allergic dogs. J. Am. Vet. Med. Assoc. 197:861, 1990.
74. Becker, A.B., et al.: Cutaneous mast cell heterogeneity: Response to antigen in atopic dogs. J. Allergy Clin. Immunol. 78:937, 1986.
75. Bevier, D.E.: Long-term management of atopic disease in the dog. Vet. Clin. North Am. [Small Anim. Pract.] 20:1487, 1990.
76. Bos, J.D., et al.: Immune dysregulation in atopic eczema. Arch. Dermatol. 128:1509, 1992.
77. Bourdeau, P., Paragon, B.M.: Alternatives aux corticoides en dermatologie des carnivores. Rev. Méd. Vét. 168:645, 1992.
78. Bruijnzeel-Koumen, C.A.F.M., et al.: New aspects in the pathogenesis of atopic dermatitis. Acta Derm. Venereol. (Stockh) [Suppl] 144:58, 1989.

79. Bruijnzeel, P.L.B., et al.: The involvement of eosinophils in the patch test reaction to aeroallergens in atopic dermatitis: Its relevance for the pathogenesis of atopic dermatitis. Clin. Exp. Allergy 23:97, 1993.

80. Butler, J.M., et al.: Pruritic dermatitis in asthmatic Basenji-Greyhound dogs: A model for human atopic dermatitis. J. Am. Acad. Dermatol. 8:33, 1983.

81. Campbell, K.L., et al.: Immunoglobulin A deficiency in the dog. Canine Pract. 16:7, 1991.

82. Carlotti, D.N., Castargent, F.: Analyse statistique de tests cutanés positifs chez 449 chiens atteints de dermatite allergique. Prat. Méd. Chirurg. Anim. Comp. 27:53, 1992.

83. Carlotti, D.: La dermatite atopique du chien. Point. Vét. 17:5, 1985.

84. Chalmers, S.A., Medleau, L.: An update on atopic dermatitis in dogs. Vet. Med. 89:326, 1994.

85. Chan, S.C., et al.: Elevated leukocyte phosphodiesterase as a basis for depressed cyclic adenosine monophosphate responses in the Basenji-Greyhound dog model of asthma. J. Allergy Clin. Immunol. 76:148, 1985.

86. Codner, E.C., et al.: Effect of tiletamine-zolazepam sedation on intradermal allergy testing in atopic dogs. J. Am. Vet. Med. Assoc. 201:1857, 1992.

87. Codner, E.C., McGrath, C.J.: The effect of tiletamine-zolazepam anesthesia on the response to intradermally injected histamine. J. Am. Anim. Hosp. Assoc. 27:189, 1991.

88. Codner, E.C., Lessard, P.: Effect of hyposensitization with irrelevant antigens on subsequent allergy skin test results in normal dogs. Vet. Dermatol. 3:209, 1992.

89. Codner, E.C., Lessard, P.: Comparison of intradermal allergy test and enzyme-linked immunosorbent assay in dogs with allergic skin disease. J. Am. Vet. Med. Assoc. 202:739, 1993.

90. Collo, M.J., et al.: A controlled trial of house dust mite eradication using natamycin in homes of patients with atopic dermatitis: Effect on clinical status and mite populations. Br. J. Dermatol. 121:199, 1989.

91. Cooper, K.D.: Atopic dermatitis: Recent trends in pathogenesis and therapy. Dermatol. Fdn. 102:128, 1994.

92. DeBoer, D.J.: Survey of intradermal skin testing practices in North America. J. Am. Vet. Med. Assoc. 195:1357, 1989.

93. Evans, A.G.: Allergic inhalant dermatitis attributable to marijuana exposure in a dog. J. Am. Vet. Med. Assoc. 195:1588, 1989.

94. Ferguson, E.A.: A review of intradermal skin testing in the UK. Vet. Dermatol. Newsl. 14:13, 1992.

95. Ferguson, E.A.: A retrospective comparison of the success of two different hyposensitization protocols in the management of canine atopy. Proc. Brit. Vet. Dermatol. Study Grp. 16:26, 1994.

96. Fontaine, J., Henroteaux, M.: Utilisation du dosage des anticorps anaphylactiques (IgG) pour le diagnostic d'atopie chez le chien. Ann. Méd. Vét. 135:57, 1991.

97. Frank, L.A., et al.: Comparison of serum cortisol concentration before and after intradermal testing in sedated and nonsedated dogs. J. Am. Vet. Med. Assoc. 200:507, 1992.

98. Frick, O.L., et al.: Immunoglobulin E antibodies to pollens augmented in dogs by virus vaccines. Am. J. Vet. Res. 44:440, 1983.

99. Frick, O.L.: Pathogenesis of chronic allergic reactions using the atopic dog as a model. Proc. Am. Acad. Vet. Allergy, 1991.

100. Griffin, C.E.: Atopic disease. Semin. Vet. Med. Surg. 6:290, 1991.

101. Griffin, C.E.: RAST and ELISA testing in canine atopy. In: Kirk, R.W. (ed): Current Veterinary Therapy X. W.B. Saunders Co., Philadelphia, 1989, p. 592.

102. Griffin, C.E., et al.: The effect of serum IgE on an *in vitro* ELISA test in the normal canine. In: von Tscharner, C., Halliwell, R.E.W. (eds): Advances in Veterinary Dermatology I. Baillière-Tindall, Philadelphia, 1990, p. 137.

103. Halliwell, R.E.W., Kunkle, G.A.: The radioallergosorbent test in the diagnosis of canine atopic disease. J. Allergy Clin. Immunol. 62:236, 1978.

104. Hanifin, J.M., et al.: Recombinant interferon gamma therapy for atopic dermatitis. J. Am. Acad. Dermatol. 28:189, 1993.

105. Héripret, D.: Les antiprurigineux non stéroidiens. Prat. Méd. Chirurg. Anim. Comp. 28:73, 1993.

106. Hill, P.B., et al.: Levels of total serum IgE, IgA, and IgG in atopic, normal, and parasitized dogs. Proc. Annu. Memb. Meet. Am. Acad. Vet. Dermatol. Am. Coll. Vet. Dermatol. 9:32, 1993.

107. Hites, M.J., et al.: Effect of immunotherapy on the serum concentrations of allergen-specific IgG antibodies in dog sera. Vet. Immunol. Immunopathol. 22:39, 1989.

108. Kapp, A., et al.: Eosinophil cationic protein in sera of patients with atopic dermatitis. J. Am. Acad. Dermatol. 24:555, 1991.

109. Kapp, A., et al.: Altered production of immunomodulating cytokines in patients with atopic dermatitis. Acta Dermatol. Venereol. (Stockh) 144:97, 1989.

110. Kleinbeck, M.L., et al.: Enzyme-linked immunosorbent assay for measurement of allergen-specific IgE antibodies in canine serum. Am. J. Vet. Res. 50:1831, 1989.

111. Leroy, B.P., et al.: A novel therapy for atopic dermatitis with allergen-antibody complexes: A double-blind, placebo-controlled study. J. Am. Acad. Dermatol. 28:232, 1993.

112. MacDonald, J.M., Angarano, D.W.: Comparison of intradermal testing with commercial *in vitro* allergy testing (ELISA) in parasitized nonallergic beagle dogs. Proc. Annu. Memb. Meet. Am. Acad. Vet. Dermatol. Am. Coll. Vet. Dermatol. 6:46, 1990.

113. Mason, I.S., Lloyd, D.H.: Factors influencing the penetration of bacterial antigens through canine skin. In: von Tscharner, C., Halliwell, R.E.W. (eds): Advances in Veterinary Dermatology I. Baillière-Tindall, Philadelphia, 1990, p. 370.

113a. McEwan, N.A.: Bacterial adherence to canine corneocytes. In: von Tscharner, C., Halliwell, R.E.W. (eds): Advances in Veterinary Dermatology I. Baillière-Tindall, Philadelphia, 1990, p. 454.

114. Miller, W.H. Jr., et al.: Evaluation of an allergy screening test for use in atopic dogs. J. Am. Vet. Med. Assoc. 200:931, 1992.

115. Miller, W.H. Jr., et al.: Evaluation of the performance of a serologic allergy system in atopic dogs. J. Am. Anim. Hosp. Assoc. 29:545, 1993.
116. Miller, W.H. Jr., et al.: The influence of oral corticosteroids or declining allergen exposure on serologic allergy test results. Vet. Dermatol. 3:327, 1992.
117. Moriello, K.A., Eicker, S.W.: Influence of sedative and anesthetic agents on intradermal skin test reactions in dogs. Am. J. Vet. Res. 52:1484, 1991.
118. Mudde, G.C., et al.: IgE positive Langerhans' cells and Th2 allergen specific T cells in atopic dermatitis. J. Invest. Dermatol. 99:103, 1992.
119. Mudde, G.C., et al.: Allergen presentation by epidermal Langerhans' cells from patients with atopic dermatitis is mediated by IgE. Immunology 69:335, 1990.
120. Nimmo Wilkie, J.S., et al.: *In vitro* lymphocyte stimulation by concanavalin A and with histamine as a co-mitogen in dogs with atopic dermatitis. Vet. Immunol. Immunopathol. 28:67, 1991.
121. Nimmo Wilkie, J.S., et al.: Abnormal cutaneous response to mitogens and a contact allergen in dogs with atopic dermatitis. Vet. Immunol. Immunopathol. 28:97, 1991.
122. Nimmo Wilkie, J.S., et al.: Altered spontaneous and histamine-induced *in vitro* suppressor-cell function in dogs with atopic dermatitis. Vet. Immunol. Immunopathol. 30:129, 1992.
123. Nimmo Wilkie, J.S., et al.: Changes in cell-mediated immune responses after experimentally-induced anaphylaxis in dogs. Vet. Immunol. Immunopathol. 32:325, 1992.
124. Nimmo Wilkie, J.S., et al.: Morphometric analyses of the skin of dogs with atopic dermatitis and correlations with cutaneous and plasma histamine and total serum IgE. Vet. Pathol. 27:179, 1990.
125. Ohlén, B.M.: Diagnostiering och behandling vid atopi hos hund i Sverige. Svensk. Veterinär. 44:299, 1992.
126. Ohlén, B.M.: Projekt allergitester i Sverige. Svensk. Veterinär. 44:365, 1992.
127. Paradis, M., Lécuyer, M.: Evaluation of an in-office allergy screening test in nonatopic dogs having various intestinal parasites. Can. Vet. J. 34:293, 1993.
127a. Paterson, S.: Use of antihistamines to control pruritus in atopic dogs. J. Small Anim. Pract. 35:415, 1994.
128. Phillips, M.K., et al.: Cutaneous histamine reactivity, histamine content of commercial allergens, and potential for false-positive skin test reactions in dogs. J. Am. Vet. Med. Assoc. 203:1288, 1993.
129. Plant, J.D.: The reproducibility of three *in vitro* canine allergy tests: A pilot study. Proc. Annu. Memb. Am. Acad. Vet. Dermatol. Am. Coll. Vet. Dermatol. 10:16, 1994.
130. Prélaud, P.: Tests cutanés d'allergie immédiate chez le chien: Minimiser erreurs et déceptions. Prat. Méd. Chirurg. Anim. Comp. 27:529, 1992.
131. Prélaud, P., Sainte-Laudy, J.: Dermatite atopique du chien. Méthodes de diagnostic *in vitro*. Prat. Méd. Chirurg. Anim. Comp. 23:441, 1988.
132. Prélaud, P., Sainte-Laudy, J.: IgG spécifiques de l'acarien de la poussière de maison, *Dermatophagoides farinae*, chez les chiens atopiques et nonatopiques. Rev. Méd. Vét. 140:1117, 1989.
133. Prélaud, P.: Traitement de l'atopie canine. Prat. Méd. Chirurg. Anim. Comp. 28:461, 1993.
134. Rachofsky, M.A.: Comments on *in vitro* allergy testing. Dermatol. Dialogue, Winter 1993/1994, p. 4.
135. Reinhold, U., et al.: Systemic interferon gamma treatment in severe atopic dermatitis. J. Am. Acad. Dermatol. 29:58, 1993.
136. Rhodes, K.H., et al.: Comparative aspects of canine and human atopic dermatitis. Semin. Vet. Med. Surg. 2:166, 1987.
137. Rhodes, K.H., et al.: Investigation into the immunopathogenesis of canine atopy. Semin. Vet. Med. Surg. 2:199, 1987.
138. Rokugo, M., et al.: Contact sensitivity to *Pityrosporum ovale* in patients with atopic dermatitis. Arch. Dermatol. 126:627, 1990.
139. Sager, N., et al.: House dust mite specific reactivity in the skin of subjects with atopic dermatitis: Frequency and lymphokine profile in the allergen patch test. J. Allergy Clin. Immunol. 89:801, 1992.
140. Schick, R.O., Fadok, V.A.: Responses of atopic dogs to regional allergens: 268 cases (1981–1984). J. Am. Vet. Med. Assoc. 189:1493, 1986.
141. Schmeitzel, L.P.: The effects of multiple intradermal skin tests on skin reactivity. Vet. Allergist, Summer, 1986, p. 1.
142. Schwartzman, R.M.: Immunologic studies of progeny of atopic dogs. Am. J. Vet. Res. 45:375, 1984.
143. Scott, D.W.: Observations on canine atopy. J. Am. Anim. Hosp. Assoc. 17:91, 1981.
144. Scott, D.W., Paradis, M.: A survey of canine and feline skin disorders seen in a university practice: Small Animal Clinic, University of Montréal, Saint-Hyacinthe, Québec, (1987–1988). Can. Vet. J. 31:830, 1990.
145. Scott, D.W., Miller, W.H. Jr.: Nonsteroidal anti-inflammatory agents in the management of canine allergic pruritus. J. S. Afr. Vet. Assoc. 64:52, 1993.
146. Scott, K.V., et al.: A retrospective study of hyposensitization in atopic dogs in a flea-scarce environment. In: Ihrke, P.J., et al. (eds): Advances in Veterinary Dermatology II. Pergamon Press, New York, 1993, p. 79.
147. Sousa, C.A.: Atopic dermatitis. Vet. Clin. North Am. [Small Anim. Pract.] 18:1049, 1988.
148. Sousa, C.A., Norton, A.L.: Advances in methodology for diagnosis of allergic skin disease. Vet. Clin. North Am. [Small Anim. Pract.] 20:1419, 1990.
149. Sporik, R., et al.: Exposure to house-dust mite allergen (der p I) and the development of asthma in childhood: A prospective study. N. Engl. J. Med. 323:502, 1990.
150. Stiller, M.J., et al.: A double-blind, placebo-controlled clinical trial to evaluate the safety and efficacy of thymopentin as an adjunctive treatment in atopic dermatitis. J. Am. Acad. Dermatol. 30:597, 1994.
151. Tanaka, Y., et al.: Immunohistochemical studies on dust mite antigen in positive reaction site of patch test. Acta Dermatol. Venereol. (Stockh) [Suppl.] 144:93, 1989.

152. van der Heijden, F.L., et al.: High frequency of IL-4 producing CD4 + allergen-specific T lymphocytes in atopic dermatitis lesional skin. J. Invest. Dermatol. 97:389, 1991.

153. van den Broek, A.H.M., Simpson, J.W.: Fat absorption in dogs with atopic dermatitis. In: von Tscharner, C., Halliwell, R.E.W. (eds): Advances in Veterinary Dermatology I. Ballière-Tindall, Philadelphia, 1990, p. 155.

154. van Joost, T., et al.: Cyclosporine in atopic dermatitis. J. Am. Acad. Dermatol. 27:922, 1992.

155. Van Stee, E.W.: Risk factors in canine atopy. Calif. Vet. 37:8, 1983.

156. Vollset, I.: Atopic dermatitis in Norwegian dogs. Nord. Vet. Med. 37:97, 1985.

157. Vollset, I., et al.: Immediate type hypersensitivity in dogs induced by storage mites. Res. Vet. Sci. 40:123, 1986.

158. Wellington, J., et al.: Determination of skin threshold concentration of an aqueous house dust mite allergen in normal dogs. Cornell Vet. 81:37, 1991.

159. Wellington, J.R., et al.: *Dermatophagoides* mites in house dust as an allergen source in atopic dogs. Cornell Vet. 81:429, 1991.

160. Willemse, T.: Hyposensitization of dogs with atopic dermatitis based on the results of *in vivo* and *in vitro* (IgGd ELISA) diagnostic tests. Proc. Annu. Memb. Meet. Am. Acad. Vet. Dermatol. Am. Coll. Vet. Dermatol. 10:61, 1994.

161. Willemse, A., van den Brom, W.E.: Evaluation of the intradermal allergy test in normal dogs. Res. Vet. Sci. 32:57, 1982.

162. Willemse, A.: Canine atopic disease: Investigations of eosinophils and the nasal mucosa. Am. J. Vet. Res. 45:1867, 1984.

163. Willemse, A., van den Brom, W.E.: Investigations of the symptomatology and the significance of immediate skin test reactivity in canine atopic dermatitis. Res. Vet. Sci. 34:261, 1983.

164. Willemse, A., et al.: Effect of hyposensitization on atopic dermatitis in dogs. J. Am. Vet. Med. Assoc. 184:277, 1984.

165. Willemse, A., et al.: Allergen specific IgGd antibodies in dogs with atopic dermatitis as determined by the enzyme linked immunosorbent assay (ELISA). Clin. Exp. Immunol. 59:359, 1985.

166. Willemse, A., et al.: Induction of non-IgE anaphylactic antibodies in dogs. Clin. Exp. Immunol. 59:351, 1985.

167. Willemse, A.: Atopic skin disease: A review and a reconsideration of diagnostic criteria. J. Small Anim. Pract. 27:771, 1986.

168. Willis, E.L.: IgE mediated insect and arachnid hypersensitivity in the dog. Proc. Annu. Memb. Meet. Am. Acad. Vet. Dermatol. Am. Coll. Vet. Dermatol. 10:33, 1994.

Feline Atopy

169. Anderson, R.K.: *In vitro* testing for feline atopic disease. Proc. Eur. Soc. Vet. Dermatol. 10:72, 1993.

170. Bettenay, S.: Diagnosing and treatment feline atopic dermatitis. Vet. Med. 86:488, 1991.

171. Bevier, D.E.: The reaction of feline skin to the intradermal injection of allergenic extracts and passive cutaneous anaphylaxis using the serum from skin test positive cats. In: von Tscharner, C., Halliwell, R.E.W. (eds): Advances in Veterinary Dermatology I. Ballière-Tindall, Philadelphia, 1990, p. 126.

172. Bevier, D.E.: Effect of methylprednisolone acetate and oral prednisone on immediate skin test reactivity in cats. Proc. Annu. Memb. Meet. Am. Acad. Vet. Dermatol. Am. Coll. Vet. Dermatol. 10:45, 1994.

173. Carlotti, D., Prost, C.: L'atopie féline. Point Vét. 20:777, 1988.

174. Chalmers, S., Medleau, L.: Recognizing the signs of feline allergic dermatoses. Vet. Med. 84:388, 1989.

175. Chalmers, S., Medleau, L.: Feline allergic dermatoses: Diagnosis and treatment. Vet. Med. 84:399, 1989.

176. Chalmers, S.A., Medleau, L.: Feline atopic dermatitis: Its diagnosis and treatment. Vet. Med. 89:342, 1994.

177. DeBoer, D.J., et al.: Feline IgE: Preliminary evidence of its existence and crossreactivity with canine IgE. In: Ihrke, P.J., et al. (eds): Advances in Veterinary Dermatology II. Pergamon Press, New York, 1993, p. 51.

178. DeBoer, D.J., et al.: Monoclonal antibodies against feline immunoglobulin E. Proc. Annu. Memb. Meet. Am. Acad. Dermatol. Am. Coll. Vet. Dermatol. 10:11, 1994.

178a. Foster, A.P., O'Dair, H.: Allergy testing for skin disease in the cat. In vivo vs in vitro tests. Vet. Dermatol. 4:111, 1993.

179. Harvey, R.G.: Effect of varying proportions of evening primrose oil and fish oil on cats with crusting dermatosis ("miliary dermatitis"). Vet. Rec. 133:208, 1993.

180. Harvey, R.G.: A comparison of evening primrose oil and sunflower oil for the management of papulocrustous dermatitis in cats. Vet. Rec. 133:571, 1993.

181. McDougal, B.J.: Allergy testing and hyposensitization for three common feline dermatoses. Mod. Vet. Pract. 67:629, 1986.

182. Miller, W.H. Jr., Scott, D.W.: Efficacy of chlorpheniramine maleate for the management of pruritus in cats. J. Am. Vet. Med. Assoc. 197:67, 1990.

183. Miller, W.H. Jr., et al.: Efficacy of DVM Derm Caps Liquid in the management of allergic and inflammatory dermatoses of the cat. J. Am. Anim. Hosp. Assoc. 29:37, 1993.

184. Miller, W.H. Jr., Scott, D.W.: Clemastine fumarate as an antipruritic agent in pruritic cats: Results of an open clinical trial. Can. Vet. J. 35:502, 1994.

185. Mueller, R.S., et al.: Effect of tiletamine-zolazepam anesthesia on the response to intradermally injected histamine in cats. Vet. Dermatol. 2:119, 1991.

186. Prost, C.: Les dermatoses allergiques du chat. Prat. Méd. Chirurg. Anim. Comp. 28:151, 1993.

187. Prost, C.: Hypersensitivity to tobacco in six dogs and two cats: A social disease. Proc. Eur. Soc. Vet. Dermatol. 10:70, 1993.

188. Reedy, L.M.: Results of allergy testing and hyposensitization in selected feline skin diseases. J. Am. Anim. Hosp. Assoc. 18:618, 1982.

189. Scott, D.W., et al.: Miliary dermatitis: A feline cutaneous reaction pattern. Proc. Annu. Kal Kan Semin. 2:11, 1986.

190. Scott, D.W., et al.: Sterile eosinophilic folliculitis in the cat: An unusual manifestation of feline allergic skin disease? Companion Anim. Pract. 19:6, 1989.
191. Scott, D.W.: Analyse du type de réaction histopathologique dans le diagnostic des dermatoses inflammatoires chez le chat: Étude sur 394 cas. Point Vét. 26:57, 1994.
192. Scott, D.W., Miller, W.H. Jr.: The combination of an antihistamine (chlorpheniramine) and an omega-3/omega-6 fatty acid–containing product (DVM Derm Caps Liquid™) for the management of pruritic cats: Results of an open clinical trial. N.Z. Vet. J. (accepted 1994).
193. Scott, D.W., Miller, W.H. Jr.: Medical management of allergic pruritus in the cat, with emphasis on feline atopy. J. S. Afr. Vet. Assoc. 64:103, 1993.
194. Willemse, T., et al.: Changes in plasma cortisol, corticotropin, and α-melanocyte–stimulating hormone concentrations in cats before and after physical restraint and intradermal testing. Am. J. Vet. Res. 54:69, 1993.

Contact Hypersensitivity

195. Baadsgaard, O., Wang, T.: Immune regulation in allergic and irritant skin reactions. Int. J. Dermatol. 30:161, 1991.
196. Calderwood Mays, M.B., et al.: Carpet deodorant contact dermatitis in a cat. Proc. Annu. Memb. Meet. Am. Acad. Vet. Dermatol. Am. Coll. Vet. Dermatol., 9:67, 1993.
197. Clark, E.G., et al.: Cedar wood–induced allergic contact dermatitis in a dog. Proc. Annu. Memb. Meet. Am. Acad. Vet. Dermatol. Am. Coll. Vet. Dermatol., 9:68, 1993.
198. Comer, K.M.: Carpet deodorizer as a contact allergen in a dog. J. Am. Vet. Med. Assoc. 193:1553, 1988.
199. Dunstan, R.W., et al.: Histologic features of allergic contact dermatitis in four dogs. Proc. Annu. Memb. Meet. Am. Acad. Vet. Dermatol. Am. Coll. Vet. Dermatol., 9:69, 1993.
200. Krawiec, D.R., Gaafar, S.M.: A comparative study of allergic and primary irritant contact dermatitis with dinitrochlorobenzene (DNCB) in dogs. J. Invest. Dermatol. 65:248, 1975.
201. Kunkle, G.A., Gross, T.L.: Allergic contact dermatitis to *Tradescantia fluminensis* (wandering Jew) in a dog. Comp. Cont. Educ. 5:925, 1983.
202. Kunkle, G.A.: Contact allergic dermatitis. Vet. Clin. North Am. [Small Anim. Pract.] 18:1061, 1988.
202a. Merchant, S.R., et al.: Eosinophilic pustules and eosinophilic dermatitis secondary to patch testing a dog with Asian jasmine. Proc. Annu. Memb. Meet. Am. Acad. Vet. Dermatol. Am. Coll. Vet. Dermatol. 9:64, 1993.
203. Michaud, A.J.: Plastic shopping bag as a possible contact allergen in a cat. Feline Pract. 19:6, 1991.
204. Nobreus, N., et al.: Induction of dinitrochlorobenzene contact sensitivity in dogs. Monogr. Allergy 8:100, 1974.
205. Olivry, T., et al.: Allergic contact dermatitis in the dog. Vet. Clin. North Am. [Small Anim. Pract.] 20:1443, 1990.
206. Olivry, T.: Allergic contact dermatitis to cement: A delayed hypersensitivity to dichromates and nickel. Proc. Annu. Memb. Meet. Am. Acad. Vet. Dermatol. Am. Coll. Vet. Dermatol. 9:63, 1993.
207. Schultz, K.T., Maguire, H.C.: Chemically-induced delayed hypersensitivity in the cat. Vet. Immunol. Immunopathol. 3:585, 1982.
208. Schultz, R.D., Adams, L.S.: Immunologic methods for the detection of humoral and cellular immunity. Vet. Clin. North Am. 8:721, 1978.
209. Schwartz, A., et al.: Pentoxifylline suppresses irritant and contact hypersensitivity reactions. J. Invest. Dermatol. 101:549, 1993.
209a. Thomsen, M.K., Kristensen, F.: Contact dermatitis in the dog: A review and clinical study. Nord. Vet. Med. 38:129, 1986.
210. Thomsen, M.K., Thomsen, H.K.: Histopathological changes in canine allergic contact dermatitis patch test reactions: A study on spontaneously hypersensitive dogs. Acta Vet. Scand. 30:379, 1989.
210a. Walton, G.S.: Allergic contact dermatitis. In: Kirk, R.W. (ed.): Current Veterinary Therapy VI. W.B. Saunders Co., Philadelphia, 1977, p. 571.
211. White, P.D.: Contact dermatitis in the dog and cat. Semin. Vet. Med. Surg. 6:303, 1991.
212. Willemse, T., Vroom, M.A.: Allergic dermatitis in a Great Dane due to contact with hippeastrum. Vet. Rec. 122:490, 1988.

Canine Food Hypersensitivity

213. August, J.R.: Dietary hypersensitivity in dogs: Cutaneous manifestations, diagnosis, and treatment. Comp. Cont. Educ. 7:469, 1985.
214. Carlotti, D.N., et al.: Food allergy in dogs and cats: A review and report of 43 cases. Vet. Dermatol. 1:55, 1990.
215. Denis, S., Paradis, M.: L'allergie alimentaire chez le chien et le chat. I: Revue de la littérature. Méd. Vét. Québec 24:11, 1994.
216. Denis, S., Paradis, M.: L'allergie alimentaire chez le chien et le chat. II: Étude rétrospective. Méd. Vét. Québec 24:15, 1994.
216a. Elmwood, C.M., et al.: Gastroscopic food sensitivity testing in 17 dogs. J. Small Anim. Pract. 35:199, 1994.
217. Ferguson, E., Scheidt, V.J.: Hypoallergenic diets and skin disease. In: Ihrke, P.J., et al. (eds): Advances in Veterinary Dermatology II. Pergamon Press, New York, 1993, p. 459.
218. Halliwell, R.E.W.: Comparative aspects of food intolerance. Vet. Med. 87:893, 1992.
219. Halliwell, R.E.W.: Management of dietary hypersensitivity in the dog. J. Small Anim. Pract. 33:156, 1993.
220. Harvey, R.G.: Food allergy and dietary intolerance in dogs: A report of 25 cases. J. Small Anim. Pract. 33:22, 1993.
221. Hillier, A., Kunkle, G.A.: Inability to demonstrate food antigen-specific IgE antibodies in the serum of food allergic dogs using the PK and oral PK tests. Proc. Annu. Memb. Meet. Am. Acad. Vet. Dermatol. Am. Coll. Vet. Dermatol. 10:28, 1994.

222. Jeffers, J.G., et al.: Diagnostic testing of dogs for food hypersensitivity. J. Am. Vet. Med. Assoc. 198:245, 1991.
223. Jeffers, J.G.: Results of dietary provocation in dogs with food hypersensitivity. Proc. Annu. Memb. Meet. Am. Acad. Vet. Dermatol. Am. Coll. Vet. Dermatol. 10:40, 1994.
224. Kunkle, G., et al.: Validity of skin testing for diagnosis of food allergy in dogs. J. Am. Vet. Med. Assoc. 200:677, 1992.
225. MacDonald, J.M.: Food allergy. In: Griffin, C.E., et al. (eds): Current Veterinary Dermatology. Mosby Year Book, St. Louis, 1993, p. 121.
226. Merchant, S.R., Taboada, J.: Food allergy and immunologic diseases of the gastrointestinal tract. Semin. Vet. Med. Surg. 6:316, 1991.
227. Olsen, J.W.: Clinical use of gastroscopic food sensitivity testing in the dog. Proc. Am. Acad. Vet. Allergy, 1991.
228. Rosser, E.J. Jr.: Diagnosis of food allergy in dogs. J. Am. Vet. Med. Assoc. 203:259, 1993.
229. Roudebush, P., et al.: Results of a hypoallergenic diet survey of veterinarians in North America with a nutritional evaluation of homemade diet prescriptions. Vet. Dermatol. 3:23, 1992.
230. Walton, G.S.: Skin responses in the dog and cat to ingested allergens: Observations of 100 confirmed cases. Vet. Rec. 81:709, 1967.
231. White, S.D., Mason, I.S.: Dietary allergy: In: von Tscharner, C., Halliwell, R.E.W. (eds): Advances in Veterinary Dermatology I. Ballière-Tindall, Philadelphia, 1990, p. 404.
232. White, S.D.: Food hypersensitivity in 30 dogs. J. Am. Vet. Med. Assoc. 188:695, 1986.

Feline Food Hypersensitivity
233. Dennis, J.S., et al.: Lymphocytic/plasmacytic colitis in cats: 14 cases (1985–1990). J. Am. Vet. Med. Assoc. 202:313, 1993.
234. Guaguère, E.: Intolérance alimentaire à manifestations cutanées: À propos de 17 cas chez le chat. Prat. Méd. Chirurg. Anim. Comp. 28:451, 1993.
235. Reedy, L.M.: Food hypersensitivity to lamb in a cat. J. Am. Vet. Med. Assoc. 204:1039, 1994.
236. Rosser, E.J.: Food allergy in the cat: A prospective study of 13 cats. In: Ihrke, P.J., et al. (eds): Advances in Veterinary Dermatology II. Pergamon Press, New York, 1993, p. 33.
237. Roudebush, P., McKeever, P.J.: Evaluation of a commercial canned lamb and rice diet for the management of cutaneous adverse reactions to foods in cats. Vet. Dermatol. 4:1, 1993.
238. White, S.D.: Food hypersensitivity in cats: 14 cases (1982–1987). J. Am. Vet. Med. Assoc. 194:692, 1989.
239. Willis, J.M.: Diagnosing and managing food sensitivity in cats. Vet. Med. 87:884, 1992.

Canine Flea Bite Hypersensitivity
240. Carlotti, D.: Diagnostic de la dermatite par allergie aux piqures de puce (DAPP) chez le chien. Ińterêt des intradermoréactions. Prat. Méd. Chirurg. Anim. Cie. 20:41, 1985.
241. Gross, T.L., Halliwell, R.E.W.: Lesions of experimental flea bite hypersensitivity in the dog. Vet. Pathol. 22:78, 1985.
242. Halliwell, R.E.W.: Hyposensitization in the treatment of flea bite hypersensitivity: Results of a double-blinded study. J. Am. Anim. Hosp. Assoc. 17:249, 1981.
243. Halliwell, R.E.W., Longino, S.J.: IgE and IgG antibodies to flea antigen in differing dog populations. Vet. Immunol. Immunopathol. 8:215, 1985.
244. Halliwell, R.E.W., Schemmer, K.R.: The role of basophils in the immunopathogenesis of hypersensitivity to fleas (*Ctenocephalides felis*) in dogs. Vet. Immunol. Immunopathol. 15:203, 1987.
245. Halliwell, R.E.W.: Clinical and immunological response to alum-precipitated flea antigen in immunotherapy of flea-allergy dogs. In: Ihrke, P.J., et al. (eds): Advances in Veterinary Dermatology II. Pergamon Press, New York, 1993, p. 41.
246. Hickey, G.J., et al.: Effects of prednisone on dermal responses in flea-allergen hypersensitized dogs. Vet. Dermatol. 4:71, 1993.
247. MacDonald, J.M.: Flea allergy dermatitis and flea control. In: Griffin, C.E., et al. (eds): Current Veterinary Dermatology. Mosby Year Book, St. Louis, 1993, p. 57.
248. Schemmer, K.R., Halliwell, R.E.W.: Efficacy of alum-precipitated flea antigen for hyposensitization of flea-allergic dogs. Semin. Vet. Med. Surg. 2:195, 1987.

Feline Flea Bite Hypersensitivity
249. Greene, W.K., et al.: Characterization of allergens of the cat flea, *Ctenocephalides felis:* Detection and frequency of IgE antibodies in canine sera. Parasite Immunol. 15:69, 1993.
250. Kunkle, G.A., Milcarsky, J.: Double-blind flea hyposensitization in cats. J. Am. Vet. Med. Assoc. 186:677, 1985.
251. Moriello, K.A., McMurdy, M.A.: The prevalence of positive intradermal skin test reactions to flea extract in clinically normal cats. Companion Anim. Pract. 19:28, 1989.
252. Plant, J.D.: Recognizing the manifestations of flea allergy in cats. Vet. Med. 86:482, 1991.

Feline Mosquito Bite Hypersensitivity
253. Johnstone, A.C., et al.: A seasonal eosinophilic dermatitis in cats. N. Z. Vet. J. 40:168, 1992.
254. Mason, K.V., Evans, A.G.: Mosquito bite caused eosinophilic dermatitis in cats. J. Am. Vet. Med. Assoc. 198:2086, 1991.
255. Wilkinson, G.T., Bates, M.J.: A possible further clinical manifestation of the eosinophilic granuloma complex. J. Am. Anim. Hosp. Assoc. 20:325, 1982.

Insect, Arachnid, and Helminth Hypersensitivity
256. Baldo, B.A., Panzani, R.C.: Detection of IgE antibodies to a wide range of insect species in subjects with suspected inhalant allergies to insects. Int. Arch. Allergy Appl. Immunol. 85:278, 1988.

257. Bornstein, S., Zakrisoon, G.: Serodiagnosis of sarcoptic mange in dogs. Proc. Eur. Soc. Vet. Dermatol. 7, 1990.
258. Griffin, C.E., et al.: Detection of insect/arachnid specific IgE in dogs: Comparison of two techniques utilizing Western blots as the standard. In: Ihrke, P.J., et al. (eds): Advances in Veterinary Dermatology II. Pergamon Press, New York, 1993, p. 263.
259. Griffin, C.E.: Insect and arachnid hypersensitivity. In: Griffin, C.E., et al. (eds): Current Veterinary Dermatology. Mosby Year Book, St. Louis, 1993, p. 133.
260. Lierl, M.B., et al.: Concentrations of airborne insect-derived particles in outdoor air (Abstract 412). J. Allergy Clin. Immunol. 85:246, 1990.
261. Moriello, K.A.: Parasitic hypersensitivity. Semin. Vet. Med. Surg. 6:286, 1991.
262. Mozos, E., et al.: Cutaneous lesions associated with canine heartworm infection. Vet. Dermatol. 3:191, 1992.
263. Powell, M.A., et al.: Reaginic hypersensitivity in *Otodectes cynotis* infestation of cats and mode of mite feeding. Am. J. Vet. Res. 41:877, 1980.
264. Thoday, K.L.: Serum immunoglobulin concentrations in canine scabies. In: Ihrke, P.J., et al. (eds): Advances in Veterinary Dermatology II. Pergamon Press, New York, 1993, p. 211.

Canine Eosinophilic Furunculosis of the Face
265. Gross, T.L.: Canine eosinophilic furunculosis of the face. In: Ihrke, P.J., et al. (eds): Advances in Veterinary Dermatology II. Pergamon Press, New York, 1993, p. 239.
266. Hotz, C.S.: Eosinophilic dermatitis in a Siberian husky. Calif. Vet. 44:11, 1990.

Bacterial Hypersensitivity
267. Miller, W.H. Jr.: Antibiotic-responsive generalized nonlesional pruritus in a dog. Cornell Vet. 81:389, 1991.
268. Pukay, B.P.: Treatment of bacterial hypersensitivity by hyposensitization with *Staphylococcus aureus* bacterin-toxoid. J. Am. Anim. Hosp. Assoc. 21:479, 1985.
269. Scott, D.W., et al.: Staphylococcal hypersensitivity in the dog. J. Am. Anim. Hosp. Assoc. 14:666, 1978.

Hormonal Hypersensitivity
270. Chamberlain, K.W.: Hormonal hypersensitivity in canines. Canine Pract. 1:18, 1974.
271. Scott, D.W., Miller, W.H. Jr.: Probable hormonal hypersensitivity in two male dogs. Canine Pract. 17:14, 1992.

Pemphigus Complex
272. August, J.R., Chickering, W.R.: Pemphigus foliaceus causing lameness in four dogs. Comp. Cont. Educ. 7:894, 1985.
273. Caciolo, P.L., et al.: Pemphigus foliaceus in eight cats and results of induction therapy using azathioprine. J. Am. Anim. Hosp. Assoc. 20:571, 1984.
274. Crameri, F.M., Suter, M.M.: Induction of acantholysis in a serum-free culture system. Proc. Annu. Memb. Meet. Am. Acad. Vet. Dermatol. Am. Coll. Vet. Dermatol. 10:63, 1994.
275. Dmochowski, M., et al.: Desmocollins I and II are recognized by certain sera from patients with various types of pemphigus, particularly Brazilian pemphigus foliaceus. J. Invest. Dermatol. 100:380, 1993.
276. Dunstan, R.W.: Controversies in immunologic diseases from a pathologist's perspective. Controversies in Veterinary Dermatology, Bad Kreuznach, 1992.
277. Greek, J.S.: Feline pemphigus foliaceus: A retrospective of 23 cases. Proc. Annu. Memb. Meet. Am. Acad. Vet. Dermatol. Am. Coll. Vet. Dermatol. 9:27, 1993.
278. Griffin, C.E.: Controversies in immunologic diseases from a clinician's standpoint. Controversies in Veterinary Dermatology, Bad Kreuznach, 1992.
279. Griffin, C.E.: Pemphigus foliaceus: Recent findings on the pathophysiology and results of treatment. Presentation, William Dick Bicentenary, Edinburgh, 1993.
280. Griffin, C.E.: Recognizing and treating pemphigus foliaceus in cats. Vet. Med. 86:513, 1991.
281. Halliwell, R.E.W., Goldschmidt, M.H.: Pemphigus foliaceus in the canine: A case report and discussion. J. Am. Anim. Hosp. Assoc. 13:431, 1977.
282. Ihrke, P.J., et al.: Pemphigus foliaceus of the footpads in three dogs. J. Am. Vet. Med. Assoc. 186:67, 1985.
283. Ihrke, P.J., et al.: Pemphigus foliaceus in dogs: A review of 37 cases. J. Am. Vet. Med. Assoc. 186:59, 1985.
284. Ioannides, D., et al.: Regional variation in the expression of pemphigus foliaceus, pemphigus erythematosus, and pemphigus vulgaris antigens in human skin. J. Invest. Dermatol. 96:15, 1991.
285. Iwatsuki, K., et al.: Ultrastructural binding site of pemphigus foliaceus antibodies: Comparison with pemphigus vulgaris. J. Cutan. Pathol. 18:160, 1991.
286. Lombardi, C., et al.: Environmental risk factors in endemic pemphigus foliaceus (fogo selvagem). J. Invest. Dermatol. 18:847, 1992.
287. Manning, T.O., et al.: Pemphigus diseases in the feline: Seven case reports and discussion. J. Am. Anim. Hosp. Assoc. 18:433, 1982.
288. Mattise, A.W.: Canine pemphigus vegetans: A report of 16 cases. Proc. Annu. Memb. Meet. Am. Acad. Vet. Dermatol. Am. Coll. Vet. Dermatol. 7:28, 1991.
289. Noxon, J.O., Myers, R.K.: Pemphigus foliaceus in two Shetland sheepdog littermates. J. Am. Vet. Med. Assoc. 194:545, 1989.
290. Olivry, T., et al.: Pemphigus vulgaris lacking mucosal involvement in a German shepherd dog: Possible response to heparin. Vet. Dermatol. 3:79, 1992.
291. Rhodes, K.H., Shoulberg, N.: Chlorambucil: Effective therapeutic options for the treatment of feline immune-mediated dermatoses. Feline Pract. 20:5, 1992.
292. Rosenkrantz, W.S.: Pemphigus foliaceus. In: Griffin, C.E., et al. (eds): Current Veterinary Dermatology. Mosby Year Book, St. Louis, 1993, p. 141.
293. Ruocco, V., Sacerdoti, G.: Pemphigus and bullous pemphigoid due to drugs. Int. J. Dermatol. 30:307, 1991.

294. Scott, D.W.: Pemphigus vegetans in a dog. Cornell Vet. 67:374, 1977.
295. Scott, D.W., et al.: Pemphigus erythematosus in the dog and cat. J. Am. Anim. Hosp. Assoc. 16:815, 1980.
296. Scott, D.W., et al.: Pemphigus vulgaris without mucosal or mucocutaneous involvement in two dogs. J. Am. Anim. Hosp. Assoc. 18:401, 1982.
297. Scott, D.W., Lewis, R.M.: Pemphigus and pemphigoid in dog and man: Comparative aspects. J. Am. Acad. Dermatol. 5:148, 1981.
298. Scott, D.W.: Pemphigus in domestic animals. Clin. Dermatol. 1:141, 1983.
299. Stannard, A.A., et al.: A mucocutaneous disease in the dog, resembling pemphigus vulgaris in man. J. Am. Vet. Med. Assoc. 166:575, 1975.
300. Suter, M.M., et al.: Ultrastructural localization of pemphigus antigens on keratinocytes *in vivo* and *in vitro*. Am. J. Vet. Res. 41:507, 1990.
301. Suter, M.M., et al.: Identification of canine pemphigus antigens. In: Ihrke, P.J., et al. (eds): Advances in Veterinary Dermatology II. Pergamon Press, New York, 1993, p. 367.
302. Wolf, R., et al.: Drug-induced versus drug-triggered pemphigus. Dermatologica 182:207, 1991.
303. Wurm, S., et al.: Comparative pathology of pemphigus in dogs and humans. Clin. Dermatol. 12:515, 1994.

Bullous Pemphigoid

304. Czech, W., et al.: Granulocyte activation in bullous diseases: Release of granular proteins in bullous pemphigoid and pemphigus vulgaris. J. Am. Acad. Dermatol. 29:210, 1993.
305. Hashimoto, T., et al.: Comparative study of bullous pemphigoid antigens among Japanese, British, and U.S. patients indicates similar antigen profiles with the 170-kD antigen present both in the basement membrane and on the keratinocyte cell membrane. J. Invest. Dermatol. 100:38S, 1993.
306. Iwasaki, T., et al.: Canine bullous pemphigoid antigen: IgG class antibody recognizes the 180 kD canine and human bullous pemphigoid antigen. Proc. Annu. Memb. Meet. Am. Acad. Vet. Dermatol. Am. Coll. Vet. Dermatol. 10:65, 1994.
307. Kunkle, G., et al.: Bullous pemphigoid in a dog: A case report with immunofluorescent findings. J. Am. Anim. Hosp. Assoc. 14:52, 1978.
308. Scott, D.W.: Pemphigoid in domestic animals. Clin. Dermatol. 5:155, 1987.
309. Thomas, I., et al.: Treatment of generalized bullous pemphigoid with oral tetracycline. J. Am. Acad. Dermatol. 28:74, 1993.

Systemic Lupus Erythematosus

310. Cohen, P.L.: T- and B-cell abnormalities in systemic lupus. J. Invest. Dermatol. 100:69S, 1993.
311. Hubert, B., et al.: Spontaneous familial systemic lupus erythematosus in a canine breeding colony. J. Comp. Pathol. 98:85, 1988.
312. Jones, D.R.E.: Canine systemic lupus erythematosus: New insights and their implications. J. Comp. Pathol. 108:215, 1993.
313. Lehmann, P., et al.: Experimental reproduction of skin lesions in lupus erythematosus by UVA and UVB radiation. J. Am. Acad. Dermatol. 22:181, 1990.
314. McVey, D.S., Shuman, W.: Use of multiple antigen substrates to detect antinuclear antibody in canine sera. Vet. Immunol. Immunopathol. 28:37, 1991.
315. Mooney, E., et al.: Characterization of the changes in matrix molecules at the dermoepidermal junction in lupus erythematosus. J. Cutan. Pathol. 18:417, 1991.
316. Norris, D.A.: Pathomechanisms of photosensitive lupus erythematosus. J. Invest. Dermatol. 100:58S, 1993.
317. Pedersen, N.C., Barlough, J.E.: Systemic lupus erythematosus in the cat. Feline Pract. 19:5, 1991.
318. Sauder, D.N., et al.: Epidermal cytokines in murine lupus. J. Invest. Dermatol. 100:42S, 1993.
319. Scott, D.W., et al.: Canine lupus erythematosus. I: Systemic lupus erythematosus. J. Am. Anim. Hosp. Assoc. 19:461, 1983.
320. Thoren-Tolling, K., Ryden, L.: Serum auto-antibodies and clinical/pathological features in German shepherd dogs with a lupus-like syndrome. Acta Vet. Scand. 32:15, 1991.
321. Velthuis, P.J., et al.: Immunohistopathology of light-induced skin lesions in lupus erythematosus. Acta Derm. Venereol. (Stockh) 70:93, 1990.
322. White, S.D., et al.: Investigation of antibodies to extractable nuclear antigens in dogs. Am. J. Vet. Res. 53:1019, 1992.

Discoid Lupus Erythematosus

323. Guaguère, E., Magnol, J.P.: Lupus érythémateux discoïde à localisation auriculaire chez le chien. Prat. Méd. Chirurg. Anim. Comp. 24:101, 1989.
324. Kalaher, K.M., Scott, D.W.: Discoid lupus erythematosus in a cat. Feline Pract. 19:7, 1991.
325. Olivry, T., et al.: Le lupus érythémateux discoïde du chien: À propos de 22 observations. Prat. Méd. Chirurg. Anim. Comp. 22:205, 1987.
326. Rosenkrantz, W.S.: Discoid lupus erythematosus. In: Griffin, C.E., et al. (eds): Current Veterinary Dermatology. Mosby Year Book, St. Louis, 1993, p. 149.
327. Scott, D.W.: Canine lupus erythematosus. II: Discoid lupus erythematosus. J. Am. Anim. Hosp. Assoc. 19:481, 1983.
327a. Scott, D.W., et al.: Unusual findings in canine pemphigus erythematosus and discoid lupus erythematosus. J. Am. Anim. Hosp. Assoc. 20:579, 1984.
328. Stanley, B.J., et al.: Bilateral rotation flaps for the treatment of chronic nasal dermatitis in four dogs. J. Am. Anim. Hosp. Assoc. 27:295, 1991.

329. Sugai, S.A., et al.: Cutaneous lupus erythematosus: Direct immunofluorescence and epidermal basement membrane study. Int. J. Dermatol. 31:260, 1992.
330. Willemse, T., et al.: Discoid lupus erythematosus in cats. Vet. Dermatol. 1:19, 1989.
331. Williams, R.E.A., et al.: The contribution of direct immunofluorescence to the diagnosis of lupus erythematosus. J. Cutan. Pathol. 16:122, 1989.

Cold Agglutinin Disease

332. Cohen, S.J., et al.: Cutaneous manifestations of cryoglobulinemia: Clinical and histopathologic study of seventy-two patients. J. Am. Acad. Dermatol. 25:21, 1991.
333. Dickson, N.J.: Cold agglutinin disease in a puppy associated with lead intoxication. J. Small Anim. Pract. 31:105, 1990.
333a. Godfrey, D.R., Anderson, R.M.: Cold agglutinin disease in a cat. J. Small Anim. Pract. 35:267, 1994.
334. Niemand, S., et al.: Kalteagglutinin-krankheit bei einer katz. Kleintierpraxis 30:259, 1985.
335. Zulty, J.C., Kociba, G.J.: Cold agglutins in cats with haemobartonellosis. J. Am. Vet. Med. Assoc. 196:907, 1990.

Uveodermatologic Syndrome

336. Boldy, K.L., et al.: Uveodermatologic syndrome in the dog: Clinical characteristics and treatment of a disorder similar to human Vogt-Koyanagi-Harada syndrome. Vet. Focus 1:112, 1989.
337. Campbell, K.L., et al.: Generalized leukoderma and poliosis following uveitis in a dog. J. Am. Anim. Hosp. Assoc. 22:121, 1986.
338. Kern, T.J., et al.: Uveitis associated with poliosis and vitiligo in six dogs. J. Am. Vet. Med. Assoc. 187:408, 1985.
339. MacDonald, J.M.: Uveodermatologic syndrome in the dog. In: Griffin, C.E., et al. (eds): Current Veterinary Dermatology. Mosby Year Book, St. Louis, 1993, p. 217.
340. Morgan, R.V.: Vogt-Koyanagi-Harada syndrome in humans and dogs. Comp. Cont. Educ. 11:1211, 1989.
341. Murphy, C.J., et al.: Antiretinal antibodies associated with Vogt-Koyanagi-Harada–like syndrome in a dog. J. Am. Anim. Hosp. Assoc. 27:399, 1991.
342. Vercelli, A., et al.: Canine Vogt-Koyanagi-Harada–like syndrome in two Siberian husky dogs. Vet. Dermatol. 1:151, 1990.

Vasculitis

343. Carpenter, J.L., et al.: Idiopathic cutaneous and renal glomerular vasculopathy of Greyhounds. Vet. Pathol. 25:401, 1988.
344. Crawford, M.A., Foil, C.S.: Vasculitis: Clinical syndromes in small animals. Comp. Cont. Educ. 11:400, 1989.
345. Griffin, C.E.: Pinnal Diseases: The Complete Manual of Ear Care. Solvay Veterinary, Inc., Princeton, 1985, p. 21.
346. Manning, T.O., Scott, D.W.: Cutaneous vasculitis in a dog. J. Am. Anim. Hosp. Assoc. 16:61, 1980.
347. Rachofsky, M.A., et al.: Probable hypersensitivity vasculitis in a dog. J. Am. Vet. Med. Assoc. 194:1592, 1989.
348. Wilcock, B.P., Yager, J.A.: Focal cutaneous vasculitis and alopecia at sites of rabies vaccination in dogs. J. Am. Vet. Med. Assoc. 188:1174, 1986.

Cutaneous Drug Reaction

349. Affolter, V.K., von Tscharner, C.: Cutaneous drug reactions: A retrospective study of histopathological changes and their correlation with the clinical disease. Vet. Dermatol. 4:79, 1993.
350. Affolter, V.K., Shaw, S.E.: Cutaneous drug eruptions. In: Ihrke, P.J., et al. (eds): Advances in Veterinary Dermatology II. Pergamon Press, New York, 1993, p. 447.
351. Baker, J.R., et al.: Pathological effects of bleomycin on the skin of dogs and monkeys. Toxicol. Appl. Pharmacol. 25:190, 1973.
352. Barthold, S.W., et al.: Reversible dermal atrophy in a cat with phenytoin. Vet. Pathol. 17:469, 1980.
353. Bureau of Veterinary Drugs: Suspected drug adverse reactions reported to the Bureau of Veterinary Drugs. Can. Vet. J. 33:237, 1992.
354. Giger, U., et al.: Sulfadiazine-induced allergy in six Doberman pinschers. J. Am. Vet. Med. Assoc. 186:479, 1985.
354a. Gupta, A.K., et al.: Lymphocytic infiltrates of the skin in association with cyclosporine therapy. J. Am. Acad. Dermatol. 23:1137, 1990.
355. Hammer, A.S., Cuoto, C.G.: Diagnosing and treating canine hemangiosarcoma. Vet. Med. 87:188, 1992.
356. Hendrick, M.J., Dunagan, C.A.: Focal necrotizing granulomatous panniculitis associated with subcutaneous injection of rabies vaccine in cats and dogs: 10 cases (1988–1989). J. Am. Vet. Med. Assoc. 198:304, 1991.
357. Henricks, P.M.: Dermatitis associated with the use of primidone in a dog. J. Am. Vet. Med. Assoc. 191:237, 1987.
358. Kunkle, G.: Adverse cutaneous reactions in cats given methimazole. Dermatol. Dialogue, Spring/Summer 1993, p. 4.
359. Mason, K.V.: Subepidermal bullous drug eruption resembling bullous pemphigoid in a dog. J. Am. Vet. Med. Assoc. 190:881, 1987.
360. Mason, K.V.: Cutaneous drug eruptions. Vet. Clin. North Am. (Small Anim. Pract.) 20:1633, 1990.
361. Mason, K.V., Rosser, E.J.: Cutaneous drug eruptions. In: von Tscharner, C., Halliwell, R.E.W. (eds): Advances in Veterinary Dermatology I. Ballière-Tindall, Philadelphia, 1990, p. 426.
362. Mason, K.V.: Fixed drug eruption in two dogs caused by diethylcarbamazine. J. Am. Anim. Hosp. Assoc. 24:301, 1988.

363. Mason, K.V., Day, M.J.: A pemphigus foliaceus–like eruption associated with the use of ampicillin in a cat. Aust. Vet. J. 64:223, 1987.
364. Mason, K.V.: Blistering drug eruptions in animals. Clin. Dermatol. 11:567, 1993.
365. Mauldin, G.N., et al.: Efficacy and toxicity of doxorubicin and cyclophosphamide used in the treatment of selected malignant tumors in 23 cats. J. Vet. Intern. Med. 2:60, 1988.
366. McEwan, N.A., et al.: Drug eruption in a cat resembling pemphigus foliaceus. J. Small Anim. Pract. 28:713, 1987.
367. Medleau, L., et al.: Trimethoprim-sulfonamide–associated drug eruptions in dogs. J. Am. Anim. Hosp. Assoc. 26:305, 1990.
368. Ogilvie, G.K., et al.: Acute and short-term toxicoses associated with the administration of doxorubicin to dogs with malignant tumors. J. Am. Vet. Med. Assoc. 195:1584, 1989.
369. Ogilvie, G.K., et al.: Hypotension and cutaneous reactions associated with intravenous administration of etoposide in the dog. Am. J. Vet. Res. 49:1367, 1988.
370. Rijlaarsdam, U., et al.: Mycosis-fungoides–like lesions associated with phenytoin and carbamazepine therapy. J. Am. Acad. Dermatol. 24:216, 1991.
371. Roche, E., Mason, K.V.: Periocular alopecia caused by a fixed drug eruption. Aust. Vet. Pract. 21:80, 1991.
372. Rosenkrantz, W.S.: Cutaneous drug reactions. In: Griffin, C.E., et al. (eds): Current Veterinary Dermatology. Mosby Year Book, St. Louis, 1993, p. 154.
373. Rosenkrantz, W.S., et al.: Cyclosporine and cutaneous immune-mediated disease. J. Am. Acad. Dermatol. 14:1088, 1986.
374. Scott, D.W., et al.: Drug eruption associated with sulfonamide treatment of vertebral osteomyelitis in a dog. J. Am. Vet. Med. Assoc. 168:1111, 1976.
375. Scott, D.W.: Drug eruption in a cat due to a miticide. Feline Pract. 7:47, 1977.
376. Stanley, R.G., Jabara, A.G.: Chronic skin reaction to a combined feline rhinotracheitis virus (herpesvirus) and calicivirus vaccine. Aust. Vet. J. 65:128, 1988.
377. Van Hees, J., et al.: Levamisole-induced drug eruptions in the dog. J. Am. Anim. Hosp. Assoc. 21:255, 1985.
378. Walder, E.: Superficial suppurative necrolytic dermatitis in miniature schnauzers. In: Ihrke, P.J., et al. (eds): Advances in Veterinary Dermatology II. Pergamon Press, New York, 1993, p. 419.

Erythema Multiforme

379. Delmage, D.A., Payne-Johnson, C.E.: Erythema multiforme in a Doberman on trimethoprim-sulphamethoxazole therapy. J. Small Anim. Pract. 32:635, 1991.
380. McMurdy, M.A.: A case resembling erythema multiforme major (Stevens-Johnson syndrome) in a dog. J. Am. Anim. Hosp. Assoc. 26:297, 1990.
381. Medleau, L., et al.: Erythema multiforme and disseminated intravascular coagulation in a dog. J. Am. Anim. Hosp. Assoc. 26:643, 1990.
382. Power, H.: Practice tip. Dermatol. Dialogue Winter 1993/1994, p. 7.
383. Scott, D.W., et al.: Erythema multiforme in the dog. J. Am. Anim. Hosp. Assoc. 19:453, 1983.

Toxic Epidermal Necrolysis

384. Frank, A.A., et al.: Toxic epidermal necrolysis associated with flea dips. Vet. Hum. Toxicol. 34:57, 1992.
385. Rachofsky, M.A., et al.: Toxic epidermal necrolysis. Comp. Cont. Educ. 11:840, 1989.
386. Scott, D.W., et al.: Toxic epidermal necrolysis in two dogs and a cat. J. Am. Anim. Hosp. Assoc. 15:271, 1979.

Linear IgA Dermatosis

387. Scott, D.W., et al.: Linear IgA dermatoses in the dog: Bullous pemphigoid, discoid lupus erythematosus and a subcorneal pustular dermatitis. Cornell Vet. 72:394, 1982.

Feline Relapsing Polychondritis

388. Bunge, M.M., et al.: Relapsing polychondritis in a cat. J. Am. Anim. Hosp. Assoc. 28:203, 1992.
389. Guaguère, E., et al.: Polychondrite auriculaire atrophiante: À propos d'un cas chez un chat. Prat. Méd. Chirurg. Anim. Comp. 27:557, 1992.

Immunoproliferative Enteropathy of Basenji Dogs

390. Breitschwerdt, E.B., et al.: Clinical and laboratory characterization of Basenjis with immunoproliferative small intestinal disease. Am. J. Vet. Res. 45:267, 1984.

Amyloidosis

391. Alhaidari, Z., et al.: Amylose cutanéomuqueuse chez un chien. Prat. Méd. Chirurg. Anim. Comp. 26:341, 1991.
392. Schwartzman, R.M.: Cutaneous amyloidosis associated with a monoclonal gammopathy in a dog. J. Am. Vet. Med. Assoc. 185:102, 1984.

Endocrine and Metabolic Diseases

■

Chapter Outline

Many hormones affect the skin and adnexa.[2-5, 235] Although this chapter is limited to a discussion of endocrine influences on the skin, hormones also affect the rest of the body. The specific actions of many proven and alleged hormonal imbalances on the skin are often poorly understood. Additionally, confusion is intensified by (1) species differences; (2) lack of adequate, standardized, or readily available diagnostic tests; (3) conflicting data in the literature; and (4) the complex physiologic and pathophysiologic interrelationships between the endocrine glands and their hormonal products. The skin must also be regarded as having endocrine functions, as it is a major site for the metabolism and interconversion of many of the steroids.[19]

Clinically, bilaterally symmetric alopecia is often the first noticeable sign of a hormonal dermatosis. The haircoat is often dull, dry, and easily epilated, and it fails to regrow after clipping. Bilaterally symmetric pigmentary disturbances (usually hyperpigmentation) may accompany the alopecia. Endocrine dermatoses are classically nonpruritic.

However, exceptions to the above clinical findings are commonplace. The alopecia and pigmentary disturbances may be focal, multifocal, and asymmetric. Secondary seborrheic skin disease, bacterial pyoderma, or both are frequent complications, resulting in varying degrees of dermatitis and pruritus.

■ FUNCTIONAL ANATOMY OF THE ENDOCRINE HYPOTHALAMUS AND HYPOPHYSIS

Anatomically and functionally, the hypothalamus and the hypophysis (pituitary gland) are most usefully thought of together as the "master gland," or the "endocrine brain."[2] The important portion of the hypophysis as it relates to dermatology is the adenohypophysis (anterior pituitary, or pars distalis).

The hypothalamus contains a number of specialized cells that combine neural and secretory activity: the endocrine neurons. The endocrine hypothalamus produces hormones (adenohypophysiotropic releasing and inhibiting factors) that are transported as unstainable neurosecretions to the pituitary portal system and then to the adenohypophysis. Important hypothalamic releasing and inhibiting factors that control the adenohypophysis include the following:

Corticotropin-releasing factor (CRF) (or adrenocorticotropic hormone–releasing factor [ACTH-RF], corticotropin-releasing hormone [CRH])

Thyrotropin-releasing hormone (TRH) (or thyroid-stimulating hormone–releasing factor [TSH-RF], thyrotropin-releasing factor [TRF])

Growth hormone–releasing factor (GHRF) (or somatotropin-releasing factor [SRF])

Growth hormone–inhibiting factor (GHIF) (or somatotropin-inhibiting factor [SIF], somatostatin)

Gonadotropin-releasing hormone (GnRH) (or follicle-stimulating hormone–releasing hormone [FSH-RH], luteinizing hormone–releasing hormone [LH-RH])

Prolactin-releasing factor (PRF)

Prolactin-inhibiting factor (PIF)

These hypophysiotropic factors are presently thought to be regulated by higher brain centers, adenohypophyseal hormones ("short-loop" feedback system), and target endocrine gland hormones ("long-loop" system).

By means of light microscopy and acidic or basic dye staining characteristics, the adenohypophysis is seen to consist of three cell types: acidophils (producing growth hormone [GH] and prolactin), basophils (producing follicle-stimulating hormone [FSH], luteinizing hormone [LH], thyrotropin [TSH], β-lipotropin, and corticotropin [ACTH]), and chromophobes (producing ACTH and β-lipotropin).[2] When electron microscopy and immunohistochemical examination are used, the adenohypophysis is observed to consist of five cell types: thyrotrophs (producing TSH), corticotrophs (producing ACTH and β-lipotropin), gonadotrophs (producing FSH and LH), somatotrophs (producing GH), and mammotrophs (producing prolactin).[2] The release of adenohypophyseal hormones is thought to be regulated by hypophysiotropic factors from the hypothalamus and negative feedback by target endocrine gland hormones.

In general, three factors determine the secretory rates of the endocrine glands: (1) humoral feedback loops, (2) neurologic stimulation or suppression, and (3) genetic influence. The effects of hormones depend on many factors, including the chemical structure, the concentration in the blood, the method of transport in the blood, the quantity of unbound target cell receptors, the integrity of target cell postreceptor mechanism, and the rate of hormonal degradation and elimination.

Most peptide hormones (e.g., ACTH, TSH, FSH, LH, and TRH) initiate their actions by activating the cell membrane enzyme adenyl cyclase and the cyclic adenosine monophosphate system. Steroid hormones (e.g., glucocorticoids and sex hormones) pass through target cell membranes and bind to cytoplasmic receptors[219]; the resultant steroid-receptor complex binds to nuclear chromatin to initiate activity. Thyroid hormones pass into target cell cytoplasm to the nucleus, where they bind chromatin receptors and initiate activity.

The basic causes of endocrine disease include the following: (1) primary hyperfunction (e.g., hyperadrenocorticism due to functional pituitary and adrenal neoplasms, and hyperestrogenism due to functional ovarian or testicular neoplasms), (2) secondary hyperfunction (e.g., hyperadrenocorticism due to bilateral adrenocortical hyperplasia), (3) primary hypofunction (e.g., congenital or acquired hypothyroidism, and hypopituitarism due to cystic Rathke's cleft), (4) secondary hypofunction (e.g., secondary hypothyroidism due to hypopituitarism), (5) ectopic hypersecretion (e.g., ectopic ACTH syndrome), (6) failure of target cell response, (7) abnormal degradation of hormone (e.g., feminization due to chronic liver disease), and (8) iatrogenic hormone excess (excessive glucocorticoids, progestogens, or estrogens).[2]

■ DIAGNOSIS OF ENDOCRINOPATHIES

The diagnosis of clinical endocrinopathies is usually based on finding an abnormal concentration of a hormone in the blood. The ideal endocrine assay does not exist. Although radioimmunoassay (RIA) and enzyme-linked immunosorbent assay (ELISA) are the most sensitive, specific, accurate, and precise available methods of measuring hormones, these techniques are usually species specific and must be specially validated for dogs and cats. Any laboratory not willing to provide validation information on request is best avoided.

Basal (resting) levels of serum and plasma hormones frequently do not distinguish normal individuals from those with an endocrinopathy. Basal blood hormone levels fluctuate in response to environmental, psychic, circadian, and drug-induced influences, and they vary with age, breed, sex, and so forth.* Thus, various stimulation and suppression tests are routinely employed to overcome this unreliability of basal blood hormone levels.

■ THYROID HORMONES

A deficiency of thyroid hormone action is the most common endocrine dermatosis of dogs, but it is rare as a naturally occurring disorder in cats.[2, 3, 73a] The etiology of canine hypothyroidism is complex, with the most important cause being lymphocytic (autoimmune) thyroiditis.

---

*See references 2, 3, 8, 13, 63, 82, 84, 103, and 120.

Thyroid Physiology

Canine thyroid physiology is a complex subject and has been exhaustively reviewed.[69] It has been shown that dogs produce 3,5,3',5'-tetraiodothyronine (thyroxine [T_4]), 3,5,3'-triiodothyronine (T_3), 3,3',5'-triiodothyronine ("reverse" T_3 [rT_3]), 3,3'-diiodothyronine (3,3'-T_2), and 3',5'-diiodothyronine (3',5'-T_2).[2, 54, 57, 66]

The thyroid gland secretes all the T_4, but up to 60 per cent of the daily T_3 requirement is formed via monodeiodination (thyroxine 5'-deiodinase) from T_4 in peripheral tissues. The preference of canine thyroid to secrete T_3 rather than T_4, is enhanced by TSH. T_3 is more potent and penetrates much faster into interstitial and intracellular spaces than does T_4. Iodine-deficient dogs show an 80 per cent reduction in their serum T_4 levels, but their serum T_3 levels remain normal, and the dogs remain eumetabolic. In addition, hypothyroid dogs being adequately maintained on only oral liothyronine (T_3) have *no* detectable serum T_4, whereas those maintained on only oral levothyroxine (T_4) show normal levels of both serum T_3 and T_4. Thus, T_3 is the major metabolically active thyroid hormone in dogs, with T_4 serving mainly as a prohormone.

In dogs, rT_3, which is metabolically inactive, is formed via monodeiodination (thyroxine 5-deiodinase) from T_4. In human beings and rodents, a number of conditions (chronic and acute illnesses, surgical trauma, fasting, starvation, fever, and glucocorticoid therapy) produce moderate to marked reduction of serum T_3 levels, mild to marked reduction of serum T_4 levels, and marked elevation of serum rT_3 levels.[27, 35, 36, 69, 99] In these circumstances, the patients are euthyroid and in no need of thyroid medication. This situation is referred to as the *euthyroid sick syndrome* and is a common source of misdiagnosis when basal T_3 and T_4 serum levels are used to diagnose hypothyroidism. The euthyroid sick syndrome also occurs in dogs and cats.* It is thought that this metabolic switch in the sick patient is protective by counteracting the excessive calorigenic effects of T_3 in catabolic states and is caused by an inhibition of one or more iodothyronine β-ring deiodinases, leading to both decreased production of T_3 from T_4 and decreased rT_3 degradation.

Studies in dogs have shown that T_2 is the major product of peripheral tissue deiodination of T_3 and rT_3. T_2 is metabolically inactive.

Information on thyroid physiology in cats is minimal, and naturally occurring feline hypothyroidism has been documented rarely. It is known that cats produce both T_3 and T_4.[12, 15, 17]

Thyroid Hormones and the Skin

Thyroid hormone plays a dominant role in controlling metabolism and is essential for normal growth and development.[2] The primary mechanisms of action of thyroid hormone are stimulation of cytoplasmic protein synthesis and increase of tissue oxygen consumption. These effects are thought to be initiated by the binding of thyroid hormone to nuclear chromatin and by augmentation of the transcription of genetic information. Available data suggest that thyroid hormone plays a pivotal role in the differentiation and maturation of mammalian skin, as well as in the maintenance of normal cutaneous function.

Hypothyroidism results in epidermal atrophy and abnormal keratinization because of decreased protein synthesis, mitotic activity, and oxygen consumption in dogs and humans.[2, 4, 5] The thyroid hormone–deficient epidermis is characterized by both abnormal lipogenesis and decreased sterol synthesis by keratinocytes.[87] Epidermal melanosis may be seen in hypothyroid dogs and humans, but the pathogenic mechanism is unclear.[12] Sebaceous gland atrophy occurs in hypothyroid dogs and humans, and sebum excretion rates are reduced in hypothyroid humans and rats.[12, 30] Hypothyroid dogs have increased triglyceride levels because of impaired plasma clearance.[88] Alterations in plasma fatty acid levels also occur with increases in oleic and linoleic

*See references 2, 3, 7, 10, 36, 46, 65, 69, 71, 83, and 96.

acids and decreases in dihomo-γ-linolenic, arachidonic, and other elongation acids.[30] Similar changes are seen in the cutaneous fatty acid concentrations. Thyroid hormones may regulate Δ-6-desaturase activity.

Thyroid hormone is necessary for the initiation of the anagen phase of the hair follicle cycle.[12] Anagen is not initiated in hypothyroid dogs, resulting in retention of the hair follicles in telogen and leading to failure of hair growth and alopecia. The oral or topical administration of T_4 to normal dogs increases both the growth rate of hair and the numbers of anagen hair follicles, especially in the flanks.[42]

In hypothyroid dogs, humans, and rats, glycosaminoglycans accumulate in the dermis, leading to an increase in the interstitial ground substance and a thick, myxedematous dermis.[4, 5] The exact cause of this tissue mucinosis is unknown, but because thyroid hormones are thought to restrain the synthesis and to increase the catabolism of glycosaminoglycans, decreased thyroid function should cause an accumulation in the dermis.

Thyroid hormone has been reported to heal the ulcers and to reduce the scarring associated with chronic radiodermatitis in humans and to improve the healing of deep dermal burns in rats.[12] These effects were thought to be due to actions of thyroid hormone on the proliferation and metabolism of fibroblasts and collagen synthesis. In humans, hypothyroidism is associated with a 50 per cent reduction in plasma fibronectin levels.[12] Not surprisingly, the skin of hypothyroid dogs and human beings exhibits poor wound healing and easy bruising.

Bacterial pyoderma is a common complication of canine hypothyroidism.[12, 21] In various animal models, it has been reported that (1) the development of lymphoid tissue depends on the integrity of the thyroid gland, (2) thyroidectomy results in hypoplasia of lymphoid organs and thymus, and (3) depletion of thyroid hormones results in impaired neutrophil functions and B and T lymphocyte functions.

Uncomplicated canine hypothyroidism is characterized by the absence of pruritus. Tissue levels of histamine are decreased in experimental canine hypothyroidism.[12] Clinically, canine hypothyroidism is characterized by (1) bilaterally symmetric alopecia; (2) a dull, dry, easily epilated haircoat that fails to grow after clipping; (3) variable hyperpigmentation; (4) skin that is often dry, cool to the touch, thick, and puffy; (5) poor wound healing; (6) easy bruising; (7) frequent seborrheic skin disease, bacterial pyoderma, or both; and (8) variable changes of coat color. Histologically, the condition is characterized by orthokeratotic hyperkeratosis, follicular keratosis, follicular dilatation, follicular atrophy, telogenization of hair follicles, epidermal melanosis, sebaceous gland atrophy, thick dermis, and increased dermal mucin (myxedema).[6, 16]

Thyroid Function Tests

No single area of veterinary diagnosis has become more misunderstood, confused, and abused than thyroid function testing. Most of this is referable to the failure to recognize (1) the significance of the euthyroid sick syndrome, (2) the unreliability of basal serum thyroid hormone levels, and (3) the unsatisfactory results obtained by sending samples to laboratories that have not validated their assays.

Classic thyroid function tests, such as basal metabolic rate, radioiodine uptake, protein-bound iodine, butanol extractable iodine, T_4 determination by competitive protein binding or column chromatography, T_3 resin uptake, and free thyroxine index (T_7 test) are inaccurate, impractical, or inferior to modern techniques and are not discussed here.

SERUM THYROID HORMONE DETERMINATIONS

RIA is the method of choice for determining serum levels of total T_4 (TT_4), free T_4 (fT_4), total T_3 (TT_3), free T_3 (fT_3), and reverse T_3 (rT_3). ELISA tests are being developed but to date they are less sensitive, with more interassay and intra-assay variability, and cannot be recommended, unless extensively validated.[70, 74a] Serum samples may be held at room temperature for at least

1 week with no significant deterioration. Reported basal serum levels of thyroid hormones in dogs are as follows: TT_4: 1.5 to 4 μg/dl; fT_4: 0.3 to 1.7 ng/dl; TT_3: 75 to 160 ng/dl: and fT_3: 0.3 to 0.6 ng/dl. However, even laboratories using RIA procedures adapted to dogs and cats may vary in their normal ranges of these hormones, so one must exercise great caution when attempting to compare published data.

The sensitivity and the specificity of TT_4 and TT_3 measurements in the diagnosis of hypothyroidism have been studied extensively. These measurements can lead to erroneous diagnoses, especially if the patient's state of health and drug history are ignored. Low levels can be seen with a variety of acute and chronic illnesses (euthyroid sick syndrome), including hyperadrenocorticism, diabetes mellitus, hypoadrenocorticism, liver disease, renal failure, various cutaneous and noncutaneous infectious diseases, and a variety of other conditions.

Drugs can decrease or falsely increase TT_3 and TT_4 levels by changing their production, binding, or metabolism. Anticonvulsants (phenobarbital, phenytoin, and diazepam) and glucocorticoids are the most common offenders, but salicylates, phenylbutazone, sulfa antimicrobials, radiocontrast agents, mitotane (o,p'-DDD), furosemide, various cardiac drugs, androgens, and estrogens, to name a few, have also been implicated.[36, 69, 70] Of special concern in dogs with dermatologic disease are corticosteroids[7, 10, 65, 96] and the potentiated sulfa antibiotics.[46, 71] Because dogs receive these or other medications because of illness, thyroid levels could be suppressed by both the disease and the drug.

Variations in TT_4 and TT_3 levels can occur with season,[2, 12] time of day,[8, 63, 67] breed,[2, 3, 13, 36, 69] body size,[12, 84] age,[13, 84] and reproductive status of bitches.[82, 97] With all these variables, it is not surprising that TT_4 and TT_3 measurements can be unreliable. Although figures vary from study to study depending on its design and inclusion or exclusion of dogs with nonthyroid illness or recent drug treatment, basal TT_4 and TT_3 measurements can be low in approximately 20 per cent of euthyroid dogs[12] and be normal in 30 to 50 per cent of hypothyroid dogs.[74]

In humans, serum thyroid hormone–binding protein levels are known to markedly influence serum thyroid hormone levels.[2, 69] Thyroid hormone–binding proteins in the dog have been identified by electrophoresis as thyroxine-binding globulin, thyroxine-binding prealbumin, albumin, inter-α-globulin, and two β-globulin regions.[2, 12, 69] Alterations in thyroid hormone–binding protein levels and resultant changes in thyroid hormone levels have not been well studied in dogs. It has been reported that glucocorticoids, phenylbutazone, salicylates, diazepam, primidone, phenytoin, androgens, and phenobarbital may decrease basal serum TT_3 and TT_4 levels by interfering with protein binding; and basal serum TT_3 and TT_4 levels may be elevated in pregnancy, pseudopregnancy, and the feminization syndrome of male dogs with functional Sertoli's cell testicular tumors, and in response to estrogen therapy, owing to increased protein-binding capacity.[2, 12, 36, 82, 97]

In summary, basal serum levels of TT_3 and TT_4 are significantly influenced by numerous conditions that have nothing to do with thyroid disease and hypothyroidism. In the absence of classic historical, clinical, and clinicopathologic evidence of thyroid hormone deficiency, low basal serum TT_3 and TT_4 levels are unreliable in diagnosing canine hypothyroidism. Basal serum TT_3 levels are a particularly poor measure of thyroid dysfunction.[24, 74] Because TT_3 is predominantly an intracellular hormone and is preferentially produced in states of thyroid deficiency, TT_4 levels drop before TT_3 levels. In addition, TT_3 levels are more severely affected by nonthyroid illnesses and drugs and are inconsistently responsive to TSH and TRH stimulation.

Because the concentration of fT_4 appears to determine hormone availability to cells, and because total hormone concentrations may change with drugs, illness, and so forth without a change in fT_4, a direct or an indirect measurement of fT_4 provides a more consistent laboratory assessment of thyroid status than does the measurement of TT_4. The standard techniques for measurement of fT_4 are RIA and equilibrium dialysis. Assays for fT_4 and fT_3 are relatively new in veterinary endocrinology and their value in diagnosis is uncertain. Depending on the definition of low fT_4 values, between 11 and 16 per cent of hypothyroid dogs with no confounding illnesses had normal fT_4 levels, whereas 0 to 8 per cent of euthyroid dogs had low levels.[24, 68, 74] Nonthyroid illness and glucocorticoids can depress fT_4 levels to the hypothyroid range.[74] Accordingly, fT_4 as a singular assessment of thyroid function appears to be of no greater value than TT_4. Preliminary data suggest that the simultaneous assessment of both TT_4 and fT_4 can increase the accuracy of basal thyroid testing by 10 to 15 per cent.[24]

In normal cats, basal serum TT_3 and TT_4 levels by RIA are reported to range from 15 to 60 ng/dl and 1.5 to 5 μg/dl, respectively.[2, 12] T_4-binding serum globulins could not be found in the cat.[2, 12]

In dogs, basal serum rT_3 levels by RIA are reported to approximate 100 ng/dl.[2] Serum rT_3 levels are expected to be elevated in the euthyroid sick syndrome.

SERUM THYROTROPIN DETERMINATION

In humans, the determination of serum TSH levels by RIA is the most sensitive and reliable indicator of hypothyroidism, often being abnormal for months before basal serum TT_4 levels and TSH stimulation test results are abnormal.[2, 12] Serum TSH levels should be elevated in primary hypothyroidism and low to normal in secondary hypothyroidism. TSH is a species-specific protein, and attempts to use human TSH kits for analyzing canine TSH levels have been unsuccessful.[2, 3]

A homologous RIA for canine serum, TSH was reported to distinguish accurately between normal dogs and dogs with experimental hypothyroidism.[79] Serum TSH levels in normal dogs were reported to range from 2.7 to 7.9 ng/dl.[51, 79] Evaluation of a commercially available, specific canine assay for serum TSH (Canine TSH assay [Canadian Bioclinical]) concluded that the test was no more predictive of hypothyroidism, normality, or response to thyroid supplementation than was basal TT_4 determination alone.[80] Another investigation of the same commercial assay found unexplained high levels of TSH in some normal dogs, and low levels in some hypothyroid dogs, also concluding that the assay could not be recommended for the diagnosis of canine hypothyroidism.[85] Serum TSH assays offer a major advancement in the area of thyroid diagnostics in dogs, and further progress in this area is awaited.

PROVOCATIVE THYROID FUNCTION TESTS

To overcome the unreliability of basal hormone measurement levels, various provocative tests of thyroid function have been developed.[100a] There is controversy about the relative efficiency and accuracy of the various tests. Results are often difficult to compare because of variation in methods (different products used at different doses, different time intervals of sampling, and different laboratories performing and interpreting the tests).

Thyrotropin Stimulation Test

TSH is a species-specific glycoprotein, with a molecular weight of about 28,000, that is produced by the adenohypophysis.[1, 2] The secretion of TSH is stimulated by hypothalamic TRH and is inhibited by hypothalamic somatostatin, thyroid hormones, glucocorticoids, dopamine, and stress. Bovine TSH is biologically active in dogs and cats.

The TSH stimulation test has been widely evaluated in dogs and is vastly superior to the determination of basal blood TT_4, TT_3, fT_4, and fT_3 levels in the diagnosis of hypothyroidism.* A commonly used procedure for conducting the TSH stimulation test in dogs is as follows: Serum samples for TT_4 determination are collected immediately before and 6 hours after the intravenous (IV) injection of 0.1 IU/kg of bovine TSH (Dermathycin or Thytropar). At Cornell University, 1 unit of TSH is administered to dogs weighing 14 kg or less and 2 units is given

---

*See references 2, 3, 24, 25, 53, 70, and 74.

to all other dogs. Single or repeated IV injections can rarely produce anaphylaxis,[48] so some investigators use the subcutaneous route.

Euthyroid dogs usually have pre-TSH serum TT_4 levels within or below the normal pre-TSH range for the laboratory performing the assay, and post-TSH serum TT_4 levels within the normal post-TSH range. Some investigators categorize the response to TSH as normal when the post-TSH TT_4 level increases by some specific amount, even if the post-TSH TT_4 value does not enter the normal post-TSH TT_4 range. The specific increase expected varies from laboratory to laboratory and cannot be used reliably elsewhere.[74] The commonly espoused criterion, that euthyroid dogs double their basal serum TT_4 levels after TSH stimulation, is unreliable. In general, measuring serum TT_3 levels before and after TSH administration is unreliable and not recommended. The value of fT_4 in this testing is currently being investigated.[74a]

The TSH stimulation test usually achieves normal poststimulation serum TT_4 levels in dogs with the euthyroid sick syndrome and drug-related low basal serum TT_4 level.[2, 12, 67, 100a] In some cases, especially in dogs with hyperadrenocorticism or dogs being treated with glucocorticoids, both the pre-TSH and post-TSH serum TT_4 levels are below the expected normal ranges.[65, 76, 96, 118] However, the slope of the response parallels that seen in normal dogs. Glucocorticoids have been reported to suppress TRH secretion, suppress pituitary responsiveness to TRH, suppress TSH secretion, depress serum thyroid hormone–binding protein levels, suppress basal serum TT_4 and TT_3 levels, inhibit the conversion of TT_4 to TT_3, and increase serum rT_3 levels.

A single TSH stimulation test does *not* reliably distinguish between primary and secondary hypothyroidism in dogs.[2, 12] If secondary hypothyroidism is suspected, bovine TSH may be administered subcutaneously or intramuscularly for 3 to 5 consecutive days. After this time, the basal serum TT_4 levels of dogs with secondary hypothyroidism should show a normal response to TSH.

If a clinician wishes to perform a TSH stimulation test on dogs receiving thyroid hormone treatment, administration of the thyroid supplement should be stopped for at least 30 days, and cessation for 60 days may give more reliable results.[2, 3, 72]

The TSH stimulation test can be conducted simultaneously with an ACTH stimulation test or a dexamethasone suppression test, with no compromise in the accuracy of either procedure.[11, 14]

In cats, the following two protocols have been reported to be accurate measurements of thyroid function: (1) serum TT_4 determinations before and 6 hours after IV injection of either 1 IU or 1 IU/kg of bovine TSH[49, 89] and (2) serum TT_4 determinations before and 10 hours after intramuscular (IM) injection of 2.5 IU of bovine TSH.[9]

Thyrotropin-Releasing Hormone Stimulation Test

TRH is a tripeptide produced by the hypothalamus.[1, 2] TRH stimulates the release of TSH and prolactin.[51] TRH secretion is enhanced by norepinephrine, histamine, serotonin, and dopamine, and it is probably inhibited by thyroid hormones.

In humans, serum TT_4 and TSH responses to exogenous TRH have been used to differentiate among primary, secondary, and tertiary hypothyroidism.[2] Patients with primary hypothyroidism have low basal serum TT_4 levels and high basal serum TSH levels, neither of which responds to TRH stimulation. Patients with secondary hypothyroidism have low basal serum TT_4 and TSH levels, neither of which responds to TRH stimulation. Patients with tertiary hypothyroidism have low basal serum TT_4 and TSH levels, both of which respond to TRH stimulation.

Detailed evaluation of the TRH stimulation test in the various forms of hypothyroidism in dogs and cats is limited. In dogs, the TRH stimulation test has been reported to distinguish reliably between euthyroid and primary hypothyroid individuals.[37a, 51, 53, 58, 70, 90] Serum TT_4 levels are determined before and 6 hours after IV injection of 200 to 500 μg or 0.05 mg/kg[37a, 100a] of TRH. Normal dogs at least double their basal serum TT_4 levels. Serum TT_3 determinations during this protocol are variable and nondiagnostic. TRH doses of greater than 900 μg or greater than 0.1 mg/kg are reported frequently to cause various cholinergic side-effects, including hypersalivation, coughing, miosis, vomiting, diarrhea, urination, tachycardia and tachypnea. Because TRH is expensive and TRH stimulation testing is not superior to the TSH stimulation test, it has limited use.

In normal cats, serum TT_4 levels were reported to show a reproducible doubling 4 hours after the IV injection of 0.1 mg/kg of TRH.[78, 89] TRH doses of 0.1 mg/kg or greater often produced the cholinergic side-effects mentioned above for dogs.

THYROID BIOPSY

The distinction between primary and secondary canine hypothyroidism can be made easily by histologic examination of a biopsy specimen of the thyroid.[2, 12] In primary hypothyroidism, there is massive loss of follicular epithelium, usually associated with lymphocytic thyroiditis.[60] In secondary hypothyroidism, the follicles are distended with colloid, the follicular epithelium is flattened, and there is no vacuolation of the colloid. Normal dogs treated with systemic glucocorticoid have increased numbers of colloid droplets per thyroid follicular cell, suggesting inhibition of thyroid lysosomal hydrolysis of colloid.[7, 12] In these dogs, basal serum TT_3 and TT_4 levels were decreased, but TSH and TRH stimulation test results were normal.

TESTS USED IN LYMPHOCYTIC THYROIDITIS

In dogs and human patients with lymphocytic thyroiditis, a number of immunologic evaluations have been conducted, including determination of serum levels of antithyroglobulin antibodies, serum levels of antimicrosomal and anticolloidal antibodies, in vitro lymphocyte blastogenesis to thyroid extract, delayed-type hypersensitivity skin test reactions to thyroid extract, and circulating immune complex levels.[2, 28, 32, 39, 54, 98] In dogs, antithyroglobulin antibodies are demonstrable in more than 50 per cent of cases of naturally occurring hypothyroidism by means of ELISA, hemagglutination, and indirect immunofluorescence techniques.[23, 34, 43–45]

Antibodies to T_3 also may be detected.[32, 38, 54] When present, these autoantibodies cause spurious elevations of the TT_3 value as measured by RIA.[66] The patient looks either normal or hypothyroid, but has TT_3 levels consistent with hyperthyroidism. Great Danes, Irish setters, borzois, Doberman pinschers, and Old English sheepdogs may be predisposed. Interestingly, antithyroglobulin antibodies are also demonstrable in more than 40 per cent of dogs with nonthyroid endocrine disorders and healthy relatives of antibody-positive patients, as well as in 13 per cent of hospitalized patients without endocrine disease. As these tests become more available, important applications may include detecting family members that might develop hypothyroidism and helping to differentiate primary immune-mediated hypothyroidism (antibody positive) from secondary and tertiary hypothyroidism (antibody negative).

■ GLUCOCORTICOIDS

Glucocorticoids are produced by the zona fasciculata of the adrenal cortex and are probably the most commonly used therapeutic agents in veterinary medicine.[2, 10, 169] Hyperglucocorticoidism may be produced by hypersecretion of ACTH or ACTH-like substances (with ectopic, idiopathic, functional pituitary neoplasm), hypersecretion of endogenous glucocorticoids (with functional adrenocortical neoplasm), and exogenous glucocorticoid administration (iatrogenic).

Glucocorticoids and the Skin

The skin is a sensitive and specific indicator of hyperglucocorticoidism, reflecting both internal disease and inappropriate therapy.[2, 4, 5] The protein catabolic, antienzymatic, and antimitotic effects of glucocorticoids are manifested in numerous ways in canine, feline, and human skin: (1) The epidermis becomes thinned and hyperkeratotic (because of suppressed deoxyribonucleic acid [DNA] synthesis, decreased mitoses, and keratinization abnormalities); (2) the basement membrane zone becomes thinned and disrupted; (3) pilosebaceous atrophy becomes pronounced; (4) the dermis becomes thinned and dermal vasculature becomes fragile (owing to inhibition of fibroblast proliferation, collagen, and ground substance production); and (5) wound healing is delayed. Unique to the dog, presumably through changes in protein structure, collagen and elastin fibers become attractive sites for mineralization, resulting in dystrophic calcinosis cutis.[66] Additionally, owing to the broad-spectrum anti-inflammatory and immunosuppressive effects of excessive glucocorticoids, patients have increased susceptibility to bacterial and fungal cutaneous infections.[2, 12]

Clinically, hyperglucocorticoidism in dogs and cats is characterized by (1) thin, hypotonic skin; (2) easy bruising (petechiae and ecchymoses); (3) poor wound healing; (4) seborrhea sicca; (5) phlebectasias; and (6) increased susceptibility to bacterial infection, demodicosis, and perhaps dermatophytosis. In dogs, calcinosis cutis, bilaterally symmetric alopecia, easy epilation, comedones, and variable hyperpigmentation are features of hyperglucocorticoidism. In human patients, but not in dogs and cats, hypertrichosis and cutaneous striae are common features of hyperglucocorticoidism.

Histologically, hyperglucocorticoidism in dogs and cats is characterized by orthokeratotic hyperkeratosis, follicular keratosis, telogenization of hair follicles, thin dermis, and telangiectasia.[6, 16] The follicular dilatation, follicular atrophy, epidermal atrophy, epidermal melanosis, sebaceous gland atrophy, and dystrophic mineralization that are seen in dogs are rare in cats.

Adrenal Function Tests

Adrenal function tests are basically of two types: those that are single measurements of basal glucocorticoid levels in blood or urine, and those that are provocative, dynamic response tests. Single measurements of basal glucocorticoid levels, although cheaper and easier to perform, are unreliable.[2, 3, 8, 153] Many dogs with hyperadrenocorticism have elevated basal glucocorticoid levels, but some dogs have normal levels.[131]

URINARY GLUCOCORTICOID DETERMINATION

In dogs, the major cortisol metabolites found in urine are cortol, 3-epiallocortol, cortolone, 3-epiallotetrahydrocortisol, and tetrahydrocortisol.[2, 12] These metabolites are excreted mainly as glucuronides, and a major portion of this fraction is represented by steroids reduced at C-20. Thus, the use of steroid assay procedures that measure only those steroids having a dihydroxyketotic side chain, such as the Porter-Silber reaction, do not measure these cortisol metabolites in dogs. In cats, virtually all glucocorticoid metabolites are excreted in bile (99 per cent), with only a small amount of Porter-Silber chromogens present as the free compounds in urine (1 per cent).[2, 15]

Assays of urinary steroids (17-ketosteroids and 17-hydroxycorticosteroids) necessitate 24-hour urine samples, metabolic cages, and collecting equipment; are easily contaminated; and must be performed before and after the administration of a provocative test agent. They are rarely used today.

The urinary cortisol to creatinine ratio was developed to avoid the need for 24-hour urine collection and to screen the patient for hyperadrenocorticism.[115, 126, 137a] Normal dogs have low values (5.7 ± 0.9), whereas dogs with hyperadrenocorticism have high values (337.6 ± 72). However, dogs with renal disease and other disorders can have values overlapping those seen in dogs with Cushing's disease, so the test is not specific. Because normal values are not seen in dogs with hyperadrenocorticism, this ratio can be a useful screening test to exclude that diagnosis.

BLOOD CORTISOL DETERMINATION

Blood cortisol levels in dogs and cats have been measured by three methods: fluorometry, competitive protein binding, and RIA.[2] RIA is the method of choice and the one in general use. Basal blood cortisol levels by RIA in normal dogs and cats approximate 0 to 8 μg/dl.[2, 3]

It has been suggested that (1) plasma should be used to assay for cortisol, (2) plasma should be separated from the blood cellular elements within 15 minutes, and (3) plasma should be kept frozen; otherwise, cortisol levels may drop by as much as 50 per cent within 6 to 8 days. However, researchers conducting other studies found no significant differences between serum and plasma cortisol levels and reported no marked decrease in cortisol levels in serum or plasma that was stored in contact with erythrocytes for up to 8 days at 4 to 20°C (39.2 to 68°F).[12] Most investigators separate the serum or plasma as quickly as possible and freeze it until the assay is performed.

Important considerations when interpreting blood cortisol levels include the following: (1) Different laboratories may vary in their normal and abnormal values, (2) stress and nonadrenal illness can markedly elevate blood cortisol levels, (3) cortisol levels can vary with the patient's age, (4) episodic cortisol secretion occurs in normal dogs and dogs with hyperadrenocorticism, and (5) single measurements of blood cortisol are of limited value in the diagnosis of hyperadrenocorticism.* The clinical significance of diurnal cortisol rhythms in dogs and cats is unclear. Most investigators found cortisol levels in dogs to be highest in the morning,[2, 12] whereas other researchers found no diurnal rhythm.[8, 12] Likewise, some investigators found cortisol levels in cats to be highest in the evening, whereas other researchers found no difference.[2, 12]

CORTISOL RESPONSE TESTS

To overcome the unreliability of basal blood cortisol levels, various provocative tests have been developed.[2, 3, 153] There is controversy about the relative efficiency and accuracy of the various tests. Results are often difficult to compare, owing to differences in methodology (the use of plasma versus serum samples, the use of different products at varying doses, different time intervals of sampling, and different laboratories performing and interpreting the tests). Cortisol response tests are traditionally begun at 8 to 10 AM.

Corticotropin (ACTH) Stimulation Test

ACTH is a polypeptide with a molecular weight of about 4500 secreted by the adenohypophysis as part of a large prohormone, pro-opiomelanocortin, which also contains in its sequence β-lipotropin and the opioid peptides β-endorphin and enkephalins.[1, 2] Secretion of ACTH is controlled by circadian rhythm and stress mechanisms inherent in the central nervous system and by negative feedback from circulating glucocorticoids.

The ACTH stimulation test (ACTH response test) reliably documents a diagnosis of hypoadrenocorticism or iatrogenic hyperadrenocorticism in dogs and cats. Basal blood cortisol levels are normal or low and show little or no response to ACTH. In addition, the ACTH stimulation test is useful for monitoring therapeutic response to o,p'-DDD.[133, 148] The ACTH stimulation test is *not* as accurate as the low-dose dexamethasone suppression test for the diagnosis of spontaneous canine hyperadrenocorticism, because about 15 per cent of the cases of pituitary-dependent hyperadrenocorticism do not have an exaggerated response, and more than 50 per cent of the cases of adrenocortical neoplasia are hyperresponsive.[125, 137a, 147, 148, 153, 185] In addition, dogs that are admitted to the hospital, are clinically stressed, or have various chronic illnesses frequently have elevated basal cortisol levels or hyperrespond to ACTH.[103, 120] Two commonly used protocols for ACTH stimulation are as follows: (1) plasma or serum cortisol samples

---

*See references 2, 8, 12, 13, 103, 120, and 165.

collected before and 2 hours after the IM injection of 2.2 IU/kg of ACTH gel or (2) plasma or serum cortisol samples collected before and 1 hour after the IV injection of 0.25 mg of synthetic ACTH (Cortrosyn). A recent study has shown that synthetic ACTH can be administered IV or IM to dogs with no difference in the results obtained.[122a] The ACTH stimulation test can be performed concurrently with the TSH stimulation test, while the accuracy of both tests is maintained.[11, 14]

The ACTH stimulation test has been studied in normal cats and in a small number of cats with spontaneous hyperadrenocorticism.* Two protocols recommended for cats are as follows: (1) plasma or serum cortisol determinations before and 90 minutes after the IM injection of 2.2 IU/kg of ACTH gel and (2) plasma or serum cortisol determinations before and 90 minutes after the IV injection of 0.125 mg of synthetic ACTH. Other investigators reported no difference in the response of the healthy cats to 0.125 mg or 0.250 mg of synthetic ACTH IM (peak cortisol responses at 30 minutes after injection).[173] It was reported that cats with diabetes mellitus may hyperrespond to ACTH,[154] but another study failed to document this finding in diabetic and nondiabetic sick cats.[191]

Low-Dose Dexamethasone Suppression Test

The low-dose dexamethasone suppression test is presently the procedure of choice for confirming a diagnosis of spontaneous canine hyperadrenocorticism.[2, 3, 125, 137a, 147, 153] In normal dogs, the low dose of dexamethasone consistently suppresses blood cortisol levels to less than 1 μg/dl for the 8-hour test period. Inadequate suppression occurs in dogs with spontaneous hyperadrenocorticism (Fig. 9:1). However, dogs that are clinically stressed or that have various chronic illnesses may also fail to demonstrate suppression with low-dose dexamethasone.[103] Dexamethasone clearance, and therefore its ability to suppress the adrenal axis, can vary in dogs with hyperadrenocorticism or nonadrenal illness, and thus the low-dose dexamethasone suppression test can give false-positive or false-negative results.[122, 130] Therefore, failure to suppress cortisol levels with low-dose dexamethasone is not pathognomonic of hyperadreno-

---

*See references 2, 9, 12, 152, 154, 156, 157, 173, and 190.

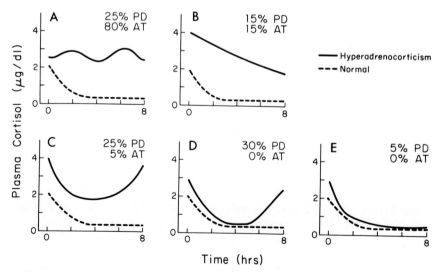

Figure 9:1. Patterns of plasma cortisol responses during low-dose dexamethasone testing in normal dogs and in dogs with hyperadrenocorticism. PD = pituitary-dependent hyperadrenocorticism, AT = adrenal tumor. (From Peterson, M. E.: Hyperadrenocorticism. Vet. Clin. North Am. [Small Anim. Pract.] 14:731, 1984.)

corticism, and the diagnosis must be supported by other clinicopathologic data.[2] A commonly used protocol for the low-dose dexamethasone suppression test is to take plasma or serum cortisol samples before and 4 and 8 hours after the IV administration of 0.01 mg/kg of dexamethasone. The dexamethasone suppression test has been performed concurrently with the TSH stimulation test, with the accuracy of both tests being preserved.[11, 14]

The dexamethasone suppression test has been studied in a few normal cats and cats with spontaneous hyperadrenocorticism.[144, 145, 154, 173] One group of investigators reported that plasma cortisol responses of healthy cats to IV injections of dexamethasone at doses of 0.01 mg/kg, 0.1 mg/kg, and 1 mg/kg were similar (with peak suppression at 6 to 10 hours after injection).[173] It was reported that the results of dexamethasone suppression testing were not different in normal, diabetic, and nondiabetic sick cats.[191]

High-Dose Dexamethasone Suppression Test

The high-dose dexamethasone suppression test is presently the procedure of choice for differentiating between pituitary-dependent hyperadrenocorticism and that caused by the adrenocortical neoplasia in dogs.[2, 3, 125, 137a, 147, 153] Suppression of blood cortisol levels to below 1.5 µg/dl is diagnostic of pituitary-dependent hyperadrenocorticism (Fig. 9:2). Such suppression should not occur with adrenocortical neoplasia. However, about 15 per cent of the dogs with pituitary-dependent hyperadrenocorticism fail to demonstrate adequate suppression with any dose of dexamethasone.[128, 153, 178] This may be because these are neoplasms arising in the intermediate lobe of the pituitary gland.[2, 128, 155, 188a] The pars intermedia is avascular and innervated by dopaminergic and serotoninergic fibers from the brain. Thus, in the dog, the intermediate lobe is under negative regulation by dopamine and somatostatin, but is relatively unresponsive to blood-borne ACTH and dexamethasone.[188a] A commonly used protocol for the high-dose dexamethasone suppression test is to take plasma or serum cortisol samples before and 4 and 8 hours after the IV injection of 0.1 mg/kg of dexamethasone. Some investigators recommended a much higher dose, 1 mg/kg.[153] Although this larger dose increases the expense of the test, it does not clearly enhance the diagnostic accuracy of the test.[2, 3, 128] In fact, it has been suggested that the 1 mg/kg dose was less reliable than the 0.1 mg/kg dose.[12, 128]

PLASMA CORTICOTROPIN (ACTH) DETERMINATION

Plasma ACTH levels have been measured by RIA in normal dogs and in dogs with spontaneous hyperadrenocorticism.* Endogenous plasma ACTH levels are extremely useful in determining the cause of spontaneous canine hyperadrenocorticism, especially when interpreted together with the results of dexamethasone suppression testing. Plasma ACTH levels range from normal to elevated (greater than 40 pg/ml) in dogs with pituitary-dependent hyperadrenocorticism and range from low to undetectable (less than 20 pg/ml) in dogs with functional adrenocortical neoplasms. As is the case with plasma cortisol levels, plasma ACTH levels fluctuate episodically throughout the day, which results in some overlap of values between normal dogs and dogs with spontaneous hyperadrenocorticism.

Plasma ACTH levels have been measured by RIA in normal cats and are reported to approximate 20 to 100 pg/ml.[2, 3, 144–154, 190] Plasma ACTH levels were markedly elevated in one cat with pituitary-dependent hyperadrenocorticism.

Accurate determination of plasma ACTH necessitates proper collection and handling of the specimen and a carefully performed, difficult RIA technique. Blood for ACTH assay must be collected in heparin- or ethylenediaminetetra-acetic–containing plastic tubes and spun within 90 minutes at 4°C (39.2°F). The plasma must be promptly separated into plastic or polypropylene tubes and kept frozen until assayed. At −20°C (−4°F), samples maintain their ACTH

---

*See references 2, 3, 12, 129, 137a, 147, 153, 161, and 185.

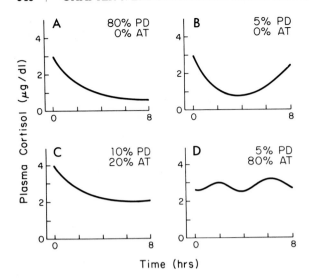

Figure 9:2. Patterns of plasma cortisol responses during high-dose dexamethasone suppression testing in dogs with hyperadrenocorticism. PD = pituitary-dependent hyperadrenocorticism, AT = adrenal tumor. (From Peterson, M. E.: Hyperadrenocorticism. Vet. Clin. North Am. [Small Anim. Pract.] 14:731, 1984.)

concentration for only 30 days, so the assay must be performed quickly.[123] At present, reliable plasma ACTH assays for dogs and cats are neither generally available nor economically feasible.

CORTICOTROPIN-RELEASING FACTOR STIMULATION TEST

CRF is a peptide secreted in pulsatile fashion by the hypothalamus.[1, 2, 104] CRF secretion is stimulated by epinephrine and serotonin, and it is inhibited by glucocorticoids and serotonin antagonists (e.g., cyproheptadine).

The isolation and synthesis of CRF makes possible an additional diagnostic test to differentiate the two causes of spontaneous hyperadrenocorticism.[2, 129, 153, 158] Synthetic ovine CRF was injected intravenously (0.1, 1, or 10 µg/kg) into normal dogs and produced peak plasma ACTH and cortisol levels within 30 to 60 minutes.[129] Preliminary information indicates that the CRF stimulation test is useful for distinguishing between canine pituitary-dependent hyperadrenocorticism (increased levels of ACTH and cortisol) and adrenocortical neoplasia (no response).[153] However, until a relatively inexpensive, single-dose, sterilized CRF preparation becomes available, the CRF stimulation test is of limited usefulness to most veterinarians.

OTHER ADRENAL FUNCTION TESTS

Attempts have been made to devise more foolproof, inexpensive, and time-efficient adrenal function tests for the dog and the cat. Tests evaluated include (1) the metyrapone response test, (2) the lysine-vasopressin test, (3) the insulin response test, (4) the glucagon response test, and (5) a combination of the ACTH response and dexamethasone suppression tests.[2, 3, 12, 109, 112, 113] However, these tests are inferior to the standard dexamethasone suppression tests and cannot be recommended.

■ GROWTH HORMONE

GH (somatotropin) is a polypeptide (molecular weight about 22,000) produced by the adenohypophysis.[1, 2] It has diametrically opposed intrinsic anabolic and catabolic activities. Its catabolic activity (enhanced lipolysis and restricted glucose transport caused by insulin resistance) is caused directly by the GH polypeptide, whereas its anabolic activity is mediated by somatomedins (insulin-like growth factors), which are primarily generated by the liver and controlled by GH.[193, 198, 199] The major function of GH is hormonal control of growth (in concert with thyroid hormones, insulin, cortisol, and sex steroids). GH is also important for the development of the thymus and T cell function.[205, 206]

The secretion of GH is episodic and labile; and it is affected by the sleep-wake cycle, physical activity, the animal's nutritional state, physical and emotional stress, and pregnancy.[1, 2] In a study of 500 normal dogs, pulsatile GH secretion was found during a 24-hour period.[194] About 30 per cent of the dogs failed to respond to clonidine and xylazine provocation, probably because the agents were administered in the postsecretory refractory period when the pituitary would not respond to further stimulation. Various neurotransmitters—norepinephrine, dopamine, and serotonin—as well as hypoglycemia, various amino acids, and progestogens stimulate GH secretion.

No significant changes occur in the concentrations of GH in whole blood held at room temperature (20 to 22°C) or in refrigeration (4°C) for 24 hours, nor in plasma held at room temperature or in refrigeration for 8 days, nor in plasma that went through four freeze/thaw cycles.[211a]

Excessive GH secretion produces acromegaly.[198, 204, 209, 210a] The skin becomes thickened, is myxedematous, and is thrown into exaggerated folds. These changes are most obvious on the face and the extremities. Hypertrichosis is common. Hyperpigmentation occurs in about 40 per cent of the human patients with acromegaly but has not been reported in dogs.[12] Histologically, acromegalic skin is characterized by increased dermal collagen and mucin and by hyperplasia of the epidermis and the appendages.[6, 16, 209]

In dogs, juvenile GH deficiency results in retention of the puppy coat, followed by bilaterally symmetric alopecia and hyperpigmentation, and by thin, hypotonic skin.[12, 199] Hyposomatotropism in the mature dog has similar cutaneous findings, but the dog has developed a normal adult coat before the hair loss starts.[199, 200, 208, 210] Histologically, both entities are characterized by orthokeratotic hyperkeratosis, follicular keratosis, follicular dilatation, follicular atrophy, telogenization of hair follicles, epidermal melanosis, sebaceous gland atrophy, thin dermis, and decreased to absent elastin fibers in chronically affected dogs.[6, 16]

Specific RIA techniques for measuring canine GH have been developed.[12, 199, 210] Basal GH levels in normal dogs and cats approximate 1 to 4.5 ng/ml.[2, 12, 194, 199, 210] No variation in normal levels has been seen by breed or sex, but age has a profound effect. Dogs younger than 1 year of age have approximately double the levels seen in dogs older than 1 year of age.[194] Young dogs also have a twofold to fourfold greater increase in their poststimulation GH levels as compared with mature dogs. Basal GH levels in pituitary dwarfs and hypophysectomized dogs may approximate these values as well. Thus, basal GH levels are inadequate for the documentation of GH deficiency.

To document GH deficiency, stimulation tests must be done.[2, 12, 202, 207] Clonidine hydrochloride (Catapres), an α-adrenergic and antihypertensive drug, has been used to stimulate GH release in dogs. Normal dogs showed a marked increase in plasma GH levels within 15 to 30 minutes after the IV injection of 20 to 30 μg/kg of clonidine, whereas pituitary dwarfs and hypophysectomized dogs fail to respond. Because some normal dogs fail to respond to clonidine or xylazine provocation,[194] this test cannot be considered diagnostic for GH deficiency. Clonidine may cause severe hypotension and shock.[18] Xylazine (Rompun), a sedative hypnotic drug, gives similar results when injected intravenously at 100 to 300 μg/kg. The 300 μg/kg xylazine dose may cause severe hypotension and shock in toy and miniature breeds of dogs.[18] More recently, testing with synthetic human or bovine GH-RF has been suggested.[192, 200] Either product is injected intravenously at 1 μg/kg, with sampling at 0, 15, and 30 minutes. Side-effects have not been reported. Proper interpretation of GH levels also necessitates the assessment of thyroid and adrenal gland function.[2, 199, 210] Both hyperglucocorticoidism and hypothyroidism impair GH secretion. In addition, pseudopregnancy, progestogen therapy, and sex hormone imbalances can cause elevation of basal plasma GH levels and poor response to xylazine.

In acromegaly, basal plasma GH levels have been markedly elevated, ranging from 11 to 1476 ng/ml.[198, 204, 209, 210a] A hallmark of acromegaly is the nonsuppressibility of plasma GH levels during the administration of an IV glucose load. In canine acromegaly, plasma GH levels were not suppressed by the IV administration of 1 gm of glucose per kilogram.[2, 198]

Somatomedins are polypeptides (molecular weight 5000 to 10,000) that can also be quantitated by RIA to assess GH status indirectly.[2, 198–200] Somatomedin C (insulin-like growth factor I) is most commonly assayed. Somatomedin C plasma levels parallel body size in dogs; normal values for Cocker spaniels are 5 to 90 ng/ml, as opposed to 230 to 330 ng/ml for normal German shepherds. Somatomedin production is impaired by glucocorticoids and estrogens. Somatomedin C levels are expected to be low or undetectable in GH-deficient states and elevated in acromegaly. Normal values have been seen in some dogs with presumed adult-onset hyposomatotropism.[200, 204a]

■ SEX HORMONES

Estrogens

Estrogens are present in both male and female animals and are produced by the ovarian follicles, the zona reticularis of the adrenal cortex, and Sertoli's and interstitial cells of the testicle.[2, 12, 235] They may also be made by peripheral aromatization of androgens. Pituitary FSH stimulates ovarian follicular growth and estrogen production in females, and spermatogenesis in males.[1, 2] Hypothalamic GnRH stimulates the pituitary to release FSH. In turn, estrogen inhibits GnRH release, and inhibin (produced by ovarian follicles and testicular Sertoli's cells) inhibits FSH release.

Estrogens are reported to stimulate epidermal mitosis, to increase epidermal thickness in mice and humans, and also to reduce epidermal thickness in rats and humans.[4, 5, 235] Epidermal atrophy was produced in dogs by daily IM injections of 1 mg of diethylstilbestrol for 400 days.

Estrogens increase skin pigmentation in the guinea pig by increasing both free melanin and melanin within melanocytes, whereas ovariectomy has the opposite effect.[12] Cutaneous hyperpigmentation is a feature of clinical dermatoses associated with hyperestrogenism in dogs.

Estrogens reduce both sebaceous gland size and sebum production in rats and humans.[12] These effects appear to result from a local action on sebaceous glands, rather than from a feedback suppression of endogenous androgens. The daily IM injection of 1 mg of diethylstilbestrol into dogs for 400 days produced marked sebaceous gland atrophy.

Estrogens suppress the initiation of anagen in rats, whereas ovariectomy has the opposite effect.[12, 235] In addition, the rate of hair growth is greater in spayed female rats than in intact normal female rats, and estradiol implanted into spayed female or castrated male rats reduces the growth rate. In dogs, estrogens administered orally, subcutaneously, intramuscularly, and topically produce alopecia. Bilaterally symmetric alopecia and easily epilated hair are striking features of clinical dermatoses associated with hyperestrogenism in dogs. There appears to be regional sensitivity of hair follicles to estrogenic abnormalities, as these dermatoses follow a predictable pattern (see below). Evidence has also been presented that suggests that these estrogen-sensitive areas of skin may have increased numbers of estrogen receptors.[215]

Estrogens are reported to increase the amount of dermal ground substance in mice and humans.[12] The daily IM injection of 1 mg of diethylstilbestrol in dogs for 400 days reduced the thickness of the subcutis.[212, 238]

Estrogens are also known to affect thymic function, to enhance antibody production, and to inhibit suppressor T cell function.[223]

Hyperestrogenism is thought to be the cause of two distinctive dermatoses in dogs: feminization of the male dog with a functional tumor of the testicle and hyperestrogenism of the intact female dog. Cutaneous changes in these syndromes include (1) bilaterally symmetric alopecia that begins in the perineal, genital, and ventral abdominal regions and spreads cranially and ventrally; (2) variable hyperpigmentation; (3) a dull, easily epilated haircoat that fails to regrow after clipping; (4) gynecomastia; (5) pendulous prepuce; (6) vulvar enlargement; and (7) variable seborrheic skin disease. In male dogs, linear preputial dermatosis appears to correlate with the presence of hyperestrogenism and testicular neoplasia. Histologically, both syndromes are characterized by orthokeratotic hyperkeratosis, follicular keratosis, follicular dilatation, follicular atrophy, telogenization of hair follicles, variable epidermal melanosis, and sebaceous gland atrophy.[6, 16]

It has been stated that adrenalectomized and ovariectomized dogs maintained on only mineralocorticoids have normal skin and haircoats, indicating that estrogens or any other sex steroids are not necessary for normal skin and haircoats in dogs. However, hypoestrogenism has been hypothesized as an etiologic consideration in the estrogen-responsive dermatosis of spayed female dogs. Clinically, the dermatosis is characterized by bilaterally symmetric alopecia that begins in the perineal, genital, and ventral abdominal areas and spreads cranially and ventrally and an easily epilated haircoat that fails to regrow after clipping. Histologically, the dermatosis is characterized by follicular keratosis and follicular dilatation with telogenization of hair follicles.[6, 16] In addition, spayed female cats with feline acquired symmetric alopecia may respond to estrogen replacement therapy.

Assays (RIA) for plasma or serum estrogens are commercially available.[2, 3] Most available assays measure only *one* type of estrogen (e.g., estradiol or estrone), and as numerous estrogenic substances are produced in the body, such assays may be unsatisfactory. Thus, one can readily understand why only 50 per cent of the dogs with feminization due to functional Sertoli's cell neoplasm of the testicle could be shown to have hyperestrogenism (only estradiol was measured). Additionally, blood estrogen levels, along with the blood levels of the other sex steroids, fluctuate markedly during the day, necessitating multiple samples and unrealistic financial considerations.[223a] Evidence has been presented that suggests that dogs can have so-called cutaneous hyperestrogenism (increased cutaneous estrogen receptors) in the *absence* of hyperestrogenism.[215] Reported values for blood estradiol in the dog and cat vary with the sex of the animal, whether it is neutered or intact, the stage of the estrous cycle, and the laboratory used.[235]

Androgens

Androgens are present in both male and female animals and they are produced by the interstitial cells of the testicle, by the zona reticularis of the adrenal cortex, and through peripheral conversion of other sex steroids.[2, 3, 235] Pituitary LH stimulates androgen secretion by testicular interstitial cells, and ovulation and corpus luteum formation and maintenance.[1, 2] Hypothalamic GnRH stimulates the pituitary release of LH. In turn, androgens and progesterone inhibit LH release, and estrogens and androgens (via hypothalamic aromatization to estrogens) inhibit GnRH release.

Androgens are reported to stimulate epidermal mitosis in mice and rats.[4, 5, 12, 235] In humans, androgens are reported to increase epidermal mitotic activity and cell turnover time and thickness.

Androgens have no effect on pigmentation in the guinea pig but are reported to stimulate pigmentation in specialized areas of the skin, such as the subcostal region of the male golden hamster and the scrotum of the ground squirrel.[12] In humans, androgens increase cutaneous pigmentation, especially in sexual skin, apparently owing to increased melanin synthesis and alteration of the packaging of melanosomes. Men with an androgen deficiency experience hypopigmentation.

Androgens enlarge the sebaceous glands in rats, rabbits, hamsters, mice, and human beings and increase sebum production in humans and rats.[12] In humans, excessive androgens produce excessively oily skin, whereas androgen deficiency produces dry skin and hair. The action of androgens involves both an increase in the rate of formation of new sebaceous cells and an increase in the size of mature cells.

In rats, androgen administration retards the initiation of anagen, whereas gonadectomy enhances it.[12] However, neither castration nor treatment with testosterone has any effect on the rate of hair growth in rats. In humans, an excess of androgens results in accelerated hair growth, whereas androgen deficiency in men causes the hair to become sparse.[219]

Androgens are reported to increase the relative and total amounts of hyaluronic acid and dermal ground substance in mice.[12] In humans, androgens cause thickening of the dermis with demonstrable increase in skin collagen content.[4, 5] Androgens also inhibit various T cell functions.[223]

In the testosterone-responsive dermatosis of male dogs, hypoandrogenism is an etiologic hypothesis. The dermatosis is characterized by (1) bilaterally symmetric alopecia that begins in the perineal, genital, and ventral abdominal areas and spreads cranially and ventrally; (2) a dull, dry, easily epilated haircoat that fails to grow after clipping; (3) thin hypotonic skin; and (4) seborrhea sicca. Alteration in coat color can be seen in some dogs. Histologically, the dermatosis is characterized by orthokeratotic hyperkeratosis, epidermal atrophy, follicular atrophy, telogenization of hair follicles, sebaceous gland atrophy, and thin dermis.[6, 16] In addition, castrated male cats with feline acquired symmetric alopecia may respond to testosterone replacement therapy. Conversely, hyperandrogenism is presumed to be the cause of seborrhea oleosa in oversexed intact male dogs, and the condition resolves with castration.[12] Hyperandrogenism has also been demonstrated in intact male animals with hyperplasia of the perianal glands and the tail gland.[236] Normal cats treated with mibolerone became virilized, showing thickening of the skin of the neck and clitoral hypertrophy.[2]

Assays (RIA) for plasma or serum androgens are commercially available and are accompanied by the same interpretational, financial, and practical considerations as previously mentioned for estrogen assays. Values for blood testosterone in normal male dogs and cats approximate 0.5 to 6 ng/ml, whereas those in normal female dogs and cats are usually less than 0.5 ng/ml.[2, 12, 17, 229a, 235]

Progesterone

Progesterone is present in both male and female animals, and it is produced by the corpus luteum of the ovary and by the zona reticularis of the adrenal cortex.[2, 3, 229a, 235] The effects of progestational compounds on the skin have not been well studied. However, with the use of these compounds (e.g., megestrol acetate and medroxyprogesterone acetate) for the management of feline and canine skin disorders, the clinician must be alerted to some possible cutaneous side-effects.

Progesterone is known to have immunosuppressive action and various progesterone analogs are known to have glucocorticoid activity.[2, 12, 177, 223] Progestational compounds have also been shown to bind to the intracellular cytosol receptor for dihydrotestosterone and to inhibit the enzyme 5-α-reductase, which converts testosterone to dihydrotestosterone. By binding androgen receptors in multiple tissues, progestational compounds may be androgenic, synandrogenic, or antiandrogenic, depending on the compound and the dose.

In the skin, topically applied progesterone was shown to suppress the sebum excretion rate significantly in women.[4, 5, 12] Medroxyprogesterone was reported to delay wound healing in rabbits. In the cat, subcutaneous injections of medroxyprogesterone acetate may produce local alopecia, atrophy, and pigmentary disturbances, and oral megestrol acetate administration can produce generalized cutaneous atrophy, alopecia, xanthomas, and poor wound healing. Bilateral flank alopecia was reported in a dog with hyperprogesteronemia and a testicular Sertoli's cell neoplasm.[217]

Assays (RIA) for plasma or serum progesterone are commercially available and are burdened by the same interpretational, financial, and practical considerations as previously mentioned for estrogen assays. Values for blood progesterone in female dogs and cats approximate less than 5 ng/ml (in anestrus, estrus, and proestrus) and 10 to 50 ng/ml (in metestrus and pregnancy), and they approximate less than 1 ng/ml in male dogs and cats.[2, 3, 235]

Sex Hormone Function Tests

As is the case with other endocrine tests, basal measurements of serum sex hormone levels can give misleading results, especially in intact dogs. Although stimulation tests with hCG[216] or GnRH[223a] to evaluate reproductive performance are available, their value in dogs with gonadal or adrenal sex hormone dermatoses is largely unknown. To date, the testing that has received widest attention in these conditions is the sex hormone ACTH response as offered by the Endocrinology Laboratory at the University of Tennessee, College of Veterinary Medicine, Knoxville, TN 37901–1071, USA.[208a] Dogs are given either synthetic ACTH (0.5 IU/kg IV) or repository ACTH (2.2 mg/kg IM). Plasma and serum are both collected in ethylenediamine-tetra-acetic acid before injection and again at 1 hour (synthetic ACTH) or 2 hours (gel ACTH) after injection. Samples are separated immediately, frozen, and mailed frozen to the laboratory by overnight mail. In addition to cortisol determinations, the laboratory measures prestimulation and poststimulation levels of progesterone, 17-hydroxyprogesterone, dehydroepiandrosterone sulfate, androstenedione, testosterone, and estradiol-17β. Normal values are available for all hormones for intact or neutered male or female animals.

Gonadotropins and Prolactin

The gonadotropins, FSH (follitropin, molecular weight about 32,000) and LH (lutropin, molecular weight about 30,000), are produced by the adenohypophysis.[1, 2] Gonadotropin secretion is stimulated by hypothalamic GnRH and inhibited by estrogens, glucocorticoids, and androgens (via aromatization to estrogens in the hypothalamus). FSH secretion is also inhibited by inhibin from the ovarian follicle and testicular Sertoli's cells. LH secretion is inhibited by progestogens and androgens. In normal dogs and cats, serum FSH levels by RIA are reported to approximate 40 to 70 ng/ml (higher in females in proestrus).[2] Serum LH levels by RIA in normal dogs and cats are reported as follows: 0 to 3 ng/ml in intact male animals, 6 to 10 ng/ml in female animals in estrus, and less than 2 ng/ml in female animals in metestrus or anestrus.[2] Gonadotropin deficiencies could be seen with hypothalamic or pituitary disorders.

Prolactin is a polypeptide (molecular weight about 22,500) produced by the adenohypophysis.[1, 2] Prolactin secretion is episodic and labile; it is stimulated by one or more hypothalamic releasing factors (including TRH) and inhibited by hypothalamic dopamine. In normal dogs and cats, serum prolactin levels by RIA are reported to approximate 1 to 10 ng/ml.[2] Hyperprolactinemia could be seen with hypothyroidism, pituitary neoplasms, and certain drug administrations (phenothiazines, cimetidine), resulting in galactorrhea, gynecomastia, and inhibition of FSH or LH secretion.

■ CLINICAL ASPECTS OF ENDOCRINE SKIN DISEASES

Canine Hyperadrenocorticism

Hyperadrenocorticism (Cushing's disease, Cushing's syndrome) is a common disorder of the dog associated with excessive endogenous or exogenous glucocorticoids and is classically characterized by polyuria and polydipsia, bilaterally symmetric alopecia, thin hypotonic skin, and skeletal muscle wasting. More than 50 per cent of cases can have nontraditional clinical findings.[184, 185]

CAUSE AND PATHOGENESIS

Canine hyperadrenocorticism may occur naturally or may be iatrogenic.[2, 3, 125, 153] The naturally occurring type may be associated with bilateral adrenocortical hyperplasia, adrenocortical neoplasia, or the ectopic ACTH syndrome. Iatrogenic canine hyperadrenocorticism results from the misuse of exogenous glucocorticoids.

In about 80 to 85 per cent of the dogs with spontaneous hyperadrenocorticism, the disorder results from excessive pituitary ACTH secretion, which produces bilateral adrenocortical hyperplasia (pituitary-dependent hyperadrenocorticism). Although some studies failed to document pituitary neoplasia as the cause of pituitary-dependent hyperadrenocorticism,[2, 111] most investigators believe that it is due to microneoplasia or macroneoplasia of the pituitary gland.[125, 151, 153] The hypersecretion of ACTH results in bilateral adrenocortical hyperplasia that may be diffuse, nodular, or both. The zona glomerulosa is usually normal in width and histologic appearance, and enlargement is due to hyperplasia of the zona fasciculata and zona reticularis. In some cases, gross enlargement of the adrenals is not seen. The adrenal cortex may be grossly and histologically normal but functionally abnormal.

When pituitary tumors cannot be demonstrated, the cause of the adrenal hyperplasia is uncertain, but the underlying defect may be in hypothalamic regulation and the negative feedback mechanism. Serotonin appears to be an excitatory transmitter with regard to ACTH release. With increased serotoninergic input, there is no hippocampal inhibition of the release of CRF, resulting in increased CRF stimulation of pituitary ACTH release. Antiserotoninergic agents, such as cyproheptadine, have been used successfully to treat human patients with hyperadrenocorticism resulting from idiopathic bilateral adrenocortical hyperplasia.[175]

Bilateral adrenocortical hyperplasia secondary to a functional pituitary tumor probably accounts for most cases of pituitary-dependent hyperadrenocorticism. Chromophobe adenomas of the pars distalis are often large, compressive, and functional, especially in brachycephalic breeds.[166] Adenomas arising from the pars intermedia are usually small, noncompressive, and nonfunctional, and are found in nonbrachycephalic breeds, but occasionally they may be functional. Canine pituitary-dependent hyperadrenocorticism has also been associated with pituitary adenocarcinomas. Except with large tumors, there appears to be no direct correlation among the size of the pituitary neoplasm, the degree of bilateral adrenocortical hyperplasia, and the severity of canine hyperadrenocorticism.[135] Large tumors tend to produce higher concentrations of ACTH. Although the rate of growth of pituitary neoplasms is variable, it is usually slow.[146]

Functional (cortisol-producing) adrenocortical neoplasms account for about 15 to 20 per cent of the cases of naturally occurring canine hyperadrenocorticism. They may be adenocarcinomas or adenomas and can occur in either gland. Older data suggested a higher frequency of occurrence in the right adrenal, but newer studies show no clear-cut predilection for one gland over the other.[150, 160, 161, 179] These neoplasms are thought to function autonomously, producing excessive amounts of cortisol, which results in negative feedback suppression of CRF (hypothalamus) and ACTH (pituitary) and in atrophy of the contralateral adrenal gland. Adrenocortical adenocarcinomas tend to be large, often extending into the adrenal vein and caudal vena cava, and they usually metastasize to the liver, lung, kidney, and lymph nodes. Dogs with bilateral adrenocortical adenomas or carcinomas have been reported rarely.[119]

The *ectopic ACTH syndrome* is a term used to describe conditions in which hyperadrenocorticism is associated with nonpituitary and nonadrenocortical neoplasia. In humans, the ectopic ACTH syndrome is most commonly seen with neoplasms of the lung and pancreas (thought to produce ACTH or an ACTH-like substance). In the dog, the ectopic ACTH syndrome appears to be rare and has been reported in association with lymphosarcoma and bronchial carcinoma.

By far, the most alarming cause of canine hyperadrenocorticism is the injudicious use of glucocorticoids for therapeutic purposes.[169] Although iatrogenic hyperadrenocorticism appears to be less common than the 50 per cent incidence rate cited in the past, it still is a problem for clinicians and pet owners. Long-term steroid use whether by mouth,[142, 169] via injection,[132, 139, 169] or topically (eyes,[108, 121, 140, 143, 164] ears,[140] skin[189]) can produce adrenocortical suppression, elevated levels of hepatic enzymes, and iatrogenic hyperadrenocorticism in dogs.

CLINICAL FEATURES

Naturally occurring canine hyperadrenocorticism is a disease of middle-aged and older dogs, but cases can be seen in young dogs. No definitive sex predilection has been documented, but many studies show a slightly higher frequency in female dogs.[147, 153, 185] Traditionally boxers, Boston terriers, Poodles, and dachshunds are predisposed, but all breeds, even dogs of mixed breeding, can be affected. The occurrence of spontaneous hyperadrenocorticism in related dachshunds,[185] Dandie Dinmont terriers,[167a] and Yorkshire terriers[168] reinforces the concept of breed predisposition. Iatrogenic canine hyperadrenocorticism knows no age, sex, or breed predilections. It occurs most commonly in dogs with chronic pruritus, because they are more likely to receive long-term systemic corticosteroids.

The clinical signs of hyperadrenocorticism are many and varied. Although some findings may be caused by the compressive or invasive effects of a pituitary or adrenal tumor, most signs are a direct result of excessive levels of cortisol and possibly other adrenal steroids. The signs at presentation depend on the dog's age, the owner's power of observation, and the cause of the hyperadrenocorticism. Old dogs are more sensitive to the catabolic effects of glucocorticoids and tend to develop signs more rapidly and markedly as compared with younger dogs. Breeders and others with a keen interest in their dog's skin may detect subtle changes in the coat and present the dog for those changes before other signs have developed. At the other end of the spectrum is the dog owner who pays little attention to the animal and presents the animal only when the disease, and therefore the signs, is well advanced. Dogs with pituitary-dependent hyperadrenocorticism resulting from pituitary adenomas or loss of feedback control tend to have signs develop gradually, whereas the rate of occurrence can be more rapid and unpredictable with pituitary adenocarcinomas or adrenal tumors.

Polyuria and polydipsia (greater than 100 ml/kg/day of water intake) are commonly the initial signs of hyperadrenocorticism and can precede easily recognized cutaneous changes by 6 to 12 months. Incidence figures vary from 32 to 82 per cent.[153, 185] Concomitant with the polyuria and polydipsia, varying degrees of polyphagia develop in approximately 50 per cent of affected dogs. In some chronic cases seen by the authors, the earliest sign of hyperadrenocorticism is apparently spontaneous improvement in the dog's allergies.

Cutaneous changes occur in most cases of hyperadrenocorticism but not all are recognized by casual inspection of the skin. The most common change occurs in the coat. Early on, the coat loses its luster and healthy appearance and is more difficult to groom (Fig. 9:3 A). Some Poodle owners comment that grooming appointments could be skipped because the hair was not growing as fast as normally. With time, hairs are lost, resulting in hypotrichosis to alopecia (Fig. 9:3 B and C). In most cases, the hair loss is symmetric and involves the trunk, sparing the head and distal extremities, but patchy hair loss or involvement of only the flank region[12] (Fig. 9:3 D) or the face[184] can also be seen. In one study of 60 dogs, 8 (13.3 per cent) had nontruncal alopecia of the legs (Fig. 9:3 E) or face.[185] Short-coated dogs, in particular, tend to have a thinned or moth-eaten coat (Fig. 9:3 F). Coat color change can be seen as the initial cutaneous sign in some dogs. Black hairs turn auburn or rust colored and brown hairs lighten to tan or blonde (Fig. 9:3 G). This change in pigmentation can involve the entire length of the hair shaft or only the distal portions. In the latter case, the color change appears to be due to solar bleaching because the hairs are not shed as rapidly as normally. Uniform color change appears to be mediated by sex hormones. In the authors' experience, coat color change with few other signs of hyperadrenocorticism is indicative of a gonadal sex hormone imbalance or adrenal neoplasia, especially adenocarcinomas.

Other cutaneous signs include thin, hypotonic skin (mimics dehydration, tends to wrinkle)

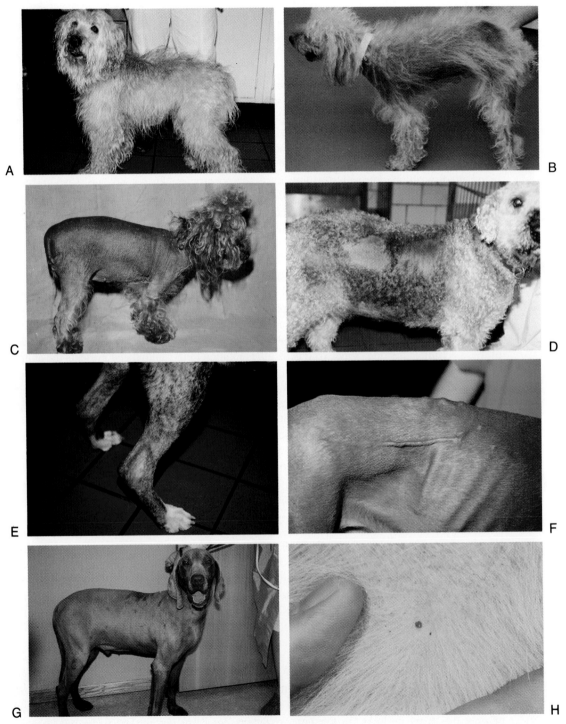

Figure 9:3. Hyperadrenocorticism. *A*, Soft-coated Wheaten terrier with an unmanageable coat. *B*, Marked truncal hypotrichosis and hyperpigmentation. *C*, Toy Poodle showing typical advanced alopecic pattern and hyperpigmented skin. This dog regrew a good haircoat with o,p′-DDD treatment. *D*, Flank alopecia secondary to an adrenal tumor. *E*, Distal extremity hair loss. *F*, Hypotrichotic and hypotonic skin. *G*, Generalized coat color change in a German shorthaired pointer. (Courtesy R. Long.) *H*, Phlebectasia.

(Fig. 9:3 *F*), hyperpigmentation, easy bruising (petechiae and ecchymoses) (Fig. 9:4), phlebectasias (see Fig. 9:3 *H*), seborrhea (dry or greasy), comedones (Fig. 9:5 *A*), poor wound healing, bacterial pyoderma (Fig. 9:5 *B*), calcinosis cutis (Fig. 9:5 *C* and *D*), and stria (Fig. 9:5 *E*). The stria may occur spontaneously or be the result of remodeling of a previous scar. Demodicosis (Fig. 9:6) may be a secondary confounding problem in more than 5 per cent of cases.[12, 185] The older veterinary literature gives incidence figures for most of the above, which can be different from those generated today. For example, a study done in the 1980s on 300 dogs[153] reported comedones in 34 per cent of the dogs, whereas a more recent study on 60 dogs showed a 5 per cent incidence rate.[185] These disparate results do not mean that the signs of hyperadrenocorticism are changing but rather that most cases are diagnosed and treated earlier before the classic cluster of changes occurs.[137a]

The skin infections seen in hyperadrenocorticism typically occur in the hypotrichotic to alopecic areas, but in some dogs, there are not other skin lesions. Typically, the infection is follicular, but large, nonfollicular superficial pustules (bullous impetigo) with minimal inflammation may be seen. The infections in these dogs respond poorly to treatment or recur shortly after treatment is discontinued. In cases in which the response to antibiotics is poor, multiple deep skin scrapings should be performed to check for demodicosis. Calcinosis cutis can be seen in up to 40 per cent of cases, but the incidence in cases presented early is much lower (1.7 to 8 per cent).[185] It occurs most commonly over the dorsal neck, on the rump, and in the axillary and inguinal regions (see Fig. 9:5 *C* and *D*). Early lesions are firm, whitish dermal papules to plaques. With time, the overlying skin reddens, ulcerates, and crusts. Old lesions can resemble pyoderma or pyotraumatic dermatitis and are often pruritic. Other causes of pruritus in hyperadrenocorticism are bacterial pyoderma, *Malassezia* dermatitis, seborrhea, and demodicosis.

Cutaneous phlebectasias are seen in up to 40 per cent of the dogs with hyperadrenocorticism, especially over the ventrum and medial thighs.[171] These vascular lesions are macular to papular, are erythematous, range up to 6 mm in diameter, are asymptomatic, and generally do not blanch with diascopy (see Fig. 9:3 *H*). These lesions do *not* regress after effective treatment. Pressure sores (decubital ulcers) are common in large dogs with hyperadrenocorticism.[3]

Musculoskeletal abnormalities are common in canine hyperadrenocorticism.[2, 3, 147, 148] Lethargy and decreased exercise tolerance are common. Skeletal muscle atrophy and weakness

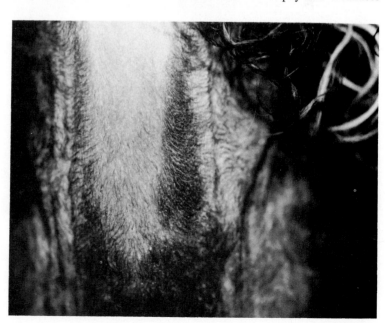

Figure 9:4. Bruising in the jugular furrow.

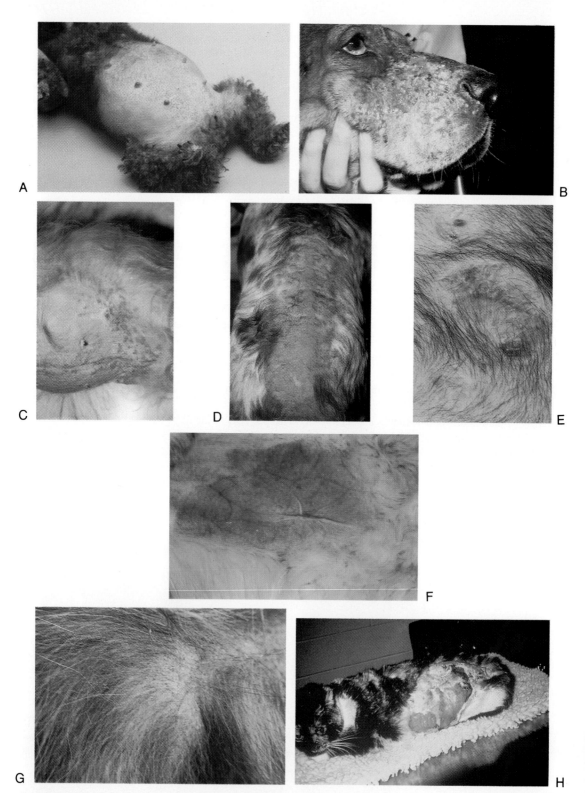

Figure 9:5. Hyperadrenocorticism. *A,* Comedones, alopecia, and potbelly. *B,* Severe facial furunculosis in a dog with Cushing's disease. *C,* Calcinosis cutis on the ventral abdomen. *D,* Calcinosis cutis along the caudal dorsum. *E,* Stria with focal ulceration. *F,* Thin, hypotonic skin with a central wrinkle, prominent vasculature, and a few petechiae in a cat with iatrogenic hyperglucocorticoidism. *G,* Hypotrichosis with scaling in a cat. *H,* Large traumatic wound in a cat with hyperadrenocorticism. (Courtesy R. Rosychuk.)

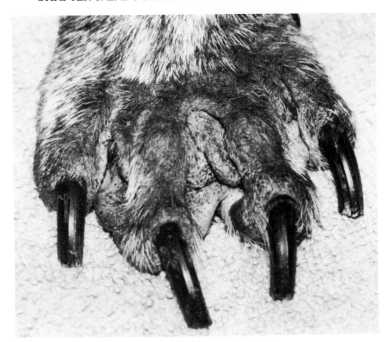

Figure 9:6. Adult-onset pododemodicosis in a cushingoid dog.

occur with atrophy being most pronounced over the head, shoulders, thighs, and pelvis. Abdominal enlargement (potbelly) is frequent (see Fig. 9:5 *A*), with the abdomen being flaccid and the dog not being able to tense the abdomen normally. In addition, a cushingoid myotonia or pseudomyotonia may be seen, which is characterized by muscle stiffness and proximal appendicular muscle enlargement. Lameness associated with osteoporosis and osteomalacia, with or without pathologic fractures, is rarely seen. Chronic hyperadrenocorticism can exaggerate common problems such as anterior cruciate ligament rupture and patellar luxation.[3]

Persistent anestrus is frequently observed in intact bitches with hyperadrenocorticism.[2, 125, 153, 229a] In addition, clitoral enlargement is not uncommon and presumably results from hypersecretion of adrenal androgens.[106] Clitoral enlargement is *not* seen with iatrogenic hyperadrenocorticism. Testicular atrophy is often seen in intact males.

Respiratory complications reported to occur with canine hyperadrenocorticism include excessive panting, bronchopneumonia, dystrophic mineralization and fibrosis, and pulmonary thrombosis.[136, 149]

Behavioral changes may also occur (aggressiveness, depression, psychoses, and self-mutilation). Neurologic signs, including ataxia, blindness, head pressing, somnolence, Horner's syndrome, anisocoria, circling, hyperesthesias, and seizures, are occasionally seen in naturally occurring canine hyperadrenocorticism and are caused by pituitary neoplasia or metastatic adrenocortical neoplasia.[107, 138, 146, 166] Exophthalmos, indolent corneal ulcers, and keratopathy have also been reported in association with canine hyperadrenocorticism.[2, 3, 182]

Palpable hepatomegaly is a common feature of canine hyperadrenocorticism. Fasting hyperglycemia can be seen in 40 to 60 per cent of cases, with overt diabetes mellitus being noted in approximately 15 per cent of dogs.[102, 141, 159] Other complications associated with hyperadrenocorticism include hypertension, recurrent urinary tract infections, urolithiasis, and acute pancreatitis.[3] Acute abdomen with or without hemoperitoneum is a rare manifestation of hemorrhage from an adrenocortical neoplasm.[175a]

DIAGNOSIS

Before the onset of the cutaneous signs, the differential diagnosis of hyperadrenocorticism is basically that of polyuria and polydipsia: chronic renal disease, chronic liver disease, diabetes mellitus, diabetes insipidus (pituitary or renal), psychogenic polydipsia, hyperthyroidism, hypercalcemia, hypernatremia, hypokalemia, hypoadrenocorticism, polycythemia vera, and pyrexia.[2, 12] With truncal alopecia and no polyuria and polydipsia, the differential diagnosis includes hypothyroidism, hyposomatotropism, and adrenal or gonadal sex hormone imbalance. Definitive diagnosis is based on history, physical examination findings, hemogram, urinalysis, serum chemistry studies, radiography, skin biopsy, and adrenal function tests.

Hemograms classically reveal leukocytosis (17,000 to 68,000/μl), neutrophilia (11,500 to 65,000/μl), lymphopenia (0 to 1000/μl), and eosinopenia (0 to 1000/μl).* Erythrocytosis (polycythemia), nucleated red blood cells, thrombocytosis, and hypersegmentation of neutrophil nuclei may also be seen.

Urinalysis usually reveals a low specific gravity (typically, 1.012). In addition, 50 per cent of the dogs have urinary tract infection, usually manifested only by bacteriuria. Proteinuria is commonly seen. About 15 per cent of the dogs have glucosuria in association with concurrent diabetes mellitus. The urinary cortisol to creatinine ratio is typically elevated in hyperadrenocorticism. However, elevations are not specific for hyperadrenocorticism.[115, 126]

Serum chemistry panel abnormalities may include mild to marked elevations in levels of cholesterol and triglycerides,[172] serum alanine transaminase, serum aspartate transaminase, and glucose and a decreased blood urea nitrogen (BUN) level. Hypophosphatemia is seen in about 33 per cent of dogs with spontaneous hyperadrenocorticism. Abnormal glucose tolerance test results and elevated serum insulin levels are common.

The serum alkaline phosphatase level is usually elevated in canine hyperadrenocorticism (80 to 95 per cent) and is mainly due to a steroid-induced isoenzyme that is hepatic in origin.[137a, 174, 188] Because this fraction can be increased in diabetes mellitus, hepatic disease, and other nonadrenal illnesses, results of this testing cannot be considered diagnostic.

Basal thyroid hormone levels (TT_4, fT_4, and TT_3) are usually low in canine hyperadrenocorticism.[2, 3, 7, 10, 118] These spuriously low thyroid hormone levels are caused by glucocorticoids and do not usually indicate concurrent hypothyroidism. The results of TSH stimulation tests are usually normal, but pre-TSH and post-TSH levels may be below the normal ranges. When the hyperadrenocorticism is corrected, thyroid hormone levels return to normal. Occasionally, a dog truly has concurrent hypothyroidism and requires thyroid hormone maintenance therapy.

Dogs with hyperadrenocorticism may also have elevated systolic (180 to 280 mm Hg; normal, 170 or less) and diastolic (110 to 180 mm Hg; normal, 100 or less) blood pressures, which may predispose to thromboembolism, glomerulosclerosis, left ventricular hypertrophy, congestive heart failure, and retinal detachment.[125, 147, 153] In dogs with cushingoid myopathies, electromyographic studies have revealed bizarre high-frequency discharges in association with histopathologic findings in skeletal muscle (atrophy, degeneration, and necrosis) and peripheral nerves (segmental demyelination).

Dogs with hyperglucocorticoidism have decreased blood GH levels, which respond poorly or not at all to xylazine or clonidine.[2, 12, 204a] Glucocorticoids can also suppress serum gonadotropin (LH and FSH) levels, prolactin levels, and testosterone, estrogen, and progesterone levels.[3, 7, 10, 229a] Serum testosterone responses to exogenous LH or human chorionic gonadotropin injections are normal in this situation.

Radiography may reveal (1) hepatomegaly; (2) osteoporosis and osteomalacia (especially of vertebrae, ribs, and flat bones), with or without pathologic fractures; (3) dystrophic mineralization of soft tissues (especially of the lung, the kidney, and the skin); and (4) adrenocortical neoplasms. The success of demonstrating adrenal tumors with routine radiographic techniques varies from 27 to 57 per cent.[137a, 150, 179, 181] Mineralization in the area of an adrenal gland indicates tumor but does not differentiate adenomas from adenocarcinomas, because the incidence of mineralization is similar for both. Special radiographic techniques (nephrotomography and x-ray computed tomography) are reported to be near perfect in detecting adrenal tumors.[137a,

---

*See references 2, 3, 12, 125, 147, 153, and 185.

[138, 160, 178, 179, 181] This testing does not differentiate adenomas from adenocarcinomas and is impractical for routine use. Ultrasonography in the hands of an experienced technician or radiologist appears to be a sensitive, relatively inexpensive, and increasingly more available test for adrenal neoplasia. When compared with other radiographic techniques, the ultrasonographic examination detected all tumors.[160, 179]

Dogs with hyperadrenocorticism may have significant elevations of coagulation factors I (fibrinogen), V, VII, IX, and X, as well as elevated levels of antithrombin III and plasminogen. These abnormalities may predispose the patient to hypercoagulability and thromboembolism.

Histopathology

Skin biopsy in canine hyperadrenocorticism may reveal many nondiagnostic changes consistent with endocrinopathy (orthokeratotic hyperkeratosis, epidermal atrophy, epidermal melanosis, follicular keratosis, follicular dilatation, follicular atrophy, telogenization of hair follicles, and sebaceous gland atrophy).[6, 16] Histopathologic findings highly suggestive of hyperadrenocorticism include dystrophic mineralization (of collagen fibers, basement membrane zone of epidermis and hair follicles), thin dermis, and absence of arrector pili muscles (Figs. 9:7 to 9:9). Histopathologic findings consistent with secondary pyoderma and foreign-body granuloma (associated with dystrophic mineralization) may be seen. Histopathologic characteristics of cutaneous phlebectasias range from marked dilatation and congestion of superficial dermal blood capillaries (macular stage) to a lobular proliferation of normal-appearing superficial dermal blood vessels, which may be encased by an epidermal collarette (papular stage).[171]

In many cases, especially with chronic disease, the tentative diagnosis of hyperadrenocorticism is straightforward and easily supported by the results of routine laboratory tests. At the other end of the spectrum is the dog with truncal alopecia, recurrent pyoderma, or seborrhea with no nondermatologic signs. Results of routine tests in these dogs often suggest a diagnosis of hyperadrenocorticism, but more than 30 per cent of these dogs have no convincing hematologic or biochemical evidence of that disease.[185] In these dogs, the diagnosis must be confirmed or refuted by adrenal function tests.

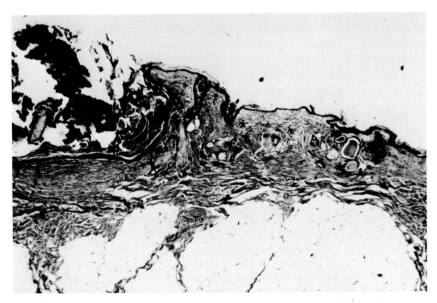

Figure 9:7. Canine hyperadrenocorticism. Note follicular keratosis and atrophy, absence of hair shafts, sebaceous gland atrophy, thin dermis, and dystrophic mineralization of dermis (right) and surface (left).

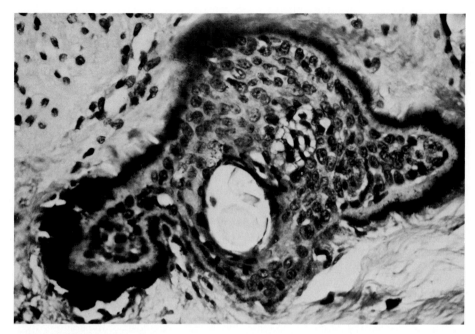

Figure 9:8. Canine hyperadrenocorticism. Dystrophic mineralization of the glassy membrane of a hair follicle.

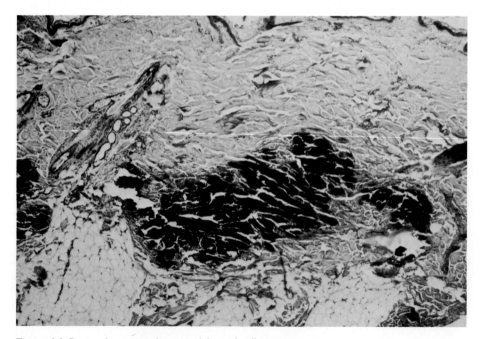

Figure 9:9. Dystrophic mineralization of dermal collagen.

Adrenal Function Tests

After spontaneous hyperadrenocorticism is suspected the diagnosis is substantiated and further defined by a two-stage protocol. The objective of the first, or screening, stage is to confirm or rule out the diagnosis of hyperadrenocorticism. After the diagnosis is confirmed, the purpose of the second stage is to differentiate pituitary-dependent hyperadrenocorticism from that caused by adrenal neoplasia.

Adrenal function tests are basically of two types: those that are single measurements of basal glucocorticoid levels in urine or blood and those that are provocative, dynamic response tests of the glucocorticoid levels in blood. Aside from the urinary cortisol to creatinine ratio test, all cortisol evaluations are currently conducted on serum or plasma. Single measurements of plasma cortisol are completely unreliable. Normal dogs, dogs recently hospitalized, and stressed dogs can have cortisol levels above normal levels, whereas up to 50 per cent of dogs with hyperadrenocorticism can have levels within the normal range.[8, 103, 120, 153] Currently, the only single cortisol assessment that can be of diagnostic significance is the urinary cortisol to creatinine ratio. Normal dogs have low values (5.7 ± 0.9), whereas dogs with hyperadrenocorticism have high values (337.6 ± 72).[115, 126] However, because dogs with renal disease and other disorders can have values that overlap those found in hyperadrenocorticism, the test is not specific for hyperadrenocorticism and performs best in excluding that diagnosis.

Single measurements of endogenous plasma ACTH levels can aid in the diagnosis of hyperadrenocorticism and the definition of its cause. Plasma ACTH levels should be normal to elevated (greater than 40 pg/ml) in dogs with pituitary-dependent hyperadrenocorticism and low to undetectable (less than 20 pg/ml) with adrenal neoplasia.[123, 153, 155] Unfortunately, not all dogs with hyperadrenocorticism have abnormal levels, and one study of 41 dogs with adrenal tumors showed that 30 per cent of the dogs had levels within the normal range.[185] Because this testing is technically difficult to perform and is not of uniform accuracy, it should be performed only with other adrenal function tests.

■ **_Tests to Diagnose Hyperadrenocorticism._** The ACTH stimulation test reliably documents a diagnosis of iatrogenic hyperadrenocorticism or hypoadrenocorticism in dogs. Basal blood cortisol levels are low or normal and show little or no response to ACTH.

In hyperadrenocorticism, dogs with pituitary-dependent bilateral adrenal hyperplasia should show an exaggerated response to the administration of ACTH.[153] Because adrenal tumors should secrete independent of ACTH, poststimulation values should show little change from the initial sample. Unfortunately, these theories do not hold in the clinical situation. In one study, 44 per cent of dogs could not be diagnosed via this testing.[185] About 15 per cent of cases of pituitary-dependent disease have a normal response, and more than 50 per cent of dogs with adrenal tumors hyperrespond.[153] In addition, stressed dogs and dogs with various chronic illnesses can hyperrespond in this testing.[103, 120, 149] With these limitations, most investigators do not rely on the ACTH stimulation test for diagnosis.

Two commonly used ACTH stimulation test protocols for dogs are as follows: (1) plasma or serum cortisol determinations are collected before and 2 hours after the IM injection of 2.2 IU/kg of ACTH gel, and (2) plasma or serum cortisol determinations are collected before and 1 hour after the IV injection of 0.25 mg of synthetic ACTH.

The low-dose dexamethasone suppression test is presently the procedure of choice for diagnosing spontaneous hyperadrenocorticism in dogs.[2, 3, 125, 137, 137a, 153, 185] Plasma or serum cortisol levels are determined before and 8 hours after an IV injection of 0.01 mg/kg of dexamethasone. Most investigators also draw a sample at 4 hours. In normal dogs, the low dose of dexamethasone consistently suppresses cortisol levels to less than 1 μg/dl for the 8-hour test period. Because of differences in dexamethasone metabolism in dogs with hyperadrenocorticism and possibly other nonadrenal illnesses, the low-dose dexamethasone suppression test does not identify all dogs with hyperadrenocorticism.[122, 130] Approximately 90 to 95 per cent of dogs with hyperadrenocorticism fail to show suppression at one or both samplings (see Fig. 9:1). With one exception, this testing does not differentiate pituitary-dependent disease from adrenal neoplasia. When results of the 4-hour sample show complete suppression but those of the 8-hour sample rise above normal levels, the pituitary-adrenal axis has escaped suppression, which indicates pituitary-dependent disease.[153] This testing can give false-positive results in uncontrolled diabetics and other chronically stressed dogs and is uninterpretable in the dog with iatrogenic hyperadrenocorticism.

■ *Tests to Differentiate the Cause of Hyperadrenocorticism.* Because the treatment of choice is different for pituitary-dependent hyperadrenocorticism and adrenal neoplasia, every effort should be made to define the cause of the hyperadrenocorticism. Unless the low-dose dexamethasone suppression test shows the diagnostic pituitary-dependent pattern or the imaging techniques (radiographs, ultrasonography, and so on) clearly demonstrate adrenal neoplasia or bilateral hyperplasia, further suppression testing is necessary.

Although various stimulation or suppression tests have been studied over the years,[12, 109, 112, 113, 137a] the only test currently used is the high-dose dexamethasone suppression test. The CRF stimulation test (discussed later) holds great promise but will not receive wide use until a clinically usable preparation of the hormone becomes available. High-dose dexamethasone suppression testing is performed with the IV injection of 0.1 mg/kg of dexamethasone with sampling points at 0, 4, and 8 hours.[125, 147, 185] Some investigators recommend a dose of 1 mg/kg,[153] but there is no clear and convincing evidence that this dose increases the accuracy of the test in most dogs. Some investigators define suppression as a decrease in cortisol to less than 50 per cent of the level at time zero, whereas other researchers use levels of less than 1.5 μg/dl. In theory, dogs with pituitary-dependent disease should demonstrate suppression completely at 4 hours and maintain or escape suppression at 8 hours (see Fig. 9:2). With adrenal neoplasia, partial or no suppression should be seen. However, 15 to 30 per cent of dogs with pituitary-dependent disease fail to have adequate suppression.[128, 153, 158, 180] In these cases, measurement of endogenous plasma ACTH levels can be helpful. However, one study showed that ACTH levels and high-dose dexamethasone testing gave contradictory results in 15 per cent of dogs tested, so some dogs cannot be categorized by this testing.[185]

CRF stimulation testing can be useful in differentiating naturally occurring hypoadrenocorticism from the iatrogenic form[104, 129, 158] and pituitary-dependent hyperadrenocorticism from adrenal neoplasia. IV injection of 1 μg/kg of CRF to normal dogs causes rapid elevations in both plasma ACTH and cortisol levels. Dogs with pituitary-dependent disease show prompt elevation in both ACTH and cortisol levels, whereas dogs with adrenal tumors should not respond. Clinically useful protocols will be developed when CRF becomes available for routine diagnostic use.

CLINICAL MANAGEMENT

The prognosis for untreated naturally occurring canine hyperadrenocorticism is poor, with death often occurring within 2 years (of septicemia, diabetes mellitus, heart failure, pancreatitis, pyelonephritis, thromboembolism, and so on).[133, 148] There is no clear and convincing evidence that treatment of the uncomplicated case prolongs survival time. However, successful treatment improves the quality of life for the dog and its owner. Death may be associated with adrenalectomy, hypophysectomy, o,p′-DDD administration, or concurrent diseases. In addition, death may occur at any time during or after therapy related to growth of a pituitary neoplasm or metastasis of an adrenocortical adenocarcinoma. Because hyperadrenocorticism is a disease of older dogs, many dogs die or are euthanized within 2 years of diagnosis as a result of any of the aforementioned conditions. Several independent studies on large numbers of dogs gave mean survival times of approximately 2 years, with ranges from 10 days to 8.2 years.[133, 153]

The cause of hyperadrenocorticism determines the treatment. Adrenocortical tumors should be surgically removed.[161, 167] When the tumor is undiagnosed, has metastasized, or cannot be removed because of the patient's health, medical treatment can be instituted, but the vigor of therapy and results seen are different from those obtained in treating pituitary-dependent disease.[114, 133a] Before any specific treatment is undertaken, all intercurrent disorders (e.g., urinary tract infection and diabetes mellitus) should be identified and treatment of these conditions should be instituted.[149] Although the problems identified may not respond completely to treatment until the hyperadrenocorticism is resolved, they can become life threatening to the patient if their control is not attempted.

Pituitary-Dependent Hyperadrenocorticism

Surgical treatment can be accomplished with either bilateral adrenalectomy or hypophysectomy.[2, 3, 110] Both procedures necessitate a skilled surgeon, intensive intraoperative and postoperative monitoring and supportive care, lifelong hormone replacement therapy, and considerable expense. Surgical techniques and management protocols have been described.[3, 110]

Radiation therapy offers a nonmedical alternative for dogs with pituitary-dependent disease.[107, 138] Because this modality is relatively new and results on its efficacy must be considered preliminary, it should be considered only in dogs refractory to medical treatment or dogs with large pituitary tumors. To date, side-effects have been minimal and response good. Response time is slow. Because pretreatment x-ray computed tomography is necessary to define the extent of the tumor and differentiate it from other nonpituitary intracranial lesions, and veterinary radiation therapy centers are limited, this form of treatment is not widely used.

Pituitary-dependent hyperadrenocorticism has been treated with drugs that act on the central nervous system, adenohypophysis, and adrenal gland.[2, 12, 153] Cyproheptadine hydrochloride (Periactin) is an antiserotonin agent that blocks serotonin-mediated CRF and ACTH release. The drug has been used to treat spontaneous canine hyperadrenocorticism (0.3 to 3 mg/kg/day orally), but most dogs were not helped.[175] Bromocriptine mesylate (Parlodel) is a potent dopamine receptor agonist that inhibits ACTH secretion. This drug has also been used to treat dogs with spontaneous hyperadrenocorticism (up to 0.1 mg/kg/day) with rare benefit.[2, 12] Side-effects seen with these drugs include vomiting, depression, behavioral changes, and changes in appetite. Because of their frequent side-effects and infrequent benefit, these drugs appear to have limited usefulness in the management of hyperadrenocorticism.[3]

Seven dogs with pituitary-dependent hyperadrenocorticism have been treated with selegiline hydrochloride (L-deprenyl) at daily oral doses of 2 mg/kg for up to 60 days.[180] This drug is a monoamine oxidase inhibitor that promotes normalization of hypothalamic dopamine levels and metabolism. In the pilot study, five of seven dogs were considered treatment successes and no clinical or laboratory side-effects were noted. More detailed studies on its safety and efficacy are underway.

Ketoconazole is an antifungal imidazole drug that also inhibits adrenocortical steroidogenesis in dogs and humans (see Chap. 3).[3, 186] Normal dogs treated with 10 to 30 mg/kg/day of ketoconazole show significant decreases in basal cortisol levels and response to exogenous ACTH.[186] Similar response is seen when dogs with pituitary-dependent hyperadrenocorticism or adrenal neoplasia are treated.[116, 117] When 9 dogs with adrenocortical neoplasia and 11 dogs with pituitary-dependent hyperadrenocorticism were treated with 15 mg/kg every 12 hours for 15 days to 12 months, 18 dogs returned to clinical normalcy.[117] Two dogs with pituitary-dependent disease did not respond. The current protocol for the use of ketoconazole recommends that the drug be given at 5 mg/kg every 12 hours for 7 days to determine whether the dog shows any idiosyncratic reactions to its administration. If none are seen, treatment is started at 10 mg/kg every 12 hours for 14 days. Response is determined by ACTH stimulation testing. Because ketoconazole is an enzyme inhibitor and not an adrenolytic agent, it is imperative that the drug be given 1 to 3 hours before testing. If this testing shows poststimulation cortisol levels above the reference range, the dosage should be increased to 15 mg/kg every 12 hours for 14 days. If this dosage produces the desired suppression, it must be maintained on a daily basis. Although ketoconazole is safe and effective in the treatment of hyperadrenocorticism, its expense precludes its long-term use in many dogs. Its primary indications are cases of adrenal neoplasia in which surgery cannot be performed or in which metastasis has occurred and dogs who cannot tolerate other medical treatments.

The drug of choice for pituitary-dependent hyperadrenocorticism in dogs is o,p′-DDD (mitotane [Lysodren]).[133, 148, 153] This drug is a chlorinated hydrocarbon derivative that causes selective necrosis and atrophy of the zona fasciculata and zona reticularis of the adrenal cortex, whereas the zona glomerulosa (mineralocorticoid-producing zone) is relatively resistant. The initial dosage of o,p′-DDD is 25 to 50 mg/kg/day for 7 to 10 days. The daily dose should be divided in half and administered every 12 hours with food.[183] Small doses of glucocorticoid (oral prednisone or prednisolone at 0.2 mg/kg/day, or oral hydrocortisone at 1 mg/kg/day) are often given during the initial 7 to 10 days of o,p′-DDD therapy to minimize the side-effects associated with acute glucocorticoid withdrawal. Some authors advise against glucocorticoid use because it makes evaluation of early responses difficult and is necessary in only about 5 per cent of the cases.[3] In dogs with concurrent diabetes mellitus, treatment with o,p′-DDD reduces the daily insulin requirement and can predispose to insulin overdosage and hypoglycemia.[102] A low initial dosage of o,p′-DDD (25 mg/kg/day) and a higher daily maintenance dose of prednisone or prednisolone (0.4 mg/kg) or hydrocortisone (2 mg/kg) prevent the rapid reduction in circulating glucocorticoid levels and daily insulin requirements and allow for easier regulation of the diabetes.

The most common side-effects observed during initial o,p′-DDD therapy include lethargy, vomiting, diarrhea, anorexia, and weakness.[133] Less common side-effects include disorientation, ataxia, and head pressing. About 25 per cent of dogs have one or more side-effects during initial therapy, but the effects are relatively mild in most dogs. Side-effects develop when plasma cortisol levels either fall below normal basal range (less than 1 μg/dl) or drop too rapidly into normal range (glucocorticoid withdrawal syndrome) and resolve promptly with glucocorticoid supplementation. If adverse signs occur during initial o,p′-DDD therapy, the drug administration should be stopped and the glucocorticoid dose doubled until the dog can be evaluated. If clinical signs persist longer than 3 days after increasing the glucocorticoid dose, other medical problems should be considered.

There are many ways to assess the effectiveness of initial o,p′-DDD therapy. Measurement of daily water consumption and eosinophil counts can be used but may be misleading, because they only indirectly reflect circulating cortisol levels and not all cushingoid dogs manifest eosinopenia or polydipsia, especially while hospitalized. A more direct approach is to perform an ACTH stimulation test. Because prednisone, prednisolone, and hydrocortisone all cross-react in most cortisol assays, glucocorticoid supplementation should not be given on the morning of ACTH stimulation testing. To ensure adequate control of hyperadrenocorticism with o,p′-DDD, both basal and post-ACTH cortisol levels should remain within the normal resting (basal) range. After o,p′-DDD induction therapy and ACTH stimulation testing, o,p′-DDD administration should be discontinued and glucocorticoid supplementation should be continued until cortisol results are available.

About 15 per cent of dogs still have exaggerated cortisol production after initial o,p′-DDD therapy.[133] In these dogs, daily o,p′-DDD therapy should be continued and ACTH stimulation tests repeated at 5- to 10-day intervals until basal and post-ACTH cortisol levels are in the normal range. This may necessitate as long as 30 to 50 days in some dogs.[133] In contrast, approximately 40 per cent of dogs have basal and post-ACTH cortisol levels below normal range after initial o,p′-DDD therapy. In these dogs, o,p′-DDD administration should be stopped and glucocorticoid supplementation continued as needed, until basal cortisol levels normalize. This usually takes about 2 to 6 weeks.

After normal cortisol levels are documented, o,p′-DDD is continued at a weekly maintenance dosage. The weekly maintenance dosage is that used for loading and should be divided in half and given twice weekly. During maintenance therapy with o,p′-DDD, glucocorticoid supplementation is rarely required. In the rare dog that manifests poor appetite, depression, weakness, and mild weight loss in spite of normal cortisol levels, alternate-morning doses of prednisone or prednisolone (0.4 mg/kg) are beneficial.

About 5 per cent of the dogs treated with maintenance o,p′-DDD therapy experience iatrogenic hypoadrenocorticism characterized by low basal and post-ACTH cortisol levels and hyperkalemia or hyponatremia. These changes can occur after weeks or years of treatment, but typically occur at about 5 months.[133] Adverse clinical signs resolve after stopping o,p′-DDD therapy and supplementation with appropriate doses of glucocorticoids and mineralocorticoids. Iatrogenic hypoadrenocorticism may be temporary or permanent, and further o,p′-DDD therapy is not indicated unless the hypoadrenocorticism resolves and basal and post-ACTH cortisol levels increase above normal range.

About 60 per cent of dogs treated with initial loading and maintenance doses of o,p′-DDD relapse within 12 months of treatment as evidenced by recurrence of clinical signs and elevated basal and post-ACTH cortisol levels.[133, 162] Control is regained by daily treatment for 5 to 14 days, and then maintenance is reinstituted with larger dosages, typically 25 to 50 per cent higher than that used previously. Approximately 40 per cent of the dogs who relapsed once do so one or more additional times.[133] Dosage adjustments allow control to be regained. In a study on 200 dogs treated with o,p′-DDD, 184 were well controlled with maintenance doses ranging from 26.8 to 330 mg/kg/week.[133] To ensure continued control and prevent serious relapse during o,p′-DDD therapy, ACTH stimulation testing should be repeated every 6 months during maintenance therapy.

An alternative protocol for the use of o,p′-DDD has been developed to minimize the occurrence of relapses and the unexpected development of hypoadrenocorticism. High doses are given for extended periods to destroy the adrenal cortex intentionally, resolving the hyperadrenocorticism but causing permanent hypoadrenocorticism.[162, 163] The o,p′-DDD is administered at 50 to 75 mg/kg/day for medium-sized to large dogs for 25 days. Dosages up to 100 mg/kg/day are recommended for toy breeds. The daily dosage is divided into three or four equal parts and is given with food. Glucocorticoid and mineralocorticoid replacement therapy is started on day 3 of treatment. Cortisone acetate is administered at 1 mg/kg every 12 hours until 1 week after the o,p′-DDD regimen is completed, and the dosage is then reduced to 0.5 mg/kg every 12 hours. Fludrocortisone (0.0125 mg/kg) and sodium chloride (0.1 mg/kg/day divided over two or three meals) is suggested therapy for the hypoadrenocorticism. Adjustments in treatment are made according to the animal's needs. Although this protocol is designed to destroy the adrenal cortex, the treatment is not uniformly successful because 11 (27 per cent) of 41 dogs relapsed within 1 year.[162] Retreatment with the original dosage for 25 days and then once-weekly administration for 5 to 6 weeks should result in another remission. Because some dogs treated by the standard o,p′-DDD protocol need nearly 70 days of loading, some of the relapses seen with this new protocol may be due to an insufficient course of treatment. An ACTH stimulation test should be performed after the 25 days of treatment to ensure that adrenal suppression has occurred. Additional loading time is indicated if the adrenals hyperrespond to ACTH.

Aside from pituitary irradiation, none of the treatments described affects pituitary tumors and their continued growth can be expected. Growth is slow but progressive. Large tumors can result in neurologic dysfunction with stupor, anorexia, and head pressing most commonly observed.[146] Other signs include pacing, circling, behavioral changes, weakness, seizures, ataxia, and adipsia. If these signs develop, pituitary irradiation is necessary for continued management.

Adrenocortical Neoplasia

The therapy of choice for adrenocortical neoplasia is unilateral adrenalectomy.[161, 167] Because the contralateral adrenal gland can be severely atrophied, these dogs usually have to be supported as glucocorticoid-deficient patients with maintenance and stress doses of glucocorticoids for 2 to 12 months. ACTH stimulation testing can be performed every 2 to 3 months to determine when the remaining adrenal gland has returned to normal function.

If the adrenal neoplasm is malignant, if the owner refuses surgery for the dog, or if the dog is considered an unsuitable surgical candidate, medical treatment may be beneficial. Although published data are limited, ketoconazole appears to be effective for both adenomas and adenocarcinomas.[117] Because ketoconazole is an enzyme blocker and not an adrenolytic agent, tumor growth continues and metastasis with all its sequelae may occur. Because o,p'-DDD is an adrenolytic agent, it can be beneficial in some dogs with adrenal tumors. Reports of success with both the standard and new protocol have been reported.[114, 162] With the standard protocol, loading often takes longer and can necessitate dosages as high as 150 mg/kg/day. Relapses are common and, in general, maintenance dosages are much higher than those needed in pituitary-dependent disease. In a study of 32 dogs, 66 per cent were considered to have a good to excellent response to o,p'-DDD, with a mean survival time of 16.4 months, and a final mean maintenance dosage of 35.3 to 1273 mg/kg/wk.[133a]

Iatrogenic Hyperadrenocorticism

Therapy for canine iatrogenic hyperadrenocorticism necessitates ceasing excessive exogenous glucocorticoid administration. When glucocorticoid therapy is withdrawn, patients may be susceptible to hypothalamic-pituitary-adrenal insufficiency for 3 to 12 months and the dog may show signs of glucocorticoid insufficiency under normal living conditions or with stress. Some investigators anticipate these problems and institute replacement therapy with hydrocortisone (0.2 to 0.5 mg/kg/day) or prednisolone (0.1 to 0.2 mg/kg/day). The glucocorticoid administration is slowly withdrawn during 7 to 14 days. Other investigators, including the authors, do not routinely use the steroid supplements unless surgery or some other known stressful situation is to occur. The glucocorticoid is dispensed and the owners are instructed to use the drug if the dog needs it, but most dogs do not. Recovery usually occurs within 3 to 4 months. Exogenous ACTH should *not* be used in iatrogenic hyperadrenocorticism. The block after prolonged glucocorticoid therapy is not at the level of the adrenocortical response to ACTH, but at the level of the ability of the hypothalamic-pituitary unit to resume release of CRF and ACTH. Therefore, ACTH supplementation may actually aggravate the problem.[2, 3, 12]

After the hyperadrenocorticism is controlled, the skin may initially show increasing scaling and pigmentation, and new hair regrowth may be different from the normal color (for example, gray hair grows in black, black grows in red) and texture. With successful therapy, the cutaneous signs of hyperadrenocorticism, including calcinosis cutis, usually regress within 3 to 4 months. Some dogs with bacterial pyoderma have recurring episodes of infection for up to 1 year after the hyperadrenocorticism has been controlled. Noncutaneous signs should resolve slowly, but some signs may remain owing to the physiologic alterations.[101, 148]

Feline Hyperadrenocorticism

Both naturally occurring and iatrogenic hyperadrenocorticism are rare in the cat.

CAUSES AND PATHOGENESIS

Naturally occurring hyperadrenocorticism has been reported in fewer than 30 cats.* Approximately 80 per cent had pituitary-dependent hyperadrenocorticism resulting from a pituitary adenoma or adenocarcinoma, whereas the remainder had functioning adrenocortical tumors.

---

*See references 105, 124, 127, 134, 144, 145, and 154.

Both adrenocortical adenomas and adenocarcinomas have been reported.[124, 127, 145] One cat had a functioning adrenocortical adenoma in its remaining adrenal gland approximately 1 year after the other gland was removed for a similar tumor. Iatrogenic hyperadrenocorticism can be produced with only great difficulty in the cat,[170] possibly because of the lower number of low-capacity, high-affinity dexamethasone-binding receptors in this species.[176]

CLINICAL FEATURES

Naturally occurring hyperadrenocorticism typically occurs in middle-aged to old cats. No breed predisposition has been noted. Females appear to be at higher risk.[124] The clinical syndrome is not as predictable as it is in the dog. The most common owner complaint is marked polyuria and polydipsia. Weight loss, anorexia, polyphagia, and depression also may be reported. On physical examination, muscle wasting and a potbelly are common findings. Skin changes occur in about one half the cases and are, in decreasing order of frequency, alopecia (see Fig. 9:5 *F* and *G*), thin skin (see Fig. 9:5 *F*), fragile skin (Fig. 9:10 *A*; also see Fig. 9:5 *H*), easy bruising (Fig. 9:10 *B*), recurrent abscessation, comedones, and hyperpigmentation.[124, 144, 145] The hair loss can be partial or complete and involve the entire trunk, the flank region, or the ventrum.[124] The increased fragility of the skin occurs in about 50 per cent of the cases and is manifested by tearing during grooming or routine handling. Although data are limited, this extreme fragility occurs more commonly in cats with adrenal tumors than in those with pituitary-dependent hyperadrenocorticism (80 per cent versus 40 per cent).[124]

Reports on cats with iatrogenic hyperadrenocorticism are rare.[170] Cutaneous signs seen include thin hypotonic skin, medial curling of the ear tips, easy bruising, mild seborrhea sicca, and spontaneous tearing of the skin. Hair loss was not reported but can be seen, especially in old cats. Because medial curling of the pinna has not been reported in the naturally occurring cases, this may be of diagnostic significance.

DIAGNOSIS

In the absence of cutaneous signs, the primary differential diagnostic consideration is diabetes mellitus. Because more than 90 per cent of cats with naturally occurring hyperadrenocorticism are prediabetic or overtly diabetic because of the insulin antagonistic action of corticosteroids, the responsiveness of the cat to insulin is of key importance.[134] The diabetes mellitus in cats with hyperadrenocorticism is difficult to impossible to regulate without treatment of the hyperadrenocorticism. With successful treatment of the hyperadrenocorticism, the diabetes responds to insulin as expected or may spontaneously resolve.

With just hair loss, the differential diagnosis includes all causes of traumatic alopecia, diabetes mellitus, advanced hyperthyroidism, and sex hormone–responsive alopecia. Cutaneous asthenia, pancreatic neoplasia, hepatic lipidosis, progestogen administration,[177] and acquired skin fragility syndrome (see Chap. 17) must be considered when extreme fragility is noted.

In cats, hemograms, serum chemistry panels, and urinalyses are of little diagnostic significance. Aside from changes associated with the diabetes, no consistent hematologic or biochemical changes are seen in cats with hyperadrenocorticism.[124, 144, 145, 190]

■ *Histopathology.* Where studied, the epidermis, adnexal glands, and hair follicles of cats with hyperadrenocorticism were normal. The most consistent abnormality is a decreased quantity of dermal collagen. The bundles in the superficial and deep dermis are thinner than normal, widely separated, and without normal organization.[6, 124] On electron microscopy, collagen fibril diameters vary in size.

■ *Adrenal Function Tests.* The ACTH stimulation test, low- and high-dose dexamethasone suppression tests, and measurement of endogenous ACTH have all been used in cats, but there

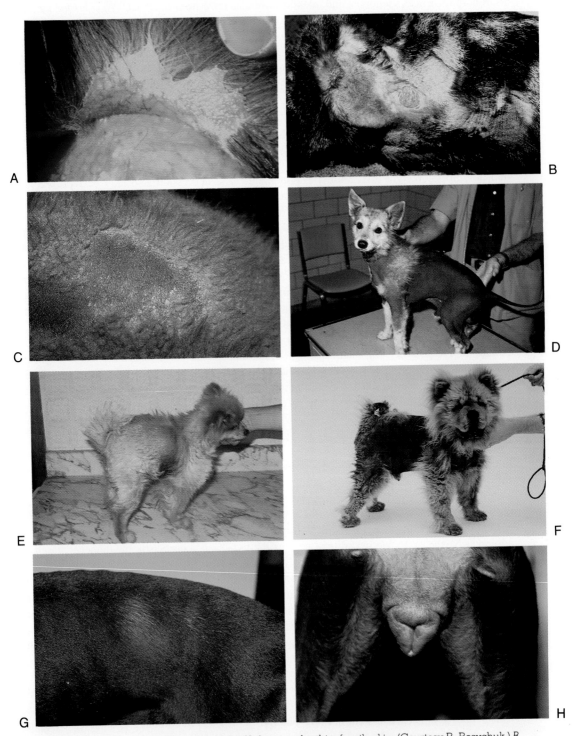

Figure 9:10. *A*, Close-up of the cat in Figure 9:5 *H* showing the thin, fragile skin. (Courtesy R. Rosychuk.) *B*, Bruising and ulceration (torn skin) on the back of a cat with iatrogenic hyperglucocorticoidism. The area has been clipped. (From Scott, D. W.: Feline dermatology 1900–1978: A monograph. J. Am. Anim. Hosp. Assoc. 16:331, 1980.) *C*, Hair loss, hyperpigmentation, and absence of primary hairs in a dwarf. *D*, Profound hair loss and hyperpigmentation in an adult dwarf. *E*, Early hyposomatotropism. Note the loss of primary hairs and early hyperpigmentation. *F*, Chronic hyposomatotropism with profound hair loss and hyperpigmentation. *G*, Hyperestrogenism. Flank hypotrichosis. *H*, Same patient as in *G* with perineal hair loss and vulvar enlargement.

are insufficient data to determine the reliability of each test or the effects of nonadrenal illness.[191] In the ACTH stimulation test, both the gel (2.2 IU/kg IM) and synthetic (125 μg IV) forms of ACTH have been used. Most protocols suggest that cortisol levels be determined before and 90 minutes after ACTH administration.[152, 156, 157, 173] Most cats with hyperadrenocorticism show an exaggerated response to ACTH, but a normal response has been seen with pituitary adenocarcinoma[144] or adrenal adenocarcinoma.[127]

Three doses of dexamethasone have been used for suppression testing.[105, 134, 144, 173] Cortisol samples are collected before and 8 hours after IV administration. Most investigators use 0.01 mg/kg for low-dose testing to confirm the diagnosis of hyperadrenocorticism. Normal cats should have their cortisol levels suppressed to less than 1 μg/dl during the test period. Where studied, all cats with hyperadrenocorticism have failed to have their cortisol levels suppressed to normal levels. High-dose testing is conducted with either 0.1 or 1 mg/kg. Suppression to 50 per cent or less of the baseline value suggests pituitary-dependent hyperadrenocorticism. Because so few cases have been studied, the accuracy of this cut-off point is open to question. Measurement of endogenous plasma ACTH levels has shown elevations in cats with pituitary-dependent hyperadrenocorticism.[105, 154, 173]

Ultrasonographic examination of the adrenal glands can be helpful in detecting unilateral or bilateral adrenal enlargement, the latter being indicative of pituitary-dependent hyperadrenocorticism. Special radiographic techniques may be of additional diagnostic value, but this is unproved in cats.[138]

CLINICAL MANAGEMENT

To date, no medical treatment has been described that has had a high degree of success in the long-term management of cats with pituitary-dependent hyperadrenocorticism. When o,p'-DDD was administered orally (12.5 to 25 mg/kg q12h) to four normal cats, two showed progressive adrenal suppression and two cats showed no response.[190] One cat developed vomiting, diarrhea, and anorexia. Data on its efficacy in clinical cases is limited, but response has not been good.[144] Ketoconazole appears to be of uncertain value. Normal cats given 30 mg/kg/day for 30 days showed no suppression of their basal cortisol levels.[187] Reports on its efficacy in clinical cases are varied. When five cats were treated with 10 to 15 mg/kg every 12 hours, two cats responded, two showed no response, and one developed thrombocytopenia.[145] Metyrapone, a blocker of adrenal conversion of 11-deoxycortisol to cortisol, has been used in five cats, with clinical response seen in three.[105, 137b, 145] At dosages of 65 mg/kg every 12 hours, adrenal suppression can be documented in 5 days. Treatment for longer than 30 days has not been reported.

Because of the limited success of medical treatments, most investigators recommend adrenalectomy as the treatment of choice. In cats with adrenal neoplasia, surgery should be curative with no need for maintenance therapy. In cats with pituitary-dependent disease, bilateral adrenalectomy must be performed and lifelong treatments for hypoadrenocorticism must be administered. Because the majority of cats with hyperadrenocorticism are poor surgical risks because of their diabetes mellitus and fragile skin, medical treatment with either ketoconazole or metyrapone should be considered. If either agent is effective, its administration should be continued until the skin is healed and the diabetes mellitus is controlled. After the cat's health is better, surgery should be performed.

There are no reports of cats with iatrogenic hyperadrenocorticism with signs of glucocorticoid or mineralocorticoid insufficiency on sudden cessation of treatment. Unless the cat is to undergo surgery near the time of glucocorticoid withdrawal, replacement therapy should not be needed.

Hypopituitarism

Hypopituitarism can be caused by failure or loss of one or more of the pituitary hormones.[1, 2, 196] The endocrine manifestations of hypopituitarism are related to the type and degree of hormonal deficiency and the stage in life at which the deficiency occurs.

Hypopituitarism may be caused by pituitary or hypothalamic deficiencies. Pituitary deficiencies may be caused by congenital hypoplasia, destructive lesions (infections, lymphocytic hypophysitis, infiltrative diseases, trauma, and neoplasms), vascular lesions, and the inherited disorder of German shepherds and carnelian bear dogs. Hypothalamic deficiencies may be caused by trauma, encephalitis, aberrant parasite migration, hamartoma, neoplasia, and neurosecretory dysfunction.

Hypopituitarism is diagnosed on the basis of various clinical signs, responses of various target organs and pituitary hormones to challenges with pituitary and hypothalamic hormones and releasing factors, and various sophisticated radiographic techniques.[1, 2]

Pituitary Dwarfism

Canine pituitary dwarfism is a hereditary hypopituitarism associated with proportionate dwarfism, bilaterally symmetric alopecia and hyperpigmentation, and variable thyroidal, adrenocortical, and gonadal abnormalities.

CAUSE AND PATHOGENESIS

In the German shepherd and carnelian bear dog, pituitary dwarfism is thought to be inherited as a simple autosomal recessive condition.[2, 12, 199] Most affected dogs appear to have a variably sized cyst (Rathke's cleft cyst) in the pituitary gland, resulting in varying degrees of anterior pituitary insufficiency. However, a few dogs have had either hypoplastic or normal anterior pituitary glands.[12, 201] The clinical signs are related to GH deficiency, with or without concurrent thyroidal, adrenocortical, and gonadal abnormalities.

Immunodeficient dwarfism has been reported in an inbred colony of Weimaraners with GH deficiency and congenital absence of the thymic cortex.[205, 206]

CLINICAL FEATURES

Canine pituitary dwarfism has been reported in many breeds, but predominantly in the German shepherd and carnelian bear dog.[2, 12, 195] No sex predilection is evident.

For the first 2 to 3 months of life, the dog may appear normal and indistinguishable from normal litter mates. After this time, the dog fails to grow, the haircoat is notably shorter, and no primary hairs develop (Fig. 9:11). The puppy coat of secondary hairs is retained. This hair

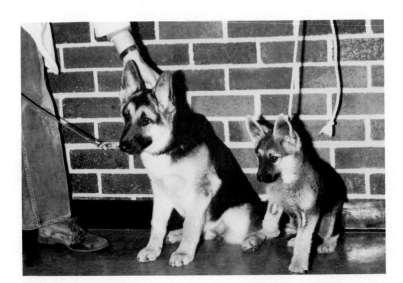

Figure 9:11. Pituitary dwarf with a normal littermate.

is soft, woolly, and easily epilated (see Fig. 9:10 *C*). Primary hairs are often present on only the face and the distal extremities. Bilaterally symmetric alopecia then develops, especially in the wear areas of the neck and caudolateral aspects of the thighs. The alopecic skin is at first normally pigmented, then progresses through increasing degrees of hyperpigmentation (see Fig. 9:10 *D*). The skin becomes thin, hypotonic, and scaly. Comedones may be numerous. These dogs may have behavioral abnormalities such as fear biting, and aggressiveness. Gonadal status may vary from atrophic testicles or absence of estrus to normal findings. If there are concurrent deficiencies of TSH or ACTH, the dogs may manifest signs of hypothyroidism and adrenocortical insufficiency. As dwarfs grow older, they often become progressively more listless, dull, and inactive, and most dwarfs die between 3 and 8 years of age owing to infections, degenerative diseases, or neurologic dysfunction.[3]

Immunodeficient dwarfism in Weimaraners is characterized by puppies that appear normal at birth, exhibiting a wasting syndrome at a few weeks of age.[205, 206] Clinical signs include unthriftiness, emaciation, lethargy, and persistent infections, usually resulting in death.

Delayed growth has been described in sibling German shepherd dogs.[203] Two dogs had histologic evidence of hypopituitarism, and two dogs had normal serum concentrations of growth hormone, T_4, and cortisol. In contrast to German shepherd dogs with pituitary dwarfism, these dogs had no dermatologic abnormalities and eventually reached normal stature.

DIAGNOSIS

The differential diagnosis includes congenital hypothyroidism with dwarfism, juvenile diabetes mellitus, gonadal dysgenesis, malnutrition, severe metabolic diseases (portacaval shunts, congenital renal disease, and congenital heart defects), and skeletal dysplasias (chondrodysplasia in Alaskan Malamutes, pseudoachondroplastic dysplasia in Miniature Poodles, and mucopolysaccharidosis).[2] Definitive diagnosis is based on history, physical examination findings, laboratory test results, skin biopsy, radiography, the presence of insulin-induced hypoglycemia, and the results of GH stimulation tests. Depending on the degree of anterior pituitary insufficiency, affected dogs may have laboratory findings consistent with hypothyroidism and secondary adrenocortical insufficiency. Immunodeficient dwarf Weimaraners have deficient lymphocyte blastogenic responses to phytomitogens, as well as thymic cortical hypoplasia.[205, 206]

Histopathologic examination of the skin reveals changes consistent with endocrinopathy (orthokeratotic hyperkeratosis, follicular keratosis, follicular dilatation, follicular atrophy, telogenization of hair follicles, sebaceous gland atrophy, epidermal melanosis, and thin dermis).[16] A highly suggestive finding is the decreased amount and size of dermal elastin fibers (see Fig. 9:14). In cases with concurrent hypothyroidism, histopathologic findings may include vacuolated or hypertrophied arrector pili muscles.

Radiography may reveal delayed closure of growth plates of long bones, delayed eruption of permanent teeth, failure of the os penis to mineralize completely by 1 year of age, open fontanelles of the skull, and smaller-than-normal heart, liver, and kidney.[2, 12, 195]

A characteristic metabolic abnormality of GH-deficient dogs is hypersensitivity to the hypoglycemic effect of insulin.[2, 12, 199] The IV injection of regular insulin at 0.025 unit/kg into GH-deficient dogs produces severe, prolonged hypoglycemia.

Basal plasma GH levels (by RIA) in normal dogs approximate 1 to 4.5 ng/ml in most reports.[2, 12] However, basal GH levels in pituitary dwarfs and hypophysectomized dogs may approximate these values. Thus, basal GH levels are inadequate for the documentation of GH deficiency. Clonidine (an α-adrenergic antihypertensive drug) and xylazine have been used to stimulate GH release in the dog and to document the existence of GH deficiency.[2, 12, 194, 199] Normal dogs show a marked increase in plasma GH levels within 15 to 30 minutes after the IV injection of 10 to 30 μg/kg of clonidine or 100 to 300 μg/kg of xylazine, whereas pituitary dwarfs and hypophysectomized dogs fail to respond.[204a] Hypothyroidism, hyperadrenocorticism, and sex hormone abnormalities must *always* be ruled out, as they can impair GH secretion.

The measurement of plasma somatomedin C levels could also be diagnostic (less than 5 ng/ml) for growth hormone deficiency but test results must be evaluated in light of the size of the dog.[2, 199] Heterozygous carriers of the pituitary dwarfism trait have intermediate levels of plasma somatomedin C, as compared with dwarfs and normal dogs. In some instances, it may be of value to assess both GH and somatomedin C levels.[2, 204a]

Human or bovine GHRF has been used to evaluate GH responses in the dog.[3, 192, 200] When administered to normal dogs at a dose of 1 μg/kg, GHRF produced a twofold to fourfold increase in GH levels, whereas there was no response in dogs with hyposomatotropism.

CLINICAL MANAGEMENT

The owner should be made aware of the chronic nature of the disease, the general unavailability of GH for treatment, and the animal's shortened life expectancy. If the owner is willing to accept these possibilities, the dwarf dog can be kept as a pet.

Bovine GH (10 IU subcutaneously, every other day for 30 days) and porcine GH (2 IU subcutaneously, every other day, or 0.1 IU/kg subcutaneously, three times weekly, for 4 to 6 weeks) have been used experimentally to treat canine pituitary dwarfism.[2, 3, 12, 195, 199] Long-term oral administration of clonidine is ineffective. A beneficial response to GH in the skin and haircoat is seen within 6 to 8 weeks. However, growth plates close rapidly, and no appreciable increase in stature is achieved. Although not reported during the treatment of canine pituitary dwarfism, repeated injections of bovine and porcine GH could result in hypersensitivity reactions[192a] or diabetes mellitus. Concurrent hypothyroidism or secondary adrenocortical insufficiency necessitate additional specific therapy with levothyroxine or glucocorticoids, respectively. If secondary adrenocortical insufficiency is present, this should always be treated first.

Hyposomatotropism in the Mature Dog

Hyposomatotropism (pseudo-Cushing's syndrome, or GH-responsive dermatosis) is a rare condition resulting in a bilaterally symmetric alopecia in the mature dog.

CAUSE AND PATHOGENESIS

The cause and the pathogenesis of this disorder are unknown.[192a, 200, 204a, 207, 208, 210] Clonidine or xylazine stimulation tests have documented inadequate or absent GH secretion in some but not all dogs.[204a] When 95 dogs with clinical signs compatible with hyposomatotropism were studied, 32 (34 per cent) had a normal GH response test result.[200] In addition, serum somatomedin C levels were normal in dogs with an abnormal GH response. Somatomedin C should be decreased with true GH deficiency. When 12 normally coated Pomeranians and 7 with hyposomatotropism were studied, all dogs showed no significant increase in GH levels after xylazine or human GHRF administration.[207] All dogs also had abnormal adrenal sex hormone synthesis, suggestive of a partial deficiency of the 21-hydroxylase enzyme. These factors, coupled with normal pituitary morphologic findings in one of two dogs at necropsy,[12] shed doubts on the primary role of GH in this condition. The GH deficiency could be induced by the abnormal adrenal steroid synthesis, or could be a coincidental endocrinopathy, which may or may not contribute to the hair loss seen in these dogs.[5, 232]

Two adult Poodles with typical clinical signs of adult-onset hyposomatotropism had fluctuating but low GH levels that showed no response to clonidine or GHRH, but normal levels of insulin-like growth factor-1.[204a] The authors suggested that both dogs had a mild and fluctuating hyperadrenocorticism with resultant glucocorticoid-caused release of somatostatin.

CLINICAL FEATURES

Hyposomatotropism has been reported predominantly in male dogs of many different breeds, but especially in Chow Chow, Keeshond, Pomeranian, Miniature Poodle, Samoyed, and Amer-

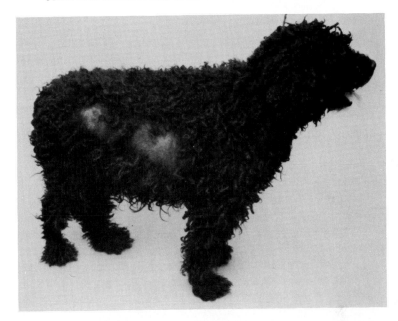

Figure 9:12.
Hyposomatotropism. Symmetric flank alopecia.

ican Water Spaniel breeds.[192a, 200] Age at onset is between 9 months and 11 years, with about 50 per cent of the affected dogs being younger than 2 years of age. The first noticeable change in the coat is a gradual loss of primary hairs with retention of secondary hairs, giving the coat a puppy-like appearance. With time, all hairs are lost around the neck, pinnae, tail, and caudomedial thighs (see Fig. 9:10 E). As those areas become alopecic, the truncal primary hairs are lost gradually and then the secondary hairs become more sparse. Complete truncal alopecia is uncommon, even in chronic cases. In many dogs, the exposed skin hyperpigments rapidly (see Fig. 9:10 F). A small number of these dogs have hair loss, with or without hyperpigmentation, restricted symmetrically to the flank region (Fig. 9:12).[211, 232] Hairs in affected areas are often easily epilated. In chronic cases, the skin may be thin and hypotonic. In cases in which skin biopsies had been performed, the hair grew back over the biopsy sites. The dogs are normal, except for the dermatologic signs.

In Airedales, boxers, and English bulldogs, a seasonal disease is seen, in which dogs develop flank alopecia and hyperpigmentation in winter or spring. The low GH levels found in these dogs may be spurious, because a seasonal follicular dysplasia is also described in these same breeds (see Chap. 10). Alternatively, the low GH levels may be caused by the hormones responsible for the hair loss, or may be real. In the last case, the GH deficiency is a cocontributor to the hair loss. By itself, it causes no hair loss but makes the hair follicles more sensitive to the effects of other hormones.

DIAGNOSIS

The differential diagnosis includes hypothyroidism, hyperadrenocorticism, and gonadal or adrenal sex hormone imbalance. Definitive diagnosis is based on history, physical examination findings, laboratory results that rule out other conditions, skin biopsy, and response to therapy. Skin biopsy reveals changes consistent with endocrinopathy (orthokeratotic hyperkeratosis, follicular keratosis, follicular dilatation, telogenization of hair follicles, epidermal melanosis, sebaceous gland atrophy, and thin dermis).[16] A highly suggestive histopathologic finding is decreased amounts and small size of dermal elastin fibers (Figs. 9:13 and 9:14), but this finding may be present only in dogs that have been clinically affected for 2 years or longer.[210] Measurements of plasma GH levels before and after the IV injection of clonidine or xylazine documents GH deficiency, but this testing is not routinely available. In dogs with seasonal GH

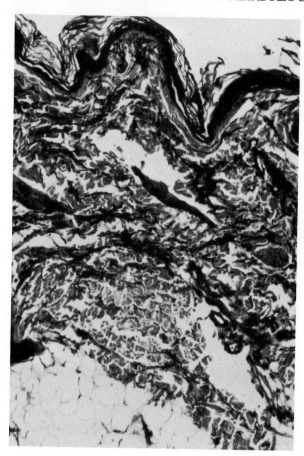

Figure 9:13. Normal canine skin. Numerous thick, long elastin bundles and fibers are present in the dermis (Verhoeff's stain). (From Parker, W. M., Scott, D. W.: Growth hormone–responsive alopecia in the mature dog: A discussion of 13 cases. J. Am. Anim. Hosp. Assoc. 16:824, 1980.)

deficiency (Airedales, boxers, and English bulldogs), xylazine responses are suppressed during the period of hair loss but become normal with hair regrowth.[18] Hypothyroidism, hyperadrenocorticism, and sex hormone abnormalities must always be ruled out before interpreting GH test results, because these conditions impair GH secretion.[2, 199, 210]

CLINICAL MANAGEMENT

Until the pathogenic mechanism of this disorder is completely defined, treatment recommendations are difficult. Some dogs with documented GH deficiency respond to GH supplementation, whereas others do not. Additionally, some dogs regrow coat with neutering, testosterone supplementation, or treatment with o,p'-DDD.[208] In light of those facts and the fact that GH is not available to veterinarians on a routine and regular basis, most investigators suggest that these animals be treated initially as if they had a gonadal or adrenal sex hormone imbalance. If there is no response to those treatments, GH supplementation is indicated.

Response to bovine, porcine, and human GH has been reported,[199, 207] although ovine GH was ineffective.[210] Original treatment protocols suggested that dogs weighing less than 14 kg be given 2.5 IU, whereas larger dogs receive 5 IU. These doses are given subcutaneously every other day for 10 treatments. Newer reports suggest dosages of 0.1 IU/kg three times weekly for 6 weeks[199] or 0.015 IU/kg twice weekly for the same period.[208a] Because GH is a diabetogenic agent, a fasting blood sugar level should be obtained before treatment and weekly thereafter. If hyperglycemia occurs, the injections should be discontinued immediately, otherwise an irreversible diabetic condition may develop. Other side-effects include acromegaly and hypersen-

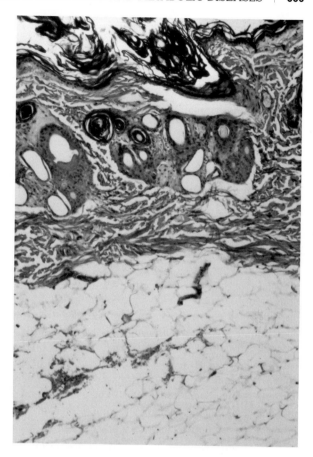

Figure 9:14. Hyposomatotropism (growth hormone–responsive dermatosis) in a dog. Marked absence of dermal elastin (Verhoeff's stain). (From Parker, W. M., Scott, D. W.: Growth hormone–responsive alopecia in the mature dog: A discussion of 13 cases. J. Am. Anim. Hosp. Assoc. 16:824, 1980.)

sitivity to the protein of origin of the GH.[204a] One author (WHM) examined a dog who had increasingly severe anaphylactic reactions at each injection of bovine GH. If response is to occur, it should be seen within 3 months. Most dogs start to lose hair again within 3 to 36 months. Retreatment should produce another remission.

Although the pathogenic mechanism of this disorder is unknown, the high number of cases within certain breeds suggest some genetic influence.[200, 211] Affected dogs should not be used for breeding.

Acromegaly

Acromegaly is due to hypersecretion of GH in the mature animal. It is a rare disease in dogs and cats.

CAUSE AND PATHOGENESIS

Acromegaly is caused by hypersecretion of GH in the mature animal (after epiphyseal closure). Hypersecretion of GH results in an overgrowth of connective tissue, bone, and viscera. In the dog, acromegaly has been reported in association with injections of anterior pituitary gland extracts, acidophilic hyperplasia or adenoma of the anterior pituitary gland, diestrus in the intact cycling bitch, and administration of progestational compounds.[2, 3, 198, 204, 209, 210a] In the cat, acromegaly has been associated with pituitary tumors.[2, 197, 204]

CLINICAL FEATURES

■ *Canine Acromegaly.* No breed or age predilections are evident, but most cases occur in middle-aged to old dogs. Because progestational stimulation is the most common cause of acromegaly in dogs, most cases occur in intact females. Male or female dogs being treated with progestational compounds are at risk. The most common signs noted include inspiratory stridor (due to soft tissue increases in the orolingual-oropharyngeal regions), increased body size (especially paws and skull) (Figs. 9:15 and 9:16), abdominal enlargement, polyuria, polydipsia, polyphagia, fatigue, frequent panting, prognathism, widening of the interdental spaces, and galactorrhea.[204] Cutaneous changes include thickened, myxedematous skin thrown into excessive folds, hypertrichosis, and thick hard claws.

■ *Feline Acromegaly.* No breed or age predilections are reported, but more than 90 per cent of cases occur in male cats. Clinical signs include increased body size (especially paws and skull), prognathism, widened interdental spaces, organomegaly, dyspnea due to cardiac failure, cardiomegaly, neurologic signs with large tumors, and polyuria and polydipsia with or without renal failure.[204] Skin changes are the same as those described for the dog but are usually not marked.

Both dogs and cats with acromegaly can have insulin-resistant diabetes mellitus. Although the diabetes occurs later than the other signs, it may be the only complaint at presentation. The changes in the skin or body may be subtle or pronounced but go unnoticed because they occurred gradually.

DIAGNOSIS

The definitive diagnosis of acromegaly is based on history, physical examination findings, serum chemistry studies, skin biopsy, persistent elevation of plasma GH levels, and the nonsuppressibility of plasma GH levels after IV glucose administration.[2, 198, 204, 209] Many acromegalic dogs have mild to moderate hyperglycemia and mild to severe elevations of serum alkaline

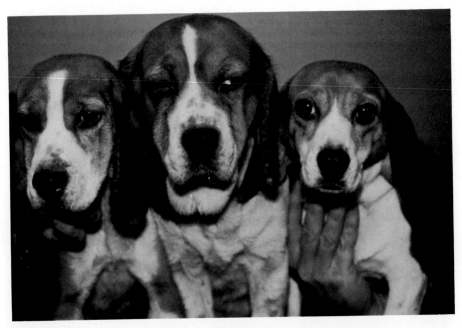

Figure 9:15. Acromegaly. Acromegalic beagle (center) and two normal littermates.

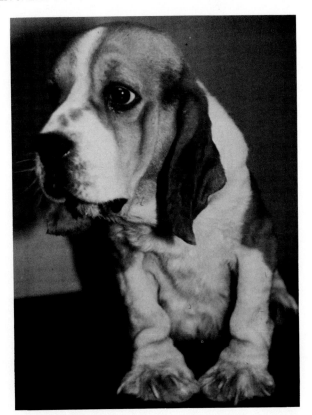

Figure 9:16. Acromegaly. Note large head and paws.

phosphatase levels. Nonsuppressibility of plasma GH levels after an IV glucose load is considered a hallmark of acromegaly. The levels of plasma GH do not always correlate with the degree of acromegaly. GH levels may also be elevated in response to stress, acute illness, chronic renal and liver disease, diabetes mellitus, and starvation.[3] The measurement of plasma somatomedin C levels (mean, 679 ± 116 ng/ml in acromegalic dogs; mean, 280 ± 23 ng/ml in normal German shepherds) could also be diagnostic, but must be evaluated in light of the size of the dog.[2, 198]

In dogs and human beings, histologic examination of acromegalic skin reveals collagenous hyperplasia, myxedema, and hyperplasia of the epidermis and appendages (Figs. 9:17 and 9:18).[209]

CLINICAL MANAGEMENT

Dogs with acromegaly associated with diestrus or with progestational compound treatment have responded well to ovariohysterectomy and to cessation of progestogen therapy, respectively.[204] Soft tissue changes should resolve, but skeletal changes are likely to be permanent. Aside from pituitary irradiation, no successful form of treatment has been described for the cat.

Sex Hormone Dermatoses

Dermatoses associated with sex hormones are uncommon and may be of gonadal or adrenal origin. Clinical signs typically include the absence of systemic signs and the presence of truncal alopecia, which may be generalized or regionalized. Regionalized, or patterned, hair loss is more common. The discussion lends itself to categorization by sex and gonadal status, but there is great overlap in each category.

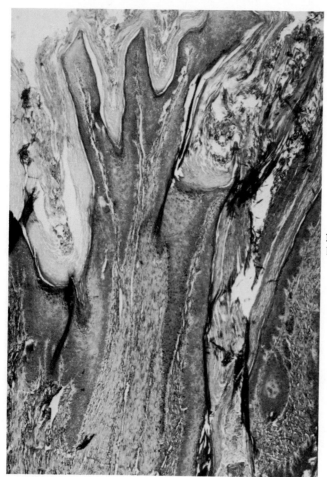

Figure 9:17. Acromegaly. Papillated hyperplasia and orthokeratotic hyperkeratosis.

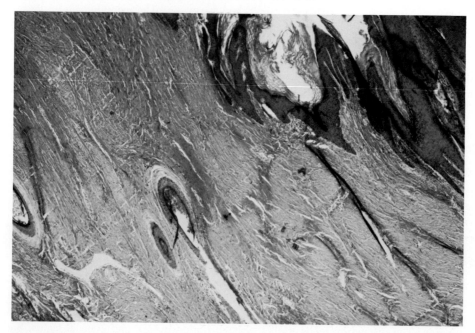

Figure 9:18. Acromegaly. Collagenous hyperplasia.

HYPERESTROGENISM IN FEMALE ANIMALS

Hyperestrogenism in the female dog is a rare disorder characterized by bilaterally symmetric alopecia, gynecomastia, vulvar enlargement, and estrous cycle abnormalities.[218, 220, 229, 234] Only one report of hyperestrogenism in the cat has been made.[225]

■ *Cause and Pathogenesis.* This disorder is usually associated with cystic ovaries and rarely with functional ovarian tumors.[220] Most estrogen-producing ovarian neoplasms are granulosa-theca cell in origin, and 10 to 20 per cent are malignant.[2] Cases have been recognized in neutered females with normal adrenal function.[208] The cause of the hyperestrogenism is unknown, but it may be due to abnormalities in peripheral conversion of sex hormones or an ectopic source of production.

Estrogenic substances have been administered to dogs by a number of investigators, resulting in cutaneous syndromes identical to the naturally occurring disease. An identical syndrome may also be seen with overdoses of estrogens used to treat mismating and urinary incontinence after ovariohysterectomy.[212, 238] Some dogs have cutaneous hyperestrogenism (normal blood estrogen levels), owing to increased numbers of cutaneous estrogen receptors.[215]

■ *Clinical Features.* Hyperestrogenism associated with polycystic ovaries is usually seen in the middle-aged intact female dog. English bulldogs may be predisposed to the disorder.[2] Hyperestrogenism associated with functional ovarian neoplasia is usually seen in older intact females, and no breed predilections are reported. The disorder is characterized by bilaterally symmetric alopecia beginning in the perineal, inguinal, and flank regions (see Fig. 9:10 *G* and *H*). The hair loss remains confined to these areas for long periods but can progress to involve the entire trunk in chronic cases. Hairs in affected areas are easily epilated. In some dogs, the hair loss is confined to the flank area and the degree of hair loss can vary with the estrous cycle.

The nipples and vulva are enlarged (Fig. 9:19 *A*), and comedones are usually numerous on the ventrum and vulvar skin. Secondary seborrheic changes can occur, but skin infections are uncommon. Estrous cycle abnormalities (irregular cycles, prolonged estrus, and nymphomania) often occur, and endometritis or pyometra may be seen. In the cat, truncal alopecia was associated with persistent estrus.[225]

■ *Diagnosis.* The primary differential diagnostic considerations include hypothyroidism, hyperadrenocorticism, and follicular dysplasia. Definitive diagnosis is based on history, physical examination findings, laboratory test results that rule out other conditions, and response to therapy. Skin biopsy differentiates hyperestrogenism from follicular dysplasia and other non-endocrine follicular disorders but does not differentiate this condition from other endocrine disorders. Changes seen include orthokeratotic hyperkeratosis, follicular keratosis, follicular dilatation, follicular atrophy, telogenization of hair follicles, epidermal melanosis, and sebaceous gland atrophy (Fig. 9:20).[16] Elevated blood estrogen levels may support the diagnosis. Ultrasonography and laparoscopy are useful for delineating ovarian neoplasms.[2, 220]

■ *Clinical Management.* Therapy for hyperestrogenism in the intact female dog consists of ovariohysterectomy. A good response is usually evident within 3 months but occasionally may not be seen for 6 months. Symptomatic therapy with topical antiseborrheic agents may be indicated. If an ovarian neoplasm is suspected, chest radiographs should be taken before surgery. No successful treatment of neutered females with nonovarian hyperestrogenism has been described.[208]

ESTROGEN-RESPONSIVE DERMATOSIS OF FEMALE ANIMALS

Estrogen-responsive dermatosis is a rare, bilaterally symmetric alopecia of unknown etiology seen in spayed female dogs.[232] The condition is extremely rare in cats.

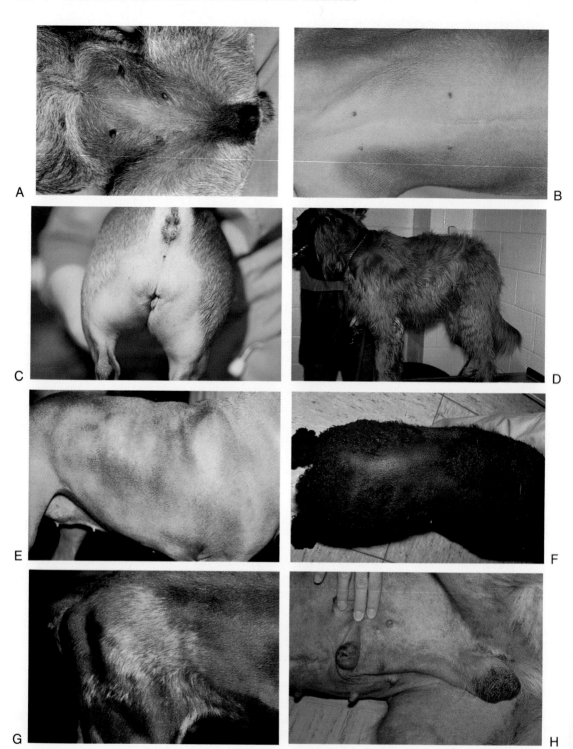

Figure 9:19. *A*, Hyperestrogenism. Note the hypertrophied, hyperpigmented vulva. *B*, Estrogen-responsive dermatosis. Ventral alopecia and juvenile nipples. *C*, Estrogen-responsive dermatosis. Perineal hair loss with small recessed vulva. *D*, Hypertrichosis in an estrogen-responsive Irish setter. *E*, Flank alopecia in an intact female with hypogonadism. *F*, Alopecia and hyperpigmentation in a bitch in overt pseudocyesis. *G*, Testosterone-responsive dermatosis. Dull dry coat with coat color change. *H*, Linear preputial dermatosis in a dog with a Sertoli's cell tumor.

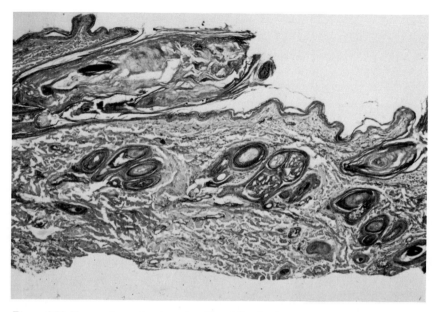

Figure 9:20. Hyperestrogenism in a dog. Note follicular keratosis and plugging, absence of hair shafts, and sebaceous gland atrophy.

■ *Cause and Pathogenesis.* The cause and the pathogenesis of estrogen-responsive dermatosis in female dogs are unknown.[98] Hypoestrogenism has been suggested as the cause of this endocrine-like dermatosis. In most cases, low estrogen levels cannot be documented. Investigators have seen positive responses to estrogen supplementation in some intact female animals that experience dermatoses before their first estrus, during pseudopregnancy, or in association with an abnormal estrous cycle. The role of estrogens in the response of those dogs is uncertain, and it is best to reserve the term estrogen-responsive dermatosis for neutered females.

■ *Clinical Features.* Estrogen-responsive dermatosis is usually first noticed when the dog is a young adult (2 to 4 years). No age or breed predilections are documented, but most reported cases involve dachshunds and boxers. In short-coated dogs, the dermatosis is characterized by hypotrichosis that begins in the perineal and genital regions. Diffuse alopecia results and can affect the caudomedial thighs, the ventral abdomen, the thorax, the neck, and the postauricular region of the head (see Fig. 9:19 *B* and *C*). Hairs in affected areas are easily epilated. The nipples and the vulva are often infantile. Some dogs have only bilateral flank alopecia (Fig. 9:21). In long-coated dogs, the first noticeable change is loss of primary hairs, giving the coat a puppy-like quality. Hair loss starts in the flank region and progresses slowly. Some Irish setters with this condition present for hypertrichosis with blonding of the retained hairs (see Fig. 9:19 *D*). Any dog with this condition can have secondary seborrheic skin disease, but this is uncommon. Dogs with estrogen-responsive dermatosis are usually normal otherwise, but concurrent estrogen-responsive urinary incontinence is occasionally seen. In cats, symmetric truncal alopecia, especially of the ventrum, may be seen.

■ *Diagnosis.* The differential diagnosis varies with the presentation. With persistent ventral hair loss, the primary differential diagnostic possibility is patterned baldness. With other presentations, hypothyroidism, hyperadrenocorticism, hyposomatotropism, adrenal sex hormone imbalance, and follicular dysplasia must be considered. Definitive diagnosis is based on history, physical examination findings, laboratory test results that rule out other conditions, and response to therapy. Skin biopsy eliminates nonendocrine causes of the hair loss, but otherwise is nondiagnostic, revealing orthokeratotic hyperkeratosis, follicular keratosis, follicular atrophy, follicular dilatation, and telogenization of hair follicles (Fig. 9:22).[6, 16]

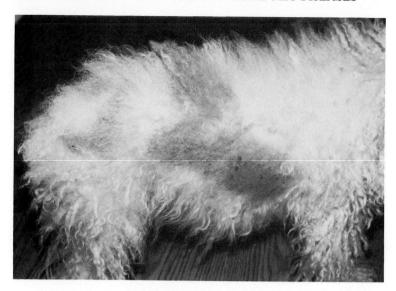

Figure 9:21. Estrogen-responsive dermatosis. Loss of primary hairs and flank alopecia.

■ *Clinical Management.* Traditionally, this condition has been treated with diethylstilbestrol, given orally at doses between 0.1 to 1 mg. Some investigators give the drug every other day, whereas other clinicians give it daily for 3 weeks, stop treatment for 1 week, and then repeat the cycle.[12] The latter scheme was developed to spare the bone marrow[233] because dogs are susceptible to sometimes irreversible bone marrow depression (thrombocytopenia, leukopenia, and anemia) with long-term administration. No data are available to indicate that either approach is safer or more effective. The drug is given as above until hair regrowth is seen, and then the frequency of administration is slowly reduced to a maintenance dose of once to twice weekly.

Diethylstilbestrol tablets are sometimes hard to obtain and the small tablet size makes division into smaller doses difficult, often thus precluding the treatment of small dogs. When

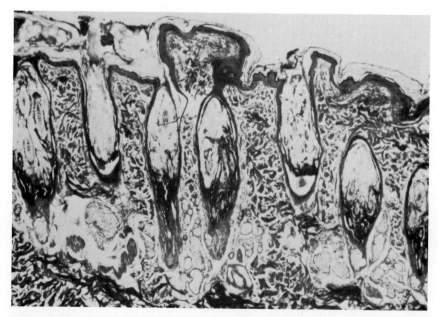

Figure 9:22. Estrogen-responsive dermatosis. Note follicular keratosis and plugging and absence of hair shafts.

diethylstilbestrol cannot be used, response may be seen with the daily administration of methyltestosterone or mibolerone (Cheque drops [Upjohn]). Methyltestosterone is given at 1 mg/kg with a maximal dose of 30 mg, whereas the mibolerone is given at 30 μg for dogs weighing less than 11 kg and at 50 μg for dogs weighing between 11 and 23 kg. The drug is given until hair regrowth is seen and then tapered to a maintenance level.

HYPOGONADISM IN INTACT FEMALE ANIMALS

The term *hypogonadism* indicates a decrease or abnormality in the functional activity of the gonads. The condition can result from primary gonadal abnormalities or irregularities in the hormonal control mechanisms. Bitches with hypogonadism can present for infertility, coat changes, or both.

■ *Cause and Pathogenesis.* A variety of disorders of sexual development (primary hypogo-nadism) have been described.[3] Many conditions have been discovered at neutering or when the bitch failed to cycle. Because the gonadal problem is identified early, coat changes are uncommon in these dogs. If the reproductive irregularity is overlooked, hair loss can occur. Miniature Poodles, terriers, and dachshunds may be predisposed.[225]

Secondary hypogonadism is much more common. The dog's history includes an irregular estrous pattern, an increasing interestrous interval, or complete anestrus. If these estral irregu-larities developed after the dog's having cycled normally for years, the hypogonadism is due to some systemic illness, typically of the endocrine system. Hypothyroidism and hyperadreno-corticism are the most common causes.[2, 3]

All nonpregnant bitches go through a phase of pseudopregnancy in diestrus. In some dogs, the pseudopregnancy becomes clinical, with the development of preparturient behaviors and mammary activity. Dogs with clinical pseudopregnancy appear to have normal diestrous hor-monal changes but, for some unknown reason, are sensitive to them.[3]

■ *Clinical Features.* The nature of the hair loss that can be seen in these dogs varies with the cause of the cyclic abnormality. With primary hypogonadism, there are no clinical or cytologic signs of estrus. Hair loss starts early in life (younger than 3 years), first in the perineal and inguinal regions, with slow progression along the ventrum and trunk.[225] With irregular cycles or increasing interestrous intervals, the hair loss starts around the heat period, gradually worsens through the cycle, and then spontaneously resolves months after the cycle is com-pleted.[225] As the interestrous interval increases, the length of the hair loss phase increases. With complete anestrus, the hair loss is persistent.

In dogs with short to medium-length coats, the hair loss associated with cyclic abnormalities occurs in the flank region and occasionally in the perineum (Fig. 9:19 E). In some dogs, the hair loss remains restricted to these areas, even with the development of complete anestrus, whereas it progresses to truncal alopecia in other dogs. The truncal alopecia is a late event and follows multiple cycles of hair loss and regrowth. In long-coated dogs, especially those with dense undercoats, the cutaneous manifestation of the cyclic abnormality is usually a change in the quality of the coat long before any hair loss is seen. The dog gradually loses its primary hairs on the trunk and has a puppy-like coat. When hair loss starts, it is usually first noted in the collar area, the flanks, and the posterior thighs. Progression to generalized truncal alopecia is slow.

In dogs with clinical pseudopregnancy, the hair loss usually is first noticed 4 to 6 weeks after estrus and involves the collar area, the rump, and the mammary region (see Fig. 9:19 F).[232] An occasional dog has flank alopecia. The hair loss can become more widespread at subsequent estrous cycles. Behavioral and physical signs (mammary development and lactation) of clinical pseudopregnancy are present.

■ *Diagnosis.* When the hair loss is cyclic and has a temporal relationship to an estrous cycle or occurs in an intact but anestrous bitch, the diagnosis of an ovarian-induced hair loss is straightforward. Other differential diagnostic possibilities include excessive shedding and seasonal flank alopecia. When the hair loss is noncyclic, hypothyroidism, hyperadrenocorticism, hyposomatotropism, adrenal sex hormone imbalance, and follicular dysplasia must be considered. Skin biopsy eliminates nonendocrine causes of the hair loss but does not indicate an ovarian cause.

Because hypogonadism in the adult dog is typically secondary to an underlying endocrine disorder, all dogs with an increasing interestrous interval should be tested for hypothyroidism and hyperadrenocorticism. If results of these tests are normal, an ovarian dysfunction is likely. The tentative diagnosis can often be supported by measurement of sex hormone levels; with abnormalities in estrogen, progesterone, or testosterone levels[224, 225]; or by response to neutering.

■ *Clinical Management.* Dogs with hypogonadism regrow coat with neutering or, if the hair loss is cyclic, do not lose coat again. If the owner does not wish to neuter the dog and there is no other intercurrent endocrine disorder, the case should be referred to a theriogenologist for evaluation and treatment. Although there are reports of hair regrowth and return to estrous function with administration of GnRH (2 µg/kg IM twice at 10-day intervals), FSH (0.75 to 2 IU/kg IM daily until signs of proestrus occur), FSH (20 IU/kg IM for 10 days) followed by weekly injections of human chorionic gonadotropin (35 IU/kg), long-term efficacy of these treatments is unknown.[214, 225] If hypothyroidism or hyperadrenocorticism is documented, correction of that condition can return the dog to normal reproductive function with subsequent hair regrowth. In some dogs, the ovarian dysfunction persists and the animal must be neutered.

HYPERANDROGENISM IN MALE DOGS

Documented hyperandrogenism in the male dog is rare and has not been reported in the cat. It can cause perianal gland and tail gland hyperplasia, with or without seborrhea oleosa, in dogs with testicular neoplasia.[232, 236] Hyperandrogenism is a suspected cause of seborrhea oleosa or truncal endocrine alopecia in oversexed intact male dogs.[12]

■ *Cause and Pathogenesis.* The circumanal glands and the tail gland of the dog are composed of the same perianal (hepatoid) gland tissue. This tissue as well as the sebaceous glands is androgen responsive. Hypertestosteronemia, usually in association with testicular neoplasia (especially interstitial cell tumors),[235] results in glandular hyperreactivity with hyperplasia and increased secretion.

■ *Clinical Features.* Dogs with idiopathic hyperandrogenism have severe seborrheic disease or, rarely, symmetric truncal hair loss. The seborrhea is greasy and is most pronounced on the face, on the ears, and in the intertriginous areas (feet, axillae, and groin). Infection and pruritus are common, which worsens the condition. The hair loss seen in some dogs mimics that seen in other endocrine conditions. All dogs with idiopathic hyperandrogenism show hypersexual behavior, aggression to other dogs or humans, or both.

Hyperandrogenism due to testicular neoplasia causes perianal gland hyperplasia. The glands around the anus enlarge uniformly, resulting in a donut-like appearance (Fig. 9:23). Tail gland hyperplasia appears as an oval enlargement of the dorsal surface of the proximal tail (Fig. 9:24). In advanced cases, the area becomes alopecic and greasy, and the glandular hyperplasia can become so severe that multiple nodules or cysts or both are seen in the area. Because perianal glands can also be found in the perineum and the inguinal area, nodular lesions can be present elsewhere. Some dogs have macular melanosis of the tail gland, the perianal area, the scrotum, the ventral tail, and the ventral abdomen (Fig. 9:25) before, simultaneously with, or after the glandular hyperplasia is seen. A testicular mass can usually be palpated in these dogs but may not be appreciable when the skin lesions are first noted.

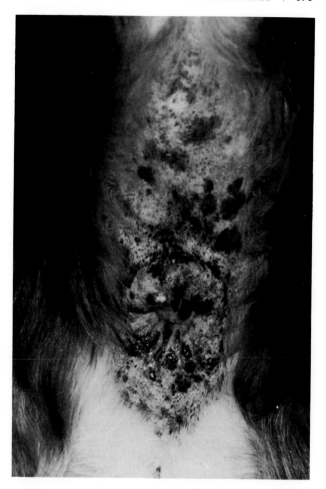

Figure 9:23. Dog with interstitial cell tumor of testicle and hypertestosteronemia. Perianal gland hyperplasia and macular melanosis.

■ *Diagnosis.*   Diagnosis is based on history, physical examination findings, determination of blood testosterone levels, and response to castration. Testicular ultrasonography may be helpful in detecting small nonpalpable tumors. Histopathologic examination of the testicular tumor usually reveals an interstitial cell neoplasm. No cause of idiopathic hyperandrogenism has been found.

■ *Clinical Management.*   Castration is indicated for these dogs. In idiopathic hyperandrogenism, the skin gradually returns to normal condition in 2 to 4 months, but the behavioral changes can last longer and may necessitate behavior modification. In seborrheic dogs, frequent bathing with an appropriate antiseborrheic shampoo hastens the dog's response. Castration of the dogs with glandular hyperplasia prevents any worsening of the condition but may not return the dog to normal status. Some of the glandular hyperplasia is irreversible, as is the overlying hair loss. The macular melanosis fades slowly during 6 months.

TESTOSTERONE-RESPONSIVE DERMATOSIS OF MALE ANIMALS

Testosterone-responsive dermatosis (hypoandrogenism) is a rare, bilaterally symmetric alopecia of unknown cause seen in castrated male dogs.[224, 232] The condition is even rarer in the cat.

■ *Cause and Pathogenesis.*   The cause and the pathogenesis of testosterone-responsive dermatosis in male dogs are unknown. Hypoandrogenism has been suggested, but not documented as the cause of this endocrine-like dermatosis.

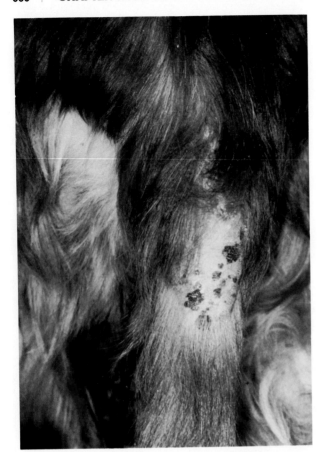

Figure 9:24. Same dog as in Figure 9:23. Alopecia, macular melanosis, and hypertrophy of tail gland.

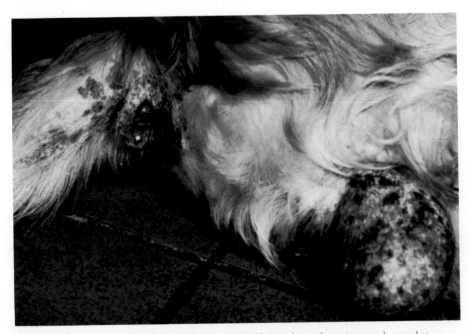

Figure 9:25. Same dog as in Figures 9:23 and 9:24. Note enlarged scrotum and macular melanosis of scrotum and perianal area.

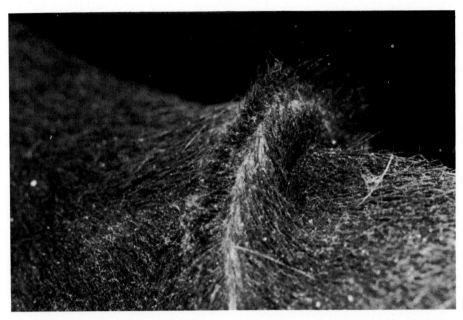

Figure 9:26. Testosterone-responsive dermatosis. Note thinning, hypotonicity, and scaling.

■ *Clinical Findings.* This condition is rare and is seen in old castrated males. Afghan hounds may be predisposed.[225] Some authors include intact dogs with testicular abnormalities or tumors in this category, because some show transient response to testosterone, but the authors believe that those cases should be described elsewhere (hypogonadism, testicular tumor) because they are not idiopathic. Castrated males with this condition first have a dull, dry coat with or without other seborrheic changes (Fig. 9:26). Dogs with dark brown or black haircoats often show coat color change to light brown or auburn, respectively, before hair loss is noted (see Fig. 9:19 *G*). The hair loss in these dogs is truncal, is slowly progressive, and mimics that seen in other endocrine disorders. Rarely, the dog has hypertrichosis.

■ *Diagnosis.* The differential diagnosis includes hypothyroidism, hyperadrenocorticism, hyposomatotropism, and adrenal sex hormone imbalance. Definitive diagnosis is made by history, physical examination findings, laboratory test results that rule out other conditions, and response to therapy. Skin biopsy is nondiagnostic, revealing orthokeratotic hyperkeratosis, epidermal atrophy, follicular keratosis, follicular atrophy, follicular dilatation, telogenization of hair follicles, thin dermis, and sebaceous gland atrophy.[16]

■ *Clinical Management.* Therapy consists of methyltestosterone given orally at 1 mg/kg, up to a maximal total dose of 30 mg, every other day.[12] A good response should be evident within 3 months. At this point, a maintenance dose may be established (once or twice weekly). Large doses of testosterone may result in seborrhea oleosa, cholestatic liver disease, and behavioral changes (aggression). Because anabolic steroids are abused substances in humans, drug use should be monitored carefully.

TESTICULAR NEOPLASIA AND THE SKIN

Testicular neoplasia is common in the dog. Data suggest an approximately equal frequency of occurrence of interstitial cell tumors, seminomas, and Sertoli's cell tumors.[13, 226a] A 10-year survey of all canine testicular tumors examined at the College of Veterinary Medicine at Cornell identified 1971 tumors with the following breakdown: interstitial cell tumor—750 (38.1

per cent), seminoma—690 (35 per cent), and Sertoli's cell tumor—531 (26.9 per cent).[18] Combinations of tumor types in the same or contralateral testicle occur in approximately 25 per cent of cases.[226a] Cryptorchid testes are more than 10 times more likely to develop tumor, especially Sertoli's cell tumor or seminoma. Canine testicular tumors, except for interstitial cell tumors, occur more frequently in the right testis in either the normal or cryptorchid location.[3, 226a]

Testicular tumors can reduce fertility by direct destruction of the testis or by the abnormal secretion of hormones, can be malignant with metastatic potential, and can cause many cutaneous abnormalities, especially endocrine alopecia. Sertoli's cell tumors and seminomas are more likely to cause hair loss than are interstitial cell tumors. When the clinician examines an old male dog with a palpable scrotal testicular tumor or a marked testicular asymmetry suggesting an unidentified tumor, the basic quandary is whether the tumor is the cause of the hair loss or a coincidental finding with no dermatologic significance. When the dog has one or more of the following abnormalities, the tumor is likely to be functionally significant and the dog should be castrated: (1) puppy-like coat, (2) patterned alopecia, (3) coat color change, (4) linear preputial dermatosis, (5) macular melanosis, (6) uniform perianal gland hyperplasia, (7) tail gland hyperplasia, and (8) numerous comedones.

Sex steroids appear to have preferential affinity for primary hair follicles. Disorders caused by sex steroids tend to cause the dog to lose its primary hairs first, while retaining the secondary hairs, giving the puppy-like coat.

Because of the presumed sex and site variation in the numbers or affinity of sex hormone receptors in the skin of dogs, sex steroid imbalances induce hair loss in certain regions of the body and the alopecia tends to be confined to these areas for long periods.[4, 5, 235] Coat color change can be explained by environmental bleaching or a direct effect of the sex hormones on pigment production and transfer. The latter is probably most important.

Linear preputial dermatosis is a term used to describe a linear narrow pigmentary change running from the preputial orifice along the ventral aspect of the prepuce to the scrotum (see Fig. 9:19 *H*).[222] The exact mechanism of the development of the lesion is unknown, but it is not associated with trauma and appears to be a cutaneous marker for testicular neoplasia, especially tumors that produce estrogens.

Dogs with macular melanosis develop multiple black macules around the anus, perineum, ventral proximal tail, inguinal area, and scrotum (see Fig. 9:25). These lesions must be differentiated from lentigines. The latter have an identical clinical appearance but are more widespread in distribution and can be seen in females. The cause of macular melanosis is unknown. Perianal and tail gland hyperplasia results from androgenic stimulation of the perianal glands (see Figs. 9:23 and 9:24). This is most commonly seen with interstitial cell tumors.[236] Comedones are not specific for a sex hormone imbalance but are commonly seen in these disorders.

The change in coat quality and color, the patterned alopecia, and comedones are not specifically seen with testicular tumor, but also can be seen in hypogonadism and adrenal sex hormone imbalance.[200, 208a, 232] Testicular tumors can be functional but not yet palpable; thus, most investigators suggest castration of the intact male dog with sex hormone signs, because it is diagnostic for neoplasia and therapeutic for both neoplasia and hypogonadism. If the patient is a poor surgical candidate or the owners refuse to neuter the dog, the condition may not be resolvable.

Sertoli's Cell Tumor

Sertoli's cell tumors were the least frequent in the Cornell review but were the most common type of tumor to cause symmetric alopecia.

■ *Cause and Pathogenesis.* A syndrome of endocrine alopecia and feminization occurs in about one third of the dogs with a testicular Sertoli's cell tumor.[2, 3, 12] An identical clinical syndrome has been reported rarely in association with testicular interstitial cell tumors and seminomas. However, more than one type of tumor may be present in the testis simultaneously and bilateral testicular neoplasia is not uncommon. In addition, a hereditary syndrome of male pseudohermaphroditism, cryptorchidism, Sertoli's cell neoplasia, and feminization has been reported in Miniature Schnauzers.[2, 213]

Many investigators demonstrated increased levels of estrogens in the peripheral blood and the neoplastic tissue of dogs with Sertoli's cell testicular neoplasia and feminization. Hyperestrogenism results in the cutaneous, prostatic, behavioral, and hematologic abnormalities. Bilateral flank alopecia has been reported in a male dog with hyperprogesteronemia and a testicular Sertoli's cell tumor.[217] Hair loss, feminization, and bone marrow suppression have been reported with hyperestrogenemia and a testicular interstitial cell tumor.[237]

■ *Clinical Features.* Functional Sertoli's cell tumors are most commonly found in cryptorchid testicles. The incidence of feminization increases from about 15 per cent with scrotally located tumors to 50 per cent in cases of inguinal and 70 per cent in cases of abdominal location. Feminization is more likely to occur with larger tumors and tends to be increasingly severe as tumor size increases. Although any breed of dog may be affected, boxers, Shetland sheepdogs, Weimaraners, Cairn terriers, Pekingese, and collies are predisposed.[2, 12, 226a, 239] The disease usually affects middle-aged to older dogs.

About 10 per cent of the dogs with Sertoli's cell tumors have one in both testicles, and about 20 per cent have another tumor type. In the Cornell review, approximately 20 per cent of the tumors had histologic features of malignancy, but metastasis occurred in only 8 per cent of those cases. Blood estrogen levels are not always elevated. In addition, the hyperestrogenism could be a local (tissue level) effect with the peripheral aromatization of androgens to estrogens.

The functional Sertoli's cell tumor feminization syndrome is characterized by varying combinations of bilaterally symmetric alopecia, gynecomastia, pendulous prepuce, and attraction of other male dogs (Fig. 9:27). It is important to emphasize that affected dogs may have alopecia, feminization, or both. The alopecia begins on the collar region, the rump, the perineum, and the genital area and progresses slowly (Fig. 9:28 *A*). In some dogs, the hair loss is restricted to the flanks (Fig. 9:28 *B*). Generalized truncal hair loss is rare. Hairs in affected

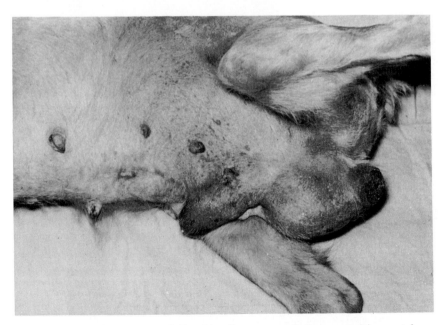

Figure 9:27. Intrascrotal testis with Sertoli's cell tumor constituting most of the scrotal mass. The small nodule at the posterior edge of the scrotum is the uninvolved but atrophied testis. Note the enlarged nipples.

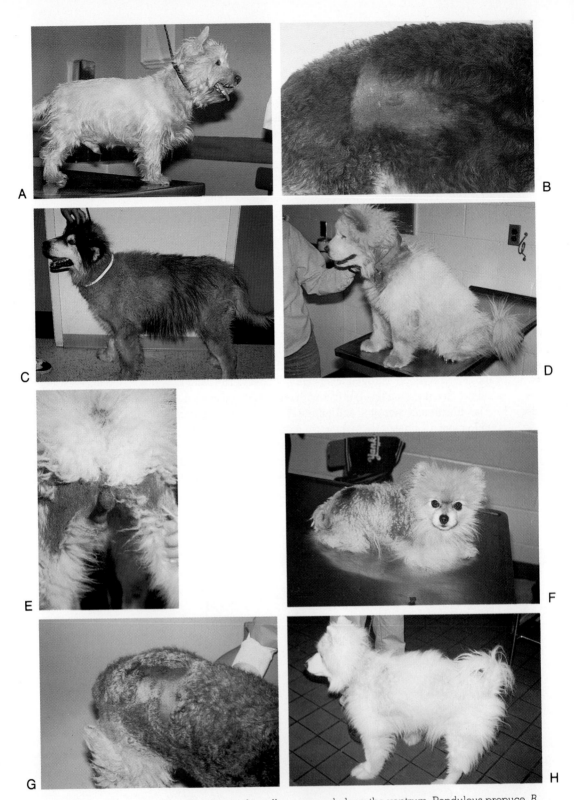

Figure 9:28. *A*, Sertoli's cell tumor. Hair loss in the collar area and along the ventrum. Pendulous prepuce. *B*, Flank alopecia in an Airedale terrier with a Sertoli's cell tumor. *C*, Male hypogonadism in a wooly Malamute. *D*, Male hypogonadism. Coat color change, loss of primary hairs, and collar region alopecia. *E*, Male hypogonadism. Pronounced hair loss and hyperpigmentation on the posterior thighs. *F*, Male hypogonadism. Incomplete hair loss after 3 years of disease. *G*, Male hypogonadism. Hair loss over the rump. *H*, Adrenal sex hormone imbalance. Loss of primary hairs and mild hypotrichosis.

areas are easily epilated. The skin may be thin or of normal thickness. Pruritus, dermatitis, and hyperpigmentation are uncommon. Linear preputial dermatosis (see Fig. 9:19 *H*) is a common but not consistent finding.

In addition to gynecomastia and attraction of other male dogs, signs of feminization may include decreased libido, aspermatogenesis, and galactorrhea. The tumor may be palpated in a retained or scrotal testicle. The non-neoplastic testicle is usually atrophied. Caution is warranted here, as functional Sertoli's cell tumors may occur in palpably normal scrotal testicles. The prostate is often enlarged (estrogen-induced squamous metaplasia) and infected, and there may be clinical signs referable to prostatomegaly, prostatitis, or both. Rarely, spermatic cord torsion with an intra-abdominal testicular Sertoli's cell tumor occurs, resulting in an acute abdomen.[227] Estrogen-induced bone marrow depression (thrombocytopenia, neutropenia, and anemia) is uncommon to rare but is a life-threatening complication.[233] Pseudohermaphroditism in Miniature Schnauzers consists of unilateral or bilateral cryptorchidism, small penis and prepuce, feminization, and endocrine alopecia.[2, 213] These dogs may also have anorexia, depression, and pyrexia with concurrent pyometra.

■ *Diagnosis.* The differential diagnosis includes hypogonadism and adrenal sex hormone imbalance. Advanced cases can mimic cases of hypothyroidism or hyperadrenocorticism, but these are rare. Definitive diagnosis is based on history, physical examination findings, laboratory tests to rule out other disorders, and response to therapy. Ultrasonographic examination may delineate scrotal tumor.[226] Skin biopsy is nondiagnostic, revealing orthokeratotic hyperkeratosis, follicular keratosis, follicular dilatation, follicular atrophy, telogenization of hair follicles, and sebaceous gland atrophy (Fig. 9:29).[16] Elevated blood estrogen levels may support the diagnosis. Diagnosis is confirmed by histopathologic examination of the neoplastic testicles.

■ *Clinical Management.* Therapy consists of bilateral castration. Although the metastatic rate of these tumors is low, all dogs should be examined carefully before surgery. If the spermatic cord is thickened or the sublumbar lymph nodes are enlarged, spread may have

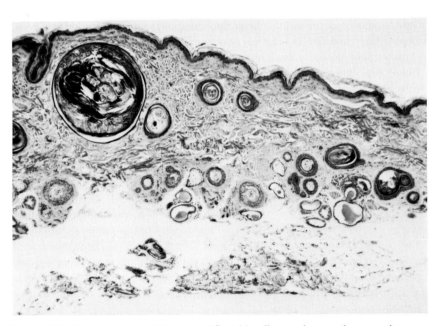

Figure 9:29. Skin from dog with functional Sertoli's cell testicular neoplasm syndrome. Note follicular keratosis and dilatation, absence of hair shafts, and sebaceous gland atrophy.

already occurred. A good clinical response is usually seen within 3 months. Remission followed by relapse indicates functional metastases.[228] Concurrent prostatic or bone marrow disease must also be treated. Aplastic anemia resulting from hyperestrogenism warrants a guarded prognosis.

Therapy of pseudohermaphroditism in Miniature Schnauzers may entail simultaneous castration and hysterectomy.

Seminomas

Seminomas are equally as common as interstitial cell tumors in dogs. They are more common in cryptorchid testes.[226a] Boxers and German shepherds are predisposed. Reports indicate a low rate of malignancy but a tendency to be locally invasive.[226a] In the Cornell study, 12.2 per cent of the seminomas had histologic features of malignancy and evidence of metastasis was recognized in 11 per cent of those cases.

Secretory activity in seminomas is rare. Most cases have no dermatologic signs. If there is secretion of estrogens, the clinical signs mimic those of Sertoli's cell tumors.

Interstitial Cell Tumors

Interstitial cell tumors are common.[226a] Boxers are predisposed. There is no tendency for cryptorchid testes to develop interstitial cell tumors, and they occur with equal frequency in the right or the left testicle. They are often multiple in the same testicle or can be found in both testes. Texts report rare evidence of malignancy, but 12.9 per cent of the tumors in the Cornell study had histologic features of malignancy. No metastatic lesions were reported.

In most cases, interstitial cell tumors cause no dermatologic abnormalities. When present, the signs include perianal gland hyperplasia, tail gland hyperplasia, macular melanosis, or combinations of these (see Fig. 9:25). Additional findings can include prostate disease, perianal adenoma, and perineal hernia. The association of perineal hernia with altered sex hormone levels has largely been disproved.[230] If estrogens or progesterone are produced in the testicle or by peripheral conversion, cutaneous signs of hyperestrogenemia may be seen.[237]

HYPOGONADISM IN INTACT MALE ANIMALS

Of all the sex hormone–related dermatoses, hypogonadism (castration-responsive dermatosis, "woolly" syndrome) in the male dog is the most poorly understood.[208, 231, 232] Dogs with this condition can either have symmetrically small and atrophic testes or palpably normal testes.

■ *Cause and Pathogenesis.* Primary, noninflammatory testicular degeneration is rare in the adult dog.[3] Dogs with symmetric atrophy have some systemic illness, especially hypothyroidism or hyperadrenocorticism, or nonpalpable bilateral secretory testicular tumors.

A syndrome of delayed gonadal maturation has been described, especially in Afghan hounds, Yorkshire terriers, and Miniature Poodles.[225] The dogs never exhibit leg-lifting behavior, show no interest in a bitch in estrus, and have hair loss early in life (younger than 3 years). The external genitalia are hypoplastic.

Most dogs with hypogonadal hair loss have palpably normal testes and can be successful stud dogs. Testicular pathologic changes are rarely seen after castration. Measurement of serum estradiol, progesterone, and testosterone levels may show abnormalities in the levels of one or more hormones,[225, 231, 232] but normal values can be found.[208, 223a] The hair loss in the dogs with normal levels may be due to abnormalities in the levels of some unmeasured sex steroid, abnormalities in peripheral conversion of the sex steroids, or some specific follicular receptor defect in which the follicle changes its sensitivity to sex hormones.

■ *Clinical Features.* There is no apparent breed predilection in dogs with atrophic hypogonadism. These dogs demonstrate a truncal alopecia, which mimics that seen in testosterone-responsive dermatosis, hypothyroidism, or hyperadrenocorticism.

Dogs with delayed gonadal maturation develop a symmetric hair loss first in the perineal and inguinal regions.[225] The hair loss spreads slowly to involve the ventrum and then the trunk.

Hypogonadism with normal testes can be seen in any breed, but Malamutes, Siberian huskies, Chow Chows, Samoyeds, Pomeranians, and Keeshonds appear to be overrepresented. Age at onset is variable, but most dogs are older than 4 years. The initial clinical sign is usually change in coat quality and color. The primary hairs on the trunk are lost slowly, while the secondary hairs are retained, giving the dog an overall puppy-like appearance (see Fig. 9:28 C). The retained secondary hairs lose their luster, become crimped and fluffy, and take on a woolly appearance. Dark hairs lighten in color down to their roots, indicating a change in pigment deposition rather than environmental bleaching (see Fig. 9:28 D). With time, hair loss is noted on the collar area, the rump, the perineum, and the caudomedial thighs (see Fig. 9:28 E). Progression of hair loss in these areas and elsewhere is slow. Rarely, dogs that have this condition for years experience complete truncal alopecia (see Fig. 9:28 F). Some dogs have hair loss restricted to the flank region (see Fig. 9:28 G). Hyperpigmentation of the skin is variable and, when present, is diffuse. The testes are normal on palpation and no other physical abnormalities are found.

■ *Diagnosis.* With atrophic hypogonadism, hypothyroidism and hyperadrenocorticism must be considered and ruled out by appropriate testing. If the dog has palpably normal testes, testicular neoplasia, adult-onset hyposomatotropism, adrenal sex hormone imbalances, and follicular dysplasia are the primary differential diagnostic possibilities. Skin biopsy is diagnostic for follicular dysplasia, but of no help in the differential diagnosis of other conditions. Castration with histopathologic evaluation of the testes is both diagnostic and therapeutic for hypogonadism and testicular neoplasia. If no response is seen within 4 months of castration, the other differential diagnostic conditions should be investigated.

If the owner is unwilling to use castration as a diagnostic test, thyroid testing and measurement of serum estradiol, progesterone, and testosterone levels should be performed. The responses to TSH in these dogs is normal, but some dogs have low or high resting TT_4 levels. Sex hormones, especially androgens, can interfere with the true measurement of TT_4 levels by changing the amount or affinity of binding proteins. With hyperandrogenemia or hypoestrogenemia, the baseline TT_4 level can be at or above normal limits. These changes are not seen in all dogs with hypogonadism and can be caused by other nongonadal disorders that alter thyroid hormone binding.

Many cases have an abnormality in one or more of the serum sex hormone levels. No consistent pattern of abnormality is reported, with some investigators reporting hyperestrogenemia,[208, 231] whereas other researchers, including the authors, often find hyperprogesteronemia.[208] Because baseline values are of questionable use in most endocrine disorders, studies on the value of GnRH stimulation in these dogs are under way.[223a]

■ *Clinical Management.* Correction of the underlying cause of the atrophic hypogonadism usually resolves the hair loss. If response is incomplete, testosterone supplementation may be necessary. Castration is curative for the dogs with normal testes, with hair regrowth in 2 to 4 months. If castration is not allowed, supplementation with testosterone[200] or treatment with human chorionic gonadotropin (50 IU/kg IM twice weekly for 6 weeks)[225] may be of some benefit. No reports are available on the long-term successful medical management of these dogs.

Most dogs who respond to castration maintain the new coat permanently, but a few dogs begin to lose hair again, 2 to 4 years after castration.[208] Not enough data are available on these dogs to characterize the reason for the relapse. The authors successfully treated several of these relapsed dogs with testosterone, but the value of this treatment needs to be proved in a larger number of dogs.

ADRENAL SEX HORMONE IMBALANCE

Dogs with this disorder have a symmetric truncal alopecia, which mimics that seen in hyposomatotropism or the gonadal sex hormone dermatoses. These dogs fail to respond to GH supplementation or neutering.[200, 208, 208a]

■ *Cause and Pathogenesis.* In a study of Pomeranians who were normal or had presumed adult-onset hyposomatotropism, abnormal sex hormone response to ACTH stimulation was seen.[207] Both groups of Pomeranians had higher post-ACTH progesterone levels when compared with those in normal control animals. Dehydroepiandrosterone sulfate and androstenedione levels were also frequently elevated. It was speculated that deficiency of 21-hydroxylase, an enzyme involved in adrenal steroidogenesis, was responsible for the abnormal adrenal sex hormone production. The investigators who made this discovery in Pomeranians termed the condition *congenital adrenal hyperplasia-like syndrome* because of its similarity to a condition in humans.[208a]

Other investigators, including the authors, tested neutered dogs from other breeds and found either elevated baseline or post-ACTH stimulation sex hormone levels, especially of the progesterone compounds.[204b, 208] Insufficient data are available to determine whether all dogs with adrenal sex hormone imbalance have enzymatic defects or whether some dogs produce higher levels of adrenocortical sex steroids than do normal dogs.

The cause of the hair loss in these dogs is uncertain but probably relates to altered sex hormone binding at the hair follicles. Because elevations in progesterone are common in these dogs and progesterone can have antiandrogenic activity,[4, 5, 235] the hair loss may be attributable to a local hypoandrogenism. Regrowth of hair in some dogs with testosterone supplementation supports this theory.[200] However, because the hair loss in these dogs does not mimic that seen in testosterone-responsive dermatoses and not all dogs respond to androgen supplementation, other mechanisms may be important.

The role of GH in this disorder also is unknown. The GH deficiency may be an intercurrent endocrinopathy, which contributes to the hair loss via changing the sensitivity of the hair follicles to sex hormones,[5, 232] or could be induced by these hormone imbalances.[2, 3] A Chow Chow examined by one author (WHM) showed an abnormal GH response to xylazine stimulation. Castration resulted in regrowth of hair and the growth hormone response returned to normal.

■ *Clinical Features.* The disorder has been recognized in many breeds, but especially in Pomeranian, Chow Chow, Keeshond, and Samoyed. Coat changes typically start between 1 and 2 years of age, but hair loss may not occur until later. Dogs of both sexes can be affected, but male dogs are overrepresented. The hair loss can start before or after neutering. If the hair loss occurs in an intact dog, regrowth may occur with neutering. This regrowth may be permanent or may last for only 1 to 2 years. Most investigators reserve consideration of adrenal sex hormone imbalance until response to neutering is poor.

The hair loss seen in these dogs mimics that seen in hyposomatotropism and gonadal sex hormone imbalance. The first clinical sign is loss of primary hair in the frictional areas of the collar, tail head region, and posteromedial thighs (see Fig. 9:28 *H*). With time, all the hairs in those areas are lost, giving a patterned alopecia. Simultaneous with the frictional hair loss, the loss of primary hairs on the trunk occurs, giving the remaining coat a puppy-like appearance (Fig. 9:30 *A*). The retained secondary hairs are lost slowly, and all exposed skin tends to

Figure 9:30. *A*, Adrenal sex hormone imbalance. Note similarities to Figures 9:10 *E* and 9:28 *F. B*, Hypothyroidism. Note symmetric truncal alopecia and hyperpigmentation. *C*, Hypothyroidism. Dull, dry, seborrheic coat. *D*, Hypothyroidism. Facial myxedema leading to a "tragic" expression. *E*, Hypothyroidism. "Rat tail." *F*, Hypothyroidism. Frictional hair loss of the distal limbs of a St. Bernard. *G*, Hypothyroidism. Truncal hypotrichosis and alopecia with secondary superficial folliculitis. *H*, Hypothyroidism. Nasal alopecia and hyperpigmentation. The area is cool to the touch.

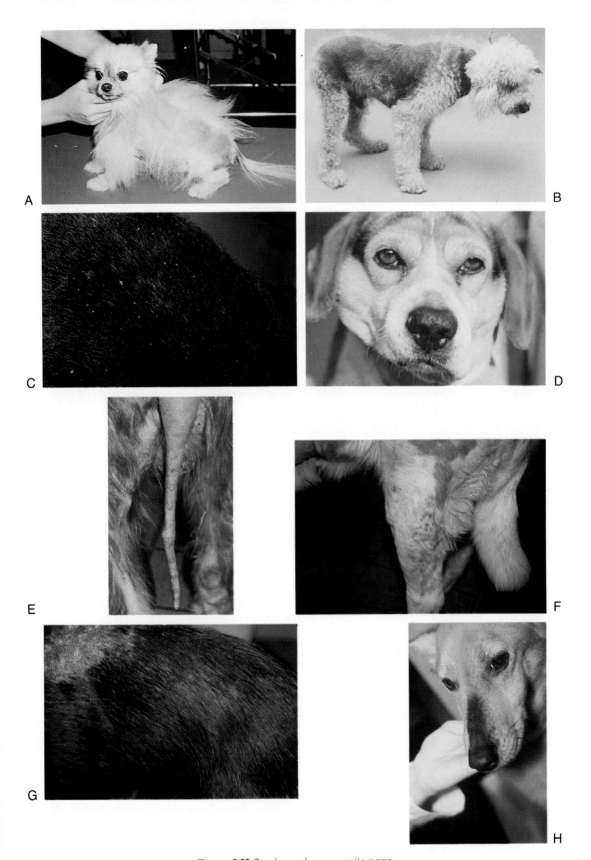

Figure 9:30 *See legend on opposite page*

become hyperpigmented quickly. Complète truncal alopecia is rare and occurs only after years of disease. These dogs tend to regrow tufts of hair at sites damaged by skin biopsy or cutting trauma. Aside from the coat problem, the dogs are otherwise healthy.

■ ***Diagnosis.*** The primary differential diagnostic possibilities if there is a persistent patterned alopecia with retention of the secondary hairs on the trunk include hyposomatotropism, gonadal sex hormone imbalance, adrenal sex hormone imbalance, and follicular dysplasia. The last disorder is excluded by skin biopsy.[6, 16] Skin biopsies in this condition show changes compatible with an endocrinopathy with no specific diagnostic features.

Results of routine laboratory tests are normal, as are those of thyroid tests and the results of low-dose dexamethasone suppression testing. The diagnosis is confirmed by the detection of abnormal concentrations of sex hormones, especially progesterone and estradiol, as determined by baseline testing[208] or in response to ACTH administration.[208a] Baseline testing is least desirable because not all dogs show abnormalities, and the testing cannot differentiate the gonadal or adrenal origin if the dog is intact. Currently, the only laboratory with well-established normal values for sex steroids before and after ACTH administration is the Endocrinology Laboratory at the University of Tennessee, College of Veterinary Medicine, Knoxville, TN 37901–1071. That laboratory requires both serum and plasma before and after conventional doses of ACTH are administered. If the dog has an adrenal sex hormone imbalance, levels of one or more of the adrenocortical sex hormones or their precursors are abnormal.

■ ***Clinical Management.*** In intact dogs, especially male dogs, neutering is the initial treatment of choice because many dogs regrow hair after surgery. If the hair loss initially occurred after neutering, recurred after regrowth occurred after surgery, or did not improve after surgery, treatment options include the administration of methyltestosterone, GH, o,p′-DDD, or ketoconazole or scientific neglect. Because GH is not readily available, and results with ketoconazole have been disappointing,[208] the options are reduced. Although response to methyltestosterone has been reported,[200] no data on its efficacy in a large number of dogs are available and the authors have had limited success with it. Current recommendations for o,p′-DDD use indicate that the drug be given at daily doses of 15 to 25 mg/kg.[208a] Response is determined by ACTH response testing for plasma cortisol at weekly intervals. The goal of therapy is to reduce the baseline cortisol concentration to a low-normal range with some response to ACTH. One investigator suggested poststimulation values of 3 to 5 μg/dl,[208a] whereas another investigator recommended 5 to 7 μg/dl.[204a, 208] After the desired adrenal suppression has been achieved, drug administration is changed to weekly and then adjusted as needed to maintain the suppression. This treatment resulted in complete hair regrowth in 10 of 12 cases treated.[204b]

Because these dogs are healthy and the o,p′-DDD treatment is expensive and not without risk, some owners elect not to treat their dog. If the hair loss does not predispose the dog to sunburn, frostbite, other environmental insults, or recurrent bacterial pyodermas, this option is acceptable.

RARE SEX HORMONE DERMATOSES

Previous editions of this text associated feline endocrine alopecia and idiopathic male feminizing syndrome with sex hormones.[12] The feline condition is discussed in Chapter 10 because the hair loss in the vast majority of cases has no endocrine basis. Occasionally, cats respond to estrogen or testosterone supplementation, but because of the hepatic sensitivity of cats to sex hormones and the rarity of the condition, all other causes of hair loss should be investigated first.

Dogs with idiopathic male feminizing syndrome have hair loss of the rump, the perineum, and the ventral abdomen, which can progress to involve the entire ventrum, the neck, and the face.[12] The exposed skin is hyperpigmented and seborrheic. Moderate to severe pruritus, ceruminous otitis, and gynecomastia are consistent findings. The testes and sex hormone levels in these dogs are normal. Skin biopsy reveals no evidence of endocrinopathy, but rather changes most consistent with hypersensitivity.[16]

Careful review of cases of presumed idiopathic male feminizing syndrome shows that pruritus precedes the skin lesions and that the gynecomastia is not true glandular development but solely hypertrophy of the nipple. In early cases, only the inguinal nipples are involved, which refutes an endocrine cause. Trauma during itching is the likely cause of the nipple hypertrophy. Most dogs with idiopathic male feminizing syndrome have hypersensitivity, with food hypersensitivity and hormonal hypersensitivity most likely. Resolution of signs with castration supports the latter diagnosis.

If the hair loss, hyperpigmentation, and seborrhea precede any pruritus and the gynecomastia is real and uniform throughout all glands, endocrine disease must be considered. Hypothyroidism and estrogen-producing testicular neoplasia are the primary differential diagnostic considerations.

Canine Hypothyroidism

Hypothyroidism is the most common endocrine disorder of the dog and is characterized by a plethora of cutaneous and noncutaneous clinical signs associated with a deficiency of thyroid hormone activity.[2, 3, 21, 36, 69] It is also the most commonly overdiagnosed endocrine disease.

CAUSE AND PATHOGENESIS

Canine hypothyroidism may be naturally occurring or iatrogenic.[2, 3, 69] Naturally occurring, acquired primary hypothyroidism accounts for more than 90 per cent of all cases of canine hypothyroidism. The two main causes of acquired primary hypothyroidism are lymphocytic thyroiditis and idiopathic thyroid necrosis and atrophy.

Lymphocytic (Hashimoto's) thyroiditis is a common cause of hypothyroidism in dogs.* Lymphocytic thyroiditis has long been recognized as a familial disorder of colony-raised beagles with polygenic inheritance. Lymphocytic thyroiditis is thought to be an autoimmune disorder in which humoral and cell-mediated autoimmunity are involved in the pathogenesis. Antithyroglobulin antibodies are demonstrable in the sera of more than 50 per cent of dogs with naturally occurring hypothyroidism, and Great Danes, Irish setters, borzois, Old English sheepdogs, and Doberman pinschers appear to be predisposed.[23, 34, 39] However, antithyroglobulin antibodies have also been found in about 40 per cent of dogs that have other nonthyroidal endocrine diseases. Antibodies have been detected in approximately 50 per cent of clinically normal dogs related to dogs with hypothyroidism and in approximately 15 per cent of randomly studied normal dogs. Dogs with various dermatoses also had an increased prevalence of antithyroglobulin antibodies.[23]

Anti-T_3 antibodies and rarely anti-T_4 antibodies can also be detected in the serum of dogs with thyroiditis.[32, 38, 54] Invariably, dogs with anti-T_3 antibodies have antithyroglobulin antibodies, but the reverse is not true.[38] These autoantibodies interfere with thyroid assays and lead to spurious results that suggest hyperthyroidism. Twenty per cent of the dogs with naturally occurring hypothyroidism also have circulating immune complexes. Lymphocytic thyroiditis has been produced in normal dogs by injections of thyroglobulin or thyroid antigens with adjuvants, intrathyroid injections of antithyroglobulin antibodies, and intrathyroid injections of allogenic lymphocytes.[39, 45] Thyroid lesions in dogs with naturally occurring lymphocytic thyroiditis are characterized by multifocal to diffuse interstitial infiltration of lymphocytes, plasma cells, and macrophages associated with destruction of thyroid follicles, and by the presence of electron-dense deposits in the follicular basement membrane that resemble antigen-antibody

---

*See references 23, 32, 38, 39, 43–45, and 54.

complexes. Because lymphocytic thyroiditis is a focal disease and because inflammation is minimal in the late stages, it has been suggested that so-called idiopathic thyroid necrosis and atrophy may be an end stage of lymphocytic thyroiditis.

Naturally occurring secondary hypothyroidism accounts for less than 10 per cent of all canine hypothyroidism and has been reported in association with pituitary dwarfism and pituitary neoplasia.[2, 12] Other causes of canine hypothyroidism are rare.

CLINICAL FEATURES

Goitrous and nongoitrous congenital hypothyroidism has been reported in the boxer, bullmastiff, German shepherd dog, Scottish deerhound, and Giant Schnauzer breeds.[31, 33, 41, 61, 64, 86] Mongrels can also be affected.[33]

Acquired hypothyroidism may affect any breed of dog. At Cornell University, breeds at risk for hypothyroidism, in decreasing order of relative risk, are the Chinese Shar Pei, Chow Chow, Great Dane, Irish wolfhound, boxer, English bulldog, dachshund, Afghan hound, Newfoundland, Malamute, Doberman pinscher, Brittany spaniel, Poodle, Golden retriever, and Miniature Schnauzer.[12, 18] Other studies include the Airedale terrier, Cocker spaniel, Irish setter, Shetland sheepdog, Old English sheepdog, and Pomeranian.[36, 69] Great Danes, Irish setters, Old English sheepdogs, and Doberman pinschers have a greater occurrence of antithyroglobulin antibodies.[23, 36] German shepherd dogs and mongrels are thought to be at lower risk.[13] Familial hypothyroidism has been suspected in Great Danes, Doberman pinschers, and German shorthaired pointers.

There is no sex predilection for canine hypothyroidism, but neutered male and female dogs may be at higher risk than intact dogs.[36, 73a] Although a dog of any age may be affected, the risk is greater for dogs between the ages of 6 and 10 years. The onset of hypothyroidism tends to occur at an earlier age (2 to 3 years old) in large and giant breeds and those breeds predisposed to the disorder.

The clinical signs associated with hypothyroidism are many and varied and involve multiple organ systems.[21, 36, 67, 69] At presentation, the dog can have only dermatologic disease, dermatologic disease plus systemic signs of illness, or systemic illness with normal skin. With this variability, hypothyroidism has rightfully been labeled ''the great impersonator.''

Although lethargy, mental depression, obesity, and thermophilia are classic manifestations of hypothyroidism, many hypothyroid dogs appear active and alert, are well-fleshed or thin, and do not exhibit heat-seeking behavior.[73a] In general, if a dog is obviously obese, it is probably not hypothyroid. The rectal temperature of most hypothyroid dogs is in the normal range.

The classic cutaneous signs of canine hypothyroidism include (1) bilaterally symmetric truncal alopecia, which tends to spare the extremities (see Fig. 9:30 B); (2) a dull, dry, brittle, easily epilated haircoat that fails to regrow after clipping (see Fig. 9:30 C); (3) thick, puffy, nonpitting skin (myxedema) that is cool to the touch (see Fig. 9:30 D); (4) variable hyperpigmentation (see Fig. 9:30 B); (5) seborrhea (see Fig. 9:30 C); (6) susceptibility to skin infections (Fig. 9:31); and (7) lack of pruritus. However, the clinical variations from this classic picture are enormous and frequent.

Most hypothyroid dogs with skin alterations have abnormal haircoats. Initially, the coat loses its normal sheen and luster and becomes dull, dry, and brittle. Shedding becomes more pronounced during nonshed periods, and the lost hairs either regrow more slowly than normally or are not replaced. Noticeable hypotrichosis or alopecia occurs first in frictional areas, especially over pressure points, the ventrum, the perineum, and the tail (see Fig. 9:30 E). Large and giant breeds often lose hair first on the lateral surface of the extremities (see Fig. 9:30 F). With time, the hair loss becomes more widespread (see Fig. 9:30 G) and involves the entire trunk in a symmetric distribution (Fig. 9:30 B). In advanced cases, all hairs except those on the head and distal extremities are lost. Most cases are presented earlier in the course of the disease and

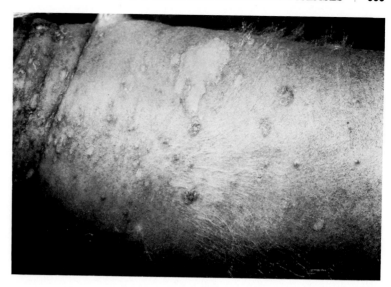

Figure 9:31. Hypothyroidism. Truncal alopecia with a secondary superficial folliculitis.

may have hypotrichosis or alopecia, which may be focal, multifocal, symmetric, or asymmetric (Figs. 9:32 to 9:34; also see Fig. 9:30 *H*). Some dogs have hair loss restricted to the flank region (Fig. 9:35). An unusual finding is hypertrichosis in which, because of the retarded turnover of the hairs, the coat becomes thick and resembles a carpet (Fig. 9:36). Hypertrichosis occurs most commonly in boxers and Irish setters. The coat can become lighter in color, especially at the tips of the hairs, because the retained hairs are more susceptible to environmental bleaching. This coat color change can be seen in nonhypertrichotic hypothyroid dogs but is more commonly noted in dogs with sex hormone imbalances.

Because thyroid hormones influence serum and cutaneous fatty acid concentrations,[30, 87, 88] seborrheic changes are common in hypothyroid dogs. The altered lipid profile can result in dryness, greasiness, or seborrheic dermatitis. These changes usually occur in the ears (ceruminous otitis) (Fig. 9:37 *A*), on the body (see Fig. 9:30 *C*), or in both locations. On the body, the seborrheic changes can be focal, multifocal, or generalized. The seborrheic changes predispose the animal to secondary staphylococcal or *Malassezia* infections, which intensify the seborrheic signs.

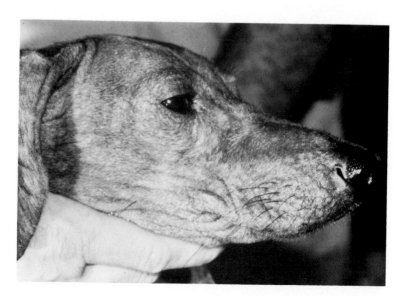

Figure 9:32. Hypothyroidism. Facial hair loss and scaling.

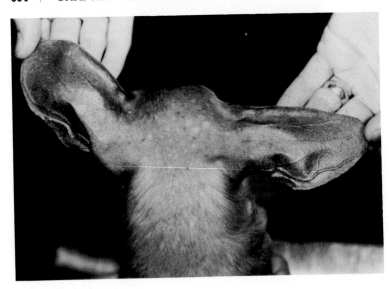

Figure 9:33. Hypothyroidism. Hair loss on the head and ears.

Bacterial pyoderma occurs frequently in hypothyroid dogs.[12, 21] The bacterial pyoderma may be localized (e.g., pododermatitis or otitis externa), multifocal, or generalized and may be superficial (folliculitis) (see Fig. 9:31) or deep (furunculosis) (Fig. 9:37 *B* and *C*). The pathogenic mechanism of this increased susceptibility to bacterial pyoderma probably relates to an altered cutaneous barrier, immunologic hyporeactivity, or a combination of both. In various laboratory animals, it has been reported that depletion of thyroid hormone results in impaired B lymphocyte and T lymphocyte functions.[12] Some dogs with bacterial pyoderma due to hypothyroidism have depressed neutrophil or T lymphocyte function as assessed by bactericidal assay or in vitro lymphocyte blastogenesis to phytomitogens, respectively.[12] The laboratory abnormalities returned to normal levels with T_4 therapy, whether or not systemic antibiotics were used concurrently. However, antibiotics are necessary to resolve the current infection, whereas T_4 therapy prevents further relapses. Some hypothyroid dogs experience a secondary *Malassezia* dermatitis in intertriginous areas or, less commonly, in a generalized distribution, or have *Malassezia* otitis externa.[21] Some cases of adult-onset generalized demodicosis have been associated with hypothyroidism.[21]

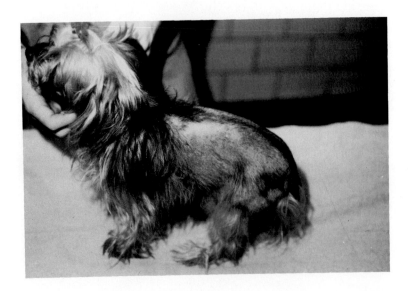

Figure 9:34. Hypothyroidism. Hair loss over the caudal dorsum.

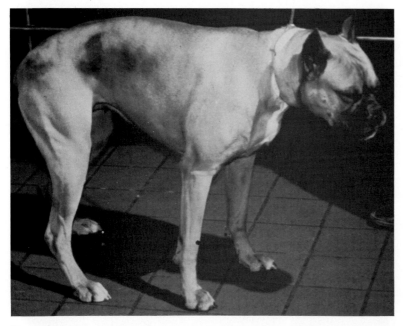

Figure 9:35. Hypothyroidism. Symmetric flank alopecia and hyperpigmentation.

When seborrhea, bacterial pyoderma, or *Malassezia* dermatitis are attributable to canine hypothyroidism, pruritus may be considerable. Poor wound healing is probably referable to defects in fibroblast function and collagen metabolism. Altered healing can be manifested by delayed healing of traumatic or surgical wounds or by the development of excessive fibrous tissue at points of minimal trauma. In the latter case, excessive scarring can occur in areas where there is a deep follicular infection, or the dog can have excessive calluses at common pressure points and other less commonly affected areas such as the tuber ischium.[18] Easy

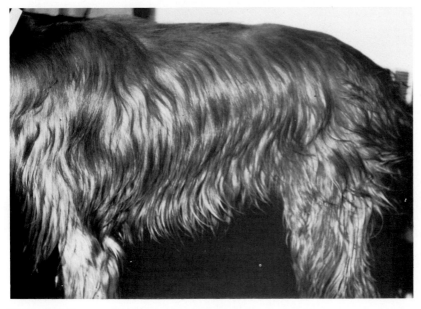

Figure 9:36. Hypertrichosis in an Irish setter with hypothyroidism.

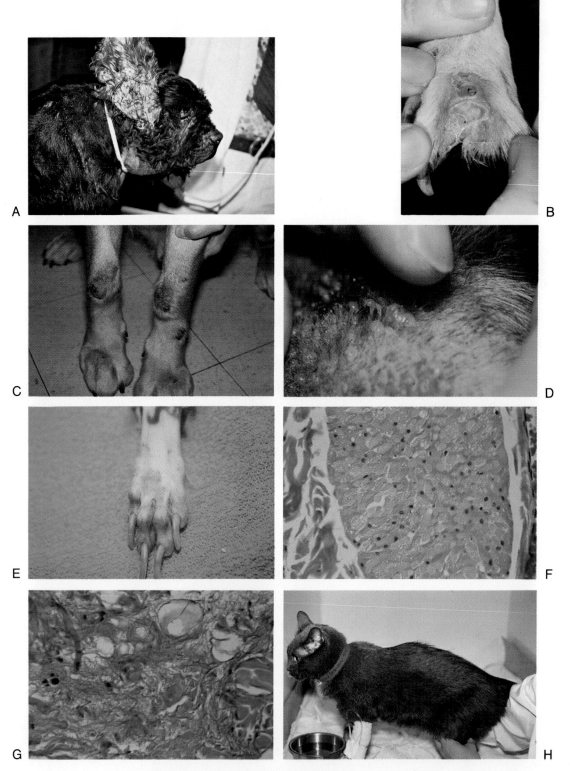

Figure 9:37. *A*, Severely hypothyroid black Cocker spaniel, showing severe chronic otitis. *B*, Hypothyroidism. Interdigital furunculosis as the only sign of disease. *C*, Hypothyroidism. Symmetric areas of furunculosis mimicking acral lick dermatitis. *D*, Hypothyroidism. Mucinous vesiculation. *E*, Hypothyroidism. Bruising secondary to trauma. *F*, Hypothyroidism. Photomicrograph showing vacuolated arrector pili muscle. *G*, Hypothyroidism. Photomicrograph showing myxedema. *H*, Traumatic dorsal hair loss and scaling in a hyperthyroid cat.

bruising may be associated with the collagen metabolism defects mentioned previously or with thrombasthenia and clotting factor defects that respond to thyroid hormone therapy.[33, 36, 69]

Other cutaneous signs commonly associated with hypothyroidism include hyperpigmentation, lichenification, comedones, and mucin accumulation.[21] The hyperpigmentation and lichenification are not specific for hypothyroidism but reflect its chronicity. Although numerous comedones can be seen on the ventral abdomen of hypothyroid dogs, they usually accompany seborrheic changes on the trunk. In the absence of other seborrheic changes, numerous comedones are more frequently associated with hyperadrenocorticism or sex hormone dermatoses. Because thyroid hormones help to regulate the production of dermal glycosaminoglycans,[4, 5] hypothyroid dogs can accumulate mucin in the dermis. This accumulation can lead to myxedema, in which the skin is thick, puffy, and cool to the touch, or rarely mucinous vesiculation (see Fig. 9:37 D).[21] The myxedematous changes are usually most pronounced on the face where the skin of the forehead, eyelids, and lips droops, producing a tragic facial expression (see Fig. 9:30 D).

The veterinary literature includes large lists of noncutaneous abnormalities associated with hypothyroidism. Aside from mental dullness, central nervous system signs are rare in primary hypothyroidism and can be caused by atherosclerotic or myxedematous changes.[52, 59, 75, 100] Signs seen can include seizures, disorientation, circling, and coma. Myxedematous coma is of most concern because death can occur rapidly.[33] Most cases have been reported in Doberman pinschers, and precoma signs include severe mental depression, hypoventilation, bradycardia, and hypothermia. Progression to coma can occur spontaneously or be precipitated by various drugs, disease, or anesthesia.

Neuromuscular disorders can be seen with or without cutaneous signs. Cranial nerve abnormalities (head tilt, ataxia, facial palsy, and laryngeal paralysis), megaesophagus, unilateral lameness, paraparesis, tetraparesis, and myopathy with weakness and atrophy have all been associated with hypothyroidism.[26, 29, 36, 69] Depending on the cause and chronicity of the problem, these changes may or may not be reversible with treatment.

The most common gastrointestinal sign of hypothyroidism in humans, but not in dogs, is constipation. In dogs, the most common gastrointestinal signs of hypothyroidism are diarrhea, vomiting, or both.[12, 36] These are occasional. Cardiovascular complications of hypothyroidism in dogs include bradycardia, weak apex beat, atherosclerosis, thrombosis, and cardiac arrhythmias associated with cardiomyopathy.[3, 67, 69]

Ocular abnormalities that may be associated with canine hypothyroidism include corneal lipidosis, corneal ulceration, keratoconjunctivitis sicca, uveitis, and retinopathy.[2, 3, 36, 69]

Hypothyroid dogs can have a mild nonregenerative anemia or an increased bleeding tendency due to platelet dysfunction[90a] or clotting factor defects (see Fig. 9:37 E). The latter is most important in dogs with von Willebrand's disease.[33, 36, 69] Because T_4 amplifies production of factor VIII and factor VIII–related antigen, hypothyroidism could induce coagulation disorders mimicking von Willebrand's disease or worsen a coexisting coagulopathy. Because there is an overlap in the breeds predisposed to von Willebrand's disease and hypothyroidism (e.g., Doberman pinscher, Shetland sheepdog, Golden retriever, and Miniature Schnauzer), no clearcut answer to the question has been developed.

Classic reproductive changes associated with hypothyroidism include infertility, altered or absent estrous cycles, abortion, high puppy mortality, decreased spermatogenesis, and testicular atrophy.[3, 22] Gynecomastia and inappropriate galactorrhea can be seen in up to 25 per cent of intact, anestrous bitches and rarely in neutered female and male animals (Fig. 9:38).[2, 12, 51] In these cases, the mammary changes are thought to be due to a hyperprolactinemia induced by elevated levels of TRH.

Renal lesions have been recognized in human beings and laboratory animals with hypothyroidism.[12] Renal lesions and renal failure have also been recognized in association with canine hypothyroidism, especially in dogs with lymphocytic thyroiditis.

Hypothyroidism can exist singularly, occur intercurrently with another endocrine disease

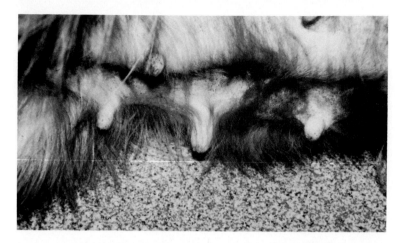

Figure 9:38. Hypothyroidism. Gynecomastia in a neutered female.

(e.g., diabetes mellitus),[37] be secondary to another endocrine disease (e.g., hyperadrenocorticism),[76] or be part of a polyglandular problem.[36] In the latter case, diabetes mellitus, hypoadrenocorticism, and thyroiditis occur simultaneously and are thought to result from an autoimmune process. With multiple intercurrent or interrelated endocrine disorders, satisfactory control of one problem (e.g., diabetes mellitus) often necessitates correction of the other intercurrent conditions.[37]

Congenital hypothyroidism has been reported in both purebred and mongrel dogs.[31, 33, 41, 61, 64, 86] It may be goitrous or nongoitrous. During the first month of life, the puppies are fairly normal but abnormalities are recognized quickly thereafter. The dogs are somnolent, mentally retarded, disproportionately dwarfed, and lame. Other signs also can be seen. Hair loss is not evident, but the coat is often different from that of the normal littermates. Early treatment is needed to prevent irreversible changes.

DIAGNOSIS

Because of the plethora of clinical signs in canine hypothyroidism, the differential diagnosis is exhaustive, as would be expected from a disease with such variable signs. Definitive diagnosis necessitates thyroid biopsy but, because that testing is impractical, most clinicians rely on the history, physical examination findings, hematology, serum chemistry determinations, urinalysis, skin biopsy, and thyroid function tests. None of these tests are specific for primary hypothyroidism, and all have some margin of error. Because no one test is diagnostic, it is important to evaluate all test results in light of the patient's history and physical examination results.

The hemogram classically reveals a normocytic, normochromic, nonregenerative anemia (packed cell volume, 25 to 36 per cent).[2, 3, 69] However, this is found in only approximately 30 per cent of the cases.[73a] In addition, macrocytic and microcytic-hypochromic anemias may be seen in canine hypothyroidism, possibly reflecting defects in vitamin B_{12} and folic acid metabolism or iron metabolism, respectively. Leptocytosis may be prominent in the anemic hypothyroid dog.

Another classic laboratory finding in hypothyroidism is hypercholesterolemia (260 to 1000 mg/dl).[2, 3, 69] However, serum cholesterol levels are greatly influenced by diet, can be evaluated in other nonthyroid disorders, and after a 24-hour fast, are significantly elevated in only about 50 to 75 per cent of the cases. They tend to be elevated with severe degrees of thyroid failure. Analysis of serum lipids in lipemic hypothyroid dogs may reveal hypercholesterolemia, hypertriglyceridemia, and intense electrophoretic bands at the origin, β_1-lipoprotein and α_2-lipoprotein positions.[30, 87, 88]

Serum creatine kinase activity is mildly to markedly elevated in less than 50 per cent of the dogs with hypothyroidism with or without concurrent clinical myopathy.[69, 73a] Other serum enzyme levels that may be mildly to markedly elevated in hypothyroidism include lactate dehydrogenase, aspartate transaminase, alanine transaminase, and alkaline phosphatase levels. These elevations presumably result from the aforementioned hypothyroid myopathy and from the degenerative hepatopathies (fatty infiltration and cirrhosis) that may accompany canine hypothyroidism.

Urinalysis is usually normal in canine hypothyroidism. A few dogs with lymphocytic thyroiditis have had proteinuria and immune complex glomerulonephritis.

Electrocardiographic examination of hypothyroid dogs may reveal bradycardia, low voltage in all leads, flat T waves, and arrhythmias.[2, 3, 69] Radiographic examination of animals with congenital hypothyroidism reveals epiphyseal dysgenesis.[2]

Skin biopsy in canine hypothyroidism may reveal many nondiagnostic changes consistent with endocrinopathy (orthokeratotic hyperkeratosis, epidermal atrophy, epidermal melanosis, follicular keratosis, follicular dilatation, follicular atrophy, telogenization of hair follicles, and sebaceous gland atrophy).[6, 16] Histopathologic findings highly suggestive of hypothyroidism include vacuolated, hypertrophied arrector pili muscles (see Fig. 9:37 *F*), increased dermal mucin (mucinosis or myxedema) (see Fig. 9:37 *G*), and a thick dermis. About 50 per cent of the biopsy specimens from hypothyroid dog skin reveal variable degrees of inflammation, reflecting the common occurrence of secondary seborrhea, bacterial pyoderma, or both.

Thyroid Testing

Except for thyroid biopsy, no one thyroid test is diagnostic for primary hypothyroidism. Because peripheral hormone levels depend on thyroid production as well as protein binding and metabolism, basal measurements are subject to a wide margin of error. Function studies (TSH or TRH stimulation tests) test the thyroid's secretory capacity and are most diagnostic, but are not infallible. All test results must be evaluated critically, and if the results do not correlate well with the history and physical examination findings, the test should be repeated.[53]

Basal serum measurements of TT_4, fT_4, TT_3, and fT_3 can be misleading. Dogs that have various nonthyroid illnesses or that are or have recently been taking drugs known to influence these tests can have spurious results and should not have basal measurements taken. Even in cases free from these confounding factors, basal testing can indicate that 30 to 50 per cent of hypothyroid dogs are euthyroid and approximately 20 per cent of euthyroid dogs are hypothyroid.[12] However, because the hormones necessary to perform function tests are expensive and unpredictably available, basal testing is routinely performed.

Most investigators suggest that measurement of TT_3 and fT_3 has limited value in the diagnosis of hypothyroidism, because normal levels are commonly found in hypothyroid dogs.[24, 53, 70] One study defined serum TT_4 and fT_4 concentrations as low, borderline, or normal by use of the mean and standard deviation of values developed in 200 euthyroid dogs.[24] Concentrations less than the mean minus two standard deviations were low; values greater than the mean minus one standard deviation were normal; and intermediate values were borderline. Using these criteria, none of the 49 euthyroid dogs with dermatologic disease had a low serum TT_4 or fT_4 level. Results for hypothyroid dogs were not as good. Six (67 per cent) of nine hypothyroid dogs had a borderline or normal TT_4 value, whereas only one (11 per cent) of nine had a borderline or normal fT_4 value. If the diagnosis of hypothyroidism was based on a low TT_4 or fT_4 finding, all nine hypothyroid dogs were identified correctly.

Another study of 24 hypothyroid and 51 euthyroid dogs used the conventional method of defining normal by giving a range of values.[74] No borderline category was defined. Among the euthyroid dogs, seven (14 per cent) had a low TT_4 and four (8 per cent) had a low fT_4 value. Seven (29 per cent) of the hypothyroid dogs had a normal TT_4 and four (17 per cent) had a normal fT_4 result. If the diagnosis of hypothyroidism had been based on finding either a low TT_4 or a low fT_4, the diagnosis of hypothyroidism would have been erroneously made in 10 (20 per cent) of 51 euthyroid dogs and missed in 2 (8 per cent) of 24 hypothyroid dogs. These studies and other reports showed that neither the TT_4 nor the fT_4 reliably detects hypothyroid dogs, especially if conventional normal ranges are used. Use of both tests together increases the accuracy of the testing, especially if specific low, borderline, and normal values are prepared.[24, 68, 70, 74] If borderline or normal results are obtained, function tests should be performed.[53] If this testing is not available, basal TT_4 and fT_4 values should be re-evaluated in 60 to 90 days. If the dog is truly hypothyroid, hormone concentration should decline.

In 1988, the K equation was introduced to improve the diagnostic precision of single-study testing.[56] The K value was defined as 0.7 times the fT_4 value (in nanomoles per liter) minus the cholesterol level (in nanomoles per liter). Values of less than -4 were diagnostic for hypothyroidism, values greater than 1 signified euthyroidism, and intermediate values were nondiagnostic. Because basal fT_4 measurements are not always low and hypercholesterolemia is not uniformly found in hypothyroid dogs, this test is expected to have some margin of error. Although euthyroid dogs rarely have low or borderline values, approximately 70 per cent of hypothyroid dogs can have borderline or normal values, so this test is of questionable value.[74]

Because immune-mediated thyroiditis is a common cause of hypothyroidism, measurement of serum antithyroglobulin or anti-T_3 antibodies can be useful in documenting this disorder. Approximately 20 per cent of euthyroid dogs have elevated values and approximately 50 per cent of hypothyroid dogs have normal levels; thus, this testing cannot be used to document hypothyroidism.

Determination of serum TSH levels, either basal values or those after TRH stimulation, could be of great diagnostic value in dogs. To date, there is no canine-specific assay that is both sensitive and specific.[79, 80, 85]

Function Studies

The TSH stimulation test is vastly superior to the determination of basal serum TT_4 and fT_4 levels for the diagnosis of hypothyroidism. Unfortunately, even after years of use, there is no standard protocol to perform the test or interpret its results. Most investigators administer the TSH by the IV route and obtain samples from the dog at 0 and either 4 or 6 hours.[25, 53, 70, 74] Because the TSH used is of bovine origin, anaphylactic signs can be seen rarely in the dog, even when the product has not been administered before.[48] To minimize the chances of these reactions, the TSH is administered by the subcutaneous route at Cornell University and results taken at 6 hours seem to be comparable to those developed with IV administration.

In the past, doses of 1, 5, or 10 IU of TSH have been suggested. Because this hormone is becoming increasingly expensive and is of unpredictable availability, most investigators use lower doses, especially in small dogs. Because reconstituted TSH maintains its potency when frozen at $-20°C$ ($-4°F$) for at least 3 months,[28, 55] these lower doses are cost effective. The most commonly suggested dose is 0.1 IU/kg.[25, 53, 70, 74] At Cornell University, 1 unit of TSH is administered to dogs weighing 14 kg or less and 2 units is given to all other dogs.

Traditionally, euthyroidism was diagnosed when the post-TSH TT_4 value was at least double the basal level. Using this system, approximately 30 per cent of euthyroid dogs can be called hypothyroid and approximately 50 per cent of hypothyroid dogs are called normal.[74] Today, most investigators base normalcy on either a rise in the post-TSH TT_4 to some predetermined value or an increase of at least some predetermined amount. Specific values for the end point of normalcy or the rise expected in normal dogs vary with the laboratory and the amount of TSH used. When one investigator used the 1.4 μg/dl rise suggested in another study[56] rather than the 1.9 μg/dl figure suggested by the testing laboratory, 4 of 75 dogs were misdiagnosed.[74] Accordingly, test results must always be interpreted in light of the normal values developed by the testing laboratory.

Another K factor was developed for dogs who underwent TSH stimulation testing. This factor was determined by taking one half of the basal TT_4 (nmoles per liter) and adding the difference between the pre-TSH and post-TSH TT_4 levels.[56] Values less than 15 were diagnostic for hypothyroidism, whereas values greater than 30 were seen in euthyroid dogs. Unfortunately, this factor can misdiagnose nearly 50 per cent of hypothyroid dogs.[74]

A single TSH stimulation test does *not* reliably distinguish between primary and secondary hypothyroidism. If secondary hypothyroidism is suspected, TSH may be administered daily for 3 to 5 days. After this period, serum TT_4 level should show a brisk response to TSH. If repeated injections of TSH are given, the IV route should be avoided to minimize the chance of anaphylaxis.

Occasionally, the clinician would like to perform a TSH stimulation test on a dog that is receiving thyroid hormone therapy. Because exogenous T_4 suppresses thyroid function,[73] the drug administration must be withdrawn for accurate testing. Most dogs can be accurately tested after a 30-day withdrawal period, but approximately 20 per cent of dogs are still under the influence of the drug.[72] An 8-week withdrawal is satisfactory in all dogs.

The TRH stimulation test was developed as a less expensive and consistently available alternative to the TSH stimulation test.[58] Because prepackaged, medical-grade TRH is expensive and poststimulation rises in TT_4 can be small, this test has received little use. Serum TT_4 levels are determined before and 6 hours after the IV injection of 0.2 to 0.5 mg or 0.05 mg/kg (maximum 1 mg)[37a, 100a] of TRH. The post-TRH TT_4 level in normal dogs should increase by 0.4 µg/dl or more or be at least 1½ times greater than the basal value.[2, 3, 58, 70] Although TRH testing in normal dogs gives good results, its accuracy in hypothyroid dogs may not be satisfactory.[37a] More detailed studies are needed before this testing should be widely used.

The diagnosis of hypothyroidism, as well as the distinction between primary and secondary hypothyroidism, can be made by thyroid biopsy.[60] Radioiodine uptake studies and other special radiographic techniques are also valuable but are not routinely available.

Although the response to thyroid hormone therapy is often listed as a diagnostic feature of hypothyroidism, it is unreliable. The metabolic effects of thyroid hormones may produce varying degrees of improvement in symptoms such as lethargy, depression, and obesity, regardless of their cause. In addition, thyroid hormone administration may produce varying degrees of hair growth in normal dogs, and hair regrowth in dogs with numerous dermatoses that are unrelated to hypothyroidism.[18, 42]

CLINICAL MANAGEMENT

After treatment of primary hypothyroidism has been started, it is continued for the remainder of the patient's life. Early regimens of thyroid hormone replacement therapy for dogs were hindered by a lack of knowledge about canine thyroid physiology and by attempts to anthropomorphize the dog. Confusion and controversy remain in regard to the dosage and the frequency of administration of thyroid hormones for canine hypothyroidism today.

In most cases, the drug of choice for treating canine hypothyroidism is levothyroxine (T_4).[2, 3, 70] An effective, commonly used regimen for canine hypothyroidism is to give levothyroxine orally at 0.02 mg/kg every 12 hours. Other clinicians use 0.01 to 0.04 mg/kg every 24 hours or divided every 12 hours. When 12 thyroidectomized dogs were treated with 0.04, 0.02, or 0.01 mg/kg of levothyroxine either once daily or divided into two equal doses every 12 hours, variability in drug absorption and elimination was noted among the dogs.[66a] Twice-daily administration resulted in drug concentrations closer to the physiologic range. Although some dogs showed satisfactory response to total daily doses of 0.01 or 0.02 mg/kg, these doses may be inadequate for many dogs. Side-effects are rare and include anxiety, panting, polydipsia, polyuria, polyphagia, diarrhea, tachycardia, heat intolerance, pruritus, and pyrexia (signs of hyperthyroidism). In dogs, it is difficult to cause an overdose with thyroid hormone because of the rapid metabolic turnover rate for T_4 (10 to 16 hours[66a] as compared with 7 days in humans), pronounced fecal excretion, and incomplete absorption from the gut.[47]

Dogs with attitudinal abnormalities (lethargy, depression, and so on) usually respond rapidly (within 2 to 4 weeks) to levothyroxine therapy. Skin changes do not usually become apparent for 4 weeks, and up to 5 months may pass before animals with skin and haircoat abnormalities show a good response. Therapy should *always* be given for a *minimum* of 3 months before any judgment about its effectiveness is rendered. Many dogs do well with 0.02 mg/kg of levothyroxine every 24 hours. A reasonable approach to therapy is first to establish that the condition being treated is responsive to thyroid hormone (levothyroxine given every 12 hours until the presenting condition is resolved), and then reduce the frequency of administration to once daily. If the patient continues to do well, once-daily treatment can be continued. If a relapse starts to occur, twice-daily administration is necessary. Although no studies have been done in which the same dogs received the levothyroxine from different manufacturers, data suggest that bioavailability does vary with the product used.[66] Accordingly, the veterinary clinician should select an effective product and use it to the exclusion of all others. Because the clinician has little control over what product a human pharmacy dispenses, prescriptions for levothyroxine should not be written.

Dogs with cardiac disease, regardless of whether it is related to their hypothyroidism, should be started on *lower* doses of levothyroxine or heart failure may be precipitated. The following protocol for levothyroxine is recommended: 0.005 mg/kg every 12 hours for 2 weeks, then 0.01 mg/kg every 12 hours for 2 weeks, then 0.015 mg/kg every 12 hours for 2 weeks, then up to routine maintenance dosage. In addition, patients with concurrent hypoadrenocorticism should not be treated for hypothyroidism until their adrenal insufficiency is corrected and stabilized with medication. Thyroid hormone therapy may also necessitate altered doses of insulin[37] and certain anticonvulsants (phenytoin and phenobarbital) in patients being managed with those agents.[36]

Liothyronine (T_3) may also be used to treat canine hypothyroidism but is rarely indicated.[2, 3, 70] It should be given orally at 4 to 6 μg/kg every 8 hours, thus necessitating more frequent administration and greater expense.

Treatment of myxedema coma is a medical emergency.[2, 33, 52] Therapy consists of administration of IV levothyroxine sodium (Synthroid for injection) or oral liothyronine sodium by gastric tube, mechanical respiratory support, administration of IV glucocorticoids and broad-spectrum antibiotics, and passive rewarming.

The reasons for therapeutic failure with thyroid hormones are multiple, and those most commonly encountered are incorrect diagnosis, failure to recognize other intercurrent endocrinopathies (e.g., hypothyroidism in a dog with a sex hormone imbalance), and insufficient therapy (e.g., insufficient course of treatment, wrong dosage, wrong frequency of administration, use of a product with poor bioavailability, and poor owner compliance). After the clinician has determined that the correct dosage of an appropriate medication was dispensed and that the clients are administering the medication appropriately, postpill testing is the next step in determining why the dog's response was poor.

In dogs, TT_4 levels peak 4 to 6 hours after oral administration of levothyroxine and decline thereafter.[66] With the administration of a satisfactory dose of an absorbable product, the TT_4 should be well within the normal range at 4 to 6 hours. Dogs given the medication once daily have higher peak values than dogs that receive that dosage divided into two equal doses.[66] If the peak TT_4 value is too high or low, dosage adjustments are necessary. The adequacy of a new dosage must be determined by additional postpill testing in 2 to 4 weeks. Because the half-life of T_4 can vary from dog to dog, an adequate peak value in a dog receiving once-daily treatment does not necessarily guarantee that normal levels are maintained during the entire 24-hour period. If this dog's response is poor or incomplete, a 24-hour postpill TT_4 value should be evaluated. If that TT_4 is well below normal, the single dose must be increased or the dog should be treated twice daily.

Postpill testing is unnecessary in dogs that show a satisfactory response to treatment with no clinical signs of overdosage. If clinical signs return later in the dog's life, testing at that point is indicated. Hypothyroid dogs rarely show clinical signs of overdosage when they are given 0.02 mg/kg of levothyroxine twice daily. If signs occur, postpill testing should be performed immediately. If the TT_4 value is greatly elevated above normal levels, the diagnosis of hypothyroidism must be questioned. Mild to moderate elevations above normal levels indicate overdosage and suggest that the half-life of levothyroxine may be longer in this dog. Some investigators decrease the dosage but maintain the twice-daily administration, whereas other researchers reduce treatment to once daily. Too few dogs are recognized with this problem to make specific recommendations.

When normal dogs are given levothyroxine, their responsiveness to TSH decreases after 4 weeks of treatment and continued treatment results in increased unresponsiveness and histologic evidence of thyroid inactivity.[72, 73] Although unproved, clinical evidence exists that unnecessary administration of levothyroxine for long periods eventually induces a secondary hypothyroidism, necessitating lifelong replacement therapy.

Treatment of secondary hypothyroidism is essentially the same as that described for primary hypothyroidism.

Dietary iodine deficiency is corrected by supplementing dogs with dietary iodine at 34 μg/kg/day, and cats with 100 μg/day.[12]

Feline Hypothyroidism

Other than congenital hypothyroidism, naturally occurring spontaneous hypothyroidism has been documented in only one cat.[80a]

CLINICAL FEATURES

Cats with congenital hypothyroidism have signs similar to those seen in the dog.[20, 50, 78] The kittens are obviously different from their littermates by 4 weeks of age. Affected cats have a decreased rate of growth, with stunting, and become disproportionate dwarfs. They are lethargic and mentally dull. Although they have full haircoats, the quality is different from that of their normal littermates, with fewer primary hairs.

When experimental adult cats underwent thyroidectomy by radiation and were followed for 96 weeks, the systemic and cutaneous signs that developed were far different from those seen in hypothyroid dogs.[93] Clinically, the cats were initially lethargic but returned to normal status spontaneously. No change in appetite or body weight was recognized. The cats groomed less than normal, which resulted in dorsal matting and seborrhea, and experienced alopecia of the pinnae, pressure points, and dorsal and lateral tail base region. With the sensitivity of the cat's thyroid axis to iodine levels,[91] iodine depletion can cause clinical signs. Experimentally deprived cats exhibited cutaneous changes more typical of the dog.[15] The coats became dry with easily epilated hairs, and symmetric alopecia developed on the lateral neck, the thorax, and the abdomen. The skin was dry, scaly, and thickened.

The cat with spontaneous adult-onset hypothyroidism resembled dogs with that disease.[80a] The cat was lethargic, thermophilic, inappetent, and obese. The cat's face was puffy and the coat was dull, dry, seborrheic, and lighter in color than normal (Fig. 9:39). Hair regrowth at clipped sites was poor. The diagnosis was confirmed by TSH response test and thyroid biopsy.

DIAGNOSIS

Because naturally occurring acquired hypothyroidism is so rare in cats, no data exist on the diagnostic value of hemograms, chemistry profiles, and other tests used in the dog. Basal measurement of TT_4 or fT_4 is completely unreliable because approximately 50 per cent of cats with diabetes mellitus, hepatopathy, renal failure, or systemic neoplasia have low levels of TT_4 or fT_4.[77, 92] To document hypothyroidism, function tests must be performed.

When either 1 IU per cat or 1 IU/kg of TSH is given intravenously, TT_4 levels peak at 6 hours. TT_3 and fT_4 peak at 7 hours. Total T_4 levels should double, and fT_4 values should triple

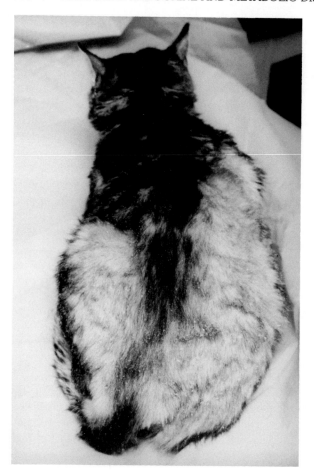

Figure 9:39. Hair loss and scaling in a cat with spontaneous hypothyroidism. (From Rand, J. S., et al.: Spontaneous adult-onset hypothyroidism in a cat. J. Vet. Intern. Med. 7:272, 1993.)

in euthyroid cats.[49, 89] When 0.1 mg per cat of TRH is given intravenously, TT_4 and fT_4 levels peak at 4 hours and increase onefold and twofold, respectively. Vomiting at the injection of TRH occurred in 4 of 13 cats.[89]

CLINICAL MANAGEMENT

Appropriate doses of thyroid hormones for cats have not been studied in detail. Cats bilaterally thyroidectomized for hyperthyroidism typically receive between 0.05 to 0.2 mg of levothyroxine every 24 hours or 30 μg of liothyronine every 8 hours.[95] These doses should be adequate for cats with congenital or acquired hypothyroidism. The cat with spontaneous adult-onset disease was treated with 0.1 mg every 24 hours and returned to normal status after 3 months of treatment.[80a] Typical of dogs, constitutional changes were noted after 1 week of treatment, whereas skin changes started about week 6 of treatment.

Feline Hyperthyroidism

Hyperthyroidism and diabetes mellitus are the most common endocrine disorders of the cat.[2, 3, 94] The cause of feline hyperthyroidism is usually a solitary thyroid adenoma or multinodular adenomatous hyperplasia of the thyroid. Thyroid carcinomas are rarely seen. Clinical signs are due to an accelerated basal metabolic rate and increased sensitivity to catecholamines.

Feline hyperthyroidism is seen in older cats, 6 to 20 years of age, with no apparent breed or sex predilections. Common clinical signs include polyphagia, polydipsia, polyuria, weight loss,

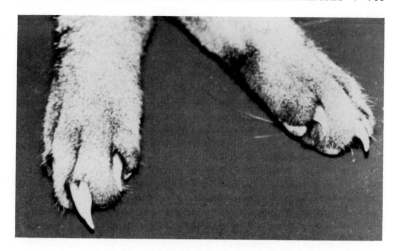

Figure 9:40. Overgrown claws in a hyperthyroid cat.

hyperactivity, tachycardia, vomiting, and diarrhea.[94] Cutaneous abnormalities can be seen in approximately 30 per cent of cases and include excessive shedding and matting of the haircoat, focal or symmetric alopecia associated with excessive grooming (see Fig. 9:37 *H*), increased rate of claw growth (Fig. 9:40), dry or greasy seborrhea, thin skin, and peripheral arteriovenous fistula.[3, 94] In chronic cases, there is complete truncal alopecia with thin, hypotonic skin, mimicking hyperadrenocorticism (Fig. 9:41).[18]

Diagnosis is based on history, physical examination findings, and elevated basal TT_4 and TT_3 levels. Common biochemical abnormalities in hyperthyroid cats include elevated levels of serum alkaline phosphatase, serum lactate dehydrogenase, and serum aspartate transaminase. More than 50 per cent of hyperthyroid cats can have TT_4 levels that overlap those seen in normal cats.[40] In these cases, the diagnosis of hyperthyroidism must be made by the T_3 suppression test or TRH stimulation test.[40] The T_3 suppression test involves the oral administration of 15 to 25 μg of liothyronine every 8 hours for seven doses.[40, 81] A sample for TT_4 and fT_4 determinations is taken before the medication administration is started and then 2 to 4 hours after the seventh dose. Hyperthyroid cats show little or no change in their TT_4 or fT_4 levels, whereas euthyroid cats show a 50 per cent reduction in TT_4 and fT_4 values. Hyperthyroid cats show no change in TT_4 levels after TRH administration.[40]

Therapy includes surgical excision, radioactive iodine treatment,[62] and the administration of antithyroid drugs (methimazole or carbimazole).[95]

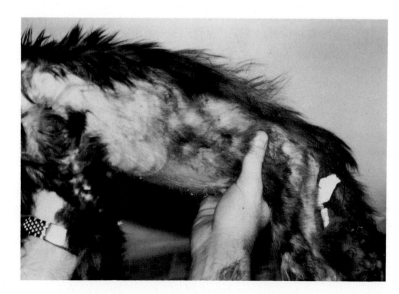

Figure 9:41. Truncal hair loss with thin hypotonic skin in a chronically hyperthyroid cat.

Diabetes Mellitus

In human beings, diabetes mellitus is associated with a number of dermatologic disorders, including vascular complications (microangiopathy and atherosclerosis), necrobiosis lipoidica, granuloma annulare, scleredema, fibrovascular papillomas, yellow nails, rubeosis, bacterial and fungal infections, diabetic neuropathy, pruritus, idiopathic bullae, alopecia, xanthomatosis, and poor wound healing.[246] Up to 30 per cent of humans with diabetes mellitus experience a skin disorder that is either an early indicator of undiagnosed diabetes or a complication of known diabetes. In dogs and cats, skin lesions have been reported to occur rarely or in as many as one third of the cases.[3, 12, 17, 240, 254, 256]

The most common dermatologic manifestations of diabetes in dogs and cats appear to be bacterial pyoderma (Fig. 9:42 *A*), seborrheic skin disease (Fig. 9:42 *B*), thin and hypotonic skin, and varying degrees of alopecia (Fig. 9:43). The thin, hypotonic skin, with or without alopecia, probably results from protein catabolism. The seborrheic skin disease (usually generalized seborrhea sicca) is probably due to protein catabolism and abnormal lipid metabolism.

Diabetics are predisposed to infections, particularly those caused by coagulase-positive staphylococci and *Candida* spp.[12, 246, 250] This susceptibility appears to be due to abnormalities in neutrophil chemotaxis, phagocytosis, intracellular killing, and cell-mediated (T cell) immune responses. These abnormalities may or may not be totally corrected by restoring normoglycemia with insulin therapy.

Rarely, pruritus vulvae, xanthomatosis, and necrobiosis lipoidica have been reported in association with diabetes mellitus in dogs.[2, 254, 256] Xanthomatosis has been reported in cats with naturally occurring and megestrol acetate–induced diabetes mellitus.

Necrolytic Migratory Erythema

Necrolytic migratory erythema is a term coined to describe the skin rash seen in humans with a glucagon-secreting pancreatic tumor (glucagonoma) or, rarely, hepatic cirrhosis and other miscellaneous gastrointestinal disorders. The rash has been recognized in dogs and possibly the cat, but because the pathogenic mechanism is incompletely understood, a standard nomenclature has not been accepted. The terms *hepatocutaneous syndrome*[12, 251, 252] and *superficial necrolytic dermatitis*[6, 245] are commonly used to describe the same condition.

CAUSE AND PATHOGENESIS

The skin lesions in necrolytic migratory erythema are due to degeneration of the keratinocytes, which results in laminar high-level epidermal edema and degeneration. The specific cause of the degeneration is still under study, but it probably results from cellular starvation or some other nutritional imbalance. Hypoproteinemia or deficiencies in biotin, essential fatty acids, or zinc have been proposed.[245, 251, 252] These nutritional deficiencies result from metabolic abnormalities caused by hyperglucagonemia, liver dysfunction, or combinations of these.

Approximately 90 per cent of cases of necrolytic migratory erythema in humans are associated with a pancreatic glucagonoma. In the veterinary literature, there are reports of approximately 70 cases of necrolytic migratory erythema in dogs and glucagonomas have been identified in only three dogs.[244, 253] The remainder have had moderate to severe liver disease with a high frequency of intercurrent pancreatic atrophy and fibrosis. Limited data are available on plasma glucagon levels in these dogs. Mildly elevated levels have been reported in four dogs with hepatic disease and one dog with a glucagonoma,[252, 253] whereas other reports found no elevations. It appears that glucagon can play a contributory role in this disorder but does not cause it in dogs. The underlying abnormality in the dogs with liver disease remains to be identified.

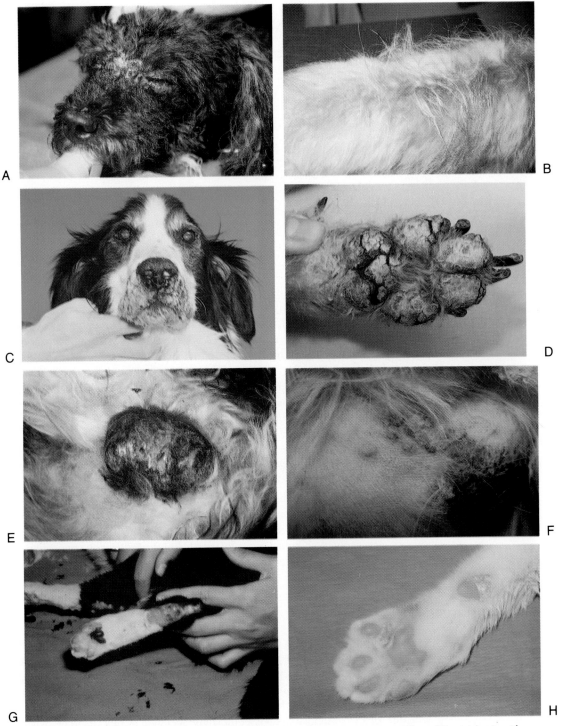

Figure 9:42. *A,* Diabetes mellitus. Severe facial bacterial pyoderma. *B,* Diabetes mellitus. Hypotrichosis with a greasy seborrhea. *C,* Necrolytic migratory erythema. Temporal muscle atrophy with crusting dermatitis of the periocular areas and muzzle. *D,* Necrolytic migratory erythema. Hyperkeratosis and fissuring of footpads. *E,* Necrolytic migratory erythema. Scrotal ulceration and crusting. *F,* Necrolytic migratory erythema. Intact and crusted vesicular lesions. *G,* Xanthomas of the hock region in a cat. (Courtesy K. Helton.) *H,* Xanthomas of the pads of a cat. (Courtesy D. Chester.)

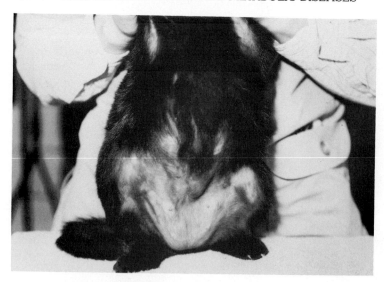

Figure 9:43. Diabetes mellitus in a cat. Abdominal hair loss.

CLINICAL FEATURES

Necrolytic migratory erythema is typically seen in old dogs.[245, 251, 252, 255] No consistent breed predisposition has been identified. Skin disease is the presenting complaint in most dogs although an occasional dog develops the eruption after systemic illness is recognized.[252] Skin lesions occur in areas of trauma, especially the muzzle, mucocutaneous areas of the face (see Fig. 9:42 *C*), distal limbs, and footpads (see Fig. 9:42 *D*). Lesions can also be seen in the mouth, on the pinnae, on the external genitalia (see Fig. 9:42 *E*), on the elbows and hocks, and along the ventrum. Most lesions are crusted with subjacent erosion or ulceration, but intact vesicular lesions (see Fig. 9:42 *F*) can occasionally be seen.

Routine laboratory evaluation of these patients usually shows normocytic, normochromic, nonregenerative anemia; borderline or frank hyperglycemia; elevations in activity of liver enzymes, especially serum alkaline phosphatase and alanine aminotransferase; and hypoalbuminemia.[252] Dogs with liver disease have increased sulfobromophthalein retention or postprandial bile acid levels. These signs of chronic liver disease are absent in dogs with glucagonoma. Positive antinuclear antibody titers can be seen.[252, 253] Bacteria, yeasts, or dermatophytes may be seen cytologically or histologically in skin specimens.

Special laboratory tests show hypoaminoacidemia, variable plasma glucagon concentrations, elevated insulin concentrations, and suggestive evidence of abnormalities in zinc metabolism and distribution.[245]

DIAGNOSIS

The differential diagnostic considerations include pemphigus foliaceus, systemic lupus erythematosus, zinc deficiency, and generic dog food dermatosis. If the laboratory evaluation is performed before skin biopsy, all differential diagnostic considerations except systemic lupus erythematosus can be excluded because dogs with pemphigus foliaceus, zinc deficiency, and generic dog food dermatosis rarely have the abnormalities described above.

Cytologic structure of the vesicular fluid is completely acellular in this disorder, whereas inflammatory cells are seen in the other differential diagnostic conditions. Skin biopsy of early lesions shows a diffuse parakeratotic hyperkeratosis, with high-level confluent vacuolation of keratinocytes resulting in a band of upper-level epidermal edema (Figs. 9:44 and 9:45).[6, 245] Dermal changes are usually minimal and include superficial edema and a perivascular accumulation of lymphocytes and plasma cells. Chronic lesions rarely show the epidermal edema

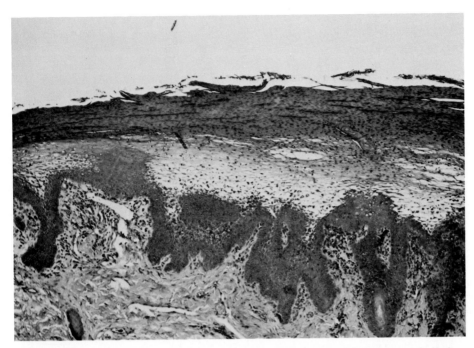

Figure 9:44. Canine necrolytic migratory erythema. Marked edema of the upper one half of epidermis with diffuse parakeratotic hyperkeratosis.

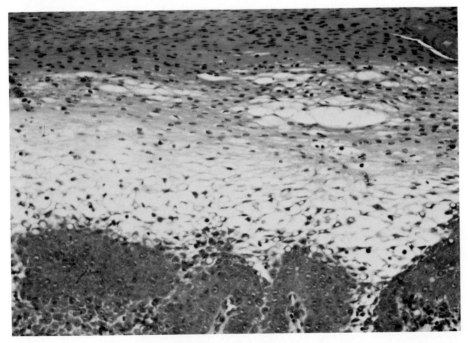

Figure 9:45. Close-up of Figure 9:44. Marked intercellular and intracellular edema with parakeratotic hyperkeratosis.

and have marked parakeratotic hyperkeratosis, epidermal hyperplasia, and surface crusting. Chronic lesions may have a superficial interstitial to lichenoid inflammatory infiltrate. Bacteria, dermatophytes, or yeast may be seen in the superficial keratin layer.

CLINICAL MANAGEMENT

Necrolytic migratory erythema is a cutaneous marker for a serious internal disease with a short survival time. One study showed that most dogs died or were euthanized within 5 months of the development of skin lesions.[252] Cases due to an identifiable and resectable glucagonoma should return to normal status with surgery. Other cases are more problematic because the pathogenesis is unknown. Treatment with corticosteroids improves the skin lesions, but eventually precipitates a diabetic crisis because these dogs are either prediabetic or overtly diabetic at diagnosis.[255] Treatment with zinc or essential fatty acid supplements has been unrewarding.[252] Work suggested that protein supplementation using egg yolks with or without zinc and pancreatic enzyme can reverse the skin lesions.[245] Because this treatment does not address the underlying problem, cure cannot be expected, but one dog has been maintained for 1 year.

Xanthomas

Xanthomas are benign granulomatous lesions associated with an abnormality in lipid metabolism. Xanthomatosis has been reported in cats with presumed hereditary hyperlipoproteinemia.[242a, 243, 248] No reports of xanthomatosis have been presented in Miniature Schnauzers with hyperlipidemia. Cases of apparently idiopathic xanthomas have been reported in the cat.[241, 242a] Most cases of xanthomatosis in dogs[242] and cats[17, 247, 249] have been associated with naturally occurring or drug (megestrol acetate)–induced diabetes mellitus in which abnormalities in fat absorption and metabolism result.[88]

Lesions consist of multiple whitish or yellow papules, nodules, or plaques, which may be ulcerated (see Fig. 9:42 *G* and *H*). The surrounding skin is erythematous, and the lesions can be painful or pruritic. The head, distal extremities, feet, and bony prominences are typically involved.

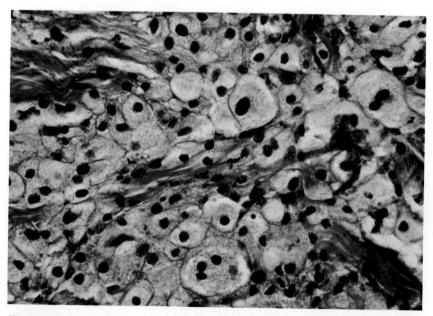

Figure 9:46. Feline xanthoma. Typical xanthoma cells.

Histopathologically, there is a nodular to diffuse infiltration of foamy macrophages and variable numbers of multinucleate histiocytic giant cells (Fig. 9:46). Granulomatous inflammation and fibroplasia may also be noted.

Lesions associated with diabetes mellitus or hyperlipoproteinemia resolve spontaneously with resolution of the underlying problem. Surgical removal without correction of the triggering cause usually results in relapse.[241] In cats with idiopathic hypertriglyceridemia and xanthomatosis,[243] feeding a low-fat commercial diet (Prescription Diet canine r/d [Hill's]) resulted in complete clinical remission within 30 days. New lesions developed each time a regular commercial cat food was given for even a short period of time.

Minoxidil in Canine Alopecia

Minoxidil is a vasodilator that has been used topically or orally to treat people with pattern baldness and alopecia areata.[254a] Although the mechanism by which it produces hair growth is unclear, minoxidil is known to increase cutaneous blood flow, have direct effects on keratinocytes (prolong life in culture, stimulate differentiation, and increase mitotic activity of matrix cells), and suppress lymphocyte-mediated immunologic phenomena.

Dogs with alopecia of undetermined cause have been treated with minoxidil.[239a, 245a] In the most detailed study,[245a] all dogs had bilaterally symmetric alopecia isolated to the flank or dorsal lumbar regions, and all dogs were breeds (boxer, Doberman pinscher, Staffordshire bull terrier, and Airedale terrier) known to develop follicular dysplasia, some of which is seasonally recurrent (see Chaps. 10 and 11). Dogs were treated with 0.1 to 0.5 mg/kg of minoxidil given orally every 24 hours. Of 12 dogs studied, 4 had a good response, 2 had a partial response, 4 had no response, and 2 dogs spontaneously regrew their hair before treatment could be given. These data are difficult to interpret and could all be explained by a spontaneously waxing and waning follicular dysplasia. In addition, 50 per cent of the treated dogs experienced moderate to severe side-effects, including weakness, lethargy, and collapse. The authors do *not* recommend the use of oral minoxidil in dogs at this time.

REFERENCES

General References

1. Abboud, C. F.: Laboratory diagnosis of hypopituitarism. Mayo Clin. Proc. 61:35, 1986.
2. Chastain, C. B., Ganjam, V. K.: Clinical Endocrinology of Companion Animals. Lea & Febiger, Philadelphia, 1986.
3. Feldman, E. C., Nelson, R. W.: Canine and Feline Endocrinology and Reproduction. W. B. Saunders Co., Philadelphia, 1987.
4. Freinkel, R. K.: Cutaneous manifestations of endocrine diseases. In: Fitzpatrick, T. B., et al. (eds.). Dermatology in General Medicine. McGraw-Hill Book Co., New York, 1993.
5. Grando, S. A.: Physiology of endocrine skin interrelations. J. Am. Acad. Dermatol. 28:981, 1993.
6. Gross, T. L., et al.: Veterinary Dermatopathology. Mosby Year Book, St. Louis, 1992.
7. Kemppainen, R. J., et al.: Effects of prednisone on thyroid and gonadal endocrine function in dogs. J. Endocrinol. 96:293, 1983.
8. Kemppainen, R. J., Sartin, J. L.: Evidence for episodic but not circadian activity in plasma concentrations of adrenocorticotrophin, cortisol, and thyroxine in dogs. J. Endocrinol. 103:219, 1984.
9. Kemppainen, R. J., et al.: Endocrine responses of normal cats to TSH and synthetic ACTH administration. J. Am. Anim. Hosp. Assoc. 20:737, 1984.
10. Kemppainen, R. J.: Effects of glucocorticoids on endocrine function in the dog. Vet. Clin. North Am. (Small Anim. Pract.) 14:721, 1984.
11. Moriello, K. A., et al.: Determination of thyroxine, triiodothyronine, and cortisol changes during simultaneous adrenal and thyroid function tests in healthy dogs. Am. J. Vet. Res. 48:458, 1987.
12. Muller, G. H., et al.: Small Animal Dermatology, 4th ed. W. B. Saunders Co., Philadelphia, 1989.
13. Quadri, S. K., Palazzolo, D. L.: How aging affects the canine endocrine system. Vet. Med. 86:692, 1991.
14. Reimers, T. J., et al.: Changes in serum thyroxine and cortisol in dogs after simultaneous injection of TSH and ACTH. J. Am. Anim. Hosp. Assoc. 18:923, 1982.
15. Scott, D. W.: Feline dermatology 1900–1978: A monograph. J. Am. Anim. Hosp. Assoc. 16:331, 1980.
16. Scott, D. W.: Histopathologic findings in the endocrine skin disorders of the dog. J. Am. Anim. Hosp. Assoc. 18:73, 1982.

17. Scott, D. W.: Feline dermatology 1979–1982: Introspective retrospections. J. Am. Anim. Hosp. Assoc. 20:537, 1984.
18. Scott, D. W., Miller, W. H.: Unpublished observations.
19. Thoday, A. J., Friedmann, P. S.: Scientific Basis of Dermatology. A Physiological Approach. Churchill Livingstone, New York, 1986.

Thyroid Physiology and Disease
20. Arnold, U., et al.: Goitrous hypothyroidism and dwarfism in a kitten. J. Am. Anim. Hosp. Assoc. 20:735, 1984.
21. Beale, K. M.: Dermatologic manifestations of hypothyroidism. In: Hypothyroidism: Diagnosis and Clinical Manifestations. Daniels Pharmaceuticals, St. Petersburg, 1993, p. 16.
22. Beale, K. M., et al.: Correlation of racing and reproductive performance in Greyhounds with response to thyroid function testing. J. Am. Anim. Hosp. Assoc. 28:263, 1992.
23. Beale, K. M., et al.: Prevalence of antithyroglobulin antibodies detected by enzyme-linked immunosorbent assay of canine serum. J. Am. Vet. Med. Assoc. 196:745, 1990.
24. Beale, K. M., et al.: Serum thyroid hormone concentrations and thyrotropin responsiveness in dogs with generalized dermatologic disease. J. Am. Vet. Med. Assoc. 201:1715, 1992.
25. Beale, K. M., et al.: Comparison of two doses of aqueous bovine thyrotropin for thyroid function testing in dogs. J. Am. Vet. Med. Assoc. 197:865, 1990.
26. Bichsel, P., et al.: Neurologic manifestations associated with hypothyroidism in four dogs. J. Am. Vet. Med. Assoc. 192:1745, 1989.
27. Brent, B. A., Hershman, J. M.: Thyroxine therapy in patients with severe nonthyroidal illnesses and low thyroxine concentration. J. Clin. Endocrinol. Metab. 63:1, 1986.
28. Bruyette, D. S., et al.: Effect of thyrotropin storage on thyroid-stimulating hormone response testing in normal dogs. J. Vet. Intern. Med. 1:91, 1987.
29. Budsberg, S. C., et al: Thyroxin-responsive unilateral forelimb lameness and generalized neuromuscular disease in four hypothyroid dogs. J. Am. Vet. Med. Assoc. 202:1859, 1993.
30. Campbell, K. L., Davis, C. A.: Effects of thyroid hormones on serum and cutaneous fatty acid concentrations in dogs. Am. J. Vet. Res. 51:752, 1990.
31. Chastain, C. B., et al.: Congenital hypothyroidism in a dog due to an iodide organification defect. Am. J. Vet. Res. 44:1257, 1983.
32. Chastain, C. B., et al.: Anti-triiodothyronine antibodies associated with hypothyroidism and lymphocytic thyroiditis in a dog. J. Am. Vet. Med. Assoc. 194:531, 1989.
33. Chastain, C. B.: Unusual manifestations of hypothyroidism in dogs. In: Kirk, R. W., Bonagura, J. D. (eds.). Kirk's Current Veterinary Therapy XI. W. B. Saunders Co., Philadelphia, 1992, p. 327.
34. Conaway, D. H., et al.: Clinical and histological features of primary progressive, familial thyroiditis in a colony of borzoi dogs. Vet. Pathol. 22:439, 1985.
35. Engler, D., Burger, A. G.: The deiodination of the iodothyronines and of their derivatives in man. Endocr. Rev. 5:151, 1984.
36. Ferguson, D. C.: An internal medical perspective of hypothyroidism. In: Hypothyroidism: Diagnosis and Clinical Manifestations. Daniels Pharmaceuticals, St. Petersburg, 1993, p. 2.
37. Ford, S. L., et al.: Insulin resistance in three dogs with hypothyroidism and diabetes mellitus. J. Am. Vet. Med. Assoc. 202:1478, 1993.
37a. Frank, L. A.: Comparison of thyrotropin-releasing hormone (TRH) and thyrotropin (TSH) stimulation tests for evaluating thyroid function in hypothyroid dogs. Proc. Am. Acad. Vet. Dermatol. Am. Coll. Vet. Dermatol 10:59, 1994.
38. Gaschen, F., et al.: Recognition of triiodothyronine-containing epitopes in canine thyroglobulin by circulating thyroglobulin autoantibodies. Am. J. Vet. Res. 54:244, 1993.
39. Gosselin, S. J., et al.: Autoimmune lymphocytic thyroiditis in dogs. Vet. Immunol. Immunopathol. 3:185, 1982.
40. Graves, T. K., Peterson, M. E.: Occult hyperthyroidism in cats. In: Kirk, R. W., Bonagura, J. D. (eds.). Kirk's Current Veterinary Therapy XI. W. B. Saunders Co., Philadelphia, 1992, p. 334.
41. Greco, D. S., et al.: Congenital hypothyroid dwarfism in a family of Giant Schnauzers. J. Vet. Intern. Med. 5:57, 1991.
42. Gunaratnam, P.: The effect of thyroxine on hair growth in the dog. J. Small Anim. Pract. 27:17, 1986.
43. Haines, D. M.: Survey of thyroglobulin autoantibodies in dogs. Am. J. Vet. Res. 45:1493, 1984.
44. Haines, D. M., et al.: The detection of canine autoantibodies to thyroid antigens by enzyme-linked immunosorbent assay, hemagglutination, and indirect immunofluorescence. Can. J. Comp. Med. 48:262, 1984.
45. Haines, D. M., Penhale, W. J.: Experimental thyroid autoimmunity in the dog. Vet. Immunol. Immunopathol. 9:221, 1985.
46. Hall, I. A., et al.: Effect of trimethoprim/sulfamethoxazole on thyroid function in dogs with pyoderma. J. Am. Vet. Med. Assoc. 202:1159, 1993.
47. Hansen, S. R., et al.: Acute overdose of levothyroxine in a dog. J. Am. Vet. Med. Assoc. 200:1512, 1992.
48. Hasler, A., Rohner, K.: Schwerwiegende Reaktionen Nach TSH-Stimulationstest Beim Hund. Schweiz. Arch. Tierheilkd. 134:423, 1992.
49. Hoenig, M., Ferguson, D. C.: Assessment of thyroid functional reserve in the cat by the thyrotropin-stimulation test. Am. J. Vet. Res. 44:1229, 1983.
50. Jones, B. R., et al.: Preliminary studies on congenital hypothyroidism in a family of Abyssinian cats. Vet. Rec. 131:145, 1992.
51. Kaufman, J., et al.: Serum concentrations of thyroxine, 3,5,3'-triiodothyronine, thyrotropin, and prolactin in dogs before and after thyrotropin-releasing hormone administration. Am. J. Vet. Res. 46:486, 1985.

52. Kelly, M. J., Hill, J. R.: Canine myxedema stupor and coma. Comp. Cont. Educ. 6:1049, 1984.
53. Kemppainen, R. J.: Laboratory diagnosis of hypothyroidism. In: Hypothyroidism: Diagnosis and Clinical Manifestations. Daniels Pharmaceuticals, St. Petersburg, 1993, p. 10.
54. Kemppainen, R. J., Young, D. W.: Canine triiodothyronine autoantibodies. In: Kirk, R. W., Bonagura, J. D. (eds.). Kirk's Current Veterinary Therapy XI. W. B. Saunders Co., Philadelphia, 1992, p. 327.
55. Kobayashi, D. L., et al.: Serum thyroid hormone concentrations in clinically normal dogs after administration of freshly reconstituted versus previously frozen and stored thyrotropin. J. Am. Vet. Med. Assoc. 197:597, 1990.
56. Larsson, M. G.: Determination of free thyroxine and cholesterol as a new screening test for canine hypothyroidism. J. Am. Anim. Hosp. Assoc. 24:209, 1988.
57. Laurberg, P.: Iodothyronine deiodination in the canine thyroid. Domest. Anim. Endocrinol. 1:1, 1984.
58. Li, W. I., et al.: Effects of thyrotropin-releasing hormone on serum concentrations of thyroxine and triiodothyronine in healthy, thyroidectomized, thyroxine-treated, and propylthiouracil-treated dogs. Am. J. Vet. Res. 47:163, 1986.
59. Liu, S. K., et al.: Clinical and pathologic findings in dogs with atherosclerosis: 21 cases (1970–1983). J. Am. Vet. Med. Assoc. 189:227, 1986.
60. Lucke, V. M., et al.: Thyroid pathology in canine hypothyroidism. J. Comp. Pathol. 93:415, 1983.
61. Medleau, L., et al.: Congenital hypothyroidism in a dog. J. Am. Anim. Hosp. Assoc. 21:341, 1985.
62. Meric, S. M., Rubin, S. I.: Serum thyroxine concentrations following fixed-dose radioactive iodine treatment in hyperthyroid cats: 62 cases (1986–1989). J. Am. Vet. Med. Assoc. 197:621, 1990.
63. Miller, A. B., et al.: Serial thyroid hormone concentrations in healthy euthyroid dogs, dogs with hypothyroidism, and euthyroid dogs with atopic dermatitis. Br. Vet. J. 148:451, 1992.
64. Mooney, C. T., Anderson, T. J.: Congenital hypothyroidism in a boxer dog. J. Small Anim. Pract. 34:31, 1993.
65. Moore, G. E., et al.: Effects of oral administration of anti-inflammatory doses of prednisolone on thyroid hormone response to thyrotropin-releasing hormone and thyrotropin in clinically normal dogs. Am. J. Vet. Res. 54:1993.
66. Nachreiner, R. F., Refsal, K. R.: Radioimmunoassay monitoring with thyroid hormone concentrations in dogs on thyroid replacement therapy: 2674 cases (1985–1987). J. Am. Vet. Med. Assoc. 201:623, 1992.
66a. Nachreiner, R. F., et al.: Pharmacokinetics of L-thyroxine after its oral administration in dogs. Am. J. Vet. Res 54:2091, 1993.
67. Nelson, R. W., Ihle, S. L.: Hypothyroidism in dogs and cats: A difficult deficiency to diagnose. Vet. Med. 82:60, 1987.
68. Nelson, R. W., et al.: Serum free thyroxine concentration in healthy dogs, dogs with hypothyroidism, and euthyroid dogs with concurrent illness. J. Am. Vet. Med. Assoc. 198:1401, 1991.
69. Panciera, D. L.: Canine hypothyroidism. Part I. Clinical findings and control of thyroid hormone secretion and metabolism. Comp. Cont. Educ. 12:689, 1990.
70. Panciera, D. L. Canine hypothyroidism. Part II. Thyroid function tests and treatment. Comp. Cont. Educ. 12:943, 1990.
71. Panciera, D. L., Post, K.: Effect of oral administration of sulfadiazine and trimethoprim in combination on thyroid function in dogs. Can. J. Vet. Res. 56:349, 1992.
72. Panciera, D. L., et al.: Thyroid function tests in euthyroid dogs treated with L-thyroxine. Am. J. Vet. Res. 51:22, 1989.
73. Panciera, D. L., et al.: Quantitative morphologic study on the pituitary and thyroid glands of dogs administered L-thyroxine. Am. J. Vet. Res. 51:27, 1990.
73a. Panciera, D. L.: Hypothyroidism in dogs: 66 cases (1987–1992). J. Am. Vet. Med. Assoc. 204:761, 1994.
74. Paradis, M., et al.: Studies of various diagnostic methods for canine hypothyroidism. Vet. Dermatol. 2:125, 1991.
74a. Paradis, M.: Serum free thyroxine concentration measured by luminescence, before and after thyrotropin administration in healthy dogs, hypothyroid dogs and euthyroid dogs with dermatopathies. Proc. Am. Acad. Vet. Dermatol. Am. Coll. Vet. Dermatol. 10:58, 1994.
75. Patterson, J. S., et al.: Neurologic manifestations of cerebrovascular atherosclerosis associated with primary hypothyroidism in a dog. J. Am. Vet. Med. Assoc. 186:499, 1985.
76. Peterson, M. E., et al.: Effects of spontaneous hyperadrenocorticism on serum thyroid hormone concentrations in the dog. Am. J. Vet. Res. 45:2034, 1984.
77. Peterson, M. E., Gamble, D. A.: Effect of nonthyroidal illness on serum thyroxine concentrations in cats: 494 cases (1988). J. Am. Vet. Med. Assoc. 197:1203, 1990.
78. Peterson, M. E.: Feline hypothyroidism. In: Kirk, R. W. (ed.). Current Veterinary Therapy X. W. B. Saunders Co., Philadelphia, 1989, p. 1000.
79. Quinlan, W. J., Michaelson, S.: Homologous radioimmunoassay for canine thyrotropin: Response of normal and x-irradiated dogs to propylthiouracil. Endocrinology 108:937, 1981.
80. Rachofsky, M. A.: Clinical relevance of results from the new canine specific endogenous TSH assay: A review of 79 cases. Proc. Am. Acad. Vet Dermatol. Am. Coll. Vet. Dermatol. 4:1988.
80a. Rand, J. S., et al.: Spontaneous adult-onset hypothyroidism in a cat. J. Vet. Intern. Med. 7:272, 1993.
81. Refsal, K. R., et al: Use of triiodothyronine suppression test for diagnosis of hyperthyroidism in ill cats that have serum concentrations of iodothyronines within normal range. J. Am. Vet. Med. Assoc. 199:1594, 1991.
82. Reimers, T. J., et al.: Effects of reproductive state on concentrations of thyroxine, 3,5,3'-triiodothyronine and cortisol in serum of dogs. Biol. Reprod. 31:148, 1984.
83. Reimers, T. J., et al.: Effect of fasting on thyroxine, 3,5,3'-triiodothyronine, and cortisol concentrations in serum of dogs. Am. J. Vet. Res 47:2485, 1986.
84. Reimers, T. J., et al.: Effects of age, sex, and body size on serum concentrations of thyroid and adrenocortical hormones in dogs. Am. J. Vet. Res. 51:454, 1990.

85. Richardson, H. W.: Evaluation of endogenous cTSH assay RIA test kit in clinically normal and suspect hypothyroid dogs. Proc. Am. Acad. Vet. Dermatol. Am. Coll. Vet. Dermatol. 4:1988.

86. Robinson, W. F., et al.: Congenital hypothyroidism in Scottish Deerhound puppies. Aust. Vet. J. 65:386, 1988.

87. Rosenberg, R. M., et al.: Abnormal lipogenesis in thyroid hormone–deficient epidermis. J. Invest. Dermatol. 86:244, 1986.

88. Simpson, J. W., van den Broek, A. H. M.: Fat absorption in dogs with diabetes mellitus or hypothyroidism. Res. Vet. Sci. 50:346, 1991.

89. Sparks, A. H., et al.: Thyroid function in the cat: Assessment by the TRH response test and thyrotropin stimulation test. J. Small Anim. Pract. 32:59, 1991.

90. Stolp, R., et al.: Plasma cortisol response to thyrotrophin releasing hormone and luteinizing hormone releasing hormone in healthy kennel dogs and in dogs with pituitary-dependent hyperadrenocorticism. J. Endocrinol. 93:365, 1982.

90a. Sullivan, P., et al.: Altered platelet indices in dogs with hypothyroidism and cats with hyperthyroidism. Am. J. Vet. Res. 54:2004, 1993.

91. Tarttelin, M. F., et al.: Serum free thyroxine levels respond inversely to changes in levels of dietary iodine in the domestic cat. N. Z. Vet. J. 40:66, 1992.

92. Thoday, K. L., et al.: Radioimmunoassay of serum total thyroxine and triiodothyronine in cats: Assay methodology and effects of age, sex, breed, heredity, and environment. J. Small Anim. Pract. 25:457, 1984.

93. Thoday, K. L.: Feline hypothyroidism: An experimental study. Vet. Dermatol. Newsl. 12(1), 1989.

94. Thoday, K. L., Mooney, C. T.: Historical, clinical and laboratory features of 126 hyperthyroid cats. Vet. Rec. 131:257, 1992.

95. Thoday, K. L., Mooney, C. T.: Medical management of feline hyperthyroidism. In: Kirk, R. W., Bonagura, J. D. (eds.). Kirk's Current Veterinary Therapy XI. W. B. Saunders Co., Philadelphia, 1992, p. 338.

96. Torres, S. M. F., et al.: Effect of oral administration of prednisolone on thyroid function in dogs. Am. J. Vet. Res. 52:416, 1991.

97. Van Der Walt, J. A., et al.: Functional endocrine modification of the thyroid following ovariectomy in the canine. J. S. Afr. Vet. Assoc. 54:225, 1983.

98. Wall, J. R., Kuroki, T.: Immunologic factors in thyroid disease. Med. Clin. North Am. 69:913, 1985.

99. Wartofsky, L., Burman, K. D.: Alterations in thyroid function in patients with systemic illness: The "euthyroid sick syndrome." Endocr. Rev. 3:164, 1982.

100. Wheatley, T., Edwards, O. M.: Mild hypothyroidism and oedema: Evidence for increased capillary permeability to protein. Clin. Endocrinol. 18:627, 1983.

100a. Yu, A. A., et al.: Comparison of the effects of endotoxin on thyrotropin and thyrotropin-releasing hormone response tests in healthy dogs. Proc. Am. Acad. Vet. Dermatol. Am. Coll. Vet. Dermatol. 10:30, 1994.

Adrenal Physiology and Disease

101. Biewenga, W. J., et al.: Persistent polyuria in two dogs following adrenocorticolysis for pituitary-dependent hyperadrenocorticism. Vet. Quart. 11:193, 1989.

102. Blaxter, A. C., Gruffydd-Jones, T. J.: Concurrent diabetes mellitus and hyperadrenocorticism in the dog: Diagnosis and management of eight cases. J. Small Anim. Pract. 31:117, 1990.

103. Chastain, C. B., et al.: Evaluation of the hypothalamic-pituitary-adrenal axis in clinically stressed dogs. J. Am. Anim. Hosp. Assoc. 22:435, 1986.

104. Chrousos, G. P., et al.: Clinical applications of corticotropin-releasing factor. Ann. Intern. Med. 102:344, 1985.

105. Daley, C. A., et al.: Use of metyrapone to treat pituitary-dependent hyperadrenocorticism in a cat with large cutaneous wounds. J. Am. Vet. Med. Assoc. 202:956, 1993.

106. Dow, S. W., et al.: Perianal adenomas and hypertestosteronemia in a spayed bitch with pituitary-dependent hyperadrenocorticism. J. Am. Vet. Med. Assoc. 192:1439, 1988.

107. Dow, S. W., et al.: Response of dogs with functional pituitary macroadenomas and macrocarcinomas to irradiation. J. Small Anim. Pract. 31:287, 1990.

108. Eichenbaum, J. D., et al.: Effect in large dogs of ophthalmic prednisolone acetate on adrenal gland and hepatic function. J. Am. Anim. Hosp. Assoc. 24:705, 1988.

109. Eiler, H., et al.: Stages of hyperadrenocorticism: Response of hyperadrenocorticoid dogs to the combined dexamethasone suppression/ACTH stimulation test. J. Am. Vet. Med. Assoc. 185:289, 1984.

110. Emms, S. G., et al.: Adrenalectomy in the management of canine hyperadrenocorticism. J. Am. Vet. Med. Assoc. 23:557, 1987.

111. Etreby, M. F. E., et al.: Functional morphology of spontaneous hyperplastic and neoplastic lesions in the canine pituitary gland. Vet. Pathol. 17:109, 1980.

112. Feldman, E. C.: Evaluation of a combined dexamethasone suppression/ACTH stimulation test in dogs with hyperadrenocorticism. J. Am. Vet. Med. Assoc. 187:49, 1985.

113. Feldman, E. C.: Evaluation of a six-hour combined dexamethasone suppression/ACTH stimulation test in dogs with hyperadrenocorticism. J. Am. Vet. Med. Assoc. 189:1562, 1986.

114. Feldman, E. C., et al.: Comparison of mitotane treatment for adrenal tumor versus pituitary-dependent hyperadrenocorticism in dogs. J. Am. Vet. Med. Assoc. 200:1642, 1992.

115. Feldman, E. C., Mack, R. E.: Urine cortisol:creatinine ratio as a screening test for hyperadrenocorticism in dogs. J. Am. Vet. Med. Assoc. 200:1637, 1992.

116. Feldman, E. C., Nelson, R. W.: Use of ketoconazole for control of canine hyperadrenocorticism. In: Kirk, R. W., Bonagura, J. D. (eds.). Kirk's Current Veterinary Therapy XI. W. B. Saunders Co., Philadelphia, 1992, p. 349.

117. Feldman, E. C., et al.: Plasma cortisol response to ketoconazole administration in dogs with hyperadrenocorticism. J. Am. Vet. Med. Assoc. 197:71, 1990.

118. Ferguson, D. C., Peterson, M. E.: Serum free and total iodothyronine concentrations in dogs with hyperadrenocorticism. Am. J. Vet. Res. 53:1636, 1992.

119. Ford, S. L., et al.: Hyperadrenocorticism caused by bilateral adrenocortical neoplasia in dogs. Four cases (1983–1988). J. Am. Vet. Med. Assoc. 202:789, 1993.

120. Garnier, F., et al.: Adrenal cortical response in clinically normal dogs before and after adaption to a housing environment. Lab. Anim. 24:40, 1990.

121. Glaze, M. R., et al.: Ophthalmic corticosteroid therapy: Systemic effects in the dog. J. Am. Vet. Med. Assoc. 192:73, 1988.

122. Greco, D. S., et al.: Dexamethasone pharmacokinetics in clinically normal dogs during low- and high-dose dexamethasone suppression testing. Am. J. Vet. Res. 54:580, 1992.

122a. Hansen, B. L., et al.: Synthetic ACTH (cosyntropin) stimulation tests in normal dogs: Comparison of intravenous and intramuscular administration. J. Am. Anim. Hosp. Assoc. 30:38, 1994.

123. Hegstad, R. L., et al.: Effect of sample handling on adrenocorticotropin concentration measured in canine plasma, using a commercially available radioimmunoassay kit. Am. J. Vet. Res. 51:1941, 1990.

124. Helton-Rhodes, K., et al.: Cutaneous manifestations of feline hyperadrenocorticism. In: Ihrke, P. J., et al. (eds.). Advances in Veterinary Dermatology, Vol. 2. Pergamon Press, New York, 1993, p. 391.

125. Jensen, R. B., DuFort, R. M.: Hyperadrenocorticism in dogs. Comp. Cont. Educ. 13:615, 1991.

126. Jones, C. A., et al.: Changes in adrenal cortisol secretion as reflected in the urinary cortisol/creatinine ratio in dogs. Dom. Anim. Endocrinol. 7:559, 1990.

127. Jones, C. A., et al.: Adrenocortical adenocarcinoma in a cat. J. Am. Anim. Hosp. Assoc. 28:59, 1992.

128. Kemppainen, R. J., Zenoble, R. D.: Nondexamethasone-suppressible, pituitary-dependent hyperadrenocorticism in a dog. J. Am. Vet. Med. Assoc. 187:276, 1985.

129. Kemppainen, R. J., et al.: Ovine corticotrophin-releasing factor in dogs: Dose-response relationships and effects of dexamethasone. Acta Endocrinol. 112:12, 1986.

130. Kemppainen, R. J., Peterson, M. E.: Circulating concentration of dexamethasone in healthy dogs, dogs with hyperadrenocorticism and dogs with nonadrenal illness during dexamethasone suppression testing. Am. J. Vet. Res. 54:1765, 1993.

131. Kemppainen, R. J., et al.: Plasma free cortisol concentrations in dogs with hyperadrenocorticism. Am. J. Vet. Res. 52:682, 1991.

132. Kemppainen, R. J., et al.: Effects of single intravenously administered doses of dexamethasone on response to the adrenocorticotropic hormone stimulation test in dogs. Am. J. Vet. Res. 50:1914, 1989.

133. Kintzer, P. P., Peterson, M. E.: Mitotane (o,p'-DDD) treatment of 200 dogs with pituitary-dependent hyperadrenocorticism. J. Vet. Intern. Med. 5:102, 1991.

133a. Kintzer, P. P., Peterson, M. E.: Mitotane treatment of 32 dogs with cortisol-secreting adrenocortical neoplasms. J. Am. Vet. Med. Assoc. 205:54, 1994.

134. Kipperman, B. S., et al.: Diabetes mellitus and exocrine pancreatic neoplasia in two cats with hyperadrenocorticism. J. Am. Anim. Hosp. Assoc. 28:415, 1992.

135. Kipperman, B. S., et al.: Pituitary tumor size, neurologic signs, and relation to endocrine test results in dogs with pituitary-dependent hyperadrenocorticism: 43 cases (1980–1990). J. Am. Vet. Med. Assoc. 201:762, 1992.

136. LaRue, M. J., Murtaugh, R. J.: Pulmonary thromboembolism in dogs: 47 cases (1986–1987). J. Am. Vet. Med. Assoc. 197:1368, 1990.

137. Mack, R. E., Feldman, E. C.: Comparison of two low-dose dexamethasone suppression protocols as screening and discriminating tests in dogs with hyperadrenocorticism. J. Am. Vet. Med. Assoc. 197:1603, 1990.

137a. Mack, R. E., et al.: Diagnosis of hyperadrenocorticism in dogs. Compend. Cont. Educ. 16:311, 1994.

137b. Mackedanz, R., Struckmann, B.: Bericht über einem Fall von Hypercortisolismus bei einer Katze. Kleintierpraxis 37:843, 1992.

138. Mauldin, G. N., Burk, R. L.: The use of diagnostic computerized tomography and radiation therapy in canine and feline hyperadrenocorticism. Probl. Vet. Med. 2:557, 1990.

139. Mbugua, S. W., et al.: Adrenocortical suppression by a glucocorticoid: Effect of a single I. M. injection of betamethasone depot versus placebo given prior to orthopaedic surgery in dogs. Acta Vet. Scand. 29:415, 1988.

140. Meyer, D. J., et al.: Effect of otic medications containing glucocorticoids in liver function tests in healthy dogs. J. Am. Vet. Med. Assoc. 196:743, 1990.

141. Moore, G. E., Hoenig, M.: Effect of orally administered prednisone on glucose tolerance and insulin secretion in clinically normal dogs. Am. J. Vet. Res. 54:126, 1993.

142. Moore, G. E., Hoenig, M.: Duration of pituitary and adrenocortical suppression after long-term administration of anti-inflammatory doses of prednisone in dogs. Am. J. Vet. Res. 53:716, 1992.

143. Murphy, C. J., et al.: Iatrogenic Cushing's syndrome in a dog caused by topical ophthalmic medication. J. Am. Anim. Hosp. Assoc. 26:640, 1990.

144. Nelson, R. W., et al.: Hyperadrenocorticism in cats. Seven cases (1978–1987). J. Am. Vet. Med. Assoc. 193:245, 1988.

145. Nelson, R. W., Feldman, E. C.: Hyperadrenocorticism. In: August, J. R. (ed.). Consultations in Feline Internal Medicine. W. B. Saunders Co., Philadelphia, 1991, p. 267.

146. Nelson, R. W., et al.: Pituitary macroadenomas and macroadenocarcinomas in dogs treated with mitotane for pituitary-dependent hyperadrenocorticism: 13 cases (1981–1986). J. Am. Vet. Med. Assoc. 194:1612, 1989.

147. Nelson, R. W., et al.: Topics in the diagnosis and treatment of canine hyperadrenocorticism. Comp. Cont. Educ. 13:1797, 1991.

148. Nichols, R.: Problems associated with medical therapy of canine hyperadrenocorticism. Probl. Vet. Med. 2:551, 1990.

149. Nichols, R.: Concurrent illness and complications associated with hyperadrenocorticism. Probl. Vet. Med. 2:565, 1990.

150. Penninek, D. G., et al.: Radiographic features of canine hyperadrenocorticism caused by autonomously functioning adrenocortical tumors: 23 cases (1978–1986). J. Am. Vet. Med. Assoc. 192:1604, 1988.

151. Peterson, M. E., et al.: Immunocytochemical study of the hypophysis in 25 dogs with pituitary-dependent hyperadrenocorticism. Acta Endocrinol. 101:15, 1982.

152. Peterson, M. E., et al.: Adrenal function in the cat: Comparison of the effects of cosyntropin (synthetic ACTH) and corticotropin gel stimulation. Res. Vet. Sci. 37:331, 1984.

153. Peterson, M. E.: Canine hyperadrenocorticism. In: Kirk, R. W. (ed.). Current Veterinary Therapy IX. W. B. Saunders Co., Philadelphia, 1986, p. 963.

154. Peterson, M. E., Steele, P.: Pituitary-dependent hyperadrenocorticism in a cat. J. Am. Vet. Med. Assoc. 189:680, 1986.

155. Peterson, M. E., et al.: Plasma immunoreactive ACTH peptides and cortisol in normal dogs and dogs with Addison's disease and Cushing's syndrome: Basal concentrations. Endocrinology 119:720, 1986.

156. Peterson, M. E., Kemppainen, R. J.: Dose-response relationship between plasma concentrations of corticotropin and cortisol after administration of incremental doses of cosyntropin for corticotropin stimulation testing in cats. Am. J. Vet. Res. 54:300, 1983.

157. Peterson, M. E., Kemppainen, R. S.: Comparison of immunoreactive plasma corticotropin and cortisol response to two synthetic corticotropin preparations (tetracosactrin and cosyntropin) in healthy cats. Am. J. Vet. Res. 53:1752, 1992.

158. Peterson, M. E., et al.: Effects of synthetic ovine corticotropin-releasing hormone on plasma concentrations of immunoreactive adrenocorticotropic, α-melanocyte-stimulating hormone and cortisol in dogs with naturally acquired adrenocortical insufficiency. Am. J. Vet. Res. 53:1636, 1992.

159. Peterson, M. E., et al.: Effect of spontaneous hyperadrenocorticism in endogenous production and utilization of glucose in the dog. Dom. Anim. Endocrinol. 3:117, 1986.

160. Poffenbarger, E. M., et al.: Gray-scale ultrasonography in the diagnosis of adrenal neoplasia in dogs: Six cases (1981–1986). J. Am. Vet. Med. Assoc. 192:228, 1988.

161. Reusch, C. E., Feldman, E. C.: Canine hyperadrenocorticism due to adrenocortical neoplasia. J. Vet. Intern. Med. 5:3, 1991.

162. Rijnberk, A., Belshaw, B. E.: An alternative protocol for the medical management of canine pituitary-dependent hyperadrenocorticism. Vet. Rec. 122:406, 1988.

163. Rijnberk, A. D., Belshaw, B. E.: o,p'-DDD treatment of canine hyperadrenocorticism: An alternative protocol. In: Kirk, R. W., Bonagura, J. D. (eds.). Kirk's Current Veterinary Therapy XI. W. B. Saunders Co., Philadelphia, 1992, p. 345.

164. Roberts, S. M., et al.: Effect of ophthalmic prednisolone acetate on the canine adrenal gland and hepatic function. Am. J. Vet. Res. 45:1711, 1984.

165. Rothuizen, J., et al.: Aging and the hypothalamus-pituitary-adrenocortical axis, with special reference to the dog. Acta Endocrinol. (Copenh.) 125:73, 1991.

166. Sarfaty, D., et al.: Neurologic, endocrinologic, and pathologic findings associated with large pituitary tumors in dogs: Eight cases (1976–1984). J. Am. Vet. Med. Assoc. 193:854, 1988.

167. Scavelli, T. D., et al.: Results of surgical treatment for hyperadrenocorticism caused by adrenocortical neoplasia in the dog: 25 cases (1980–1984). J. Am. Vet. Med. Assoc. 189:1360, 1986.

167a. Scholten-Sloof, B. E., et al.: Pituitary-dependent hyperadrenocorticism in a family of Dandie-Dinmont terriers. J. Endocrinol. 135:535, 1992.

168. Schulman, J., Johnston, S. D.: Hyperadrenocorticism in two related Yorkshire terriers. J. Am. Vet. Med. Assoc. 182:524, 1983.

169. Scott, D. W.: Dermatologic use of glucocorticoids: Systemic and topical. Vet. Clin. North Am. 12:19, 1982.

170. Scott, D. W., et al.: Iatrogenic Cushing's syndrome in the cat. Feline Pract. 12:30, 1982.

171. Scott, D. W.: Cutaneous phlebectasias in cushingoid dogs. J. Am. Anim. Hosp. Assoc. 21:351, 1985.

172. Simpson, J. W., van den Brock, A. H. M.: Assessment of fat absorption in normal dogs and dogs with hyperadrenocorticalism. Res. Vet. Sci. 48:38, 1990.

173. Smith, M. C., Feldman, E. C.: Plasma endogenous ACTH concentrations and plasma cortisol responses to synthetic ACTH and dexamethasone sodium phosphate in healthy cats. Am. J. Vet. Res. 48:1719, 1987.

174. Solter, P. F., et al.: Assessment of corticosteroid-induced alkaline phosphatase isoenzyme as a screening test for hyperadrenocorticism in dogs. J. Am. Vet. Med. Assoc. 203:534, 1993.

175. Stolp, R., et al.: Results of cyproheptadine treatment in dogs with pituitary-dependent hyperadrenocorticism. J. Endocrinol. 101:311, 1984.

175a. Vandenbergh, A. G. G. D., et al.: Haemorrhage from a canine adrenocortical tumour: A clinical emergency. Vet. Rec. 131:539, 1992.

176. van den Broek, A. H. M., Stafford, W. L.: Epidermal and hepatic glucocorticoid receptors in cats and dogs. Res. Vet. Sci. 52:312, 1992.

177. Vollset, I., Jakobsen, G.: Feline endocrine alopecia-like disease probably induced by medroxyprogesterone acetate. Feline Pract. 16:16, 1986.

178. Voorhout, G., et al.: Computed tomography in the diagnosis of canine hyperadrenocorticism not suppressible by dexamethasone. J. Am. Vet. Med. Assoc. 192:641, 1988.

179. Voorhout, G., et al.: Nephrotomography and ultrasonography for the localization of hyperfunctioning adrenocortical tumors in dogs. Am. J. Vet. Res. 51:1280, 1990.

180. Bruyette, D. S., et al.: L-Deprenyl therapy of canine pituitary dependent hyperadrenocorticism. Poster, ACVIM Forum, Washington, DC, 1993.

181. Voorhout, G., et al.: Assessment of survey radiography and comparison with x-ray computed tomography for detection of hyperfunctioning adrenocortical tumors in dogs. J. Am. Vet. Med. Assoc. 196:1799, 1990.

182. Ward, D. A., et al.: Band keratopathy associated with hyperadrenocorticism in the dog. J. Am. Anim. Hosp. Assoc. 25:583, 1989.

183. Watson, A. D. J., et al.: Systemic availability of o,p'-DDD in normal dogs, fasted and fed, and in dogs with hyperadrenocorticism. Res. Vet. Sci. 43:160, 1987.

184. White, S. D.: Facial dermatosis in four dogs with hyperadrenocorticism. J. Am. Vet. Med. Assoc. 188:1441, 1986.

185. White, S. D., et al.: Cutaneous markers of canine hyperadrenocorticism. Comp. Cont. Educ. 11:446, 1989.

186. Willard, M. D., et al.: Ketoconazole-induced changes in selected canine hormone concentrations. Am. J. Vet. Res. 47:2504, 1986.

187. Willard, M. D., et al.: Effects of long-term administration of ketoconazole in cats. Am. J. Vet. Res. 47:2510, 1986.

188. Wilson, S. M., Feldman, E. C.: Diagnostic value of the steroid-induced isoenzyme of alkaline phosphatase in the dog. J. Am. Anim. Hosp. Assoc. 28:245, 1992.

188a. Young, D. W., Kemppainen, R. J.: Molecular forms of β-endorphin in the canine pituitary gland. Am. J. Vet. Res. 55:567, 1994.

189. Zenoble, R. D., Kemppainen, R. J.: Adrenocortical suppression by topically applied corticosteroids in healthy dogs. J. Am. Vet. Med. Assoc. 191:685, 1987.

190. Zerbe, C. A., et al.: Hyperadrenocorticism in a cat. J. Am. Vet. Med. Assoc. 190:559, 1987.

191. Zerbe, C. A., et al.: Effect of nonadrenal illness on adrenal function in the cat. Am. J. Vet. Res. 48:451, 1987.

Growth Hormone Physiology and Disease

192. Aribat, T., et al.: Growth hormone response induced by synthetic human growth hormone–releasing factor (1-44) in healthy dogs. J. Am. Vet. Med. Assoc. 36:367, 1989.

192a. Bell, A. G., et al.: Growth hormone responsive dermatosis in three dogs. N. Z. Vet. J. 41:195, 1993.

193. Bercu, B. B., Diamond, F. B.: Growth hormone neurosecretory dysfunction. Clin. Endocrinol. Metab. 15:537, 1986.

194. Bourdin, M., et al.: Exploration functionnelle biochimique des troubles de la sécrétion de GH. Proc. Gr. Etud. Dermatol. Anim. Cie. 7:20, 1991.

195. DeBowes, L. J.: Pituitary dwarfism in a German shepherd puppy. Comp. Cont. Educ. 9:931, 1987.

196. Eigenmann, J. E., et al.: Panhypopituitarism caused by a suprasellar tumor in a dog. J. Am. Anim. Hosp. Assoc. 19:377, 1983.

197. Eigenmann, J. E., et al.: Elevated growth hormone levels and diabetes mellitus in a cat with acromegalic features. J. Am. Anim. Hosp. Assoc. 20:747, 1984.

198. Eigenmann, J. E.: Disorders associated with growth hormone oversecretion: Diabetes mellitus and acromegaly. In: Kirk, R. W. (ed.). Current Veterinary Therapy IX. W. B. Saunders Co., Philadelphia, 1986, p. 1006.

199. Eigenmann, J. E.: Growth hormone–deficient disorders associated with alopecia in the dog. In: Kirk, R. W. (ed.). Current Veterinary Therapy IX. W. B. Saunders Co., Philadelphia, 1986, p. 1015.

200. Lothrop, C. D., Schmeitzel, L. P.: Growth hormone–responsive alopecia in dogs. Vet. Med. Rep. 2:82, 1990.

201. Lund-Larsen, T. R., Grondalen, J.: Atelotic dwarfism in the German shepherd dog. Low somatomedin activity associated with apparently normal pituitary function (two cases) and with panadenopituitary dysfunction (one case). Acta Vet. Scand. 17:298, 1976.

202. Morrison, W. B., et al.: Orally administered clonidine as a secretagogue of growth hormone and as a thymotropic agent in dogs of various ages. Am. J. Vet. Res. 51:65, 1990.

203. Randolph, J. F., et al.: Delayed growth in two German shepherd dog littermates with normal serum concentrations of growth hormone, thyroxine, and cortisol. J. Am. Vet. Med. Assoc. 196:77, 1990.

204. Randolph, J. F., Peterson, M. E.: Acromegaly (growth hormone excess) syndromes in dogs and cats. In: Kirk, R. W., Bonagura, J. D. (eds.). Kirk's Current Veterinary Therapy XI. W. B. Saunders Co., Philadelphia, 1992, p. 322.

204a. Rijnberk, A., et al.: Disturbed release of growth hormone in mature dogs: A comparison with congenital growth hormone deficiency. Vet. Rec. 133:542, 1993.

204b. Rosenkrantz, W., Griffin, C. E.: Lysodren therapy in suspect adrenal sex hormone dermatosis. Proc. Wld. Cong. Vet. Dermatol. 2:121, 1992.

205. Roth, J. A., et al.: Thymic abnormalities and growth hormone deficiency in dogs. Am. J. Vet. Res. 41:1256, 1980.

206. Roth, J. A., et al.: Improvement in clinical condition and thymus morphologic features associated with growth hormone treatment of immunodeficient dwarf dogs. Am. J. Vet. Res. 45:1151, 1984.

207. Schmeitzel, L. P., Lothrop, C. D.: Hormonal abnormalities in Pomeranians with normal coat and in Pomeranians with growth hormone–responsive dermatosis. J. Am. Vet. Med. Assoc. 197:1333, 1990.

208. Schmeitzel, L. P., Parker, W.: Growth hormone and sex hormone alopecia. In: Ihrke, P. J., et al. (eds.). Advances in Veterinary Dermatology, Vol. 2. Pergamon Press, New York, 1993, p. 451.

208a. Schmeitzel, L. P., et al.: Congenital adrenal hyperplasia–like syndrome. In: Bonagura, J. D. (ed.). Kirk's Current Veterinary Therapy XII. W. B. Saunders Co., Philadelphia, 1995.

209. Scott, D. W., Concannon, P. W.: Gross and microscopic changes in the skin of dogs with progestogen-induced acromegaly and elevated growth hormone levels. J. Am. Anim. Hosp. Assoc. 19:523, 1983.

210. Scott, D. W., Walton, D. K.: Hyposomatotropism in the mature dog: A discussion of 22 cases. J. Am. Anim. Hosp. Assoc. 22:467, 1986.

210a. Selman, P. J., et al.: Progestins and growth hormone excess in the dog. Acta Endocrinol. 125:42, 1991.

211. Shanley, K. J., Miller, W. H.: Adult-onset growth hormone deficiency in sibling Airedale terriers. Comp. Cont. Educ. 9:1076, 1987.

211a. Trotot, V., et al.: Effets des conditions de conservation du sang total et du plasma de chien sur la concentration plasmatique en hormone de croissance. Rev. Méd. Vét. 144:909, 1993.

Sex Hormone Physiology and Disease

212. Barsanti, J. A., et al.: Diethylstilbestrol-induced alopecia in a dog. J. Am. Vet. Med. Assoc. 182:63, 1983.
213. Bruinsma, D. L., Ackerman, L. A.: Male pseudohermaphroditism in a Miniature Schnauzer. Vet. Med. (S.A.C.) 78:1568, 1983.
214. Carlson, R. A.: Endocrine alopecia in a dog showing response to FSH administration. J. Am. Anim. Hosp. Assoc. 21:735, 1985.
215. Eigenmann, J. E.: Estrogen-induced flank alopecia in the female dog: Evidence for local rather than systemic hyperestrogenism. J. Am. Anim. Hosp. Assoc. 20:621, 1984.
216. England, G. C. W., et al.: Evaluation of the testosterone response to hCG and the identification of a presumed anorchid dog. J. Small Anim. Pract. 30:441, 1989.
217. Fadok, V. A., et al.: Hyperprogesteronemia associated with Sertoli cell tumor and alopecia in a dog. J. Am. Vet. Med. Assoc. 188:1058, 1986.
218. Fayrer-Hosken, R. A., et al.: Follicular cystic ovaries and cystic endometrial hyperplasia in a bitch. J. Am. Vet. Med. Assoc. 201:107, 1992.
219. Feldman, S. R.: Androgen insensitivity syndrome (testicular feminization): A model for understanding steroid hormone receptors. J. Am. Acad. Dermatol. 27:615, 1992.
220. Fiorito, D. A.: Hyperestrogenism in bitches. Comp. Cont. Educ. 14:727, 1992.
221. Fourrier, P., Lepesant, V.: Dysendocrinie sexuelle chez un caniche mâle agé de 5 ans. Prat. Méd. Chirurg. Anim. Comp. 22:395, 1987.
222. Griffin, C.: Linear prepucial erythema. Proc. Am. Acad. Vet. Dermatol. Am. Coll. Vet. Dermatol. 2:35, 1986.
223. Grossman, C. J.: Regulation of the immune system by sex steroids. Endocr. Rev. 5:435, 1984.
223a. Hammerling, R., et al.: Is there a role for estradiol in the etiology of dermatoses in the male dog? Proc. Am. Acad. Vet. Dermatol. Am. Coll. Vet. Dermatol. 10:82, 1994.
224. Hubert, B., Olivry, T.: Dermatologie et hormones sexuelles chez les carnivores domestiques 1re partie: Physio-pathologie. Prat. Méd. Chirurg. Anim. Cie. 25:477, 1990.
225. Hubert, B., Olivry, T.: Dermatologie et hormones sexuelles chez les carnivores domestiques 2e partie: Étude clinique. Prat. Méd. Chirurg. Anim. Cie. 25:483, 1990.
226. Johnson, G. R., et al.: Ultrasonographic features of testicular neoplasia in dogs: 16 cases (1980–1988). J. Am. Vet. Med. Assoc. 198:1779, 1991.
226a. Ladds, P. W.: The male genital system. In: Jubb, K. V., et al. (eds.). Pathology of Domestic Animals, 4th ed., Vol. 3. Academic Press, New York, 1993, p. 471.
227. Laing, E. J., et al.: Spermatic cord torsion and Sertoli cell tumor in a dog. J. Am. Vet. Med. Assoc. 183:879, 1983.
228. Lanore, D., et al.: Métastase sécrétante d'un sertolinome. Prat. Méd. Chirurg. Anim. Cie. 27:727, 1992.
229. Lecomte, R.: Hyperoestrogenisme spontané ou iatrogène et ses répercussions cliniques et hématologiques. Prat. Méd. Chirurg. Anim. Cie. 24:73, 1989.
229a. Leyva-Ocariz, H.: Effect of hyperadrenocorticism and diabetes mellitus on serum progesterone concentrations during early metoestrus of pregnant and nonpregnant cycles induced by pregnant mares' serum gonadotrophin in domestic dogs. J. Reprod. Fert. (suppl.) 47:371, 1993.
230. Mann, F. A., et al.: Serum testosterone and estradiol 17-beta concentrations in 15 dogs with perineal hernia. J. Am. Vet. Med. Assoc. 194:1578, 1989.
231. Medleau, L.: Sex hormone–associated endocrine alopecias in dogs. J. Am. Anim. Hosp. Assoc. 25:689, 1989.
232. Miller, W. H., Jr.: Sex hormone–related dermatoses in dogs. In: Kirk, R. W. (ed.). Current Veterinary Therapy X. W. B. Saunders, Co., 1989, p. 595.
233. Morris, B. J.: Fatal bone marrow suppression as a result of Sertoli cell tumor. Vet. Med. (S. A. C.) 78:1070, 1983.
234. Nemzek, J. A., et al.: Cystic ovaries and hyperestrogenism in a canine female pseudohermaphrodite. J. Am. Anim. Hosp. Assoc. 28:402, 1992.
235. Schmeitzel, L. P., Lothrop, C. D.: Sex hormones and skin disease. Vet. Med. Rep. 2:28, 1990.
236. Scott, D. W., Reimers, T. J.: Tail gland and perianal gland hyperplasia associated with testicular neoplasia and hypertestosteronemia in a dog. Canine Pract. 13:15, 1986.
237. Suess, R. P., et al.: Bone marrow hypoplasia in a feminized dog with an interstitial cell tumor. J. Am. Vet. Med. Assoc. 200:1346, 1992.
238. Watson, A. D. J.: Oestrogen-induced alopecia in a bitch. J. Small Anim. Pract. 26:17, 1985.
239. Weaver, A. D.: Survey with follow-up of 67 dogs with testicular Sertoli cell tumours. Vet. Rec. 113:105, 1983.

Miscellaneous

239a. Bussiéras, J., et al.: Intérêt possible du minoxidil dans le traitement de certaines alopécies canines. Prat. Méd. Chirurg. Anim. Cie. 22:25, 1987.
240. Camy, G.: Alopécie endocrinienne associée à un diabète chez un chien. Point. Vét. 20:501, 1988.
241. Carpenter, J. L., et al.: Cutaneous xanthogranuloma and viral papilloma on an eyelid of a cat. Vet. Dermatol. 3:1987, 1992.
242. Chastain, C. B., Graham, C. L.: Xanthomatosis secondary to diabetes mellitus in a dog. J. Am. Vet. Med. Assoc. 172:1209, 1978.
242a. Denerolle, P. J.: Three cases of feline cutaneous xanthomas. Proc. Wld. Cong. Vet. Dermatol. 2:84, 1992.
243. Grieshaber, T. L., et al.: Spontaneous cutaneous (eruptive) xanthomatosis in two cats. J. Am. Anim. Hosp. Assoc. 27:509, 1991.

244. Gross, T. E., et al.: Glucagon-producing pancreatic endocrine tumors in two dogs with superficial necrolytic dermatitis. J. Am. Vet. Med. Assoc. 197:1619, 1990.

245. Gross, T. L., et al.: Superficial necrolytic dermatitis (necrolytic migratory erythema) in dogs. Vet. Pathol. 30:75, 1993.

245a. Harvey, R. G.: The use of minoxidil (Loniten, Upjohn), in selected cases of canine alopecia. A report of an open trial. Vet. Dermatol. Newsl. 12:36, 1990.

246. Huntley, A. C.: The cutaneous manifestations of diabetes mellitus. J. Am. Acad. Dermatol. 7:427, 1982.

247. Jones, B. R., et al.: Cutaneous xanthomata associated with diabetes mellitus in a cat. J. Small Anim. Pract. 26:33, 1985.

248. Jones, B. R., et al.: Inherited hyperchylomicronemia in the cat. Feline Pract. 16:7, 1986.

249. Kwochka, K. W., Short, B. G.: Cutaneous xanthomatosis and diabetes mellitus following long-term therapy with megestrol acetate in a cat. Comp. Cont. Educ. 6:185, 1984.

250. Latimer, K. S., Mahaffey, E. A.: Neutrophil adherence and movement in poorly and well-controlled diabetic dogs. Am. J. Vet. Res. 45:1498, 1984.

251. McNeil, P. E.: The underlying pathology of the hepatocutaneous syndrome: A report of 18 cases. In: Ihrke, P. J., et al. (eds.). Advances in Veterinary Dermatology, Vol. 2. Pergamon Press, New York, 1993, p. 113.

252. Miller, W. H., Jr., et al.: Necrolytic migratory erythema in dogs. A hepatocutaneous syndrome. J. Am. Anim. Hosp. Assoc. 26:573, 1990.

253. Miller, W. H., Jr., et al.: Necrolytic migratory erythema in a dog with a glucagon-secreting endocrine tumor. Vet. Dermatol. 2:179, 1991.

254. Niemand, H. G.: Bildbericht. Kleintierpraxis 16:193, 1971.

254a. Price, V. H. (ed.): Rogaine (topical minoxidil, 2%) in the management of male pattern baldness and alopecia areata. J. Am. Acad. Dermatol. 16(3 Pt. 2), 1987.

255. Walton, D. K., et al.: Ulcerative dermatosis associated with diabetes mellitus in the dog: A report of four cases. J. Am. Anim. Hosp. Assoc. 22:79, 1986.

256. Wilkinson, J. S.: Spontaneous diabetes mellitus. Vet. Rec. 72:548, 1960.

Acquired Alopecias

■

Chapter Outline

An acquired alopecia is a hair loss that develops sometime during the life of an animal. The hereditary alopecias (see Chap. 11) and hair losses that develop as a result of specific disease processes, such as dermatophytosis, endocrine abnormalities, immunologic diseases, or self-inflicted hair loss from hypersensitivity or parasitism are discussed elsewhere in this book. The conditions presented here include canine and feline pinnal alopecia, feline acquired symmetric alopecia, short hair syndrome of silky breeds, preauricular alopecia of cats, excessive shedding, anagen and telogen defluxion, traction alopecia, trichorrhexis nodosa, cyclic follicular dysplasia, injection reactions, and cicatricial alopecia.

■ CANINE ACQUIRED ALOPECIAS

Canine Pinnal Alopecia

Pinnal alopecia is most common in dachshunds but has also been observed in other breeds, such as Chihuahuas, Boston terriers, Whippets, and Italian Greyhounds. The pinnal alopecia is seldom noticed in animals less than 1 year of age. If it is, a genetic alopecia is likely. At first, the haircoat is thinner and the hairs become smaller than normal on the pinnae. Progressive diminution of the hairs makes the alopecia more prevalent as the dog ages. With close observation, however, the clinician notes that very small vellus hairs are still present (Fig. 10:1*A*). Uncommonly, the condition may progress to total pinnal alopecia when the dog reaches 8 to 9 years of age. The remainder of the dog's coat is normal. Diagnosis is facilitated by dermatopathologic examination, which helps rule out other diseases. Changes similar to those of pattern baldness may be seen; these include hair follicles that are often in anagen but are reduced in length and diameter. No treatment is available.

It is important to differentiate such spontaneous alopecias from dermatoses that cause hair loss on the pinnae. Hair follicle dysplasias, estrogen-responsive dermatosis, rare cases of hypothyroidism, hyperadrenocorticism, dermatophytosis, and alopecia areata may also cause pinnal alopecia. However, these other differentials do not feature miniaturization of hairs. Vasculitis can occur on the pinnae and cause alopecia with severe erythema, scaling, crusting, and eventually ulceration and tissue loss at the pinna margin. Other inflammatory diseases may cause alopecia and are differentiated by the history of inflammation or previous pruritus.

Pattern Baldness

Pattern baldness is most commonly seen in dachshunds but may be seen in breeds such as the Manchester terrier, Miniature Doberman pinscher, and Chihuahua.[8] The cause is unknown, but the alopecia is probably genetically determined (see Chap. 11).

Canine Follicular Dysplasia

There is a group of diseases characterized by coat changes, including alopecia, that are referred to as follicular dysplasia. Color dilution alopecia is a well-documented hereditary follicular dysplasia (see Chap. 11). Among certain breeds, including Siberian husky, Irish water spaniel, Portuguese water dog, curly coated retriever, boxer, Airedale terrier, English and French bulldogs and Miniature Schnauzers, there is a marked predilection, suggesting a genetic basis (see Chap. 11) (Fig. 10:2).[4] In addition, there are several endocrine syndromes (adrenal sex hormone imbalances) that may also have abnormalities in follicular receptors, indicating a component of the disease that may be considered a dysplasia. These syndromes also have predisposed breeds, the Pomeranian, the Samoyed, and the Chow Chow (see Chap. 9). Clinical findings in these dogs include poor, dry, frizzy haircoats, changes in coat color, loss of primary

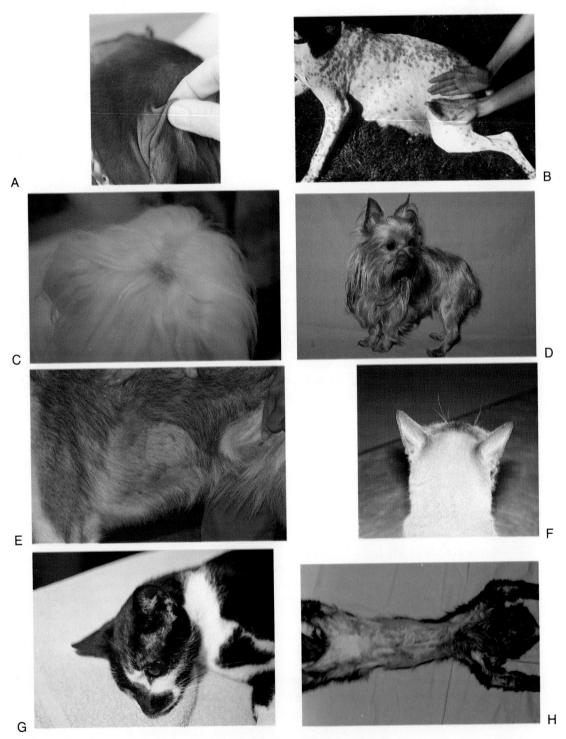

Figure 10:1 *See legend on opposite page*

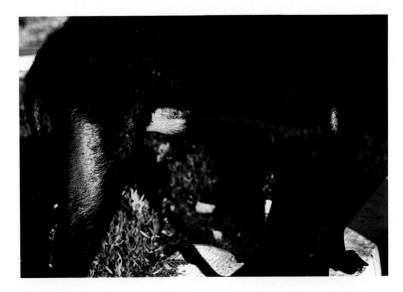

Figure 10:2. Curly coated retriever with pattern alopecia from a hair follicle dysplasia. The condition stopped progressing when the dog became 2 years old.

hairs and retention of secondary hairs, development of curly or twisted hairshafts, and varying degrees of alopecia. Some cases have presented for failure to regrow their coat following clipping (Fig. 10:3). These dogs were usually clipped because of a poor or dull coat that the owner believed would improve with regrowth after clipping. In general, changes are most pronounced on the truncal part of the body; however, the neck and proximal extremities are often involved as well.

Diagnosis is based on histopathologic examination. Different features may be seen in the various breeds, suggesting that multiple abnormalities may be occurring and vary from breed to breed or syndrome to syndrome. Histologic changes can include macromelanosomes, distortion of hairshafts or follicle shape, follicular hyperkeratosis, distorted anagen hair bulbs, abnormal tricholemmal keratinization, and a predominance of catagen or telogen follicles.[4, 20] Treatment of these disorders has not been very successful, nor has much been reported. Synthetic retinoids, particularly etretinate, may be helpful in some cases.[2, 3, 9]

Anagen and Telogen Defluxion

In *anagen defluxion,* a special circumstance (e.g., antimitotic drugs, infectious diseases, endocrine disorders, or metabolic diseases) interferes with anagen, resulting in abnormalities of the hair follicle and hair shaft. Hair loss occurs suddenly, within days of the insult, as the growth phase continues (Fig. 10:4*A* and *B*).[1c, 7] In *telogen defluxion,* a stressful circumstance (e.g., high fever, pregnancy, shock, severe illness, surgery, or anesthesia) causes the abrupt, premature cessation of growth of many anagen hair follicles and the synchronization of these hair follicles in catagen, then in telogen.[1c, 7] Within 1 to 3 months of the initial insult, a large number of telogen hairs are shed as a new wave of hair follicle cyclic activity begins (see Fig. 10:1*B*).

Figure 10:1. *A*, Pinnal alopecia in a dachshund. Note the small vellus hairs still present on folded skin margins. *B*, Telogen defluxion. Postpartum shedding resulting from the physiologic stress of gestation and lactation. *C*, Traction alopecia in a Maltese. Note the oval erythematous alopecic patch caused by a barrette used to pull the hair snugly forward. *D*, Yorkshire terrier with short hair syndrome. This dog previously had long, silky hair that reached the floor. *E*, Area of alopecia that persisted for 3½ months in a Siberian husky before hair regrowth occurred. *F*, Periodic alopecia of the pinnae of a Siamese cat. Hair will regrow spontaneously. The cause is unknown. *G*, Preauricular feline alopecia. Note normal sparseness of hair between the eye and the ear. *H*, Feline symmetric alopecia. Ventral view showing characteristic bilateral alopecia without skin reaction or lesions.

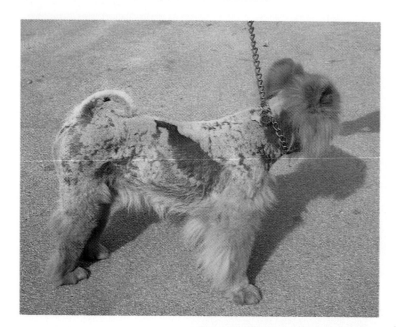

Figure 10:3. A Chow Chow that had been clipped because of a poor haircoat. The truncal hair did not regrow after the clipping.

Figure 10:4. *A*, Anagen defluxion in a kitten during the course of an acute viral upper respiratory infection. Note the widespread disheveled and fractured appearance of the haircoat. *B*, Hairs from a dog with anagen defluxion. Note the focal area of transient metabolic arrest and the structural defect that is susceptible to fracture *(arrow)*.

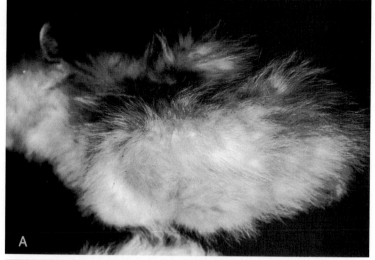

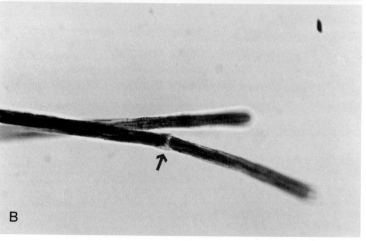

Diagnosis is based on history, physical examination, and direct hair examination. Telogen hairs are characterized by a uniform shaft diameter and a slightly clubbed, nonpigmented root end that lacks root sheaths (see Chap. 2). Anagen defluxion hairs are characterized by irregularities and dysplastic changes. The diameter of the shaft may be irregularly narrowed and deformed, and breaking often occurs at such structurally weakened sites, resulting in ragged points (see Chap. 2). Skin biopsy is only rarely helpful. When the alopecia due to telogen defluxion begins, histopathologic examination shows only normal skin. In anagen defluxion, the characteristic changes are usually most evident in the affected hairs, and these are usually lost when the skin is clipped for biopsy. Typical histopathologic findings in anagen defluxion include apoptosis and fragmented cell nuclei in the hair matrix of anagen hair follicles, and eosinophilic dysplastic hair shafts within the pilar canal.[20]

Both anagen and telogen defluxion spontaneously resolve when the inciting factor is relieved.

Excessive Shedding

Owners often ask ''Why does my dog (or cat) shed so much?'' They are naturally concerned about large amounts of hair getting on their rugs, furniture, and clothing. If excessively shed hairs are not associated with gross alopecia, the condition may cause inconvenience to the owner, but it is probably normal or at least causes no problem for the animal. The hair growth cycle is controlled by a number of factors (see Chap. 1), and the questions about shedding are often difficult to answer. Very little information about it is available in the literature. In the northern hemisphere, many outdoor dogs and cats shed to varying degrees in spring and fall; indoor pets may shed all year long. When animals are shedding excessively, many hairs can be easily epilated, but areas of actual alopecia *cannot* be created. In contrast, the clinician can usually create alopecia by gentle manual epilation in animals with hair loss due to endocrine disorders and follicular dysplasias. When there is no obvious clinical disease, modification of diet or adjustment of light and temperature can be considered treatment. If no abnormal conditions can be discovered, the only treatment is to remove the dead telogen hairs from the animal by combing, brushing, or, in some cases, vacuuming.

Traction Alopecia

Traction alopecia has been described in dogs that have had barrettes, rubber bands, or other methods used to tie up their hair.[10, 20] When these devices have been applied too tightly or for too much time, alopecia may result. Initially, an inflammatory plaque may occur, but it progresses to an atrophic scarred patch. Invariably, lesions are present on the top or lateral aspects of the cranium. If the disease is allowed to progress too long, the alopecia becomes permanent (see Fig. 10:1 C).

Diagnosis is based on the characteristic history and physical examination findings. In the late stages, there are few differentials because of the atrophic nature and location of the alopecia. Early lesions should be differentiated from alopecia areata and dermatophytosis. Biopsy findings depend on the stage of the lesion that is sampled.[10, 20] Early lesions may show variable mononuclear cell infiltrates, edema, and vasodilatation. Hydropic degeneration of epidermal basal cells and apoptosis may be seen. Chronic cases may be characterized by fibrosing dermatitis and scarring alopecia or a ''cell–poor'' hydropic interface dermatosis with marked pilosebaceous atrophy (''faded'' follicles).

Treatment consists of instructing the owner regarding proper placement of hair-holding devices. Atrophic scars do not respond to medical therapy; if treatment is desired for cosmetic purposes, surgical excision is required.

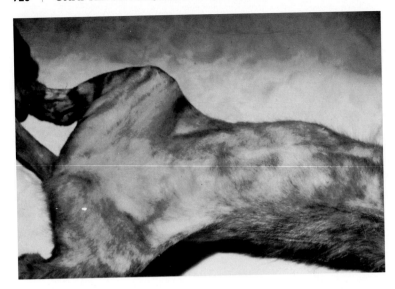

Figure 10:5. Trichorrhexis nodosa associated with chronic use of flea shampoo on a cat. Note the generalized hypotrichosis and broken hairs of varying lengths.

Figure 10:6. *A,* Trichorrhexis nodosa. Hair from the cat in Figure 10:5. Note the nodular area in the center of the hair shaft, where breakage will occur. *B,* Trichorrhexis nodosa. Hair from the cat in Figure 10:5. This hair has fractured at a nodule, giving the appearance of two brooms end to end.

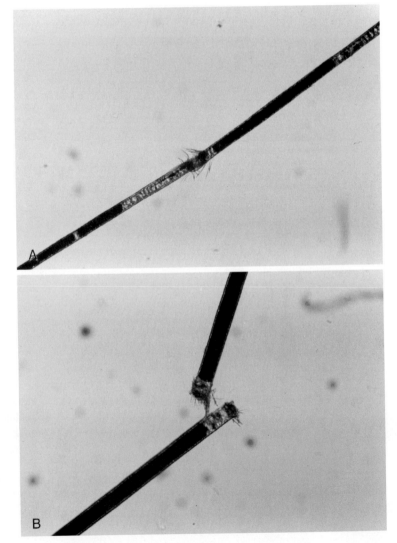

Trichorrhexis Nodosa

Trichorrhexis nodosa appears along the hair shaft as small, beaded swellings associated with a loss of cuticle.[5, 18] The expanded areas are composed of frayed cortical fibers through which the hair readily fractures. The basic cause is trauma, and a contributing factor is inherent weakness of the hair shaft. Examples of physical trauma include excessive brushing, back combing, application of heat, and prolonged ultraviolet light exposure. Sources of chemical trauma include bathing in excessively salty water or chlorinated swimming pools, shampooing, and insecticidal or acaricidal dips.

Clinical signs include multifocal or generalized hypotrichosis, wherein affected areas show broken, stubby hairs (Fig. 10:5). Trichogram reveals hairs with nodular areas of cortical splitting that resemble two brooms pushed together (Fig. 10:6 *A* and *B*).

Treatment requires eliminating the source of physical or chemical trauma.

Cyclic Follicular Dysplasia

Dogs occasionally develop a temporary pattern alopecia. Typically, truncal alopecia or marked thinning of the haircoat is present, but associated scaling and inflammation are absent. Most commonly, lesions involve the trunk, especially the flank region. In some cases, the problem is a seasonal one, with hair loss occurring primarily in the winter or spring months. This kind of alopecia appears to be more of a problem in Alaska, where it has been seen in Labrador retrievers, mixed breeds, Yorkshire terriers, and an Airedale terrier[11]; therefore, duration of light exposure may be important. Some dogs may experience only one or two episodes, whereas others develop some degree of alopecia every year. In a sense, this condition may be considered an abnormal shedding pattern.

SEASONAL FLANK ALOPECIA

Seasonal flank alopecia is a more localized cyclic follicular dysplasia that also tends to occur in the fall or spring.[1b, 4, 6, 13] Some dogs lose hair in the late fall and regrow it spontaneously in the spring; others do the reverse and lose hair in the spring. Airedale terriers, English bulldogs and boxers are at higher risk, but the condition has been described in Miniature Schnauzers, Miniature Poodles, Doberman pinschers, Bouvier de Flanders, Scottish terriers, and French bulldogs.[6, 13, 20] These dogs develop a nonscarring alopecia most often confined to the thoracolumbar region (Fig. 10:7). The lesions are bilaterally symmetric, annular to polycyclic in shape

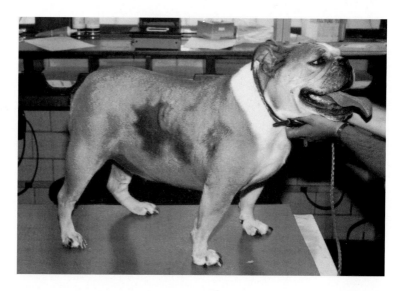

Figure 10:7. English bulldog with recurrent seasonal flank alopecia (follicular dysplasia). Note alopecia and hyperpigmentation.

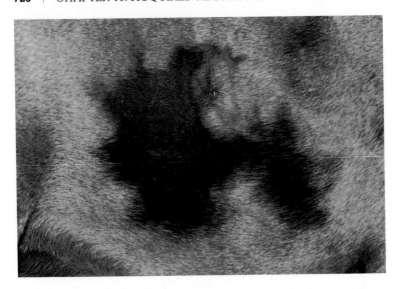

Figure 10:8. Close-up of the dog in Figure 10:7. Note the generally well-circumscribed scalloped margins of alopecia.

and have well-demarcated borders; in addition, the alopecic skin is usually markedly hyperpigmented (Fig. 10:8). Scaling and bacterial folliculitis may occur in the alopecic areas. In some dogs, only one side of the body is affected, or one side is more severely affected than the other.[6] The spontaneous regrowth of hair that occurs in 3 to 4 months may consist of completely normal hair, or hair that is a different color, texture, or both. In over half the cases, the hair

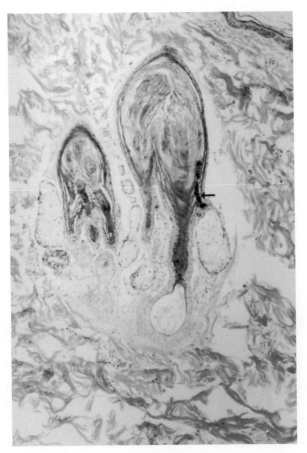

Figure 10:9. Seasonal flank alopecia. Note the dysplastic, keratin-filled hair follicles with tentacular projections into underlying dermis (octopus- or jelly fish–like appearance). Note also the melanin cast in the sebaceous duct *(arrow).*

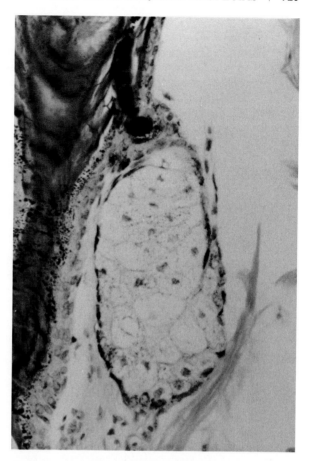

Figure 10:10. Close-up of Figure 10:9. Note the fine stippling of the sebaceous gland with melanin and the melanin cast within the associated sebaceous duct.

loss occurs at least twice in successive years.[6] To date, underlying causes, such as common endocrinopathies, have not been identified.

Histologically, the fully developed lesions reveal follicular atrophy and infundibular hyperkeratosis, which extends into the opening of secondary follicles and sebaceous ducts, giving the appearance of a malformed foot.[6] Dysplastic follicles usually have an octopus– or jelly fish–like appearance (Fig. 10:9); the hyperkeratotic, distended infundibulum is the body and the subjacent secondary follicles are the tentacles. Sebaceous glands are melanized (Fig. 10:10). As melanin-containing sebocytes undergo their normal degenerative process, plugs of melanin are formed in sebaceous ducts and extruded as casts into the distended hair follicle infundibulum (see Fig. 10:9).[13]

There is currently no effective treatment for seasonal or cyclic follicular dysplasia. The prognosis is unpredictable in any given dog. Some dogs continue to develop recurrent seasonal hair loss for years; other dogs have an occasional year when the alopecia does not recur; still other dogs eventually develop permanent alopecia.[6, 13] The degree of alopecia is also variable with some dogs developing a virtually identical hair loss year after year, and other dogs developing larger areas of hair loss as years go by.[6]

Injection Reactions

Injection reactions may induce focal areas of alopecia. Two types may be seen. In the first, there is an inflammatory reaction that is usually either a panniculitis or a vasculitis. Rabies vaccines (particularly those licensed for subcutaneous use) are most commonly associated with the vasculitic form of this disease.[12, 19, 20] In the second type, there is no gross inflammation and the hair just falls out. There may be associated pigment changes and dermal and epidermal atrophy. This form of reaction most commonly occurs with subcutaneous injections of glucocorticoid or progestational compounds.

Lesions are most commonly seen over the shoulders, back, and posterolateral thighs, at sites where injections are given. The inflammatory reactions initially present as a circular to oval erythematous plaque. It is firm when palpated and may extend into the deeper tissues. In some cases, the skin is not erythematous but just thickened and firm. Chronically, the alopecic area becomes hyperpigmented and shiny, with or without mild scaling. The noninflammatory form presents as an atrophic hypopigmented oval to circular patch (Fig. 10:11). With both forms, the first signs of the lesions usually occur 2 to 4 months after an injection.

Diagnosis is based on the presence of typical lesions with a compatible history. Differential diagnoses are dermatophytosis, folliculitis, cellulitis, demodicosis, alopecia areata, and localized scleroderma. Dermatopathologic examination is useful for establishing the diagnosis and ruling out the other differentials. In the inflammatory form, varying degrees of panniculitis are present, and lymphoid nodules are often prominent.[4, 20] Vasculitis may or may not be evident. The overlying hair follicles are telogenized, atrophic, and occasionally miniaturized. In the noninflammatory form, varying degrees of dermal and pilosebaceous atrophy are present.

Treatment is not usually required, although it may take months to over a year before hair regrowth occurs. In some cases, the alopecia is permanent. When hair regrowth does occur, the new hairs are often a different color. When hair growth does not recur, surgical excision is effective. For the inflammatory form, intralesional or systemic glucocorticoids may be beneficial.

Short Hair Syndrome of Silky Breeds

Yorkshire terriers and silky terriers normally have long, silky hair coats. The luxurious coat was achieved by many generations of selective breeding, and it is a source of great pride to the

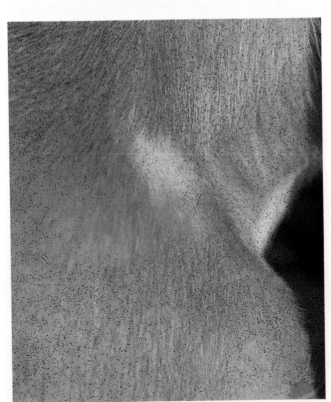

Figure 10:11. Focal area of noninflammatory alopecia following a glucocorticoid injection.

pet's owner. Occasionally, an apparently normal-coated mature dog loses its coat, and the coat is replaced with hairs that never grow to their former full length (see Fig. 10:1 *D*).[8] The owner is distressed by this and seeks help, often after unsuccessfully trying vitamin and mineral supplements or coat conditioners containing fatty acids. The affected dogs have no itching, erythema, or scaling of the skin. Onset occurs when the dog is 1 to 5 years of age. There are no broken or bitten hairs. Because the long silky hairs are gone, the remaining haircoat would be adequate for a mixed-breed dog or a purebred dog with shorter hair. The condition also occurs in younger dogs. In such cases, the puppy coat is normal, but it is replaced with a permanent shorter coat. The abnormal new coat is apparent when the dog is 5 months of age. The hair on the head is of normal length; however, the posterior abdominal area, hind legs, and chest have hairs that are shorter than normal. There is no scaliness or inflammation of the skin.

It can only be theorized that the hair cycle has been shortened by some unknown factor, such that the hairs are shed before they reach their normal full length. The most important differential diagnoses are hair follicle dysplasias, endocrine (especially hypothyroidism) and congenital disorders, and psychogenic alopecia. There is no known treatment.

Post-Clipping Alopecia

Failure to regrow hair following clipping has been termed *post-clipping alopecia*.[4] The hairs may not regrow for up to 24 months, but they usually regrow within 1 year. Although this condition has been described as relatively common, the authors consider it uncommon in their clinical experiences and discussion with groomers and surgeons. It is seen more often in breeds with long, thick coats, such as Siberian huskies and Chow Chows, but it may occur in any dog (see Fig. 10:1 *E*). The condition is most commonly seen following clipping for surgical procedures or for the removal of mats. The clinical appearance is typical; in the affected areas, the coat looks exactly as it did after it was clipped several months previously. The rest of the coat is usually normal. It has been proposed that this syndrome may occur as the result of vascular perfusion changes in response to cutaneous temperature changes.[4] Another possibility, however, is that these dogs are in their normal catagen stage of hair growth, between losing and growing a new haircoat. This theory is supported by the discovery of similar histologic changes in biopsies from normal-haired and affected areas[2]; both can show catagen arrest. Most of these dogs regrow hair in the clipped area after they go through a heavy shedding or so-called blowing of their coat.[2]

Cicatricial Alopecia

A variety of diseases may result in a scarring alopecia. Once adnexal units are replaced by scar tissue, hair loss becomes permanent.[4] In addition to the scarring diseases, deep physical, thermal, and chemical injury may result in scarring alopecia.

■ FELINE ACQUIRED ALOPECIAS

Feline Pinnal Alopecia

Some Siamese cats develop a spontaneous periodic alopecia of the ears (see Fig. 10:1 *F*). Lesions are typically present on both pinnae. The alopecia may be patchy or involve most of the pinnal surface, and the affected skin is clinically normal. After several months, the hair regrows without treatment. The cause is unknown.[15]

Feline Preauricular Alopecia

The temporal region between the ear and eye of cats is more sparsely haired than are other parts of the head (see Fig. 10:1 *G*). This is a physiologic, not a pathologic, condition.[15] In longhaired or densely coated cats, this area is not noticeable; however, in cats with short or less dense haircoats, it can look like an alopecia. When cat owners ask their veterinarians about the condition, they can be told that the condition is normal and neither requires nor would respond to treatment. In typical cases, skin scrapings, fungal cultures, and biopsies are totally unnecessary. If inflammation, excessive scale, or follicular casts are present, diagnostic tests for other diseases should be considered.

Feline Acquired Symmetric Alopecia

Feline acquired symmetric alopecia (formerly feline endocrine alopecia) is a rare acquired bilaterally symmetric hypotrichosis of unknown origin.[7, 14, 16]

CAUSE AND PATHOGENESIS

The exact cause and pathogenesis of feline acquired symmetric alopecia are unknown. The name was changed in the last edition of this book because no true endocrine cause had been proved.[8] Recently, however, there has been a study that suggests there may be abnormal thyroid function and 73 per cent of affected cats responded to liothyronine (T_3) therapy.[16, 17] One theory suggested that these cats may have had a decreased thyroid reserve. The results were based on basal changes in group averages. Individual cases can have normal total thyroxine (TT_4) or TT_3 levels or a normal response to thyroid-stimulating hormone (TSH). However, as groups, these cats had a depressed response to TSH.[17] It has also been observed that an identical pattern of alopecia can be self-inflicted. Because cats are sometimes secret groomers, the owners may not be aware that they are licking or pulling excessively at the hairs. Hair regrowth that occurs with gonadal or thyroid hormones in these cats may be due to psychological or other changes not related to treatment of a true deficiency. In this syndrome, placement of an Elizabethan collar or bucket on the cat's head for several weeks will demonstrate whether the alopecia was self-inflicted. If hair regrowth does not occur, traumatic causes can be excluded and this syndrome should then be considered.

CLINICAL FEATURES

Feline acquired symmetric alopecia is a rare disease seen mostly in neutered male and female cats. No breed predilection has been reported, but purebred cats are rarely affected. The age of affected cats ranges from 2 to 12 years, with an average of 6 years.

Feline acquired symmetric alopecia is characterized by bilaterally symmetric hypotrichosis, which begins in the genital and perineal regions (see Fig. 10:1 *H*). Diffuse thinning of the hair, rather than complete baldness, affects the anogenital region, proximal tail, caudomedial thighs, and ventral abdomen. Long-standing cases may have hypotrichosis of the lateral thorax and flanks, but the dorsum is spared. Hairs in the affected areas are easily epilated. Pruritus and skin lesions are usually absent.

DIAGNOSIS

The first diagnostic question is whether the cat has bitten or licked the hairs, and thereby caused the alopecia, or the hairs have fallen out by themselves. Close examination by rolling the skin reveals normal numbers of hairs in cats that lick off the hair (Fig. 10:12). Trichogram helps because the distal hair tips are intact and pointed, and the proximal (bulbar) ends are telogenized in this syndrome. If the distal end of the hair shows a broken or chewed off edge, the cat is creating the hair loss. It must be emphasized here that most cats with a symmetric alopecia that appears noninflammatory *are* causing it by licking and chewing and do *not* have acquired symmetric alopecia.[7]

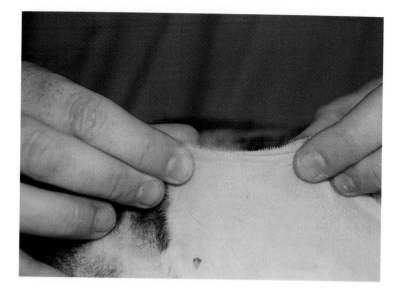

Figure 10:12. Atopic cat with skin being rolled between fingers, revealing normal numbers of short, barbed off hairs.

The differential diagnosis includes the pruritic causes of alopecia such as flea bite hypersensitivity, atopy, food hypersensitivity, psychogenic alopecia, dermatophytosis, feline demodicosis (rare), and ectoparasites such as *Otodectes cynotis* and *Cheyletiella blakei*. Nonpruritic causes of alopecia include hypothyroidism (extremely rare), hyperadrenocorticism (extremely rare), excessive shedding, trichorrhexis nodosa, and telogen and anagen defluxion. Definitive diagnosis is based on history, physical examination, results of laboratory studies, and response to therapy. Hemogram, serum chemistries, urinalysis, and tests of thyroid and adrenal function are normal. Skin biopsy reveals telogenization of hair follicles.[20]

CLINICAL MANAGEMENT

The client should be counseled about the benign nature of this condition and informed that treatment may not be necessary. If treatment is elected, liothyronine should be tried initially. Liothyronine given orally at 20 μg/cat q12h slowly increasing to 50 μg/cat should be administered for 12 weeks.[16] The most significant side-effects to consider are cardiac arrhythmias, including premature ventricular beats.

Alternatively, combined androgen-estrogen therapy appears to be more effective than either sex hormone alone.[15] Excellent results have been obtained with intramuscular injections of repositol testosterone (12.5 mg/cat) and repositol diethylstilbestrol (0.625 mg/cat). If diethylstilbestrol is unavailable, one can use estradiol (0.5 mg/cat). The cats are re-examined in 6 weeks, and if new hair growth is not evident, a second injection is given. Relapse occurs after a variable period of time (6 months to 2 years) in about 50 per cent of the cats, and retreatment is usually effective. The occasional transient side-effects that are seen with androgen-estrogen therapy are signs of estrus in females and aggressiveness, urine spraying, or both in males. These signs are seen during the first week of therapy. Overdose of either testosterone or estrogen can result in severe hepatobiliary disease and death. Repositol testosterone, repositol diethylstilbestrol, and repositol estradiol are not licensed for use in cats in the United States.

Progestational compounds are also effective for the treatment of feline acquired symmetric alopecia.[15] Repositol progesterone (2.2 to 22 mg/kg) or medroxyprogesterone acetate (50 to 175 mg/cat) may be administered intramuscularly or subcutaneously. The cats are re-examined in 6 weeks, and a second injection is given if hair regrowth is not evident. Megestrol acetate may be given orally (2.5 to 5 mg/cat), once every other day, until hair growth is evident. A maintenance dose of 2.5 to 5 mg/cat, once every 1 to 2 weeks, is usually required. Because potential side-effects of progestational compounds in the cat are numerous and occasionally severe, the previously mentioned treatments, or *no* treatments are recommended (see Chap. 3). Progestational compounds are not licensed for use in cats in the United States. Interestingly, they can produce feline symmetric alopecia–like hair loss.

Injection Reactions

Cats may also react to various subcutaneous injections, though less frequently. Rabies reactions similar to those in dogs have been described.[12] Praziquantel (Droncit) has been incriminated in multiple cases. Besides the inflammatory alopecic form, a pruritic ulcerative form may also occur (Fig. 10:13). These reactions can be very difficult to manage, and the cats often develop secondary infections. Because most of these lesions occur in the dorsocervical or shoulder region, the major differential diagnosis is feline ulcerative linear fibrosing dermatitis (see Chap. 17). Chronic vaccine reactions have been incriminated as a cause of neoplasia, especially fibrosarcomas, in the cat (see Chap. 19).

Pancreatic Paraneoplastic Alopecia

This recently recognized syndrome has been seen in old cats that present with a 2-week to 2-month history of inappetance, lethargy, weight loss, and progressive alopecia.[1a] The alopecia involves the ventrum and the legs, and focal areas of scaling may be present. Hair is easily epilated from all over the body. The footpads are painful, and the cats are reluctant to walk. Skin biopsy reveals telogenization of hair follicles and focal areas of epidermal hyperplasia, alternating orthokeratotic and parakeratotic hyperkeratosis, and a mild superficial lymphocytic perivascular dermatitis. All cats had a pancreatic carcinoma of either acinar cell or pancreatic duct origin.

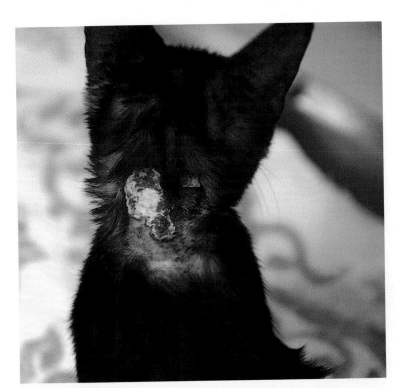

Figure 10:13. Injection reaction due to subcutaneous administration of Droncit.

REFERENCES

1a. Brooks, D. G., et al.: Pancreatic paraneoplastic alopecia in 3 cats. J. Am. Anim. Hosp. Assoc. (accepted 1993).

1b. Cieslowski, D., Paradis, M.: Alopécie saisonnière canine. Méd. Vét. Québec 24:98, 1993.

1c. Fadok, V. A.: The dynamics of hair growth and development. Dermatol. Rep. 4:1, 1985.

2. Griffin, C. E.: Personal observation, 1993.

3. Griffin, C. E.: Open forum. Etretinate—how is it being used in veterinary dermatology? Dermatol. Dialogue, 1993.

4. Gross, T. L., et al.: Veterinary Dermatopathology. Mosby–Year Book, St. Louis, 1992.

5. Kral, F., Schwartzman, R. M.: Veterinary and Comparative Dermatology. J. B. Lippincott Co., Philadelphia, 1964.

6. Miller, M. A., Dunstan, R. W.: Seasonal flank alopecia in boxers and airedale terriers: 24 cases (1985–1992). J. Am. Vet. Med. Assoc. 203:1567, 1993.

7. Miller, W. H., Jr.: Symmetrical truncal hair loss in cats. Comp. Cont. Educ. 12:461, 1990.

8. Muller, G. H., et al. (eds.): Small Animal Dermatology, 3rd ed. W. B. Saunders Co., Philadelphia, 1983.

9. Power, H.: Personal communication, 1993.

10. Rosenkrantz, W. S., et al.: Traction alopecia in the canine: Four case reports. Calif. Vet. 43:7, 1989.

11. Rosenkrantz, W. S., Griffin, C. E.: Unpublished observations.

12. Schmeitzel, L. P., et al.: Focal cutaneous reactions at vaccination sites in a cat and four dogs. Am. Acad. Vet. Dermatol. Am. Coll. Vet. Dermatol. 2:39, 1986.

13. Scott, D. W.: Seasonal flank alopecia in ovariohysterectomized dogs. Cornell Vet. 80:187, 1990.

14. Scott, D. W.: Thyroid function in feline endocrine alopecia. J. Am. Anim. Hosp. Assoc. 11:798, 1975.

15. Scott, D. W.: Feline dermatology, 1900–1978: A monograph. J. Am. Anim. Hosp. Assoc. 16:331, 1980.

16. Thoday, K. L.: Differential diagnosis of symmetrical alopecia in the cat. In Kirk, R. W. (ed.). Current Veterinary Therapy IX. W. B. Saunders Co., Philadelphia, 1986, p. 545.

17. Thoday, K. L.: Aspects of feline symmetric alopecia. In: von Tscharner, C., Halliwell, R. E. W. (eds.). Advances in Veterinary Dermatology I. Baillière-Tindall, Philadelphia, 1990, p. 47.

18. Whiting, D. A.: Structural abnormalities of the hair shaft. J. Am. Acad. Dermatol. 16:1, 1987.

19. Wilcock, B. P., Yager, J. A.: Focal cutaneous vasculitis and alopecia at sites of rabies vaccination in dogs. J. Am. Vet. Med. Assoc. 188:1174, 1986.

20. Yager, J. A., Wilcock, B. P.: Color Atlas and Text of Surgical Pathology of the Dog and Cat. Dermatopathology and Skin Tumors. Wolfe Publishing, London, 1994.

Congenital and Hereditary Defects

■

Chapter Outline

Congenital and hereditary defects appear to be occurring more commonly. Some of this apparent increase in frequency no doubt reflects an enhanced ability to diagnose these conditions. However, this does not explain all cases. Many of the disorders discussed have an unproven mode of inheritance or are transmitted as recessive traits. Breeding of apparently normal parents or siblings of an affected dog or cat distributes the gene more widely, with the eventual production of new cases. Breeders of animals with suspected or proven genodermatoses should be instructed to avoid breeding of all close relatives of the affected animal.

■ DISORDERS OF THE SURFACE AND FOLLICULAR EPITHELIUM

A variety of disorders of keratinization or cornification are recognized in dogs and cats. Those with a known or suspected inherited basis are discussed in this chapter, and the remainder are covered in Chapter 13. Also included here are developmental defects and inflammatory disorders with a hereditary basis.

Primary Seborrhea in Dogs

Primary seborrhea is used to describe animals with an inherited disorder of keratinization or cornification. The epidermis, the follicular epithelium, the hair cuticle, and the claw can all be involved.

CAUSE AND PATHOGENESIS

Primary seborrhea is most commonly recognized in the American Cocker spaniel, English Springer spaniel, West Highland white terrier, and Basset hound.[5, 32, 42] Other breeds affected include the Irish setter, German shepherd dog, dachshund, Doberman pinscher, Chinese Shar Pei, and Labrador retriever.[2, 3, 5, 10] Other seborrheic breeds (e.g., English bulldogs)[4] are seen in certain hospital populations because of breeding practices in the surrounding area. This disorder has been studied most extensively in the American Cocker spaniel[29–34] and the West Highland white terrier.[42, 43, 51] Data from these breeds may or may not apply to other breeds.

A variety of cellular kinetic studies have been performed in normal beagles, normal Cocker spaniels, and Cocker spaniels with primary seborrhea.[29–34] When the seborrheic Cocker spaniels were compared with normal dogs, their basal cell labeling indices were three to four times greater than normal values. The epidermis, the hair follicle infundibulum, and the sebaceous glands were all hyperproliferative, but the hair root matrix was normal.[29, 30] The calculated epidermal cell renewal time for these dogs was approximately 8 days[30] as compared with 21 days for normal Cocker spaniels.[31] Similar kinetic abnormalities have been demonstrated in seborrheic Irish setters.[10] The hyperproliferative nature of the Cocker spaniels' skin appears to be due to some as yet uncharacterized primary cellular defect because the hyperproliferation remains in cell culture and persists when seborrheic skin is grafted onto normal dogs.[30, 33, 34]

In an extensive study of 100 West Highland white terriers over 12 generations, the inheritance of primary seborrhea was proved and it was probably transmitted as an autosomal recessive trait.[43] This mode of inheritance probably applies to other breeds because single affected dogs can be recognized in litters by clinically normal parents. Although labeled index studies were not performed in the seborrheic West Highland white terriers, histologic and ultrastructural studies indicated epidermal hyperproliferation.

CLINICAL FEATURES

Because of the inherited basis of the disease, signs occur early in life and become more severe with advancing age. Affected West Highland White terriers demonstrate clinical changes at 10 weeks of age.[43] In most dogs, early changes such as mild flaking or dullness of the coat are overlooked or attributed to intestinal parasites, inadequate nutrition, or other puppyhood problems. Usually by 12 to 18 months of age, the dog is presented for its seborrhea.

The presenting complaint varies from dog to dog. Common seborrheic findings include ceruminous, hyperplastic otitis externa (Fig. 11:1A); a dull coat with excessive flaking of the skin; greasy malodorous skin, which is marked in body folds or intertriginous areas; follicular casts; multiple discrete to coalescent, scaly or crusty pruritic patches (seborrheic dermatitis) (Fig. 11:1B and C); digital hyperkeratosis; and dry, brittle claws (Fig. 11:1D).

Most seborrheic dogs have all of the seborrheic abnormalities described previously, but the severity of each varies from case to case. Irish setters and Doberman pinschers tend to have dry flaky skin, whereas Cocker spaniels, Springer spaniels, West Highland white terriers, Basset hounds, Chinese Shar Peis, and Labrador retrievers usually exhibit otitis, greasy seborrhea, seborrheic dermatitis, or typically some combination of these. The greasiness and seborrheic dermatitis involve most or all of the body but are most pronounced on the face, the ventral neck, the feet (especially interdigitally), the perineum, and the ventral body. Basset hounds and Chinese Shar Peis also have signs of the disorder in their various body folds. The caudodorsum of these greasy dogs is often dry and flaky.

Aside from the visual and olfactory findings, pruritus occurs in many of these dogs. This is especially true when the dog is greasy or has seborrheic dermatitis. The pruritus follows the development of skin lesions, although it precedes the skin lesions in many secondarily seborrheic dogs. Dogs with seborrhea are prone to secondary bacterial infections and *Malassezia* dermatitis (see Chap. 13). When dogs with primary seborrhea have either condition, their skin lesions worsen rapidly and their pruritus increases dramatically, especially when *Malassezia* dermatitis is present. In some cases, the lesions of the secondary infections are so severe and widespread that the seborrheic lesions cannot be appreciated until the staphylococcal or *Malassezia* component is resolved.

DIAGNOSIS

The clinical lesions seen in primary or secondary seborrhea (see Chap. 13) are identical, and thus, the diagnosis of primary seborrhea is made by exclusion. In dogs younger than 1 year, the list of differential diagnostic possibilities is short and includes demodicosis, cheyletiellosis, nutritional deficiency, ichthyosis, epidermal dysplasia, and food hypersensitivity. In adult dogs, the list is much longer.

Figure 11:1. *A,* Primary seborrhea in a Cocker spaniel. Hyperplastic ceruminous otitis externa. *B,* Primary seborrhea in a Cocker spaniel. Seborrheic plaques in the intertriginous area of the ventral neck. *C,* Primary seborrhea in a Cocker spaniel. Erythema, alopecia, and seborrheic plaques on the abdomen. *D,* Primary seborrhea in a Cocker spaniel. Hyperkeratosis of the footpads and dystrophic claws in a 1-year-old dog. *E,* Primary seborrhea in a Persian cat. Kitten with a greasy, matted haircoat and patchy alopecia. *F,* Canine ichthyosis in a terrier-cross with generalized dry, hyperkeratotic, alopecic skin. The dog has appeared this way since birth. *G,* Congenital ichthyosis in a dog. Marked hyperkeratosis and mild erythema in a pinna. *H,* Pinna and periocular region of a dog with epidermal dysplasia. Chronic alopecia, hyperpigmentation, and lichenification.

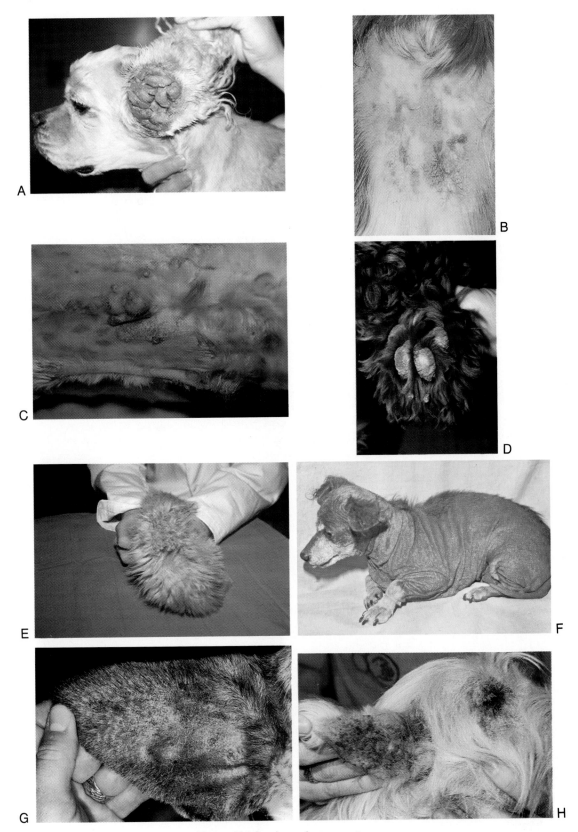

Figure 11:1 *See legend on opposite page*

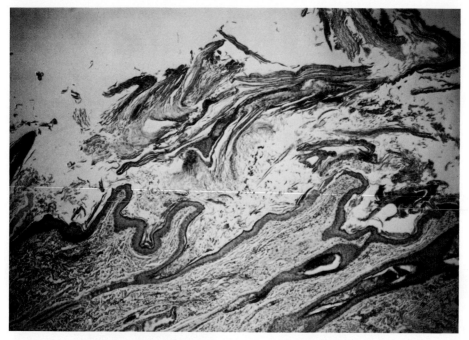

Figure 11:2. Canine seborrheic dermatitis. Hyperplastic superficial perivascular dermatitis with a marked keratinization defect and parakeratotic capping.

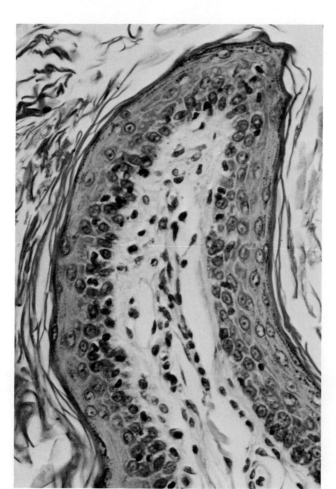

Figure 11:3. Close-up of Figure 11:2. Papillary squirting.

The diagnosis of primary seborrhea is supported by biopsy. In noninfected flaky or greasy areas, one sees a hyperplastic superficial perivascular dermatitis. There is usually a marked keratinization defect, characterized by orthokeratotic or parakeratotic hyperkeratosis, follicular keratosis, and variable dyskeratosis (Fig. 11:2). In many cases, the epidermis is normal to slightly increased in thickness. In uninflamed lesions, the perivascular cellular infiltrate is mild and consists of lymphocytes and plasma cells. In inflamed lesions, the perivascular inflammation becomes more intense, and one sees papillomatosis and focal areas of parakeratotic hyperkeratosis (parakeratotic ''caps'') overlying edematous dermal papillae (papillary ''squirting'') (Fig. 11:3). This capping is commonly seen at the follicular ostia.[3] Bacteria are numerous in the surface and follicular debris and yeast may be seen. Evidence of secondary bacterial infection (e.g., intraepidermal pustular dermatitis or folliculitis) is commonly found.

CLINICAL MANAGEMENT

Primary seborrhea cannot be cured, and the ease of control varies from dog to dog. The seborrheic changes in these dogs worsen significantly with dietary inadequacies, external parasites, or endocrine or metabolic diseases, so these dogs should be monitored carefully for the development of any intercurrent disease. Seborrheic dogs are prone to secondary staphylococcal infections or *Malassezia* dermatitis. Administration of an appropriate antibiotic or ketoconazole is often necessary at the onset of antiseborrheic therapy to resolve pre-existing infections. During maintenance therapy, a sudden worsening of the dog's seborrhea may indicate that the infection has returned and the dog should be examined.

The mainstay of treatment of these dogs involves the use of antiseborrheic shampoos and moisturizers. The shampoo selection and the vigor of treatment depend on the nature of the seborrhea.[27] Dogs with dry, uninflamed skin are easier to manage than those that are greasy. Many dogs are both dry and greasy, especially in the intertriginous regions and between the toes and the pads. Long hair impedes the thorough cleaning of the skin, especially when the area is greasy, so owners should be encouraged to keep the coat cut short.

Dogs with dry skin with mild to moderate scaling usually require a bath once or twice weekly to return the skin to near-normal condition. Dogs with heavy scaling need to be bathed two or three times a week. This intense bathing is done for 2 to 3 weeks to reduce the corneocyte count to near normal,[15a] and then the frequency of bathing is gradually decreased to some maintenance level. Some investigators set a frequency (e.g., once weekly), whereas other clinicians allow the client to decide on the basis of the individual dog's needs. As long as the dog is not prone to secondary bacterial infections, the latter method is most appropriate. Overbathing any dog, but especially one with dry seborrhea, can result in seborrhea.

A large number of grooming or antiseborrheic shampoos are appropriate for the bathing of dry skin. Product selection depends on client and veterinarian preference. It is advisable to start with the mildest product and change to a stronger one only if the initial product is unsatisfactory. For mildly flaky skin, moisturizing hypoallergenic shampoos (HyLyt*efa hypoallergenic moisturizing shampoo, Allergroom hypoallergenic emollient shampoo), colloidal oatmeal shampoos (Epi-Soothe), or emollient-based chlorhexidine products (ChlorhexiDerm shampoo and Nolvasan shampoo) are commonly used. For more severe flaking, sulfur and salicylic acid products (Micro Pearls sulfur shampoo, Sebolux shampoo, SebaLyt antiseborrheic shampoo) are appropriate. For recalcitrant cases, mild tar products (Clear Tar shampoo, Nu Sal T shampoo, T-Lux shampoo) might be appropriate but, because all tar products are degreasing agents, they should be used cautiously. Strong tars, selenium sulfides, and benzoyl peroxide shampoos are contraindicated in these patients.

If the dog's coat is dirty, a rapid shampooing with a nonmedicated grooming product is indicated before the antiseborrheic bath. After the dog is lathered with the antiseborrheic product, the shampoo must remain in contact with the skin for 10 to 15 minutes for maximal effect. Gentle manipulation of the dog's skin during this waiting period tends to keep the dog happy and increases the cleaning action of the shampoo. After 10 to 15 minutes, the dog is rinsed thoroughly. Rinsing should take two to three times longer than lathering. Prolonged rinsing not only removes the debris and shampoo but also aids in hydration of the skin. The dry skin of many of these dogs becomes flaky again soon after the bath, especially when the humidity is low. The application of an afterbath rinse (Alpha–Sesame Oil dry skin rinse, Humilac dry skin spray and rinse, HyLyt*efa bath oil coat conditioner, Micro Pearls cream rinse) helps to provide a barrier to transepidermal water loss and its associated drying. Although any afterbath rinse can be effective, studies have shown that those containing oils, especially linoleic acid, are most effective in decreasing transepidermal water loss.[11] If the client keeps some diluted product in a misting bottle and sprays it on the dog as needed, the frequency of bathing can often be reduced.

For dogs with greasy skin, the shampoos must be stronger and need to be used more often. These dogs are prone to bacterial or yeast infections and often have to be treated with antibiotics or antifungal agents to control these secondary problems. Dogs with mildly to moderately greasy skin can be treated with sulfur and salicylic acid or mild tar products. Dogs with very greasy skin are often bathed with stronger tars (LyTar shampoo and Allerset-T shampoo), selenium sulfides (Selsun Blue dandruff shampoo), or benzoyl peroxides (OxyDex shampoo, Pyoben shampoo, and Micro Pearls benzoyl peroxide shampoo). All these products are excellent degreasers and create a dry seborrhea if used excessively. After the presenting greasiness is resolved, many investigators switch to a less potent product or alternate between a strong and a mild product. Greasy dogs often need an afterbath rinse, especially if the dog's environment has low humidity. Most strong shampoos can disrupt the epidermal barrier and increase transepidermal water loss, with resultant worsening of the seborrhea.[11a] An afterbath rinse can prevent this, but it may make the dog too greasy, so each case must be approached on its own merits.

Seborrheic dogs usually have a ceruminous otitis externa, which must be treated on a routine and regular basis. Instead of antiseborrheic shampoos, ceruminolytic ear flushes are employed (see Chap. 18). The frequency of maintenance use is best determined by having the client smell the ears. When the waxy odor is first noticed, the ears should be cleaned. Despite vigorous cleaning, many of these dogs experience recurrent secondary bacterial or yeast infections. These infections are heralded by the sudden need to clean the ears frequently, otic pruritus, otic malodor, or combinations of these. Appropriate medications should be dispensed promptly and used for 2 to 3 weeks. Ear surgery should be considered for dogs that have frequent infections.

If the client is unable or unwilling to bathe the seborrheic dog, it becomes an unacceptable house pet. Some dogs, especially those that are greasy, have recurrent bacterial or yeast infections despite the most diligent efforts of their owners. These dogs are candidates for systemic treatment. Although omega-3 and omega-6 fatty acid supplements can be beneficial in these dogs,[4, 5] they rarely provide complete control and should be used as an adjunct to other treatments. Because primary seborrhea is a hyperproliferative disorder, drugs that inhibit cell replication may be beneficial. Corticosteroids and cytotoxic drugs have application here. Because these drugs have severe side-effects and are needed lifelong, they should be reserved for cases in which all other measures have failed.

Retinoic acids have been used extensively in seborrheic dogs, with varying results from dog to dog and investigator to investigator. Although some dogs respond to isotretinoin (1 to 3 mg/kg q12h orally), results are usually disappointing.[13] Most favorable results have been obtained with etretinate. When 16 Cocker spaniels with severe seborrhea were given etretinate at a dosage of 1 mg/kg every 24 hours orally for 120 days, 15 dogs had a moderate to excellent response.[42] In moderately affected dogs, marked improvement was noted by day 60 of treatment. Severely affected dogs required longer courses of treatment for maximal responses. This treatment has no effect on the hyperplastic otitis that these dogs have, and this must be managed by other means.[6] Five West Highland white terriers and 4 Basset hounds also studied showed no response to treatment.[42] Ten of the 25 dogs treated experienced side-effects, including increased pruritus, reluctance to eat hard food, vomiting, stiff gait, conjunctivitis, and exfoliative dermatitis. The side-effects disappeared with withdrawal of drug administration and did not recur with alternate-day drug administration.

If a response is seen to etretinate, treatment should be lifelong. Alternate-day treatment is usually not satisfactory, and suggested regimens include administration for 5 of 7 days; 1 week on, 1 week off; or daily use during alternate months.[6] With long-term administration, some dogs may have keratoconjunctivitis sicca and should be monitored for this condition. If it occurs, drug withdrawal may result in the regaining of tear function. Topical cyclosporine is usually effective if the etretinate administration cannot be stopped.[6] Both isotretinoin and etretinate can alter fat metabolism and liver function. Alterations usually occur early in treatment and are mild and transitory.[6] Long-term administration of etretinate has not resulted in severe metabolic changes in normal dogs, but cases should be monitored periodically.

Seborrheic dogs unresponsive to bathing or etretinate administration are usually destroyed by their owners. Most of those dogs have greasy seborrhea, which predisposes them to near-constant bacterial or yeast infections. Maintenance treatment with antibiotics or ketoconazole often makes these dogs more acceptable to their owners and less malodorous. The expense of these drugs often precludes their use in all but small dogs. As a last resort, long-term corticosteroid or cytotoxic treatment is considered. Corticosteroids can be beneficial in greasy dogs because of their atrophic effects on the epidermis and sebaceous glands. Prednisolone is administered daily at 1 to 2 mg/kg until the greasiness is controlled and then adjusted slowly to the lowest alternate-day dosage that is effective. Some dogs require daily treatment. Because these dogs are already prone to secondary infections and corticosteroids aggravate that predisposition, these patients must be examined frequently. Most of these dogs have signs of iatrogenic hyperadrenocorticism at some point in treatment. If the corticosteroids administration is stopped, a severe rebound in the seborrhea can be expected. Although the authors are aware of cases apparently well controlled with methotrexate,[4] specific details on protocols, efficacy, and side-effects are not available. Because this drug is used in hyperproliferative disorders of humans,[1] it should be of some benefit in dogs. One author (WHM) treated a seborrheic Cocker spaniel for pemphigus foliaceus with azathioprine. While the dog was receiving maintenance treatment (2.2 mg/kg q48h), its seborrhea improved markedly. This suggests that drugs other than methotrexate may be beneficial. No details are available to support or refute that supposition.

Primary Seborrhea in Cats

Seborrhea is rare in cats and primary seborrhea has been reported in only Persian cats.[40] An autosomal recessive mode of inheritance was demonstrated. Cats of either sex or any coat color can be affected. Among affected cats, the severity of the seborrheic signs is variable. Severe seborrhea is obvious in affected kittens by 2 to 3 days of age because their hairs paste together and they look dirty (see Fig. 11:1E). With time, the whole body becomes scaly and greasy and hair is lost (Fig. 11:4). Waxy debris accumulates in the face folds and ears (Fig. 11:5) and the cats have a rancid waxy odor. Mildly affected cats have similar signs, which are much milder and do not appear until about 6 weeks of age.

Biopsy of noninfected skin shows a marked keratinization defect, characterized by orthokeratotic hyperkeratosis and papillomatosis (Fig. 11:6). The perivascular cellular infiltrate is mild and consists predominantly of lymphocytes.

No effective treatment has been reported for severely affected cats. Retinoic acids have been used safely in cats[6] but are untried in primary seborrhea. A commercial omega-3 and omega-6 fatty acid–containing product (DVM Derm Caps) was used unsuccessfully in two cats.[4] Mildly affected cats can be kept fairly normal by good grooming, periodic clipping, and occasional bathing with antiseborrheic shampoos. Tar products should not be used on cats.

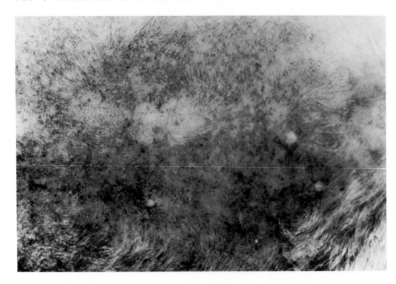

Figure 11:4. Primary seborrhea in a Persian kitten. Alopecia and marked comedone formation on the ventral thorax and abdomen.

Figure 11:5. Primary seborrhea in a Persian kitten. Marked accumulation of cerumen on a pinna.

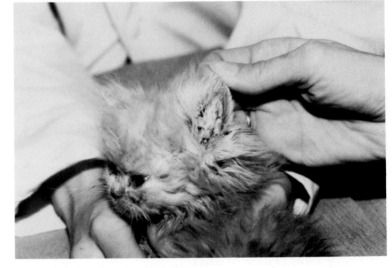

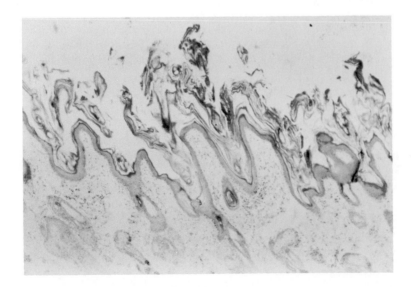

Figure 11:6. Primary seborrhea in a Persian kitten. Marked orthokeratotic hyperkeratosis, papillomatosis, and mild lymphocytic perivascular dermatitis.

Ichthyosis

Ichthyosis (fish scale disease) is a rare congenital skin disease and has been reported in dogs. It has been seen in one litter of cats.[4] It is characterized by extreme hyperkeratosis on all or part of the skin and by exaggerated thickening of the digital, carpal, and tarsal pads.

CAUSE AND PATHOGENESIS

Canine ichthyosis resembles human ichthyosis, although not enough cases have been reported to reveal whether different forms of the disease occur in dogs.[2, 9, 37, 46]

In humans, there are a variety of hereditary ichthyosiform dermatoses characterized by the accumulation of large amounts of scales on the skin's surface.[1] The major forms of ichthyosis are ichthyosis vulgaris (autosomal dominant), X-linked ichthyosis (X-linked recessive), lamellar ichthyosis (autosomal recessive or dominant), and epidermolytic hyperkeratosis (autosomal dominant). Ichthyosis vulgaris begins in early childhood, whereas the other forms are present at or near birth. All forms persist for the animal's liftime. Lamellar ichthyosis and epidermolytic hyperkeratosis are associated with an increased epidermal transit rate, and ichthyosis vulgaris and X-linked ichthyosis appear to be due to some as yet incompletely defined barrier defect.[28]

Too few dogs with ichthyosis have been reported in veterinary medicine to characterize the disorder. Because the parents of affected dogs have been normal, cases have been recognized in both sexes, and single cases have occurred in litters of five puppies or more, an autosomal recessive mode of inheritance is most likely.[4, 7] Most cases in dogs resemble lamellar ichthyosis. Labeled index studies performed on three West Highland white terriers with lamellar ichthyosis by one author (WHM) had an average epidermal basal cell labeling index of 11.87 per cent and an epidermal nucleated cell labeling index of 7.2 per cent. The average calculated epidermal cell renewal time was 3.56 days. These values suggest that lamellar ichthyosis in dogs is also due to epidermal hyperproliferation. Ultrastructural studies in Cavalier King Charles spaniels support the findings from West Highland White terriers.[7]

CLINICAL FEATURES

Ichthyosis appears to be most common in West Highland white terriers but has also been recognized in the Doberman pinscher, Irish setter, collie, bull terrier, American Staffordshire terrier (pit bull), Labrador retriever, Jack Russell terrier, Cavalier King Charles spaniel, English Springer spaniel, Yorkshire terrier, Rottweiler, and mongrels.[2, 3, 5, 36a] Either sex may be involved, and all dogs are abnormal at birth. Affected West Highland white terriers tend to be born with black skin, which cracks and peels off at about 2 weeks of age.[4]

Much of the body of these dogs is covered with tightly adhering, verrucous, tannish gray scales (see Fig. 11:1F) and feathered keratinous projections, which give a rough texture to the skin (Fig. 11:7). Although some of these projections adhere to the skin, others constantly flake off, often riding up hair shafts in large sheets (see Fig. 11:1G). Large quantities of scaly, seborrheic-smelling debris accumulate on the skin surface. Scaly, erythematous dry patches are particularly prominent in the flexural creases and intertriginous areas. Marked thickening of the horny layer of the nasal planum and digital pads is observed (Fig. 11:8). Masses of hard keratin accumulate at the margins of the pads and often extend upward from the margin in winglike projections. The entire paw of some individuals appears grossly enlarged, and the whole foot seems heavier than normal. There is pain and discomfort of the feet. Hyperkeratosis may surround the mucocutaneous junctions of the face. Some dogs may have severe erythroderma or hair loss.[46] Intercurrent ocular disease and noninflammatory myopathy has been reported in Rottweilers.[36a]

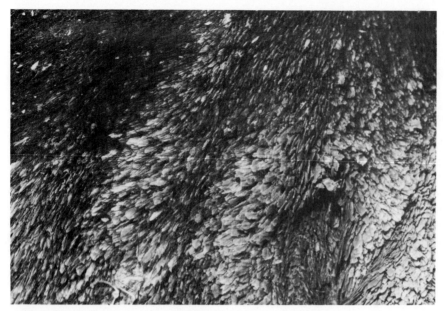

Figure 11:7. Close-up of skin from the chest of a 5-month-old Doberman pinscher with canine ichthyosis, showing the laminated, tightly adhering scales.

DIAGNOSIS

If the dog is presented in early puppyhood, no other diagnoses are appropriate. If the dog is presented as an adult with no prior history, all causes of seborrhea or exfoliative dermatitis must be considered (see Chap. 13). The diagnosis is confirmed by biopsy, which usually reveals characteristic histopathologic changes, especially the prominent granular layer and the presence of many mitotic figures in keratinocytes. Marked orthokeratotic hyperkeratosis (Fig. 11:9) and focal digitate projections of hyperkeratosis may be seen. Follicular keratosis and plugging are

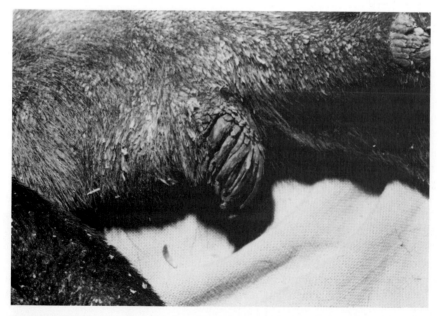

Figure 11:8. Carpal pad of the dog in Figure 11:7. Note the feather-like hyperkeratosis of the carpal pad.

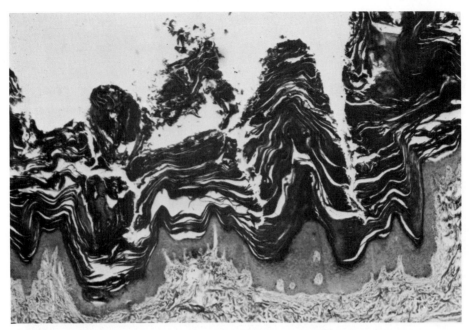

Figure 11:9. Congenital canine lamellar ichthyosis. Marked laminated orthokeratotic hyperkeratosis.

common. The epidermis may or may not be hyperplastic. One of the most characteristic histopathologic changes is marked hypergranulosis, but this layer may be normal,[3] thin,[46] or irregular.[7] Mitotic figures may be numerous. The superficial epidermis may contain numerous vacuolated keratinocytes,[36a] which may rupture and result in reticular degeneration. Severe reticular degeneration may lead to microvesicle formation.

CLINICAL MANAGEMENT

The owner should understand the chronic nature, incurability, and difficult treatment of ichthyosis. Although the affected dog's general health seems to be good, the skin changes are so severe and their management so difficult that the patients are troublesome house pets. Still, a devoted owner may be capable of tolerating the burden of caring for these dogs.

Frequent bathing and the use of emollient rinses helps these dogs. To facilitate the cleaning and moisturization of the skin, the coat should be kept short. Harsh shampoos (selenium sulfides, strong tar products, and benzoyl peroxides) should be used cautiously, as they can worsen the condition. In humans, ointments or solutions of 3 to 12 per cent lactic acid, 60 per cent propylene glycol, or both are beneficial, especially if the skin is hydrated before the agent is applied.[1] One author (WHM) successfully used a 5 per cent lactic acid spray or ointment, and a 50 per cent propylene glycol solution has been reported to be beneficial.[46] Commercial moisturizers (Humilac [Allerderm], Hylyt*efa [DVM], Micro Pearls cream rinse [EVSCO]) can also be beneficial.

Because of the intensity of topical treatment, most affected dogs are euthanized. When tried, oral administration of isotretinoin (1 to 2 mg/kg q12h) has been uniformly successful.[4, 6, 46] Because of the expense of this product, long-term results with this drug are not known.

Epidermal Dysplasia in West Highland White Terriers

Epidermal dysplasia in West Highland white terriers (Armadillo Westie syndrome) is an uncommon condition, which tends to occur in families in this breed.[47] The mode of inheritance is unknown, but it is probably transmitted as an autosomal recessive trait.

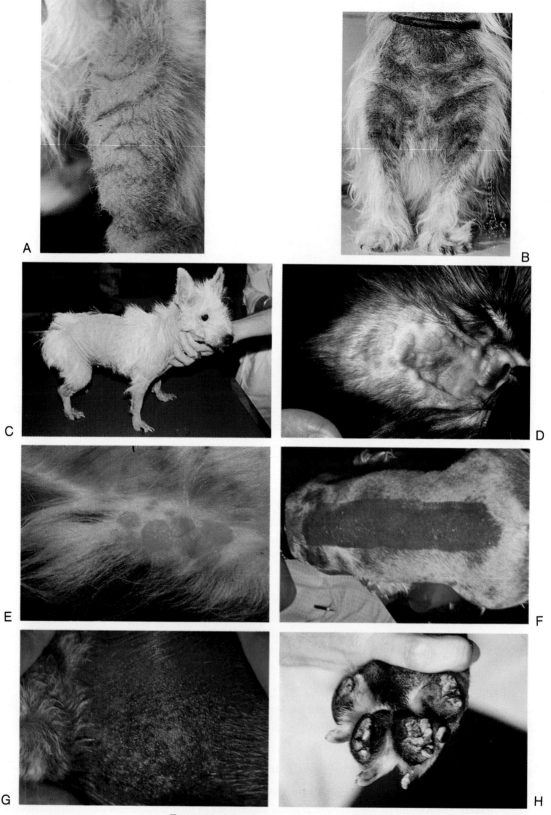

Figure 11:10 *See legend on opposite page*

CAUSE AND PATHOGENESIS

Dogs with this condition have a dysplastic epidermis and an inflammatory perivascular dermatitis associated with *Malassezia* infection. Resolution of the *Malassezia* infection results in the elimination of the inflammation but not the dysplasia. These findings, coupled with an early age at onset, suggest that the dysplasia is an inherited disorder of keratinization that predisposes the dog to *Malassezia* dermatitis and possibly hypersensitivity to the organism.

CLINICAL FEATURES

Dogs of either sex can be affected, and signs usually begin between 6 and 12 months of age, although some adult-onset cases have been recognized.[47] Typically, affected dogs have a somewhat greasy coat before pruritus, the primary sign of this disorder, is recognized. The pruritus is initially focused at the face, the ears (see Fig. 11:1H), the legs (Fig. 11:10A), the feet, and the ventrum (Fig. 11:10B) and is mild to moderate. The involved skin is inflamed, is greasy, and has large amounts of keratosebaceous debris on the surface. With time, the pruritus becomes intense and the lesions more widespread. Animals with advanced cases are greasy, nearly bald, lichenified, and often hyperpigmented (see Fig. 11:1C). Early on, there may be some improvement with large doses of corticosteroids, but response to these drugs is soon lost. There is no response to antihistamines, antibiotics, and antiseborrheic shampoos.

DIAGNOSIS

In the absence of cytologic evidence of a secondary *Malassezia* dermatitis, the primary differential diagnostic considerations are food hypersensitivity, scabies, and cheyletiellosis. When yeast are present, atopy, primary seborrhea, and ichthyosis must also be considered. The demonstration of *Malassezia* yeast via cytologic examination of the keratosebaceous debris is not sufficient to make the diagnosis of epidermal dysplasia, as yeast are commonly found in some West Highland White terriers.[39] Biopsy is necessary to confirm the diagnosis. Areas sampled should not have the surface debris removed by close clipping or presurgical cleaning.

Histopathologic findings include variable degrees of hyperplastic perivascular dermatitis with epidermal dysplasia (Fig. 11:11).[3, 47] The epidermis shows varying degrees of hyperchromasia, excessive keratinocyte mitoses, crowding of basilar keratinocytes, epidermal "buds," and loss of polarity (Fig. 11:12). Lymphocytic exocytosis and diffuse spongiosis are prominent (Fig. 11:13). In properly taken samples, marked parakeratotic surface and follicular hyperkeratosis is seen. In most cases, numerous spherical to oval single budding yeasts (Fig. 11:14) are seen in the surface and superficial follicular keratin. Yeast are absent in some cases.[3]

CLINICAL MANAGEMENT

This condition is frustrating to manage. Resolution of the *Malassezia* dermatitis eliminates the pruritus and returns the dog to near-normal status. A mild keratinization defect (scaling, minor crusting) persists. However, because the treatments of yeast infection do not completely eliminate the organism, the *Malassezia* dermatitis recurs after treatment is discontinued.

Figure 11:10. *A,* Epidermal dysplasia. Marked thickening and folding of erythematous, alopecic skin on a limb. *B,* Epidermal dysplasia. Chronic alopecia, hyperpigmentation, and lichenification. *C,* Epidermal dysplasia in a West Highland white terrier. Early erythroderma. *D,* Psoriasiform-lichenoid dermatosis in an English Springer spaniel. Erythematous lichenoid plaques on a pinna. (Courtesy K. Mason.) *E,* Same dog as in *D.* Erythematous lichenoid papules and plaques on prepuce. (Courtesy K. Mason.) *F,* Miniature Schnauzer whose back has been clipped to expose the area affected with lesions. *G,* Prominent, soft comedones on the skin of another Schnauzer. *H,* Marked hyperkeratosis of the footpads in a Dogue de Bordeaux. (Courtesy M. Paradis.)

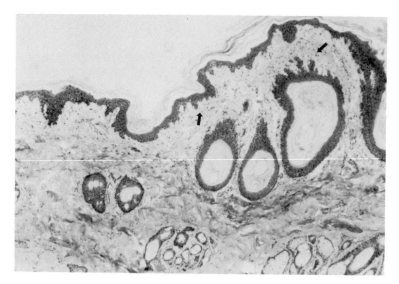

Figure 11:11. Epidermal dysplasia and *Malassezia pachydermatis* infection in a West Highland white terrier. Note marked epithelial budding of the epidermis and the hair follicle's outer root sheath *(arrows).*

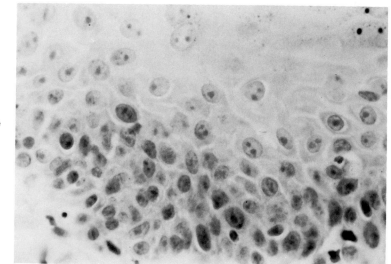

Figure 11:12. Close-up of Figure 11:11. Epidermal dysplasia.

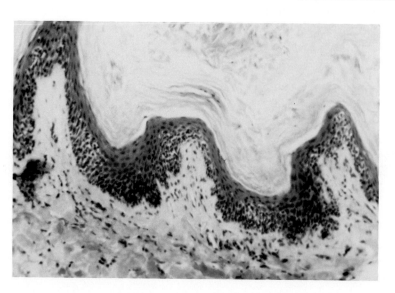

Figure 11:13. Close-up of Figure 11:11. Note diffuse spongiosis, lymphocytic exocytosis, and focal parakeratotic hyperkeratosis.

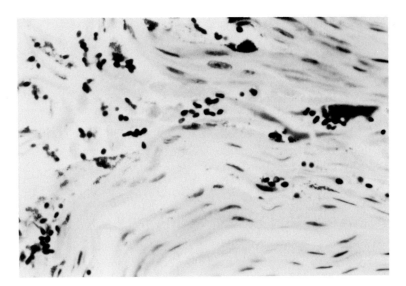

Figure 11:14. Close-up of Figure 11:11. Numerous yeasts in parakeratotic follicular keratin.

Although various shampoos can be beneficial in the treatment of *Malassezia* dermatitis (see Chap. 5), these dogs respond poorly to those treatments. Ketoconazole (10 mg/kg q12h to q24h) for 30 to 45 days is necessary to induce remission. Enilconazole (Imaverol [Jannsen]) rinses are also effective in those countries where the product is available. Because the epidermal dysplasia persists, the *Malassezia* dermatitis and its associated signs recurs. Attempts to prevent reinfection by the frequent use of antiseborrheic or antifungal shampoos has been unrewarding. The use of these shampoos or a 50 per cent white vinegar and water rinse once or twice weekly can decrease the frequency of severe infections, but episodic or constant use of ketoconazole or enilconazole is necessary.

Treating the epidermal dysplasia with fatty acid supplements (DVM Derm Caps [DVM]) or retinoic acids (isotretinoin or etretinate) have been unrewarding in the few cases in which it was attempted.[4, 47] The only method of control that the authors have found to be effective is the daily or alternate-day administration of ketoconazole. This has been successful in two dogs for longer than 3 years. Because of the expense of this treatment and poor prognosis for cure, most affected dogs are euthanized.

Psoriasiform-Lichenoid Dermatosis in English Springer Spaniels

Psoriasiform-lichenoid dermatosis is uncommon to rare and is recognized in only English Springer spaniels.[16, 36] The dermatosis begins in young dogs (4 to 18 months of age) of both sexes. Asymptomatic, generally symmetric, erythematous, lichenoid papules and plaques are initially noted on the pinnae (see Fig. 11:10D), in the external ear canal, and in the inguinal region (see Fig. 11:10E). With time, lesions become increasingly hyperkeratotic (some, almost papillomatous), and spread to involve the face, the ventral trunk, and the perineal area. Chronic cases resemble severe seborrhea. The exclusive occurrence of this dermatosis in English Springer spaniels suggests a genetic predilection. It has been proposed that affected dogs develop a distinct and exaggerated reaction to a superficial staphylococcal infection.[10a]

Skin biopsy reveals a superficial perivascular to interstitial dermatitis with psoriasiform epidermal hyperplasia, and areas of lichenoid interface dermatitis, intraepidermal microabscesses (containing eosinophils and neutrophils), and Munro's microabscesses (Figs. 11:15 and 11:16).[3] Chronic hyperkeratotic lesions frequently show papillated epidermal hyperplasia and papillomatosis.

This dermatosis is characterized by a waxing and waning course for 1 to 3 years. Spontaneous remissions are not reported. Various medicaments, including anti-inflammatory doses of

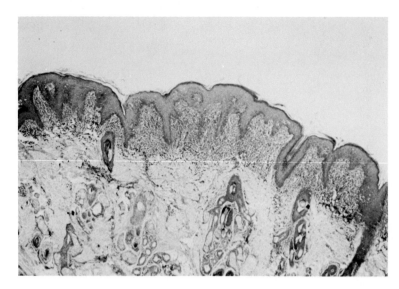

Figure 11:15. Psoriasiform-lichenoid dermatosis in an English Springer spaniel. Psoriasiform epidermal hyperplasia and lichenoid cellular infiltrate. (Courtesy K. Mason.)

glucocorticoids, oral vitamin A, levamisole, dapsone, autogenous vaccine, and antiseborrheic shampoos, are of little or no help. Four cases treated with cephalexin (20 mg/kg q12h) showed an excellent response with complete resolution of lesions.[10a] Retinoic acid derivatives might be useful, but no information is available.

Schnauzer Comedo Syndrome

The Schnauzer comedo syndrome affects the backs of some Miniature Schnauzer dogs and is typified by multiple comedones that may become crusted, nonpainful papules.

CAUSE AND PATHOGENESIS

This condition has been observed exclusively in Miniature Schnauzers. It seems to be a seborrheic or acneiform disorder and occurs in only certain predisposed individuals. The exclusive occurrence in Schnauzers and the clinicopathologic similarity to nevus comedonicus in humans[1] suggest that this syndrome may be a developmental dysplasia of hair follicles with

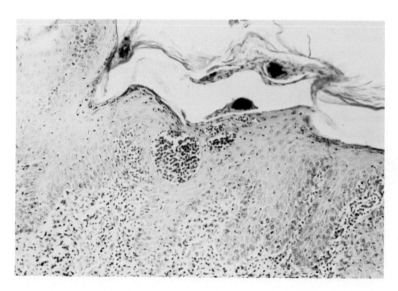

Figure 11:16. Psoriasiform-lichenoid dermatosis in an English Springer spaniel. Epidermal microabscess containing neutrophils and eosinophils. (Courtesy K. Mason.)

an inherited basis. After it is recognized, Schnauzer comedo syndrome can usually be treated and easily controlled, but recurrences are common. However, there is much variability, with some cases responding more favorably to therapy than others.

CLINICAL FEATURES

The predisposed individual tends to form comedones (blackheads) over the back. These can be felt as sharp, crusted, papular projections above the surface of the skin. Some comedones are soft and waxy.

The lesions are most numerous at the midspinal area of the back, fanning out laterally and extending from the neck to the sacrum (see Fig. 11:10F). Schnauzer comedo syndrome is seldom noted in the early stage before the comedo extrudes from the follicular orifice. At that stage, there is no pain or discomfort. In some individuals, the comedo changes into a soft, small, acne-like pustule and causes slight irritation (see Fig. 11:10G). Dogs do not usually display visible pain or itching. In some dogs, the plugged follicles become infected. In these cases, the number of papular lesions increases rapidly; they become much more widespread and can involve the entire trunk. If secondary staphylococcal infection occurs, especially when it is widespread, the lesions tend to be pruritic or painful.

DIAGNOSIS

Clipping a small spot on the back exposes the skin so the individual comedones and papules can be seen. The restriction of these lesions to the caudal dorsum of a Schnauzer with no other signs of disease is virtually pathognomonic of the condition. The diagnosis can be confirmed by biopsy in which a section through one of the noninfected comedones reveals a keratinous plug blocking the hair follicle and sebaceous gland. A small cystic cavity is formed, lined by thin, stretched follicular epithelium and filled with keratin and sebum (Fig. 11:17). Sebum secretion accumulates behind the plug, which further dilates the cyst. If the follicle ruptures, a perifollicular inflammatory infiltrate appears. If a secondary bacterial infection is present, perifolliculitis, folliculitis, or furunculosis may be seen.

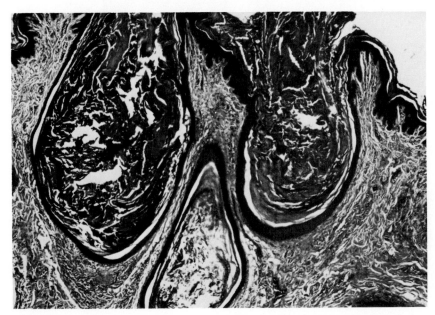

Figure 11:17. Comedones (acne) are dilated follicles with keratin plugs blocking the follicular opening.

CLINICAL MANAGEMENT

The owner should be informed that, because of its genetic basis, the condition can be controlled but not cured. Mild cases require no treatment and become apparent only when the coat is clipped or plucked. If the owner finds the lesions objectionable, or they bother the dog or become infected repeatedly, topical antiseborrheic therapy should be instituted. If a secondary infection is present, systemic antibiotics should be administered for 3 to 4 weeks.

In mild cases, daily or alternate-day wiping of the area with various human acne cleaning pads, alcohol, or Listerine antiseptic (contains 0.06 per cent thymol, 0.09 per cent eucalyptol, 0.06 per cent methyl salicylate, and 0.04 per cent menthol) loosens or dissolves the comedones. Benzoyl peroxide gel also can be used but may be irritating with repeated application. In more severe cases, antiseborrheic shampoos are indicated. Because these plugged follicles are easily inflamed by harsh agents, the mildest shampoo should be used first and only replaced by a stronger one if the first product is ineffective. Sulfur, tar and sulfur, benzoyl peroxide, and benzoyl peroxide plus sulfur shampoos are most commonly used. Bathing the dorsum twice weekly for 1 to 3 weeks removes the comedones, and then the frequency is adjusted to the patient's needs. The rare case that is refractory to topical therapy may benefit from the administration of isotretinoin at a dosage of 1 mg/kg every 12 hours.[6]

Footpad Hyperkeratosis

Familial footpad hyperkeratosis has been reported in Irish terriers[26] and the Dogue de Bordeaux.[41] Single cases have been recognized in several related Kerry blue terriers,[5] the Labrador retriever, the Golden retriever, and mongrels.[4]

All cases develop severe hyperkeratosis by 6 months of age. All pads of all feet are involved. The entire surface of the pad is involved, but the keratin is more compacted in certain regions and forms horns (see Fig. 11:10*H*).[4, 41] With severe hyperkeratosis, fissures and secondary infection can occur and cause lameness. No other skin lesions are present.

Histopathologic findings include moderate to severe epidermal hyperplasia with marked

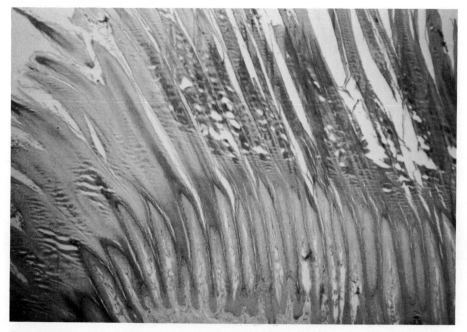

Figure 11:18. Digital hyperkeratosis in an Irish terrier. Marked papillated hyperplasia and orthokeratotic hyperkeratosis.

papillated and diffuse orthokeratotic hyperkeratosis (Fig. 11:18).[41] Some fusion of the conical papillae by keratin can be seen.

Treatment is symptomatic. Daily soaks in 50 per cent propylene glycol cause significant improvement within 5 days, but treatment must be continued to maintain the response.[41] Treatment with retinoic acids has been proposed but not tested. The mode of inheritance has not been established.

Aplasia Cutis

Aplasia cutis (epitheliogenesis imperfecta) is a congenital inherited discontinuity of squamous epithelium.[17, 22, 38] It is considered an autosomal recessive trait in cattle, horses, sheep, and pigs, but little is known of its inheritance in dogs and cats. The condition is characterized by areas of abrupt absence of epithelium, with resultant ulcers. Histologically, the ulcerated areas are distinguished by the complete absence of epidermis, hair follicles, and glands. The lesions of aplasia cutis in the newborn rapidly become infected, and septicemia soon results in death. Small lesions may, with supportive therapy, heal by scar formation. Skin grafting may be beneficial.

Dermoid Sinus

A dermoid sinus is a neural tube defect resulting from incomplete separation of the skin and neural tube during embryonic development. The sinus is a tubular indentation of skin extending from the dorsal midline as a blind sac ending in the subcutaneous tissue or extending through the spinal canal to the dura mater. The lumen becomes filled with sebum, keratin debris, and hair. It may become cystic and is often inflamed. If infected, it may produce meningomyelitis and neurologic clinical abnormalities.

Dermoid sinus has been reported in multiple Rhodesian Ridgeback dogs and in a Shih tzu and a boxer.[2, 8, 15, 35, 48] A case in an English bulldog has also been seen.[4] The dermoid sinus of Rhodesian Ridgeback dogs may be caused by a gene complex; if so, most individuals of this breed carry some of the genetic factors. The only available data concerning inheritance of the dermoid sinus suggested that the factor may be inherited as a simple recessive gene.[35] If this is so, complete eradication of the problem can be achieved by only a program of progeny testing. However, by not breeding from affected individuals, the incidence can be rapidly reduced. When additional cases occur, breeders should extend that policy by not using either parent or any sibling of an affected pup for breeding. The problem is complicated further because dermoid sinus is not always easy to detect in a young pup.

CLINICAL FEATURES

Lesions are often noted in young dogs. Whorled hair may be seen along the topline (normal in the Rhodesian Ridgeback), or isolated whorls may appear at the dorsal midline at the cervicothoracic or lumbothoracic junction. A tuft of hair may protrude from single or multiple small openings in the skin and a cord of tissue may be palpated, descending from the skin toward the spine (Fig. 11:19).

Diagnosis can be suspected on the basis of the anamnesis and the clinical appearance, but it is confirmed by a fistulogram. A tract may be delineated from the skin to the dorsal processes of the thoracic vertebrae. Lumbar myelograms may demonstrate attenuation of the subarachnoid space near the termination of the fistula.

CLINICAL MANAGEMENT

Sinuses that are quiescent need no treatment other than observation. If drainage or neurologic signs are present, surgical dissection is the treatment of choice, but because of the deep

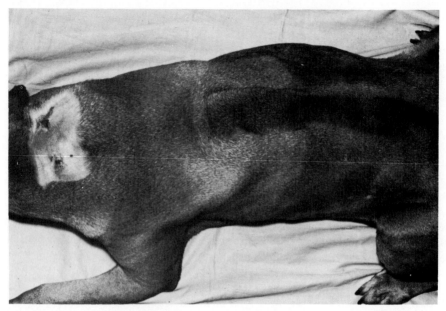

Figure 11:19. Dual fistulae opening on either side of the midline in the cervical region of the Rhodesian Ridgeback dog are typical lesions of a dermoid sinus. (Neck has been clipped.) Notice the whorled ridge of hair on the lower back from which the breed derived its name.

attachments of the dermoid sinus, complete removal is not always possible. The tissue at the base is often fibrous, and careful blunt dissection is needed. Meningitis may complicate these cases; therefore, extreme care should be taken to ensure an aseptic technique during surgery. Successful surgery often results in complete recovery. Affected individuals should not be bred.

Epidermolysis Bullosa

In humans, the term *epidermolysis bullosa* refers to a group of hereditary mechanobullous diseases.[1] Classification is by mode of inheritance and histopathologic features. In all forms, cutaneous blistering occurs in response to trauma. The pathogenesis is not completely described but focuses on abnormal keratin production and anchoring fibril defects.

The first reports of epidermolysis bullosa in dogs were in collies[45] and Shetland sheepdogs.[36b] Those cases may have had dermatomyositis as the skin lesions mimicked those seen in dermatomyositis. The authors and others[117] have examined multiple collies and Shetland sheepdogs with the classic skin lesions of dermatomyositis but have been unable to demonstrate muscle disease by electromyography (EMG) or multiple biopsies. These cases may have dermatomyositis without muscular involvement[19, 50] or epidermolysis bullosa simplex.

Junctional epidermolysis bullosa has been described in a Toy Poodle,[12] multiple Beaucerons,[14] and multiple Siamese cats.[24] The poodle had multiple vesicles and bullae within 24 hours of birth and was euthanized at 3 days of age. Lesions occurred on all footpads, in the oral cavity, and in the glabrous skin of the ventrum. The Beaucerons developed crusted papules and erosions in the genital region and at mucocutaneous junctions at 6 weeks of age.[14] By 16 weeks of age, erosive and ulcerative lesions were present on the face, the pinnae, the medial thighs, the perianal and perivulvar regions, the ventral aspect of the tail, and the feet. Pedigree analysis suggested an autosomal recessive mode of transmission. Skin biopsy specimens from the dogs showed numerous subbasilar vacuoles and clefts without inflammation (Fig. 11:20). Ultrastructural studies showed cleavage of the basement membrane through the lamina lucida, leaving the lamina densa attached to the dermis (Fig. 11:21). The cats were presented for shedding of

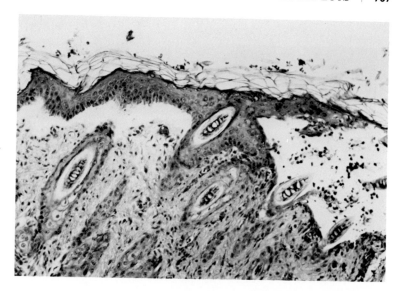

Figure 11:20. Junctional epidermolysis bullosa in a puppy. Subepidermal vesicle. (Courtesy R. Dunstan.)

all claws with secondary bacterial paronychia at 5 weeks of age. The sire of the kittens was affected. Biopsy results were similar to those reported for the dog, but ultrastructural studies were not performed. An autosomal recessive mode of inheritance was suggested.

Dystrophic (dermolytic) epidermolysis bullosa has been described in a domestic shorthair cat[55] and multiple Beaucerons.[25] The cat had disease from 3 months of age, which included paronychia and claw loss on all feet; ulceration of the gums, tongue, palate, and oropharynx (Fig. 11:22A); and ulceration with crusting of the metacarpus, metatarsus, and digital pads (Fig. 11:22B). Skin biopsy showed subbasilar dermal-epidermal separation. Ultrastructural studies showed clefting below the lamina densa. Multiple Beauceron pups from three separate litters were examined for the early development of erosive crusty lesions around mucocutaneous junctions and over pressure points and sloughing of claws. The dogs also had defects in tooth enamel, retarded growth, and an abnormal stance. Biopsy showed subbasilar clefting, but ultrastructural studies were not performed. These dogs may have had junctional epidermolysis bullosa.

No specific treatment of epidermolysis bullosa exists. Environmental management to minimize trauma and appropriate treatment for secondary infections may allow mildly affected animals to lead a reasonably normal life.

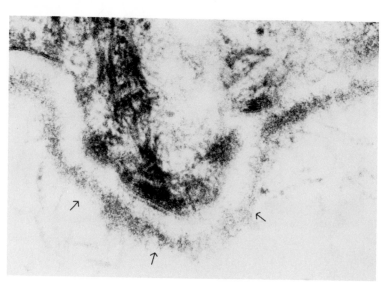

Figure 11:21. Junctional epidermolysis bullosa in a puppy. Electron microscopy reveals smaller than normal hemidesmosomes and decreased electron density in the underlying lamina lucida (arrows). (Courtesy R. Dunstan.)

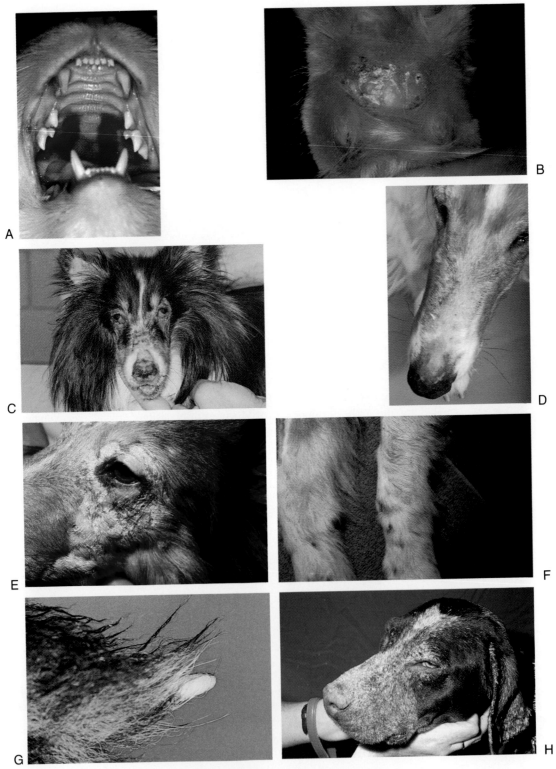

Figure 11:22 *See legend on opposite page*

Familial Canine Dermatomyositis

Familial canine dermatomyositis is a hereditary, idiopathic inflammatory condition of the skin and muscles of young collies, Shetland sheepdogs, and their crosses.[18, 19] It has also been reported in the Welsh corgi, Chow Chow, German shepherd dog, and Kuvasz[3, 54] and recognized in other purebred dogs. The familial basis in these other breeds is unproved.

CAUSE AND PATHOGENESIS

The cause of dermatomyositis in humans or dogs is unknown.[1, 19] An immune-mediated pathogenesis is suspected because of detectable immunologic abnormalities,[20] but it is unclear whether this immunologic reaction causes all of the changes seen or is in response to some pre-existing muscle or skin damage. Although dermatomyositis could be induced by drugs, infections (especially viral ones), toxins, or internal malignancies, their causal relationship in dermatomyositis remains unproved.[1]

A familial history is rare in humans, but common in collies and Shetland sheepdogs. Breeding studies in collies support an autosomal dominant mode of inheritance with variable expressivity.[19] Limited studies in the Shetland sheepdog conducted by one author (WHM) suggest a similar mode of inheritance in this breed.

CLINICAL FEATURES

In collies and Shetland sheepdogs, there is no sex, coat color, or coat length association with dermatomyositis. This may or may not be true for other breeds. Because of the familial predisposition, lesions occur early in life, typically before 6 months of age. Signs in some dogs appear as early as 7 to 11 weeks of age. The progression of lesions is variable. Some mildly affected dogs have few lesions, which heal rapidly without scarring. Most dogs have new lesions after the first ones are recognized, but the rate of progression is variable. The extent of the skin lesions is known by 1 year of age. Unless management changes occur, lesions usually decrease in number and severity from that point on.

Skin lesions occur in areas of mechanical trauma and are commonly seen on the face (see Fig. 11:22 *C* and *D*), especially around the eyes (Fig. 11:22*E*); on the tips of the ears; on carpal and tarsal regions (Fig. 11:22*F*); on the digits; and on the tip of the tail (Fig. 11:22*G*). Oral and footpad lesions can be seen but are rare. Although intact vesicles can be seen in some dogs, primary lesions are usually absent. Typical skin lesions are characterized by alopecia, erythema, scaling, and mild crusting. Ulceration can be seen in severely affected dogs. Skin lesions are usually not pruritic unless a secondary staphylococcal infection has occurred. In mildly to moderately affected dogs, large areas of normal skin remain, whereas severely affected dogs have involvement of the entire face, distal limbs, and tail. Some dogs have long, soft claws.

The myositis typically occurs after the skin lesions are recognized and correlates with the severity of the skin lesions. Mildly affected dogs have no clinical muscle disease and convincing evidence of this may not be found on EMG testing or muscle biopsy. These cases may have epidermolysis bullosa, dermatomyositis with focal but undetected myositis, or dermatomyositis without the myositis.[50] In humans, the diagnosis of amyopathic dermatomyositis can

Figure 11:22. *A*, Dystrophic epidermolysis bullosa in a kitten. Oral ulceration. (Courtesy S. White.) *B*, Dystrophic epidermolysis bullosa in a kitten. Ulcerated carpal footpad. (Courtesy S. White.) *C*, Shetland sheepdog with dermatomyositis. Severe facial scarring and drop-jaw. *D*, Dermatomyositis in a collie. Chronic case with scarring alopecia on the bridge of the nose. *E*, Shetland sheepdog with severe, typical lesions on cheek and eyelids. *F*, Dermatomyositis in a collie. Patchy alopecia and erythema over the cranial aspect of the carpi. *G*, Collie with dermatomyositis. Alopecia of the tip of the tail. *H*, Hereditary lupoid dermatosis in a German shorthaired pointer. Marked scaling and hyperkeratosis of the face and pinna. (Courtesy M. Song.)

be made only when no muscle changes are detected for 4 years or longer after the skin lesions have occurred. To the authors' knowledge, this type of follow-up testing has not been done in dogs. The rare dog related to dogs with classic dermatomyositis has EMG changes of myositis with no skin lesions. The significance of these findings is unknown.

Clinical signs of myositis are variable. A common finding is a dirty water bowl that contains food particles. These dogs do not have trouble chewing their food but do not swallow it completely, so residual pieces are washed from the mouth during drinking. Some dogs have a peculiar high-stepping gait. Severely affected dogs drink, chew, and swallow with difficulty; have a stiff gait; have megaesophagus; and often have secondary aspiration pneumonia. The most common sign of the myositis is asymptomatic atrophy, especially of the muscles of mastication and distal limbs.

The rare dog has skin lesions only in adulthood.[19, 54] The lesions can be the classic superficial lesions of dermatomyositis or be more deeply ulcerated (see Idiopathic Ulcerative Dermatosis in Shetland Sheepdogs and Collies in this chapter). These cases could represent an adult-onset variant of the diseases or be dogs who had mild, unrecognized disease as puppies.

DIAGNOSIS

The differential diagnostic considerations should include demodicosis, staphylococcal folliculitis, dermatophytosis, discoid lupus erythematosus, and epidermolysis bullosa. The latter might be considered if there are no muscle signs or lesions and if vesicles are present.

Diagnosis is made by history, physical examination findings, biopsy of affected skin and muscle, EMG, and laboratory tests to rule out other conditions. Biopsy of affected skin shows scattered vacuolar change of the surface and follicular basal cells (Fig. 11:23).[3] Occasional apoptotic basal cells (Civatte's bodies) may be seen. With confluent hydropic change, intrabasal or subepidermal clefting may be seen (Fig. 11:24). Dermal inflammation can be absent. Most cases show a mild perivascular to interstitial dermatitis in which lymphocytes, plasma cells, and histiocytes predominate. Mild pigmentary incontinence may be present in the superficial

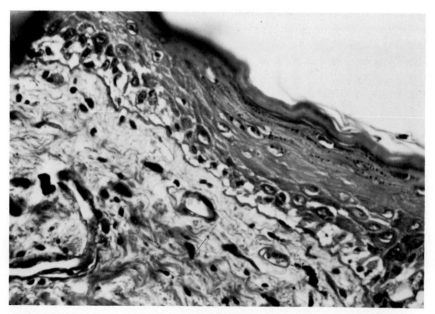

Figure 11:23. Dermatomyositis (epidermolysis bullosa simplex) in a collie. Marked hydropic degeneration of epidermal basal cells without inflammation. (From Scott, D. W., Schultz, R. D.: Epidermolysis bullosa simplex in the collie dog. J.A.V.M.A. 171:721, 1977.)

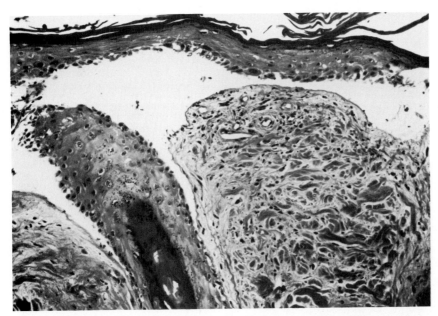

Figure 11:24. Dermatomyositis (epidermolysis bullosa simplex) in a collie. Subepidermal vesicle due to hydropic degeneration of epidermal basal cells. (From Scott, D. W., Schultz, R. D.: Epidermolysis bullosa simplex in the collie dog. J.A.V.M.A. 171:721, 1977.)

dermis. Follicular atrophy and fibrosis are common findings (Figs. 11:25 and 11:26). Vasculitis may occasionally be seen in the skin. Muscle biopsy may show mixed inflammatory exudates, accompanied by muscle fiber necrosis and atrophy.[19] In some cases, a vasculitis may be found. Needle EMG abnormalities include positive sharp waves and fibrillation potentials in muscles of the head and of distal extremities.

Hemograms and serum chemistry profiles are usually unremarkable. Creatine kinase levels are normal or slightly increased. Neurologic examination and nerve conduction studies are usually normal. Elevated concentrations of immunoglobulin G and circulating immune complexes may be found in active disease.[20] The magnitude of the elevations in immunoglobulin G and circulating immune complex levels correlates with the severity of the skin disease.[19]

CLINICAL MANAGEMENT

The skin lesions of dermatomyositis are worsened by trauma and prolonged solar exposure. Management changes to avoid these secondary insults should be instituted. Mildly affected dogs usually require no additional treatment, as their skin lesions heal spontaneously. Severely affected dogs are difficult to manage. These dogs have widespread skin lesions and a generalized myopathy, which results in lameness and difficulty in drinking and eating. These dogs often have aspiration pneumonia. Although large doses of prednisolone (1 mg/kg q24h) improve the skin lesions, the disease is progressive and euthanasia should be encouraged.

Mildly to moderately affected dogs can usually be maintained as acceptable pets for extended periods. Some skin lesions remain and muscle atrophy, especially of the muscles of mastication, is noted. Oral doses of vitamin E (200 to 800 IU/day) or marine lipid supplements (e.g., DVM Derm Caps) appear to be beneficial for the skin but not the muscle lesions. Occasional use of prednisolone (1 mg/kg q24h) is necessary in some dogs for traumatic flares. Continued use of glucocorticoids should be discouraged because the muscle atrophy may be aggravated.

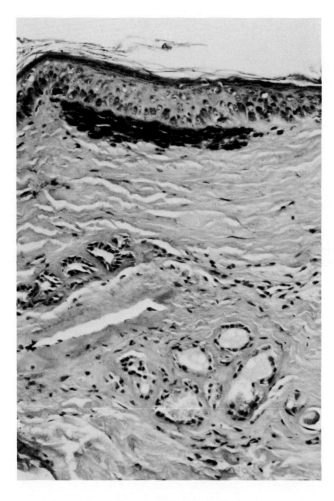

Figure 11:25. Canine dermatomyositis. Fibrosing dermatitis, with orphaned apocrine glands and pigmentary incontinence.

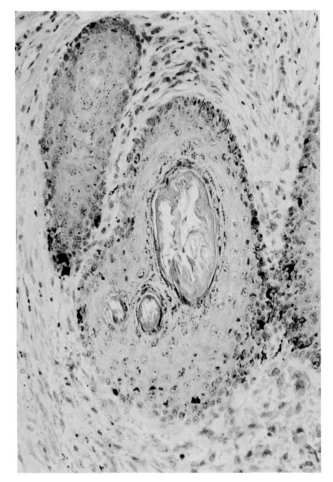

Figure 11:26. Canine dermatomyositis. Perifollicular fibrosis.

Treatment with pentoxifylline (Trental [Hoecsht-Roussel]) has been recommended.[19] This drug increases tissue oxygenation by increasing microvascular blood flow. It is a gastric irritant and must be given with food. Dosages of 400 mg every 24 to 48 hours have been suggested.[19, 23] Response is slow, and 2 to 3 months of treatment are necessary before efficacy can be determined. No data are available on the efficacy of this treatment.

The above treatments usually minimize the development of new skin lesions, and those that do occur tend to be milder. Muscle disease progresses, and old dogs have profound atrophy of the muscles of the head, the distal limbs, and sometimes the body. With severe atrophy, the animal's ability to eat and drink can be compromised and dietary manipulations are necessary. The limb and body atrophy can cause an abnormal gait, but locomotion is still possible. Amyloidosis can occur in some chronically affected dogs.[21]

Idiopathic Ulcerative Dermatosis in Shetland Sheepdogs and Collies

The ulcerative dermatosis described in Shetland sheepdogs and collies is of unknown etiology but may be a variant of dermatomyositis.[23]

CLINICAL FEATURES

Lesions occur in middle-aged to older dogs with no antecedent history of skin disease. The disease appears to be more prevalent in Shetland sheepdogs. No sex predilection is noted, but relapses or exacerbations can be seen with estrus. In all dogs, there can be cyclic recrudescence.

The initial lesions are vesiculobullous and are seen in the groin and then axillary regions. Lesions coalesce and ulcerate to form large serpiginous lesions with distinct borders between normal and abnormal skin. In rare cases, lesions can be found on the eyelids, the pinnae, the oral mucosa, the external genitalia, the anus, and the footpads. The lesions are painful, especially if secondarily infected.

DIAGNOSIS

The differential diagnostic considerations include bullous pemphigoid, erythema multiforme, systemic lupus erythematosus, and pemphigus vulgaris. Skin biopsy shows hydropic degeneration of basal cells and extensive individual keratinocyte necrosis, which can extend into the stratum spinosum.[3] In the dermis, there is a superficial perivascular to partially lichenoid dermatitis. No follicular atrophy is seen. Direct immunofluorescence testing and antinuclear antibody tests are negative. Some dogs have EMG abnormalities typical of those seen in dermatomyositis.

CLINICAL MANAGEMENT

Because lesions may be triggered or worsened by trauma, management changes to minimize trauma are appropriate. Antibiotic therapy is indicated in cases with secondary infections. Medications used in dermatomyositis (e.g., corticosteroids, vitamin E, and pentoxifylline) are reported to be effective. The cyclic nature of the disease can make maintenance management more difficult.

Canine Benign Familial Chronic Pemphigus

In humans, benign familial pemphigus is an autosomal dominant disorder of cellular cohesion among keratinocytes.[1] Because of the defect, the epidermis cannot withstand trauma and vesiculobullous lesions develop in response to friction or infection. A similar disorder has been reported in English setters and their crosses.[49] The disorder has also been recognized in a Doberman pinscher.[4]

CLINICAL FEATURES

Lesions occur in dogs at about 6 months of age and occur over pressure points on the limbs[49] or on the pinnae.[4] Lesions are first characterized by alopecia, erythema, and slight scaling. Increased scaling and crusting occur later. Vesicopustules are rarely seen. Lesions remain localized and cannot be easily induced.

DIAGNOSES

The differential diagnosis is limited and includes pressure point irritation and superficial bacterial folliculitis. Skin biopsy shows acanthosis with orthokeratotic and parakeratotic hyperkeratosis and marked, diffuse, incomplete acantholysis of the lower and middle portions of the epidermis and follicular outer root sheath.[49] Acantholytic dyskeratotic cells (corps ronds) may be seen. Immunofluorescence testing is negative.

CLINICAL MANAGEMENT

In humans, treatment of infections and avoidance of trauma usually provide good results.[1] Severe cases can be helped by the administration of systemic glucocorticoids or methotrexate. Because the lesions in dogs are asymptomatic and localized, no treatment has been attempted.

Hereditary Lupoid Dermatosis of German Shorthaired Pointers

The lupoid dermatosis of German shorthaired pointers is a newly described disorder. Cases have been recognized in the United States[53] and Europe.[44, 50a, 52] Aside from a familial predisposition, no cause of the dermatosis has been determined.

CLINICAL FEATURES

Lesions are first noted at about 6 months of age. Scaling and crusting are seen first on the face, the ears, and the back and then in a more generalized distribution (Fig. 11:22 *H*). The hocks and the scrotum may be severely involved. The lesions are variably painful or pruritic. Pyrexia and lymphadenopathy may accompany the skin lesions. Lesions may have a waxing and waning course[44] or be persistent.[53]

DIAGNOSIS

The differential diagnostic possibilities include nutritional disorders, a primary keratinization disorder, drug eruption, sebaceous adenitis, and systemic lupus erythematosus. The rare dog has laboratory evidence (proteinuria and positive antinuclear antibody titer) of the latter disorder.[53] Skin biopsy shows mild to moderate acanthosis, orthokeratotic and parakeratotic hyperkeratosis, hydropic degeneration of basal cells, and extensive individual keratinocyte necrosis with occasional satellitosis (Fig. 11:27).[53] The individual keratinocyte necrosis is found throughout the stratum spinosum and may be confluent. Basilar clefting may be present. The dermis shows a mixed cellular mild to moderate interface dermatitis, and sebaceous glands may be normal, small, or absent.

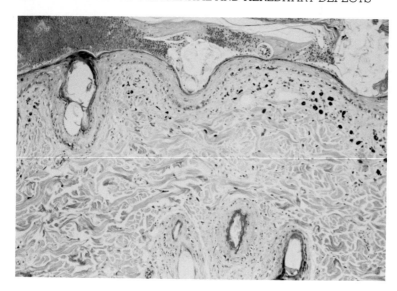

Figure 11:27. Hereditary lupoid dermatosis of German shorthaired pointer. Hydropic interface dermatitis. (Courtesy T. Gross.)

CLINICAL MANAGEMENT

To date, no uniformly successful treatment has been reported. Antiseborrheic baths and immunosuppressive doses of corticosteroids have given poor results. Fatty acid supplements may be beneficial,[50a, 52] but most cases show no response to this treatment.[53] Treatment with retinoids has been suggested but remains unproved.

■ DISORDERS OF HAIRS AND HAIR GROWTH

A variety of inherited disorders of the hair shaft or hair growth are reported in dogs and cats. Congenital conditions are easily recognized because they occur near birth, when they are easy to differentiate from endocrine and other acquired alopecias. Inherited disorders with tardive onset are more difficult and can mimic a variety of other disorders. Careful inspection of hairs via a trichogram or a skin biopsy differentiates inherited disorders from other acquired alopecias. These tests should be performed routinely in animals with abnormal hairs, for hair loss early in life, or for hair loss with an unusual distribution.

Inherited hair disorders have no specific treatment. Nutritional supplements, special diets, and so forth, as espoused by some breeders, are of minimal benefit. Good gentle grooming is imperative to minimize secondary infections and seborrhea. Without the normal protection of their coat, affected animals are susceptible to frostbite, sunburn, the effects of low environmental humidity, and other environmental insults. With appropriate management changes, these animals can lead nearly normal lives.

Structural Defects of the Hair Shaft

In humans, a variety of inherited or acquired conditions affect the shape, composition, and strength of the hair shafts.[1] Depending on the condition, the defect can be recognized because the scalp hairs are unmanageable or unusual in appearance or because the hairs break easily with routine brushing or combing. Diagnosis is made by light and scanning electron microscopic examination of affected hairs.

Coat abnormalities are common in veterinary medicine, but only four hair shaft defects have been reported. Undoubtedly, more occur but have gone unrecognized because microscopic examination of hair shafts was not a routine part of the clinical evaluation of patients with abnormal coats.

TRICHORRHEXIS NODOSA

In humans and animals, trichorrhexis nodosa is most often an acquired defect in which external insults damage the cuticle and weaken the hair shaft (see Chap. 10). In humans, some cases have an inherited basis.[1] The authors (WHM and DWS) have examined two unrelated young Golden retrievers for a poor coat. At examination, there was no hair loss, but the hairs were uneven in length. Trichograms showed nodular hair fracture typical of trichorrhexis nodosa (Fig. 11:28). No systemic or topical cause of the problem could be identified, and the condition persisted. These cases suggest that inherited trichorrhexis nodosa may occur in animals.

PILI TORTI

Pili torti is a condition in which curvature of the hair follicle leads to flattening and rotation of the hair shaft. In humans, most cases have a hereditary basis and the patients often experience other cutaneous and systemic abnormalities.[1] Localized acquired pili torti can result from follicular inflammation.

Pili torti has been reported in a litter of kittens[66] and in some bull terriers with acrodermatitis.[130] In the dogs, most hairs were normal, suggesting that the affected hairs resulted from follicular inflammation. In the cats, all hairs were affected by 10 days of age (Fig. 11:29A). In addition to the generalized hair loss, the kittens had a periocular and pedal dermatitis and paronychia. All secondary hairs showed the flattening and rotation typical of pili torti (Fig. 11:30), but primary hairs were not involved. On biopsy, follicular hyperkeratosis with occasional cystic dilatation was the only notable finding.

SHAFT DISORDER OF ABYSSINIAN CATS

Shaft disorder is an uncommon to rare condition of Abyssinian cats.[88] Only whiskers and primary hairs are affected. These hairs are rough and lusterless and have an onion-shaped swelling visible with the naked eye, usually at the tip of the hair (Fig. 11:31). Hair fracture can occur at the swelling. Skin biopsy shows no follicular abnormalities. The cause of the condition is unknown, but because of its restriction to Abyssinian cats, it must be considered an inherited disorder. No details on treatment are available.

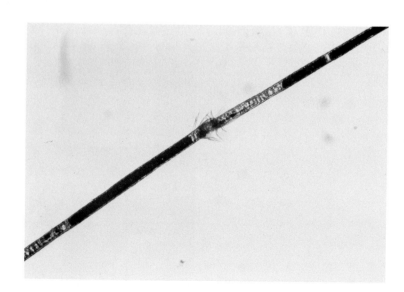

Figure 11:28. Trichorrhexis nodosa. Discrete splintering of hair.

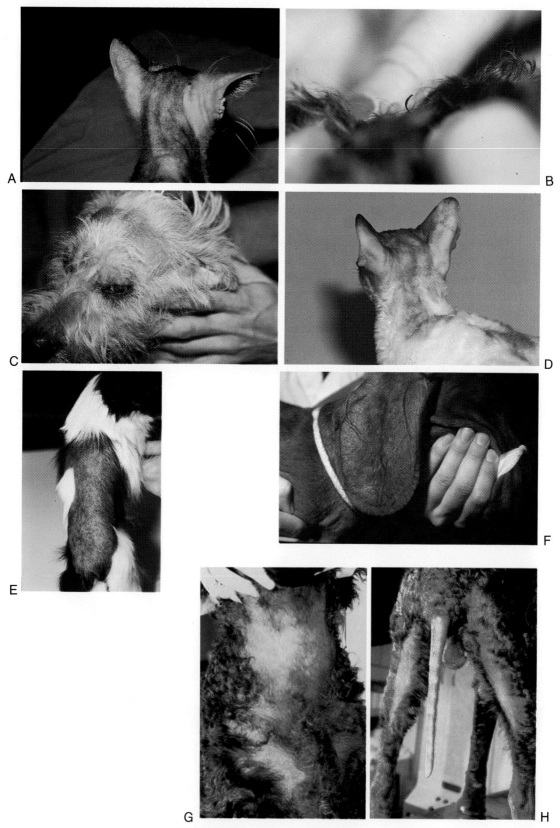

Figure 11:29 *See legend on opposite page*

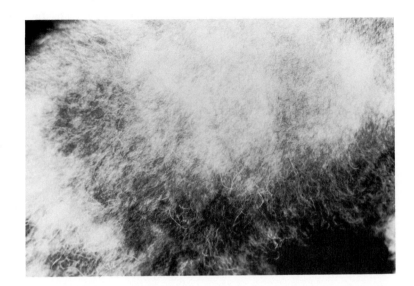

Figure 11:30. Pili torti in a cat. Note hypotrichosis and twisted hairs. (Courtesy C. Foil.)

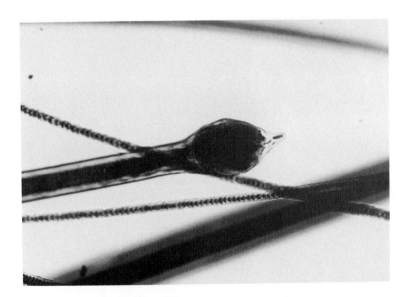

Figure 11:31. Shaft disorder of Abyssinian cats. Note the onion-shaped swelling at the tip of the hair.

Figure 11:29. *A*, Pili torti in a cat. (Courtesy C. Foil.) *B*, Spiculosis in a Kerry blue terrier. (Courtesy H. Raue.) *C*, Congenital hypotrichosis in a dog. *D*, Congenital hypotrichosis in a Devon rex cat. *E*, Black hair follicular dysplasia. Note the marked hypotrichosis over the dorsum that spares white-coated areas. (Courtesy C. Foil.) *F*, Pattern baldness on the pinna of a 7-year-old dachshund. *G*, Pattern baldness on the ventral neck of an Irish water spaniel. *H*, Pattern baldness on the tail and thighs of an Irish water spaniel.

SPICULOSIS

Spiculosis is a rare disorder of young intact male Kerry blue terriers.[73a] Affected dogs have multiple, hard, brittle follicular spicules (see Fig. 11:29 B), which are 1 to 2.5 mm in diameter and 0.5 to 3 cm in length. The spicules can be found on any haired surface but are most common over the lateral hock region. Although the spicules can be asymptomatic, most dogs lick or chew at them.

Biopsy shows follicular dysplasia with premature keratinization.[73a] This defect results in an amorphous mass of keratin, which is shaped into the spicule by the outer root sheath and the follicular wall (Fig. 11:32).

In asymptomatic dogs, no treatment is indicated and the spicules persist. In pruritic animals, the only effective treatment has been with isotretinoin (1 mg/kg orally q24h). After 3 to 4 months of treatment, the spicules disappear. With discontinuation of the drug regimen, the dog may remain normal or the spicules may redevelop. In the latter case, maintenance therapy with isotretinoin is indicated.

Congenital Hypotrichosis or Alopecia

With congenital hair loss, the hypotrichosis or alopecia is obvious at birth or develops during the first 2 to 4 weeks of life. Some animals have only hair follicle disease, whereas other animals also have involvement of other skin appendages. Additional ectodermal defects such

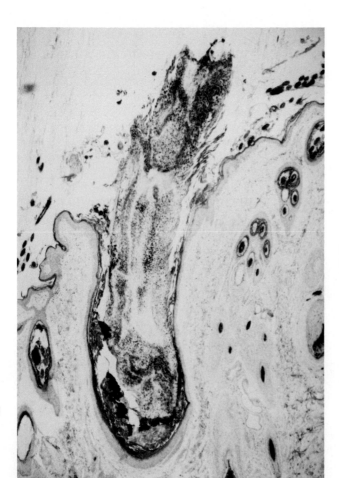

Figure 11:32. Spiculosis in a Kerry blue terrier.

as abnormal dentition or tear production may also be noted. To categorize these animals accurately, Foil[2] proposed a numerical classification scheme, noting changes in hair, teeth, claws, adnexal glands, or other ectodermal structures. Classification of newly recognized cases according to this scheme should help to categorize these disorders and remove some of the confusion or misclassification that currently exists in the veterinary literature.

ALOPECIC BREEDS

The best known examples of hairless dog breeds are the Mexican hairless dog and the Chinese crested dog (Fig. 11:33). Other hairless breeds include the Inca hairless dog, Peruvian Inca Orchid, and American hairless terrier.[2, 70, 71] In cats, the sphinx is bred for its hairlessness (Fig. 11:34).[82]

These hairless breeds resulted from the intentional breeding of animals with a spontaneous mutation. In the Mexican hairless, an autosomal dominant mode of inheritance has been demonstrated.[71] The American hairless terrier was developed from American rat terriers with an autosomal recessive hairless trait.[2] The hairless Mexican hairless dogs have a shorter survival time than their haired relatives.[70] This decreased survival may be due to a familial immunoincompetence linked to the hairlessness.

CONGENITAL HYPOTRICHOSIS

Congenital hypotrichosis is the term used to describe animals born without their normal pelage or who develop non–color-linked hair loss within the first month of life. Some animals have only hair follicle involvement, whereas other animals have additional ectodermal defects. Many cases are not well characterized.

Dogs

Congenital hypotrichosis has been described in the American Cocker spaniel, Belgian shepherd, Toy and Miniature Poodles, whippet, beagle, French bulldog, Rottweiler, Yorkshire terrier,

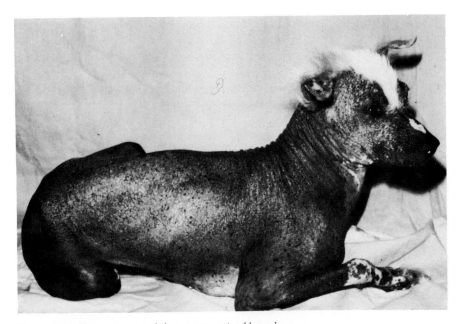

Figure 11:33. Chinese crested dog, a recognized breed.

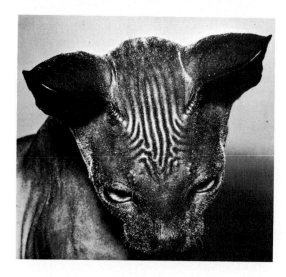

Figure 11:34. Feline alopecia universalis. (From Scott, D. W.: Feline dermatology 1900–1978: A monograph. J.A.A.H.A. 16:331, 1980.)

Labrador retriever, Bichon frisé, Lhasa apso, and Basset hound.* It has been recognized by the authors in Cocker spaniel–Miniature Poodle crossbreeds.[4] Most cases have been recognized in male animals, suggesting some sex linkage.

Most affected animals are born with noticeable hair loss, which progresses over the next month or so. Some dogs are born normally haired but lose it shortly thereafter.[2, 65] The hair loss is symmetric in distribution and typically involves the temporal regions, the ear pinnae, the caudal dorsum, and the entire ventrum (Figs. 11:35 and 11:36; also see Fig. 11:29C). Some cases are born nearly bald[70a, 84] or experience near-total hair loss by 12 to 14 weeks of age.[65] When the hair loss is regionalized, it is well-delineated from the adjacent normal skin. Early on, the hairless skin is clinically normal, but it can become hyperpigmented and seborrheic with advancing time. If the dog is examined after its puppy teeth have been replaced by adult teeth, abnormalities in dentition may be recognized.

Cats

Congenital hypotrichosis has been reported in Birman,[62] Burmese,[58] Devon rex[86] and Siamese[83] cats. Multiple kittens in the litter are involved, and no sex linkage has been described. In Birman and Siamese cats, the condition is an autosomal recessive trait.

Affected cats either are born hairless or have a thin downy coat that is lost in the first weeks of life (see Fig. 11:29D). Affected Burmese cats have no whiskers, claws, or papillae on the tongue.[58] At necropsy of affected Birman kittens, no thymus was found.[62]

The tentative diagnosis of congenital hypotrichosis in dogs or cats is straightforward and is confirmed by skin biopsy (Figs. 11:37 to 11:39). In all cases, hair follicle involvement is marked. In some cases, there is complete absence of follicles,[62] whereas hair follicles are hypoplastic and decreased in number in other cases.[57, 83] Adnexae (sebaceous glands, sweat glands, and arrector pili muscles) are reduced in number, hypoplastic, or absent.

BLACK HAIR FOLLICULAR DYSPLASIA

Black hair follicular dysplasia is a rare disorder in which dogs with bicolor or tricolor coats lose hairs in the black areas only at an early age.

---

*See references 2, 3, 5, 63–65, 67, 70a, 72, 73, 75, 84, and 87.

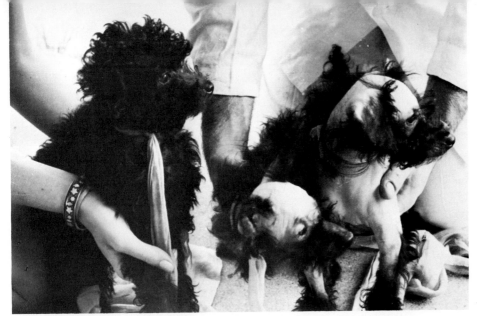

Figure 11:35. The partially alopecic males compared with a full-coated sister. The pattern of alopecia, which is bilaterally symmetric and includes about two thirds of the body surface, is the same in both males. (From Selmanowitz, V. J., et al.: Congenital ectodermal defect in Miniature Poodles. J. Hered. 61:196, 1970.)

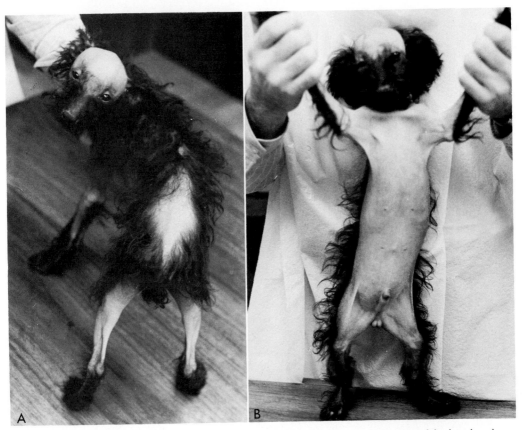

Figure 11:36. *A,* Diamond-shaped alopecic region over the dorsal pelvis and alopecia of the head and limbs. *B,* Ventral view of affected male, showing the pattern of alopecia on the trunk and legs. (From Selmanowitz, V. J., et al.: Congenital ectodermal defect in Miniature Poodles. J. Hered. 61:196, 1970.)

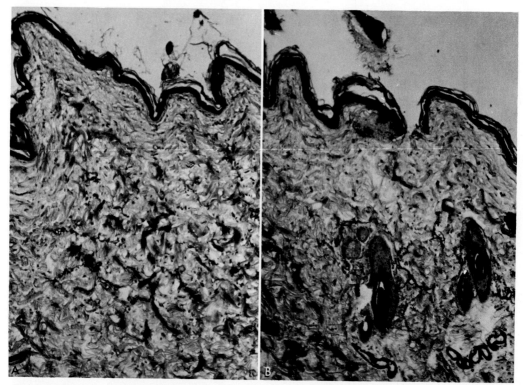

Figure 11:37. *A,* Appendage-free skin from the head; hair follicles, sebaceous glands and sweat glands are absent. (Acid orcein elastica stain ×70.) *B,* Transition zone of appendage-free and appendage-containing skin. Hair follicles, sweat glands, and sebaceous gland cells (near the upper portion of the section of the follicle in the center of the photograph) appear normal. The portion of dermis lacking appendages marks the beginning of a large area of alopecia. There is no overt difference in the appearance of the epidermis and connective tissue on either side of the transition. (From Selmanowitz, V. J., et al.: Congenital ectodermal defect in Miniature Poodles. J. Hered. 61:196, 1970.)

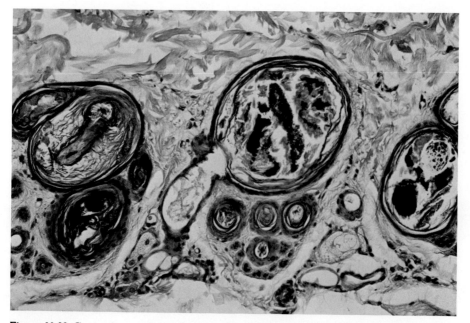

Figure 11:38. Canine hypotrichosis. Dystrophic hair follicles and abortive hair shafts.

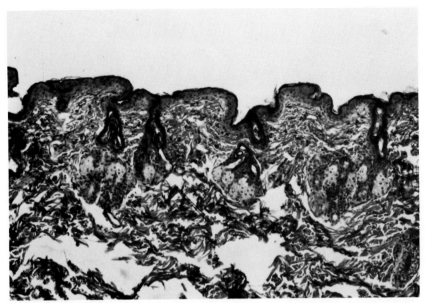

Figure 11:39. Hereditary hypotrichosis in a Siamese cat. The poorly developed hair follicles are devoid of hair shafts. (From Scott, D. W.: Feline dermatology 1900–1978: A monograph. J.A.A.H.A. 16:331, 1980.)

■ *Cause and Pathogenesis.* Black hair follicular dysplasia is a familial disorder with near-uniform involvement of the puppies with black coats. Histologic and ultrastructural studies show disorders of pigment transfer and cuticular abnormalities of the affected and some normal hairs.[69] The early age at onset suggests that the defect in hair formation plays a significant role in the hair loss. With disorderly proliferation of hair matrix cells, normal pigment transfer to the developing hairs is not expected and the hairs are weakened even further. Some undetermined coat color genetic influence or possibly a deficiency in melanocyte-stimulating hormone could contribute to the pigmentary changes.[61]

■ *Clinical Features.* Black hair follicular dysplasia has been recognized in mongrels and purebred dogs of many breeds, including the bearded collie, Basset hound, Papillon, Saluki, beagle, American Cocker spaniel, Schipperke, dachshund, Gordon setter, and Pointer.[2, 3, 5, 61, 69, 85] Dogs are born normal but show coat changes by 4 weeks of age. Only the black hairs are affected (see Fig. 11:29E). The first noticeable change is loss of luster of the black hairs, followed by progressive hair loss until all black hairs are lost. Because the hair loss is due to shaft fracture, stubble can remain. Excessive scaliness occurs in the involved areas. The rate of hair loss is variable, but near-total alopecia occurs by 6 to 9 months of age.

■ *Diagnosis.* The color-linked nature and early age at onset of the hair loss make the diagnosis straightforward. Biopsy specimens from nonblack areas are normal, whereas black areas show clumped melanin in epidermal and follicular basal cells and hair matrix cells.[3, 69] Large melanin granules (macromelanosomes) are seen within hair shafts, and the follicles are irregular, are dilated, and are filled with keratin, fragments of hair shafts, and large clumps of free melanin. Numerous peribulbar melanophages occur in the dermis. The pigmentary changes seen are less pronounced than they are in color dilution alopecia.

Tardive Hypotrichosis or Alopecia

Animals with tardive hypotrichosis or alopecia are born with normal coats. Focal, regionalized, or generalized hair loss occurs either about the time when the puppy coat is replaced by the adult coat or when the animal is a young adult.

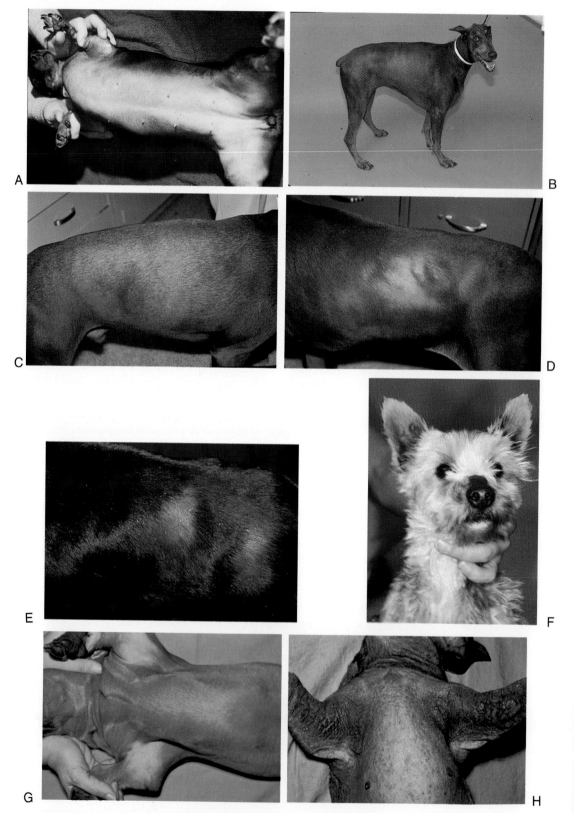

Figure 11:40 *See legend on opposite page*

PATTERN BALDNESS

Pattern baldness has been reported in only dogs, and three syndromes are recognized. The first is pinnal alopecia of male and, rarely, female dachshunds. Affected dogs slowly start to lose hair from both pinnae at about 6 to 9 months of age, and the hair loss progresses slowly to complete pinnal alopecia (see Fig. 11:29 F). Complete baldness usually occurs by 8 or 9 years of age. As the hair loss progresses, the exposed skin hyperpigments. Aside from the pinnal hair loss, the dogs have normal coats.

The second syndrome occurs in American water spaniels and Portuguese water dogs. Hair loss in these dogs typically is noted at about 6 months of age and is restricted to the ventral neck, the caudomedial thighs, and the tail (Fig. 11:29 G and H). Recognition of this problem by the respective breed clubs has sharply reduced the frequency of occurrence.

The third and most common syndrome is seen primarily in dachshunds but also is recognized in Boston terriers, Chihuahuas, whippets, Manchester terriers, Greyhounds, and Italian Greyhounds.[2, 3] The condition is recognized almost exclusively in female animals. At approximately 6 months of age, affected dogs gradually begin to lose hair in the postauricular regions and along the ventral neck, on the entire ventrum (Fig. 11:40A), and on the caudomedial thighs. Hair loss is gradual over the next 12 months but remains restricted to the described areas. Close inspection of the hairless skin reveals multiple small fine hairs. The primary differential diagnostic consideration for this syndrome is estrogen-responsive dermatosis (see Chap. 9). In estrogen-responsive dermatosis, the hair loss begins later in life and leaves no residual hairs.

Histologically, pattern baldness is characterized by a decrease in size (miniaturization) of the hair follicles with normal adnexal structures.[3] The follicles are shorter and thinner, have smaller hair bulbs, and produce fine hair shafts.

COLOR DILUTION ALOPECIA

Color dilution alopecia (color mutant alopecia) occurs in some dogs with blue or fawn coat colors. These colors are dilutions of black or brown, respectively, and result from the influence of coat color genes at the D locus and possibly others.[78, 79] Color dilution alopecia does not occur in all dogs with blue or fawn coats and the frequency within affected breeds varies.

■ *Cause and Pathogenesis.* The cause of color dilution alopecia is unknown, but coat color genes play a significant role in the condition. Under the influence of genes at the D locus and possibly others, dilute hairs have larger pigment granules (macromelanosomes) than their nondilute counterparts. Although the hairs are lighter in color, they contain as much or more melanin than nondilute black or brown hairs.

Only one allele, d, is recognized at the D locus in dogs.[78, 79] If this gene was solely responsible for color dilution alopecia, all dogs with dilute coat colors would lose hair, but they do not. Unrecognized, deleterious alleles may be present within certain breeds and cause lethal pigmentary changes, which result in the hair loss. This is supported by the absence of cuticular abnormalities, except at the points of pigmentary clumping in some dogs, the accumulation of stage IV melanosomes, and the visualization of vacuoles in melanocytes in hair bulb cells, suggesting a degenerative process.[68] The finding of cuticular changes in some normal, nondilute hairs from affected dogs suggests that a duel defect may exist in some dogs.[59]

Figure 11:40. A, Pattern baldness on the ventrum of a 2-year-old dachshund. B, Color dilution alopecia in a blue Doberman pinscher. C, Color dilution alopecia in a fawn Doberman pinscher. D, Follicular dysplasia in an adult red Doberman pinscher. E, Follicular dysplasia in an adult black Doberman pinscher. F, Facial and pinnal hyperpigmentation and alopecia in a Yorkshire terrier. G, Acanthosis nigricans, juvenile stage. Note the small hyperpigmented patches in the axillae of this 6-month-old dachshund. H, Acanthosis nigricans, severe hyperpigmentation, and lichenification in a 5-year-old dachshund.

■ *Clinical Features.* Color dilution alopecia is most widely recognized and reported in blue or fawn Doberman pinschers.[68, 78] It also has been reported in dachshunds, Great Danes, whippets, Italian Greyhounds, Chow Chows, Standard Poodles, Miniature Doberman pinscher, Yorkshire terriers, Silky terrier, Chihuahua, Boston terrier, Salukis, Newfoundlands, Shetland sheepdogs, Schipperkes, Burmese Mountain dogs, and mongrels with dilute coat colors.* It has also been reported in cream Chow Chow and blond Irish setters, but these cases may represent some other condition.[5] The frequency of the disease in blue or fawn Doberman pinschers can be as high as 93 per cent in blues and 75 per cent in fawns.[77] Incidence figures for other breeds are unknown but are probably much lower than they are in Doberman pinschers. Some breeds with a dilute coat color (e.g., Weimaraners) do not lose hair.

Color dilution alopecia can be first manifested by a dorsally oriented recurrent bacterial folliculitis or hypotrichosis. Only hairs or hair follicles in the dilute areas are involved. The onset of signs is tardive, and the starting point depends on management factors and the depth of the coat color. Dogs with light blue (e.g., gray) coats are usually affected at approximately 6 months of age, whereas dogs with less dilution (e.g., steel blue) may not have noticeable signs until 2 to 3 years of age or later. Vigorous grooming can accelerate the process.

In the recurrent folliculitis form, papules and pustules are seen and disappear with appropriate antibiotic treatment. The involved follicles tend to remain hairless or regrow hair slowly. With repeated bouts of infection, the hypotrichosis becomes more widespread and persistent. In the hair loss form, secondary pyodermas can also occur, but the history and physical examination findings clearly show that hair loss preceded the infection. Dogs with the hair loss form typically lose hairs first over the dorsum and then from the rest of the body (Fig. 11:40 *B* and *C*). The rate of hair loss is variable, but most light-colored dogs are almost completely alopecic by 2 to 3 years of age.

The initial hair loss in these dogs is due to shaft fracture, and some broken hairs regrow. With time, the tendency to regrow decreases. Exposed skin is subject to environmental insults and scaliness is commonly seen.

■ *Diagnosis.* The differential diagnosis varies with the age at onset. In the young dog, only other inherited hair defects or demodicosis should be investigated. With onset at 2 to 3 years or later, endocrine disorders, especially hypothyroidism, are considered for dogs with just hair loss. All causes of superficial folliculitis should be considered in that presentation.

Microscopic examination of plucked hairs shows numerous macromelanosomes, of irregular shapes and sizes, unevenly distributed along the shaft. In some cases, the macromelanosomes are huge and distort the hair shaft (Fig. 11:41). The cuticle may be absent or fractured over the bulging pigment clumps (Fig. 11:42). Histopathologic study initially shows melanin clumping in epidermal and follicular basal cells (Fig. 11:43) and hair matrix cells; numerous macromelanosomes in hair shafts; hair follicles in various stages of growth with follicular hyperkeratosis, fractured hair shafts, and free clumps of melanin (Fig. 11:44); and numerous peribulbar melanophages.[3, 78] With time, all follicular activity ceases and the follicles are dilated and cystic.

■ *Clinical Management.* Early on, hair loss is due to shaft fracture, so every effort should be made to avoid the use of harsh shampoos and topical agents and vigorous grooming techniques. These measures should slow but not prevent hair loss. Anecdotal reports suggest that treatment with oral retinoic acids can be of benefit, but specific details are unavailable.[6] Etretinate was reported to occasionally help dogs with color dilution alopecia, resulting in decreased scaling, and decreased frequency and severity of bacterial pyoderma.[67a] However, any hair regrowth was partial and characterized by fine hairs.

---

*See references 2, 3, 5, 57, 59, 61, 74, and 79.

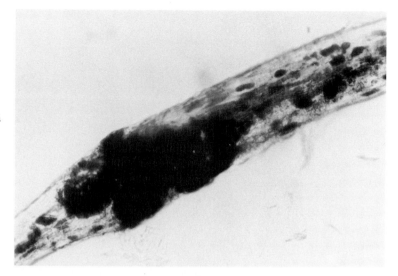

Figure 11:41. Color dilution alopecia. Marked melanin clumping and distortion of cuticular-cortical anatomy.

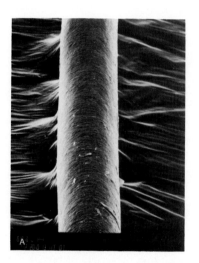

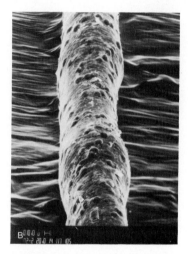

Figure 11:42. Color dilution alopecia. Scanning electron microscopic views (SEMs) of hairs from a normal black *(A)* and affected blue *(B)* Doberman pinscher. The cortical irregularities in *B* are due to macromelanosomes. (Courtesy D. Prieur.)

Figure 11:43. Color dilution alopecia. Melanin clumping in surface epidermis.

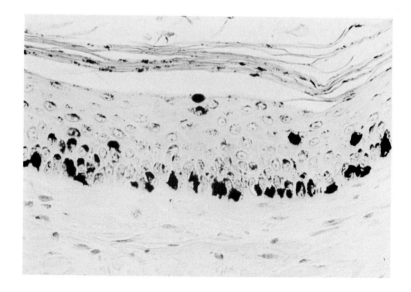

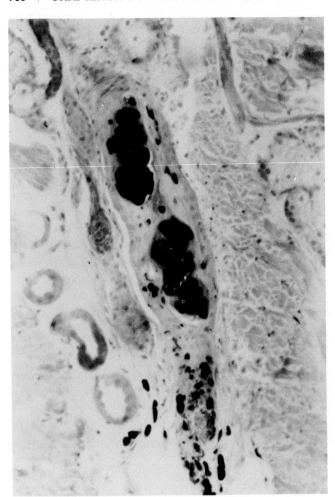

Figure 11:44. Color dilution alopecia. Marked clumping of melanin ("melanotic mush") in the pilar canal of a hair follicle.

FOLLICULAR DYSPLASIA

Non–color-linked follicular dysplasia is a newly recognized condition. A variety of breeds are affected. Onset can be during puppyhood or early adult life, and progression is slow.

■ *Clinical Features.* Follicular dysplasia has been seen or reported in many different breeds, including the Siberian husky, English Springer spaniel, Airedale terrier, Malamute, German shorthaired and wirehaired pointer, Rottweiler, Irish water spaniel, Portuguese water dog, Curly-coated retriever, Chesapeake Bay retriever, Miniature Schnauzer, Doberman pinscher, boxer, Bouvier des Flandres, English bulldog, Staffordshire terrier, and French bulldog.[2–4] Features of the disorder vary somewhat with the breed involved.

■ *Siberian Husky and Malamute.* Multiple dogs in a litter can be affected.[80, 81] At 3 to 4 months of age, the guard hairs on the trunk are lost in a slowly progressive fashion and the coat turns a reddish color. The head and the distal limbs are spared. Areas clipped for biopsy do not regrow hair. Secondary hairs are less frequently involved.

■ *Doberman Pinschers.* Black or red dogs can be affected, and the hair loss is noted between 1 and 4 years of age.[77] Hair loss begins in the flank region and progresses slowly to involve the caudal dorsum and entire flank region (Fig. 11:40 *D* and *E*). Complete truncal hair loss has not been recognized.

■ *Airedale Terrier, Boxer, English Bulldog, and Staffordshire Terrier.* Hair loss begins between 2 and 4 years of age and is restricted to the flank or saddle regions.[76] In some dogs, the hair loss persists, whereas cyclic loss and regrowth occurs in other dogs (see Chap. 10).

■ *Irish Water Spaniels, Portuguese Water Dogs, and Curly-Coated Retrievers.* The hair loss in these dogs is due to hair fracture.[3] Alopecia is usually not recognized until 2 to 4 years of age, but excessive hairs in grooming tools is recognized from an early age. Hair loss occurs first over the caudal dorsum and spreads slowly to involve most of the trunk. Early on, spontaneous hair regrowth can occur, but the new hairs are not of normal quality and texture. These, plus other hairs, are lost eventually, and the hair loss persists.

■ *Other Dogs.* Insufficient details are available to determine whether the hair loss is different from that discussed above.

■ *Diagnosis.* The primary differential diagnostic consideration in these dogs is endocrine hair loss, especially that associated with the sex hormones. Histopathologic examination shows surface and follicular orthokeratotic hyperkeratosis, variation in follicular activity with a high frequency of catagen arrest, melanin clumping within hairs and hair bulbs, fractured hair shafts with clumps of free melanin in hair follicle lumina, and peribulbar melanophages.[3] Huskies have tortuous glassy membranes and follicular epithelial cell disarray.[81] Portuguese water dogs occasionally have one or more severely malformed hairs.[4]

Melanoderma and Alopecia in Yorkshire Terriers

Melanoderma and alopecia in Yorkshire terriers is a well-recognized, but poorly studied syndrome.[5, 56, 60] It is probably a genetic dermatosis, but the mode of inheritance is unknown. The cause is unknown, but one investigator demonstrated decreased dermal elastin and abnormal growth hormone response to clonidine administration in eight dogs.[60] Typically, the syndrome affects Yorkshire terriers, of either sex, beginning at 6 months to 3 years of age.

The dogs have a symmetric alopecia and marked hyperpigmentation over the bridge of the nose, on the pinnae, and occasionally on the tail and feet (Fig. 11:40 *F*). Affected skin is smooth and shiny. There is no pruritus or pain, and affected dogs are otherwise healthy.

Skin biopsy specimens are reported to show orthokeratotic hyperkeratosis of the epidermal surface and of the hair follicles and epidermal melanosis.

Some dogs with mild lesions appear to recover spontaneously. Most dogs remain affected throughout their lifetime. Three dogs treated with growth hormone regrew hair but lost it again.[60]

■ DISORDERS OF PIGMENTATION

Hypopigmentary Disorders

Loss of skin pigment (leukoderma) or hair pigment (leukotrichia) has a variety of inflammatory or metabolic causes. Idiopathic cases occur with some regularity and have been reported in dogs of various breeds.[3] The high frequency of these changes in the Belgian Tervurens, German shepherd dog, Rottweiler, and Doberman pinscher suggests a hereditary influence in these breeds (see Chap. 12).

Hyperpigmentary Disorders

Aside from lentigines (see Chap. 12) or macular melanosis associated with testicular neoplasia (see Chap. 9), the hyperpigmentation seen in dogs and rarely in cats is poorly demarcated, involves large areas, and has a variety of inflammatory or endocrine causes. Acanthosis nigricans in some dachshunds probably has a hereditary basis.

ACANTHOSIS NIGRICANS

Canine acanthosis nigricans is an uncommon cutaneous reaction pattern characterized by axillary hyperpigmentation, lichenification, and alopecia in association with various known and unknown causes.

■ *Cause and Pathogenesis.* Canine acanthosis nigricans is best thought of as a cutaneous reaction pattern with multiple causes.[2, 5, 89, 96] The pathogenesis of the reaction pattern is poorly understood. Canine acanthosis nigricans may be divided into primary (idiopathic) and secondary types.

Primary (idiopathic) canine acanthosis nigricans is almost exclusively a disease of dachshunds. The striking breed predilection and early age at onset strongly suggest that this type of canine acanthosis nigricans is a genodermatosis. Indeed, one form of acanthosis nigricans in humans is known to be inherited.[1]

Secondary canine acanthosis nigricans is associated with underlying disorders, including (1) friction or intertrigo (conformational abnormalities, obesity, or both, resulting in excessive axillary friction and dermatitis), (2) endocrinopathy (underlying hypothyroidism, hyperadrenocorticism, sex hormone imbalances, and so on), and (3) hypersensitivity (chronic axillary pruritus and dermatitis associated with canine atopy, food hypersensitivity, or contact dermatitis). In humans, acanthosis nigricans has been associated with tissue resistance to insulin, drugs (e.g., nicotinic acid, diethylstilbestrol, and glucocorticoids), and internal malignancy (especially of the gastrointestinal or female reproductive tract).[1, 93] Drug-induced acanthosis nigricans has not been reported in animals, and the cases in dogs associated with malignancy may have had other causes.[95]

■ *Clinical Features.* Although primary canine acanthosis nigricans has been reported in several breeds, dachshunds are overwhelmingly the breed at risk. Primary canine acanthosis nigricans occurs in either sex and begins in dogs younger than 1 year of age. Secondary canine acanthosis nigricans may occur in any breed and is more commonly recognized in those predisposed to the various underlying diseases described previously. Secondary canine acanthosis nigricans generally mimics any sex or age predilection inherent in the underlying diseases.

The earliest sign of primary canine acanthosis nigricans is usually bilateral axillary hyperpigmentation (Fig. 11:40 *G*). With time, lichenification, alopecia, and seborrheic changes develop (Fig. 11:40 *H*). In severe cases, the dermatosis may spread to involve the forelimbs, the ventral neck, the chest, the abdomen, the groin, the perineum, the hocks, the periocular area, and the pinnae. Seborrheic skin disease (greasy with rancid odor) and secondary bacterial pyoderma or *Malassezia* dermatitis are common complicating factors. Pruritus is variable and is usually most severe when seborrheic changes, bacterial pyoderma, or *Malassezia* dermatitis is present.

■ *Diagnosis.* The differential diagnosis of canine acanthosis nigricans includes the previously mentioned causes of primary and secondary disease. Definitive diagnosis is based on history, physical examination findings, laboratory tests that rule out other conditions, skin biopsy, and response to therapy. Juvenile-onset acanthosis nigricans in a dachshund is most likely to be primary and genetic. Thyroid function is usually normal in dachshunds with acanthosis nigricans. Histopathologic examination is nondiagnostic, revealing hyperplastic superficial perivascular dermatitis with focal parakeratosis, epidermal melanosis, pigmentary incontinence, and follicular keratosis (Fig. 11:45). The perivascular inflammatory infiltrate is usually mixed

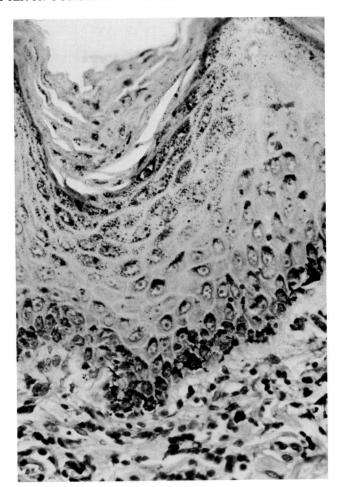

Figure 11:45. Canine acanthosis nigricans. Epidermal hyperplasia and full-thickness hypermelanosis.

mononuclear cells and neutrophils. A similar histopathologic pattern may be seen with many chronic inflammatory dermatoses.[3]

■ *Clinical Management.* The prognosis for cure in canine acanthosis nigricans varies with the underlying cause. When the acanthosis nigricans is due to some definable and correctable disorder, the lesions need no specific treatment and resolve spontaneously as the primary disease is treated. Response may be slow. Primary canine acanthosis nigricans in the dachshund is a controllable, but not a curable, disease.

Early cases of acanthosis nigricans need no treatment. As the lesions become more widespread and hyperplastic, the resultant seborrheic changes necessitate treatment. Antiseborrheic bathing and the frequent application of talc to the intertriginous areas is beneficial but provides only short-term improvement. When the lesions are confined to small areas, the application of a potent topical glucocorticoid (e.g., betamethasone valerate ointment) can be beneficial for some time. Eventually, the lesions become too widespread for the safe use of these topical products. Advanced cases can be treated with melatonin, systemic glucocorticoids, or vitamin E.

Melatonin, a pineal gland hormone, has been effective in the treatment of canine acanthosis nigricans.[89, 94] It has been postulated that melatonin may be a physiologic antagonist to melanocyte-stimulating hormone (MSH) and that the acanthosis nigricans may represent an imbalance between melatonin and MSH. Melatonin (Rickards Research Foundation, 18001 Euclid Avenue, Cleveland, OH 44112) is given subcutaneously at 2 mg per dog, daily for 3 to 5 days, then weekly or monthly, as needed.

Systemic glucocorticoids are effective in the treatment of canine acanthosis nigricans,[89] presumably via their anti-inflammatory, antiseborrheic, and anti-MSH effects. Prednisolone or prednisone is given orally at 1 mg/kg every 24 hours for 7 to 10 days, and then on an alternate-morning regimen.

Vitamin E acetate (*dl*-α-tocopherol acetate), 200 IU given orally every 12 hours as the only treatment, produced improvement within 30 to 60 days in eight cases of primary acanthosis nigricans.[96] Hyperpigmentation was not reduced, but inflammation, lichenification, pruritus, greasiness, and objectionable odor all subsided. There were no side-effects, and improvement was maintained while treatment continued.

Disorders of Atypical Coloration

Coat color is controlled by multiple genes with various known or presumed alleles at each locus. In mice, in which coat color genetics is best known, certain coat colors are external markers for serious internal disease. The importance of coat color in certain dermatologic or systemic illnesses in pets is of increased interest.

CONGENITAL DISORDERS

Animals born with a dilute coat color (e.g., blue or beige) are at risk for color dilution alopecia. Although the authors are aware of several neonatal Rhodesian Ridgebacks in which a chocolate coat color was associated with a congenital cerebellar disorder, the best known examples of linkage of coat color with internal disease are cyclic hematopoiesis and the Chédiak-Higashi syndrome.

Chédiak-Higashi Syndrome

The Chédiak-Higashi syndrome is an inherited disorder of Persian cats, white tigers, Hereford cattle, Aleutian mink, and humans.[91] In cats, it is an autosomal recessive disorder seen in only Persian cats with blue smoke hair color and yellow eyes. Microscopic examination of unstained hairs reveals multiple large, elongated, irregular clumps of melanin (macromelanosomes).[92] Affected cats have giant lysosomes in the cytoplasm of various cells, including neutrophils and macrophages.[90] On blood smears, these lysosomes appear as large eosinophilic granules.

Chédiak-Higashi syndrome is characterized by increased susceptibility to infection, partial oculocutaneous albinism, photophobia, and bleeding disorders. The cats have red fundic light reflection instead of yellow-green. Because of the immunologic deficiency, affected cats are at increased risk for infection. Most cases of dermatophytic pseudomycetoma have occurred in smoke-colored Persian cats.

There is no specific treatment. Affected animals should not be used for breeding.

Canine Cyclic Hematopoiesis

Cyclic hematopoiesis (gray collie syndrome, or canine cyclic neutropenia) is a lethal autosomal recessive syndrome in which collie puppies are born with a silver gray haircoat that differs from the normal sable or tricolor coat.[91, 98] In some of these puppies, a slight yellow pigmentation may be present, which produces a mixture of light beige and light gray hair. The light-colored nose is a characteristic and diagnostic feature.

In addition to the hair color change, gray collie puppies are usually smaller and weaker than their littermates, a difference observable by 1 week of age. By 8 to 12 weeks of age, signs of clinical illness appear, including fever, diarrhea, lymphadenopathy, infections, conjunctivitis, and arthralgia. The term *cyclic neutropenia* reflects the appearance of neutropenia alternating with rebounding neutrophilia. This cycle continues at 10- to 12-day intervals until death. Other hematologic abnormalities include nonregenerative anemia as well as cyclic reticulocytosis, monocytosis, and thrombocytosis.[5, 98] Other clinicopathologic abnormalities include hyperglobulinemia, depressed mitogenic responses of lymphocytes, and cyclic hormonogenesis.[5]

There is no effective treatment, and parents and littermates should not be used for breeding. Affected animals usually die before 6 months of age without supportive care. Even with optimal care, most die before 2 years of age because of hepatic or renal failure associated with amyloidosis. Bone marrow transplantation is effective but impractical.[98] In differential diagnosis, this syndrome must not be mistaken for the dominant or Maltese gray collie and a transient dilution called *powder puff.*

Acquired Disorders

Coat color change in adult animals can be focal, regionalized, or generalized. Change can be due to reversion to puppy coloration after trauma or endocrine disorders, temperature effects, topical insults (e.g., sunlight and bleaching shampoos), nutritional disorders, drugs, and endocrine diseases (especially hyperadrenocorticism and sex hormone imbalances). Most of the above can occur in any breed. A peculiar gilding syndrome has been described in Miniature Schnauzers.

Acquired Aurotrichia in Miniature Schnauzers

This syndrome was first reported in 1991 and appears to be uncommon.[97] Dogs of either sex can be affected, and the disorder is recognized in young adult dogs, typically between 2 and 3 years of age. More than half of the reported cases started in warm weather, but the condition can start in periods with minimal solar exposure. The cause of the alteration in hair color is unknown, but because of the restriction to the Miniature Schnauzer breed, there must be some genetic influence.

Affected dogs typically have patchy color change of the hairs over the dorsal thorax and along the abdomen (see Chap. 12).[97] The affected hairs are golden in color. In a few dogs, the color change is diffuse in those areas and may involve the periocular region or ears. Concomitant with the gilding, the number of secondary hairs in the area is decreased. The dogs are otherwise healthy. Aside from some pigmentary changes in the guard hairs, there is no histologic explanation for the gilding.

No treatment is indicated or should be effective. The condition resolves spontaneously in 6 to 24 months. Both the coloration and the density of the undercoat return to normal. Relapses are uncommon.

■ DISORDERS OF COLLAGEN

The best known example of a congenital disorder of collagen is cutaneous asthenia in which abnormal production or degradation results in abnormally fragile skin. The other conditions discussed are less clear-cut. They have a high incidence in certain breeds, which suggests an inherited predisposition and abnormalities in dermal collagen are seen in biopsy specimens. However, it is not clear whether the collagen changes are primary or secondary to some as yet described condition. Because of the striking breed predisposition, the conditions are considered here.

Cutaneous Asthenia

Cutaneous asthenia (Ehlers-Danlos syndrome, or dermatosparaxis) is a group of inherited, congenital connective tissue diseases characterized by loose, hyperextensible, and abnormally fragile skin that is easily torn by minor trauma.

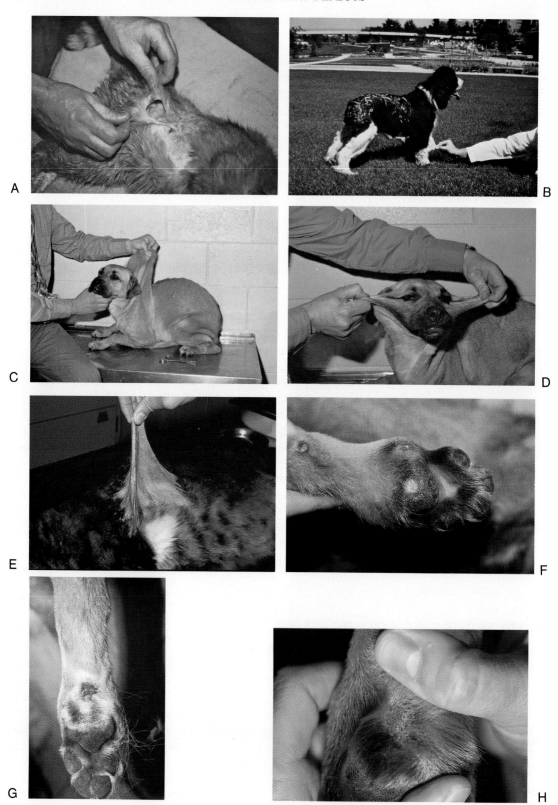

Figure 11:46 *See legend on opposite page*

CAUSE AND PATHOGENESIS

This disease complex resembles the Ehlers-Danlos syndrome of humans, which consists of at least 10 different disorders that are usually distinguishable clinically, biochemically, and genetically.[1, 104] Most forms in humans have a dominant mode of inheritance but recessive and X-linked inheritance also occurs. Depending on the form studied, the defect can result from deficient synthesis of $\alpha2(I)$ collagen chains or type III collagen, mutations in the helical structure of type III collagen, abnormal conversion of type I procollagen to collagen, or various enzymatic abnormalities.[1]

Dermatosparaxis means "torn skin"; because of the collagen defects the skin of affected animals often tears easily resulting in large, gaping "fish mouth" wounds (Fig. 11:46A). These lacerations heal readily but leave thin, highly visible "cigarette paper" scars (Fig. 11:46B). The tensile strength of the skin of affected dogs is reduced 40-fold, whereas that of affected cats is reduced 10-fold.[106, 109] Cutaneous asthenia has been reported in sheep, cattle mink, dogs, and cats, as well as in human beings.[106, 107, 109] Cases have been reported in various purebred and mongrel dogs and cats with varying modes of inheritance.[108]

Recessive cutaneous asthenia has been absolutely confirmed in only cats,[101–103, 114, 117, 118] but the occurrence of the disease in a mongrel dog with apparently normal parents suggests a recessive form in dogs.[100] Affected collagen forms twisted ribbons rather than cylindric fibrils and fibers (see Figs. 11:48 and 11:49). These structural changes are due to abnormalities in formation or maintenance of collagen fibrils and fibers.[102, 110, 114] Biochemical studies have demonstrated a procollagen processing defect in which there is decreased activity of procollagen peptidase and an accumulation of partially processed type I procollagen containing N-terminal propeptides.[114] Collagenase activity typically is increased $2\frac{1}{2}$ times above normal levels.[114]

Dominant cutaneous asthenia is a simple autosomal trait in dogs and cats. Changes are recognizable in the fetus, and the trait is probably lethal in the homozygous state.[113, 119] The defect can cause focal or diffuse changes in the dermal collagen and results from abnormalities in the packing of collagen into fibrils and fibers owing to mutations of structural proteins. Unlike normal fibers in which the fibrils are uniform in diameter, cylindric, and packed in uniform parallel arrays, the fibers here are severely disorganized with many larger-than-normal fibrils.[114] A mixture of abnormal and normal fibers is found in heterozygous animals. Biochemical studies show a decrease in proteodermatan sulfate levels, an increase in hyaluronic acid levels, and an altered iduronic to glucuronic acid ratio.[114]

Dermal thickness in dogs can be thinner than normal (1.21 mm versus 1.71 mm)[106] or normal.[104] The dermis in cats can also be thinned (0.25 mm versus 1.71 mm)[104] or normal.[5] Normal dermal thickness is usually a result of an increased thickness of individual collagen bundles.

Ehlers-Danlos syndrome has been reported in the beagle, dachshund, boxer, St. Bernard, German shepherd dog, English Springer spaniel, Greyhound, Manchester terrier, Welsh corgi, Red kelpi, soft-coated Wheaton terrier, and mongrels.[2, 100, 119a] The authors have recognized it in the Irish setter, Keeshond, and English setter.[4] Most cases in the cat occur in domestic shorthaired or longhaired breeds or Himalayan cats.

Figure 11:46. A, Cutaneous asthenia in a cat. Hyperfragility of the skin. B, Typical appearance of a Springer spaniel with cutaneous asthenia. Note the numerous scars on the back. (Courtesy G. A. Hegreberg.) C, Cutaneous asthenia in a dog. Hyperextensibility of the skin. (Courtesy G. Ackland.) D, Cutaneous asthenia in a dog. Same dog as in C. (Courtesy G. Ackland.) E, Cutaneous asthenia in a cat. Hyperextensibility of the skin. (Courtesy P. McKeever.) F, Collagen disorder of the footpads of a German shepherd. G, Solitary fistula on the caudal metatarsal area of a German shepherd. H, Fluctuant swelling on the caudal metatarsal area of a German shepherd.

CLINICAL FEATURES

The skin is soft, pliable, and thin; it is loosely attached to underlying tissues and is hyperextensible. It has decreased elasticity and a moist, blanched appearance. The skin can be stretched to extreme lengths (see Fig. 11:46 C to E) and may hang loosely in folds, especially on the legs and the throat. In long-coated dogs, the excessive folding may be noticed on only the face and may result in the need for repeated eyelid surgeries. Minimal trauma from traction or scratching may produce skin tears, with little or no bleeding. Healing is rapid, but irregular thin white scars are prominent disfiguring features (see Fig. 11:46 B). Widening of the bridge of the nose, subcutaneous hematomas, elbow hygromas, and epicanthal folds are additional signs in some affected animals. Some animals manifest only cutaneous hyperextensibility or only fragility, whereas other animals exhibit both features. Some animals may have concurrent joint laxity and ocular changes (microcornea, sclerocornea, lens luxation, and cataracts).[100, 112]

DIAGNOSIS

The clinical syndromes of excessively folded skin, hyperextensible skin, easily torn skin, or excessively scarred skin in a young animal with no history of severe trauma are highly suggestive of cutaneous asthenia. Complete documentation may necessitate biopsies for ultrastructural and biochemical study. The skin extensibility index devised by Patterson and Minor[116] is helpful. Extensibility is quantified by manually extending a fold of dorsolumbar skin to the maximal distance above the spine that can be attained without pain. This distance is measured, as is the body length from the base of the tail to the occipital crest. Extensibility is calculated as follows:

$$\text{Extensibility index} = \frac{\text{vertical height of skin fold}}{\text{body length}} \times 100$$

In affected dogs, the skin extensibility index is greater than 14.5 per cent, whereas in affected cats, it is greater than 19 per cent.[106]

Skin biopsy may reveal striking dermal abnormalities or normal skin. Collagen fibers may

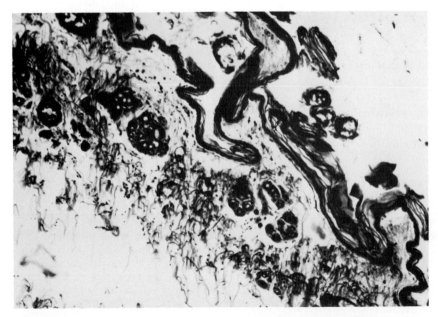

Figure 11:47. Cutaneous asthenia. Histopathologic view showing fragmented collagen fibrils that are shortened and disoriented.

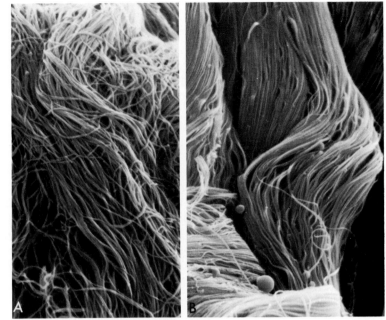

Figure 11:48. SEMs of collagen fibrils in a fiber bundle from the dermis of a dermatosparactic cat *(A)*, and a normal cat *(B)* (×6000). (From Holbrook, K. A., et al.: Dermatosparaxis in a Himalayan cat: II. Ultrastructural studies of dermal collagen. J. Invest. Dermatol. 74:100, 1980.)

be more eosinophilic than normal and blurred in appearance, fragmented, shortened, and disoriented (Fig. 11:47). Additionally, collagen fibers may form irregularly sized bundles, may demonstrate improper interweaving, and may be surrounded by mucinosis (Figs. 11:48 and 11:49).[109] Alternatively, the collagen may appear normal on light microscopic examination.[116]

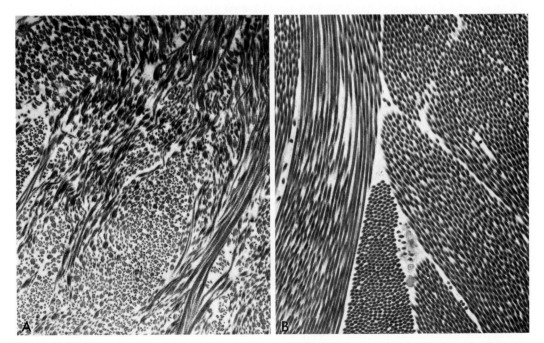

Figure 11:49. *A,* Transmission electron microscopic view (TEM) of a collagen fiber bundle from the dermis of the dermatosparactic cat showing fibers and fibrils in various planes of a section within the bundle (×10,000). *B,* TEM of a dermal collagen fiber bundle from the normal control cat. All fibrils within a fiber are organized in the same plane (×6200). (From Holbrook, K. A., et al.: Dermatosparaxis in a Himalayan cat: II. Ultrastructural studies of dermal collagen. J. Invest. Dermatol. 74:100, 1980.)

One special stain is useful, even in those animals with histologically normal skin. Collagen stains blue with Masson trichrome stain but has segmental red staining abnormalities in animals with cutaneous asthenia.[114]

CLINICAL MANAGEMENT

The clinician should inform the owner of the nature, heritability, and chronic incurable course of the disease. The animal should not be used for breeding. Most affected animals are euthanized.

With appropriate lifestyle and housing modifications and prompt veterinary attention to wounds and intercurrent skin diseases, pets without joint laxity can lead long lives. Cats should be declawed to prevent wounding during grooming or scratching. The affected animal cannot play with other animals and must be leash walked away from woody trees and shrubs. All visitors to the pet's household must be aware of the defect lest a sudden grab for restraint results in a large skin wound. Households contain numerous items with sharp corners or rough surfaces, which can rip the affected pet's skin. These must be removed or padded. Because these animals are prone to hygromas, floors and all resting places should be well padded. Any skin disease, especially conditions that result in pruritus, must be addressed and resolved quickly. Wounds should be sutured promptly.

Because vitamin C is necessary in collagen synthesis, the authors (WHM and DWS) treated one affected Irish setter and one domestic shorthair cat with 500 mg and 50 mg, respectively, of vitamin C orally every 12 hours. The owners and referring veterinarian of the dog reported that the skin was much less stretchy and less fragile, whereas no change was seen in the cat. The improvement in the dog may have been spurious or the result of some other factor, but further investigations with vitamin C are warranted.

Disorder of the Footpads in German Shepherd Dogs

The cause of this condition is unknown. Signs occur early in life, and multiple dogs of a litter are typically affected. The condition shows some clinical and histologic features of the familial vasculopathy of German shepherd dogs, suggesting some common etiopathogenesis.

CLINICAL FEATURES

German shepherd dogs of either sex are affected at a few weeks to a few months of age.[5, 99] One case in an 11-month-old dog has been reported.[99] Usually, multiple dogs in the litter are involved. The pads of all feet are softer than normal. Swelling, depigmentation, ulceration, and crusting can develop on one or more pads (see Fig. 11:46*F*), especially the metacarpal and metatarsal pads. When ulcerated, the pads are tender and can cause lameness. The dogs are otherwise healthy.

DIAGNOSIS

In the absence of a drug history to induce a drug eruption or skin lesions elsewhere, the clinical signs are typical of this disorder. Diagnosis is by biopsy, which shows a deep diffuse dermatitis focused around multifocal areas of collagenolysis (Fig. 11:50). The inflammation can be neutrophilic[5] (Fig. 11:51) or lymphoplasmacytic.[99]

CLINICAL MANAGEMENT

Treatment with antibiotics, glucocorticoids, and topical agents has been unrewarding. With foot protection and good wound care, the ulcers heal spontaneously by 1 year of age. The pad

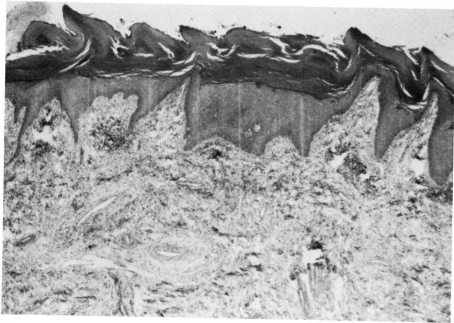

Figure 11:50. Collagen disorder of the footpads of German shepherds. Diffuse to nodular dermatitis.

softness remains. Long-term follow-up of most dogs has not been reported, but some dogs have renal amyloidosis and die by 2 to 3 years of age.[5]

Focal Metatarsal Fistulation of German Shepherd Dogs

Metatarsal fistulation is an uncommon disorder of German shepherd dogs of unknown etiology.[111] The condition appears to be most common in dogs of direct German ancestry.[4] Where

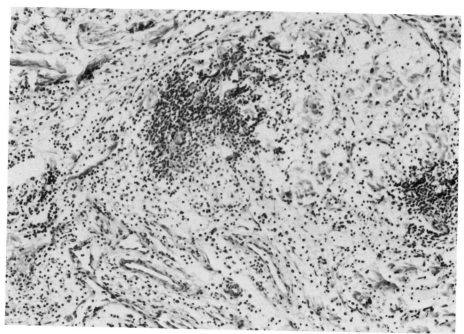

Figure 11:51. Close-up of Figure 11:50. Focal accumulations of neutrophils and mononuclear cells around degenerate collagen.

studied, all affected dogs have had significantly elevated antibody levels against type I and II collagen.[4, 115] These latter findings suggest some familial disorder of collagen.

CLINICAL FEATURES

With the exception of one German shepherd dog crossbred, all cases have occurred in German shepherd dogs between the ages of 2½ and 4 years.[4, 111] The dogs examined by the authors have all been of direct German ancestry and are low at the carpi and tarsi (flat-footed). Lesions are initially asymptomatic, and the owners become aware of them only because the dog licks the area or because bloody spots are seen on the floor.

Lesions occur on the central plantar surface of the metatarsus just proximal to the metatarsal pad (see Fig. 11:46*G*). Typically, both hindlegs are involved, and the occasional dog has similar lesions above one or both metacarpal pads.[111] At examination, a well-demarcated fistula with serosanguineous discharge is seen. Palpation identifies a fibrous tract to deeper tissues. Early lesions have an intact epithelium, with fluid accumulating beneath the surface, yielding a smooth, rounded, fluctuant cystic structure (Fig. 11:46*H*). No other skin lesions are identified.

DIAGNOSIS

With a single lesion, the differential diagnostic considerations include foreign body or a focal bacterial or fungal infection. Bilaterally symmetric lesions in a German shepherd dog are pathognomonic.

Cytologic evaluation of the draining fluid shows a pyogranulomatous inflammation with or without intracellular bacteria. Closed lesions are sterile, whereas open lesions may be secondarily infected by staphylococci. Biopsy shows a deep nodular to diffuse deep dermatitis with fibrosis and fistulous tracts (Fig. 11:52). The cellular infiltrate is predominantly pyogranulomatous. Hair follicle rupture with endogenous foreign body reaction to follicular keratin and hair shafts is common.

Routine laboratory evaluations are noncontributory and antinuclear antibody titers are negative. Eleven dogs tested for circulating antibodies to type I and II[4] collagen had significantly elevated titers.[115] Because nonaffected German shepherd dogs have yet to be tested, the significance of these anticollagen antibodies is unknown.

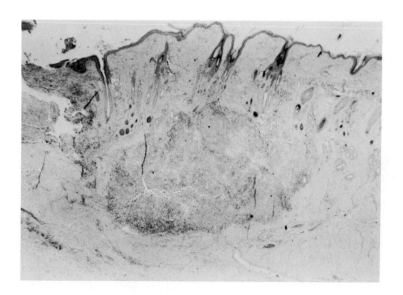

Figure 11:52. Metatarsal fistula in a German shepherd. Deep dermal pyogranulomatous nodule.

CLINICAL MANAGEMENT

Surgical removal of the fistula and deep tissues provides temporary improvement, but new lesions reform weeks to months later. Systemic antibiotic treatment improves secondarily infected lesions but has no effect on early lesions. Prednisolone administration at 1.1 to 2.2 mg/kg every 24 hours results in resolution of the lesions in most dogs in 14 to 28 days. Spontaneous resolution in one dog has been reported.[111] After resolution, the lesions may never recur[111] or episodic relapses may be seen. The authors' cases are in this latter category. In these cases, repeated treatments with prednisolone are effective but can induce signs of iatrogenic hyperadrenocorticism. In a limited number of cases the twice daily application of a 0.1 per cent fluocinolone acetonide in dimethyl sulfoxide solution (Synotic [Syntex]) to early lesions has prevented fistulation and has been satisfactory for long-term control.[4]

Multiple Collagenous Nevi

Solitary collagenous nevi (see Chap. 19) can occur in any breed of dog. In some German shepherd dogs, multiple collagenous nevi develop between 3 to 5 years of age. These skin lesions are a cutaneous marker for renal cystadenocarcinomas or uterine leiomyomas. This trait appears to have an autosomal dominant mode of inheritance.

■ DISORDERS OF VESSELS

Aside from the rare case of congenital hemangioma or arteriovenous fistula, inherited disorders of blood vessels are rare. Most cases of vascular disease are due to an acquired vasculitis (see Chap. 8), but an idiopathic and apparently familial vasculopathy has been described in four breeds of dogs.

Familial Vasculopathy

Beagles

A systemic necrotizing vasculitis of small to medium-sized arteries is well described in colony-bred beagles.[127] No sex predilection is noted, and signs occur early in life (4 to 10 months of age). Signs are cyclic and include fever, lethargy, unwillingness to move, and a hunched stance. No skin lesions have been described.

German Shepherd Dogs

Affected dogs have signs at 4 to 7 weeks of age within 7 to 10 days of their first immuniza-tion.[129] No sex predilection is noted. The dogs are lethargic and pyrexic and have a peripheral lymphadenopathy and skin lesions. The bridge of the nose is swollen and crusted, ulcerated lesions occur on the ear margins, the nasal planum, and the tail tip. All footpads are soft and swollen with variable depigmentation. In severe cases, the central portion of the pads can ulcerate.

Skin biopsy shows a nodular to diffuse mononuclear dermatitis around degenerated collagen bundles and subtle vascular alteration, especially of postcapillary venules.[129] Depigmented lesions have a hydropic interface dermatitis with pigmentary incontinence. At necropsy, colla-genolyis of footpads, peritendinous sheaths and deep fascia of the distal limbs, and ventrum is seen.

Treatment with antibiotics or glucocorticoids causes minimal to no improvement. Dogs recover spontaneously by 5 to 6 months of age, with residual scarring at points of ulceration. The pads remain soft. Pyrexia, lethargy, or panosteitis can occur at each subsequent immuni-zation.

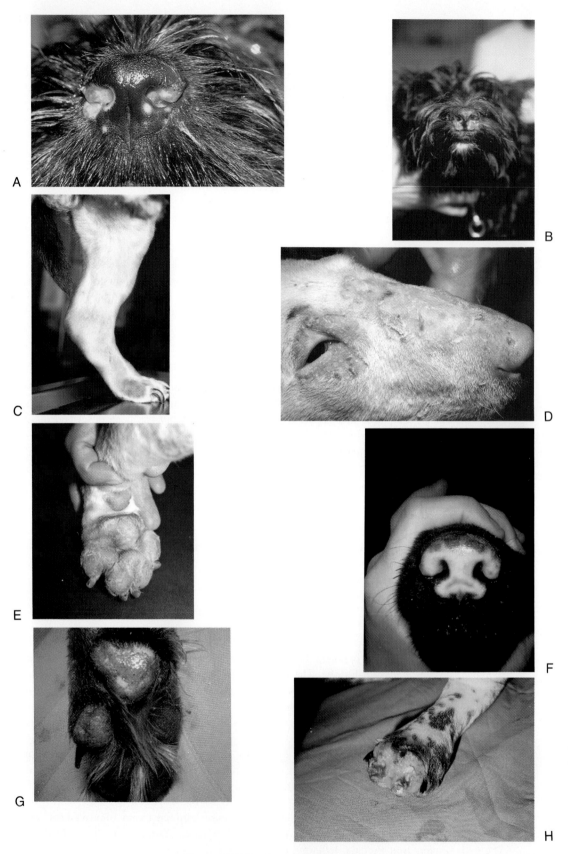

Figure 11:53 *See legend on opposite page*

To date, no cause of the condition has been defined. It is unclear whether there is some systemic immunologic abnormality that results in the vasculitis or whether the vessels are abnormal. The condition appears to have an autosomal recessive mode of inheritance.

Greyhounds

Large numbers of racing Greyhounds have manifested this condition (see Chap. 8).[120] No sex predilection is noted, and signs can occur in dogs 6 to 72 months of age. Approximately 75 per cent of cases have only skin lesions, whereas the remainder have renal plus cutaneous signs. In the latter situation, signs of renal disease are typically noted when the skin lesions are found, but they can precede or follow the skin lesions.

Skin lesions occur primarily over the tarsus, the stifle, or the inner thigh. Occasionally, the forelimb is involved. The first sign noted is swelling and tenderness, followed by sharply demarcated deep ulcerations. Lesions vary in size from 1 mm to 10 cm in diameter. Lesions heal slowly but spontaneously with routine wound care.

Skin biopsy shows dermal thrombosis of arterioles, venules, and capillaries in the superficial or deep dermis.[120] No cause of the condition is known. The mode of inheritance is unknown.

Scottish Terriers

This condition has been reported in five Scottish terrier puppies, and no additional cases have been reported with the withdrawal of their parents from the breeding program.[126] Affected dogs first had a bilateral nasal discharge at 3 to 4 weeks of age, followed by progressive ulceration and destruction of the nasal planum, the nostrils, and the nasal mucosa by 5 to 6 months of age (Fig. 11:53A and B). No treatments were effective. Skin biopsy showed a nodular to diffuse pyogranulomatous dermatitis with a leukocytoclastic vasculitis (Fig. 11:54). The condition probably had an autosomal dominant mode of inheritance.

Lymphedema

Lymphedema is swelling of some part of the body due to abnormal lymph flow.

CAUSE AND PATHOGENESIS

Lymphedema can be primary or secondary.[121] Primary lymphedema is caused by developmental defects in lymphatics and lymph nodes. Secondary lymphedema results from the obstruction of lymphatics or lymphatic flow by inflammatory or neoplastic disease, surgery, or trauma. In some dogs, primary lymphedema has been shown to be inherited as an autosomal dominant trait with variable expressivity.[121, 124, 125] Canine primary lymphedema has been classified by lymphangiography and histopathologic study into two basic structural defects: (1) lymphatic hypoplasia, with or without hypoplasia or absence of the regional lymph nodes, and (2) lymphatic hyperplasia and dilatation.[121, 122, 124]

Figure 11:53. *A,* Hereditary pyogranulomatous disease with vasculitis in Scottish terriers. Bilateral ulceration of the nostrils. *B,* Hereditary pyogranulomatous disease with vasculitis in Scottish terriers. Focal ulcerated granulomas, depigmentation, and loss of the surface architecture of the nasal planum. *C,* Congenital lymphedema in a dog. The hindleg is swollen, edematous, and pits easily. *D,* Lethal acrodermatitis in a bull terrier. Erythema, alopecia, and peeling skin on the face. *E,* Lethal acrodermatitis in a bull terrier. Hyperkeratotic footpads and pedal erythema. *F,* Canine tyrosinemia. Depigmentation and ulceration of the nose. (Courtesy G. A. Kunkle.) *G,* Canine tyrosinemia. Ulceration of footpads. (Courtesy G. A. Kunkle.) *H,* Acral mutilation in an English pointer.

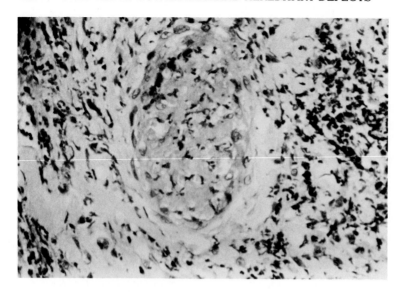

Figure 11:54. Hereditary pyogranulomatous disease with vasculitis in Scottish terriers. Leukocytoclastic vasculitis surrounded by pyogranulomatous dermatitis.

CLINICAL FEATURES

Primary lymphedema has been recognized in several breeds of dogs, including the English bulldog, German shepherd, borzoi, Belgian Tervuren, Old English sheepdog, Labrador retriever, Great Dane, Poodle, and Old English sheepdog–Labrador retriever crosses.[121] There appears to be no sex predilection. The onset of disease is usually within the first 12 weeks of life.

The hindlimbs are the most commonly affected, although the front limbs, the ventrum, the tail, and the pinnae may be involved.[122] Affected skin is usually normal in surface appearance but is thickened and spongy and pits with digital pressure (see Fig. 11:53 C). The swollen skin is not warm, tender, or inflamed. Regional lymph nodes may not be palpable, and the dogs are usually healthy otherwise. Because lymphedema predisposes affected tissues to secondary bacterial infection and delayed healing, these complications may be clinically apparent.

DIAGNOSIS

Differential diagnosis includes other causes of obstructive, inflammatory, and hypoproteinemic edema. Definitive diagnosis is based on history, physical examination findings, laboratory tests to rule out other conditions, skin biopsy, and lymphangiography.[122] Skin biopsy reveals variable degrees of subcutaneous and dermal edema (Fig. 11:55).[128] Lymphatics may be dilated and hyperplastic or may be hypoplastic. Chronic cases may show variable degrees of fibrosis and epidermal hyperplasia. Inflammatory cells are usually few in number to absent, unless secondary infection is present.

CLINICAL MANAGEMENT

The prognosis and the indicated therapy vary with the severity of the lymphedema.[122] Mild cases may wax and wane, spontaneously regress, or persist indefinitely with no adverse consequences to the patient. More severe cases may require (1) frequent bandaging (e.g., modified Robert Jones splint) to reduce the lymphedema,[128] (2) surgical extirpation of the edematous tissues, (3) reconstructive surgery, or (4) amputation of the affected part. No successful form of medical management has been reported for dogs. The benzopyrene group of drugs has proven benefit in humans.[122] Dogs with severe primary lymphedema often die shortly after birth because of pleural and abdominal effusions.[123]

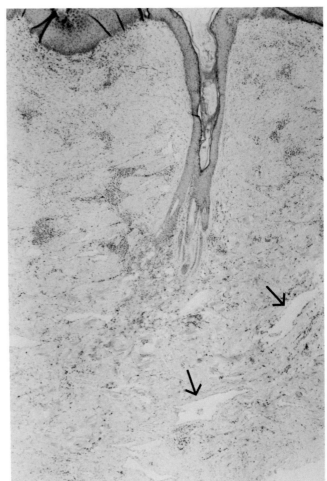

Figure 11:55. Congenital lymphedema. Fibrosing dermatitis and marked dilatation of dermal lymphatics (arrows).

■ ENDOCRINE, METABOLIC, AND IMMUNOLOGIC DISORDERS

Endocrine, metabolic, or immunologic diseases can occur in any animal. Certain breeds or specific families within a breed are at greater risk for a particular disease, suggesting a heritable influence. The reader is referred to Chapters 8 and 9 for a complete discussion of these disorders. The disorders discussed subsequently have each been recognized in only one breed of dog and therefore are included in this chapter.

Acrodermatitis

Acrodermatitis has been reported as an inherited, autosomal recessive trait that produces a lethal syndrome in bull terriers.[131, 133, 136] The clinical, pathologic, and genetic features of the syndrome resemble acrodermatitis enteropathica in humans, lethal trait A46 in Black Pied Danish cattle, and experimental zinc deficiency in dogs. Although affected bull terriers had significantly lowered serum zinc levels, they did not respond to high-dose zinc replacement therapy.[131, 136] The specific cause of the condition is as yet incompletely defined, but affected dogs have defective zinc metabolism.[135, 136]

CLINICAL FEATURES

At birth, affected pups have skin pigmentation that is lighter than normal, and the coat in some dogs is dull, brittle, and fluffy.[130] The pups are weaker than their normal littermates, and they cannot chew or swallow well because of their high-arched hard palate. Their growth is retarded.[131] By 6 weeks of age, their feet are splayed, the footpads are cracked, and crusted skin lesions appear between the toes. Ulcerated, exudative crusted lesions are also found on the ears and the muzzle (Fig. 11:53D). Papular or pustular dermatitis may be found around all body orifices but most notably around those of the head. The foot lesions (Fig. 11:53E) progress rapidly to severe interdigital pyoderma and paronychia. Later, there is onychodystrophy and frondlike keratinization of the noncontact areas of the footpads. A generalized bacterial folliculitis may develop, being most severe in areas prone to frictional trauma, such as the elbows and the hocks. Affected animals may have diarrhea and respiratory infections with chronic nasal discharges. At weaning time, they appear especially aggressive, but by 14 to 16 weeks, they become less active, less responsive to external stimuli, and sleep a great deal. Many have ocular abnormalities. The average survival time is 7 months, but conventional treatments may prolong this time.

DIAGNOSIS

If multiple puppies are presented at one time, no other differential diagnoses are appropriate. In individual cases, drug eruption, pemphigus foliaceus, and staphylococcal or *Malassezia* infection secondary to some congenital immunodeficiency may be considered. There is a high incidence (75 to 100 per cent) of secondary yeast infection in bull terriers with acrodermatitis.[130, 134] Skin biopsies should be performed in all cases.

Histopathology shows diffuse parakeratotic hyperkeratosis with focal crusting and intraepidermal pustules.[3] The superficial epidermis may show laminar pallor as is seen in necrolytic migratory erythema (see Chap. 9) but the keratinocytes are viable and not degenerating. There is severe reduction in lymphocytes in T-cell areas of lymphoid tissues.

Routine laboratory tests show no consistent abnormalities specific for this disorder.[131, 136] Serum zinc levels may be low or normal.[131, 135, 136] *Malassezia* yeasts can be isolated in most cases by scraping, by the Mackenzie toothbrush technique, on acetate tape preparations, or by biopsy.[130, 134]

CLINICAL MANAGEMENT

Efforts to return these dogs to normal status with oral or parenteral zinc supplementation have been unrewarding.[131, 136] Treatment with systemic antibiotics resolves cutaneous and systemic infections but provides no long-term solution, as infections return. If *Malassezia* infection is present, the administration of ketoconazole (10 mg/kg q12h) results in marked improvement.[130] One animal has been maintained well for nearly 2 years with ketoconazole.

Parents of affected dogs are carriers for the disorder, as are more than one half of the clinically normal siblings of affected dogs. No relatives of the affected dogs should be used for breeding. Some of the apparently normal littermates may develop a zinc-responsive dermatitis (see Chap. 16).

Tyrosinemia

A single case of congenital tyrosinemia in a young dog has been reported.[132] It appeared to be similar to tyrosinemia type II in humans or pseudodistemper in mink. Tyrosinemia, inherited as an autosomal recessive trait, is a group of distinct metabolic diseases with five phenotypes in humans.[1] The case reported in the dog was characterized by an early age at onset of characteristic eye and skin lesions with varying degrees of mental retardation.

CAUSE AND PATHOGENESIS

The tyrosinemia in the dog was apparently hereditary, as both parents had elevated serum tyrosinase levels. The serum tyrosinase levels were elevated because of the deficiency of cytosolic hepatic tyrosine aminotransferase. The pathophysiologic change is considered an inflammatory response to tyrosine crystals deposited in tissues. This appears to be the case with the corneal lesions, but many skin lesions have no crystals. Instead, there may be increased numbers of highly condensed tonofibrils and increased numbers of keratohyaline granules in the granular layer. Tyrosine is known to influence the number of microtubules in the tonofibrils.

CLINICAL FEATURES

The 7-week-old German shepherd puppy was small for its age when it first had conjunctivitis and cloudy corneas. The globes were small, and cataracts and corneal granulation were present, but no ulceration. There was ulceration of the nose, the tongue, and central portions of the footpads (see Fig. 11:53*F* and *G*). As the disease progressed, ulcers involved the metatarsal pads and the claw folds, and claws were broken. Erythematous bullae were found on the abdomen. The nasal planum developed erythema, focal ulceration with marginal crusting, and hypopigmentation.

DIAGNOSIS

Diagnosis of a metabolic defect was suspected because of the historical and physical examination findings and confirmed by metabolic screening tests. High levels of tyrosine in the serum and urine were identified.

Histopathologic examination of ulcerated skin lesions revealed pyogranulomatous inflammation associated with large, dark brown granules (110 to 170 mm in diameter) of tyrosine surrounded by an eosinophilic, amorphous material, which resembled the Splendore-Hoeppli reaction. The granules gave a positive orange reaction when stained with Millon's reaction for tyrosine.

CLINICAL MANAGEMENT

The prognosis for a cure is not good. In humans, dramatic reduction of plasma tyrosine levels with subsequent clearing of skin and eye lesions occurs in patients receiving diets low in tyrosine and phenylalanine. Symptoms recur when a regular diet is resumed. Dietary manipulation also resulted in clearing of the dog's skin lesions.

■ MISCELLANEOUS DISORDERS

Acral Mutilation Syndrome

Acral mutilation and analgesia is an unusual hereditary sensory neuropathy of dogs that results in progressive mutilation of the distal extremities.

CAUSE AND PATHOGENESIS

The disorder has been reported in German shorthaired pointers[138] and English pointer dogs. It is probably inherited in an autosomal recessive manner.[140] Pathologic lesions are identified at the level of the primary sensory neuron. Necropsy changes are seen grossly as a decrease in prominence of the spinal ganglia and dorsal roots. The nerve cell bodies of the subcapsular mantle zone are decreased in number (by 22 to 50 per cent), and the neuron mantle is decreased in thickness. The number of small neurons (20 μm or less) in the affected ganglia is disproportionately increased in affected dogs. The spinal cord changes occur in the dorsolateral fasciculus, where reduced fiber density correlates well with the loss of pain perception that is seen clinically. Light and electron microscopic examinations of spinal roots, ganglia, and peripheral nerves show myelinated and unmyelinated fiber degeneration. Neuronal degeneration does not account for the deficiency of sensory cell bodies. This mutilation acropathy is a manifestation of a sensory neuropathy in which the neuronal deficiency results from insufficient development and slowly progressive postnatal degeneration.[138]

CLINICAL FEATURES

The syndrome appears first in affected pups at 3 to 5 months of age. Both sexes and more than one pup per litter may be affected. The pups may be smaller than littermates. They begin to bite and lick their paws. There is total loss of temperature and pain sensation in the toes and in some cases in the proximal legs and trunk. Usually, the hindlegs are most severely involved, and occasionally, only the toes of the rear legs are affected.

The toes and feet become swollen and the skin of the footpads, the plantar surface, and the area over the tuber calcis may be ulcerated. Paronychia is present, and autoamputation of the toes may be noted. The puppies walk unflinchingly on the mutilated feet (see Fig. 11:53 *H*). Proprioception is normal, tendon reflexes are intact, and no motor or autonomic impairment is present. EMG studies reveal no denervation potentials.

DIAGNOSIS

History and a thorough clinical examination of puppies of predisposed breeds provides a presumptive diagnosis. Histopathologic examination of nerve tissues at necropsy establishes a definitive diagnosis.

CLINICAL MANAGEMENT

Attempts to prevent further mutilation by means of bandages, restraint collars, or sedation are of little benefit, and euthanasia is usually requested by the owners.

The hereditary aspects of this syndrome are important, as it has been seen in several strains of English pointers.[5] Parents of affected pups should not be used as breeders. Siblings should not be used either until the mode of inheritance is firmly established. Even then, the breeding of siblings should probably be discouraged unless some test is developed to identify carriers of the disorder.

Cutaneous Mucinosis

Mucin is a component of the normal dermal ground substance.[1] Excessive accumulation, be it focal, regionalized, or generalized, can be seen in hypothyroidism, acromegaly, alopecia mucinosa, dermatomyositis, or discoid lupus erythematosus[141] or can be idiopathic.[137] The Chinese Shar Pei is prone to the latter.[139, 142]

Shar Peis have more dermal mucin than do other breeds.[65, 139] Some dogs have exaggerated amounts and exhibit pronounced folding (see Fig. 15:11 *C*), mucinous vesiculation (see Fig. 9:37 *D*), or a combination of both. The exaggerated folding is most pronounced on the head, the ventrum, and the distal extremities, and some of these dogs snore and snort owing to involvement of tissues in the oropharynx. The vesicles vary in size and can occur in normal-appearing or edematous skin.

DIAGNOSIS

The tentative diagnosis of diffuse mucinosis is made by the clinical findings of exaggerated folds and is confirmed by skin biopsy, in which the dermis contains excessive mucin with no other abnormalities.[65, 137, 141] Visually, the vesicles mimic those seen in the various autoimmune and immune-mediated disorders, but clinical evalution of the vesicle's contents quickly identifies the mucinous nature of the fluid. Mucinous vesicles do not discharge fluid with puncture by a small-gauge needle. The fluid must be expressed by digital pressure and then is thick, clear, and sticky. Biopsy of these lesions shows focal accumulation of mucin in the superficial dermis. To date, the mucinosis seen in Shar Peis has occurred in euthyroid dogs. Because this breed is prone to hypothyroidism,[142] an intercurrent thyroid abnormality could lead to very severe mucinosis.

CLINICAL MANAGEMENT

In most cases, the excessive mucinosis seen in Shar Peis is a cosmetic problem only. Most animals seem to outgrow it by 2 to 5 years of age.[139] Dogs with oropharyngeal involvement may warrant treatment, as they can experience respiratory arrest with anesthesia.[142] High levels of prednisolone (2.2 mg/kg) for 6 days, followed by a slow reduction to no medication in 30 days should reduce the amount of mucin.[139] Most animals require only one course of treatment to remain normal. A few dogs require repeated or continuous treatment. These dogs should be evaluated for hypothyroidism.

REFERENCES

General References

1. Fitzpatrick, T. B., et al.: Dermatology in General Medicine, 4th ed. McGraw Hill Book Co., New York, 1993.
2. Foil, C. S.: The skin. In: Hoskins, J. D. (ed.). Veterinary Pediatrics, 2nd ed. W. B. Saunders Co., Philadelphia, 1995.
3. Gross, T. L., et al.: Veterinary Dermatopathology. Mosby Year Book, St. Louis, 1992.
4. Miller, W. H., Jr., Scott, D. W.: Unpublished observations, 1994.
5. Muller, G. H., et al.: Small Animal Dermatology, 4th ed. W. B. Saunders Co., Philadelphia, 1989.
6. Power, H. T., Ihrke, P. J.: The use of synthetic retinoids in veterinary medicine. In: Bonagura, J. D. (ed.). Kirk's Current Veterinary Therapy XII. W. B. Saunders Co., Philadelphia, 1995.

Disorders of the Surface and Follicular Epithelium

7. Alhaidari, Z., Ortonne, J. P. Congenital ichthyosis in two Cavalier King Charles littermates. Proc. Wld. Cong. Vet. Dermatol. 2:68, 1992.
8. Antin, I. P.: Dermoid sinus in a Rhodesian Ridge-back dog. J. Am. Vet. Med. Assoc. 157:961, 1970.
9. August, J. R., et al.: Congenital ichthyosis in a dog: Comparison with the human ichthyosiform dermatoses. Comp. Cont. Educ. 10:40, 1988.
10. Baker, B. B., Maibach, H. I.: Epidermal cell renewal in seborrheic skin of dogs. Am. J. Vet. Res. 48:726, 1987.
10a. Burrows, A., Mason, K. V.: Observations of the pathogenesis and treatment of lichenoid-psoriasiform dermatitis of Springer spaniels. Proc. Am. Acad. Vet. Dermatol. Am. Coll. Vet. Dermatol. 10:81, 1994.
11. Campbell, K. L., Kirkwood, A. R.: Effect of topical oils on transepidermal water loss with seborrhea sicca. In: Ihrke, P. J., et al. (eds.). Advances in Veterinary Dermatology, Vol. 2. Pergamon Press, New York, 1993, p. 157.
11a. Campbell, K. L., et al.: Effects of four anti-seborrheic shampoos on transepidermal water losses, hydration of the stratum corneum, skin surface lipid concentration, skin surface pH, and corneocyte counts in dogs. Proc. Am. Acad. Vet. Dermatol. Am. Coll. Vet. Dermatol. 10:85, 1994.
12. Dunstan, R. W., et al.: A disease resembling junctional epidermolysis bullosa in a Toy Poodle. Am. J. Dermatopathol. 10:442, 1988.
13. Fadok, V. A. Treatment of canine idiopathic seborrhea with isotretinoin. Am. J. Vet. Res. 47:1730, 1986.
14. Fontaine, J., et al.: Familial junctional epidermolysis bullosa in Beauceron dogs. Vet. Dermatol. (In press.)
15. Gammie, J. S. Dermoid sinus removal in a Rhodesian Ridgeback dog. Can. Vet. J. 27:250, 1986.
15a. Gordon, J. G., Kwochka, K. W.: Corneocyte counts for evaluation of antiseborrheic shampoos in dogs. Vet. Dermatol. 4:57, 1993.
16. Gross, T. L., et al.: Psoriasiform lichenoid dermatitis in the Springer spaniel. Vet. Pathol. 23:76, 1986.
17. Gupta, B. N.: Epitheliogenesis imperfecta in a dog. Am. J. Res. 34:443, 1973.
18. Hargis, A. M., et al.: A skin disorder in three Shetland sheepdogs. Comparison with familial canine dermatomyositis of collies. Comp. Cont. Educ. 7:306, 1985.
19. Hargis, A. M., Mundell, A. C.: Familial canine dermatomyositis. Comp. Cont. Educ. 14:855, 1992.

20. Hargis, A. M., et al.: Complement levels in dogs with familial canine dermatomyositis. Vet. Immunol. Immuno-pathol. 20:95, 1985.
21. Hargis, A. M., et al.: Severe secondary amyloidosis in a dog with dermatomyositis. J. Comp. Pathol. 100:427, 1989.
22. Hewitt, M. P., et al.: Epitheliogenesis imperfecta in a black Labrador puppy. Can. Vet. J. 16:371, 1975.
23. Ihrke, P. J., Gross, T. L.: Ulcerative dermatosis of Shetland sheepdogs and collies. In: Bonagura, J. D. (ed.). Kirk's Current Veterinary Therapy XII. W. B. Saunders Co., Philadelphia, 1995.
24. Johnstone, I., et al.: A hereditary junctional mechanobullous disease in the cat. Proc. Wld. Cong. Vet. Dermatol. 2:111, 1992.
25. Koch, H., Walder, E.: Epidermolysis bullosa dystrophia in Beaucerons. In: von Tscharner, C., Halliwell, R. E. W. (eds.). Advances in Veterinary Dermatology, Vol. 1. Baillière Tindall, Philadelphia, 1990, p. 441.
26. Kral, F., Schwartzman, R. M.: Veterinary and Comparative Dermatology. J. B. Lippincott Co., Philadelphia, 1964.
27. Kwochka, K. W.: Shampoos and moisturizing rinses in veterinary dermatology. In: Bonagura, J. D. (ed.). Kirk's Current Veterinary Therapy XII. W. B. Saunders Co., Philadelphia. (In press.)
28. Kwochka, K. W.: Keratinization abnormalities: Understanding the mechanism of scale formation. In: Ihrke, P. J., et al. (eds.). Advances in Veterinary Dermatology, Vol. 2. Pergamon Press, New York, 1993, p. 91.
29. Kwochka, K. W.: Cell proliferation kinetics in the hair root matrix of dogs with healthy skin and dogs with idiopathic seborrhea. Am. J. Vet. Res. 51:1570, 1990.
30. Kwochka, K. W.: In vivo and in vitro examination of cell proliferation kinetics in the normal and seborrheic canine epidermis. Proc. Am. Acad. Vet. Dermatol. Am. Coll. Vet. Dermatol. 7:46, 1991.
31. Kwochka, K. W., Rademakers, A. M.: Cell proliferation of epidermis, hair follicles, and sebaceous glands of beagles and Cocker spaniels with healthy skin. Am. J. Vet. Res. 50:587, 1989.
32. Kwochka, K. W., Rademakers, A. M.: Cell proliferation kinetics of epidermis, hair follicles, and sebaceous glands of Cocker spaniels with idiopathic seborrhea. Am. J. Vet. Res. 50:1918, 1989.
33. Kwochka, K. W., Smeak, D. D.: The cellular defect in idiopathic seborrhea of Cocker spaniels. In: von Tscharner, C., Halliwell, R. E. W. (eds.). Advances in Veterinary Dermatology, Vol. 1. Ballière Tindall, Philadelphia, 1990, p. 265.
34. Kwochka, K. W., et al.: Development and characterization of an in vitro cell culture system for the canine epidermis. Proc. Am. Acad. Vet. Dermatol. Am. Coll. Vet. Dermatol. 3:9, 1987.
35. Mann, G. E., Stratton, J.: Dermoid sinus in the Rhodesian Ridgeback. J. Small Anim. Pract. 7:631, 1966.
36. Mason, K. V., et al.: Characterization of lichenoid-psoriasiform dermatosis of Springer spaniels. J. Am. Vet. Med. Assoc. 189:897, 1986.
36a. Messinger, L. M., et al.: Investigation of physical, histological, ultrastructural, and biochemical abnormalities of related Rottweiler dogs with a congenital disorder of cornification. Proc. Am. Acad. Vet. Dermatol. Am. Coll. Vet. Dermatol. 10:12, 1994.
36b. Miller, W. H., Jr.: Canine facial dermatoses. Comp. Cont. Educ. 1:640, 1979.
37. Muller, G. H.: Ichthyosis in two dogs. J. Am. Vet. Med. Assoc. 169:1313, 1976.
38. Munday, B. L.: Epitheliogenesis imperfecta in lambs and kittens. Br. Vet. J. 126:47, 1970.
39. Palshof, P., Christoffersen, E.: *Malassezia pachydermatis* on the skin of normal and seborrheic West Highland white terriers. Proc. Eur. Soc. Vet. Dermatol. 10:269, 1993.
40. Paradis, M., Scott, D. W.: Hereditary primary seborrhea oleosa in Persian cats. Feline Pract. 19:17, 1990.
41. Paradis, M.: Footpad hyperkeratosis in a family of Dogues de Bordeaux. Vet. Dermatol. 3:75, 1992.
42. Power, H. T., et al.: Use of etretinate for treatment of primary keratinization disorders (idiopathic seborrhea) in Cocker spaniels, West Highland white terriers, and Basset hounds. J. Am. Vet. Med. Assoc. 201:419, 1992.
43. Raczkowski, J. J.: Pathogenetic Studies of Canine Seborrheic Skin Disease in the West Highland White Terrier Breed. Masters thesis, Kansas State University, 1984.
44. Rest, J. R., Theaker, A. J.: Lupoid dermatosis in a German shorthaired pointer. Proc. Eur. Soc. Vet. Dermatol. 10:271, 1993.
45. Scott, D. W., Schultz, R. D.: Epidermolysis bullosa simplex in a collie dog. J. Am. Vet. Med. Assoc. 171:721, 1977.
46. Scott, D. W.: Congenital ichthyosis in a dog. Companion Anim. Pract. 19:7, 1987.
47. Scott, D. W., Miller, W. H., Jr.: Epidermal dysplasia and *Malassezia pachydermatis* infection in West Highland white terriers. Vet. Dermatol. 1:25, 1989.
48. Selcer, E. A., et al.: Dermoid sinus in a Shih tzu and a boxer. J. Am. Anim. Hosp. Assoc. 20:634, 1984.
49. Shanley, K. J., et al.: Canine benign familial chronic pemphigus. In: Ihrke, P. J., et al. (eds.). Advances in Veterinary Dermatology, Vol 2. Pergamon Press, New York, 1993, p. 353.
50. Stonecipher, M. R., et al.: Cutaneous changes of dermatomyositis in patients with normal muscle enzymes. Dermatomyositis sine myositis? J. Am. Acad. Dermatol. 28:951, 1993.
50a. Theaker, A. J.: A case of lupoid dermatosis in a German short-haired pointer. Proc. Br. Vet. Dermatol. Study Grp. 16:5, 1994.
51. Vroom, M. W.: A retrospective study of 43 West Highland white terriers. Proc. Wld. Cong. Vet. Dermatol. 2:70, 1992.
52. Vroom, M. W.: Three cases with hereditary lupoid dermatosis of the German shorthaired pointer. Proc. Eur. Soc. Vet. Dermatol. 10:67, 1993.
53. White, S. D., Gross, T. L.: Hereditary lupoid dermatosis of the German shorthaired pointer. In: Bonagura, J. D. (ed.). Kirk's Current Veterinary Therapy XII. W. B. Saunders Co., Philadelphia, 1995.

54. White, S. D., et al.: Dermatomyositis in an adult Pembroke Welsh corgi. J. Am. Anim. Hosp. Assoc. 28:398, 1992.
55. White, S. D., et al.: Dystrophic (dermolytic) epidermolysis bullosa in a cat. Vet. Dermatol. 4:91, 1993.

Disorders of Hairs and Hair Growth
56. Allen, L. S. S.: Skin condition in Yorkshire terriers. Canine Pract. 12:29, 1985.
57. Beco, L., et al.: Color mutant alopecia in seven dachshunds (five with dead leaf coat color). Proc. Eur. Soc. Vet. Dermatol. 10:61, 1993.
58. Bourdeau, P., et al.: Alopécie héréditaire généralisée féline. Rec. Med. Vet. 164:17, 1988.
59. Brignac, M., et al.: Microscopy of color mutant alopecia. In: von Tscharner, C., Halliwell, R. E. W. (eds.). Advances in Veterinary Dermatology, Vol. 1. Baillière Tindall, Philadelphia, 1990, p. 448.
60. Carlotti, D.: A propos des alopécies auriculaires. Point Vet. 25:8, 1993.
61. Carlotti, D. N. Canine hereditary black hair follicular dysplasia and color mutant alopecia: Clinical and histopathological aspects. In: von Tscharner, C., Halliwell, R. E. W. (eds.). Advances in Veterinary Dermatology, Vol. 1. Baillière Tindall, Philadelphia, 1990, p. 43.
62. Casal, M., et al.: Congenital hypotrichosis with thymic aplasia in nine Birman kittens. ACVIM Abstract No. 68, Washington, DC, 1993.
63. Chastain, C. B., Sawyer, D. E.: Congenital hypotrichosis in male Basset hound littermates. J. Am. Vet. Med. Assoc. 187:845, 1985.
64. Conroy, J. D.: Hypotrichosis in Miniature Poodle siblings. J. Am. Vet. Med. Assoc. 166:697, 1975.
65. Dunstan, R. W., Rosser, E. J.: Newly recognized and emerging genodermatoses in domestic animals. Curr. Probl. Dermatol. 17:216, 1987.
66. Geary, M. R., Baker, K. P.: The occurrence of pili torti in a litter of kittens in England. J. Small Anim. Pract. 27:85, 1986.
67. Grieshaber, T. L., et al.: Congenital alopecia in a Bichon frisé. J. Am. Vet. Med. Assoc. 188:1053, 1986.
67a. Griffin, C. E.: Etretinate—how is it being used in veterinary dermatology? Derm. Dialogue, Spring/Summer 1993, p. 4.
68. Guaguère, E.: Aspects histopathologiques et ultrastructuraux de l'alopécie des robes diluées: A propos d'un cos chez un Doberman pinscher bleu. Prat. Med. Chirurg. Anim. Cie. 26:537, 1991.
69. Hargis, A. M., et al.: Black hair follicular dysplasia in black and white Saluki dogs. Vet. Dermatol. 2:69, 1991.
70. Hirota, Y., et al.: Immunologic features in hairless descendants derived from Mexican hairless dogs. Jpn. J. Vet. Sci. 52:1217, 1990.
70a. Ihrke, P. J., et al.: Generalized congenital hypotrichosis in a female Rottweiler. Vet. Dermatol. 4:65, 1993.
71. Kimura, T., et al.: The inheritance and breeding results of hairless descendants of Mexican hairless dogs. Lab. Anim. 27:55, 1993.
72. Kral, F., Schwartzman, R. M.: Veterinary and Comparative Dermatology. J. B. Lippincott Co., Philadelphia, 1964.
73. Kunkle, G. A.: Congenital hypotrichosis in two dogs. J. Am. Vet. Med. Assoc. 185:84, 1984.
73a. McKeever, P. J., et al.: Spiculosis. J. Am. Anim. Hosp. Assoc. 28:257, 1992.
74. Malik, R., France, M. P.: Hyperpigmentation and symmetrical alopecia in three Silky terriers. Aust. Vet. Pract. 21:135, 1991.
75. Marks, A., et al.: Congenital hypotrichosis in a French bulldog. J. Small Anim. Pract. 33:450, 1992.
76. Miller, M. A., Dunstan, R. W.: Seasonal flank alopecia in boxers and Airedale terriers: 24 cases (1985–1992). J. Am. Vet. Med. Assoc. 203:1567, 1993.
77. Miller, W. H., Jr.: Follicular dysplasia in adult black and red Doberman pinschers. Vet. Dermatol. 1:181, 1990.
78. Miller, W. H., Jr.: Color dilution alopecia in Doberman pinschers with blue or fawn coat colors: A study on the incidence and histopathology of this disorder. Vet. Dermatol. 1:113, 1990.
79. Miller, W. H., Jr.: Alopecia associated with coat color dilution in two Yorkshire terriers, one Saluki, and one mix-breed dog. J. Am. Anim. Hosp. Assoc. 27:39, 1991.
80. Post, K., et al.: Clinical and histopathologic changes as seen in Siberian husky follicular dysplasia. In: von Tscharner, C., Halliwell, R. E. W. (eds.). Advances in Veterinary Dermatology, Vol. 1. Baillière-Tindall, Philadelphia, 1990, p. 446.
81. Post, K., et al.: Hair follicle dysplasia in a Siberian husky. J. Am. Anim. Hosp. Assoc. 24:659, 1988.
82. Robinson, R.: The Canadian hairless or sphinx cat. J. Hered. 64:47, 1973.
83. Scott, D. W.: Feline dermatology 1900–1978: A monograph. J. Am. Anim. Hosp. Assoc. 16:313, 1980.
84. Selmanowitz, V. J., et al.: Congenital ectodermal defect in Poodles. J. Hered. 61:196, 1970.
85. Selmanowitz, V. J., et al.: Black hair follicular dysplasia in dogs. J. Am. Vet. Med. Assoc. 171:1079, 1977.
86. Thoday, K.: Skin diseases of the cat. In Pract. 3:21, 1981.
87. Thomsett, L. R. Congenital hypotrichia in the dog. Vet. Rec. 73:915, 1961.
88. Wilkinson, G. T., Kristensen, T. S.: A hair abnormality in Abyssinian cats. J. Small Anim. Pract. 30:27, 1989.

Disorders of Pigmentation
89. Anderson, R. K.: Canine acanthosis nigricans. Comp. Cont. Educ. 1:466, 1979.
90. Colgan, S. P., et al.: Defective in vitro motility of polymorphonuclear leukocytes of homozygote and heterozygote Chédiak-Higashi cats. Vet. Immunol. Immunopathol. 31:205, 1992.
91. Halliwell, R. E. W., Gorman, N. T.: Veterinary Clinical Immunology. W. B. Saunders Co., Philadelphia, 1989.
92. Prieur, D. J., Collier, L. L.: Morphologic basis of inherited coat-color dilutions of cats. J. Hered. 72:178, 1981.
93. Rendon, M. I., et al.: Acanthosis nigricans: A cutaneous marker for tissue resistance to insulin. J. Am. Acad. Dermatol. 21:461, 1989.

94. Rickards, R. A.: A new treatment for canine melanosis. Mod. Vet. Pract. 47:38, 1966.
95. Schwartzman, R. M., Orkin, M.: A Comparative Study of Skin Diseases of Dog and Man. Charles C Thomas, Springfield, IL, 1962, pp. 313–318.
96. Scott, D. W., Walton, D. K.: Clinical evaluation of oral vitamin E for the treatment of primary acanthosis nigricans. J. Am. Anim. Hosp. Assoc. 21:345, 1985.
97. White, S. D., et al.: Acquired aurotrichia (''gilding syndrome'') of Miniature Schnauzers. Vet. Dermatol. 3:37, 1991.
98. Yang, T.: Gray collie syndrome. J. Am. Vet. Med. Assoc. 191:390, 1987.

Disorders of Collagen

99. Affolter, V.: Collagen disorder of the footpads of three German shepherd dogs. In: Ihrke, P. J., et al. (eds.). Advances in Veterinary Dermatology, Vol. 2. Pergamon Press, New York, 1993, p. 418.
100. Barnett, K. C., Cottrell, B. D.: Ehlers-Danlos syndrome in a dog: Ocular, cutaneous and articular abnormalities. J. Small Anim. Pract. 28:941, 1987.
101. Collier, L. A., et al.: A clinical description of dermatosparaxis in a Himalayan cat. Feline Pract. 10:25, 1980.
102. Counts, D. F., et al.: Dermatosparaxis in a Himalayan cat. I. Biochemical studies of dermal collagen. J. Invest. Dermatol. 74:96, 1980.
103. Fontaine, J., et al.: Anomalie du collagene dermique: Dermatosparaxie chez un chat europeén. Point Vet. 24:255, 1992.
104. Ducatelle, R., et al.: A morphometric classification of dermatosparaxis in the dog and cat. Vlaams Diergeneesk. Tudschr. 56:107, 1987.
105. Duvic, M., Pinnell, S. R.: Ehlers-Danlos syndrome. In: Thiers, B. H., Dobson, R. L. (eds.). Pathogenesis of Skin Disease. Churchill Livingstone, New York, 1988, p. 565.
106. Freeman, L. J., et al.: Ehlers-Danlos syndrome in dogs and cats. Semin. Vet. Med. Surg. 2:221, 1987.
107. Hegreberg, G. A., Padgett, G. A.: Ehlers-Danlos syndrome in animals. Bull. Pathol. 8:247, 1967.
108. Hegreberg, G. A., et al.: A heritable connective tissue disease of dogs and mink resembling the Ehlers-Danlos syndrome of man. II. Mode of inheritance. J. Hered. 60:249, 1969.
109. Hegreberg, G. A., et al.: A heritable connective tissue disease of dogs and mink resembling the Ehlers-Danlos syndrome of man. III. Histopathologic changes of the skin. Arch. Pathol. 90:159, 1970.
110. Holbrook, K. A., et al.: Dermatosparaxis in the Himalayan cat. II. Ultrastructural studies of dermal collagen. J. Invest. Dermatol. 74:100, 1980.
111. Kunkle, G. A., et al.: Focal metatarsal fistulas in five dogs. J. Am. Vet. Med. Assoc. 202:756, 1993.
112. Matthews, B. R., Lewis, G. T.: Ehlers-Danlos syndrome in a dog. Can. Vet. J. 31:389, 1990.
113. Minor, R. R.: Animal models of heritable diseases of the skin. In: Goldsmith, E. L. (ed.). Biochemistry and Physiology of Skin. Oxford University Press, New York, 1982.
114. Minor, R. R., et al.: Genetic diseases of connective tissues in animals. Curr. Probl. Dermatol. 17:199, 1987.
115. Neibauerer, G. W., et al.: Antibodies to canine collagen types I and II with spontaneous cruciate ligament rupture and osteoarthritis. Arthritis Rheum. 30:319, 1987.
116. Patterson, D. F., Minor, R. R.: Hereditary fragility and hyper-extensibility of the skin of cats. Lab. Invest. 37:170, 1977.
117. Rest, J. R.: Pathology of two possible genodermatoses. J. Small Anim. Pract. 30:230, 1989.
118. Scott, D. W.: Cutaneous asthenia in a cat. Vet. Med. (S.A.C.) 69:1256, 1974.
119. Scott, D. W.: Feline dermatology. Introspective retrospections. J. Am. Anim. Hosp. Assoc. 20:537, 1984.
119a. Sousa, C.: Soft-coated Wheaten terriers and E.D.S. Derm. Dialogue 1:3, 1982.

Disorders of Vessels

120. Carpenter, J. L., et al.: Idiopathic cutaneous and renal glomerular vasculopathy of Greyhounds. Vet. Pathol. 35:401, 1988.
121. Fossum, T. W., Miller, M. W.: Lymphedema-etiopathogenesis. J. Vet. Intern. Med. 6:238, 1992.
122. Fossum, T. W., et al.: Lymphedema—Clinical signs, diagnosis and treatment. J. Vet. Intern. Med. 6:312, 1992.
123. Ladds, P. W., et al.: Lethal congenital edema in bulldog pups. J. Am. Vet. Med. Assoc. 155:81, 1971.
124. Luginbuhl, H., et al.: Congenital hereditary lymphedema in the dog, part II. Pathological studies. J. Med. Genet. 4:153, 1967.
125. Patterson, D. F., et al.: Congenital hereditary lymphedema in the dog, part I. Clinical and genetic studies. J. Med. Genet. 4:145, 1967.
126. Pedersen, K., Scott, D. W.: Idiopathic pyogranulomatous inflammation and leukocytoelastic vasculitis of the nasal planum, nostrils, and nasal mucosa in Scottish terriers in Denmark. Vet. Dermatol. 2:85, 1991.
127. Scott-Moncrieff, J. C. R., et al.: Systemic necrotizing vasculitis in nine young beagles. J. Am. Vet. Med. Assoc. 201:1553, 1992.
128. Takahashi, J. L., et al.: Primary lymphedema in a dog: A case report. J. Am. Anim. Hosp. Assoc. 20:849, 1984.
129. Weir, J. A. M., et al.: Familial cutaneous vasculopathy of German shepherd dogs: Clinical, genetic, and preliminary pathological and immunologic studies. Can. Vet. J. (In press.)

Endocrine, Metabolic, and Immunologic Disorders

130. Bettenay, S. V.: Acrodermatitis of bull terriers—Long term management. Proc. Wld. Cong. Vet. Dermatol. 2:69, 1992.
131. Jezyk, P. F., et al.: Lethal acrodermatitis in bull terriers. J. Am. Vet. Med. Assoc. 188:833, 1986.
132. Kunkle, G. A., et al.: Tyrosinemia in a dog. J. Am. Anim. Hosp. Assoc. 20:615, 1984.
133. McEwan, N. A.: Confirmation and investigation of lethal acrodermatitis of bull terriers in Britain. In: Ihrke, P. J., et al. (eds.). Advances in Veterinary Dermatology, Vol. 2. Pergamon Press, New York, 1993, p. 151.

134. McEwan, N. A.: Isolation of yeasts from bull terriers suffering from lethal acrodermatitis. Proc. Eur. Soc. Vet. Dermatol. 10:277, 1993.
135. Mundell, A. C.: Mineral analysis in bull terriers with lethal acrodermatitis. Proc. Am. Acad. Vet. Dermatol. Am. Coll. Vet. Dermatol. 4:22, 1988.
136. Smits, B., et al.: Lethal acrodermatitis in bull terriers: A problem of defective zinc metabolism. Vet. Dermatol. 2:91, 1991.

Miscellaneous Disorders
137. Beale, K. M., et al.: Papular and plaque-like mucinosis in a puppy. Vet. Dermatol. 2:29, 1991.
138. Cummings, J. F., et al.: Acral mutilation and nociceptive loss in English Pointer dogs. Acta Neuropathol. 53:119, 1981.
139. Griffin, C. E., Rosenkrantz, W. S.: Skin disorders of the Shar Pei. In: Kirk, R. W., Bonagura, J. D. (eds.). Kirk's Current Veterinary Therapy XI. W. B. Saunders Co., Philadelphia, 1991, p. 519.
140. Hutt, F. B.: Necrosis of the toes. In: Genetics for Dog Breeders. W. H. Freeman, San Francisco, 1979.
141. Miller, W. H., Jr., Buerger, R. G.: Cutaneous mucinous vesiculation in a dog with hypothyroidism. J. Am. Vet. Med. Assoc. 196:757, 1990.
142. Miller, W. H., Jr., et al.: Dermatologic disorders of Chinese Shar-Peis: 58 cases (1981–1989). J. Am. Vet. Med. Assoc. 200:986, 1992.

Pigmentary Abnormalities

■

Chapter Outline

■ THE NORMAL PROCESS OF SKIN PIGMENTATION

The color of normal skin depends primarily on the amount of melanin, carotene, and oxyhemoglobin or reduced hemoglobin that it contains and the location of the pigments within the subcutis, vessels, dermis, epidermis, and hair.[6, 15a] Epidermal and hair pigmentation results primarily from melanin, which has two forms and imparts four basic colors. Black and brown pigments are derived from eumelanins. The phaeomelanins are yellow and red pigments and contain cysteine thiol groups that react to form 5-S-cysteinyl dopa. Intermediate melanins are a blend of eumelanin and phaeomelanin. A lack of melanin results in white hair or skin. The pigment melanin is formed in melanocytes within a membrane-bound organelle called the melanosome. (For a complete description, see Chap. 1.) The melanosome is formed by the fusion of two different membrane-bound vesicles that arise from the Golgi-associated smooth endoplasmic reticulum and the rough endoplasmic reticulum. Melanosomes contain the enzyme tyrosinase, which has an important regulatory role in melanin synthesis; the level of its activity correlates with the degree of pigment production. Tyrosinase, which contains copper, converts tyrosine to dopa and dopa to dopa quinone. This process begins the production of both types of melanin. Intermediates in melanin synthesis are known to be cytotoxic,[25] and their release from melanosomes could result in cellular death.

Melanosomes have been subcategorized into four stages of development. Stages I and II are developing the structural configuration and localization of precursors but have no melanin deposition. Stage III melanosomes have some melanin and are actively producing melanin, as evidenced by very high levels of tyrosinase activity. Stage IV melanosomes are the most mature; they have large amounts of melanin and low levels of tyrosinase activity. As melanosomes migrate toward the end of the melanocyte dendrite, they pass through these stages of development.

Light-colored skin has melanocytes with more stage I, II, and III melanosomes and fewer stage IV melanosomes than does dark skin. The tips of the melanocyte dendrites are phagocytized by keratinocytes, completing the transfer of pigment to the epidermal cells. In humans, there is one melanocyte for approximately 36 keratinocytes. This association of one melanocyte with a group of keratinocytes has been referred to as the *epidermal melanin unit*. In lower animals, melatonin and possibly other endocrine hormones are believed to play a major regulatory role in cutaneous pigmentation. It may be, however, that the interaction between keratinocytes and melanocytes is more important in the pigmentation of humans, dogs, and cats. At least in humans, keratinocytes are known to produce multiple factors that influence the growth, differentiation, tyrosinase activity, pigmentation, and morphology of melanocytes.[39] Basic fibroblast growth factor and endothelin-1 are produced by cultured human keratinocytes.[40] Both of these factors are melanocyte mitogens, and endothelin-1 also increases tyrosinase activity in vitro. These local factors would better explain the patterns and localized control of the pigment changes seen in animals.

Hair pigmentation is separate from the skin, and a follicular melanin unit has also been described.[24] In the hair, melanocytes are found in the hair bulb. In contrast to epidermal melanocytes, which are always active, hair melanocytes are active only during anagen. The controlling mechanism for hair pigmentation is still unknown.[24] Follicular melanocytes produce larger melanin granules. Variation in hair coloration reflects the melanosome size, type, shape, and dispersion. The color of these hair melanosomes may be modulated in vivo by hydrogen peroxide.

Visible pigmentation depends on which stage of melanosomes is transferred, the size of the melanosomes, and how the melanosomes are dispersed within the keratinocyte. Melanosomes larger than 0.5 to 0.7 μm are dispersed individually within keratinocytes, and smaller melanosomes are grouped into melanosome complexes. As keratinocytes migrate to the surface of the skin, melanosomes may be degraded at different rates. Lighter skin has higher levels of melanosome degradation than darker skin does. If one considers all the factors involved in normal pigmentation, it becomes apparent that defects may occur at many different levels of pigmentation.

In small animals, coat color is more varied than skin color is. Hair color is controlled by multiple coat color genes; various alleles at each locus influence the relative amounts of eumelanin, phaeomelanin, and mixed type or intermediate melanins as well as granule size and dispersion within the hair shaft.

Alterations in cutaneous pigmentation are very common in canine and feline dermatoses.[10, 13, 17] In most cases, the pigmentation changes are the result of another disease process, especially one of an inflammatory nature. Hyperpigmentation and hypopigmentation are most prominent. Epidermal hyperplasia and diseases that affect the basal cell layer of the epidermis and anagen hair bulb often alter pigmentation. Although secondary pigmentary changes are most common, there are diseases that primarily affect pigmentation or present with nothing other than abnormal or unacceptable pigmentation.

■ HYPERPIGMENTATION

Hyperpigmentation *(hypermelanosis)* occurs when the pigmentation is greater than normal for the area of skin in question.[15a] This occurs as a result of increased amounts of melanin in the dermis, epidermis, or both. Excess pigment in the skin is called *melanoderma;* in the hair, *melanotrichia.* Melanin within dermal melanophages or melanosomes causes a slate or steel blue color. Macromelanosomes in hair are associated with diluted coat colors (e.g., blue or fawn).

Hyperpigmentation in animals may be genetic, acquired, or associated with pigmented neoplasms.

Genetic Hyperpigmentation

LENTIGO

Lentigo (pl., lentigines) is a genetic cause of hyperpigmentation.[15a] In dogs, the condition is a macular melanosis that is intensely black and usually occurs as multiple lesions that are most common on the ventrum. Lentigines appear in mature dogs. They often increase in number and size over a period of several months; subsequently, they become static and remain unchanged for the life of the dog. These sharply circumscribed macules do not itch and are of no consequence to the patient. They have been referred to as *tar spots* (Fig. 12:1). The lesions are sometimes grouped in clusters or may spread rather diffusely over the ventral surface of the body. Occasionally, the lesions have a hyperkeratotic surface; they should not be confused with the pigmented epithelial nevus, however, which is rough and has a slightly raised lesion (see Chap. 19).[6, 7, 12, 35]

A hereditary form of lentigo called *lentiginosis profusa* has been reported in pugs.[4] The mating of two unrelated dogs affected with the disorder produced one with the same condition. As a result, there was thought to be an autosomal dominant mode of inheritance, as is found in humans.[4] Many of the lesions described in these dogs were clinically and histologically hyperplastic,[34] however, so it is likely that the authors were actually describing pigmented epidermal nevi.[12] Similarly, generalized lentigines—probably epidermal nevi—were reported in a cat.[21]

Histologically, early lentigines are characterized by a sharply localized increase in the number of melanocytes and melanosomes.[28, 34] The epidermal pigmentation is greatly increased, because almost every keratinocyte contains melanosomes. Usually, no structural changes or only mild structural changes occur in the epidermis. As the lesion develops, the epidermis may thicken, hyperkeratosis may occur, and slight rete ridges may form.

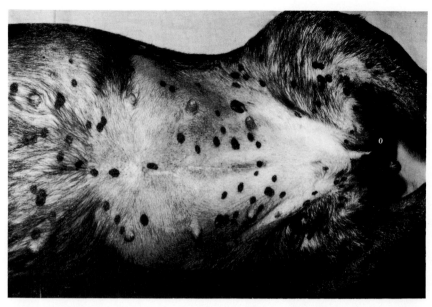

Figure 12:1. Close-up view of a 7-year-old French bulldog with multiple lentigines. Note the intensity of the pigmentation and the sharply demarcated borders.

The significance of lentigo lies in its diagnostic differentiation from pigmented tumors, especially melanomas. In humans, lentigines may become malignant, but to our knowledge, no malignancy in dogs or cats has been reported. No clinical management of these lesions is required. If the clinician or the client is concerned about the lesions, a biopsy is indicated to establish a definitive diagnosis. No treatment is required. If the client wishes to eliminate the lesions, surgical excision is necessary because no medical therapy is currently available.

LENTIGO SIMPLEX IN ORANGE CATS

Lentigo simplex has been described in orange cats.[29] The condition is characterized by asymptomatic macular melanosis, usually beginning in cats younger than 1 year of age.

The lesions start on the lips and begin as tiny, black, asymptomatic spots that gradually enlarge and become more numerous with time. There can be lesions on the nose, gingiva, and eyelids in addition to the lip. Well-circumscribed, generally circular areas of intense, uniform macular melanosis, ranging from 1 to 9 mm in diameter and occasionally coalescent, are present in variable numbers (Fig. 12:2 *A*). Surrounding tissue is normal. The lesions do not vary in the intensity of hyperpigmentation with the time of year. They are asymptomatic, do not develop into melanoma, and have no identified cause.

Histopathologic findings include marked hypermelanosis, predominantly of the basal cell layer of the epithelium, that is caused by the increased numbers of melanocytes and by hypermelanosis of the neighboring basal keratinocytes (Fig. 12:3). Occasionally, melanophages are seen in the superficial dermis.

Lentigo simplex is a cosmetic defect. Because no nonsurgical treatment is known, lesions are left untreated. Their elimination would require surgical excision.

Acquired Hyperpigmentation

The most common form of hyperpigmentation is postinflammatory. Many dogs and some cats produce more pigment in or around areas of inflammation. Many diseases characterized by chronic erythematous papular lesions may undergo hyperpigmentation. Often this type of

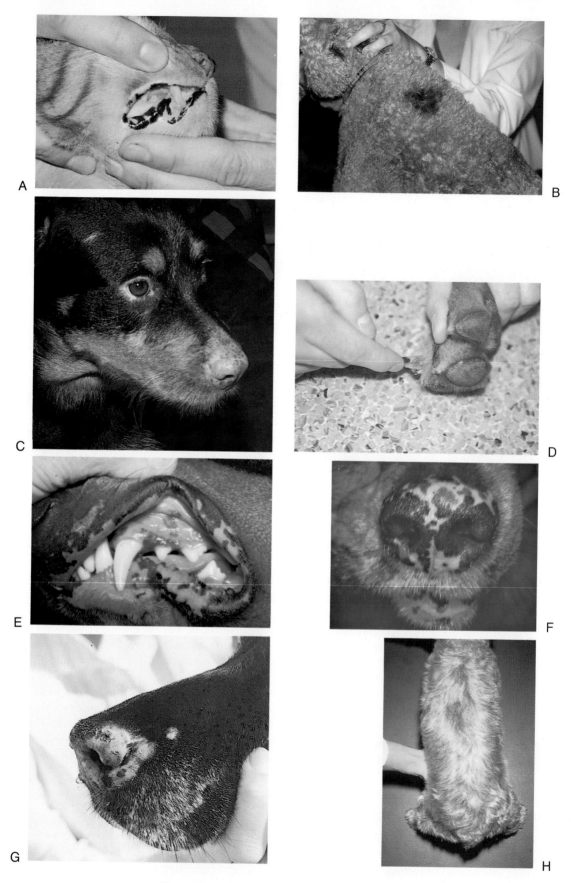

Figure 12:2 *See figure legend on opposite page*

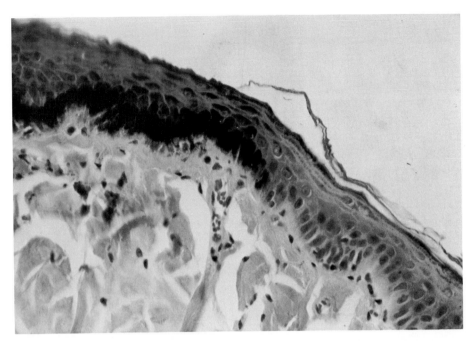

Figure 12:3. Feline lentigo simplex. Note the abrupt transition between the melanotic area (left) and normal epithelium (right).

postinflammatory hyperpigmentation has a lattice-like appearance (Fig. 12:4) and is most commonly seen with superficial bacterial pyodermas. Many other chronic inflammatory diseases also result in hyperpigmentation; examples include the chronic or healing lesions of canine demodicosis, canine scabies, the center of healing circular dermatophytosis, acanthosis nigricans, and food hypersensitivity. Occasionally, a patch of pigmented comedones appears as a hyperpigmented patch or plaque. These patches or plaques may be from slate blue to gray in color and should raise the suspicion of *Demodex*, hyperadrenocorticism,[17] or comedo nevus.

More diffuse hyperpigmentation may result from the chronic exposure to ultraviolet light of skin that has lost hair or from chronic irritation due to cutaneous friction (Fig. 12:5). Most pruritic diseases may be incriminated because both friction and inflammation may lead to hyperpigmentation. It is common to see hyperpigmentation in dogs with hypersensitivity diseases. Diffuse hyperpigmentation may also result from some metabolic or hormonal disorders such as hyperadrenocorticism, hypothyroidism, and the sex hormone dermatoses (see Chap. 9). The mechanism is unknown, although it has been suggested that the hyperpigmentation may result from direct effects of the hormonal changes on the melanocytes. However, the direct actions of these hormones on the melanocytes have not been well defined.[13] The possibility of indirect effects through keratinocyte changes has not been investigated. In some cases, it also appears that ultraviolet exposure may play a role. When alopecia precedes the hyperpigmentation, skin is exposed to light, which can contribute to the pigment changes that occur. Protection of the skin decreases the hyperpigmentation.

Figure 12:2. Pigment abnormalities. *A*, Lentigo simplex in an orange cat with marked macular melanosis of the lips. *B*, Melanotrichia patches in a Poodle with sebaceous adenitis. *C*, Vitiligo in a Rottweiler. Note the nasal and eyelid depigmentation and patch leukotrichia on the head. *D*, Vitiligo of the claws concurrent with onychodystrophy. *E*, Patchy, hypopigmentation present from birth on the lips of a mature Doberman pinscher. *F*, A 2-year-old Newfoundland that had a normal black color at birth but gradually developed patchy hypopigmentation evident in skin and hairs. *G*, Epitheliotropic lymphoma affecting the nasal planum. *H*, Acquired aurotrichia in a miniature Schnauzer. (Courtesy S. White.)

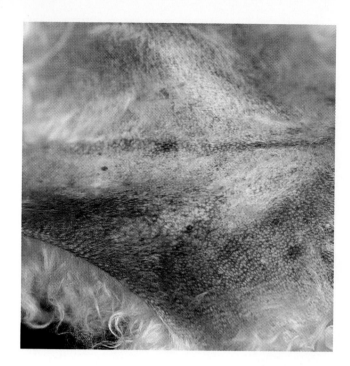

Figure 12:4. Area of lattice-like hyperpigmentation in a dog with chronic superficial folliculitis.

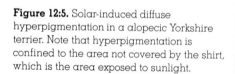**Figure 12:5.** Solar-induced diffuse hyperpigmentation in a alopecic Yorkshire terrier. Note that hyperpigmentation is confined to the area not covered by the shirt, which is the area exposed to sunlight.

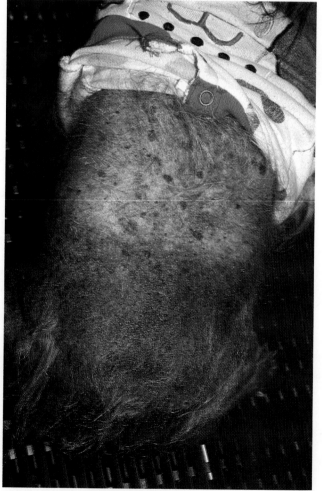

Melanotrichia may also occur in animals after the healing of areas of deep inflammation (e.g., panniculitis, vaccine reaction). This is seen more in certain breeds such as the Yorkshire terrier, Silky terrier, Bedlington terrier, Old English sheepdog, and Poodle (Fig. 12:6). In some dogs, especially Poodles with sebaceous adenitis, multifocal areas of melanotrichia may be seen. (see Fig. 12:2*B*). Because the inflammatory lesions of sebaceous adenitis occur even in areas without melanotrichia, it is possible that this alteration is not due to inflammation but occurs as a result of some other pathomechanism. Multifocal areas of melanotrichia have been seen in Poodles following bouts of intervertebral disk disease. The exact mechanism of hyperpigmentation in these inflammatory diseases is unknown.

The focal postinflammatory melanotrichia seen in adult dogs with silver or gray haircoats may be the result of reversion to a puppy coat under the influence of genes at the graying (G) locus. Silver dogs are usually born with dark coats that lighten when the adult hairs develop. If the melanotrichia is due to G locus influences, the hairs revert to their normal adult color at the next shedding. In other dogs, the melanotrichia may be due to the influence of melanocyte-stimulating factors.

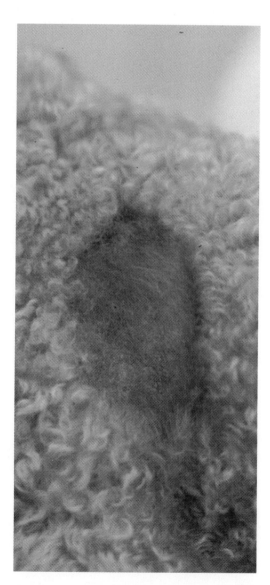

Figure 12:6. Melanotrichia following the healing of an alopecic lesion that resulted from a subcutaneous triamcinolone acetonide injection.

Recent studies suggest that keratinocytes may be able to stimulate melanogenesis by releasing melanocyte-stimulating factors. It is possible that these factors are present at low levels in normal epidermis, but their levels and activity are increased in response to stimulation or keratinocyte stress.[40] This is an attractive hypothesis to explain the local pigment changes that occur in the wide variety of diseases that result in stimulation of keratinocyte proliferation by inflammation. Melanotrichia may also occur following the resolution of metabolic or hormonal disorders; it is commonly noted in dogs with hyperadrenocorticism that are treated with mitotane (o,p'-DDD) (Fig. 12:7). The mechanism is unknown, but G locus influences are probably important in dogs with silver coats.

Hyperpigmentation from drugs, although rare, may also cause pigment changes. O,p'-DDD therapy (or the control of the disease being treated) may be associated with hypermelanosis and melanotrichia. Because this change is usually temporary, even when o,p'-DDD therapy is continued, it is possibly caused by hormonal changes and not by the drug. Experimentally, the drug minocycline has been shown to cause hyperpigmentation in dogs,[1] and the effect was believed to be attributable to iron deposition. In humans, a variety of other metallic substances may cause cutaneous pigment changes; for example, changes may be acquired by parenteral or topical absorption of metals such as silver, gold, and mercury.[2]

CANINE ACANTHOSIS NIGRICANS

This primary disease is seen most commonly in dachshunds. It begins when the dog is less than 1 year of age and starts as hyperpigmented macules or patches in the axilla and inguinal region. This condition is discussed in Chapter 11.

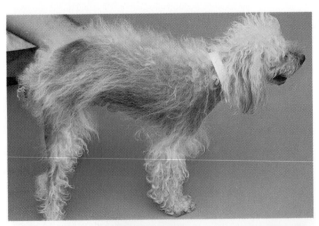

A

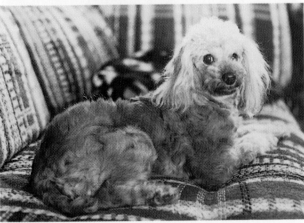

B

Figure 12:7. Apricot Poodle that developed melanotrichia following treatment of its Cushing's disease with mitotane (o,p'-DDD.) A, Before treatment. B, After treatment. Usually the normal coat color returns, even with continued o,p'-DDD maintenance therapy.

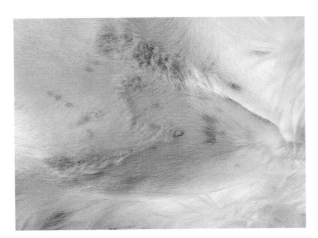

Figure 12:8. Inflammatory linear verrucous epidermal nevi.

FELINE ACROMELANISM

Siamese, Himalayan, Balinese, and Burmese kittens are born white and develop points as adults owing to the influence of external temperature[26, 28]; high environmental temperatures produce light hairs, and low temperatures produce dark hairs. Coat color also appears to be affected by physiologic factors that determine heat production and loss (e.g., inflammation, alopecia). These color change phenomena appear to be associated with a temperature-dependent enzyme involved in melanin synthesis. The changes in coat color are usually temporary, and the normal color returns with the next hair cycle, if the temperature influences are remedied.

TUMOR HYPERMELANOSIS

The common hyperpigmented tumors are the melanocytoma and melanoma; however, a variety of tumors may occur with hyperpigmentation (see Chap. 19). A very rare form of canine acanthosis nigricans may be associated with the following malignant neoplasms: hepatic carcinoma, thyroid adenocarcinoma, primary pulmonary carcinoma, ovarian and testicular tumors, and mammary adenocarcinoma with pulmonary metastasis. Basal cell tumors, trichoblastomas, epidermal nevi, and epithelial nevi (Fig. 12:8) may also commonly occur as hyperpigmented lesions.[8, 35, 37]

■ HYPOPIGMENTATION

Hypopigmentation *(Hypomelanosis)* refers to a lack or decrease of pigment in the skin or haircoat in areas that should normally be pigmented.[3, 15a] The disorder may be congenital or acquired. Lack of melanin pigment in hair is called *leukotrichia,* and lack of pigment in the skin is referred to as *leukoderma.*

Genetic Hypopigmentation

A variety of pigmentary conditions are known or suspected to be inherited disorders and are associated with atypical coat color from birth (e.g., Chédiak-Higashi syndrome, cyclic hematopoiesis) or very narrow breed predisposition (e.g., acanthosis nigricans, aurotrichia of Miniature Schnauzers). Some of these are covered in Chapter 11, and the remainder are considered here.

CHÉDIAK-HIGASHI SYNDROME

This is an autosomal recessive disorder reported in Persian cats with yellow eyes and a blue smoke haircoat color.[15] It is characterized by partial oculocutaneous albinism (see Chap. 11).

VITILIGO

Vitiligo is a hereditary leukoderma of human beings that may have an autoimmune or neurogenic pathogenesis.[3, 6, 15a, 23] A presumptive hereditary vitiligo has been described in Belgian Tervuren dogs, German shepherds, collies, Siamese cats, Rottweilers, Doberman pinschers, and Giant Schnauzers. It has also been described in a bull mastiff, Old English sheepdogs, and a dachshund with adult-onset diabetes mellitus.[13, 14, 18, 19, 22, 30, 31] Antimelanocyte antibodies were demonstrated in the serum of all 17 Belgian Tervuren dogs with vitiligo, and in none of 11 normal Belgian Tervuren dogs tested.[22] Also, three affected Siamese cats had autoantibodies, but four normal Siamese cats did not. The animals develop somewhat symmetric macular depigmentation, especially of the nose, lips, buccal mucosa, and facial skin. The footpads and claws, as well as the haircoat, may be affected (see Fig. 12:2 *C* and *D*). The onset of the condition is usually in young adulthood. In some cases, pigment returns to affected areas; in others, however, the depigmentation is permanent. Diagnosis is based on history, physical examination, and histopathologic evaluation. Late lesions of vitiligo are characterized by a relatively normal epidermis and dermis, except that no melanocytes are seen (Fig. 12:9 *A* and *B*). In some cases (possibly early lesions) a mild lymphocytic interface dermatitis and occasional lymphocyte exocytosis may be seen.[12] Successful treatment has not been reported.

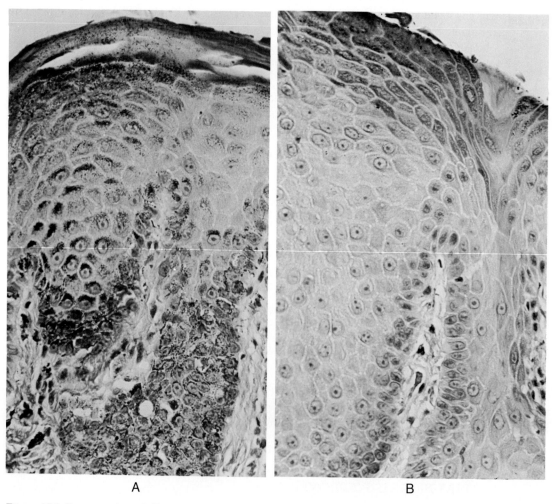

A B

Figure 12:9. Canine vitiligo. *A,* Normal skin adjacent to a vitiliginous macule. *B,* Complete absence of melanin in a vitiliginous area.

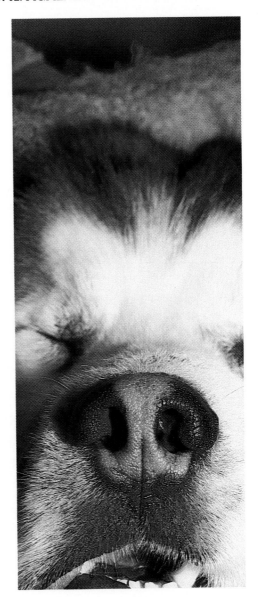

Figure 12:10. Canine snow nose (black and white).

NASAL DEPIGMENTATION

Nasal depigmentation, also called *Dudley nose,* is a syndrome of unknown origin that may be a form of vitiligo.[12] It has been reported in Afghan hounds, Samoyeds, Siberian huskies, yellow Labrador retrievers, white German shepherds, Golden retrievers, Poodles, Doberman pinschers, Irish setters, and Pointers.[12] The dogs are normal at birth, but the black of the nasal planum gradually fades to a chocolate brown or whitish color. The cause is unknown, and no treatment has yet worked effectively. A few patients recover spontaneously; in others, the degree of pigmentation waxes and wanes, sometimes seasonally. Because this discoloration is a show ring fault, breeders of show animals are understandably concerned. A distinction between noses that depigment almost entirely and those that only lighten should be made. A common syndrome of seasonal nasal hypopigmentation is seen in Siberian huskies, Golden retrievers, Labrador retrievers, and Bernese Mountain dogs (Fig. 12:10).[10, 18] It has been referred to as *snow nose* and is characterized by a decrease in the nasal pigment, typically during the winter months. The pigment gets darker again in the spring or summer. Complete depigmentation is not noted. The lips, pads, eyelids, claws, and haircoat are not normally affected.[11]

ALBINISM

Albinism is a hereditary lack of pigmentation that is transmitted as an autosomal recessive trait.[7, 13, 15a] Albino individuals have a normal complement of melanocytes, but they lack tyrosinase for melanin synthesis and therefore have a biochemical inability to produce melanin. Therefore, histopathologic studies reveal a normal epidermis with no pigment, but clear basal cells representing melanocytes are still seen. Skin, hair, and mucous membranes are amelanotic. Although humans have unpigmented (pink) irides, dogs typically have milder ocular changes, with blue eyes.[14] These dogs should not be used as breeders.

PIEBALDISM

Genetically determined white spotting is referred to as piebaldism. It is common in dogs and is transmitted as a completely dominant trait. Melanocytes are absent or incompletely differentiated in affected sites.

WAARDENBURG-KLEIN SYNDROME

This syndrome has been described in cats, bull terriers, Seelyham terriers, collies, and Dalmatians. In addition to blue eyes and amelanotic skin and hair, the affected animals are deaf and have heterochromia of the irides.[14] The defect is in the migration and differentiation of melanoblasts. Therefore, the affected skin has no melanocytes present. The syndrome is transmitted as an autosomal dominant trait with incomplete penetrance, so these animals should not be used for breeding.

MUCOCUTANEOUS HYPOPIGMENTATION

Leukoderma or hypopigmentation of the nasal planum, lips, or eyelids or in the tongue and oral cavity is considered a fault in most breeds of dogs. The nasal form is a particularly common problem in Australian shepherds, Siberian huskies, and Golden and Labrador retrievers. Some of these dogs also have seasonal nasal hypopigmentation. Although they have lightly pigmented noses, there is still enough pigment to prevent sunburn. Dogs with complete leukoderma of the nasal planum are prone to sunburn, which may develop into nasal solar dermatitis (see below, Acquired Hypopigmentation).

Hypopigmentation of the lips and nose occurs as a congenital condition in Doberman pinschers, Rottweilers, and occasionally, other breeds (see Fig. 12:2 E).[7] It is present from birth and is static in contrast to vitiligo, which is acquired in mature dogs and often progresses or changes over time. The cause of congenital hypopigmentation is unknown. Many owners object to the cosmetic appearance, but no treatment is effective.

CANINE CYCLIC HEMATOPOIESIS

Canine cyclic hematopoiesis (also known as *gray collie syndrome* and *canine cyclic neutropenia*) is a lethal autosomal recessive syndrome wherein collie puppies are born with a silver-gray haircoat that differs from the normal sable or tricolor coat (see Chap. 11).[13, 16, 33] In some of these puppies, a slight yellow pigmentation may be present, which produces a mixture of light beige and light gray hair. The light-colored nose is a characteristic and diagnostic lesion.

TYROSINASE DEFICIENCY

Tyrosinase deficiency has been reported in Chow Chows, but the condition is extremely rare. Puppies with this condition exhibit a dramatic color change. The normally bluish black tongue turns pink, and portions of the hair shafts turn white. The buccal mucosa may also rapidly depigment.

The change in color is the result of a deficiency of tyrosinase, the enzyme necessary to produce melanin. Tyrosinase deficiency can be confirmed by skin biopsy. After tyrosine is added to histologic preparations, the specimen is incubated, and the melanin is measured after tissue staining.[5]

There is no effective treatment; however, melanin reappears spontaneously in 2 to 4 months. Chow Chow breeders have claimed success with the use of vitamins, unsaturated oils, and dietary changes, but the improvement was probably spontaneous.

Acquired Hypopigmentation

Acquired depigmentation of previously normal skin and hair can result from many factors that destroy melanocytes or inhibit melanocyte function.[3] Trauma, burns, infections, and ionizing irradiation may have potent local effects. Acquired depigmentation of the nose and lips can result from contact dermatitis from plastic or rubber food dishes (see Chap. 8). It may also be idiopathic (see Fig. 12:2 *F*). Dogs that sunbathe frequently or swim in chlorine pools and dry themselves in the sun may develop lighter and coarser haircoats. Inflammation may cause hypopigmentation. This postinflammatory hypopigmentation is less common than hyperpigmentation. We have seen a red Irish setter puppy that had severe pustular dermatitis and developed white bands around the hair shafts, presumably as a result of the effects on pigment production in the hair bulb during the infection. Postinflammatory hypopigmentation is most evident in the groin and inguinal region following folliculitis. Multiple circular hypopigmented macules may be seen, or they can coalesce into variably shaped macules. Other infections, such as blastomycosis, sporotrichosis, and leishmaniasis, may cause hypopigmentation.[13, 18] Hypomelanosis due to drugs has been seen with subcutaneous injections of glucocorticoids and progestational drugs and with topical glucocorticoids. Some dogs that receive ketoconazole for mycotic infections or procainamide for cardiac disease develop diffuse lightening of their coats. Chemical hypomelanosis may occur following the administration of potent antioxidants such as dihydroquinone and monobenzyl ether.[13, 18]

Some chronic metabolic diseases may affect haircoat color. This cause appears to be particularly prominent in the sex hormone dermatoses of male dogs. Deficiencies of nutrients such as zinc, pyridoxine, pantothenic acid, and lysine have produced graying of the hair. Copper deficiency is said to cause black hair to develop a reddish brown hue. Hypomelanosis associated with neoplastic conditions has been seen in dogs. Leukoderma or leukotrichia (Fig. 12:11; also see Fig. 12:2 *G*), especially of the nasal planum, lips, and face, may occur as an

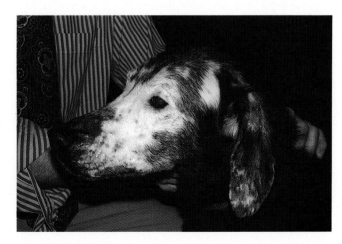

Figure 12:11. Leukotrichia in a dog with epitheliotropic lymphoma. The white hairs grew in after a favorable response to treatment with isotretinoin (Accutane). This photo was taken 18 months after the initiation of isotretinoin therapy.

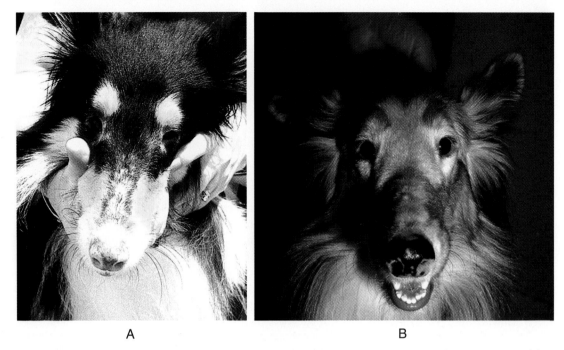

Figure 12:12. Leukotrichia following vitamin E therapy in a dog with lupus erythematosus. Repigmentation of the nasal planum preceded the development of leukotrichia. *A,* Before treatment. *B,* After treatment.

early sign of epitheliotropic lymphoma (mycosis fungoides).[18] Nasal depigmentation has also been seen with pagetoid reticulosis and squamous cell carcinoma.[18] A peritumoral melanotic halo has been seen around basal cell tumors.[13] Leukoderma or leukotrichia may be seen with mammary adenocarcinoma or gastric carcinoma.[13]

Normal black Newfoundlands 18 months of age may develop patches of depigmentation on the nose, lips, and eyelids (see Fig. 12:2 *F*). The lesions steadily progress, affecting the hair follicles in a diffuse manner. The animals become ''gray roans.'' Supplementation with trace minerals, vitamins, and zinc produces no improvement.

One tricolor collie with lupus erythematosus developed leukotrichia following vitamin E therapy[11] (Fig. 12:12 *A* and *B*). A cause for the leukotrichia was not determined, although it was speculated that there was an association with vitamin E because the mucocutaneous depigmentation attributed to lupus was reversed with therapy before the leukotrichia developed. A litter of chocolate Labrador retrievers puppies developed idiopathic leukotrichia that was reversible.[36] In this litter, 7 of 10 puppies were affected with varying degrees of leukotrichia, which was initially noted at 8 weeks of age on the face but then spread. By the time the puppies were 14 weeks of age, one owner reported that pigmentation was returning. Eventually, all the affected puppies developed normal coat colors, and no recurrences were noted over the following 18 months.

PERIOCULAR LEUKOTRICHIA

Bilateral periocular leukotrichia (goggles) occurs in Siamese cats.[28] There is no apparent age predilection, but the condition is seen more commonly in females. Commonly recognized precipitating factors include pregnancy, dietary deficiency, and systemic illnesses. The condition is characterized by patchy or complete lightening of the hairs of the mask in a halo-like appearance around both eyes (Fig. 12:13). The condition is transient and usually resolves within the succeeding two hair cycles.

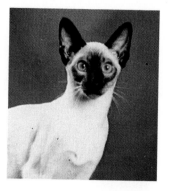

Figure 12:13. Periocular leukotrichia (goggles) in a Siamese cat after estrus.

A syndrome of unilateral periocular depigmentation, called *Aguirre syndrome,* has been described in Siamese cats. This condition is associated with Horner's syndrome, or corneal necrosis with uveitis, and upper respiratory tract infections.[15, 32]

NASAL SOLAR DERMATITIS

Nasal solar dermatitis may develop on the noses of dogs that are normally amelanotic (e.g., Australian shepherd). If the dog has one of the preceding diseases, depigmentation precedes the inflammation and is limited to nonhaired amelanotic lesions. Nasal solar dermatitis must be differentiated from other diseases in which nasal depigmentation results from inflammation. Depigmentation and inflammatory nasal lesions occur in many disorders but especially in discoid lupus erythematosus, systemic lupus erythematosus, pemphigus erythematosus and foliaceus, Uveodermatologic syndrome, drug eruption, epithelioptropic lymphoma (mycosis fungoides), and bullous pemphigoid. Cases of nasal solar dermatitis and early cases of these disorders are sometimes difficult to differentiate clinically. Careful observation of nasal architecture can be useful. Initially, the hypopigmentary disease does not affect the architecture and does not cause scaling or crusting; these effects occur only with secondary solar damage. The solar damage is limited to the amelanotic areas. The other disorders often cause scaling, crusting, or loss of normal architecture early in the course of the disease. Histopathologic evaluation can usually establish the correct diagnosis.

■ MISCELLANEOUS PIGMENT CHANGES

Acquired Aurotrichia

This syndrome occurs in Miniature Schnauzers of either sex.[38] The primary guard hairs turn from silver or black to gold (see Fig. 12:2 *H*). These gold hairs occur primarily in patches on the dorsal thorax and abdomen, although periocular and pinnal involvement occur in some cases. An associated thinning of the secondary hair in the affected areas may be noted (see Chap. 11 for details).

Red Hair

A variety of conditions can cause hair to become reddish in color. Lightly colored hair exposed to saliva or tears becomes stained by porphyrins. When seen in areas other than around the oral cavity or ventral to the eyes, this change usually indicates excessive licking. Poor-quality protein diets have been associated with the development of red hair; the condition resolves when a proper diet is followed.[9] This color change was associated with indicanuria and indicanemia. Diets deficient in copper may also cause red hair.

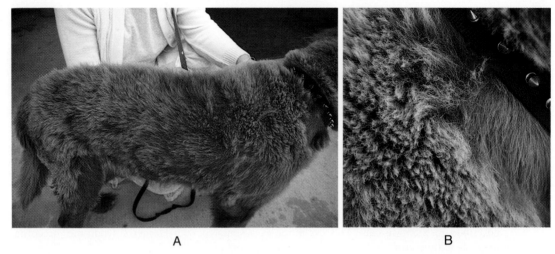

Figure 12:14. Laborador retriever that was castrated because of a large testicular tumor. Two months after the dog's castration, the client noted hair loss. The old coat, which the client described as having been that way for years, was replaced by a new brown coat that was the same color as the dog's coat when it was young. *A*, Patches of alopecia present on the trunk. *B*, Close-up of the neck area.

A variety of endocrinopathies may cause lightening of the haircoat or result in dark hair turning red. Although it is reported with hypothyroidism and hyperadrenocorticism, this change seems especially common with Sertoli's cell tumors and in cases of hyperestrogenism or hyperprogesteronism. Some dogs with Sertoli's cell tumors fail to shed their coat normally, and hairs are actually retained in catagen or telogen. The hairs remain for years; the lightened, red, dry, frizzy coat may be partly caused by chronic ultraviolet and environmental exposure (Fig. 12:14). The potential effects of sun, chlorine, detergents, and environmental factors should be considered any time the coat color has changed.

FLUSHING

Cutaneous flushing, in which the skin turns varying shades of red, is due to vasodilatation of cutaneous blood vessels. Flushing can be persistent or paroxysmal; it is caused by emotional, autonomic, or endocrine influences or by the direct action of vasoactive compounds in the blood vessels.[6, 20] In humans, widespread flushing can be caused by a variety of physiologic and pathologic conditions, especially the carcinoid syndrome, systemic mastocytosis, Zollinger-Ellison syndrome, or pheochromocytoma. In dogs, persistent flushing has been attributed to drug reactions and mast cell tumors. Paroxysmal flushing has been associated with pheochromocytoma and mast cell tumors.[20]

REFERENCES

1. Benitz, K.F., et al.: Morphologic effects of minocycline in laboratory animals. Toxicol. Appl. Pharmacol. 11:150, 1967.
2. Bergfeld, W.F., McMahon, J.T: Identification of foreign metallic substances inducing hypopigmentation of skin. Light microscopy, electron microscopy, and x-ray energy spectroscopic examination. In: Callen J.P., et al. (eds). Advances in Dermatology—Vol 2. Year Book Medical Publishers, Chicago, 1987, p. 171.
3. Bolognia, J.L., Pawelek, J.M.: Biology of hypopigmentation. J. Am. Acad. Dermatol. 19:217, 1988.
4. Briggs, O.M.: Lentiginosis profusa in the pug: Three case reports. J. Small Anim. Pract. 26:675, 1985.
5. Engstrom, D.: Tyrosinase deficiency in the chow chow. In: Kirk, R. W. (ed.) Current Veterinary Therapy II. W.B. Saunders Co., Philadelphia, 1966, p. 352.
6. Fitzpatrick, T.B., et al.: Dermatology in General Medicine, 3rd ed. McGraw-Hill Book Co., New York, 1987.
7. Foil, C.S.: Comparative genodermatoses. Clin. Dermatol. 3:175, 1985.

8. Goldschmidt, M.H., Shoffer, F.S.: Skin Tumors of the Dog and Cat. Pergamon Press, Tarrytown, N.Y., 1992.
9. Griess, D., Guaguère, E.: Variations de l'indicanémie et de l'indicanurie dans le syndrome rubra-pilaire du chien. Rev. Méd. Vét. 132:12, 1981.
10. Griffin, C.E.: Nasal dermatitis. Dermatol. Rep. 2:1, 1983.
11. Griffin, C.E.: Personal observations.
12. Gross, T.L., et al.: Veterinary Dermatopathology: Gross and Microscopic Pathology of Skin Diseases. Mosby–Year Book, St. Louis, 1992.
13. Guaguère, E., Alhaidari, Z.: Disorders of melanin pigmentation in the skin of dogs and cats. Proc. Wld. Sm. Anim. Vet. Assoc. 8:47, 1991.
14. Guaguère, E., Alhaidari, Z.: Pigmentary disturbances. Adv. Vet. Dermatol. 1:395, 1990.
15. Holzworth, J.: Diseases of the Cat: Medicine and Surgery, Vol. I. W. B. Saunders Co., Philadelphia, 1987.
15a. Levine, N., Maibach, H. I.: Pigmentation and Pigmentary Disorders. CRC Press, Boca Raton, Fla., 1993.
16. Lothrop, C.D., et al.: Cyclic hormonogenesis in gray collie dogs: Interactions of hematopoietic and endocrine systems. Endocrinology 120:1027, 1987.
17. MacDonald, J.M.: Hyperpigmentation. In: Griffin C.E., et al. (eds.). Current Veterinary Dermatology. Mosby–Year Book, St. Louis, 1993, p. 234.
18. MacDonald, J.M.: Nasal depigmentation. In: Griffin, C.E., et al. (eds.). Current Veterinary Dermatology, Mosby–Year Book, St. Louis, 1993, p. 223.
19. Mahaffey, M.B., et al.: Focal loss of pigment in the Belgian Tervuren dog. J. Am. Vet. Med. Assoc. 173:390, 1978.
20. Miller, W.H., Jr.: Cutaneous flushing associated with intrathoracic neoplasia in a dog. J. Am. Anim. Hosp. Assoc. 28:217, 1992.
21. Nash, S., Paulsen, D.: Generalized lentigines in a silver cat. J. Am. Vet. Med. Assoc. 196:1500, 1990.
22. Naughton, G.K., et al.: Antibodies to surface antigens of pigmented cells in animals with vitiligo. Proc. Soc. Exp. Biol. Med. 181:423, 1986.
23. Nordlund, J.J.: Vitiligo. In: Thiers, B.H., Dobson, R.L. (eds.). Pathogenesis of Skin Disease. Churchill Livingstone, New York, 1986, p. 99.
24. Ortonne, J.P., Prota, G.: Hair melanins and hair color: Ultrastructural and biochemical aspects. J. Invest. Dermatol. 101:82S, 1993.
25. Pawelek, J., et al.: New regulators of melanin biosynthesis and the autodestruction of melanin cells. Nature 286:617, 1980.
26. Scott, D.W.: Feline dermatology 1900–1978: A monograph. J. Am. Anim. Hosp. Assoc. 16:331, 1980.
27. Scott, D.W.: Unpublished observations, 1987.
28. Scott, D.W.: Feline dermatology 1983–1985: The secret sits. J. Am. Anim. Hosp. Assoc. 23:255, 1987.
29. Scott, D.W.: Lentigo simplex in orange cats. Companion Anim. Pract. 1:23, 1987.
30. Scott, D.W., Randolph, J.F.: Vitiligo in two old English Sheepdog littermates and a dachshund with juvenile-onset diabetes mellitus. Companion Anim. Pract. 19:18, 1989.
31. Scott, D.W.: Vitiligo in the rottweiler. Canine Pract. 15(3):22, 1990.
32. Simon, M.: Observation clinique. Depigmentation perioculaire chez deux chats siamois. Prat. Med. Chirurg. Anim. Comp. 20:49, 1985.
33. Trail, P.A., Yang, T.J.: Canine cyclic hematopoiesis: Alterations in T lymphocyte populations in peripheral blood, lymph nodes, and thymus of gray collie dogs. Clin. Immunol. Immunopathol. 41:216, 1986.
34. VanRensburg, I.B.J., Briggs, O.M.: Pathology of canine lentiginosis profusa. J. S. Afr. Vet. Assoc. 57:159, 1986.
35. Walder, E.: Epithelial tumors. In: Gross, T. L., et al. (eds). Veterinary Dermatopathology: Gross and Microscopic Pathology of Skin Diseases. Mosby-Year Book, St. Louis, 1992, p. 330.
36. White, S.D., Butch, S. Leukotrichia in a litter of Labrador retrievers. J. Am. Anim. Hosp. Assoc. 26:319, 1990.
37. White, S.D., et al. Inflammatory linear verrucous epidermal nevus in four dogs. Vet. Dermatol. 3:107, 1993.
38. White, S.D., et al.: Acquired aurotrichia ("Gilding syndrome") of miniature schnauzers. Vet. Dermatol. 3:37, 1992.
39. Yaar, M., Gilchrest, B.A.: Human melanocyte growth and differentiation: A decade of new data. J. Invest. Dermatol. 97:611, 1991.
40. Yohn, J.J., et al.: Cultured human keratinocytes synthesize and secrete endothelin-1. J. Invest. Dermatol. 100:23, 1993.

Keratinization
Defects

■

Chapter Outline

Keratinization defects are those that alter the surface appearance of the skin. The epidermis of animals is being replaced constantly by new cells. The epidermal cell renewal time in normal dogs is approximately 22 days.[14] Despite this high turnover rate, the epidermis maintains its normal thickness, has a barely perceptible surface keratin layer, and loses its dead cells invisibly into the environment. If the delicate balance between cell death and renewal is altered, the epidermal thickness changes, the stratum corneum becomes noticeable, and the normally invisible sloughed cells of the stratum corneum become obvious. The causes of keratinization defects are numerous; they produce clinical signs by altering proliferation, differentiation, desquamation, or some combination of these.[15]

The keratinization defects include hyperkeratosis, hypokeratosis, and dyskeratosis. Hyperkeratosis is common in chronic dermatoses. It is further distinguished histopathologically into *parakeratotic* (nucleated) and *orthokeratotic* (anuclear) types.[10, 20] Hypokeratosis is not as common, but it is seen histologically in some cases, presumably as a result of very rapid exfoliation. Another fault in epidermopoiesis is dyskeratosis, which is seen in neoplastic skin diseases (such as squamous cell carcinoma), pemphigus, lichenoid reactions, and some types of seborrhea.

Keratinization defects can be congenital or acquired. The congenital defects (e.g., primary seborrhea, ichthyosis, epidermal dysplasia of West Highland White terriers, psoriasiform-lichenoid dermatosis of English Springer spaniels, and Schnauzer comedo syndrome) are covered in Chapter 11. The most common acquired keratinization defect is the callus, which is covered in Chapter 15. The remainder are considered here.

■ CANINE SEBORRHEA

Seborrhea is a chronic skin disease of dogs that is characterized by a defect in keratinization with increased scale formation, excessive greasiness of the skin and haircoat, and sometimes by secondary inflammation. Some patients are both flaky and greasy, depending on the region of the body involved. Ingrained in the veterinary literature are the terms seborrhea sicca, seborrhea oleosa, and seborrheic dermatitis. *Seborrhea sicca* denotes dryness of the skin and coat. There is focal or diffuse scaling of the skin with the accumulation of white to gray nonadherent scales, and the coat is dull and dry (Fig. 13:1*A*). *Seborrhea oleosa* is the opposite; the skin and hairs are greasy (Fig. 13:1*B*). The greasy keratosebaceous debris is best appreciated by touch and smell. The malodor of dogs with severe seborrhea oleosa is tremendous. *Seborrheic dermatitis* is characterized by scaling and greasiness with gross evidence of local or diffuse inflammation (Fig. 13:1*C*). It is often associated with folliculitis. Classic *localized* seborrheic dermatitis has circular lesions with alopecia, erythema, marginal epidermal scaling, and later, hyperpigmentation (Fig. 13:1*D*). This must be differentiated from other disorders that cause similar lesions.

These three terms appropriately describe the dog's clinical appearance and aid in initial shampoo selection, but they cannot be used to direct the diagnostic effort to find the cause for the seborrhea. Individuals respond to the same seborrheic insult in different manners. Although most fatty acid–deficient dogs have dull, dry, and flaky coats, some are greasy, and a dog with early generalized demodicosis may be either flaky or greasy. Regardless of the nature of the seborrhea, all causes of seborrhea should be considered and excluded only by the appropriate testing.

Etiologically, seborrhea is classified into primary and secondary types. *Primary seborrhea* is an inherited disorder of epidermal hyperproliferation and is covered in Chapter 11. It is most commonly seen in American Cocker spaniels, English Springer spaniels, West Highland White

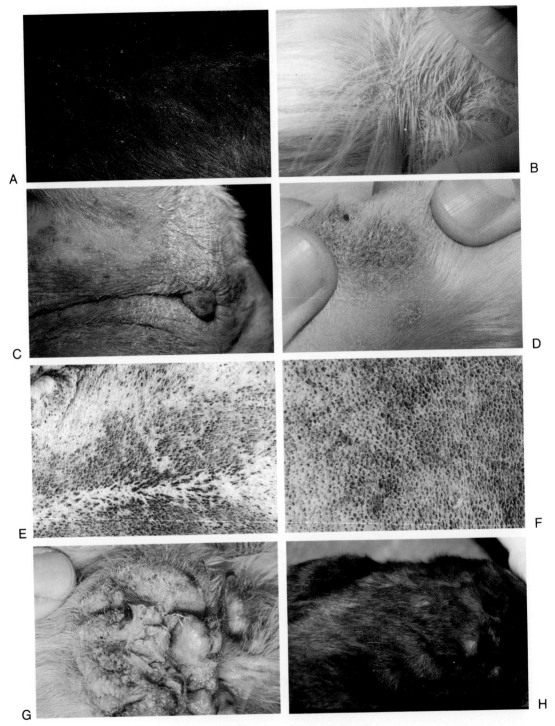

Figure 13:1 *See legend on opposite page*

terriers, and Basset hounds, but Irish setters, Doberman pinschers, Chinese Shar Peis, dachshunds, Labrador retrievers, and German Shepherds are at increased risk.[16, 20] However, not all individuals within those breeds are affected. A veterinarian does the owner and animal a great injustice if seborrheic signs in a dog of those breeds are immediately classified as primary seborrhea. The diagnosis of primary seborrhea is tenable only if the signs started early in life and appropriate diagnostic tests have failed to reveal a cause for the keratinization defect.

Secondary seborrheas are those caused by some external or internal insult that alters the proliferation, differentiation, or desquamation of the surface and follicular epithelium.[15] Virtually any disorder discussed in this textbook can result in seborrheic signs during the acute or healing phase of the disease.

Cause and Pathogenesis

Any disorder that alters cellular proliferation, differentiation, or desquamation produces seborrheic signs. In most instances, the mechanisms by which the following seborrhea-inducing factors cause their changes are incompletely understood.

■ *Inflammation.* Inflammatory skin diseases are typically characterized by epidermal hyperplasia,[10] which probably results from the release or production of dermal eicosanoids, histamine, and cytokines. Leukotriene B_4 concentrations have been reported to be increased in the skin lesions of dogs with seborrhea.[13a] If the inflammation is mild, seborrheic signs can develop in the absence of pruritus. Examples include grooming that is too vigorous,[2] demodicosis, dermatophytosis, cheyletiellosis, lice, low-grade contact dermatitis, and early epitheliotropic lymphoma.

■ *Endocrine Factors.* Hormones influence cellular proliferation[20] and serum and cutaneous lipid profiles.[6, 30] Although all hormonal imbalances can cause seborrhea, spontaneous or iatrogenic hyperadrenocorticism and hypothyroidism are the most common causes. In hyperadrenocorticism, other signs of the disease are usually present; in contrast, some hypothyroid dogs are perfectly normal aside from the seborrhea.

■ *Nutritional Factors.* Glucose, protein, essential fatty acids, and various vitamins and trace minerals are necessary for normal cellular proliferation and differentiation. Deficiency, excess, or imbalance in one or more of these nutrients can produce seborrhea. Fat-deficiency seborrhea is the most common nutritional seborrhea; it can be the result of dietary inadequacy,[6] malabsorption or maldigestion,[12] or endocrine disease (especially hypothyroidism).[5]

■ *Environmental Factors.* The water and lipid content of the skin is important to maintain normal invisible desquamation.[6-8, 15] If transepidermal water loss increases, desquamation changes and the squames (packets of dead cells) become visible. Low environmental humidity, excessive bathing (especially with harsh products), and fatty acid deficiency can produce this change.

As can be seen from the above-mentioned factors, virtually any disease can cause seborrhea and can do so by many different mechanisms.

Figure 13:1. *A*, Severe flaking in a dog with a fatty acid deficiency. *B*, Greasy seborrhea in a dog with chronic liver disease. Note that the greasy material adheres to the hairs and stains them. *C*, Diffuse seborrheic dermatitis in a hypothyroid dog. *D*, Focal seborrheic dermatitis in a dog with vitamin A–responsive dermatosis. *E*, Vitamin A–responsive dermatosis in a Cocker spaniel. Marked comedo formation on the abdomen. *F*, Vitamin A–responsive dermatosis. Same dog as in *E*. Close-up of follicular plugging. *G*, Vitamin A–responsive dermatosis. Same dog as in *E* and *F*. Severe ceruminous otitis externa. *H*, Flaking in a cat caused by too low an environmental humidity level.

Clinical Features

The clinical signs of secondary seborrhea include flakiness, greasiness, seborrheic dermatitis, ceruminous otitis externa, or some combination of these. The nature, distribution, and severity of the signs depend on the cause of the seborrhea and the individual patient. In general, systemic causes (e.g., endocrine disease, dietary deficiency, hepatic or gastrointestinal disease, and primary or secondary lipid abnormalities) result in generalized signs that are not pruritic at their onset. These animals can become pruritic, however, as the seborrhea worsens, and they often have more pronounced seborrheic changes around the face, feet (especially interdigitally) intertriginous areas, and perineum. Allergic disorders, although systemic diseases, tend to cause regionalized seborrheic changes, and pruritus precedes the seborrheic changes.

Except for low environmental humidity and overzealous or inappropriate topical treatments (e.g., excessive bathing, dipping, or powdering, contact dermatitis to a shampoo), external causes (e.g., cheyletiellosis, demodicosis, dermatophytosis) result in focal, multifocal, or regionalized signs of secondary seborrhea. At examination, these dogs have areas of normal skin.

Diagnosis

The diagnosis of seborrhea is straightforward and is based on the characteristic lesions. Determining the cause of the seborrhea is far more difficult. Beyond the mandatory history, dietary review, skin scrapings, *trichography,* and fecal examinations for intestinal parasites and evidence of malabsorption or maldigestion, the specific diagnostic approach varies from case to case.

Some investigators perform skin biopsies early in the diagnostic effort; others perform routine laboratory and endocrine testing first. If the seborrhea is focal, multifocal, or regionalized, an early biopsy may be indicated to characterize the external insult. When the seborrhea is generalized and probably attributable to some systemic disease, an early biopsy is not necessary. In this case, the tissues would show the characteristic changes of a keratinization defect; for example, a variably hyperplastic superficial perivascular dermatitis with orthokeratotic or parakeratotic hyperkeratosis may be found (Fig. 13:2), but biopsy would be unlikely to reveal the cause of such changes.

Dogs with a generalized seborrhea, especially older dogs whose symptoms are of recent onset, should have *hemography,* a chemistry profile, and urinalysis performed to aid in the initial characterization of any systemic disease. Any abnormality detected should be followed in an appropriate manner. If that testing and the basic in-office tests are noncontributory, a thyroid evaluation, preferably by thyroid-stimulating hormone (TSH) response test, should be performed.

If the seborrheic lesions are focal, multifocal, or regionalized, an external cause is likely. If the history and physical examination do not result in a short list of differential diagnoses, a skin biopsy is useful in categorizing the disorder.

As mentioned before, seborrheic dogs are prone to secondary staphylococcal infections and *Malassezia* dermatitis. If either of these conditions is identified by physical examination and exudative cytologic examination, they should be resolved before skin biopsies are taken because the inflammation caused by these infections can mask some of the subtle histologic features of the underlying disease.

Clinical Management

The primary aim of treatment in secondary seborrhea is the correction of its cause. With treatment, the seborrheic signs should resolve spontaneously in 30 to 60 days; in chronic cases, however, a complete response may not occur for 3 to 4 months. Since seborrheic dogs are prone to secondary staphylococcal infections or *Malassezia* dermatitis, appropriate treatment

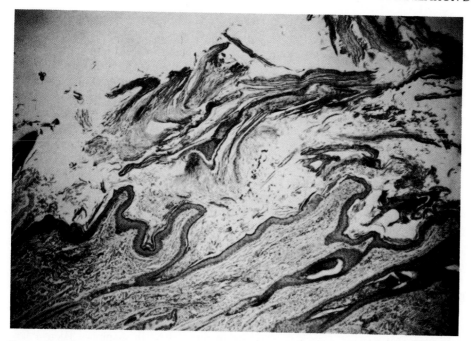

Figure 13:2. Canine seborrheic dermatitis. Hyperplastic superficial perivascular dermatitis with a marked keratinization defect and parakeratotic capping.

may be necessary if the dog is infected. Resolution of these secondary infections and the underlying cause of the seborrhea can result in very rapid improvement.

The topical agents used in primary seborrhea are also used here, but treatment protocols in correctable secondary seborrhea are less intense. Typically, the dog is bathed, with or without moisturization, twice weekly for 1 to 2 weeks. Very greasy dogs may require alternate-day bathing for 2 to 3 weeks. No specific protocol should be mandated, as the response of secondarily seborrheic dogs is quite variable once treatment of the underlying cause has been instituted. As in primary seborrhea, overbathing a dog with secondary seborrhea exacerbates the seborrhea. The client is in the best position to determine when the dog needs a treatment. If the dog is not too flaky or greasy on its scheduled bath day, the treatment should be postponed until the surface debris builds up to an unacceptable level. As the treatment for the underlying disease progresses, the bathing interval increases. The baths can often be stopped after 30 days. At that point, the dog may not be entirely normal, but many owners find the residual disease acceptable, especially if bathing the dog has been very difficult.

There are a large number of grooming or antiseborrheic shampoos that are appropriate for the bathing of dry dogs.[17] Product selection depends on client and veterinarian preference. It is advisable to start with the mildest product and change to a stronger one only if the initial product is unsatisfactory. For mildly flaky dogs, moisturizing hypoallergenic shampoos (HyLyt*efa hypoallergenic moisturizing shampoo, Allergroom hypoallergenic emollient shampoo), colloidal oatmeal shampoos (Epi-Soothe), or emollient-based chlorhexidine products (ChlorhexiDerm shampoo, Nolvasan shampoo) are commonly used. For more severe flaking, sulfur-salicylic acid products (Micro Pearls sulfur–salicylic acid shampoo, Sebolux shampoo, SebaLyt antiseborrheic shampoo) are appropriate. For very recalcitrant cases, mild tar products (Clear Tar shampoo, NuSal-T shampoo, T-Lux shampoo) might be appropriate; these should be used cautiously, however, because all tar products are degreasing agents. They should not increase transepidermal water loss and therefore could be used in the winter.[7] Strong tars, selenium sulfides, and benzoyl peroxide shampoos can increase transepidermal water loss and decrease surface lipids, so they are contraindicated in these patients because they are too drying.[8a, 29]

If the dog's coat is dirty, a rapid shampooing with a nonmedicated grooming product is indicated before the antiseborrheic bath. After the dog has been lathered with the antiseborrheic product, the shampoo must remain in contact with the skin for 10 to 15 minutes for maximum effect. Gentle manipulation of the dog's skin during this waiting period tends to keep the dog happy and increases the cleansing action of the shampoo. After 10 to 15 minutes, the dog should be rinsed thoroughly. It should take 2 to 3 times longer for the rinsing than it did for the lathering. Prolonged rinsing not only removes the debris and shampoo but also aids in hydration of the skin. Many of these dry dogs become flaky again soon after the bath, especially when the environmental humidity is low. The application of an afterbath rinse (Alpha-Sesame Oil dry skin rinse, Humilac dry skin spray and rinse, HyLyt*efa bath oil coat conditioner, Micro Pearls cream rinse) helps provide a barrier to transepidermal water loss and its associated drying.[28] Although any afterbath rinse can be effective, studies have shown that those containing oils, and especially linoleic acid, are most effective in decreasing transepidermal water loss.[8] If the client keeps some diluted product in a misting bottle and sprays it on the dog as needed, the frequency of bathing can often be reduced.

For greasy dogs, the shampoos used are stronger.[9a, 17] Dogs that are mildly to moderately greasy can be treated with sulfur–salicylic acid or mild tar products. Very greasy dogs are often bathed with stronger tars (LyTar shampoo, Allerset-T shampoo), selenium sulfides (Selsun Blue dandruff shampoo), or benzoyl peroxides (OxyDex shampoo, Pyoben shampoo, Micro Pearls benzoyl peroxide shampoo). All these products are excellent degreasers but create a dry seborrhea if used excessively. Greasy dogs often need an afterbath rinse, especially if the humidity level is low. All strong shampoos can disrupt the epidermal barrier and increase transepidermal water loss, with resultant worsening of the seborrhea.[8] An afterbath rinse can prevent this, but it may make the dog too greasy. Each case must be approached on its own merits.

In occasional cases, the cause of the secondary seborrhea can be identified but not corrected; common examples include low winter humidity and intentional fatty acid deficiency for weight loss or control of pancreatitis or abnormalities in lipid metabolism. In these cases, bathing and moisturizing must be continued at some maintenance level. The application of moisturizers containing fat can be beneficial in these animals.[7]

■ VITAMIN A–RESPONSIVE DERMATOSIS

A vitamin A–responsive dermatosis has been described primarily in Cocker spaniels but it has also been recognized in a Labrador retriever and a Miniature Schnauzer.[11, 13, 22, 26] The condition is characterized by an adult-onset, medically refractory seborrheic skin disease, wherein marked follicular plugging and hyperkeratotic plaques with surface fronds are typically seen (see Fig. 13:1 *E* and *F*). The follicular plugging and hyperkeratotic plaques are especially prominent on the ventral and lateral chest and abdomen. Other lesions include varying degrees of focal crusting, scaling, alopecia, and follicular papules. A ceruminous otitis externa is usually present (Fig. 13:1 *G*). A generally dry, dull, disheveled, easily epilated haircoat is present along with a rancid skin odor and mild to moderate pruritus. Except for the skin disease, the dogs are generally healthy.

The marked follicular plugging that occurs in these dogs is highly suggestive of this disease. In the absence of systemic signs of hyperadrenocorticism, only sebaceous adenitis (see Chap. 17), true vitamin A deficiency or hypervitaminosis A (see Chap. 16), and atypical generalized demodicosis produce such profound follicular changes. The clinical lesions are characterized histologically by profound, disproportionately marked follicular orthokeratotic hyperkeratosis (Fig. 13:3). At present, the final diagnosis of vitamin A–responsive dermatosis can be confirmed only by response to treatment.

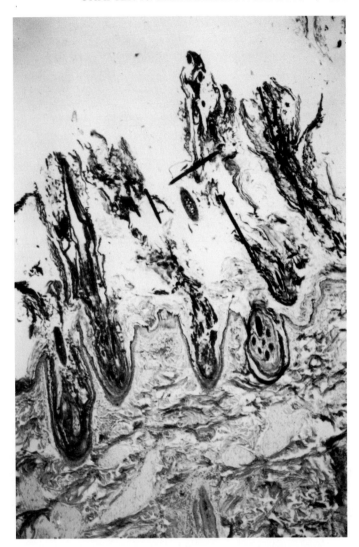

Figure 13:3. Vitamin A–responsive dermatosis. Disproportionate orthokeratotic hyperkeratosis of multiple hair follicles.

Treatment consists of 10,000 U vitamin A (retinol) given orally, once daily with a fatty meal. Improvement can be expected in 3 weeks, with complete clinical remission in 8 to 10 weeks. Treatment should be continued for life because the lesions and symptoms reappear when treatment is discontinued.

■ FELINE SEBORRHEA

Primary seborrhea is very rare in cats (see Chap. 11). Although cats suffer from many of the disorders that cause secondary seborrhea in dogs,[25] seborrheic signs are uncommon in this species. Cats' fastidious grooming habits, which remove scales quickly, may be partially responsible for this lower incidence.

When cats do become seborrheic, they usually have seborrhea sicca with fine white or gray flakes and scales in the coat (see Fig. 13:1 *H*). When the signs are fairly generalized and the cat is not pruritic, dietary deficiency, intestinal parasitism, low environmental humidity, diabetes mellitus, hyperthyroidism, cheyletiellosis, and pediculosis are the primary differentials.[19, 20, 25] Contact dermatitis and overzealous shampooing or powdering could be added to the list, but these causes are easily excluded through the history. With pruritus or more localized

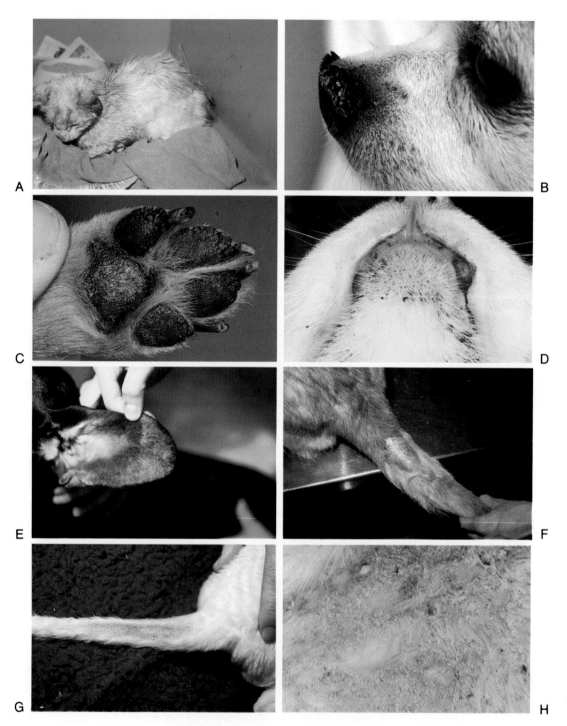

Figure 13:4 *See legend on opposite page*

lesions, demodicosis, dermatophytosis, and allergy must be considered. Greasy seborrheic signs (seborrhea oleosa) (Fig. 13:4*A*) are extraordinarily rare in the cat and usually indicate severe chronic hepatic, pancreatic, or intestinal disease, drug eruption, or systemic lupus erythematosus.[19, 25]

As in dogs, correction of the cause for the seborrhea results in spontaneous resolution of the signs. Bathing can help hasten the cat's response, but is not widely done because most cats are intolerant of repeated bathing. With the exception of products that contain tar, selenium, quaternary ammonium compounds, or phenol, shampoos used on dogs can also be used on cats.

■ NASODIGITAL HYPERKERATOSIS

Nasodigital hyperkeratosis is characterized by increased amounts of horny tissue originating from and tightly adherent to the epidermis of the footpads or nasal planum.

Cause and Pathogenesis

Hyperkeratosis of the nose, footpads, or both can occur as an idiopathic entity or as a coexistent feature of a variety of disorders. The idiopathic form occurs most commonly in old dogs. It shows no breed or sex predilection and is probably a senile change.[10, 16, 20]

Nasodigital hyperkeratosis can be seen in a variety of disorders but especially in the congenitohereditary disorders of keratinization (Chap. 11), distemper or leishmaniasis (Chap. 7), pemphigus foliaceous or systemic lupus erythematosus (Chap. 8), zinc-responsive and generic dog food dermatosis (Chap. 16), and cutaneous lymphoma (Chap. 19). With nasal hyperkeratosis only, discoid lupus erythematosus and pemphigus erythematosus (Chap. 8) must be considered. If lesions are restricted to the pads, familial pad hyperkeratosis[21] (Chap. 11) and papillomavirus infection (Chap. 19) enter the list of differential diagnoses. Except for the latter two, all of the aforementioned disorders usually have lesions in the haired skin and often produce systemic signs of illness. However, some cases have lesions restricted to the nose, footpads, or both, either at their onset or during their entire course.

Clinical Features

The hyperplastic keratin that develops in senile nasodigital hyperkeratosis grows in a variety of shapes, depending on its location, its stage of development, and the variation among individual animals. At times, small verrucous keratin growths appear in a regular pattern. At other times, the keratin is ridged, grooved, or feathered. Dryness is the characteristic common to all lesions. The nasal planum, which is moist, black, soft, and shiny in normal dogs, becomes hard, dry, rough, and hyperkeratotic, especially on the dorsum of the nose (see Fig. 13:4*B*). Fissures, erosions, and ulcers develop in the dry epidermal tissue.

The digital hyperkeratosis involves the entire surface of all pads but is most pronounced at the edges of weightbearing pads (Fig. 13:4*C*) and on the accessory carpal and tarsal pads. The contact surfaces of weightbearing pads are less involved because friction during walking wears down the keratin. The hard, cracked pads contain excess keratin tissue, which makes walking painful, especially for heavy dogs. Fissures and erosions add significantly to the discomfort.

Figure 13:4. *A,* Greasy seborrhea in a cat with pancreatic insufficiency. *B,* Nasodigital hyperkeratosis. Note the frondlike hyperkeratosis on the dorsum of the nasal planum. *C,* Nasodigital hyperkeratosis. Same dog as in *B.* Keratin accumulation is most marked at the edges of the pads. *D,* Feline acne. Multiple comedones on the chin. *E,* Ear margin dermatosis with marginal hypotrichosis and scaling. *F,* Canine tail gland hyperplasia. *G,* Feline tail gland hyperplasia. *H,* Parapsoriasis. Coalescent erythematous, scaly plaques on the abdomen of a dog. A small island of normal skin is visible.

Corns form in the feet of some individuals as excess keratin develops into deep, circular plaques.[20] These press into the surrounding footpad and cause pain when pressure is created as the animal walks.

Diagnosis

The diagnosis of simple nasodigital hyperkeratosis can be straightforward or very complicated. If the typical lesions occur in an old dog with no other skin or systemic problems, the diagnosis can be made on the basis of the clinical findings. If the nasodigital hyperkeratosis is present along with other skin lesions in a young to middle-aged dog, or if it occurs with nasal or pedal depigmentation, erythema, erosion, and crusting, all of the disorders mentioned previously must be considered and excluded by means of the appropriate testing.

The diagnosis is confirmed by a biopsy that reveals the characteristic features of idiopathic nasodigital hyperkeratosis and none of the features for the other differential diagnoses. Histopathologic findings in idiopathic nasodigital hyperkeratosis include irregular to papillated epidermal hyperplasia and marked orthokeratotic to parakeratotic hyperkeratosis.

Clinical Management

Because the formation of excess keratin cannot be stopped, treatment must be lifelong and directed toward the softening and removal of the excessive keratin. Since these measures are time consuming and somewhat messy, they are usually reserved for cases in which the hyperkeratosis causes discomfort or fissuring.

Dogs with profound hyperkeratosis should have the excess keratin removed with scissors or a razor blade. After appropriate instruction, many clients can perform the trimming at home and may choose to use it as the sole method of treatment for asymptomatic dogs. In most cases, the trimming is necessary only at the onset of treatment because further keratin buildup is minimized by the application of hydrating and softening agents.

Topical treatment must include hydration and the application of a keratolytic agent. Hydration of the pads is easily accomplished by soaking the feet in water and applying wet compresses to the nose. After 5 to 10 minutes of hydration, the areas are covered with keratolytic agent. Petroleum jelly, ichthammol ointment, various human dry skin lotions, 50 per cent propylene glycol, 6.6 per cent salicylic acid, 5 per cent sodium lactate, and 5 per cent urea in propylene glycol gel (KeraSolv gel, DVM Pharmaceuticals, Inc.), and tretinoin gel (Retin-A-Ortho) can all be effective.[16, 20, 21] If petroleum jelly or ichthammol are used, the animal must be confined to a crate or the feet must be bandaged so that floors, carpets and furniture will not be stained. When the nose or pads are fissured, ointments containing antibiotics and corticosteroids are indicated.

Typically, daily hydration and softening must be performed for 7 to 10 days to return the nose and pads to near normal. The owners should be warned not to try to remove all of the keratin because overzealous treatment can remove the normal protective keratin layer and predispose the nose and pads to lacerations and frictional ulcers. When the nose and pads are near normal, some clients prefer to stop all treatments until significant buildup occurs; others prefer to continue treatment once or twice weekly to prevent buildup. Each case must be managed on its own merits. When topical treatment is impossible, isotretinoin or etretinate therapy may be of some benefit, but their efficacy remains unproven.[23]

■ ACNE

In humans, acne is a multifactorial disease of the pilosebaceous unit.[9] Acne-prone individuals have an alteration in the pattern of follicular keratinization and produce more sebum than do their normal counterparts. The levels of linoleic acid in sebum from an acne patient are low, and free fatty acids are prevalent. Bacteria (*Propionibacterium acnes, Propionibacterium granulosum,* and micrococci) and yeast (*Pityrosporum ovale*) play an important contributory role through their lipolytic action on sebum to produce free fatty acids, the production of inflammatory enzymes (e.g., proteases), and the induction of follicular inflammation. Because androgens stimulate sebum production, patients with systemic or cutaneous hormonal imbalances can have severe acne. However, there is no evidence that the androgenic influence occurs in all human acne patients.

Treatment of the human acne patient varies with the severity of the disease. Medications used include topical comedolytic agents (vitamin A acid, benzoyl peroxide, various antibiotic solutions), systemic antibiotics (tetracycline, minocycline, erythromycin, clindamycin), and isotretinoin for severe cases.

Acne in dogs and cats is uncommon and has not been thoroughly studied.[4, 24] Pets with acne have abnormal follicular keratinization; beyond that, however, there may be little pathomechanistic similarity to human acne. For example, the comedonal lipid profiles from hairless dogs showed a predominance of free sterols, ceramides, and free fatty acids.[3] These lipids are of epidermal rather than sebaceous origin and suggest that the sebaceous glands are minimally important in acne in dogs.

Canine Acne

Although skin lesions are fairly common in the acne-prone skin of the chin and lips of young dogs, it is doubtful that this is a true acne in which the defect in follicular keratinization arises de novo. Previous editions of this text,[20] other textbooks on veterinary dermatology,[16] and review papers have characterized canine acne as a papulopustular eruption that develops from comedones.[4] However, careful inspection of the involved skin rarely reveals comedones; instead, sterile or secondarily infected papules or furuncles are the primary lesions seen. In all likelihood, canine acne is due to a traumatic follicular insult with resultant folliculitis. The subject is discussed in detail under muzzle folliculitis and furunculosis in Chapter 4.

Feline Acne

Feline acne is an uncommon condition that affects cats of either sex and is not confined to adolescence.

CAUSE AND PATHOGENESIS

Feline acne is an idiopathic disorder of follicular keratinization.[4, 24, 25] Although some cats experience only one episode during their lives, many affected cats have cyclic or near constant disease. Poor grooming habits, an underlying seborrheic predisposition, the production of abnormal sebum, hair cycle influences, stress, direct viral influences, and immunosuppression have all been considered in the pathogenesis.[24] Although each of these would be an aggravating factor, none has been proven causal. Hormonal influences probably play little or no role in the pathogenesis, for cases are recognized with equal frequency in males and females.[19]

CLINICAL FEATURES

The earliest lesions are comedones on the chin, the lower lip, and occasionally the upper lip (Fig. 13:4*D*). At this stage, there are no symptoms associated with the lesions, so they are often overlooked or ignored by the client. Some cases remain in the comedonal stage, but others progress and develop papules and pustules. In severe cases, a suppurative folliculitis, furunculosis, or cellulitis may develop (Fig. 4:6*A*) (*Pasteurella multocida*, β-hemolytic streptococci, staphylococci). In severe cases, the chin and lips can become edematous and thickened, and the cat often scratches or rubs the chin on furniture or other rough surfaces. Regional lymphadenopathy may be prominent. Cysts of variable sizes and scarring are commonplace in chronic cases.

DIAGNOSIS

In most cases, the diagnosis of feline acne is straightforward and is based on the presence of classic lesions on the chin and lips. In the comedonal stage, demodicosis, dermatophytosis, and *Malassezia* infection should be excluded by the appropriate tests. With furuncular lesions, primary or secondary bacterial or fungal infections should be considered and documented by appropriate cytologic and cultural techniques. With pronounced chin edema (the so-called fat chin), an eosinophilic granuloma with collagen degeneration must be considered (see Chap. 17).

Histopathologic findings in feline acne include follicular keratosis, plugging, and dilatation (comedo).[10] In advanced cases, perifolliculitis, folliculitis, and furunculosis may be seen (Fig. 13:5).

CLINICAL MANAGEMENT

The need for treatment and intensity of treatment vary from case to case. If the owner does not object to the presence of asymptomatic comedones, no treatment is required. If the lesions are visually objectionable or if they progress to sterile or secondarily infected papules or furuncles or induce pruritus, treatment is required.

Topical therapy is beneficial in all cases and is directed towards the dislodgement and dissolution of the comedone. In many cases, the ease and efficacy of treatment can be increased by clipping the area before treating it. If draining papules and furuncles are admixed with the comedones, the area should be hot packed in a magnesium sulfate (Epsom salt) solution (2 tbsp or 30 ml/L warm water) for 5 to 10 minutes. Soaking promotes drainage and softens the surrounding comedones. Because drainage typically indicates secondary bacterial infection, appropriate antibiotics should be administered orally for 14 to 21 days. Antibiotic selection

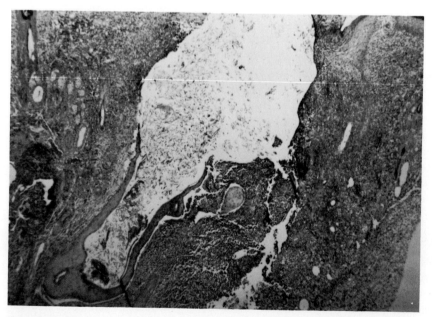

Figure 13:5. Feline acne. Ruptured comedo (follicular plug) with surrounding pyogranulomatous dermatitis.

depends on the invading organism, but clavulanated amoxicillin, enrofloxacin, or a cephalosporin are good empiric choices.

Although alcohol, various human acne cleaning pads, or Listerine antiseptic can be effective comedolytic agents in cats, most investigators dispense antiseborrheic shampoos for daily to twice weekly use. Sulfur-salicylic acid, ethyl lactate, or benzoyl peroxide products receive the most use.[4, 24] Benzoyl peroxide has pronounced follicular flushing properties but may be too irritating for some cats. Other topical products used in cats include vitamin A acid (Retin-A 0.05 per cent cream) and topical clindamycin, tetracycline, or erythromycin solutions or ointments.[24] Topical metronidazole 0.75 per cent gel (Metrogel, Curatek Pharmaceuticals) has been reported to be useful, perhaps through its combined antibacterial and anti-inflammatory properties.[4a]

After all the papules and comedones have been eliminated, treatment should be discontinued gradually over several weeks. Some cats remain free of lesions for extended periods and others relapse. Once the amount of time that passes before relapse is known, a maintenance cleaning program can be instituted. These cats with recurrent acne may benefit from fatty acid supplementation.[24]

Aside from antibiotics and fat supplements, systemic therapy is rarely indicated. In cats with severe inflammation, a 10- to 14-day course of oral prednisolone (1 to 2 mg/kg q24h) can be beneficial and may reduce scar tissue formation. Any bacterial infection should be resolved before the corticosteroid is administered. Cats that do not allow topical treatment or are refractory to it may benefit from the oral administration of isotretinoin (2 mg/kg/day).[23, 24] If response is to occur, it should be seen in 30 days. Approximately one third of treated cats respond.[24] Responders require long-term treatment, but the frequency of administration can often be reduced to every 2 or 3 days.

■ CANINE EAR MARGIN DERMATOSIS

Marginal seborrhea affecting the pinna of the ear is characterized by numerous small, greasy plugs (follicular casts) adhering to the skin and hairs of the medial and lateral margins. It is most common in dachshunds but also occurs in other breeds with pendulous ears (see Fig. 13:4*E*). The small particles can be easily removed for diagnosis with the thumbnail or a flat instrument. These particles are soft, irregular, and greasy. With time, the scaling becomes more confluent and can involve the entire ear margin, and the condition can be accompanied by partial alopecia of the pinna. In chronic cases, the seborrheic debris on the ear margins, especially at the tips, can become very thick and hard. With head shaking, scratching, or blunt trauma, the hard crust and its subjacent viable tissues can crack and result in an ear fissure (see Chap. 18). The fissure is painful and causes the dog to shake its head, which accelerates the fissuring.

In early cases, the diagnosis of ear margin dermatosis is straightforward. Seborrheic changes are restricted to the ear margin of a dog with pendulous ears. Pruritus and pain are absent. With heavy crusting and fissures, all the causes of vasculitis (Fig. 13:6) must be considered (see Chap. 8). Histopathologic examination shows marked surface and follicular orthokeratotic or parakeratotic hyperkeratosis (Fig. 13:7).

Ear margin dermatosis is an incurable condition that can be controlled with antiseborrheic treatments. Coupled with these treatments, management changes should be considered. Affected dogs should not be allowed to sleep near forced air heating ducts, wood stoves, or other dry heat sources, because these will worsen the seborrhea.[19] In addition, the dog's diet should be reviewed and improved if necessary.

Because of the follicular nature of the seborrhea, sulfur-salicylic, benzoyl peroxide, or benzoyl peroxide–sulfur shampoos are most commonly used to remove the accumulated debris. In chronic cases in which the debris is hard, the areas should be soaked in warm water for 5 to 10 minutes before the shampoo is applied. The areas are shampooed every 24 to 48 hours until

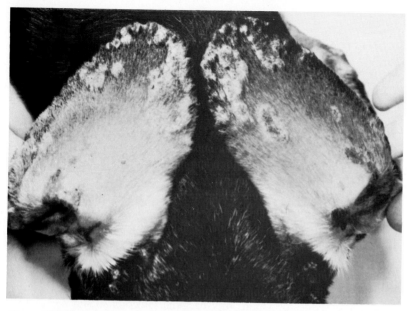

Figure 13:6. Ear margin scaling and crusting in a dachshund. Lesions away from the ear margins suggest an underlying vasculopathy.

the debris is completely removed. Severe cases can take 10 to 14 days for this to occur. After the cleaning, a moisturizer should be applied to minimize transepidermal water loss. When the ears are near normal, the frequency of shampooing is reduced to an as-needed basis.

In some cases, removal of the debris results in pinnal inflammation. In most instances, however, this inflammation is mild and requires no treatment. Moderately inflamed lesions benefit from the application of a 1 per cent hydrocortisone cream or ointment.[16] With severe inflammation or early fissures, prednisolone (1 mg/kg q24h orally) is needed for 7 to 10 days.

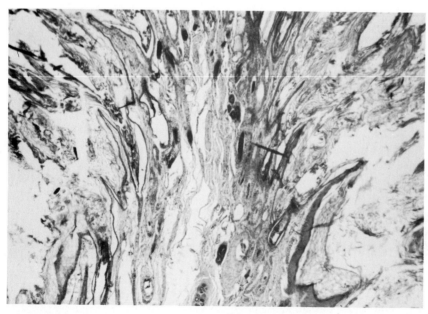

Figure 13:7. Histopathologic section of ear margin dermatosis. Tangential section shows a papillated epidermis with orthokeratotic hyperkeratosis.

With extensive fissuring, pinnal surgery is required. With multiple fissures, a cosmetic ear crop should be performed. Appropriate diagnostic tests should be performed before surgery to assure that the fissure was not caused by some underlying vasculitic process.

■ CANINE TAIL GLAND HYPERPLASIA

All dogs have an oval spot on the dorsal surface of the tail, about 2.5 to 5 cm distal to the anus, that is different from other skin. The area has simple instead of compound hair follicles and numerous large sebaceous and perianal (hepatoid) glands.

Some dogs with primary or secondary seborrhea or with relative or absolute elevated blood androgen levels develop hyperplasia of the sebaceous glands, perianal glands in the tail gland, or both. When the androgen levels are elevated, the perianal glands around the anus and elsewhere are also typically hyperplastic. Early tail gland hyperplasia usually goes unnoticed because the overlying hairs hide the defect. With time, however, the area becomes hairless because of friction and compression of the hair follicles by the hyperplastic glands. At this stage, the owner notices an oval, bulging, hairless area on the tail (see Fig. 13:4 *F*). The overlying skin may be scaly, greasy, hyperpigmented, or some combination thereof. In advanced cases, the area can have a nodular appearance because of nonuniform glandular hypertrophy and cystic dilatation or secondary infection.

The area of the tail gland hyperplasia may become infected, although this is uncommon. Grouped or single pustules may develop, with each pustule representing an acne-like sebaceous or perianal gland infection. Puncturing the pustules, expressing the contents, and administering systemic antibiotics usually provide relief. In some cases, the infection may recur.

Tail gland hyperplasia is usually a strictly cosmetic defect requiring no treatment. Because many cases are caused by hyperandrogenism, castration should be offered to prevent further enlargement. When this is performed, a beneficial response usually occurs within 2 months. The owner should be warned that castration may not lead to complete resolution of the existing lesion. Although the glands should become less hyperplastic, the alopecia may be permanent as a result of prolonged glandular pressure on the hair follicles. In the past, medical treatment with estrogens or progestational compounds has been recommended because of their anti-androgenic effects. As a result of their potential serious side effects, however (e.g., bone marrow suppression, diabetes mellitus), these agents are no longer suggested.

Animals that do not respond sufficiently to castration or are not neutered may benefit from surgery. An elliptic piece of skin is removed from the dorsal area of the tail over the enlargement. Blunt dissection and curettage are then performed to remove the excess glandular material under and lateral to the incision. Before the wound is sutured, additional loose skin can usually be removed to provide a normal conformation of skin around the tail. The area should be bandaged to prevent self-damage or suture removal by the dog. Excellent cosmetic correction usually results, with only a small scar remaining visible. Without castration, recurrence can be expected in 1 to 3 years.

■ FELINE TAIL GLAND HYPERPLASIA

Cats have the same tail gland area as dogs, but it is located in a line along the dorsal aspect of the tail and is commonly called the *supracaudal organ*. As in dogs, this area is rich in sebaceous and apocrine glands (Fig. 13:8), and a waxy secretion accumulates on the surface.

In some cats, especially those kept in catteries or small enclosures, unusually large amounts of excess secretions accumulate and cause matting of the hair and the formation of scales and crusts (Fig. 13:9). In some cases, the overlying hair coat is thinned, and the skin may become hyperpigmented (see Fig. 13:4 *G*). Rarely, secondary bacterial folliculitis and furunculosis complicate the condition. This condition is of great concern to owners of uncastrated male show cats, which accounts for the popular name *stud tail*[25]; however, it has also been observed

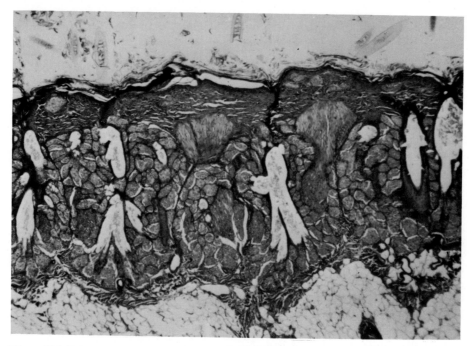

Figure 13:8. Feline stud tail. Marked sebaceous gland hyperplasia.

in females and altered males. Castration does not resolve the condition but may help stop its progression.[19]

Treatment consists of clipping the affected area and washing it with antiseborrheic shampoos. Benzoyl peroxide shampoo can be very useful. This treatment can be followed by daily cleaning with alcohol or a milder antiseborrheic shampoo (e.g., sulfur-salicylic acid). It is advisable to provide affected cats with as little confinement as possible, because fresh air and sunshine may help prevent recurrence. The unconfined cat usually resumes cleaning itself and the tail gland area with the customary fastidiousness characteristic of healthy, well-adjusted cats. Progestational compounds may be helpful; because of their common side-effects, however, their advisability as therapy for a benign, asymptomatic disease is questionable. Retinoids have not been used in this condition, but they may be of some value in recalcitrant cases.

If the cat fails to care for the problem, the owner must carefully and frequently comb and groom the area to prevent recurrence.

■ EXFOLIATIVE DERMATOSES

Virtually every surface or superficial follicular skin lesion in dogs and cats exfoliates (falls off in scales and layers) during its development, maturation, or involution. With the coalescence of adjacent lesions, large areas of exfoliation can occur, making the list of possible exfoliative dermatoses large indeed. True exfoliative dermatoses, however, are characterized by generalized severe desquamation with or without generalized erythema (erythroderma). Although affected animals may have some unaffected areas on the body, those that are involved are uniformly affected, with no visible normal skin.

In animals receiving no medications for a systemic or skin disease, the following must be considered as causes of the exfoliative dermatitis: ichthyosis, contact dermatitis to a topical agent (shampoo, dip, and so forth), pemphigus foliaceus, systemic lupus erythematosus, erythema multiforme or toxic epidermal necrolysis, epitheliotropic lymphoma, the disorders that cause cutaneous flushing, and parapsoriasis.[1, 18, 19, 27] When an animal is receiving nonsteroidal

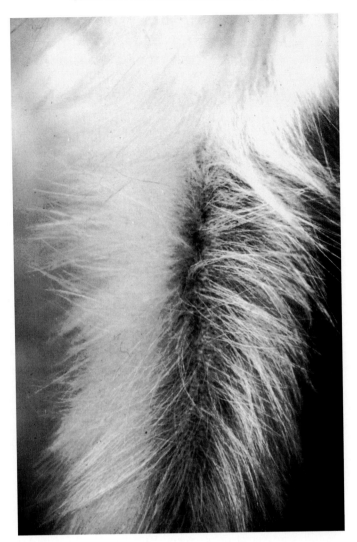

Figure 13:9. Feline tail gland hyperplasia with accumulation of greasy material in the hairs.

medications, drug eruption and unexpected physiologic response to the drug must be added to the list. Corticosteroids from internal (e.g., hyperadrenocorticism) or external sources increase the number of possibilities. In these animals, widespread superficial bacterial folliculitis, dermatophytosis, *Malassezia* dermatitis, demodicosis, cheyletiellosis, and occasionally scabies must be considered. Idiopathic cases are reported.[1]

With careful consideration of the history, physical findings, and routine in-office diagnostic tests (e.g., skin scrapings, trichography, cytologic tests), the list of differential diagnoses for an exfoliative dermatosis becomes considerably shorter. Definitive diagnosis is often made by skin biopsy. Most causes of exfoliative dermatosis are covered elsewhere in this textbook. Parapsoriasis, cutaneous flushing, and physiologic response to a drug are considered here.

■ PARAPSORIASIS

In humans, parapsoriasis (resembling psoriasis) is grouped into three major entities, each of which has several morphologic variants. To date, only large plaque parapsoriasis has been reported in animals and only in one dog and one cat.[27] The dermatoses were characterized by widespread erythematous, scaly plaques that spared the head, pinnae, and distal limbs (see Fig. 13:4 *H*). Irregular hair loss occurred in the involved areas. In the dog, many of the plaques

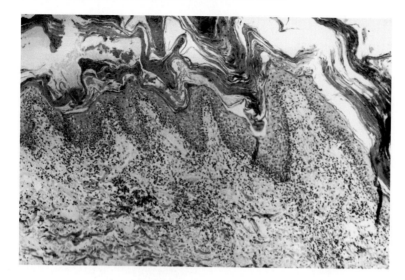

Figure 13:10. Parapsoriasis. Superficial perivascular to lichenoid dermatitis with parakeratotic hyperkeratosis and diffuse exocytosis of lymphocytes.

were studded with large, superficial, flaccid, yellow pustules, annular erosions, and epidermal collarettes that were a result of a secondary staphylococcal infection.

Biopsy of affected skin showed a focally parakeratotic, regularly hyperplastic, superficial perivascular to lichenoid interface dermatitis with diffuse exocytosis of normal lymphocytes (Fig. 13:10). A striking finding was a diffuse accumulation of lymphocytes arranged in a line within the basal cell layer of the epidermis and hair follicle outer root sheaths (Fig. 13:11).

Both animals were treated with high levels of corticosteroids, the dog with oral prednisolone (2.2 mg/kg q24h) and the cat with methylprednisolone acetate injections (5 mg/kg q2wk). Marked healing occurred in 8 to 10 days, with complete resolution of all lesions in 6 to 10 weeks. Both cases required maintenance therapy to prevent relapse.

■ CUTANEOUS FLUSHING

Cutaneous flushing is due to vasodilation of the cutaneous blood vessels and is manifested by the skin turning various shades of red.[9] The flushing can be regionalized or generalized and paroxysmal or persistent. Pathologic flushing is due to the direct action of vasoactive com-

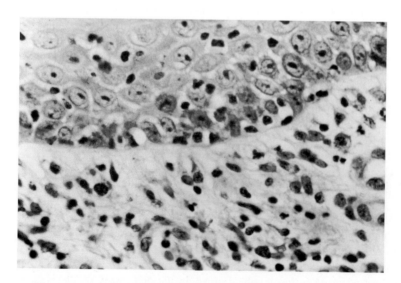

Figure 13:11. Parapsoriasis. Diffuse spongiosis and exocytosis of lymphocytes. Note the row of lymphocytes within the basal layer.

pounds on the blood vessels. Because some vasoactive compounds (e.g., histamine) are pruritogenic, some flushing disorders can be pruritic, but the flushing precedes the pruritus.

In dogs, persistent, widespread erythema (erythroderma) can be a feature of systemic lupus erythematosus, demodicosis, drug reaction, thallium toxicosis, mast cell tumor, or systemic mastocytosis.[18, 31] Paroxysmal flushing has been associated with pheochromocytoma, drug reaction, mast cell tumor, and the carcinoid syndrome.[18]

In humans, the carcinoid syndrome refers to an uncommon condition associated with slow-growing malignant carcinoid tumors derived from enterochromaffin cells, which produce a variety of vasoactive compounds.[9] In most instances, the tumor is located in the gastrointestinal tract, but it can also be found in the ovary, testis, skin, or bronchus. In dogs, the carcinoid syndrome has been reported in association with a pulmonary adenocarcinoma[18] and has been recognized in several dogs with intestinal lesions.[19]

At their onset, flushing disorders in dogs have no associated exfoliation. In chronic cases, especially when the flushing is persistent, desquamation occurs but remains overshadowed by the erythroderma. All animals with such a presentation should have a thorough evaluation for an internal malignancy.

■ PHYSIOLOGIC RESPONSE TO DRUGS

As mentioned earlier, virtually all surface or superficial follicular skin lesions exfoliate at some point, especially during their involution. Accordingly, the drugs used to treat the lesions cause exfoliation in effect. If the skin lesions are widespread and numerous, an exfoliative dermatosis will result. Because clients are aware of the initial lesions, most recognize that the exfoliation is a sign of healing and are not concerned by it.

Drugs that influence epidermal turnover (e.g., hormones, cytotoxic agents, retinoic acids) can cause an exfoliative dermatitis near the onset of treatment or after discontinuation of the drug. Exfoliation at the termination of treatment with a cytostatic agent should be expected, and the client should be made aware of this expectation. The most common example is the profound scaling that occurs when an animal is withdrawn from a chronic course of treatment with moderate to high doses of a corticosteroid. Similar changes can occur in dogs with spontaneous hyperadrenocorticism that are being treated with mitotane (o,p'-DDD) and in hypothyroid dogs within the first few weeks of treatment with thyroid hormone. Much more problematic is the exfoliation that occurs 1 to 2 weeks after treatment with a nonsteroidal agent is instituted (Fig. 13:12). The basic quandary is whether the exfoliation represents a drug

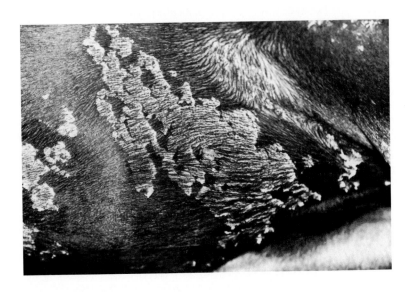

Figure 13:12. Exfoliative dermatosis in a hypothyroid Doberman pinscher resulting from the institution of thyroid hormone replacement therapy.

eruption or clinical evidence of increased epidermal turnover. If the pharmacology of the drug allows this change and the animal is showing no clinical or laboratory evidence of systemic illness, the question can be answered by observing the animal carefully for 7 to 10 days. Pharmacologic exfoliation will lessen or stop within this time, but a drug eruption will persist or worsen.

REFERENCES

1. Anderson, R. K.: Exfoliative dermatitis in the dog. Comp. Cont. Educ. 3:885, 1981.
2. Baker, B. B., et al.: Epidermal cell renewal in dogs after clipping the hair. Am. J. Vet. Res. 35:445, 1974.
3. Bedford, C. J. Young, J. M.: A comparison of comedonal and skin surface lipids from hairless dogs showing clinical signs of acne. J. Invest. Dermatol. 77:341, 1981.
4. Bond, R.: Canine and feline acne. Vet. Ann. 33:230, 1993.
4a. Breen, P., Jeromin, A.: Practice tips. Dermatol. Dialogue. Winter 93/94, p. 7.
5. Campbell, K. L., Davis, C. A.: Effects of thyroid hormones on serum and cutaneous fatty acid concentrations in dogs. Am. J. Vet. Res. 51:752, 1990.
6. Campbell, K. L., et al.: Effects of oral sunflower oil on serum and cutaneous fatty acid concentration profiles in seborrheic dogs. Vet. Dermatol. 3:29, 1992.
7. Campbell, K. L., Schaeffer, D. J.: Effects of four veterinary shampoos on transepidermal water losses, hydration of the stratum corneum, skin surface lipid concentrations, and corneocyte counts in dogs. Proc. Am. Acad. Vet. Dermatol. Am. Coll. Vet. Dermatol. 9:96, 1993.
8. Campbell, K. L., Kirkwood, A. R.: Effect of topical oils on transepidermal water loss in dogs with seborrhea sicca. Advances in Veterinary Dermatology, Vol. 2. Pergamon Press, Oxford, 1993, p. 157.
8a. Campbell, K. L., et al.: Effects of four anti-seborrheic shampoos on transepidermal water losses, hydration of the stratum corneum, skin surface lipid concentration, skin surface pH, and corneocyte counts in dogs. Proc. Am. Acad. Vet. Dermatol. Am. Coll. Vet. Dermatol. 10:85, 1994.
9. Fitzpatrick, T. B., et al.: Dermatology in General Medicine, 4th ed. McGraw-Hill Book Co., New York, 1993.
9a. Gordon, J. G., Kwochka, K. W.: Corneocyte counts for evaluation of antiseborrheic shampoos in dogs. Vet. Dermatol. 4:57, 1993.
10. Gross, T. L., et al.: Veterinary Dermatopathology. Mosby–Year Book, St. Louis, 1992.
11. Guaguère, E.: Cas clinique: Séborrhée primaire répondant à l'administration de vitamine A. Point. Vét. 16:689, 1984.
12. Guaguère, E.: Quel est votre diagnostic? Point. Vét. 18:245, 1986.
13. Ihrke, P. J., Goldschmidt, M. H.: Vitamin A–responsive dermatosis in the dog. J. Am. Vet. Med. Assoc. 182:682, 1983.
13a. Kietzmann, M.: Eicosanoid levels in canine inflammatory skin diseases. In: von Tscharner, C., Halliwell, R. E. W. (eds.). Advances in Veterinary Dermatology I. Baillière-Tindall, London, 1990, p. 211.
14. Kwochka, K. W., Rademakers, A. M.: Cell proliferation of epidermis, hair follicles, and sebaceous glands of Beagles and Cocker spaniels with healthy skin. Am. J. Vet. Res. 50:587, 1989.
15. Kwochka, K. W.: Keratinization abnormalities: Understanding the mechanism of scale formation. Advances in Veterinary Dermatology, Vol. 2. Pergamon Press, Oxford, 1993, p. 91.
16. Kwochka, K. W.: Keratinization Disorders. Current Veterinary Dermatology. Mosby–Year Book, St. Louis, 1993, p. 167.
17. Kwochka, K. W.: Shampoos and moisturizing rinses in veterinary dermatology. In: Bonagura, J. D. (ed.): Kirk's Current Veterinary Therapy XII. W. B. Saunders Co., Philadelphia (in press, 1994).
18. Miller, W. H., Jr.: Cutaneous flushing associated with intrathoracic neoplasia in a dog. J. Am. Anim. Hosp. Assoc. 28:217, 1992.
19. Miller, W. H., Jr., Scott, D. W.: Unpublished observations, 1994.
20. Muller, G. H., et al.: Small Animal Dermatology, 4th ed. W. B. Saunders Co., Philadelphia, 1989.
21. Paradis, M.: Footpad hyperkeratosis in a family of Dogues de Bordeaux. Vet. Dermatol. 3:75, 1992.
22. Parker, W., et al.: Vitamin A–responsive seborrheic dermatitis in the dog: A case report. J. Am. Anim. Hosp. Assoc. 19:546, 1983.
23. Power, H. T., Ihrke, P. J.: The use of synthetic retinoids in veterinary medicine. In: Bonagura, J. D. (ed.). Kirk's Current Veterinary Therapy XII. W. B. Saunders Co., Philadelphia (in press, 1994).
24. Rosenkrantz, W. S.: The pathogenesis, diagnosis, and management of feline acne. Vet. Med. 86:504, 1991.
25. Scott, D. W.: Feline dermatology 1900–1978: A monograph. J. Am. Anim. Hosp. Assoc. 16:331, 1980.
26. Scott, D. W.: Vitamin A–responsive dermatosis in the cocker spaniel. J. Am. Anim. Hosp. Assoc. 22:125, 1986.
27. Scott, D. W.: Exfoliative dermatoses in a dog and a cat resembling large plaque parapsoriasis in humans. Comp. Anim. Pract. 2:22, 1986.
28. Scott, D. W., et al.: A clinical study on the efficacy of two commercial veterinary emollients (Micropearls and Humilac) in the management of wintertime dry skin in dogs. Cornell Vet. 81:419, 1991.
29. Scott, D. W., et al.: A clinical study on the effect of two commercial veterinary benzoyl peroxide shampoos in dogs. Canine Pract. 19:7, 1994.
30. Simpson, J. W., van den Brock, A. H. M.: Fat absorption in dogs with diabetes mellitus or hypothyroidism. Res. Vet. Sci. 50:346, 1991.
31. White, S. D. The skin as a sensor of internal medical disorders. In: Ettinger, S. J. (ed.). Textbook of Veterinary Internal Medicine, 3rd ed. W. B. Saunders Co., Philadelphia, 1989, p. 5.

Psychogenic
Skin Diseases

■

Chapter Outline

Psychodermatology, also known as psychocutaneous medicine and dermatopsychosomatics, is a growing field of interest in human medicine.[10] Workers in this field believe that the body (soma) and mind (psyche) have been treated separately for too long and constitute a single unit. It is believed that the role of emotional factors in diseases of the skin is of such significance that if it is ignored, effective management of at least 40 per cent of the patients who come to departments of dermatology is impossible. Research in laboratory animals and humans indicates that the central nervous system, through the effects of neurohormones, can significantly modulate immune responses and pruritus. The relationship between the hypothalamus and the immune system seems to involve (1) neurohormones secreted by the hypothalamus (thyrotropin releasing factor, prolactin releasing factor, gonadotropin releasing hormone); (2) the neurotransmitters norepinephrine, serotonin, dopamine, acetylcholine, γ-aminobutyric acid; and (3) the polypeptide neuroregulators somatostatin, vasoactive intestinal peptide, substance P, neurotensin, enkephalins, and endorphins.[10]

The role of neurotransmitters and neuroregulators in veterinary dermatology is unknown. Recent studies with drugs that block serotonin or endorphin actions suggest that they play some role. Part of the effect may be related to the decrease in the effects of endorphin-induced histamine release.

Studies in laboratory animals have shown that the central nervous system can interact with the immune system. Guinea pigs sensitized to bovine serum albumin were conditioned by repeatedly being exposed to the allergen and an odor simultaneously.[13] They eventually experienced the allergic reaction when exposed to the odor alone, without the allergen.

In humans, psychodermatologic conditions are divided into (1) *psychophysiologic disorders* in which there is a bona fide skin disorder (allergy, urticaria) that can be exacerbated by emotional stress; (2) *primary psychiatric disorders* in which there is anxiety, depression, delusion, and obsessive-compulsive behavior; and (3) *secondary psychiatric disorders*.[6a]

Most lesions of psychogenic dermatoses in animals are the result of self-induced damage. There is good clinical evidence that psychological disturbances are the cause.[2, 8, 12] Obsessive-compulsive disorders are characterized by repetitive, stereotypic, ritualistic behaviors in excess of what is required for normal function; the execution of these behaviors interferes with normal daily activities and functioning.[2, 8] Behavioral conditions that can be present in obsessive-compulsive animals include boredom, attention-seeking, hyperactivity, and anxiety. Three general factors are involved in the etiopathogenesis:

1. Breed predisposition. Breeds that are emotional and nervous develop more psychogenic dermatoses. Abyssinian and Siamese cats are especially at risk. Among dogs, the predisposed breeds include Doberman pinschers, Great Danes, Irish setters, Labrador retrievers, and German shepherds.[8b, 15, 20]
2. The lifestyle of the animal can be causative or contributory. When individuals not of predisposed breeds are forced into stressful, isolated, or boring situations and are without human or canine companionship, they may develop psychogenic dermatoses. Long confinement in crates, continual chain restraint, small pen housing, or domination by a forceful or inconsiderate owner may precipitate problems. A rival animal in the same house or an aggressive neighborhood animal can trigger a psychogenic disturbance.
3. The individual animal, regardless of breed or lifestyle, can be particularly nervous, hyperesthetic, fearful, or shy.

The diagnosis of a psychogenic dermatosis is by exclusion and generally cannot be well documented. The diagnosis is also occasionally used for those frustrating cases that do not respond to treatment even when a thorough work-up has not been performed. Physical causes must always be eliminated before a diagnosis of psychogenic dermatosis is made. This process includes ruling out such causative factors as trauma, neuropathy, local pain, parasites, allergy, bacterial or fungal infections, or internal diseases. The problem of accurate diagnosis can be compounded by the fact that psychogenic factors may play a partial role in a disease; a work-up may reveal an organic disease, but the psychological component may be significant enough that treatment of it is necessary for adequate control of the whole condition.

Dermatoses thought to be psychogenic in origin or to have a significant psychogenic component include acral lick dermatitis *(lick granuloma),* tail dock neuroma, feline psychogenic alopecia and dermatitis, and miscellaneous psychogenic manifestations such as tail sucking (feline), tail biting (canine), flank sucking, foot licking, self-nursing, and anal licking.

■ CANINE PSYCHOGENIC DERMATOSES

Acral Lick Dermatitis

Acral lick dermatitis, also known as *lick granuloma* results from an urge to lick the lower cranial portion of a leg, producing a thickened, firm, oval plaque. The condition may be organic or psychogenic in origin.[15, 20] In the past, many authors thought that most cases that presented with lesions and a history compatible with acral lick dermatitis were of psychogenic origin; today, however, it is believed that organic disease is commonly present (see Chap. 4, Acral Lick Furunculosis). Potential organic causes should always be excluded. At the very minimum, bacterial or fungal disease, demodicosis, previous trauma, allergy (inhalant, food, flea), and underlying joint disease should be ruled out before diagnosing a case as purely psychogenic in origin.

CAUSE AND PATHOGENESIS

Boredom is often the major cause of a dog's habit of licking its leg. A carefully taken history reveals that the dog is alone much of the day. The classic patient is a large, active dog whose owners work and have no children at home. Either there is no companion dog or another dog in the household provides no play activity. Unusual restrictions on the dog's freedom can be a causative factor. Dogs kept in crates for long periods or dogs that are chained can become bored and relieve their frustrations by constantly licking a leg. In other dogs, a pre-existing focal dermatosis (e.g., an infection, neoplasm, or wound) precipitates a vicious circle.

The constant licking produces an eroded area on the skin that itches exquisitely. An itch-lick cycle is established until a firm, ulcerated lesion results. Possibly, a wound may initiate the licking, or the licking may occur in response to stress or boredom. The licking of the erosion or wound leads to ulceration and to the exposure of deeper skin layers. The licking prevents the ulcer from healing and predisposes the animal to secondary infection. Epidermal hyperplasia and dermal fibrosis account for the nodular plaque that is characteristic of the disease. The lesion at this stage used to be called a granuloma or tumor, but it is neither neoplastic nor granulomatous.

Excessive licking may cause the production and release of endorphins, making the animal feel better (euphoric) and at the same time producing an analgesic effect that decreases the animal's pain perception. This process essentially addicts the dog to the compulsive licking.

Electrophysiologic studies have suggested that a mild distal sensory axonal polyneuropathy may be present in some cases of acral lick dermatitis.[18]

On the basis of the phenomenology of the condition and the pharmacologic response, it has been proposed that canine acral lick dermatitis is an animal model of obsessive-compulsive disorder.[8, 12]

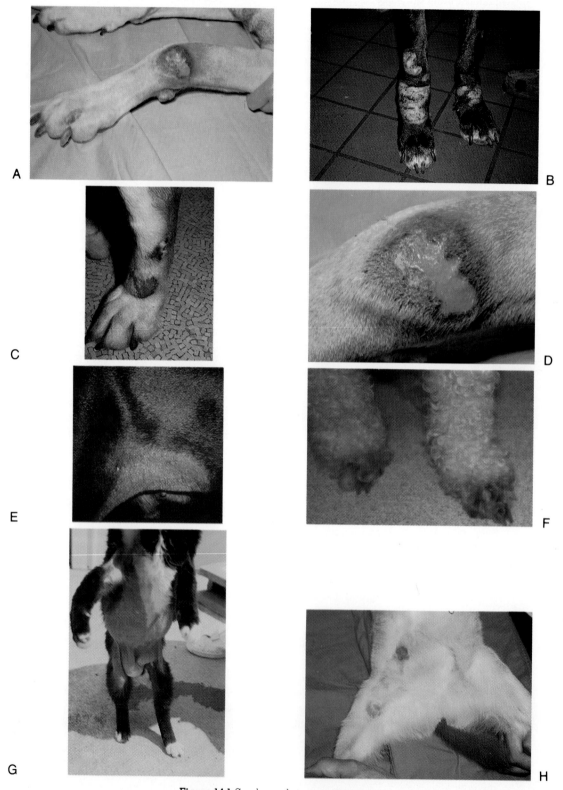

Figure 14:1 *See legend on opposite page*

CLINICAL FEATURES

Predisposed breeds include the Doberman pinscher, Great Dane, Labrador retriever, Irish setter, Golden retriever, and German shepherd.[8b, 12, 15, 20] Other breeds, including smaller dogs, can also develop acral lick dermatitis. It can occur at any age, although most dogs are over 5 years of age when presented for treatment. Males with the disorder outnumber females two to one.

In almost all cases, the lesion is single and unilateral (Fig. 14:1 *A*). In some cases, multiple legs may be affected, and these cases may respond poorly to treatment because there is often an organic disease, such as staphylococcal furunculosis, or an allergy that must be addressed. One clue that there may be a psychogenic component to the condition is the development of a newly licked area when the original lesion has been covered by a bandage or wrap. The most common site for a lesion is the cranial carpal or metacarpal area (Fig. 14:1 *B* and *C*). The next most frequent sites are the cranial radial, metatarsal, or tibial regions. Chronic lesions become hard, thickened plaques or nodules that have an ulcerated surface and a hyperpigmented halo (Fig. 14:1*D*). Extremely large lesions on the joints that have been present for years may be associated with arthritis or ankylosis of the underlying joint.

DIAGNOSIS

A tentative diagnosis can usually be made from the clinical examination and history. A definitive diagnosis requires ruling out the other differential diagnoses, which include neoplasia, pressure point granulomas, calcinosis circumscripta, bacterial furunculosis, demodicosis, dermatophytosis, mycotic or mycobacterial granulomas, and underlying hypersensitivity disorders. Histiocytomas and mastocytomas may be mistaken for acral lick dermatitis if they occur on the cranial surface of the leg. Fungal cultures confirm the diagnosis of lesions induced by mycoses; exfoliative cytologic findings and biopsy provide the basis for diagnosis. However, hypoallergenic diets and intradermal tests are often indicated to detect a causative or concurrent allergic disease.

Histopathologically, the lesions usually show features that are characteristic of the disorder but are not diagnostic by themselves.[15] An ulcerated surface is bordered by irregular epidermal hyperplasia, which may be papillated and is usually marked. A mild perivascular accumulation of neutrophils and mononuclear cells is usually present. The dermis shows varying degrees of fibroplasia, and dermal papillae often show vertical streaking of fibroblasts and collagen fibrils (Fig. 14:2). Common findings include moderate to marked numbers of plasma cells around the apocrine sweat glands and inferior segments of hair follicles and sebaceous gland hyperplasia (Fig. 14:3). Folliculitis or furunculosis may coexist.

Radiographs usually reveal a secondary periosteal reaction of bones that underlie large chronic acral lick dermatitis lesions.[15] Joint disease is not induced by the licking; if present, it may be the cause of the excessive licking.

CLINICAL MANAGEMENT

Psychological counseling with the client should be the first step in the management of acral lick dermatitis of psychogenic origin. The client needs to understand that the dog's problem is

Figure 14:1. *A,* Acral lick dermatitis. The carpal area is commonly affected. *B,* Bilateral acral lick dermatitis in a Great Dane. *C,* Metatarsal acral lick dermatitis demonstrating characteristic location and appearance. *D,* Close-up of *A* shows the thickened nodule with the characteristic ulcerated epidermis surrounded by a hyperpigmented halo. *E,* Flank sucking. Focal area of alopecia, lichenification, and hyperpigmentation in the flank of a Doberman pinscher. *F,* Salivary staining of a paw associated with *Malassezia* pododermatitis in an atopic dog. *G,* Typical pattern in feline psychogenic alopecia with self-inflicted alopecia of the abdomen, groin, and inguinal regions. Note the alopecia on the medial forelegs and the mammary enlargement in this cat that were caused by megestrol acetate. *H,* Erosive plaque of dermatitis in a cat from self-licking. Alopecia is also present.

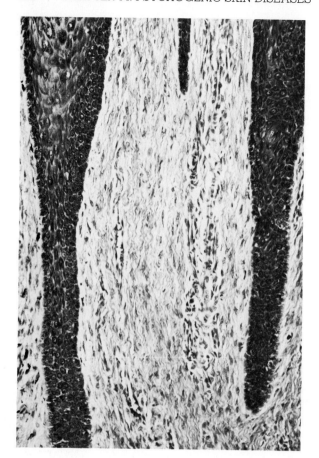

Figure 14:2. Vertical streaking of collagen fibrils between rete ridges.

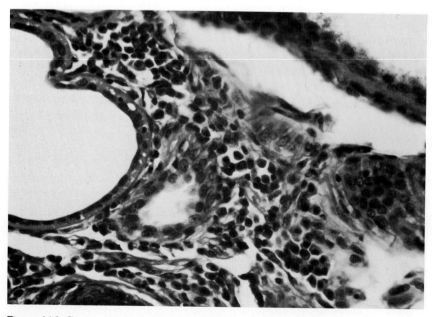

Figure 14:3. Canine acral lick dermatitis. Periapocrine plasma cells.

in his head and not just on the leg. Together, the clinician and client must become psychological detectives to find what caused the dog to lick its leg. Examples of causes include the following:

1. The dog is left alone all day.
2. The dog is confined for long periods to a crate, kennel, cage, or run.
3. There is a new pet in the home.
4. There is a new baby in the home.
5. A female dog is in heat nearby but not accessible to the male dog.
6. A new dog has come to the neighborhood.
7. A death has occurred in the family.
8. A long-time companion of the dog has died.

The first step in treatment is to recognize the cause and eliminate it, if possible. Sometimes a change in the dog's lifestyle is the answer. Each situation differs, but the following are examples of successful corrective measures.

1. More walks and human companionship are very helpful. Some owners can take their dog to work if they own a small shop or business.
2. For a kennel dog, avoidance of confinement to cages, kennels, or runs can be beneficial. The owner can make a house pet of the afflicted dog. Even nightly confinement to a cage may cause enough frustration to trigger acral lick dermatitis.
3. A new puppy as a companion can act as a diversion that may discourage further licking. The success of this method depends on the extent to which a friendship develops between the two dogs. For a male dog, a spayed female is very suitable. The owner should be aware that obtaining a companion dog is not a guaranteed cure.
4. Freedom to leave the house and premises can enable the dog to develop a life of his own in the neighborhood. This suggestion is suitable for some rural areas, but is usually impossible in suburban or urban areas where leash laws are in effect.

Once the lesion is present, therapy for the psychological component alone may not be effective. Systemic, topical, and surgical treatment may be required along with psychotherapy. One or more of the following approaches may be useful.[8a, 8b]

■ *Psychological Drug Therapy.* A variety of drugs that affect central nervous system neurotransmitters or endorphins or that have other sedative, antidepressant, or antianxiety effects may be beneficial in these cases. The psychological drugs may be needed for only a short while, until the habit is broken by behavior modification or the underlying boredom or stress is eliminated. In other cases, long-term treatment may be required. The older drugs are often less expensive and can be used when long-term treatment is required. In some cases, an expensive drug may be needed initially, but maintenance with a less expensive drug may be possible.

Anxiolytic oral drugs (especially benzodiazepines and antihistamines) that may be helpful are

Phenobarbital, 2.2 to 6.6 mg/kg q12h
Diazepam (Valium), 0.2 mg/kg q12h
Hydroxyzine (Atarax), 2.2 mg/kg q8h

Tricyclic antidepressant oral drugs, and especially those with serotonin re-uptake inhibitor properties, have been shown to be efficacious in some very resistant cases:

Fluoxetine (Prozac), 1 mg/kg q24h can be used.[12, 16] The problem is that it is very expensive.
Amitriptyline (Elavil), 1 to 3 mg/kg q12h[8, 19]
Imipramine (Tofranil), 2 to 4 mg/kg q24h[8]
Clomipramine (Anafranil), 1 to 3 mg/kg q24h[3, 12]

Fluoxetine and clomipramine can both cause lethargy, anorexia, hyperactivity, personality changes, and diarrhea.[12]

Endorphin blockers may also be effective. Naltrexone (Trexan) has been used in dogs with severe chronic acral lick dermatitis.[2, 21] Dogs were treated with 2.2 mg/kg orally every 24 hours. Of 10 dogs, 7 responded well, but 4 dogs relapsed when the drug was discontinued. Long-term control may be accomplished with reduced doses or longer intervals between doses. No significant side-effects have been seen. The drug is very expensive.

Endorphin substitution by the administration of an exogenous source of opiate may decrease dogs' desire to stimulate the release of endorphins. Hydrocodone (Hycodan) at 0.25 mg/kg q8h improved all of three dogs within 3 weeks.[1] Two were 100 per cent better after 16 weeks of treatment.

Progestagens have a calming effect, especially on male dogs. An injection of repositol progesterone (Depo-Provera, 20 mg/kg every 3 weeks) has been successful in selected cases. Megestrol acetate (Megace, Ovaban) has been used orally at 1 mg/kg q24h then tapered to minimal maintenance doses and frequencies. These agents have to be continued for several months and should not be used in intact female dogs.

■ ***Treating the Lesion.*** Along with the psychological treatment, the skin lesion should be treated until it is healed; treatment of the lesion alone yields disappointing results. Attempts at preventing licking mechanically by the use of Elizabethan collars, buckets, muzzles, bandages, casts, and wire-cloth devices may be helpful in allowing initial healing but are usually unsuccessful alone. Repellent liquids and creams have shown only limited success and usually only with early and mild lesions.

■ *Topical Applications.* *Topical corticosteroids* may be helpful, but their use is limited to the mild early lesion. One commercially available product, Synotic, contains fluocinolone acetonide 0.01 per cent in 60 per cent dimethyl sulfoxide (DMSO). This product is applied twice a day.

Dissolved in DMSO, corticosteroids can penetrate the lesion. One homemade formula uses equal parts of 90 per cent DMSO solution and a solution of 1 per cent hydrocortisone acetate and 2 per cent Burow's solution in propylene glycol (Hydro B-1020, Hydro-Plus). This solution is applied to the lesion twice a day for several weeks. Rubber gloves should be worn by the dog's owner when handling this and all other products containing DMSO.

A combination of fluocinolone in DMSO (Synotic) and flunixin meglumine (Banamine) has been reported to be effective in many cases.[15] Three milliliters of flunixine meglumine are added to an 8-ml vial of Synotic. This solution is applied twice a day until the lesion has healed. The treatment time varies from 3 to 8 weeks.

The *analgesic* capsaicin (HEET) mixed with Bitter Apple (isopropyl alcohol, water, bitter extract), one part HEET (capsaicin 0.25 per cent, methyl salicylate 15 per cent, camphor 3.6 per cent, acetone, alcohol) to two parts Bitter Apple, has also been reported to be effective in early lesions.[5] This solution is applied initially two to three times per day, then it is tapered as needed.

■ *Intralesional Injections.* Triamcinolone acetonide (Vetalog) or methylprednisolone acetate (Depo-Medrol) injections have also been recommended. These agents are helpful in lesions smaller than 3 cm in diameter. They are useless in large chronic lesions.

■ *Surgical Removal.* In some cases, surgical excision of the entire lesion is the treatment of choice. This is easily and quickly accomplished if the lesion is small enough to allow surgical repair without undue skin tension. The clinician should always close the incision with mattress sutures and use bandages or protective devices to prevent removal of the sutures or self-inflicted trauma by the dog before healing is complete, which requires at least 2 to 3 weeks. If the animal traumatizes the surgical site before complete healing has occurred, the resulting wound will be very difficult to manage. Systemic antibiotics should always be prescribed postoperatively.

In extreme cases, excision of the lesion and replacement with a full-thickness skin graft can be performed.

■ *Radiation Therapy.* The occasional effectiveness of radiation therapy has, in general, been shown to correlate with the duration and size of the lesion.[7, 9, 12a] Large chronic lesions are much less likely to respond favorably. Only 35 per cent of the cases have sustained excellent responses to radiation therapy.[12a]

■ *Cryosurgery.* Cryosurgery may be used as a last resort for lesions that are so large that they cannot be removed surgically, cannot be grafted with a full-thickness skin flap, and have not responded to other treatment. When properly performed, the hardened mass of tissue is frozen and sloughs over a period of several weeks. New healthy skin begins to grow from the wound margins. Freezing destroys nerve endings, thereby blocking the itch-lick cycle. The procedure must usually be repeated two or three times. It should be attempted only by those familiar with cryosurgical techniques.

■ *Acupuncture.* Acupuncture has been reported to be effective, but its usefulness must be further documented.

In summary, a guarded prognosis should be given to the client before beginning any treatment. Acral lick dermatitis is one of the most obstinate skin disorders, but at least it is not a life-threatening one.

Miscellaneous Psychogenic Manifestations

There is a group of six psychogenic manifestations or obsessive-compulsive disorders that involve sucking or licking a specifically selected anatomic area.[2, 8] The animal concentrates on one area to which it habitually returns. The treatment regimens that can be tried are those discussed for canine acral lick dermatitis and feline psychogenic alopecia and dermatitis.

■ *Tail Biting.* Tail biting is seen mostly in young, long-tailed, long-haired dogs. These dogs chase their tail and then bite the tip (Fig. 14:4). Many of the afflicted dogs stop this habit when they get older. These *tail chasers* must be differentiated from the dog that traumatizes the tail

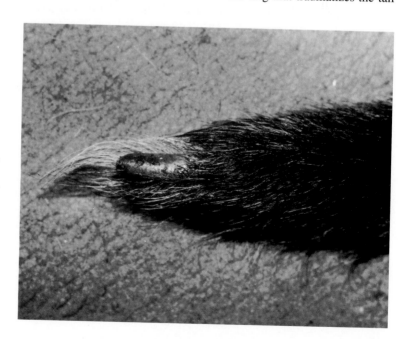

Figure 14:4. Tail biting in a dog. Notice the alopecia and excoriation on the tip of the tail.

tip when it becomes infected and pruritic or when the tail's normal sensations are altered by lumbosacral stenosis or a tail dock neuroma.

■ *Tail Dock Neuroma.* This is a rare disorder that follows some tail dockings.[4] Cocker spaniels may be predisposed. The nerves attempt to regrow in a haphazard fashion, and a neuroma develops. This is palpable as a firm, deep nodule that is usually adhered to the skin in the scarred tail tip. Histologically, the nodule is characterized by fibrous tissue with thick collagen bundles and multiple small nerve bundles randomly located throughout the nodule (see Chap. 19). This neuroma appears to stimulate pain or some sensation that causes the dog to lick or chew at its tail. Surgical removal of the neuroma is the treatment of choice.

■ *Flank Sucking.* Flank sucking in dogs is similar, in most respects, to tail sucking in cats, but it is more common and is especially prevalent in Doberman pinschers (see Fig. 14:1*E*). At one time, trichuriasis was thought to be a cause of the disorder, but this has not been documented. In fact, treatment for whipworms or surgical removal of the cecum (typhlectomy) were rarely successful. It has been suggested that tail biters and flank suckers may have a form of psychomotor epilepsy. This condition should be differentiated from localized folliculitis that is pruritic. Folliculitis usually is associated with inflammation and alopecia, and it may demonstrate hyperpigmentation and lichenification. These conditions respond to antibiotics. Atopy and food hypersensitivity should also be ruled out. Biopsies should be taken before a diagnosis of psychogenic flank sucking is made because the presence of dermatopathologic abnormalities suggests that an underlying organic disease is present. Therapy with phenobarbital or primidone may be helpful. One investigator has suggested a single intramuscular injection of medroxyprogesterone acetate (20 mg/kg) as possible therapy.[11]

■ *Self-Nursing.* This is virtually restricted to female dogs and cats but can occasionally be seen in males. Usually the self-nursing is confined to one nipple, and the animal repeatedly suckles that nipple. The nipple may become enlarged through inflammation and lichenification. Spaying the animal seems to be helpful in correcting this annoying habit in some animals. Sedation and psychological training to break the habit may also be useful.

■ *Anal Licking.* This habit, which is almost impossible to break, occurs only in dogs, and a breed predilection exists for Poodles. Many dogs, and particularly poodles, lick the anal area because of anal sac disease and even perianal *Malassezia* dermatitis. However, if these causes, atopy, and food hypersensitivity are ruled out, the possibility of psychogenic anal licking becomes much more likely. Removal of the anal sacs is not curative in this syndrome. Anorectal disease, particularly inflammation of the lower colon and rectal mucosa, should also be ruled out. Neurotic poodles that lick the anal area cause their owners much anguish. When this condition is chronic, the perianal skin becomes thickened, hyperpigmented, verrucous, and lichenified. Secondary bacterial pyoderma or *Malassezia* dermatitis is likely, and some response to antibiotics or anti-yeast medication occurs. The specific therapy is to try to identify and remove the cause or to administer antianxiety or antidepressant drugs as for acral lick dermatitis.

■ *Foot Licking.* This condition is usually associated with atopy, other hypersensitivities, or *Malassezia* dermatitis (see Fig. 14:1 *F*); rarely, foot licking alone is seen. It is a difficult habit to break.

■ FELINE PSYCHOGENIC DERMATOSES

Psychogenic Alopecia and Dermatitis

Psychogenic alopecia or dermatitis *(neurodermatitis)* is an alopecia or a chronic skin inflammation produced by constant licking. When dermatitis is not present, the complaint may be of excessive grooming.[6, 14] The dermatitic form results from more severe grooming.

CAUSE AND PATHOGENESIS

The primary abnormality is thought to be excessive grooming that may result from an anxiety neurosis. The anxiety may be caused by psychological factors such as displacement phenomena (e.g., a new pet or baby in the household, a move to new surroundings, boarding, hospitalization, loss of a favorite bed or companion, or competition for a social hierarchy position with other pets in the household or in response to other cats entering the affected cat's territory). There is a breed predilection for the more emotional breeds such as Siamese and Abyssinian.

Feline psychogenic alopecia and dermatitis may be expressed in many ways. Some cats lick vigorously at a particular area until the sharp barbs on the tongue produce alopecia, abrasion, ulceration, and secondary infection. Other cats lick and chew more gently or over a more widespread area, so alopecia is the predominant lesion. Some cats actually chew at their hair or skin, whereas others chew and pull their hair out.

It has been proposed that the stress may induce an elevation in the levels of adrenocorticotropin hormone and melanocyte-stimulating hormone, which then causes increased endorphin production.[22] The endorphins protect the animal from abnormalities associated with chronic stress. However, their narcotic, addictive-like effect may act to reinforce the abnormal grooming behavior.

CLINICAL FEATURES

Areas that the cat can lick easily are the most common sites: medial forelegs, the inside of the thigh, the caudal abdomen, and the inguinal region (Fig. 14:5; also see Fig. 14:1 *G*). Less

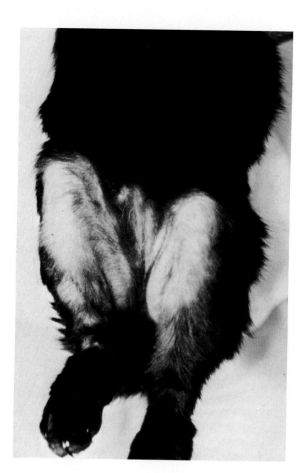

Figure 14:5. Feline psychogenic alopecia. Hair has been removed from the inguinal area by the cat's licking and biting.

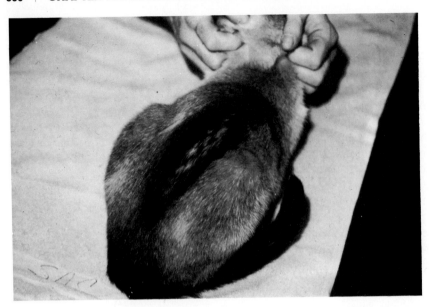

Figure 14:6. Constant licking removed hair from the back, reducing the skin temperature and causing the hair to grow in dark in color.

commonly, the dorsal lumbar, sacral, or tail regions may be involved. This pattern should raise one's index of suspicion about flea bite hypersensitivity. A symmetric alopecia may also involve the caudomedial thighs and ventrum. The characteristic lesion of the dermatitic form is a bright red, elongated, oval plaque or red streak (see Fig. 14:1 *H*). Eosinophilic plaques may result. Animals with chronic cases develop lichenification and hyperpigmentation. The course is long and progresses slowly, sometimes remaining static for months. Siamese or Siamese-cross cats often lick out the hair in a localized area of the back, the ventral abdomen, or a leg without causing a skin reaction. Because the temperature-labile enzymes that convert melanin precursors into melanin are active (high temperatures produce white hair, low temperatures produce pigmented hair, and the hairless area is cool), the hair becomes dark (Fig. 14:6). After the next shedding, the hair is usually replaced by normal-colored hair.

DIAGNOSIS

Lesions of the dermatitic form may be confused with or possibly develop into eosinophilic plaques. The alopecic forms may be confused with dermatophytosis, demodicosis, atopy, food or flea bite hypersensitivity, and feline acquired symmetric alopecia. Because cats are often reclusive groomers, owners may not know that the cat is licking or chewing excessively. Several helpful techniques are available to answer the question, "Does the cat groom excessively?" Tufts of hair may have been found in the cat's favorite hiding places. Alternatively, the cat may be vomiting hair balls, or hair may be visible in the feces. With cats that use litter boxes, the client can inspect the feces over the next several days and find that they contain hair. Physical examination reveals short stubby hairs that are readily palpated by rubbing the fingertips against the normal angle of hair growth. Another method is to roll the skin and view the folded skin perpendicularly to reveal numerous shorn off hairs. Placing an Elizabethan collar on the cat will result in hair growth in areas that cannot be groomed. This time-consuming procedure is rarely needed to establish excessive grooming as a cause of the hair loss. A simple laboratory test for differentiating between self-induced hair loss and spontaneous alopecia is the epilation and microscopic examination of hairs from the affected areas. In psychogenic alopecia, hairs do *not* epilate easily; they appear to be broken off when examined microscopically, and the hairs regrow while the cat is wearing an Elizabethan collar. In addition, cats that are fur-mowing as a result of a hypersensitivity often respond to an injection of methylprednisolone acetate, whereas cats with psychogenic disease do not.

Because feline psychogenic alopecia is diagnosed primarily by ruling out other differential diagnoses, an accurate diagnosis involves a complete work-up. Skin scrapings, fungal cultures, biopsies (which should show normal skin in nondermatitic areas), and a complete blood count constitute the minimal data base that should be obtained. If an eosinophilia is present or the biopsy reveals an inflammatory or endocrine appearance, the diagnosis of psychogenic alopecia is not warranted. Further tests should include hypoallergenic diet trials, trial ectoparasite therapy for *Cheyletiella* and *Otodectes,* intradermal allergen testing, and endocrine function testing. An initial alternative to the endocrine function test may be a 30-day trial with an Elizabethan collar. Cats that respond to liothyronine supplementation do not regrow their hair when grooming is prevented.[17]

CLINICAL MANAGEMENT

Many of the treatments for psychogenic dermatitis have potential side-effects, require frequent administration, and are expensive. Therefore, cats with the alopecic form of the disease may best be served by no treatment other than attempts at relieving the stressful situation.

Cats are such territorial creatures that a change in the pecking order of animals in the territory has tremendous anxiety potential. One needs to look for a new cat that entered the household or invaded the cat's territory. Other factors are barking dogs, a new baby, moving to a new home, or major changes in the present home. If these problems can be modified or removed, the cat may improve without any therapy or with just a 30-day course of antianxiety drugs to break the habit.

Topical medications are of little value because the cat immediately licks them off. The alopecic form may be successfully managed with phenobarbital (2.2 to 6.6 mg/kg q12h orally) or diazepam (total dose of 1 to 2 mg orally q12h to q24h). Some authors have reported occasional success with 12.5 to 25 mg primidone administered orally q8h to q24h.[6] Treatment with the endorphin blocker naloxone 1 mg/kg subcutaneously has been shown to have some efficacy, with one injection lasting up to several weeks.[22] If a thorough diagnostic work-up was not performed or if previous treatments proved ineffective, trial therapy with chlorpheniramine 2 mg/cat q12h or systemic glucocorticoids is warranted. A response may be seen in some cases of psychogenic alopecia; however, allergic dermatitis may also respond. Aggressive flea control may help in cats that are not intradermal test–positive to fleas. Whether this response to flea control reflects an undetected flea allergy or that the presence of fleas stresses the cat is unknown. In cases of dermatitis, if cytologic tests reveal intracellular bacteria, concurrent antibiotic therapy is indicated. Progestational compounds (a total dose of 2.5 to 5.0 mg megestrol acetate (Ovaban) administered orally every other day then weekly, or 100 mg medroxyprogesterone acetate (Depo-Provera) administered subcutaneously as needed) have also been recommended. Again, the side-effects of these drugs can be striking, so one must weigh the gravity of the disease against the possible drug toxicities.

Tail Sucking

Tail sucking occurs mostly in cats and specifically in Siamese cats. It is easily recognized by a wetness of the distal 2 to 3 cm of the tail. Close examination of the skin reveals normal skin without inflammation or scaling. Whenever the cat ceases to lick the tail and the hair dries, the condition can no longer be detected. Drying occurs when the cat's attention is focused on interesting activities; when bored, the cat resumes licking its tail. Treatment is not successful until the cat's boredom is relieved, possibly by changes in its lifestyle.

REFERENCES

1. Brignac, M.M.: Hydrocodone treatment of acral lick dermatitis. Proc. 2nd Wld. Cong. Vet. Dermatol. 2:50, 1992.
2. Dodman, N.H., et al.: Use of narcotic antagonists to modify stereotypic self-licking, self-chewing, and scratching behavior in dogs. J. Am. Vet. Med. Assoc. 193:815, 1988.
3. Goldberger, E., Rapoport, J.L.: Canine acral lick dermatitis: Response to the antiobsessional drug clomipramine. J. Am. Anim. Hosp. Assoc. 27:179, 1991.
4. Gross, T.L., Carr, S.H.: Amputation neuroma of docked tails in dogs. Vet. Pathol. 27:61, 1990.
5. Helton-Rhodes, K.: Bitter Apple: HEET combination topical therapy in the dog. Dermatol. Dialogue Spring/ Summer, 1993, p. 5.
6. Holzworth, J.: Diseases of the Cat: Medicine and Surgery, Vol. I. W.B. Saunders Co., Philadelphia, 1987.
6a. Koo, J.Y.M., Pham, C.T.: Psychodermatology. Practical guidelines in pharmacotherapy. Arch. Dermatol. 128:381, 1992.
7. MacDonald, J.M.: Personal communication, 1991.
8. Overall, K.L.: Recognition, diagnosis, and management of obsessive-compulsive disorders. Part 1: Canine Pract. 17:40, 1992.
8a. Overall, K.L.: Recognition, diagnosis, and management of obsessive-compulsive disorders. Part 2: A rational approach. Canine Pract. 17:25, 1992.
8b. Overall, K.L.: Recognition, diagnosis, and management of obsessive-compulsive disorders. Part 3: A rational approach. Canine Pract. 17:39, 1992.
9. Owen, L.N.: Canine lick granuloma treated with radiotherapy. J. Small Anim. Pract. 30:454, 1989.
10. Panconesi, E.: Stress and skin diseases: Psychosomatic dermatology. Clin. Dermatol. 2:4, 1984.
11. Pemberton, P.L.: Canine and feline behavior control: Progestin therapy. In: Kirk, R.W. (ed.): Current Veterinary Therapy VIII. W.B. Saunders Co., Philadelphia, 1983, p. 62.
12. Rapoport, J.L., et al: Drug treatment of canine acral lick: An animal model of obsessive-compulsive disorder. Arch. Gen. Psychiatr. 49:517, 1992.
12a. Rivers, B., et al.: Treatment of canine acral lick dermatitis with radiation therapy: 17 cases (1979–1991). J. Am. Anim. Hosp. Assoc. 29:541, 1993.
13. Russell, M., et al.: Learned histamine release. Science 225:733, 1984.
14. Scott, D.W.: Feline dermatology 1900–1978: A monograph. J. Am. Anim. Hosp. Assoc. 16:331, 1980.
15. Scott, D.W., Walton, D.K.: Clinical evaluation of a topical treatment for canine acral lick dermatitis. J. Am. Anim. Hosp. Assoc. 20:562, 1984.
16. Shoulberg, N.: The efficacy of fluoxetine (Prozac) in the treatment of acral lick and allergic-inhalant dermatitis in canines. Proc. Annu. Memb. Meet. AAVD and ACVD 6:31, 1990.
17. Thoday, K.L.: Aspects of feline symmetric alopecia. In: von Tscharner, C., Halliwell, R.E.W. (eds.). Advances in Veterinary Dermatology I. Baillère Tindall, London, 1990, p. 47.
18. van Nes, J.J.: Electrophysiological evidence of sensory nerve dysfunction in 10 dogs with acral lick dermatitis. J. Am. Anim. Hosp. Assoc. 22:157, 1986.
19. Voith, V.L.: Behavioral disorders. In: Davis, L.E. (ed.). Handbook of Small Animal Therapeutics. Churchill Livingstone, New York, 1985, p. 519.
20. Walton, D.K.: Psychodermatoses. In: Kirk, R.W. (ed.). Current Veterinary Therapy IX. W.B. Saunders Co., Philadelphia, 1986, p. 557.
21. White, S.D.: Naltrexone for treatment of acral lick dermatitis in dogs. J. Am. Vet. Med. Assoc. 196:1075, 1990.
22. Willemse, T., et al: Feline psychogenic alopecia and the role of the opioid system. In: von Tscharner, C., Halliwell, R.E.W. (eds.). Advances in Veterinary Dermatology I. Baillère Tindall, London, 1990, p. 195.

Environmental Skin Diseases

■

Chapter Outline

■ PHOTODERMATITIS

Electromagnetic radiation comprises a continuous spectrum of wavelengths varying from fractions of angstroms to thousands of meters. The ultraviolet (UV) spectrum is of particular importance in dermatology.[13] UVC (less than 290 nm) is damaging to cells and does not typically reach the earth's surface because of the ozone layer. UVB (290 to 320 nm) is often referred to as the sunburn, or erythema, spectrum and is about 1000 times more erythemogenic than UVA. UVA (320 to 400 nm) is the spectrum associated with photosensitivity reactions.

Incident ultraviolet light (UVL) is partially reflected, absorbed, and transmitted inward. Absorbed light raises the energy level of light-absorbing molecules (chromophores), resulting in various biochemical processes that can damage virtually any component of a cell. This damage can result in cellular hyperproliferation, mutagenesis, alteration of cell surface markers, and toxicity. Chromophores in the skin include keratin proteins, blood, hemoglobin, porphyrin, carotene, nucleic acids, melanin, lipoproteins, peptide bonds, and aromatic amino acids, such as tyrosine, tryptophan, and histidine.[27a] Natural barriers to UVL damage include the stratum corneum, melanin, blood, and carotenes. These barriers can easily be overcome by prolonged, repeated exposure to sunlight.

Photodermatology is an ever-expanding field in human medicine and includes photodynamic mechanisms and various specific diseases not recognized in veterinary medicine.[13, 27b] Phototoxicity and photosensitivity are of primary concern to veterinary clinicians.[46] *Phototoxicity* is the classic sunburn reaction and is a dose-related response to light exposure. *Photosensitivity* occurs when the skin has increased susceptibility to the damaging effects of UVL because of the production, ingestion, and injection of or contact with a photodynamic agent. Photosensitivity is most important in farm animals, but cases are recognized in dogs.[11, 19]

■ SOLAR DERMATITIS

Solar dermatitis occurs from an actinic reaction on white skin, light skin, or damaged skin (e.g., depigmented or scarred areas) that is not sufficiently covered by hair.[14a, 46] The condition develops when such skin is exposed to direct or reflected sunshine. The rapidity of onset and the severity of the reaction depend on various factors related to the animal, the duration of sun exposure, and the intensity of the sunlight. The sun's rays are most intense during the summer months from 9 AM to 3 PM but especially from 11 AM to 2 PM. Altitude influences solar intensity. For every 300 m (1000 ft) increase in elevation, the sun's intensity increases by 4 per cent.[13] The dermatitis is purely a phototoxic reaction (sunburn) and has no apparent relationship to a hypersensitivity state. The pathogenesis of phototoxicity is incompletely understood, but it involves the epidermis and blood vessels of the superficial and deeper vascular plexus. Exposure to UVB and UVC results in the formation of clusters of vacuolated keratinocytes in the superficial epidermis (so-called sunburn cells), as well as dyskeratotic keratinocytes, vascular dilatation and leakage, and depletion of mast cells with an increase in tissue levels of histamine, prostaglandins, leukotrienes, other vasoactive compounds, inflammatory cytokines, adhesion molecules, and reactive oxygen species.[13, 18a, 24a] These latter changes could be the direct result of the UVB or could be mediated by cytokines released by the epidermal cells. Solar dermatitis in companion animals is divided into canine nasal solar dermatitis, feline solar dermatitis, and canine solar dermatitis of the trunk and extremities. The nasal and feline forms are the most common entities and therefore are discussed in the greatest detail.

Canine Nasal Solar Dermatitis

Canine nasal solar dermatitis is an actinic reaction in poorly pigmented nasal skin of dogs.[14a, 21, 37, 46]

CAUSE AND PATHOGENESIS

This is a phototoxic reaction occurring in poorly pigmented skin. Affected dogs may be born without pigment, or the nose may have undergone spontaneous noninflammatory depigmentation (see Chap. 12). Australian shepherds appear to be at increased risk.[34, 46] Any dog with an active or resolved traumatic or inflammatory condition that causes hair loss, depigmentation, or scarring of the nasal area is also susceptible to this photodermatitis. The condition is more frequently seen in sunny climates.

CLINICAL FEATURES

The lesions are found principally at the junction of the haired and hairless skin of the nose (Fig. 15:1 *A*), but any area on the nasal planum or the face can be affected if it is sparsely haired and lightly pigmented. Initially, the area that was devoid of pigment becomes erythematous and scaly. If sun exposure continues, perilesional hair loss occurs, with resultant involvement of the newly exposed skin. Exudation and crusting follow and ulceration may be seen, especially if the dog rubs the area. If intense photoprotection is started early, the area can heal completely. In most cases, these measures are adopted too late, and the lesion heals by scarring. The healed area is larger than the original lesion, and the scarred skin is more susceptible to solar and traumatic damage. Progression and enlargement of the lesions are evident with the passage of each year but are especially rapid during periods of prolonged exposure to intense sunlight. This usually occurs during the summer months but may be seen during the winter as a result of reflection from snow. In chronic cases, deep ulcers form and tissues of the nares and nasal tip disappear, exposing unsightly nasal tissues that bleed easily. Sometimes, vertical fissures occur at the nasal tip, dorsal to and involving the nares. After they are established, these fissures are often permanent. Although rare, squamous cell carcinomas can occur.

DIAGNOSIS

The diagnosis of nasal solar dermatitis can be straightforward or complicated, depending on the chronicity of the condition. The key features of the diagnosis are the restriction of lesions to sun-exposed, nonpigmented, sparsely haired skin; the onset of signs after solar exposure; the absence of skin lesions in the affected area before the current condition began; and the complete or near-complete resolution of the lesions with removal from sunlight. In early cases, the affected area is red and scaly, but the architecture should be normal and adjacent areas of black skin should be perfectly normal. If all of the above are true, the diagnosis of solar dermatitis is warranted.

Because of the scarring nature of solar dermatitis, the diagnosis of chronic cases is more problematic. These cases start with abnormal skin from previously unrecognized or unreported episodes and do not heal completely with strict photoisolation. The basic quandary here is whether the dog has chronic solar dermatitis or some other nasal skin disease with a secondary photodermatitis. If the animal has identical lesions in areas not exposed to sun or lesions that are heavily pigmented, the latter case is true. However, many dogs with underlying disease have lesions restricted to the face.

The list of facial dermatoses (those that start on, remain confined to, or have their most pronounced lesions on the face) is extensive. The ones germane to this discussion are discoid lupus erythematosus, systemic lupus erythematosus, dermatomyositis and epidermolysis bullosa, pemphigus foliaceus, pemphigus erythematosus, drug reaction, and infectious folliculitis and furunculosis due to bacterial, dermatophyte, yeast, or leishmanial infection. Except for discoid lupus erythematosus (see Chap. 8), which tends to start on and remain restricted to the perinasal area, these diseases tend to start in the haired skin on the bridge of the nose and work

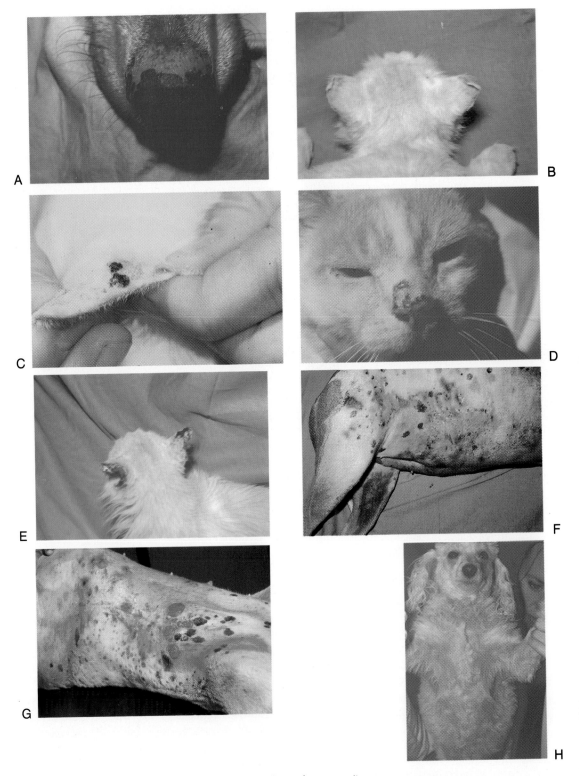

Figure 15:1 *See legend on opposite page*

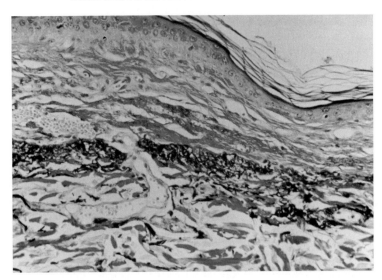

Figure 15:2. Solar elastosis. Degeneration of elastin fibers. (Courtesy A. Hargis.)

toward the nasal planum. They also tend to involve the pinnae and the mucocutaneous junctions and have no predilection for nonpigmented skin. When the nasal planum is extensively ulcerated, fissured, and friable, vasculitis, neoplasia (especially basal cell tumors, squamous cell carcinomas, fibrosarcomas, and lymphomas), and granulomatous diseases (especially sterile pyogranuloma syndrome) must be considered.

The diagnosis of solar dermatitis is confirmed by biopsy. The early depigmented areas of the nose show fewer melanocytes and less melanin pigment than are seen in normal skin. After exposure to solar radiation, epidermal hyperplasia with intraepidermal edema is observed. Vacuolated (sunburn cells) and dyskeratotic keratinocytes may be seen. Perivascular accumulations of inflammatory cells are seen in the upper dermis, and vascular dilatation is noted in the lower dermis. Solar elastosis (basophilic degeneration of elastin) may or may not be seen (Fig. 15:2).[14a] Ulceration can cause disappearance of the epidermis and even of the dermis and underlying cartilages. In rare advanced cases, activity in the cells of the basal layer is increased, and large, polyhedral tumor cells that invade the dermis and subcutaneous tissue are formed. A squamous cell carcinoma forms, and cords of neoplastic cells invade the tissue to the level of the nasal cartilage.

CLINICAL MANAGEMENT

After the diagnosis is confirmed, the pre-existing lesions must be treated, and most importantly, new lesions must be prevented. In early cases, photoprotection allows the lesions to heal spontaneously. In more advanced cases, corticosteroids are necessary to decrease the inflammation. Although topical products are most beneficial, many dogs resent their thorough application, and thus the oral route is commonly used. Prednisolone (1.1 mg/kg q24h) administered

Figure 15:1. *A*, Nasal solar dermatitis. Note sharp margin of erythematous, sunburned depigmented area. Negative direct immunofluorescent test. *B*, Feline solar dermatitis. Sunburned erythematous margins of the pinnae precede the more serious stage of the disease. Note the characteristic curling of the tips. *C*, Actinic keratoses on the pinnal margin. *D*, Actinic keratoses on the nasal area. *E*, This 14-year-old cat had the disease for several years until a squamous cell carcinoma developed on both ears. *F*, Truncal solar dermatitis. Squamous cell carcinoma has developed on the posterior abdomen of sun-loving brown and white Staffordshire terrier. *G*, Close-up of the same dog as in *F*. *H*, Contact dermatitis due to a carpet deodorizer.

for 7 to 10 days should be sufficient. If the lesions shows cytologic evidence of bacterial infection, antibiotics should be administered.

Avoidance of direct or reflected sunlight is paramount, especially in chronic cases in which solar sensitivity is extreme.[46] During the summer, the most dangerous photoperiod is from 9 AM to 3 PM, with the peak from 11 AM to 2 PM. Affected dogs should be kept indoors or in the shade during these times. When indoors, the dog can sunbathe beneath a closed window because glass effectively filters UVB, but open windows or doors defeat the purpose of the animal's being kept indoors.[13] Reflections from white concrete sidewalks or run flooring must also be avoided.

Strict photoisolation is usually impossible, and sunblocks or sunscreens can allow some sun exposure.[13] Sunblocks are opaque agents that reflect and scatter incident light. White or colored zinc oxide preparations are most commonly used in humans and may be of benefit in dogs that do not lick the area. Most clients prefer sunscreens that are clear and absorb incident light. Most products absorb only UVB, but some agents contain ingredients to screen UVA as well. Various formulations are available for individuals sensitive to para-aminobenzoic acid, the most common ingredient in sunscreens. Waterproof products with a sun protective factor (SPF) of 15 or higher should be used.[46] For maximal efficacy, the product should be applied and gently rubbed into the area 15 to 30 minutes before sun exposure. When solar exposure is unpredictable, the sunscreen should be applied twice daily on a regular basis.[46]

The addition of artificial pigmentation to the area can be beneficial but does not negate the need for other measures, as black skin can still absorb some sunlight. Black ink can be applied to the skin's surface with felt-tipped markers or by a cotton-tipped applicator (Q-tip) with permanent laundry or stamp pad ink. Markers are easiest to use, but the solvents can be irritating. Permanent coloring can be achieved by tattooing.[21, 41] Tattooing was popular, but poor early results, the expense of the equipment, the need for multiple treatments under general anesthesia, and rare adverse reactions to the tattoo ink[35] have limited its use. Most of the early treatment failures were because skin with an active immune-mediated disorder (e.g., discoid lupus erythematosus) and not true solar dermatitis was tattooed. Tattooing should be considered when other photoprotection measures are ineffective.

Although some benefit may be seen with the administration of β-carotene,[32] treatment with systemic agents usually is unrewarding. Preliminary work has shown that topically applied vitamin C can help protect pig skin against UVL damage when the vitamin C is applied after irradiation.[8] This treatment or the oral administration of vitamin C may or may not be beneficial in dogs.

When the solar dermatitis progresses to an actinic keratosis or squamous cell carcinoma or results in massive tissue destruction, treatments with retinoic acids, hyperthermia, cryosurgery, surgical excision, photochemotherapy, or radiotherapy may be of some benefit, but efficacy data are limited.[46] Patients requiring these treatments have a poor prognosis.

Feline Solar Dermatitis

Feline solar dermatitis is a chronic actinic dermatitis of the white ears and, occasionally, the eyelids, the nose, and the lips of cats, which is caused by repeated sun exposure.[37, 46, 51] It can develop into an actinic keratosis or true squamous cell carcinoma.

CAUSE AND PATHOGENESIS

The disease occurs in white cats or in colored cats with white-haired areas on the face or ears. Blue-eyed white cats are most susceptible. Actinic damage to the ear tip occurs from repeated exposure to UVB light. Early lesions are often ignored or unrecognized, but the damage done makes the area more susceptible to further actinic insults. The disease occurs mostly in warm, sunny climates such as those of California, Florida, Hawaii, Australia, and South Africa. Sixteen cats with solar dermatitis were examined for heme biosynthesis abnormalities, but none were demonstrated.[22]

CLINICAL FEATURES

The earliest sign is erythema and fine scaling of the margin of the pinna. The hair is lost in this area, making it even more accessible to solar radiation. There is almost no discomfort to the cat at this stage. In susceptible cats, the first lesions can occur as early as 3 months of age. Lesions become progressively more severe each summer. The advancing lesions consist of severe erythema of the pinna, peeling of the skin, and formation of marginal crusts (see Fig. 15:1 *B*). At this stage many cats show pain and further damage their ears by scratching. The margins of the pinnae may be curled. The margins of the lower eyelids, nose, and lips may be affected, especially in white, blue-eyed cats. An actinic keratosis or invasive squamous cell carcinoma can develop in some cases on the ears, the nose, or other areas (see Fig. 15:1 *C* and *D*). Carcinomatous change may occur, usually after 6 years of age, but sometimes as early as 3 years. The squamous cell carcinoma appears as an ulcerating, hemorrhagic, and locally invasive lesion. It is partially crusted and, in advanced cases, destroys the pinna (see Fig. 15:1 *E*).

DIAGNOSIS

A tentative diagnosis of feline solar dermatitis can be made from the clinical appearance, the color of the cat, and the history. As in the dog, the question remains as to whether the cat has a primary or secondary solar dermatitis. For pinnal lesions, the primary differential diagnostic considerations include dermatophytosis, early notoedric mange, fight wounds, vasculitis, and possibly frostbite or cold agglutinin disease. Discoid or systemic lupus erythematosus and pemphigus erythematosus or foliaceus may have to be considered. The differential diagnostic possibilities are excluded by skin biopsy, which also detects dysplastic or neoplastic changes.

Histopathologic study shows that, in the early stages, superficial perivascular dermatitis (spongiotic, hyperplastic changes) is present. Vacuolated (sunburn cells) or dyskeratotic keratinocytes may be seen. Solar elastosis may be noted in the superficial dermal connective tissue. With the formation of squamous cell carcinoma, the epidermal surface is ulcerated and the dermis is invaded by nests of polyhedral epithelial tumor cells. In a disorganized manner, these cells resemble the stratum spinosum. Their nuclei vary moderately in size, and mitotic figures are frequent. In advanced cases, the masses of tumor tissue extend to the level of the cartilage.

CLINICAL MANAGEMENT

Affected cats should be kept indoors from 9 AM to 3 PM and should not be allowed to sunbathe by open doors or windows. During the summer, the ears should be protected with a waterproof sunscreen. β-Carotene and canthaxanthin (25-mg doses of active carotenoids) are administered orally to treat feline solar dermatitis.[22] Only the most severely affected cats fail to respond. Carotenoids are thought to quench the triplet state of singlet oxygen and free radicals and possibly to form a lipid-carotene complex in skin that absorbs the damaging solar radiation.

After early irreversible lesions develop, serious consideration should be given to a cosmetic amputation of the ear tips. This merely rounds off the ears, removes the thinly haired tips, and allows hair to cover and protect the pinna. Results are usually excellent, cosmetically and prophylactically. Photoprotection is necessary to prevent new lesions.

Cats with actinic keratoses who are not candidates for surgery may benefit from treatment with retinoic acids. Although isotretinoin at 3 mg/kg was ineffective,[9] more recent studies with etretinate (10 mg per cat q24h) have shown some promise.[43] If the etretinate is ineffective, superficial irradiation (plesiotherapy) with a hand-held strontium probe can be beneficial.[33] If all of the above fail or the cat has advanced disease at presentation, radical amputation of the pinna is necessary.

Canine Solar Dermatitis of the Trunk and Extremities

Although the nose and the ears are the areas most exposed and are therefore most susceptible to actinic damage, other regions of the body can also be affected. A combination of factors is necessary for sun damage to occur. First, the skin must be unpigmented or poorly pigmented. Second, only a sparse haircoat covers the skin, allowing the ultraviolet rays of the sun to reach the epidermis. Third, the areas so predisposed must be regularly and frequently exposed to the sun. This occurs in dogs that like to sunbathe or that are confined to areas where no sun shelter is available during the middle of the day, especially if the ground cover is highly reflective. As is true of the other types of solar dermatitis, the chance of actinic disease is increased in sunny climates.

Breeds predisposed to truncal solar dermatitis include the Dalmatian, American Staffordshire terrier, German shorthaired pointers, white boxers, whippets, beagles, and white bull terriers.[32, 37, 46] There are multiple reports of photosensitization in dogs in which affected animals had ulcerative and necrotic skin lesions in white-haired, sun-exposed skin.[12, 19] The onset of signs was sudden, and the affected areas were heavily haired so photosensitization was more likely than phototoxicity. The sensitizing agent in these cases was not identified.

The flank and the abdomen are the areas most severely affected (Fig. 15:1 *F* and *G*). In dogs who sunbathe in right or left lateral recumbency, the flanks and the ventrolateral abdomen are most commonly affected, but lesions can be seen on the nose, the ears, the tail tip, or the distal limbs. Dogs that sunbathe on their back or that are caged on wire above white concrete can have the entire ventrum involved. At first, regular sunburning occurs and the affected areas are erythematous and scaly. Running a hand over affected areas of skin may produce a bumpy feeling, as the white areas of skin are thickened, whereas the black areas are normal. At this stage, biopsy reveals variable degrees of superficial perivascular dermatitis with necrotic keratinocytes. Superficial dermal fibrosis may be prominent. Solar elastosis may be seen (see Fig. 15:2).

After two summers or more, the sunburned areas become thicker and develop erosion, ulceration, crusting, and comedones, and they occasionally develop necrosis, fistulae, and scarring. At this stage, a skin biopsy may reveal follicular cysts, pyogranulomatous inflammation, and premalignant actinic keratosis. Finally, a squamous cell carcinoma can develop, especially if the dog continues to be exposed to direct sunlight. Such squamous cell carcinomas should be removed surgically, and the procedure should be repeated if necessary. There is always a danger of metastasis to the regional lymph nodes and internal structures. Skin with solar damage is also more likely to develop a hemangioma or hemangiosarcoma.[46]

Therapy involves photoprotection by keeping the animal out of the sun and by using topical sunscreens if practical. It has been reported that β-carotene (30 mg orally q12h for 30 days, then q24h for life), in combination with anti-inflammatory doses of prednisone or prednisolone, is effective in early cases.[32] Etretinate at 1 mg/kg every 24 hours or divided every 12 hours is effective when dysplastic change has occurred.[43]

Actinic Keratosis

Actinic keratoses may be seen in dogs and cats and are premalignant epithelial dysplasias (see Chap. 19).

Miscellaneous Effects of Solar Exposure

Exposure to UVL is an important factor in precipitating or potentiating a number of skin lesions and may also exacerbate generalized systemic disease activity.[27a, 27b] Although the role of UVL is clearly defined in some conditions, its pathogenic role in other disorders is less well understood. For example, UVL exposure may induce or exacerbate the lesions of discoid lupus erythematosus, systemic lupus erythematosus, pemphigus (especially pemphigus erythematosus), and pemphigoid (see Chap. 8).

In addition, UVL exposure of skin has important local and systemic immunologic consequences (photoimmunologic changes).[27a] For example, exposure to UVB or UVA changes Langerhans' cell morphologic features and function and influences cutaneous cytokine production. Impaired antigen recognition and processing and impaired immune responses may influence susceptibility to cutaneous neoplasms and infections. The damaging effects on cutaneous immunity of low-dose UVB are genetically determined in mice.[53a] This UVB susceptibility is mediated almost exclusively by tumor necrosis factor-α (TNF-α), and the trait appears to be a risk factor for the development of squamous cell carcinoma and basal cell carcinoma.

■ IRRITANT CONTACT DERMATITIS

Contact dermatitis is an inflammatory skin reaction caused by direct contact with an offending substance.[13, 36, 37]

CAUSE AND PATHOGENESIS

The disease is divided into two types: primary irritant contact dermatitis and contact hypersensitivity (see Chap. 8).

Primary irritant contact dermatitis causes cutaneous inflammation in most exposed dogs and cats without any antecedent period of sensitization. The rapidity of onset and the intensity of the reaction depend on the nature of the contactant, its concentration, and the duration of the contact. Corrosive substances such as strong acids and alkalies injure the skin immediately and produce lesions of varying severity. Severe reactions should be classified as chemical burns. Less potent contactants need prolonged or repeated contact to produce irritation. A number of primary irritants such as soaps, detergents, disinfectants, hair-coloring agents, weed and insecticidal sprays, fertilizers, strong acids and alkalies, and flea collars are potential causative agents.[1, 2, 36, 37] Although most primary irritants are chemicals, similar skin lesions can be produced by thermal injuries, solar overexposure, and contact with living organisms.

CLINICAL FEATURES

Environmental irritants such as fertilizers and carpet cleaners typically produce dermatitis in areas where the haircoat is thin or missing. The abdomen, the chest, the axillae, the flanks, the interdigital spaces, the legs, the perianal area, and the ventral surface of the tail are the most susceptible areas (Fig. 15:3 *A* and *B*; also see Fig. 15:1 *H*). When the offending agent is a liquid (e.g., shampoo and flea dip solution) or a topical medication (Fig. 15:3 *C*) or is bound to a collar (Fig. 15:3 *D* and *E*), the reaction occurs where the substance touches the skin. Licking of the contactant can cause oral lesions (Fig. 15:3 *F*) and spread the agent to other areas of the body.

Patches of erythema and papules represent primary lesions (Fig. 15:3 *A*). Vesicles are rarely present in dogs and cats (Fig. 15:3 *C*). As the disease progresses, crusts, excoriations, hyperpigmentation, and lichenification occur. Intense pruritus may promote severe scratching and biting. Pyotraumatic dermatitis and eventual ulceration may obliterate primary lesions.

Single episodes are common in primary irritant contact dermatitis, as in scrotal involvement from soap that is not rinsed off (Fig. 15:3 *G*). Seasonal recurrence results from exposure to plants, lawn fertilizer, herbicides, and ice-melting substances.

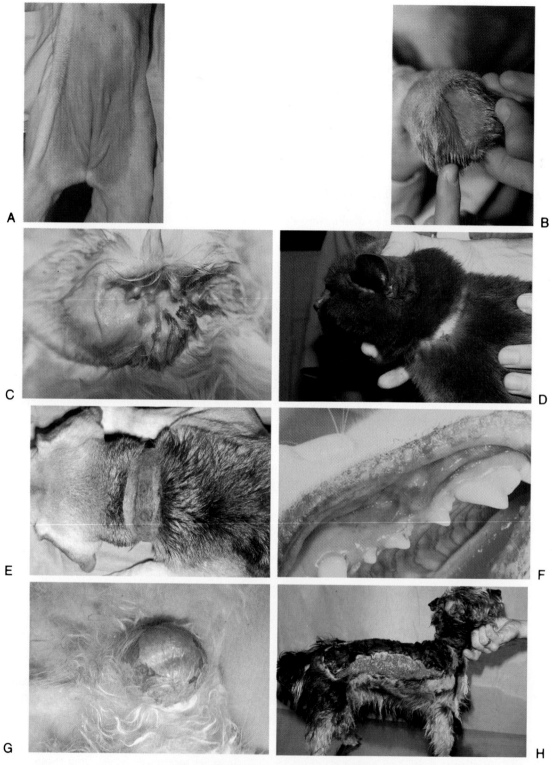

Figure 15:3 *See legend on opposite page*

DIAGNOSIS

The tentative diagnosis of contact dermatitis is based on historical and physical findings. If multiple animals in a household are affected, primary irritant contact dermatitis is much more likely than contact hypersensitivity. When the contactant is harsh and produces immediate reactions or is applied intentionally (e.g., medication), the diagnosis is straightforward. With low-grade environmental contactants, identification is more difficult, and atopy, food hypersensitivity, drug hypersensitivity, *Malassezia* dermatitis, and early scabies must be considered.

In most clinical cases, the histopathologic changes of primary irritant contact dermatitis consist of nondiagnostic superficial perivascular dermatitis (spongiotic, hyperplastic changes). The exact appearance depends on the stage of contact dermatitis and the effects of secondary infection and excoriation. Neutrophils or mononuclear cells may predominate in a given case.

The confirmation of irritant contact dermatitis can be made by provocative exposure testing, in which the agent is applied to normal and diseased skin. With low-grade irritants, one application to normal skin may not be sufficient to cause irritation so diseased skin should also be challenged. With harsh irritants, which cause ulceration and necrosis, provocative exposure testing should be avoided. Patch testing is of unproven value in the diagnosis of irritant contact dermatitis.

CLINICAL MANAGEMENT

The difficult task of discovering and eliminating offending substances depends on the correlation of a detailed history and a careful examination of the environment of the dog. Soap, flea collars, grasses, pollens, insecticides, petrolatum, paint, wool, carpets, rubber, and wood preservatives are examples of contact irritants. If the location of the initial inflammation can be correlated with an agent that came in contact with that area, the cause can sometimes be found. With removal of the irritant, the lesions should heal spontaneously. For pruritic patients, a 5- to 7-day course of prednisolone (1.1 mg/kg q24h) can be beneficial.

When the contactant cannot be found, relief depends on systemic and topical therapy. The involved areas should be bathed frequently with plain water or a mild, nonirritating shampoo. Drying must be complete, as macerated tissue is more susceptible to the irritant. For localized lesions, topical corticosteroids may be beneficial in controlling the inflammation. For animals with widespread lesions, repeated 7- to 10-day courses or alternate-day administration of oral steroids is necessary.

■ BURNS

Superficial and deep burns are painful, often produce scarring, and are an important cause of sepsis. Burn management is long and arduous.

CAUSE AND PATHOGENESIS

Burns can be caused by strong chemicals, electric currents, solar and microwave radiation, and heat.[2, 7, 37, 44, 47, 54] Most cases in small animals are caused by heat from fires, boiling liquids, electric heating pads, animal driers, and hot metals (e.g., mufflers and wood stoves). The length of exposure and the temperature of the heat source are key in determining the extent of the

---

Figure 15:3. *A*, Contact dermatitis due to a floor cleaner. *B*, Contact dermatitis caused by a caustic cage cleaner. *C*, Acute vesicular eruption due to an ear medication. *D*, Contact dermatitis caused by a leather collar. *E*, Acute erythema and erosion due to flea collar dermatitis. *F*, Cheilitis and gingivitis due to contact with a lawn fertilizer. *G*, Irritant contact dermatitis affecting the delicate scrotal skin. *H*, Full-thickness thermal burn in a Silky terrier, with sloughing and infection.

burn. In pigs, water at 44°C (111.2°F) needed 6 hours of contact to cause a burn, whereas temperatures of 70°C (158°F) or greater caused transepidermal necrosis in less than 1 second.[54] The temperature of flames, boiling liquids, and common hot metal sources greatly exceeds 70°C (158°F), and burns occur instantaneously with exposure.

Electric heating pads are a common unexpected cause of burns in small animals. Heat output can vary from pad to pad and can fluctuate during use. At the lowest setting, temperatures as high as 44°C (111.2°F) can be achieved, whereas temperatures of 56°C (132.8°F) can be obtained at the medium setting.[54] The burn potential of these pads is modified by the padding surrounding the unit, the nature of the animal's coat, and several other factors, but, clearly, animals kept on these pads for prolonged periods are at great risk.

Burns of dogs and cats have been categorized into two types: partial-thickness burns and full-thickness burns.[37] *Partial-thickness burns* involve the epidermis and the superficial dermis. Healing of the burned area can be complete with little or no scarring because of re-epithelialization from the hair follicles and sebaceous glands.[13] In *full-thickness burns*, there is complete destruction of all cutaneous structures. Without surgical intervention, healing occurs via second intention with extensive scarring.

The cause of the burn and the percentage of body involvement has great impact on the patient's survival. Patients burned by fire are at great risk for damage to the respiratory tract, and chemicals can burn the mouth or other tissues if spread by licking or careless handling by the owner.[47] Heat causes capillary leakage at and distant to the burn site. Patients with large burns experience fluid and electrolyte imbalances and can die rapidly if not treated appropriately.[13, 47]

Loss of the skin as a protective barrier opens the underlying tissue to invasive infection. Although microcirculation is restored within 48 hours to areas of partial-thickness injury, the full-thickness burn is characterized by complete occlusion of the local vascular supply. The avascular, necrotic tissue of the full-thickness burn, with impaired delivery of humoral and cellular defense mechanisms, provides an excellent medium for bacterial proliferation, with the ever-present potential for life-threatening sepsis. Initial colonization of the burn wound surface by gram-positive organisms shifts by the third to fifth day after the burn to an invasive gram-negative flora (especially *Pseudomonas aeruginosa*).

CLINICAL FEATURES

Burns caused by fire or contact with hot metal are obvious from the outset but may not reach their full extent for 24 to 48 hours. Burns from microwave radiation, electric currents, chemicals, and electric heating pads or cage driers can be more insidious, as the haircoat may hide the trauma and the owner may be aware of only the animal's apparent pain and its accompanying behavioral changes.[7, 44, 54] When the animal is presented for treatment of skin burned by heating pads or cage driers, the affected skin is usually hard and dry. Chemical, electric, or microwave burns are erosive to necrotic in nature.[2, 7, 44] These burns may also not be maximally expressed for an additional 24 to 48 hours. Infection causes a purulent discharge and sometimes an unpleasant odor. Large areas of necrotic skin may slough and reveal a deep, suppurating wound (see Fig. 15:3 *H*). If the skin is debrided and sutured, temporary closure may be achieved. However, the sutured area almost always sloughs, leaving a large, raw surface.

If 25 per cent of the body is involved in the burn, there are usually systemic manifestations, including septicemia, shock, renal failure, and anemia.[14, 47]

DIAGNOSIS

The diagnosis is straightforward if the client has observed the accidental burning. If the burn was not observed or was malicious, the diagnosis can be more difficult, especially if the burn is superficial. The histologic findings of a gradually tapering coagulation necrosis of the epidermis and deeper tissues confirm a thermal or chemical burn. With microwave burns, there is full-thickness coagulation necrosis.[44] Electric burns may show a diagnostic histologic feature of a fringe of elongated, degenerated cytoplasmic processes that protrudes from the lower end of the detached basal cells into the space separating the epidermis and the dermis. The nuclei of the basal cells and often of the higher-lying epidermal cells appear stretched in the same direction as the fringe of cytoplasmic processes. This gives the image of keratinocytes that are "standing at attention."

CLINICAL MANAGEMENT

For minor and major burns, the initial wound management, after evaluation and stabilization as needed, is the same.[14, 37, 47] For extensive burns, prompt attention to the patient's fluid and electrolyte balance is crucial for survival. Patients with chemical burns should be bathed when possible to remove any residual agent. After the patient is stabilized, wound management can begin. The best treatment of burns is the prompt surgical excision of the diseased tissue with sutured wound closure. Except for small burns, this is impractical in pets. Regardless of the location or the depth of the wound, removal of all debris, loose skin, and necrotic tissue is imperative. The wound is thoroughly cleaned with povidone-iodine or some other suitable antiseptic cleaner and debrided as needed. Daily hydrotherapy is used for complete cleaning of all burn wounds. Suturing is seldom necessary, because the sutured area almost always sloughs. After all burn wounds have been adequately cleaned and debrided, local care consists of the application of topical antimicrobial agents. Occlusive burn wound dressings are avoided because of their tendency to produce a closed wound with bacterial proliferation and to delay healing. Nonocclusive dressings, changed frequently, can be useful in certain cases. The wound should be cleaned two or three times daily and the topical product should be reapplied.

In human patients with burns, a 0.5 per cent silver nitrate solution, silver sulfadiazine, mafenide acetate (Sulfamylon) cream, and iodophors receive wide use.[13] The silver nitrate solution is used as a wet dressing and is considered effective. Because most veterinary patients do not tolerate wet dressings, silver sulfadiazine is probably the most commonly used burn cream.[34, 37] It is nonstaining, painless, and has fair penetration of an eschar. Practioners report excellent results with mupirocin ointment (Bactoderm [SmithKline Beecham]).[34] The technical information on this product warns of nephrotoxicity due to absorption of the polyethylene glycol in the base. Treatment of large deep burns could result in renal failure. Systemic antibiotics are not effective in preventing burn wound infection and may allow invasion by resistant organisms.

Burn healing is slow, with weeks to months of treatment. Most burns that receive veterinary attention are full-thickness and heal hairless with scarring (Fig. 15:4 A). In some cases, the scarring impedes function and various plastic surgical procedures must be performed. After all these obstacles are overcome, most patients lead a normal life. Because the scarred skin is hairless and often nonpigmented, solar exposure should be limited. Burn scar malignancies have been reported in dogs, so the areas should be examined periodically.[15]

■ FROSTBITE

CAUSE AND PATHOGENESIS

Frostbite is an uncommon condition in healthy animals who have been acclimatized to the cold. Ill animals or those that have recently moved from a warm climate to a cold one are more susceptible. Frostbite is due to prolonged exposure to freezing temperatures or contact with frozen metal objects. The lower the temperature is, the greater the risk. Lack of shelter, blowing wind, and wetting decrease the amount of exposure time necessary for frostbite to develop.

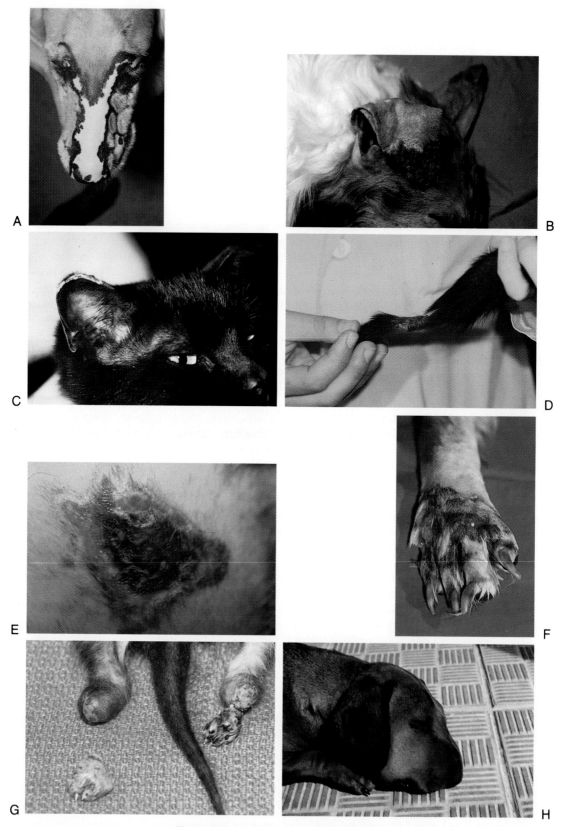

Figure 15:4 *See legend on opposite page*

CLINICAL FEATURES

Frostbite typically affects the tips of the ears, the digits, the scrotum, and the tail tip because these areas are not well insulated by hair and the blood vessels are not well protected.[37, 51] While frozen, the skin appears pale and is hypoesthetic and cool to the touch. After thawing, there may be mild erythema, edema, pain, and eventual scaliness of the skin. In mild cases, the hair of affected areas may turn white. Later, the tips and margins of the pinnae may curl. In severe cases, the skin becomes necrotic and sloughs (Fig. 15:4 *B* to *D*). Healing proceeds slowly; but if the tips of the ears are lost, the remaining pinna of the ear has a rounded contour that is usually so cosmetically acceptable as to be unnoticed. Often, the lesions look similar to burns.

CLINICAL MANAGEMENT

One should rapidly thaw frozen tissues by the *gentle* application of warm water.[13] *Tissues must be handled gently.* In mild cases, the thawed skin is red and scaly with little or no necrosis. Healing occurs spontaneously. In severe cases, necrosis occurs and the affected tissue should be amputated, but not too early, because more tissue may actually be viable than is initially suspected. Once frozen, tissues may be more susceptible to subsequent damage by the cold. Ear tips that are permanently scarred and alopecic could be treated beneficially by plastic surgery. This should remove the hairless portion and leave the remaining pinna well covered with hair for protection from the cold. Every effort should be made to keep these patients in protected quarters during cold weather.

■ MISCELLANEOUS CAUSES OF NECROSIS AND SLOUGHING OF THE EXTREMITIES

There are many well-documented causes of peripheral cutaneous necrosis in small animals, including solar dermatitis, frostbite, severe burns, exposure to caustic contactants, cold agglutinin disease, drug eruption, systemic lupus erythematosus, vasculitis (Fig. 15:4 *E*), snake bite, septicemia, and vascular insufficiency due to pressure (pressure sore), traps, and elastic bands.[11]

There are also some rare, often poorly documented or poorly understood associations. Dogs may rarely have peripheral necrosis with ergotism and leptospirosis.[27] Dry gangrene of the pinnae was reported in cats fed decomposed scallops.[37] Peripheral necrosis and sloughing have been reported in dogs and cats with disseminated intravascular coagulation (Fig. 15:4 *F*).[37, 52] Necrosis and sloughing of the digits have been reported as sequelae of hepatitis in dogs.[31] Necrosis and sloughing of the digits have also been seen in puppies and kittens (Fig. 15:4 *G*) fed highly concentrated formulas containing evaporated milk.[23, 34] Necrosis has been associated with sensory nerve damage either because it induces self-trauma (e.g., cauda equina syndrome and so-called chilblains)[24, 25] or because it interferes with proprioception (e.g., trophic ulcer of the footpad).[20]

■ SNAKE BITE

Two subfamilies of venomous snakes are indigenous to the United States: *Crotalidae* and *Elapidae. Crotalidae*, commonly called pit vipers, include the copperhead, the cottonmouth

Figure 15:4. *A,* Permanent scarring and depigmentation from a healed burn. The dog is now susceptible to solar dermatitis. *B,* Frostbite. Pinnal necrosis and ulceration. *C,* Frostbite. The tip of the pinna has sloughed. *D,* Frostbite. Necrosis of the distal tail. *E,* Tissue slough secondary to deep vascular occlusion. *F,* Pedal necrosis secondary to disseminated intravascular coagulation. *G,* Pedal necrosis in a kitten fed an inappropriate milk replacement. *H,* Profound facial edema secondary to a puff adder bite. (Courtesy P. Bland.)

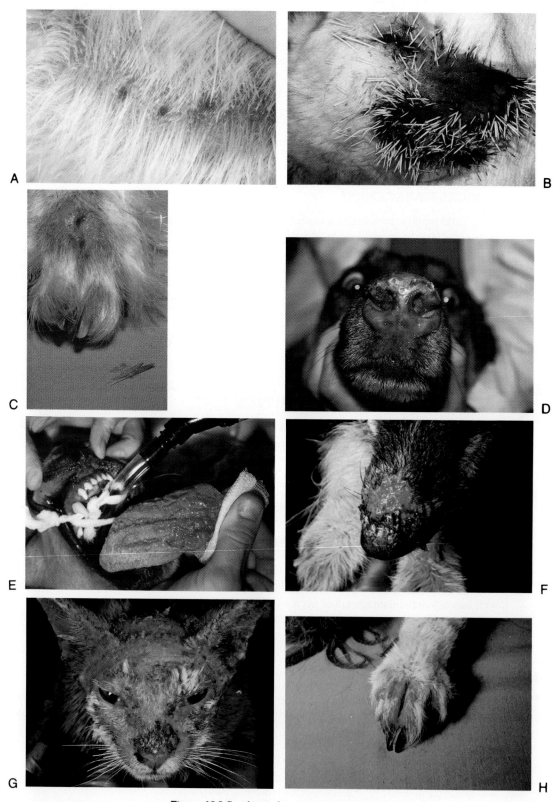

Figure 15:5 *See legend on opposite page*

moccasin, and the rattlesnake. One or more species of this subfamily are found in virtually all of the 48 contiguous states. *Elapidae* are represented in this country by two genera of coral snakes, which are found in only the southeastern and southwestern United States.

Snake venoms contain many toxic polypeptides, low molecular weight proteins, and enzymes.[26, 29, 30, 42, 48, 53] In general, venoms produce alterations in the resistance and integrity of blood vessels, changes in blood cells and blood coagulation mechanisms, direct or indirect changes in cardiac dynamics, alterations of nervous system function, depression of respiration, and necrosis at the site of envenomation. Necrosis is much more common with pit viper bites than with coral snake bites.[26, 30] The severity of a poisonous snake bite depends on the type and size of the snake, the amount of venom injected in relation to the victim's weight, the site of venom injection, and the time interval between the venom injection and the onset of medical therapy.[42]

Most snake bites occur during spring and summer. The face and legs are most commonly involved. Bites around the face are potentially serious because of rapid swelling and respiratory embarrassment (Fig. 15:4 *H*). Cutaneous manifestations of snake bites include rapid, progressive edema, which usually obliterates the fang marks (Fig. 15:5 *A*), pain, and, occasionally, local hemorrhage. Ecchymosis and discoloration become apparent several hours later, and this area often becomes necrotic and sloughs.

All snake bites are potentially lethal, especially in small dogs or cats, and specific wound treatments should be postponed until the patient is stable. Although there can be some benefit to removal of local venom by suction, the stress to the dog or cat can outweigh any potential benefits. Antivenin should be administered when available.[26, 30, 42] Because these antisera contain horse serum, the patient should undergo skin testing with the product before administration. Even with a negative test, reactions can occur, so the patient should be monitored carefully for signs of anaphylaxis. Because snake bites are contaminated by the oral flora, which often includes *Clostridium tetani*,[42] broad-spectrum antibiotics should be administered.

Beyond the above measures, treatment recommendations are controversial. Some investigators administer antihistamines, whereas other researchers do not.[26, 30, 42] Corticosteroids, unless used to treat shock, are not currently recommended. With pit viper bites, tissue slough can be expected, and the resulting wound should be managed similarly to a burn.[26]

■ FOREIGN BODIES

Foreign bodies occasionally cause skin lesions in dogs and cats. Although porcupine quills (Figs. 15:5 *B* and 15:6), air rifle pellets, and road gravel are common foreign bodies, most are of plant origin (seeds and awns, wood slivers). One of the most notorious plants in the United States in this regard is the foxtail *(Hordeum jubatum)*.[5] A related plant *(Hordeum murinum)* causes problems in France.[1a]

In a retrospective study of 182 cases of grass awn migration in dogs and cats in California, younger dogs (with increased activity) and hunting and working breeds (with increased exposure) were at greater risk.[5] The most common site of grass awn localization was the external ear canal (51 per cent of cases), with the other common cutaneous sites being the interdigital webs (see Fig. 15:5 *C*). Lesions consist of nodules, abscesses, and draining tracts. Secondary bacterial infection is exceedingly common.

Figure 15:5. *A*, Snake fang marks. (Courtesy D. Carlotti.) *B*, Porcupine quills. *C*, Digital draining tract secondary to foxtail penetration. (Courtesy S. White.) *D*, Burdock dermatitis of the nose and muzzle. *E*, Burdock glossitis. *F*, Thallium intoxication. Severe ulceration and crusting of the skin of the nasal region. A purulent exudate is present. *G*, Thallium intoxication. The skin of the entire head is affected; the superficial epidermis is loosened and peeling over extensive areas. (From Zook, B. C., et al.: Thallium poisoning in cats. J.A.V.M.A. 153:285, 1968.) *H*, Thallium intoxication. Erythema, alopecia, and erosion of the digits and interdigital spaces.

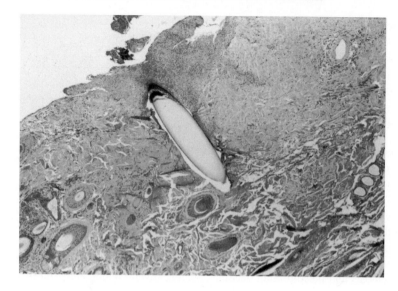

Figure 15:6. Porcupine quill lodged in a necrotic dermatitis.

Another common plant foreign body in the United States is the burdock (*Arctium* spp.).[14b] The burs of these common weeds become trapped in the haircoat, where they often cause local irritation and mat formation. Dogs generally do not tolerate the burs well and chew and lick them from their fur. In doing so, the dogs may produce focal skin lesions (see Fig. 15:5 *D*) or, more commonly, oral lesions. The lesions of typical burdock stomatitis are seen as (1) multiple 2- to 3-mm, whitish, shiny papules along the junction of the upper buccal and gingival mucosa or (2) multiple, erythematous, granular papules and plaques on the dorsal surface of the tongue (see Fig. 15:5 *E*). Some dogs with burdock stomatitis are remarkably asymptomatic, whereas other animals show typical signs of stomatitis. Biopsies reveal nodular to diffuse pyogranulomatous inflammation centered on plant material (Fig. 15:7).

The only effective treatment is surgical removal of the foreign body.

■ ARTERIOVENOUS FISTULA

An *arteriovenous fistula* is a vascular abnormality, defined as a direct communication between an adjacent artery and a vein that bypasses the capillary circulation.[18] Arteriovenous fistulae

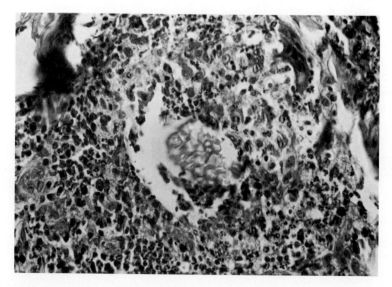

Figure 15:7. Burdock surrounded by mixed inflammatory infiltrate.

may be congenital or acquired and are rarely reported in dogs and cats.[4, 6, 16, 18, 37] Most clinically relevant cutaneous arteriovenous fistulae are acquired, and most of these result from penetrating wounds or blunt trauma, although they may also be secondary to infection, neoplasia, and iatrogenic factors (surgical declaw procedures and extravascular injections of irritating substances). Recurrent peripheral arteriovenous fistula has been reported in a cat with hyperthyroidism.[16]

Acquired arteriovenous fistulae most commonly involve the paws (after dewclaw procedures or injury) and the neck (secondary to neoplasms), but they have involved the temporal region, the pinnae, the legs, the flank, and the tongue. Affected areas show persistent or recurrent edema, pain, and occasionally, secondary infection and hemorrhage. Superficial blood vessels proximal to the fistula may be distinct and tortuous. Arteriovenous fistulae are generally characterized by pulsating vessels, palpable thrills, and continuous machinery murmurs. Occlusion of the artery proximal to the fistula results in a sudden decrease in heart rate and disappearance of the murmur and thrill.[18]

Diagnosis is based on the history, physical examination findings, and demonstration of the arteriovenous fistula by contrast radiography. Therapy includes surgical extirpation of the fistula or, in some instances, amputation of the affected part.

■ MYOSPHERULOSIS

Myospherulosis is a rare granulomatous reaction thought to be due to the interaction of ointments, antibiotics, or endogenous fat with erythrocytes.[17, 56] It is associated with small saclike structures (parent bodies) filled with endobodies (spherules) and has been reported in humans and dogs. The condition has been induced experimentally in laboratory animals. Myospherulosis is most commonly reported after injections of oil medicaments or after the topical application of oily products to open wounds. Because muscle is not always involved, it has been suggested that *spherulocytosis* or *spherulocytic disease* might be a better designation for this entity.[27c]

Patients are usually presented for solitary subcutaneous or dermal nodules, which may or may not be discharging.[17, 34] Histologic examination reveals several solid and cystic masses. The walls of the cystic area and most solid areas are composed of histiocytes with abundant vacuolated cytoplasm. Histiocytes surround parent bodies (30 to 350 μm) composed of thin eosinophilic walls and filled with homogeneous eosinophilic, 3- to 7-μm spherules (Fig. 15:8). Parent bodies and spherules do not stain with periodic acid–Schiff, Gomori's methenamine silver, or Ziehl-Neelsen stains but are positive for endogenous peroxidase (diaminobenzidine reaction) and hemoglobin, indicating that the spherules are erythrocytes.[56]

The only effective treatment is surgical excision.

■ THALLIUM TOXICOSIS

Thallium is a cumulative, general cell poison that may produce skin lesions or systemic toxicity.[39, 55, 57]

CAUSE AND PATHOGENESIS

The use of thallium as a rodenticide and roach poison in the United States was banned more than 20 years ago because of its toxicity. Despite the unavailability of thallium for all these years, cases are still occasionally recognized in the United States from baits found in house walls, garages, and barns.[55, 57] With doses of more than 20 mg/kg of body weight, the fatality rate is 100 per cent, and the clinical signs are those of damage to the central nervous system and circulatory system.[39] Nervousness, convulsions, tremors, salivation, weakness, and paralysis, together with a rapid weak pulse, are seen. Reliable early signs of less acute toxicity include

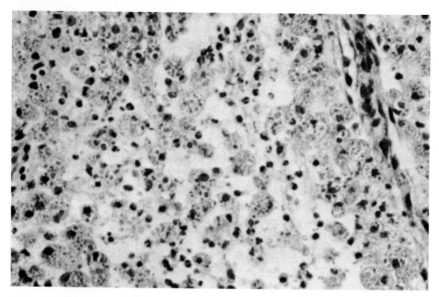

Figure 15:8. Myospherulosis. Macrophages containing many intracytoplasmic inclusions (fragments of erythrocytes).

vomiting, hemorrhagic gastroenteritis, polydipsia, pyrexia, and brick red mucous membranes. Colic and dyspnea are often apparent. Smaller doses of thallium may be cumulative and may produce the subacute or a chronic syndrome. Even with the best of care, the mortality rate can be extremely high (70 per cent); therefore, the prognosis is poor. Thallium is rapidly absorbed through the oral and intestinal mucosa and through the skin. It is mainly excreted in the urine, but it may persist in various tissues for up to 3 months. Thallium and potassium move together through cell walls and are excreted together in the urine. Therefore, increased turnover of one substance increases the secretion of the other. In rats, cystine and methionine seem to protect against the alopecic and toxic effects of thallium.

Researchers emphasize that thallium poisoning may be commonly unrecognized in cats that do not show cutaneous involvement.[37] Although the syndrome with skin lesions is classic and highly suggestive, cases of poisoning without skin lesions exhibit multisystemic problems that necessitate a detailed case work-up and laboratory support for accurate diagnosis. Even with intensive supportive care, only 19 per cent of the feline patients in one study recovered; thus, a poor prognosis must be given.[37] Many of the antidotal drugs suggested for other species are highly toxic to cats, and consequently, the clinician is further handicapped in treating this species.

CLINICAL FEATURES

Thallium poisoning is divided into two syndromes. In acute toxicity, the onset of signs is delayed by 12 to 96 hours after ingestion, but the length of the course until death is only 4 to 5 days. Skin lesions are not seen in acute intoxication. If the animal ingests smaller amounts or survives the peracute signs, severe gastrointestinal signs occur, which necessitate intensive supportive care. With ingestion of small amounts over some time, chronic intoxication occurs. Signs may not develop for 7 to 21 days after ingestion and may not reach their peak for an additional 21 days. Chronically intoxicated animals have hyperemic mucous membranes, mild to moderate gastrointestinal signs, and skin lesions characterized by erythema and hair loss. The hair loss is first noted in frictional areas, and ulceration may follow the hair loss. Advanced cases have involvement of the face (see Fig. 15:5 *F* and *G*), the ears, the ventrum, the perineum, the feet (see Fig. 15:5 *H*), and the mucocutaneous junctions (Fig. 15:9 *A*). The footpads become hyperkeratotic and ulcerated. Signs of other organ involvement are common.

DIAGNOSIS

Because thallium intoxication is rare, it often is not suspected. The primary differential diagnostic possibilities to explain the systemic and cutaneous signs include drug eruption, systemic lupus erythematosus, necrolytic migratory erythema, toxic epidermal necrolysis, erythema multiforme major, lymphoreticular neoplasia, and the various rickettsial and protozoal diseases. The diagnosis is confirmed by the detection of thallium in the urine by a rapid colorimetric spot test (Gabriel-Dubin test) or absorption spectrophotometry.[39] The spot test is inexpensive and more readily available than absorption spectrophotometry but is less sensitive, with both false-positive and false-negative reactions reported. In most cases, these urine tests are performed after skin biopsy results suggest thallotoxicosis.

Thallium exerts a local toxic effect on epidermal cells in the process of differentiation leading to keratin formation. Degenerative changes are evident in the hair follicle and in the surface epidermis.[50] The direct insult to the hair follicle is especially noteworthy in anagen hairs; the hair shaft is converted to an amorphous mass, the bulb degenerates, and the hair is lost. Follicular plugging and parakeratosis are prominent. The surface epidermis shows massive parakeratotic hyperkeratosis and dyskeratosis with vacuolar degeneration of keratinocytes (Fig. 15:10). Multiple spongiform microabscesses are present in the superficial epidermis and the hair follicle's outer root sheath. The superficial dermis shows edema, vascular dilatation, and extravasation of erythrocytes.

CLINICAL MANAGEMENT

The prognosis in all cases of thallitoxicosis is grave, and most animals die. In mildly intoxicated cases, supportive care with the administration of appropriate fluids, electrolytes, antibiotics, and so forth is paramount and may be the only treatment needed, as the thallium is slowly eliminated from the body via the bile and urine. Various specific treatments have been suggested, but none is without hazard. Aside from specific adverse reactions for each agent, all can precipitate a thallium crises by drawing thallium from tissues into the blood. Because of this rebound, chelators such as dithizone (diphenylthiocarbazone) (70 mg/kg q8h) or dithiocarb sodium (diethyldithiocarbamate sodium) (30 mg/kg q8h) are no longer recommended.[55, 57] Gastrointestinal trapping of the thallium with Prussian blue or activated charcoal may be of some benefit. The charcoal appears to be more effective. Potassium chloride supplementation (1 to 2 gm q8 to 12h) promotes renal elimination by competing with thallium for distal tubular reabsorption. Patients should be monitored for signs of cardiac and renal toxicity. Combination treatment with charcoal and potassium chloride has been suggested.[55, 57]

If the animal survives the intoxication, the skin lesions heal spontaneously with complete hair regrowth. Bathing with mild shampoos or hydrotherapy can accelerate the skin's healing but may unduly stress the animal.

■ MISCELLANEOUS TOXICOSES

Veterinary textbooks on toxicology mention skin changes for many compounds.[39] Most cases involve farm animals, but pets can be equally as susceptible. The agents can cause skin lesions by direct action on the skin, by altering levels of vital nutrients, or by altering the function of other organs. The number of cases of reported cutaneous toxicoses in small animals is small, but these are probably underreported.

Arsenic is a general tissue poison that combines with and inactivates sulfhydryl groups in tissue enzymes.[10, 38] Sources of arsenic include herbicides, rodenticides, pesticides, and arsenical

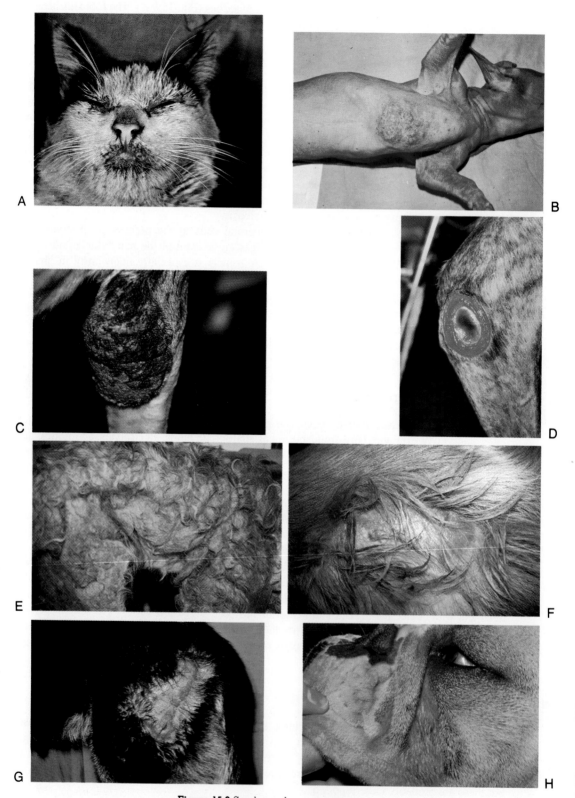

Figure 15:9 *See legend on opposite page*

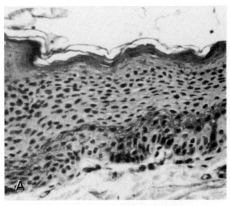

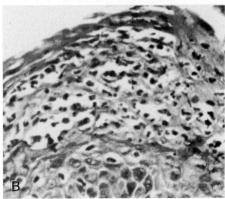

Figure 15:10. Histologic sections of skin from canine axilla. *A*, Note hyperkeratosis and parakeratotic scale, constituting approximately 65 per cent of epidermis. Epidermal cells are vacuolated (×195, H & E stain). *B*, Higher magnification of spongiform abscesses, showing multilocular spaces containing neutrophils (×360, H & E stain). (From Schwartzman, R. M., Kirschbaum, J. O.: The cutaneous histopathology of thallium poisoning. J. Invest. Dermatol. 39:169, 1962.)

medicaments. Signs of arsenic toxicosis vary according to the dose, the physical form, the route of administration, and the composition (organic or inorganic).

Arsenic toxicosis was reported in a mature dog presented for listlessness, anorexia, weight loss, rough coat, swollen muzzle, and necrosis and ulceration of the pinnae, feet, lips, and prepuce.[10] A container of liquid insecticide (44 per cent sodium arsenite) was found to be leaking into the dog's house. Arsenic concentrations were found at toxic levels in urine, blood, feces, and hair. Bathing the dog and cleaning up its environment resulted in complete remission within 1 month. Chronic arsenic toxicosis is a known cause of Bowen's disease in humans.[13] Although cases in animals (see Chap. 19) do not appear to be associated with arsenic poisoning, it should be considered, especially when the animal has intercurrent gastrointestinal signs.

Mycotoxins are toxic metabolites produced by molds. Intoxication occurs by ingestion of spoiled grain or grain products. Ergotism was the first recognized mycotoxicosis and has been reported to cause necrotizing skin lesions in dogs.[50] A case of necrolytic migratory erythema (see Chap. 9) was reported in a dog that ate moldy biscuit meal containing ochratoxin A, citrinin, and sterigmatocystin.[28] As most owners do not feed obviously spoiled foods, this may be an isolated case. However, it does demonstrate that agents that produce no direct skin signs can do so by altering the function of other organs.

Figure 15:9. *A*, Early inflammation and crusting of the eyelids and lips of a cat with thallium poisoning. (From Zook, B. C., et al.: Thallium poisoning in cats. J.A.V.M.A. 153:285, 1968.) *B*, Sternal callus in a dachshund. *C*, Callus dermatitis. Note intertriginous folds in the thick, rugose callus. *D*, Pressure sore in the hock region. *E*, Severe matting predisposes the animal to pyotraumatic dermatitis. *F*, Pyotraumatic dermatitis with sharp margins. *G*, Pyotraumatic dermatitis typically develops rapidly into a glistening, suppurative, hairless lesion bordered by a band of erythematous skin. *H*, Facial fold intertrigo. The thumb is pulling the lip forward to expose the erythematous, infected crevice hidden in the fold.

■ CALLUS AND HYGROMA

A *callus* is a round or oval hyperkeratotic plaque that develops on the skin, typically over bony pressure points. The elbow and the hock are the most common sites. Dogs with deep chests often develop sternal lesions. Large breeds are especially susceptible if the dog sleeps on cement, brick, or wood. Many adult dogs develop varying degrees of callus. Dogs that sleep in unusual positions because of orthopedic disease or that are hypothyroid can have calluses in unusual locations. Callosities are a normal, protective response to pressure-induced ischemia and inflammation.[37] The callus is hairless and gray and has a wrinkled surface (see Fig. 15:9 B). Histologically there is irregular to papillated epidermal hyperplasia and orthokeratotic to parakeratotic hyperkeratosis. Small follicular cysts are seen in the dermis.

Although calluses, especially those in unusual locations, can be mistaken for lesions of ringworm, demodicosis, or other inflammatory disorders, diagnosis in most cases is straightforward. Most callosities need no treatment, but some calluses necessitate treatment because the owner finds them objectionable or because they are extremely hyperplastic and become ulcerated or easily infected. Environmental modification is mandatory.

Padding (e.g., foam rubber pads, air mattresses, and straw bedding) must be provided, and the dog must use it consistently. Padding efforts often frustrate the client because the dog avoids the padding or destroys it. If the environment cannot be padded, the individual lesions can be protected by making pads for affected areas (e.g., elbow pads). With some ingenuity, virtually any callus can be padded. Again, the dog can frustrate the effort by removing the pad. After padding is provided, the callus can be softened with any good hand cream. In extreme cases, the callus can be removed surgically. This has to be performed carefully because there can be excessive hemorrhage and sutures often do not hold. Wound dehiscence is a possible complication of surgery.

Hygroma is a false or acquired bursa that develops subcutaneously over bony prominences.[37] Hygromas develop after repeated trauma-induced necrosis and inflammation over pressure points. They are initially soft to fluctuant (fluid filled) but may become abscesses or granulomas with or without fistulous tracts, especially if they are secondarily infected.

Histologically, hygromas are characterized by cystic spaces surrounded by dense walls of granulation tissue, the inner layer of which is a flattened layer of fibroblasts. Early lesions usually respond well to loose, padded bandages applied for 2 to 3 weeks and corrective housing. More severe lesions may necessitate extensive drainage, extirpation, or skin grafting procedures.

■ CALLUS DERMATITIS AND PYODERMA

Callus dermatitis is a secondary infection of a callus subjected to repeated trauma or softened without the obligatory environmental modifications.

CAUSE AND CLINICAL FEATURES

The callus is the initial response to trauma. Continued trauma and the proliferative skin reaction that follows produce crevices in the callus and intertriginous areas, which results in a fold dermatitis. Additional trauma causes epidermal breakdown, ulceration of pressure points, and fistulae. The lesions are most common over the hock and elbow joints of giant breeds such as Great Danes, St. Bernards, Newfoundlands, and Irish wolfhounds (see Fig. 15:9 C). Sternal calluses on the chest of dachshunds, setters, Pointers, boxers, and Doberman pinschers may also become secondarily ulcerated and infected. Often, there is no specific bacterial flora involved in this infection, although staphylococci are commonly isolated. Pressure point granulomas, which contain free hair shafts, may develop.

Ulcerated or fistulated lesions may be deeply infected, and exudative cytologic examination should be performed in all cases. The surface should be scrubbed, and the lesion should be squeezed firmly before samples are collected. In many cases, pieces of hair shafts pop to the surface. Infection usually results in a pyogranulomatous inflammation.

CLINICAL MANAGEMENT

Primary attention must be given to relieving the trauma so the tissue can heal. This can be accomplished through the use of waterbeds, special bedding, pads for various body parts, or a combination of these measures. In severe cases, surgical excision of the callus may be indicated. This is major surgery with a difficult postoperative course, and the reader is referred to texts on soft tissue surgery for details of treatment.

Mild surface inflammation and fold dermatitis can be relieved by daily whirlpool baths in warm water. Distal lesions may be amenable to soaking in a bucket. With imbedded hair shafts, a mildly hypertonic drawing solution of magnesium sulfate (Epsom salts) (30 ml/L or 2 tbsp/qt of warm water) can be beneficial. In noninfected lesions, hydrotherapy is typically sufficient to cause healing. When this is not possible, the topical application of an antibiotic cream or Preparation H, a human hemorrhoid preparation containing live yeast extract and shark liver oil, can be beneficial.

Infected lesions necessitate a prolonged course with antibiotics. Six weeks or longer of treatment is usually necessary. Because the infected tissue cannot return to normal condition with antibiotic treatment, the client is not able to determine when the infection is resolved. Cytologic examinations should be performed every second week. When no sign of infection is present, treatment should be continued for an additional 7 to 14 days. Relapses are prevented by management changes.

■ PRESSURE SORES

Pressure sores (decubital ulcers) result from prolonged application of pressure concentrated over a bony prominence in a relatively small area of the body. The pressure is sufficient to compress the capillary circulation, causing tissue damage or frank necrosis.[11, 13, 37] Tissue anoxia and full-thickness skin loss rapidly progress from a small localized area to a conical ulcer widest at the skin surface. Pressure sores almost invariably become infected with a variety of pathogenic bacteria. Within 24 to 48 hours, the edges of the ulcerated area are undermined. The ulceration may extend to the underlying bone. Because of the area of capillary and venous congestion at the base of the ulcer and tissue margins, systemic antibiotics do not penetrate well.

Animals that are recumbent for prolonged periods on hard surfaces are at increased risk for pressure sores. Emaciation increases the susceptibility. Lesions are initially characterized by an erythematous to reddish purple discoloration. This progresses to oozing, necrosis, and ulceration. The resultant ulcers tend to be deep, to be undermined at the edges, to be secondarily infected, and to heal slowly (Fig. 15:9 D).

Prevention is paramount. All recumbent animals should be kept on a waterbed or eggcrate foam rubber pad, be turned frequently, and receive a daily whirlpool bath. If a pressure sore develops, additional padding should be supplied in that area. The wound should be cleaned frequently with an appropriate antiseptic solution. If the patient recovers from its disease fairly quickly, the pressure sore should heal spontaneously but slowly. Application of Preparation H or a raw honey[3] may accelerate healing. Surgical repair should be reserved as a last resort because wound dehiscence is common.

■ PYOTRAUMATIC DERMATITIS

Pyotraumatic dermatitis (acute moist dermatitis, or ''hot spots'') is produced by self-induced trauma as the patient bites or scratches at a part of its body in an attempt to alleviate some pain or itch.[37] The majority of cases are complications of flea bite hypersensitivity, but allergic skin diseases, other ectoparasites, anal sac problems, inflammations such as otitis externa, foreign bodies in the coat, irritant substances, dirty unkempt coats (Fig. 15:9 E), psychoses, and painful musculoskeletal disorders may be underlying causes. These factors initiate the itch-scratch cycle, which varies in intensity with individuals. The intense trauma produces severe large lesions in a few hours. Animals particularly disposed to this problem are those with a heavy pelage that has a dense undercoat, such as Golden and Labrador retrievers, collies, German shepherds, and St. Bernards. The problem is much more common in hot, humid weather and may be related to lack of ventilation in the coat.

A typical lesion is red, moist, and exudative. There is a coagulum of proteinaceous exudate in the center of the area surrounded by a red halo of erythematous skin. The hair is lost from the area, but the margins are sharply defined from the surrounding normal skin and hair (Fig. 15:9 F). The lesion progresses rapidly if appropriate therapy is not started at once (Fig. 15:9 G). Much pain is associated with the local area, and this may eventually deter the animal from further self-trauma. Lesions are often located in close proximity to the primary painful process (e.g., near infected ears, anal sacs, and flea bites on the rump).

True hot spots have bacteria colonizing the surface of the lesion but are not skin infections. This is in contrast to pyotraumatic folliculitis (see Chap. 4) in which the dog traumatizes the skin over a staphylococcal folliculitis or furunculosis.[45] Without clipping and palpating the lesion, it can be difficult (if not impossible) to differentiate pyotraumatic dermatitis from pyotraumatic folliculitis.

Diagnosis is made by the history of acute onset, the physical appearance, and some association with a primary cause. True pyotraumatic dermatitis is a relatively flat, eroded to ulcerated lesion. Lesions that are thickened, are plaquelike, and are bordered by papules or pustules (satellite lesions) should always suggest a primary eruptive process, especially a staphylococcal infection, which the dog has traumatized.[45]

Therapy is effective if applied promptly and vigorously. Sedation or anesthesia may be needed to allow thorough cleaning of the area. Cleaning with povidone-iodine or chlorhexidine is the first and most important step in local therapy. Cleaning is more rapid and effective when the hair is clipped, but clipping is not always possible in show dogs. In unclipped areas, the shampoo formulation of the antiseptic should be used, whereas solutions are applied on clipped lesions. After cleaning, a drying agent should be applied. Many such products are marketed today, and no studies suggest that one product is superior to another. The authors routinely use a 2 per cent aluminum acetate solution (Domeboro solution) or an aluminum acetate and 1 per cent hydrocortisone solution with good results. The solution is dabbed on the lesion every 8 to 12 hours and allowed to dry on.

Most cases benefit from 5 to 7 days of treatment with a corticosteroid. In mild cases, the hydrocortisone in the aluminum acetate and hydrocortisone solution may be sufficient. In more inflamed cases, a more potent topical agent (e.g., betamethasone valerate cream) or oral prednisolone (1.1 mg/kg q24h) can be used. If oral corticosteroids are not contraindicated, that route of treatment is most satisfactory because the owner does not have to manipulate a tender lesion repeatedly. After the inflammation and exudation have disappeared, treatment can be discontinued. The residual scaling and crusting can be removed with a mild antiseborrheic shampoo. In most instances, this step is skipped, and the skin returns to normal condition in 7 to 10 days.

At the time of the initial treatment, it is most important to find the predisposing factor and to eliminate or modify it to stop the patient's reflex self-trauma. The treatment to accomplish this varies, depending on the primary cause. Some unfortunate dogs have repeated problems. There is no simple prophylaxis. Constant attention to grooming, hygiene, baths, and parasite control and periodic cleaning of the ears and anal sacs helps. Owners should be particularly vigilant during periods of hot, humid weather. Although diet (e.g., high protein content) is often suggested as a cause, except for severe fatty acid deficiency or food hypersensitivity, this has never been proved.

■ INTERTRIGO

Intertrigo (skin fold dermatitis) is a frictional dermatitis that occurs in areas where two skin surfaces are intimately apposed. The apposition results from the intentional breeding of certain dogs (e.g., English bulldog and Chinese Shar Pei) for pronounced folding, congenital or acquired anatomic defects; it may also result from thickening of the dermis or subcutis caused by obesity, hormonal influences, or inflammatory skin disease. Skin rubbing against skin is irritating, and the areas where this occurs have poor air circulation. If moisture, sebum, glandular secretions, and excretions such as tears, saliva, and urine are present, these areas provide an environment that favors skin maceration and bacterial overgrowth. Although bacteria play a central role in the pathogenesis of fold dermatitis, they rarely invade viable tissues, so the old designation of fold pyoderma is inaccurate. The surface bacteria act on the trapped secretions and sebum and produce breakdown products, which are irritating and odoriferous. As the irritants are rubbed on the apposed surface, inflammation results and produces the clinical signs of the disease and causes the increased production of more irritants. A vicious cycle is created. In some dogs, numerous *Malassezia* yeast can be found in the surface material and no doubt contribute to the symptoms.

Satisfactory treatment of an intertrigo necessitates resolution of the inflammation and exudation and elimination of the tissue apposition that triggered the intertrigo. If the folding cannot be eliminated because the anatomic defect is uncorrectable or would destroy the desired appearance of the dog, cure cannot be achieved and a long-term control regimen should be instituted. When the folding can be eliminated, only a short course of treatment is necessary to resolve the dermatitis.

Removal of the bacteria and the entrapped surface debris is essential and necessitates the use of antiseborrheic products. Benzoyl peroxide– or sulfur-based products, in gel, ointment, or shampoo formulations, are most commonly used. Although the gels and ointments have better residual activity, they can be irritating and worsen the inflammation if used at the onset of treatment. Most investigators use shampoos to gain control and reserve the other formulations for maintenance treatments.

After the surface debris is removed, tissue inflammation can be eliminated by the topical application of a corticosteroid cream or the oral administration of prednisolone (1.1 mg/kg q24h). A 5- to 7-day course of treatment should be sufficient. In mild cases, an aluminum acetate and hydrocortisone solution is very effective.

If the skin apposition cannot be eliminated (e.g., by surgery or weight loss), the dermatitis recurs unless maintenance cleaning with an antiseborrheic product is instituted. For folds of the face, the body, or the vulva, the daily application of a plain or medicated talc can be beneficial and reduce the amount of bathing required. Lip, vulvar, and tail folds are usually not amenable to talcing. The talc is applied carefully to the crevice of each fold. Before the next application, the previous day's dose must be removed by brushing with a dry cloth or by washing. If the area is washed, it should be dried completely before the talc is reapplied. In many cases, the talcing can reduce the frequency of washing from once daily to once or twice weekly. Where talcing is ineffective, prophylactic application of a benzoyl peroxide gel can be extremely beneficial.

Facial fold intertrigo is seen in brachycephalic breeds, especially Pekingese, English bulldogs, and pugs (Fig. 15:9 *H*).[37] The fold may rub on the cornea and cause severe keratitis and ulceration. The breed standards in some cases require a facial fold, so even though its presence may damage the eye, one should be careful to explain the ramifications of surgical correction to owners and should obtain their approval before ablating the folds.

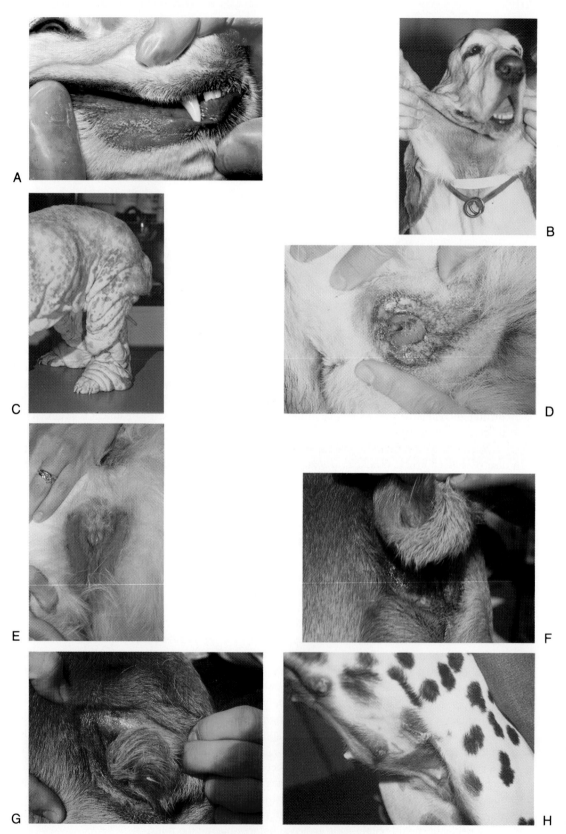

Figure 15:11 *See legend on opposite page*

Lip fold intertrigo is primarily an aesthetic problem to owners, because it produces severe halitosis.[37] Owners may need to be convinced that the small lip fold can produce all that odor. This problem is prevalent in dogs with a large lip flap, such as spaniels and St. Bernards (Fig. 15:11 A). Cheiloplasty is curative.

Body fold intertrigo occurs primarily in obese individuals, and in certain basset hounds and Chinese Shar Pei dogs (Fig. 15:11 B and C).[37] It is most common in Shar Pei puppies that have an increased number of folds and in those with a tendency to seborrhea. As the puppies mature, they do grow out of their folds on parts of the body, and therefore fold dermatitis in the adult Shar Pei is more concentrated on the head and face, where the folds persist. It may also be seen on the ventral midline of female dogs and cats with intertrigo between pendulous mammary glands or with rolls of body fat.

Vulvar fold intertrigo is common in obese older female animals that have infantile vulvae as a result of spaying at a young age (Fig. 15:11 D).[37] The vulva is recessed, and vaginal secretions and drops of urine may accumulate in the folds of the perivulvar region. This is a special stimulus to ulceration and bacterial growth, and the odors produced are especially unpleasant. Licking is a near-constant feature and worsens the dermatitis (Fig. 15:11 E). Ascending bacterial urinary tract infections are a common sequela to vulvar fold intertrigo. Several methods of management may help. Because obesity is usually present, weight reduction is indicated. Modest doses of oral diethylstilbestrol or estrogenic hormone injections cause vulvar enlargement and may reduce the folds. The potential danger of such endocrine therapy must be considered. Surgical vulvopasty (episioplasty), with fixation of the dorsal vulvar commissure to elevate the vulva out of the crevice, is curative. Squamous cell carcinoma has been reported to arise from chronic vulvar fold dermatitis.[37]

Tail fold intertrigo results from pressure of corkscrew tails on the skin of the perineum (Fig. 15:11 F and G). It is seen in English bulldogs, pugs, Boston terriers, and other breeds with that type of tail.[37] In addition, a rump fold intertrigo may be seen in certain Manx cats. In some cases, the tail may partially obstruct the anus, so that feces, anal sac secretions, and other skin gland products enhance the skin maceration from the intertrigo. Amputation resolves the problem, but the surgery is complicated.

■ CALCINOSIS CUTIS

Calcinosis cutis involves the deposition of calcium salts in dermal tissues. Lesions can be localized (see Chap. 19) or widespread. In dogs, widespread calcinosis cutis typically occurs in spontaneous or iatrogenic hyperadrenocorticism (see Chap. 9), but several reports describe ventral calcinosis caused by percutaneous penetration of calcium carbonate or calcium chloride.[40, 49] Lesions consisted of multiple erythematous, crusted, ulcerated papules and plaques on the glabrous skin of the ventral abdomen, the inguinal region, and the medial thighs (Fig. 15:11 H). Lesions resolved spontaneously with avoidance of further contact.

The nature and location of the lesions described mimicked the calcinosis cutis seen in hyperadrenocorticism, but the dogs had no other signs of that disease. When calcinosis cutis is recognized in glabrous areas, the owner should be questioned carefully about possible exposure to bone meal, landscaping products, or barn dusts before adrenal function tests are performed.

Figure 15:11. A, Lip fold intertrigo characterized by erythema, exudation, and fetid odor. B, Neck fold intertrigo. C, Profound folding predisposes this Shar Pei to fold dermatitis. D, Vulvar fold intertrigo with erosion. E, Vulvar fold intertrigo. Severe dermatitis due to constant licking. F, Tail fold intertrigo in a dog with screw tail conformation. (Courtesy P. Ihrke.) G, Close-up of the dog in F. (Courtesy P. Ihrke.) H, Calcinosis cutis secondary to percutaneous penetration of calcium carbonate.

REFERENCES

1. Al-Bagdadi, F. K., et al.: Hair dye effects on the hair coat and skin of the dog: A scanning electron microscopic study. Anat. Histol. Embryol. 17:349, 1988.
1a. Bergeaud, P.: Pathologies liées aux épillets. Point Vét. 26:105, 1994.
2. Bilbrey, S. A., et al.: Chemical burn caused by benzalkonium chloride in eight surgical cases. J. Am. Anim. Hosp. Assoc. 25:31, 1989.
3. Borum, T.: Management of decubital ulcers with the topical application of raw honey. Mississippi Vet. J. Summer 1986, p. 16.
4. Bouayad, H., et al.: Peripheral acquired arteriovenous fistula: A report of four cases and literature review. J. Am. Anim. Hosp. Assoc. 23:205, 1987.
5. Brennan, K. E., Ihrke, P. J.: Grass awn migration in dogs and cats: A retrospective study of 182 cases. J. Am. Vet. Med. Assoc. 182:1201, 1983.
6. Butterfield, A. B., et al.: Acquired peripheral arteriovenous fistula in a dog. J. Am. Vet. Med. Assoc. 176:445, 1980.
7. Coyne, B. E., et al.: Thermoelectric burns from improper grounding of electrocautery units: Two case reports. J. Am. Anim. Hosp. Assoc. 29:7, 1993.
8. Darr, D., et al.: Protection against UVB damage to porcine skin with topical application of vitamin C. In: von Tscharner, C., Halliwell, R. E. W. (eds.). Advances in Veterinary Dermatology, Vol. 1. Baillière Tindall, London, 1990, p. 463.
9. Evans, A. G., et al.: A trial of 13-*cis*-retinoic acid for treatment of squamous cell carcinoma and preneoplastic lesions of the head in cats. Am. J. Vet. Res. 46:2553, 1985.
10. Evinger, J. V., Blakemore, J. C.: Dermatitis in a dog associated with exposure to an arsenic compound. J. Am. Vet. Med. Assoc. 184:1281, 1984.
11. Fadok, V. W.: Necrotizing skin diseases. In: Kirk, R. W. (ed.). Current Veterinary Therapy VIII. W. B. Saunders Co., Philadelphia, 1983, p. 473.
12. Fairley, R. A.: Photosensitivity dermatitis in two collie working dogs. N. Z. Vet. J. 30:61, 1982.
13. Fitzpatrick, T. B., et al.: Dermatology in General Medicine IV. McGraw-Hill Book Co., New York, 1993.
14. Fox, S. M.: Management of thermal burns—Part I. Comp. Cont. Educ. 7:631, 1985.
14a. Frank, L. A., Calderwood-Mays, M. B.: Solar dermatitis in dogs. Compend. Cont. Educ. 16:465, 1994.
14b. Georgi, M. E., et al.: Pappus bristles: The cause of burdock stomatitis in dogs. Cornell Vet. 72:43, 1982.
15. Gourley, I. M., et al.: Burn scar malignancy in a dog. J. Am. Anim. Hosp. Assoc. 180:109, 1982.
16. Harari, J., et al.: Recurrent peripheral arteriovenous fistula and hyperthyroidism in a cat. J. Am. Anim. Hosp. Assoc. 20:759, 1984.
17. Hargis, A. M., et al.: Myospherulosis in the subcutis of a dog. Vet. Pathol. 21:248, 1984.
18. Hosgood, G.: Arteriovenous fistulas: Pathophysiology, diagnosis and treatment. Comp. Cont. Educ. 11:625, 1989.
18a. Hruza, L. L., Pentland, A. P.: Mechanisms of UV-induced inflammation. J. Invest. Dermatol. 100:35S, 1993.
19. Hudson, W. E., Florax, M. J. H.: Photosensitization in foxhounds. Vet. Rec. 128:618, 1991.
20. Hunt, G. B., Chapman, B. L.: "Trophic" ulceration of two digital pads. Aust. Vet. Pract. 21:196, 1991.
21. Ihrke, P.: Nasal solar dermatitis. In: Kirk, R. W. (ed.). Current Veterinary Therapy VII. W. B. Saunders Co., Philadelphia, 1981, p. 440.
22. Irving, R. A., et al.: Porphyrin values and treatment of feline solar dermatitis. Am. J. Vet. Res. 43:2067, 1982.
23. Israel, E., et al.: Microangiopathic hemolytic anemia in a puppy: Grand Rounds Conference. J. Am. Anim. Hosp. Assoc. 14:521, 1978.
24. Jepson, P. G. H.: Chilblain syndrome in dogs. Vet. Rec. 108:392, 1981.
24a. Kimura, T., Doi, K.: Responses of the skin over the dorsum to sunlight in hairless descendants of Mexican hairless dogs. Am. J. Vet. Res. 55:199, 1994.
25. Komarek, J. V.: Fallbericht: Verfolgung der Rute beim Hund-Cauda-equina-syndrome. Kleintier-Prax. 33:25, 1988.
26. Kostolich, M.: Reconstructive surgery of a snakebite wound. Canine Pract. 15:15, 1990.
27. Kral, F., Schwartzman, R. M.: Veterinary and Comparative Dermatology. J. B. Lippincott Co., Philadelphia, 1964.
27a. Ledo, E.: Photodermatosis. Part I: Photobiology, photoimmunology, and idiopathic photodermatoses. Int. J. Dermatol. 32:387, 1993.
27b. Ledo, E.: Photodermatoses. Part II: Chemical photodermatoses and dermatoses that can be exacerbated, precipitated, or provoked by light. Int. J. Dermatol. 32:480, 1993.
27c. Lazarov, A., et al.: Dermal spherulosis (myospherulosis) after topical treatment for psoriasis. J. Am. Acad. Dermatol. 30(Part 1):265, 1994.
28. Little, C. J. L., et al.: Hepatopathy and dermatitis in a dog associated with the ingestion of mycotoxins. J. Small Anim. Pract. 32:23, 1991.
29. Mansfield, P. D.: The management of snake venom poisoning in dogs. Comp. Cont. Educ. 6:988, 1984.
30. Marks, S. L., et al.: Coral snake envenomation in the dog: Report of four cases and review of the literature. J. Am. Anim. Hosp. Assoc. 26:629, 1990.
31. Mason, B. J. E.: Necrosis of a dog's toes following hepatitis. Vet. Rec. 101:286, 1977.
32. Mason, K. V.: The pathogenesis of solar induced skin lesions in bull terriers. Proc. Annu. Memb. Meet. Am. Acad. Vet. Dermatol. Am. Coll. Vet. Dermatol. 4:12, 1987.
33. Miller, W. H., Jr.: Epidermal dysplastic disorders of dogs and cats. In: Bonagura, J. D. (ed.). Kirk's Current Veterinary Therapy XII. W. B. Saunders Co., Philadelphia, 1995.
34. Miller, W. J., Jr., Scott, D. W.: Unpublished observations, 1994.

35. Mills, B. C.: Feline deaths following tattooing with Indian ink. Univ. Sydney Post-Grad Comm. Vet. Sci. Control and Therapy 134:2355, 1987.
36. Muller, G. H.: Contact dermatitis in animals. Arch. Dermatol. 96:423, 1967.
37. Muller, G. H., et al.: Small Animal Dermatology IV. W. B. Saunders Co., Philadelphia, 1989.
38. Neiger, R. D.: Arsenic poisoning. In: Kirk, R. W. (ed.). Current Veterinary Therapy X. W. B. Saunders Co., Philadelphia, 1989, p. 159.
39. Osweiler, G. D., et al.: Clinical and Diagnostic Veterinary Toxicology, 3rd ed. Kendall/Hunt Publishing Co., Dubuque, IA, 1985.
40. Paradis, M., Scott, D. W.: Calcinosis cutis secondary to percutaneous penetration of calcium carbonate in a Dalmatian. Can. Vet. J. 30:57, 1989.
41. Patterson, J. M.: Nasal solar dermatitis in the dog—A method of tattooing. J. Am. Anim. Hosp. Assoc. 14:370, 1978.
42. Peterson, M. E., Meerdink, G. L.: Bites and stings of venomous animals. In: Kirk, R. W. (ed.). Current Veterinary Therapy X. W. B. Saunders Co., Philadelphia, 1989, p. 177.
43. Power, H. T., Ihrke, P. J.: The use of synthetic retinoids in veterinary medicine. In: Bonagura, J. D. (ed.). Kirk's Current Veterinary Therapy XII. W. B. Saunders Co., Philadelphia, 1995.
44. Reedy, L. M., Clubb, F. J.: Microwave burn in a Toy Poodle: A case report. J. Am. Anim. Hosp. Assoc. 27:497, 1991.
45. Reinke, S. I., et al.: Histopathologic features of pyotraumatic dermatitis. J. Am. Vet. Med. Assoc. 190:57, 1987.
46. Rosenkrantz, W. S.: Solar dermatitis. In: Griffin, C. E., et al.: Current Veterinary Dermatology. Mosby-Year Book, St. Louis, 1993, p. 309.
47. Saxon, W. D., Kirby, R.: Treatment of acute burn injury and smoke inhalation. In: Kirk, R. W., Bonagura, J. D. (eds.). Kirk's Current Veterinary Therapy XI. W. B. Saunders Co., Philadelphia, 1992, p. 146.
48. Schaer, M.: Eastern diamondback rattlesnake envenomation of 20 dogs. Comp. Cont. Educ. 6:997, 1984.
49. Schick, M. P., et al.: Calcinosis cutis secondary to percutaneous penetration of calcium chloride in dogs. J. Am. Vet. Med. Assoc. 190:207, 1987.
50. Schwartzman, R. M., Kirschbaum, J. O.: The cutaneous histopathology of thallium poisoning. J. Invest. Dermatol. 39:169, 1962.
51. Scott, D. W.: Feline dermatology, 1900–1978: A monograph. J. Am. Anim. Hosp. Assoc. 16:331, 1980.
52. Shakespeare, A. C., et al.: Infarction of the digits and tail secondary to disseminated intravascular coagulation and metastic hemangiosarcoma in a dog. J. Am. Anim. Hosp. Assoc. 24:517, 1988.
53. Springer, T. R., Bailey, W. J.: Snake bite treatment in the United States. Int. J. Dermatol. 25:479, 1986.
53a. Streilein, J. W.: Sunlight and skin-associated lymphoid tissues (SALT). J. Invest. Dermatol. 100:47S, 1993.
54. Swaim, S. F., et al.: Heating pad and thermal burns in small animals. J. Am. Anim. Hosp. Assoc. 25:156, 1989.
55. Thomas, M. L., et al.: Chronic thallium toxicosis in a dog. J. Am. Anim. Hosp. Assoc. 29:211, 1993.
56. Waldman, J. S., et al.: Subcutaneous myospherulosis. J. Am. Acad. Dermatol. 21:400, 1989.
57. Water, C. B., et al.: Acute thallium toxicosis in a dog. J. Am. Anim. Hosp. Assoc. 201:883, 1992.

Nutritional Skin Diseases

■

Dermatoses may result from numerous nutritional deficiencies, excesses, or imbalances, but the skin responds with only a few types of clinical reactions and lesions. These include scaling, crusting, alopecia, and a dry, dull haircoat. Consequently, physical examinations alone can seldom reveal a specific nutritional cause.

It is useful to know the nutritional requirements of dogs and cats[1, 10] but it is difficult to prove that a specific deficiency causes a specific skin disease. Since the 1980s, a few new skin diseases were described that were definitely connected to nutritional factors, and it became fashionable to name them in terms of their response to a nutrient rather than in terms of a deficiency. Notable examples of these are the zinc-responsive dermatoses and the vitamin A–responsive dermatoses (rather than zinc deficiency and vitamin A deficiency). In many instances, these entities may represent genetically related inabilities to absorb or metabolize the nutrients rather than true nutritional deficiencies; in others, the response obtained may be the result of presently unknown effects of supraphysiologic doses of the nutrients.

Major nutritional problems of concern are deficiencies of essential fatty acids, protein, the minerals zinc and copper, and vitamins A, B, and E, as well as excessive levels of vitamin A. (see Chap. 3, Systemic Therapy). Food hypersensitivity may also produce dermatoses (see Chap. 8).

■ FATTY ACID DEFICIENCY

Fatty acid deficiency is uncommon to rare and seen only in animals that are fed dry rations, commercial food that has been poorly preserved (storage, temperature, preservative problems), or homemade foods.[1, 5, 10, 16] A deficiency may occur because fat was left out of the food to save costs, because it leaked from the bag during storage, or because it became rancid. Fatty acid deficiency also may occur from diets that contain fat but have inadequate antioxidants, such as vitamin E. Signs of fatty acid deficiency can be seen in dogs that are fed high-quality reducing dog foods in which the fat content has been lowered.

Dog food should have a minimum of 3 per cent fat in canned food and 7 to 8 per cent fat in dry food. Cats usually have 35 to 40 per cent of their calories provided by fat—a much higher amount—because they need a dense caloric formula. The oxidation of fat during storage is a great concern because when fat becomes rancid, the essential fatty acids as well as vitamins D, E, and biotin are destroyed. Oxidation may occur in canned food after 1 year and in dry food after 6 months, especially if the food is stored at high temperatures. Animals may also develop fatty acid deficiency in association with intestinal malabsorption, pancreatic disease, and chronic hepatic disease.

Animals must be on a diet deficient in essential fatty acids for several months before skin problems become evident.[3, 4, 5, 10, 17, 18] There is an early decrease in lipid production with resultant fine scaling of the skin and loss of the luster and sheen of the hair (Fig. 16:1 *A*). This dry phase can last for months and can have associated hair loss and secondary bacterial infections. Eventually, the skin thickens and becomes greasy, especially in the ears, in the intertriginous areas, and between the toes. The dryness of the coat is replaced by greasiness, and many animals become pruritic. Secondary bacterial or *Malassezia* infections can occur, with intensification of the seborrheic changes and pruritus.

Fatty acid deficiency in a number of species produces abnormal keratinization, resulting in epidermal hyperplasia, hypergranulosis, and orthokeratotic or parakeratotic hyperkeratosis. This abnormal keratinization is thought to result from arachidonic acid deficiency with resultant prostaglandin E deficiency, which causes aberrations in the ratios of epidermal cyclic adenosine monophosphate (cyclic AMP) to cyclic guanosine monophosphate (cyclic GMP) and in DNA synthesis.

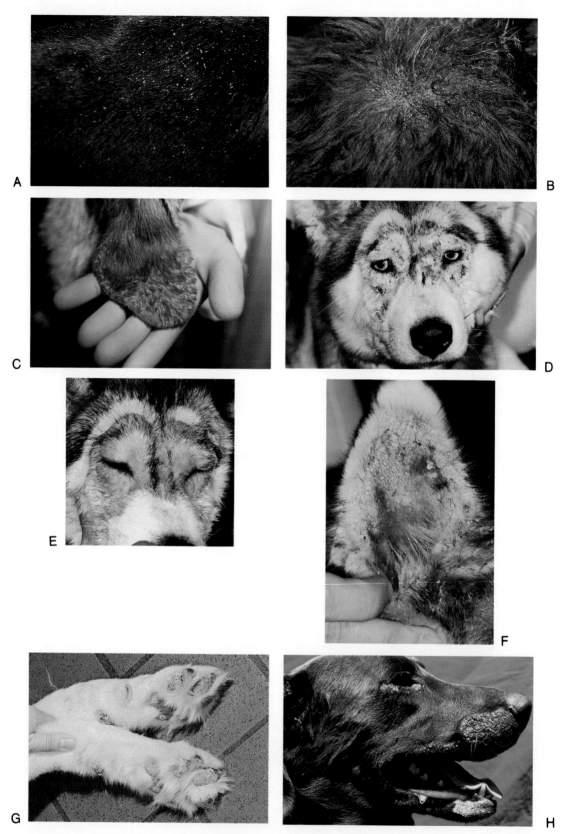

Figure 16:1 See legend on opposite page

The polyunsaturated fatty acid linoleic acid is essential in the diet of all animals. Arachidonic and linolenic acids are also required; however, with the exception of arachidonic acid in the cat, these acids can be synthesized from linoleic acid. Cats seems to lack an active Δ-6-desaturase to initiate the conversion of linoleic acid to arachidonic acid and thus are obligate carnivores.[1, 5, 11]

Therapy produces visible responses after 3 to 8 weeks of fatty acid supplementation if the dermatosis is indeed an essential fatty acid deficiency. In such cases, the coats may develop more luster. Fatty acid deficiency can be corrected by changing the dog's ration to one of higher quality and fat content, through the administration of various veterinary fatty acid supplements, or by the addition of household fats to the diet. If fats are to be added, equal parts of vegetable and animal fats are recommended; even though dogs can convert linoleic acid to arachidonic acid, conversion is unnecessary if it is provided in the diet. Animal fats contain arachidonic acid, but vegetable fats do not. The concentration of unsaturated essential fatty acids in various fats is as follows: safflower oil, 70 per cent; pork fat, 29 per cent; soybean oil, 50 per cent; poultry fat, 24 per cent; corn oil, 59 per cent; beef and butter fat, 3 per cent. Palm oil, olive oil, and coconut oil are low in linoleic acid and should not be used.[11]

The animal's diet should not be supplemented with more than 2 teaspoons (10 ml) of oil per cup (226 gm) or can of food, because this amount increases the caloric intake by 25 per cent. Usually one half this amount (1 teaspoon or 5 ml) of equal parts animal and vegetable fat per cup or can of food is a reasonable and effective supplement.

Although household fat supplementation can be effective, it is more beneficial to upgrade the basic diet or to use balanced nutritional supplements. If the fatty acid deficiency is compounded by intercurrent vitamin or mineral imbalances, household supplements will not correct them and may aggravate a vitamin E deficiency. Most prescription supplements contain all the necessary vitamins and minerals for the skin in addition to the essential fatty acids. Although most supplements are reasonably priced, the cost of using them continually in a normal dog or cat usually exceeds the cost of a better quality pet food.

Excessive fat supplementation is contraindicated in cases in which the fatty acid deficiency is intentional, such as in the management of obesity, pancreatic disease, or hyperlipidemia disorders. In these cases, treatment with balanced omega-6 and omega-3 fatty acid supplements (Derm Caps, DVM Pharmaceuticals; EFA Caps, Allerderm; Efa Vet, Efamol Vet) may be of some benefit.[11b] These supplements contain linoleic acid plus the marine lipids, eicosapentaenoic and docosahexaenoic acid. They are thought to modulate arachidonic acid metabolism with the production of various leukotrienes and prostaglandins, which can alter the inflammatory cascade and epidermal proliferation.[1a] These products have received the most attention in the treatment of allergic disorders (see Chaps. 3 and 8), but those reports indicate that improvement in coat quality also occurs with their use. It is unknown whether the improvement is due to the modulation of epidermal proliferation or to some other mechanism. The products supply high-quality fats in small volumes with low caloric density (fewer than 5 calories for every 9.1 kg of body weight); therefore, their use in obese animals should not significantly slow the weight loss. No data are available on the safety and efficacy of these supplements in dogs with pancreatitis or other disorders of lipid metabolism. The authors are aware of cases of flare-ups in pancreatitis when the full recommended dosage was initiated suddenly; with gradual introduction over 2 weeks, however, some dogs with pancreatitis have been able to tolerate the supplement.

Figure 16:1. A, Fatty acid deficiency in a dog. Dull, dry, brittle haircoat and diffuse scaling. B, Vitamin A deficiency in a dog. Marked follicular hyperkeratosis and follicular casts. C, Vitamin E deficiency in a dog. Marked exfoliative erythroderma on the pinna. D, Zinc-responsive dermatosis. Facial crusting. E, Same dog as in D. Severe erythema underlying crusts. F, Same dog as in D and E. Erythematous, crusted pinna. G, Same dog as in D, E, and F. Hyperkeratosis of footpads. H, Generic dog food dermatosis. Hyperkeratotic, crusted plaques with peripheral erythema in a mucocutaneous distribution. (Courtesy P. Ihrke.)

When dietary fat supplementation is impossible, topical application of essential fatty acids may be of some benefit. Studies in mice have shown that topically applied fats can correct the cutaneous changes of fatty acid deficiency.[11b] No data are available to support or refute this mechanism in dogs. Some of these dogs do very well when bathed with shampoos containing fatty acids (e.g., HyLyt*efa, DVM Pharmaceuticals) or rinsed with after-bath products containing fatty acids (e.g., Alpha-Sesame Oil-VR). The response seen in these animals may be due to mechanisms other than transepidermal fat absorption.

Fatty acid deficiency responds gradually to supplementation. Mild cases should return to normal in 4 to 8 weeks, but severe cases can take up to 6 months. Shampooing with antiseborrheic products hastens the clinical improvement, but these products should be used only when absolutely necessary. There is no specific laboratory test for fatty acid deficiency; the diagnosis is confirmed by response to treatment. If seborrheic changes are controlled by bathing, it may be impossible to determine whether the supplementation is of any benefit.

■ PROTEIN DEFICIENCY

Protein deficiency may be produced by inanition, starvation, feeding kittens commercial dog food, or feeding dogs special or very low-protein diets. Many commercial pet foods are actually extremely high in protein; as a result, protein deficiency is rare.

Hair is 95 per cent protein with a high percentage of amino acids that contain sulfur. The normal growth of hair (the sum of growth in all follicles being 100 feet per day) and the keratinization of skin require 25 to 30 per cent of the animal's daily protein requirement.[5, 10, 11] Animals with protein deficiency have hyperkeratosis, epidermal hyperpigmentation, and loss of hair pigment. There is patchy alopecia in which hairs become thinner, rough, dry, dull, and brittle. They are easily broken and grow slowly; shedding is prolonged. These lesions, together with scales and crusts, may appear symmetrically on the head, back, thorax, and abdomen, and on the feet and legs. Lesions are more prominent in young, growing dogs whose protein requirements are higher. In humans, a mean hair root diameter of less then 0.06 mm suggests protein deficiency, but no similar specifications are available for animals. An analysis of the diet and the provision of protein on a dry matter basis (25 per cent for dogs and 33 per cent for cats) should be therapeutic. High-quality protein from eggs, meat, or milk is important in supplementation.

■ VITAMIN DEFICIENCIES

Vitamin A

This vitamin functions to maintain healthy skin and epithelial cells; therefore, deficiency and toxicity signs, which are similar, are manifested cutaneously.[5, 10, 11, 16] There is hyperkeratinization of the epithelial surfaces. Hyperkeratosis occurs in the sebaceous glands, occluding their ducts and blocking secretion. Localized or generalized firm papular eruptions with a firm center are formed. A poor coat, alopecia, scaling of the skin, and an increased susceptibility to bacterial infection are also observed. A single injection of 6000 IU aqueous vitamin A solution per kg of body weight for 2 months is adequate therapy for a serious deficiency.

True vitamin A deficiency has been recognized in a mongrel dog.[11c] The dog had severe seborrheic skin lesions, nyctalopia, and diarrhea since puppyhood. The skin was thickened, hyperpigmented, and alopecic, with marked follicular hyperkeratosis (Fig. 16:1 *B*). Antiseborrheic shampoos were of no benefit, and the dog responded only partially to low-dose supplementation of vitamin A.

Because vitamin A is stored so well, toxicity may be of greater concern than deficiency. There is real danger of oversupplementation or toxicity from excess liver in the diet. A level 30 times the requirement for 2 to 3 months can produce toxicity. The dosage of retinol for dogs and cats should not exceed 400 IU/kg/day orally.

Hypervitaminosis A is best described in cats fed large amounts of liver.[7b] Among their other signs, these cats have disheveled, seborrheic coats probably as a result of their inability to groom themselves properly. Reports of this condition in dogs are rare.[7b, 11c] Affected dogs show pain when manipulated owing to vertebral changes, and they have seborrheic skin lesions identical to those seen in hypovitaminosis A or vitamin A–responsive dermatosis.

Vitamin A–Responsive Dermatosis

Some cases of severe seborrhea in Cocker spaniels and several other breeds have responded to vitamin A supplementation[6] and are discussed in detail in Chapter 13.

Vitamin E

Vitamin E, selenium, and fatty acids have a balanced relationship. Experimental vitamin E deficiency in dogs also results in severe suppression of in vitro lymphocyte blastogenesis.[9] In cats, a similar imbalance produces pansteatitis.[5, 7a, 16] This syndrome results when high-fat foods, such as canned red tuna, are fed almost exclusively. If food processing or fat oxidation has inactivated the vitamin E, the imbalance results. Cats show pain on gentle palpation and are anorectic, lethargic, and excitable. They may die in several weeks. There are large, firm lumps in the subcutaneous tissues and abdominal cavity. Diagnosis can be made at biopsy or autopsy by finding yellow fat and steatitis. Biopsy reveals lobular panniculitis and *ceroid* within lipocytes, macrophages, and giant cells. Ceroid is a pink to yellow homogenous material on H & E stain and deep crimson on acid-fast stain.

Naturally occurring vitamin E deficiency has not been reported in dogs, but experimentally induced vitamin E deficiency has been studied.[19] Researchers showed that skin lesions can be produced. They consisted of an early keratinization defect (seborrhea sicca), a later greasy and inflammatory stage (erythroderma and seborrhea oleosa) (Fig. 16:1 *C*); in addition, the dogs tended to develop secondary bacterial pyoderma. The dermatohistopathologic findings in dogs with experimentally produced vitamin E deficiency are nondiagnostic. Morphologically, the findings are characterized by hyperplastic superficial perivascular dermatitis. This is a common reaction pattern in canine skin, one most commonly seen in hypersensitivity reactions, ectoparasitisms, and seborrheic disorders. When the experimental dogs that had been fed a vitamin E–deficient diet were provided a vitamin E supplement equal to or double the National Research Council recommendations, the dermatosis responded dramatically. The erythema and greasiness subsided within 3 to 6 weeks, and the scaling resolved within 8 to 10 weeks.

Vitamin E deficiency induces T cell dysfunction in dogs and has been associated as a causal factor in generalized demodicosis in dogs.[2a, 2b] Research has not been able to substantiate this claim. Megadose vitamin supplementation, although of some probable benefit, has not been curative.[2d]

A number of dermatoses in dogs and humans have been treated successfully with oral vitamin E, including discoid lupus erythematosus, acanthosis nigricans, and epidermolysis bullosa or dermatomyositis. It is unlikely that vitamin E deficiency would occur in dogs on commercial diets. It would enter into the differential diagnosis of a dog with seborrhea or erythroderma. Diagnosis would be based on dietary history, physical examination, the ruling out of more common canine dermatoses, compatible skin biopsy results, and response to vitamin E therapy.

Vitamin E is used in doses of 10 mg (13.5 IU)/kg/day as an antioxidant and for the therapy of pansteatitis in cats (resulting from excess tuna or fat in the diet). In severe cases, it is mandatory to use systemic corticosteroids during the painful period of treatment (2 to 3 weeks).[7a] Vitamin E in doses of 400 to 800 IU q12h has been used successfully in discoid lupus erythematosus, systemic lupus erythematosus, and in disorders involving the basement membrane zone.

Vitamin B

B-complex vitamins are considered as a group because deficiencies of single B vitamins are very rare and the clinical syndromes are similar.[5, 10, 11] These vitamins are synthesized by intestinal bacteria; because they are water soluble and not stored, a constant supply is needed, and toxicities do not occur. It is possible for biotin, riboflavin, niacin, and pyridoxine deficiencies to have clinical ramifications.

Biotin can be inactivated by feeding the animal a diet high in uncooked eggs.[5, 10, 11] The whites contain avidin, which binds biotin so that it cannot be absorbed. Biotin deficiency can also result from prolonged oral antibiotic therapy. The most striking sign is a "spectacle eye" of alopecia around the face and eyes. Biotin deficiency should be differentiated from demodicosis, dermatophytosis, and other facial dermatoses (discoid lupus erythematosus, pemphigus, dermatomyositis, epidermolysis bullosa). In severe cases, crusted lesions of the face, neck, body, and legs are present. There may also be lethargy, emaciation, and diarrhea. Biotin deficiency has been shown to cause a widespread papulocrustous dermatitis in cats.[4]

Riboflavin deficiency may produce a dry, flaky dermatitis (seborrhea), especially around the eyes and ventrum; the outstanding sign, however, is cheilosis.[10, 11] The deficiency also produces alopecia on the head of cats.[5] Riboflavin deficiency is all but impossible if any meat or dairy products are present in the diet.

Niacin deficiency is manifested as pellagra and is characterized by ulcerated mucous membranes, diarrhea, and emaciation. It may produce a pruritic dermatitis of the rear legs and abdomen.[10, 11] For a deficiency to be produced, the diet must be low in animal protein and high in corn. Corn and all cereals are low in tryptophan, which is converted to niacin by all animals except cats. Commercial pet foods contain more than enough niacin; therefore, supplementation is not needed.

Pyridoxine deficiency, produced experimentally in cats, causes a dull, waxy, unkept haircoat with generalized and fine white scales.[12] In some experimental cats, it caused multiple areas of alopecia in the temporal and periauricular area, on the dorsum of the muzzle, periorally, and on the extremities. When these experimental pyridoxine-deficient cats were fed a balanced diet, all of the skin lesions resolved. This condition has not been observed clinically and remains a laboratory phenomenon.

The most common signs of B-complex deficiencies are a dry, flaky seborrhea with alopecia, anorexia, and weight loss. Effective treatment consists of brewer's yeast, B-complex injections, or both. Supplementation may be needed only if the animals are anorectic or have problems that cause excess water turnover.

When 119 dogs with dull coat, brittle hair, loss of hair, scaly skin, pruritus, or dermatitis were given biotin (0.5 mg/10 kg body weight/day) for 3 to 5 weeks, 108 (91 per cent) were cured or improved significantly.[2c] Insufficient data were supplied to determine whether these dogs were truly deficient in biotin or responded by some other therapeutic effect. This report highlights the need for broad-based vitamin supplementation when a nutritional deficiency is suspected or when fatty acids are added to a seborrheic dog's diet.

■ MINERAL IMBALANCES

Zinc, copper, and calcium are three minerals that influence iodine metabolism and each other; abnormal levels of any one of them may be reflected in the skin. Because of the great variation among individuals, only one or several of a group of animals may develop lesions, even though all have been fed and managed alike.

Copper deficiency should appear as a balance problem only if excess zinc is added to the diet.[10, 11] Copper is needed by enzymes that convert L-tyrosine to melanin and by the follicular cells in the conversion of prekeratin to keratin. A deficiency is manifested by hypopigmentation and faulty keratinization of the skin and hair follicles, with the hair becoming dull and rough. Because commercial pet foods have adequate copper levels, supplements are not needed.

■ ZINC-RESPONSIVE DERMATOSIS

Zinc is an important cofactor and modulator of many critical biological functions.[11d, 13a] Although zinc deficiency was thought to play a role in many dermatoses of the dog, recent work[11a] indicates that zinc deficiency is rare in the dog. Zinc deficiency has been documented in bull terriers with acrodermatitis (see Chap. 11), and relative or absolute deficiency is suspected in two other dermatologic syndromes.[2, 8, 13]

Syndrome I occurs in Siberian huskies and Alaskan malamutes primarily, but bull terriers may also be affected.[11a] Skin lesions in these breeds develop despite well-balanced, diets with sufficient zinc. Lesions develop early in adulthood (at 1 to 3 years of age) and progress at a variable rate. There is early erythema followed by alopecia, crusting, scaling, and underlying suppuration around the mouth, chin, eyes and ears (see Fig. 16:1 *D* to *F*). Other body openings and the scrotum, prepuce, and vulva may be affected. Although the coat is dull, there is excess sebum production. Thick crusts may appear on the elbows and other pressure points. The skin may be inelastic and the legs stiff, as a result of hardened crusts. Secondary bacterial or *Malassezia* infections are common. The footpads may become hyperkeratotic (Fig. 16:1 *G*). In chronic cases, hyperpigmentation occurs in the area of the lesions. There may be a decreased sense of smell (hyposmia) and taste (hypogeusia). Clinical signs may be precipitated or intensified by stress and estrus.

It has been shown that Malamutes have a genetic defect of decreased capability for zinc absorption from the intestines.[8, 11] In some Siberian huskies, hypothyroidism and a decreased serum zinc level have been reported, but the significance of these is unknown.[8] Dogs on high-calcium or high-cereal diets, which have high levels of phytate, show poor zinc absorption, owing to binding of the zinc. Prolonged enteritis and diarrhea also prevent normal absorption. A severe deficiency may cause poor growth and weight loss in young puppies and poor wound healing in any animal.[14, 15]

Syndrome II occurs in rapidly growing puppies that are fed zinc-deficient diets, diets high in phytates or minerals such as calcium (which interfere with zinc absorption), or diets that are oversupplemented with minerals and vitamins. Many breeds may be abnormal, but Great Danes, Doberman pinschers, beagles, German shepherds, German shorthaired pointers, Labrador retrievers, Rhodesian Ridgebacks, and standard poodles have been reported.[6, 8, 13, 22] The severity of lesions can vary greatly within a litter. Some animals may be normal, whereas others are stunted, depressed, and anorectic. The skin lesions are hyperkeratotic plaques over areas of repeated trauma or where calluses might normally occur. The footpads and nasal planum may be affected, and any thickened area may have deep fissures. There may be secondary infection of the crusts and an associated lymphadenopathy. Severely affected dogs can look as though they have canine distemper.

In both syndromes, serum or hair zinc levels may be abnormal. Proper analysis for zinc is difficult and can be unreliable, however, because samples may be contaminated by zinc in glassware or rubber stoppers, and by the influences of various environmental, physiologic, and disease-related factors.[11a, 22, 24]

Diagnosis may be made by history taking, physical examination, and skin biopsy. Hyperplastic superficial perivascular dermatitis, with marked diffuse and follicular parakeratotic hyperkeratosis, is suggestive of zinc deficiency (Figs. 16:2 and 16:3). Papillomatosis and diffuse spongiosis are also common findings. Eosinophils are often prominent in the perivascular cellular infiltrate. Intraepidermal pustular dermatitis and suppurative folliculitis reflect secondary bacterial infection.

Treatment involves the inspection and correction of any inadequacy in the diet, including the base diet, water, and any treats or supplements given to the animal. In Syndrome II, dietary adjustments alone can resolve the skin lesions in 2 to 6 weeks. Zinc supplementation is necessary in Syndrome I and can hasten the animal's response in Syndrome II. In the latter case, the supplement need be given for only a few weeks to restore the zinc stores in the animal; in Syndrome I, the supplementation must be lifelong.

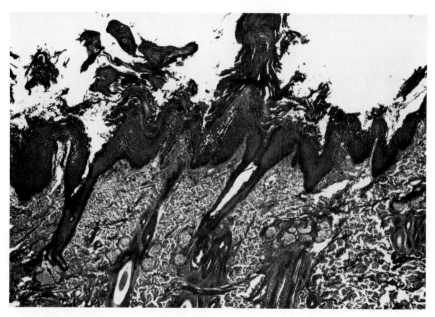

Figure 16:2. Zinc-responsive dermatosis in a Siberian husky. Hyperplastic perivascular dermatitis with marked diffuse parakeratotic hyperkeratosis.

Oral zinc supplementation with zinc sulfate (10 mg/kg/day) or zinc methionine (1.7 mg/kg/day) is adequate in most cases. If zinc sulfate is used, the tablets should be crushed and mixed with food to enhance absorption and decrease gastric irritation. In Syndrome II, the supplement can be withdrawn when the skin has returned to normal, if the nutritional problem has been corrected. In Syndrome I, zinc administration is lifelong and dosage adjustments may be necessary. In both syndromes, existing skin lesions can be improved by hydrating the crusts with wet dressings or whole-body warm water soakings for 5 to 10 minutes and then bathing the animal with an antiseborrheic shampoo. Lesions on the face and elsewhere improve with the application of petrolatum or an ointment-based topical agent. Topical agents are less messy, and the active ingredient—an antibiotic or keratolytic agent—provides additional benefits.

Some dogs, especially Siberian huskies, do not respond to oral zinc supplementation.

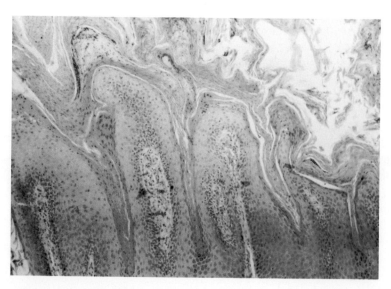

Figure 16:3. Close-up of Figure 16:2. Papillomatosis and diffuse parakeratotic hyperkeratosis that also involves hair follicles.

Intravenous injection with sterile zinc sulfate solutions at dosages of 10 to 15 mg/kg has been effective.[22a] Weekly injections for at least 4 weeks are necessary to resolve the lesions, and maintenance injections every 1 to 6 months are necessary to prevent relapses. Dogs that require intravenous treatment should not be used for breeding. The same recommendation should be made for all dogs with Syndrome I.

In kittens, dietary zinc deficiency was reported to cause thinning of the haircoat, slow hair growth, scaly skin, and ulceration of the buccal margins.[7] The cat's requirement for dietary zinc was estimated at between 15 and 50 ppm.

■ GENERIC DOG FOOD SKIN DISEASE

Dogs fed only generic dog foods for 2 to 4 weeks developed bilateral symmetric scaling and crusting dermatoses.[20, 21] The lesions involved the bridge of the nose, mucocutaneous junctions, pressure points, and distal extremities (Fig. 16:1 *H*). Well-demarcated, older lesions had erythematous borders with scales, crusts, and variable hyperpigmentation and lichenification. A few dogs had alopecia, focal erosions, papules, and pustules; most had fever, depression, lymphadenopathy, and pitting edema of dependent areas.

Skin biopsies showed hyperplastic superficial perivascular dermatitis with diffuse parakeratotic hyperkeratosis and focal epidermal dyskeratosis and a mixed dermal cellular infiltrate (Fig. 16:4). Although the clinical and histopathologic findings are similar to those seen in the zinc-responsive dermatoses, the acuteness of onset and the frequent occurrence of systemic illness suggest that other nutritional imbalances may play a role.

The differential diagnosis should include relative or absolute zinc deficiency, immune-mediated skin diseases (especially pemphigus foliaceous and systemic lupus erythematosus), staphylococcal folliculitis, and necrolytic migratory erythema. Treatment with antibiotics or corticosteroids was unsuccessful, but rapid response occurred 1 week after simply changing the dogs' diet to a national brand of dog food that met National Research Council requirements.

Since the original reports on this disorder, no additional cases have been reported. Improvements in the formulation of generic pet foods must have been made, because they are still marketed.

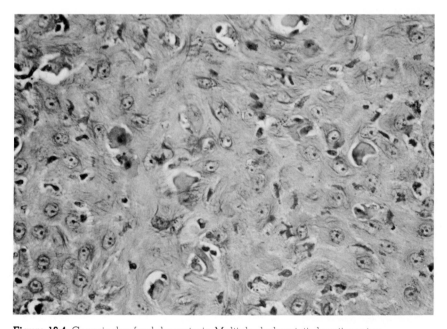

Figure 16:4. Generic dog food dermatosis. Multiple dyskeratotic keratinocytes.

■ NUTRITIONAL SUPPLEMENTS

Pets that are fed high-quality commercial foods typically receive no benefits from additional supplements. When disease results from the animal eating low-quality food or from inherent metabolic defects that alter the digestion or absorption of one or more nutrients, one can choose to supplement the existing diet or upgrade the base diet with a higher quality food. It is more appropriate and cost effective to upgrade the base diet because all nutrients should be in the correct proportion. If the owners are reluctant to change foods without absolute proof of the benefit of doing so, or if the animal refuses to eat anything different, a supplement proposed by Lewis can be beneficial.[10, 11] For every 9 to 14 kg of body weight, the dog should be given 1 teaspoon (5 ml) of corn oil or safflower oil, 2 ounces (56 gm) of cooked liver, 100 mg of zinc sulfate, and 1 drop of tincture of iodine. Most owners find it convenient to make large batches of the supplement. Problems with thorough mixing of the ingredients and giving the dog the correct amount can be overcome by making a purée of the mixture in a blender and freezing the supplement in ice cube trays. At each meal, the owner can thaw the appropriate number of cubes and add them to the diet. Because this supplement provides fat, protein, vitamins A and E, biotin, riboflavin, niacin, iodine, and zinc, it should resolve all nutritional dermatoses unless they have a genetic basis (e.g., Syndrome I zinc-responsive dermatoses) or are secondary to severe gastrointestinal disorders. If no change is seen after 8 weeks of supplementation, nutritional causes can be discounted; if a good response is seen, the supplement can be continued or a new base diet can be selected.

REFERENCES

1. Anderson, R.W. (ed.): Nutrition of the Dog and Cat: Proceedings of an International Symposium. Elmsford, New York, Pergamon Press, 1980, p. 67.
1a. Campbell, K.L.: Fatty acid supplementation and skin disease. Vet. Clin. North. Am. (Small Anim Pract.) 20:1475, 1990.
2. Fadok, V.A.: Nutritional therapy in veterinary dermatology. In: Kirk, R.W. (ed.). Current Veterinary Therapy IX. W.B. Saunders Co., Philadelphia, 1986, p. 591.
2a. Figueiredo, C.: Vitamin E serum contents, erythrocyte and lymphocyte counts, PCV and Hg determination in normal dogs, dogs with scabies, and dogs with demodicosis. Proc. Annu. Memb. Meet. Am. Acad. Vet. Dermatol. 1, 1985.
2b. Figueiredo, C., et al.: Clinical evaluation of the effect of vitamin E in the treatment of generalized canine demodicosis. Adv. Vet. Dermatol., 2:247, 1993.
2c. Frigg, M., et al.: Clinical study on the effect of biotin on skin conditions in dogs. Schweiz Arch Tierheilk 131:621, 1989.
2d. Gilbert, P.A., et al.: Serum vitamin E levels in dogs with pyoderma and generalized demodicosis. J. Am. Anim. Hosp. Assoc. 28:407, 1992.
3. Hansen, A.E., Weise, H.F.: Fat in the diet in relation to nutrition of the dog. I. Characteristic appearance and gross changes of animals fed diets with and without fat. Tex. Rep. Biol. Med. 52:205, 1951.
4. Hansen, A.E., Weise, H.F.: Studies with dogs maintained on diets low in fat. Proc. Soc. Exp. Biol. Med. 52:205, 1943.
5. Holzworth, J.: Diseases of the Cat: Medicine and Surgery. W.B. Saunders Co., Philadelphia, 1987.
6. Ihrke, P.J., Goldschmidt, M.H.: Vitamin A–responsive dermatosis in the dog. J. Am. Vet. Med. Assoc. 182:687, 1983.
7. Kane, E., et al.: Zinc deficiency in the cat. J. Nutr. 111:488, 1981.
7a. Koutinas, A.F., et al.: Pansteatitis (steatitis, "yellow fat disease") in the cat: A review article and report of 4 spontaneous cases. Vet. Dermatol. 3:101, 1993.
7b. Kronfeld, D.S.: Vitamin and Mineral Supplementation for Dogs and Cats. Veterinary Practice Publishing Co., Santa Barbara, 1989.
8. Kunkle, G.A.: Zinc-responsive dermatoses in dogs. In: Kirk, R.W. (ed.). Current Veterinary Therapy VII. W.B. Saunders Co., Philadelphia, 1980, p. 472.
9. Langweiler, M., et al.: Effect of vitamin E deficiency on the proliferative response of canine lymphocytes. Am. J. Vet. Res. 42:1681, 1981.
10. Lewis, L.D.: Cutaneous manifestations of nutritional imbalances. Proceedings, Am. Anim. Hosp. Assoc. 48:263, 1981.
11. Lewis, L.D., Morris, M.L., Jr.: Small Animal Clinical Nutrition, 2nd ed. Topeka, Mark Morris Associates, 1984.
11a. Logas, D.L., et al.: Comparison of serum zinc levels in healthy, systemically ill, and dermatologically diseased dogs. Vet. Dermatol. 4:61, 1993.
11b. Miller, W.H. Jr.: Nutritional considerations in small animal dermatology. Vet. Clin. North Am. 19:497, 1989.

11c. Miller, W.H. Jr.: Unpublished observations, 1994.

11d. Norris, D.: Zinc and cutaneous inflammation. Arch. Dermatol. 121:985, 1985.

12. Norton, A.: Skin lesions seen in cats with vitamin B (pyroxidine) deficiency. Proc. Annu. Memb. Meet. Am. Acad. Vet. Dermatol. and Am. Coll. Vet. Dermatol. 3:24, 1987.

13. Ohlen, B., Scott, D.W.: Zinc responsive dermatitis in puppies. Canine Pract. 13:2, 1986.

13a. Russell, R.M., et al: Zinc and the special senses. Ann. Intern. Med. 99:227, 1983.

14. Sanecki, R.K., et al.: Tissue changes in dogs fed a zinc-deficient ration. Am. J. Vet. Res. 43:1642, 1982.

15. Sanecki, R.K., et al.: Extracutaneous histologic changes accompanying zinc deficiency in pups. Am. J. Vet. Res. 46:2119, 1985.

16. Scott, D.W.: Feline dermatology 1900–1978: A monograph. J. Am. Anim. Hosp. Assoc. 16:331, 1980.

17. Scott, D.W.: Feline dermatology 1979–1982: Introspective retrospections. J. Am. Anim. Hosp. Assoc. 20:537, 1984.

18. Scott, D.W.: Feline dermatology 1983–1985: "The secret sits." J. Am. Anim. Hosp. Assoc. 23:255, 1987.

19. Scott, D.W., Sheffy, B.E.: Dermatosis in dogs caused by vitamin E deficiency. Comp. Anim. Pract. 1:42, 1987.

20. Sousa, C.A., et al.: Dermatosis associated with feeding generic dog food: 13 cases (1981–1982). J. Am. Vet. Med. Assoc. 192:676, 1988.

21. Sousa, C.A.: Nutritional dermatoses. In: Nesbit, G. H. (ed.). Dermatology: Contemporary Issues in Small Animal Practice. Churchill Livingstone, Inc., New York, 1987.

22. van den Broek, A.H.M., Thoday, K.L.: Skin disease in dogs associated with zinc deficiency: A report of 5 cases. J. Small Anim. Pract. 27:313, 1986.

22a. Willemse, T.: Zinc-responsive disorders of the dog. In: Kirk, R.W., Bonagura, J.D. (eds.). Kirk's Current Veterinary Therapy XI. W.B. Saunders Co., Philadelphia, 1992, p. 532.

23. Wolf, A.M.: Zinc-responsive dermatosis in a Rhodesian Ridgeback. Vet. Med. 80:37, 1985.

24. Wright, R.P.: Identification of zinc-responsive dermatoses. Vet. Med. 80:37, 1985.

Miscellaneous
Skin Diseases

∎

■ CANINE SUBCORNEAL PUSTULAR DERMATOSIS

Subcorneal pustular dermatosis is a very rare, idiopathic, sterile, superficial pustular dermatosis of dogs.[2, 5, 6]

Cause and Pathogenesis

The cause of subcorneal pustular dermatosis is unknown. In humans, it has been postulated that immunologic mechanisms may play a role.[4, 6] Immune complexes and immunoglobulin (Ig)A that could be chemoattractant to neutrophils have been demonstrated in vivo in the stratum corneum. Elevated levels of tumor necrosis factor α have been demonstrated in the serum and pustules of a human with subcorneal pustular dermatosis.[8] Some cases of human subcorneal pustular dermatosis are associated with the presence or development of paraproteinemia (usually the IgA type), with or without myeloma, but this condition has not been reported in dogs.[6]

Clinical Features

No apparent age (6 months to 14 years old) or sex predilection exists. Although many breeds have been affected, miniature Schnauzers have accounted for about 40 per cent of the cases.

Affected dogs usually have a multifocal to generalized, pustular to seborrhea-like dermatitis. The head and trunk, particularly, are affected in a symmetric fashion. Intact pustules are usually nonfollicular, greenish yellow in color, and transient in nature, persisting for only 2 to 4 hours at a time (Fig. 17:1 A and B). Thus, the affected dogs often have only circular areas of alopecia, erosion, scaling, crusting, and epidermal collarettes. Lesions tend to heal centrally, often with hyperpigmentation, and to spread peripherally, producing annular and serpiginous configurations. Rarely, the footpads may be affected and show a superficial peeling. Pruritus varies from nonexistent to extreme. The course of the dermatosis is often to erupt and regress. Usually, the dogs are otherwise healthy. Occasional dogs have peripheral lymphadenopathy; rarely, they have pyrexia, anorexia, and depression.

Diagnosis

Because this dermatosis is diagnosed by the exclusion of other conditions, improved diagnostic techniques should make it a rare entity.

The differential diagnosis includes bacterial folliculitis, pemphigus foliaceus, systemic lupus erythematosus, sterile eosinophilic pustulosis, seborrheic skin disease, scabies, atopy, and food hypersensitivity. Definitive diagnosis is based on history, physical examination, exclusion through laboratory testing, and response to therapy. Subcorneal pustular dermatosis responds poorly to systemic antibiotics, systemic glucocorticoids, and topical agents. Direct smears from intact pustules usually reveal numerous nondegenerate neutrophils, occasional acantholytic keratinocytes, and no microorganisms (Fig. 17:2). Carefully performed cultures from intact pustules are usually negative, but a few colonies of coagulase-negative or coagulase-positive staphylococci are occasionally isolated. Immunofluorescence testing is negative. Skin biopsy reveals intraepidermal (subcorneal) pustular dermatitis.[2, 6] Acantholysis is usually minimal, but it is occasionally marked. Neutrophils do not show degenerative changes. Hair follicles are rarely involved (Figs. 17:3 and 17:4).

Up to one half of affected dogs may have a mild to moderate mature neutrophilia (13.8 to 21.1×10^3/ml).[6] Serum protein electrophoresis occasionally reveals increased amounts of α_1, α_2, and β globulins.[6]

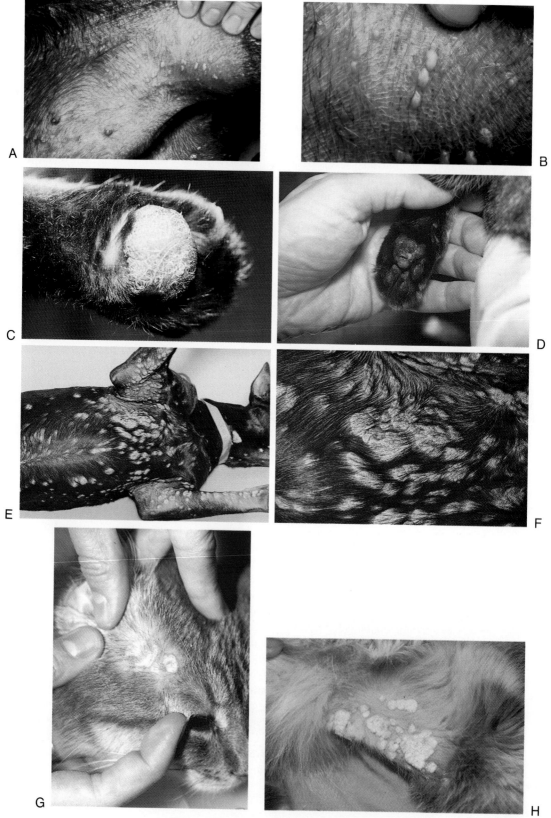

Figure 17:1 See legend on opposite page

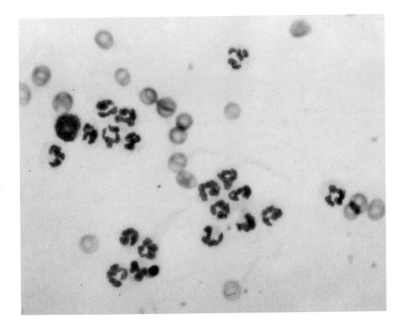

Figure 17:2. Canine subcorneal pustular dermatosis. Cytologic examination reveals nondegenerate neutrophils and no microorganisms.

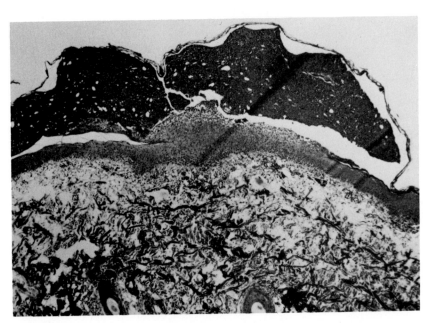

Figure 17:3. Canine subcorneal pustular dermatosis. A large subcorneal pustule.

Figure 17:1. *A*, Multiple nonfollicular pustules on the abdomen of a dog with subcorneal pustular dermatosis. *B*, Close-up view of *A*. *C*, Feline plasma cell pododermatitis. Swollen footpad with cross-hatched white striae. *D*, Feline plasma cell pododermatitis. Ulcerated nodule projecting from a footpad. *E*, Lichenoid dermatitis on the chest and forelegs of a dog. *F*, Same dog as in *E*. Lichenoid papules and plaques on the chest. *G*, Idiopathic lichenoid dermatitis in a cat. Cluster of lichenoid papules in the preauricular area. *H*, Same cat as in *G*. Cluster of lichenoid papules and plaques in the axillary area.

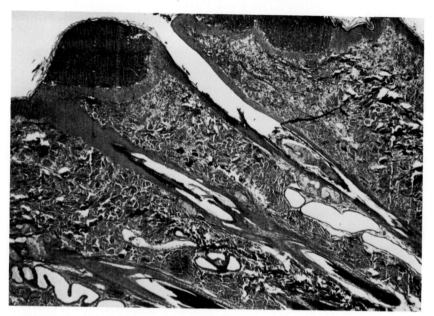

Figure 17:4. Canine subcorneal pustular dermatosis. Subcorneal pustules that do not involve hair follicles.

Clinical Management

The drug of choice in subcorneal pustular dermatosis is dapsone (see Chap. 3), which is given orally at 1 mg/kg q8h. A beneficial response is usually seen in 1 to 4 weeks. In a minority of cases, the therapy can be stopped and long-term remission may result; more often, however, the drug is tapered to maintenance levels, with the dosage varying from dog to dog (from 1 mg/kg q24h to twice a week).

In dogs, the major side-effects of dapsone have been hematologic and hepatic. Many dogs develop mild nonregenerative anemia and leukopenia, and mild to moderate elevations of serum alanine aminotransferase during induction therapy. If these laboratory abnormalities are not associated with clinical signs, it is not necessary to stop therapy; the levels will return to normal when maintenance doses are achieved. Dapsone has also caused fatal thrombocytopenia in one dog, profound leukopenia in one dog, occasional vomiting and diarrhea, and generalized, pruritic erythematous maculopapular skin eruptions.[6] Dapsone is *not* licensed for use in dogs.

Very rarely, dogs have apparently become resistant to dapsone. These dogs may or may not benefit from the oral administration of sulfasalazine (Azulfidine), 10 to 20 mg/kg q8h until the dermatosis is controlled, and then as needed. Chronic administration of sulfasalazine may be associated with keratoconjunctivitis sicca. One dog that did not respond to dapsone was successfully managed with injectable gold.[7]

■ FELINE PLASMA CELL PODODERMATITIS

Plasma cell pododermatitis is a rare cutaneous disorder of cats.[2, 9, 10]

Cause and Pathogenesis

The cause and pathogenesis of this disorder are unknown. However, the tissue plasmacytosis, the consistent hypergammaglobulinemia, and the beneficial response to immunomodulating drugs suggest an immune-mediated pathogenesis. In addition, some cases have recurred on a seasonal basis, suggesting that the condition is an allergic response.

Clinical Features

No age, breed, or sex predilections are apparent. Clinically, plasma cell pododermatitis begins as a soft, painless swelling of multiple footpads on multiple paws (see Fig. 17:1 C). The central metacarpal or metatarsal pads are usually affected. Lightly pigmented pads may take on a violaceous hue. The surface of affected pads is cross-hatched with white scaly striae. Affected pads feel mushy. The cats are usually otherwise healthy. In some cases, one or more pads may become ulcerated and secondarily infected, which occasionally results in pain, lameness, and regional lymphadenopathy. Occasional cats develop recurring hemorrhage from ulcerated or nodular areas of a footpad (see Fig. 17:1 D).[11]

A minority of cats with plasma cell pododermatitis also have plasma cell stomatitis, which is characterized by ulceroproliferative gingivitis and symmetric vegetative plaques at the palatine arches.[9] In addition, an occasional cat has immune-mediated glomerulonephritis or renal amyloidosis.[10]

Diagnosis

The differential diagnosis includes infectious or sterile granulomas and pyogranulomas, or neoplasia, all of which typically affect only one footpad. Definitive diagnosis is based on history, physical examination, aspiration cytologic study, culture, and biopsy. Neutrophilia and lymphocytosis may be seen, and hypergammaglobulinemia is typical. Serum protein electrophoresis reveals a polyclonal gammopathy. Carefully performed cultures are negative. Aspiration cytologic study reveals numerous plasma cells with smaller numbers of lymphocytes and neutrophils. Antinuclear antibody tests are occasionally positive, and direct immunofluorescence testing rarely reveals Ig at the basement membrane zone. However, these latter two immunologic findings are nondiagnostic. Most cats are feline leukemia virus (FeLV) and feline immunodeficiency virus (FIV) negative.[9, 10, 11]

Skin biopsy of early lesions is characterized by superficial and deep perivascular dermatitis with plasma cells predominating. Later lesions are characterized by diffuse plasmacytic dermatitis (Figs. 17:5 and 17:6).[1, 2] Many plasma cells contain Russell bodies (Mott cells). Variable numbers of neutrophils are present, reflecting the absence or presence of ulceration and secondary infection. Rarely, leukocytoclastic vasculitis is also present.

Clinical Management

The therapy of choice is not clear. Because plasma cell pododermatitis is usually asymptomatic and may spontaneously regress, treatment may not be indicated in most cases. When treatment is necessary, both large doses of systemic glucocorticoid (prednisone or prednisolone administered orally at 4.4 mg/kg q24h) or chrysotherapy may be effective.[9, 10, 11] A clear response to therapy is evident in 2 to 3 weeks, and maximum improvement is seen in 10 to 14 weeks. Footpads may remain slightly enlarged. Focal ulcers or nodules that hemorrhage usually require surgical correction.[11]

■ LICHENOID DERMATOSES

Lichenoid dermatoses are rare, usually idiopathic skin disorders of dogs and cats.[12-15]

Cause and Pathogenesis

The cause and pathogenesis of most of these dermatoses are unclear; their clinical and histopathologic features suggest an immune-mediated pathomechanism.[4]

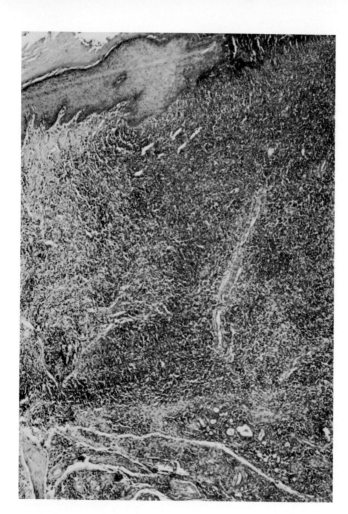

Figure 17:5. Feline plasma cell pododermatitis. Diffuse plasmacytic dermatitis.

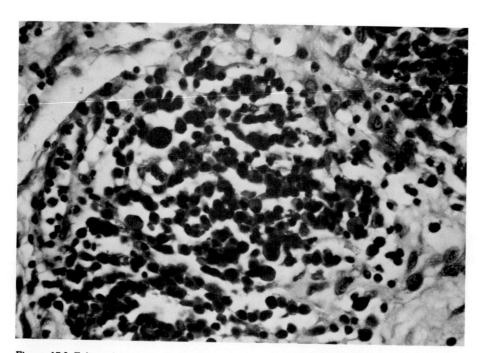

Figure 17:6. Feline plasma cell pododermatitis. Numerous plasma cells.

Clinical Features

There are no apparent age, breed, or sex predilections. Lichenoid dermatoses are characterized by the usually asymptomatic, symmetric onset of grouped, angular, flat-topped papules that develop a scaly to markedly hyperkeratotic surface (see Fig. 17:1 *E* to *H*). Lesions may coalesce to form hyperkeratotic, alopecic plaques, and they may occur anywhere on the body. Affected animals are usually otherwise healthy.

Diagnosis

The differential diagnosis includes staphylococcal folliculitis, dermatophytosis, and various granulomatous and neoplastic conditions. Definitive diagnosis is based on history, physical examination, exclusion through laboratory testing, and skin biopsy. Carefully performed cultures are negative. Skin biopsy reveals hyperkeratotic and hyperplastic lichenoid and hydropic interface dermatitis (Fig. 17:7). The inflammatory infiltrate is characteristically lymphoplasmacytic. If intraepidermal pustular dermatitis, suppurative folliculitis, or both are present, one should suspect a lichenoid tissue reaction in response to staphylococcal infection. Such cases respond to appropriate systemic antibiotic therapy. If eosinophilic microabscesses are present, one should suspect a lichenoid tissue reaction in response to an ectoparasite (especially scabies or cheyletiellosis).

Clinical Management

The prognosis for canine and feline idiopathic lichenoid dermatoses appears to be good. All cases have undergone spontaneous remission after a course of 6 months to 2 years. No form of therapy has been shown to be beneficial. In humans, oral retinoids have been useful in many cases.[4]

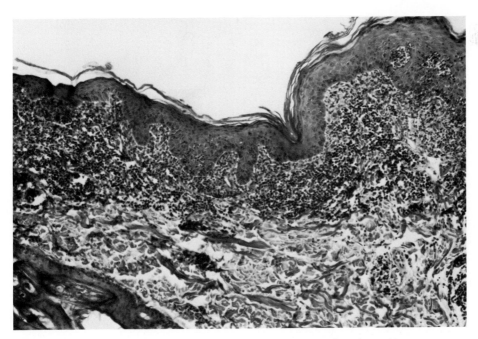

Figure 17:7. Canine idiopathic lichenoid dermatitis. Lichenoid interface dermatitis.

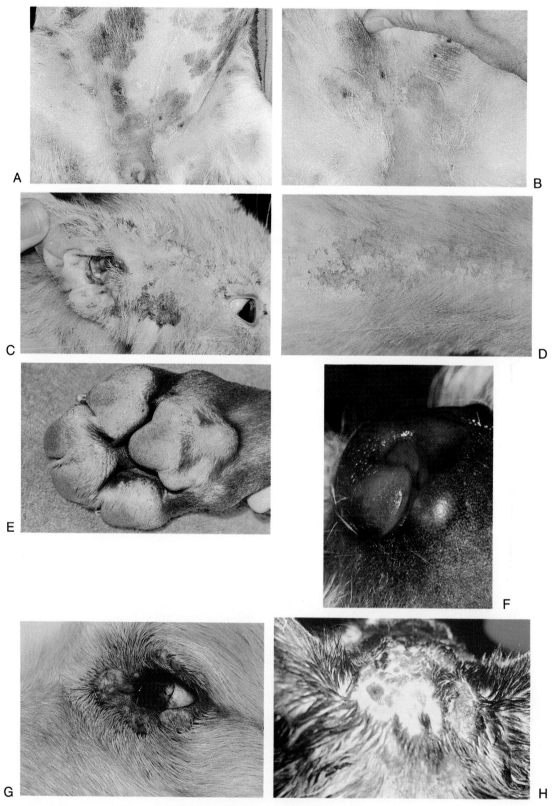

Figure 17:8 See legend on opposite page

■ CANINE STERILE EOSINOPHILIC PUSTULOSIS

Sterile eosinophilic pustulosis is a rare idiopathic dermatosis of dogs.[16–20]

Cause and Pathogenesis

The cause and pathogenesis are unknown. The peripheral eosinophilia, sterile tissue eosinophilia, and responsiveness to systemic glucocorticoids that characterize this syndrome suggest that it may be immune-mediated. However, intradermal skin testing, hypoallergenic diets, and immunopathologic studies have not been helpful in elucidating the etiopathogenesis. Cats also rarely develop a clinical and pathologic sterile eosinophilic folliculitis; the clinical presentation is different, however, and the lesions are associated with an underlying hypersensitivity such as atopy, food hypersensitivity, flea bite hypersensitivity, and mosquito bite hypersensitivity (see Chap. 8).[21]

Clinical Features

No apparent age, breed, or sex predilections exist. The onset of clinical signs is often acute, and the distribution of lesions is multifocal (especially involving the trunk) or generalized. Pruritic, erythematous, follicular and nonfollicular papules and pustules evolve into annular erosions with epidermal collarettes (Fig. 17:8 *A* and *B*). Peripheral spread, central healing, and hyperpigmentation of lesions result in numerous target lesions. Although most dogs are otherwise healthy, fever, anorexia, depression, and peripheral lymphadenopathy may be present.

Diagnosis

The differential diagnosis includes staphylococcal folliculitis, pemphigus foliaceus, and subcorneal pustular dermatosis. Definitive diagnosis is based on history, physical examination, hemogram, direct smears, cultures, and skin biopsy. Most dogs have peripheral eosinophilia (up to 5.6 $\times$ 10^3/ml). Direct smears reveal numerous eosinophils, nondegenerative neutrophils, occasional acanthocytes, and no microorganisms (Fig. 17:9). Carefully performed cultures are negative. Biopsy reveals intraepidermal eosinophilic pustular dermatitis and eosinophilic folliculitis and furunculosis (Fig. 17:10). Flame figures are occasionally seen in the surrounding dermis. Direct and indirect immunofluorescence testing is negative. Serum alpha, beta, and gamma globulins may be elevated.

Clinical Management

Most dogs respond well to systemic glucocorticoids (oral prednisone or prednisolone 2.2 to 4.4 mg/kg q24h) in 5 to 10 days; however, stopping treatment consistently results in relapses. Thus, long-term, alternate-morning therapy is indicated, and cure is unlikely. In two dogs that could not be treated with glucocorticoids, the authors had good success with dapsone or the combination of an antihistamine (diphenhydramine) and an omega-6 and omega-3 fatty acid supplement (Derm Caps, DVM Pharmaceuticals).

Figure 17:8. *A,* Canine sterile eosinophilic pustulosis. Pustules and annular erosions on the abdomen. *B,* Close-up of the dog in *A.* Annular erosion with epidermal collarettes. *C,* Feline hypereosinophilic syndrome. Erythema and excoriation of the face and pinna. *D,* Same cat as in *C.* Erythema, alopecia, and excoriation over the back. *E,* Canine sterile pyogranuloma. Erythematous nodules bordering footpads. *F,* Canine sterile pyogranuloma. Erythematous nodules bordering nostrils. *G,* Canine sterile pyogranuloma. Multiple erythematosus, ulcerated, crusted papules around the eye. *H,* Idiopathic sterile pyogranulomas in a cat. Violaceous papules and nodules on the top of the head (the area has been clipped).

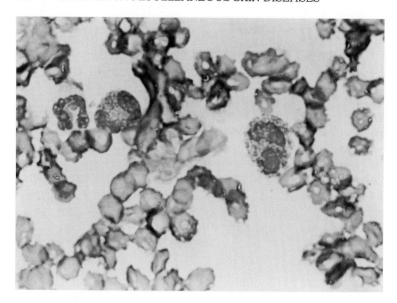

Figure 17:9. Canine sterile eosinophilic pustulosis. Cytologic examination reveals numerous eosinophils.

■ FELINE HYPEREOSINOPHILIC SYNDROME

The hypereosinophilic syndrome is a rare disorder of cats.[22–24] It is characterized by persistent idiopathic eosinophilia associated with a diffuse infiltration of various organs by mature eosinophils.

Cause and Pathogenesis

The cause and pathogenesis of this syndrome are unknown, but it is believed to be immune-mediated.

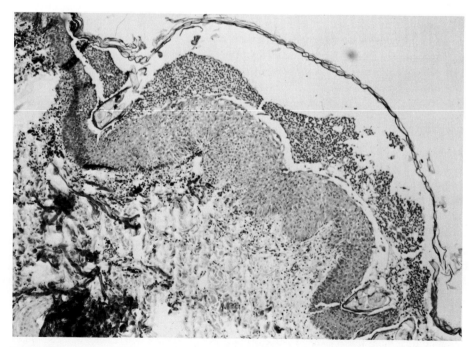

Figure 17:10. Canine sterile eosinophilic pustulosis. Subcorneal eosinophilic pustular dermatitis and eosinophilic folliculitis.

Clinical Features

There are no apparent age, breed, or sex predilections. Tissue infiltration with mature eosinophils results in multisystemic organ dysfunction. The bone marrow, lymph nodes, liver, spleen, and gastrointestinal tract are typically involved. The most common clinical signs include diarrhea, weight loss, vomiting, and anorexia.[24] Physical examination often reveals thickened bowel loops, lymphadenopathy, and hepatosplenomegaly. Rarely, affected cats may have dermatosis characterized by generalized maculopapular erythema, severe pruritus, marked excoriation, and possibly, wheals (see Fig 17:8 *C* and *D*).

Diagnosis

Diagnosis is based on history, physical examination, exclusion through laboratory testing, and skin biopsy. Moderate to marked peripheral eosinophilia (average 42.6×10^3/ml) is characteristic. Direct smears of skin lesions reveal a predominance of eosinophils and basophils. Skin biopsy reveals variable degrees of superficial and deep perivascular dermatitis, with eosinophils predominating.

Clinical Management

The prognosis is poor; most cases exhibit short survival times and fail to respond to any treatment. Cats with cutaneous lesions may have slowly progressive disease and longer survival times (2 to 4 years).[22, 23] These cats may show a favorable, but transient, response to high doses of glucocorticoids.

■ IDIOPATHIC STERILE GRANULOMA AND PYOGRANULOMA

Idiopathic, sterile, granulomatous to pyogranulomatous skin disease is uncommon in dogs but very rare in cats.[25–27]

Cause and Pathogenesis

The cause and pathogenesis of the condition are unknown. The characteristic granulomatous histopathologic appearance, absence of microbial agents and foreign material, and good response to systemic glucocorticoids suggest an immune-mediated pathogenesis.

Clinical Features

DOG

The disorder may occur in dogs of all ages, breeds, and sexes, but collies, Weimaraners, Great Danes, boxers, and Golden retrievers may be predisposed.[25] Lesions are usually multiple and typically affect the head (especially the bridge of the nose, the muzzle, and the periocular region), the pinnae, and the paws. Firm, painless, nonpruritic, dermal papules, plaques, and nodules are found (see Fig. 17:8 *E* to *G*). The lesions may become alopecic, ulcerated, and secondarily infected, especially on the paws. Animals are usually otherwise healthy.

CAT

In cats, two clinical syndromes have been described.[2, 27] Some animals develop pruritic papules and nodules on the head and pinnae (see Fig. 17:8 *H*) Lesions are usually erythematous to

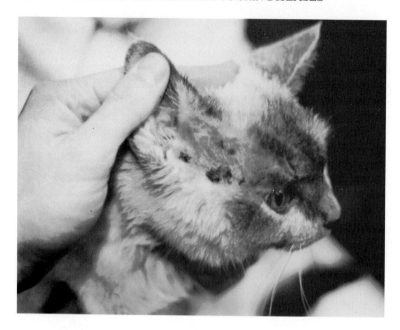

Figure 17:11. Idiopathic sterile granulomas in a cat. Preauricular plaque.

violaceous in color. Other cats present with pruritic, symmetric preauricular plaques (preauricular xanthogranulomas) (Fig. 17:11).[2, 27] Papules and wheal-like lesions coalesce to form orange-yellow, friable, well-circumscribed plaques. These plaques become reddish purple on palpation.

Diagnosis

The differential diagnosis includes other granulomatous and pyogranulomatous (bacterial, mycotic, foreign body) and neoplastic disorders. Definitive diagnosis is based on history, physical examination, cultures, and biopsy. Cytologic examination reveals pyogranulomatous or granulomatous inflammation with no microorganisms (Fig. 17:12). Cultures are best made from

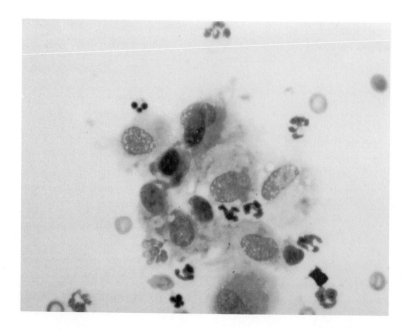

Figure 17:12. Canine sterile pyogranuloma. Cytologic examination reveals macrophages, nondegenerate neutrophils, and no microorganisms.

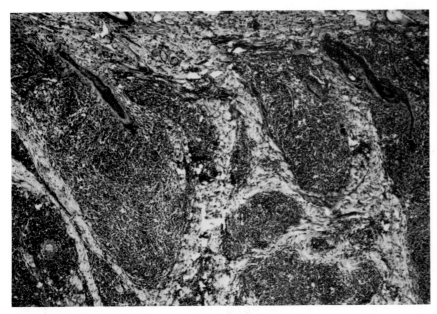

Figure 17:13. Canine idiopathic sterile granuloma. Granulomatous dermatitis that tends to track appendages (AOG stain).

tissue taken by aseptic surgical biopsy techniques, and they are negative. In dogs, biopsy usually reveals a nodular to diffuse, granulomatous to pyogranulomatous dermatitis. Early lesions show a characteristic vertical orientation of oblong (sausage-shaped) perifollicular granulomas or pyogranulomas that track, but do not initially involve, the hair follicles (Figs. 17:13 to 17:15). Special stains and polarization reveal no microorganisms or foreign material. Rarely, dogs have a diffuse sarcoidal granulomatous dermatitis (Fig 17:16).[28]

In cats, biopsy of the papulonodular lesions on the head and pinnae reveals perifollicular pyogranulomatous dermatitis.[27] Biopsy of the preauricular plaques reveals a diffuse granulomatous dermatitis that is separated from epithelial structures by a narrow grenz zone, contains

Figure 17:14. Canine sterile granuloma. Granulomatous dermatitis.

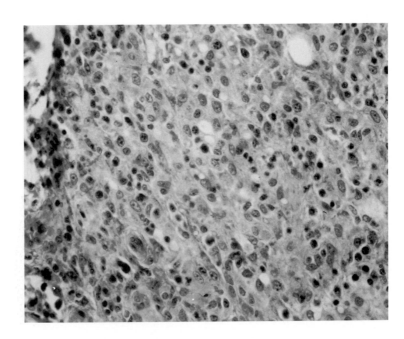

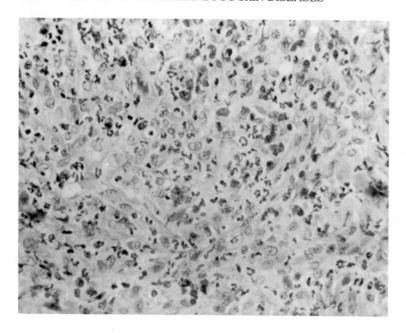

Figure 17:15. Canine sterile pyogranuloma. Pyogranulomatous dermatitis.

numerous multinucleated histiocytic giant cells, and exhibits unexplained purpura (Figs. 17:17 and 17:18).[2, 27]

Clinical Management

Therapy may consist of surgical excision of solitary lesions, if feasible, or of systemic glucocorticoids if multiple lesions are present or surgery is impractical. In dogs, prednisone or prednisolone is administered orally at 2.2 to 4.4 mg/kg q24h until the lesions have regressed in 7 to 14 days. About 60 per cent of dogs then require prolonged alternate-morning glucocorticoid therapy. Occasionally, dogs are unresponsive to glucocorticoids or become refractory after variable periods of remission. Azathioprine (Imuran) is useful in such cases and is administered orally at 2.2 mg/kg q24h until remission, then on alternate days. The oral administration of

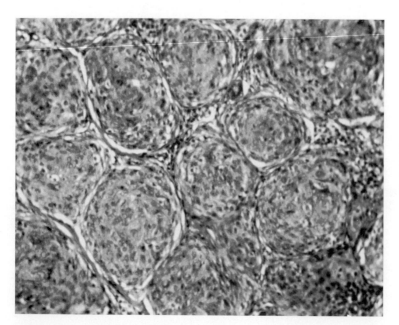

Figure 17:16. Canine sterile sarcoidal granuloma. Confluent sarcoidal (naked epithelioid) granulomas.

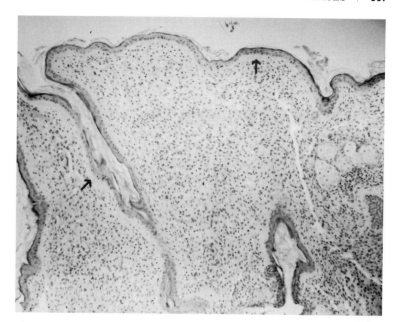

Figure 17:17. Feline preauricular granuloma. Diffuse granulomatous dermatitis with narrow grenz zone *(arrows)*.

sodium iodide has been reported useful in some cases[1] but not in others.[25] In cats, lesions often spontaneously resolve after about 9 months.[27]

■ GRANULOMATOUS SEBACEOUS ADENITIS

Granulomatous sebaceous adenitis is an uncommon idiopathic dermatosis of dogs, and is rare in cats.[3, 29, 30, 33, 36]

Cause and Pathogenesis

The cause and pathogenesis of the disorder are unknown, but speculations include the following: (1) sebaceous gland destruction is a developmental and inherited defect; (2) sebaceous

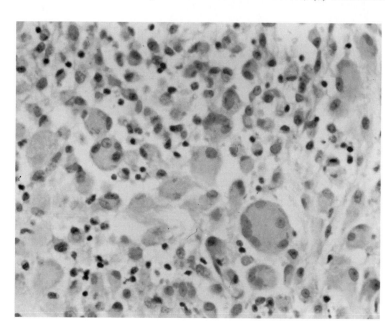

Figure 17:18. Feline preauricular granuloma. Numerous histiocytes and multinucleated histiocytic giant cells.

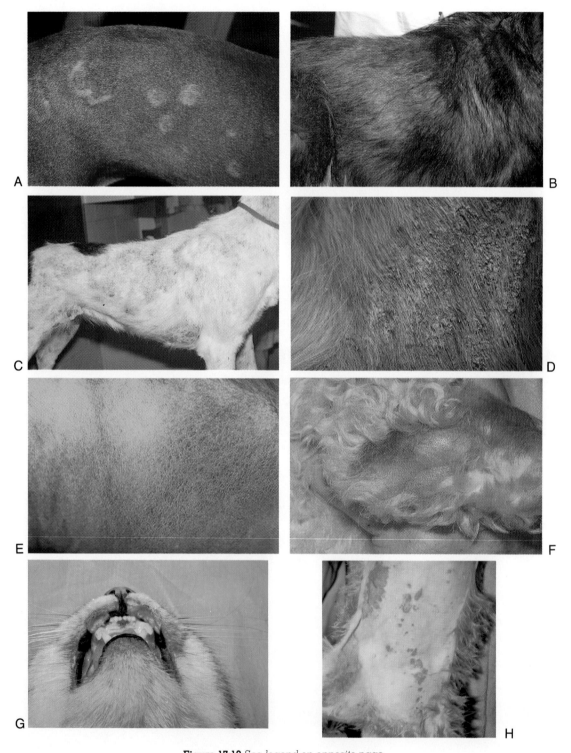

Figure 17:19 *See legend on opposite page*

gland destruction is an immune-mediated disease directed against a component of the gland; (3) the initial defect is a keratinization abnormality with subsequent obstruction of the sebaceous ducts resulting in inflammation of the glands; and (4) the sebaceous adenitis and keratinization defects are the result of an abnormality in lipid metabolism.[3, 36, 36a]

Preliminary pedigree analysis of affected and related Standard Poodles suggests an autosomal recessive mode of inheritance.[36a] However, because over 25 per cent of affected dogs may have subclinical disease, breeding studies are being undertaken to confirm the mode of inheritance.

Clinical Features

DOG

There is no apparent sex predilection, and the disorder tends to appear in young adult to middle-aged dogs. Although many breeds may be affected, there are breed predilections for Vizslas, Akitas, Samoyeds, and Standard Poodles.[3, 36] In general, the dermatologic abnormalities are bilaterally symmetric; prominent on the face, head, pinnae, and trunk; and dominated by abnormal keratinization. The cutaneous changes are somewhat dependent on haircoat type and breed.

In short-coated dogs, such as Vizslas, lesions begin as generally annular areas of scaling and alopecia that tend to enlarge peripherally, to become polycyclic, and occasionally, to coalesce (Fig. 17:19 A). The scales are usually fine, white, and nonadherent. Lesions are usually asymptomatic, unless secondary staphylococcal infection occurs. Intermittent edematous swelling of the muzzle, lips, and eyelids is occasionally seen.[34, 35]

The Standard Poodle manifests marked hyperkeratosis, followed by alopecia. The hairs are dull and brittle, with tightly adherent, silver-white scale that incorporates small tufts of matted hairs. Lesions often begin on the face and pinnae, but progressively involve the neck and dorsal trunk.

Akitas tend to have fairly generalized, erythematous and greasy skin changes (Figs 17:19 B to D). Papules, pustules, scales, matting of the hair, and yellow-brown greasy keratosebaceous debris are usually prominent. Severe hair loss, especially of the undercoat, is often present. Some animals may show signs of systemic illness, such as fever, malaise, and weight loss.

Samoyeds develop moderate to severe, predominantly truncal alopecia and scaling. Hairs are dull, brittle, and broken. Follicular casts are prominent.

In German shepherds, lesions may begin on the tail and progress cranially on the body.

Dogs with granulomatous sebaceous adenitis are generally nonpruritic. However, secondary staphylococcal infection is a frequent complication, and affected animals may then be pruritic.

CAT

Lesions consist of multifocal annular areas of scale, crust, broken hairs, follicular casts, and alopecia (Fig 17:19 E).[31, 36] Lesions begin on the head, pinnae, and neck, then spread caudally on the body.

Figure 17:19. *A,* Canine granulomatous sebaceous adenitis. Annular and arciform areas of alopecia and scaling in a Viszla. *B,* Canine sebaceous adenitis. Early disease in an Akita with a thin, broken, dishevelled haircoat. *C,* Canine sebaceous adenitis. Advanced disease in an Akita, with pronounced hair loss, hyperkeratosis, and dermatitic areas. *D,* Canine sebaceous adenitis. Marked hyperkeratosis, follicular casting, and broken hairs. *E,* Feline sebaceous adenitis. Marked follicular hyperkeratosis, broken hairs, and alopecia. *F,* Canine morphea. Alopecic, shiny plaque on lateral elbow. *G,* Feline indolent ulcer. Bilateral lip ulcers that are chronic and necrotic. *H,* Eosinophilic plaque in scattered patches on the cat's abdomen and chest. Hair has been clipped away. Lesions are well demarcated, red, moist, and raised and have been licked incessantly.

Diagnosis

The differential diagnosis includes staphylococcal folliculitis, demodicosis, dermatophytosis, keratinization defects (especially seborrhea and ichthyosis), follicular dysplasia, and endocrinopathies. Skin scrapings and carefully performed cultures are negative. Prominent follicular casts are most likely associated with granulomatous sebaceous adenitis, seborrhea, vitamin A–responsive dermatosis, demodicosis, and follicular dysplasia. Microscopic examination of affected hairs reveals casts or collars of yellow-brown keratosebaceous material surrounding hair shafts at varying intervals (Fig. 17:20).

Dermatohistopathologic findings are variable in intensity. They vary with the chronicity of the lesion and, to some extent, with the haircoat type and breed of animal.[2, 3, 36] In general, early lesions are characterized by variable degrees of sebaceous adenitis (granulomatous to pyogranulomatous). In most cases, sebocytes are no longer visible within the granulomas, and the diagnosis is based on the finding of discrete perifollicular granulomas in areas in which sebaceous glands are normally found (Figs. 17:21 and 17:22). The other adnexae are spared.

Chronic lesions are characterized by a hyperplastic superficial perivascular dermatitis with prominent orthokeratotic or parakeratotic hyperkeratosis of epidermis and hair follicles and variable degrees of perifollicular fibrosis and follicular atrophy. Sebaceous glands are absent. Standard Poodles may have only a scanty lymphocytic inflammation at the level of the sebaceous duct, but no sebaceous glands are present.

It has been reported that biopsies from clinically normal Standard Poodles that were still normal 2 years later may contain focal areas of mild granulomatous sebaceous adenitis.[36, 36a] Animals with secondary staphylococcal infections may have areas of neutrophilic intraepidermal pustular dermatitis, suppurative folliculitis and furunculosis, and nodular to diffuse pyogranulomatous dermatitis or panniculitis.

Clinical Management

Response to therapy varies somewhat, depending on the severity or chronicity of the disease and on the breed of animal.[3, 36] Further confusion is created by the fact that some dogs have cyclic patterns of spontaneous improvement and worsening, independent of any therapy.[3] Prognosis is poorest when sebaceous glands have been completely lost.

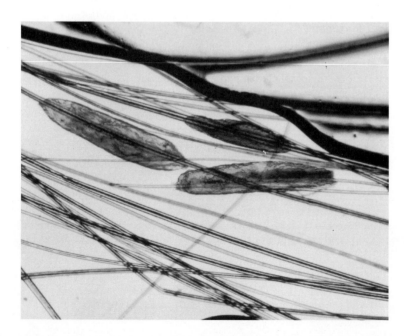

Figure 17:20. Canine sebaceous adenitis. Trichogram reveals prominent casts of keratosebaceous debris surrounding numerous hair shafts.

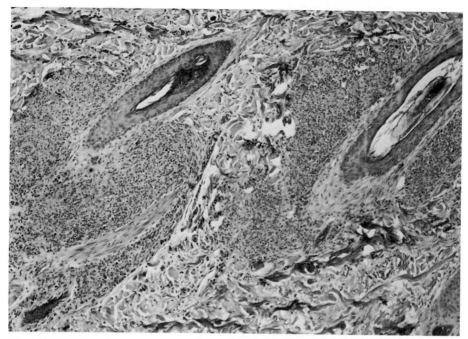

Figure 17:21. Sebaceous adenitis. Perifollicular granulomas where sebaceous glands should be.

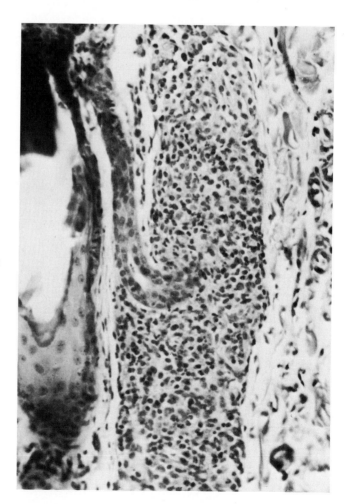

Figure 17:22. Canine granulomatous sebaceous adenitis. Sebaceous duct exiting a granuloma.

Mild cases may be satisfactorily controlled with keratolytic shampoos and emollient rinses. More stubborn cases may benefit from the topical application of 50 to 75 per cent propylene glycol in water as a spray or rinse once daily then two to three times weekly as needed.[3, 36] Some dogs respond to the oral administration of products containing omega-6 and omega-3 fatty acids; others do not.[3, 34, 36]

In severe or refractory cases, synthetic retinoids may be useful. Isotretinoin (1 to 2 mg/kg/day orally) has been reported to be very effective in Vizslas, but it is usually ineffective or minimally effective in other breeds.[32, 34, 36] Etretinate (1 to 2 mg/kg/day orally) has been reported to be ineffective or occasionally to result in a maximum of 50 per cent improvement.[34, 36] Responses to synthetic retinoids generally require 4 to 8 weeks of therapy, and therapy must usually be continued for life. The potential side-effects of synthetic retinoids are legion (see Chap. 3), but they are uncommon and are usually mild when they do occur.[34]

Cyclosporine (Sandimmune, Sandoz, 5mg/kg q12h orally) has been reported effective in dogs that failed to respond to synthetic retinoids.[3, 35] Cyclosporine commonly produces side-effects in dogs: gastrointestinal irritation, gingival hyperplasia, hirsutism, nephrotoxicity, hepatotoxicity, papillomatosis, increased frequency of bacterial and viral infections, and a lympho-plasmacytoid dermatitis.

Rarely, dogs have been observed to undergo spontaneous remission.[33, 36] Because of the possible hereditary nature of granulomatous sebaceous adenitis in certain breeds, it would be wise to discourage the use of affected animals for breeding purposes. No information on the treatment of granulomatous sebaceous adenitis in cats has been published.

■ CANINE LOCALIZED SCLERODERMA

Localized scleroderma (morphea) is a rare disease of dogs.[37, 38]

Cause and Pathogenesis

In humans, the cause and pathogenesis of localized scleroderma are unknown.[4] Three predominant theories on pathogenesis have emerged: (1) the vascular theory (early endothelial injury, perivascular fibrosis, hypoxia, and abnormal vascular reactivity), (2) the abnormal collagen metabolism theory (increased production of collagen and reduced collagenase activity), and (3) the immunologic theory (humoral and cell-mediated autoimmunity).

Clinical Features

In dogs, no age, breed, or sex predilections are apparent. Canine localized scleroderma is characterized by asymptomatic, well-demarcated, sclerotic plaques that are alopecic, smooth, and shiny (see Fig. 17:19 *F*). Lesions tend to be linear and to occur on the trunk and limbs. Affected dogs are otherwise healthy.

Diagnosis

The diagnosis is based on history, physical examination, and skin biopsy. Histopathologically, a fibrosing dermatitis is seen. The overlying epidermis is unremarkable (Fig. 17:23). The entire dermis and subcutis are replaced by collagenous tissue (Fig. 17:24). The normal loosely woven, fine-fibered appearance of the superficial dermis is replaced by dense collagen bundles. Pilosebaceous units are essentially absent. A mild superficial and deep perivascular accumulation of lymphohistiocytic cells is present (Fig. 17:25).

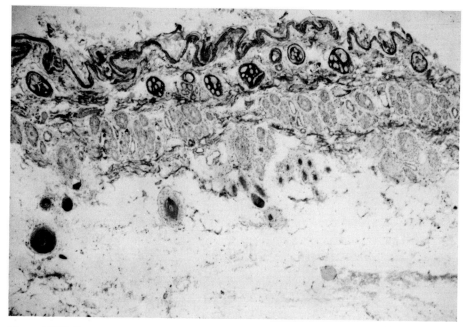

Figure 17:23. Canine morphea. Normal skin peripheral to a lesion.

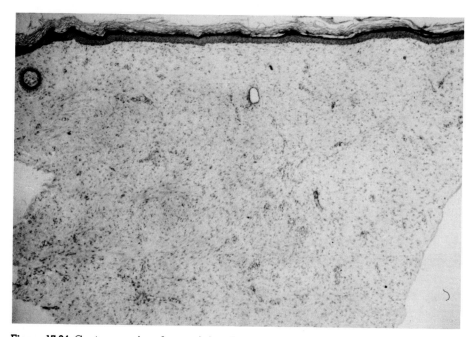

Figure 17:24. Canine morphea. Lesional skin. Fibrosing dermatitis.

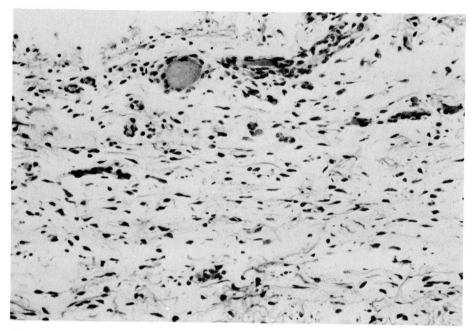

Figure 17:25. Canine morphea. Perivascular accumulation of lymphoid cells within subcutaneous fat.

Clinical Management

The prognosis appears to be good. Spontaneous remission may occur over a course of several weeks,[37] or permanent scarring may result.[38] When regrowth occurs, the hair is usually thinner and finer than normal, and it may be a slightly different color.[38] In humans, no forms of topical or systemic therapy are known to be of regular benefit to patients with localized scleroderma.

■ FELINE EOSINOPHILIC GRANULOMA COMPLEX

The eosinophilic granuloma complex includes a group of lesions that affect the skin, mucocutaneous junctions, and oral cavity of cats. The term itself is often used as a final diagnosis; in fact, however, there is another primary cause. It is essential to realize that the eosinophilic granuloma complex is nothing more than a mucocutaneous reaction pattern in cats—*not* a specific disease.

Three lesions have traditionally been recognized: (1) the indolent ulcer, (2) the eosinophilic plaque, and (3) the eosinophilic granuloma. These lesions are common, and are most frequently seen in cats that have hypersensitivities (allergies) to inhalants, foods, or insects, especially to fleas and mosquitoes (see Chapter 8).[1, 3, 39, 40, 42] However, bacterial involvement may occasionally be a factor, because antibiotic therapy resolves or markedly improves some lesions.[3]

In some instances, these lesions may be heritable;[3, 43] therefore, when no hypersensitivity can be documented, a heritable form of the disorder should be considered. In contrast to what had been reported in earlier veterinary literature, more recent attempts to transmit eosinophilic plaques by autologous tissue techniques have been unsuccessful.[41]

Feline Indolent Ulcer

Indolent ulcer (eosinophilic ulcer, rodent ulcer) is a common cutaneous, mucocutaneous, and oral mucosal lesion of cats. Clinically, most indolent ulcers occur unilaterally on the upper lip (see Fig. 17:19 *G*). However, lesions also occur in the oral cavity, in other areas of the skin, and bilaterally. The lesions are usually well circumscribed, red-brown in color, alopecic, and glistening; they have a raised border. Pruritus and pain are rare, and peripheral lymphadenopathy may be present. There are no age or breed predilections, but females may be predisposed. Lip ulcers appear to be precancerous and may rarely undergo malignant transformation into squamous cell carcinoma (see Chap. 19). Cats with indolent ulcers may also have eosinophilic plaques, eosinophilic granulomas, or both.

The differential diagnosis includes infectious ulcers (bacterial, fungal, FeLV-associated), trauma, and neoplasia (squamous cell carcinoma, mast cell tumor, lymphoma). Carefully performed cultures are negative. Biopsy is nondiagnostic, revealing hyperplastic, ulcerated, superficial perivascular to interstitial dermatitis (with neutrophils and mononuclear cells usually predominating) and fibrosing dermatitis (Fig. 17:26). Blood eosinophilia and tissue eosinophilia are rare. Chronic, recurrent, medically refractory cases should be evaluated for underlying flea bite hypersensitivity, atopy, and food hypersensitivity.

Therapy with systemic glucocorticoids is often effective. Prednisone or prednisolone is administered orally (4.4 mg/kg q24h) until the lesions are healed. Alternatively, methylprednisolone acetate (Depo-Medrol) may be administered subcutaneously at 20 mg/cat every 2 weeks until the lesions are healed, or either dexamethasone (0.4 mg/kg q24h) or triamcinolone (0.8 mg/kg q24h) may be administered orally. Recurrent lesions may be managed with alternate-evening oral glucocorticoids or repeated subcutaneous injections of methylprednisolone (*never* more frequently than every 2 months). Medically refractory lesions should be evaluated for underlying hypersensitivity disorders and managed appropriately. Some refractory lesions respond to systemic antibiotics (e.g., amoxicillin clavulanate, cefadroxil, enrofloxacin).[3] Other methods of treatment reported to be occasionally successful in feline indolent ulcer include radiotherapy, cryosurgery, laser therapy, surgical excision, mixed bacterial vaccines, and immunomodulating drugs such as levamisole, thiabendazole, and aurothioglucose (Solganal).[1, 3] Progestational compounds, such as megestrol acetate (Ovaban, Megace) or medroxyprogesterone acetate (Depo-Provera), have also been effective in many cases of feline indolent ulcer. However, because of the side-effects resulting from these drugs, they are *not* recommended.

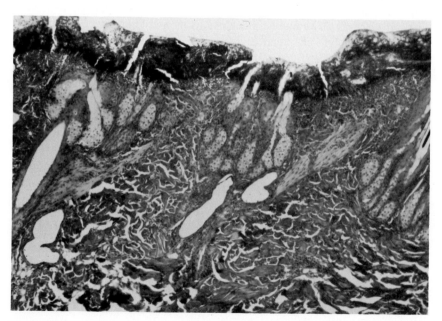

Figure 17:26. Histologic section of indolent ulcer. There is surface ulceration with fibrin covering the necrotic surface and a dense mononuclear cellular infiltrate in the dermis. Note the ulcerative perivascular dermatitis. (From Scott, D. W.: Feline dermatology 1900–1978: A monograph, J. Am. Anim. Hosp. Assoc. 16:331, 1980.)

Feline Eosinophilic Plaque

Eosinophilic plaque is a common cutaneous lesion of cats. Clinically, most eosinophilic plaques occur on the abdomen and medial thighs (Fig. 17:27 *A*; also see Fig. 17:19 *H*). Lesions may be single or multiple, and they may also occur on mucocutaneous junctions or in other areas of the skin. Eosinophilic plaques are well circumscribed, raised, round to oval, red, oozing, often ulcerated, and 0.5 to 7 cm in diameter. Pruritus is usually severe. Peripheral lymphadenopathy may be present. Cats with eosinophilic plaque may also have indolent ulcers, eosinophilic granulomas, or both. Lesions that are histologically similar to eosinophilic plaques occasionally occur in the conjunctiva[45] and cornea.[44] There are no age or breed predilections, but females may be predisposed.

The differential diagnosis includes infectious granulomas (bacterial, fungal) and neoplasia (mast cell tumor, lymphoma). Carefully performed cultures are negative. Biopsy reveals hyperplastic superficial and deep perivascular dermatitis with eosinophilia, to interstitial or diffuse eosinophilic dermatitis (Figs. 17:28 and 17:29). Flame figures may be seen. Diffuse spongiosis, which involves hair follicle outer root sheaths, and eosinophilic microvesicles and microabscesses may be seen. Some lesions have remarkable mucinosis of the epidermis and hair follicle outer root sheath,[3] and some involve the subcutaneous fat. Direct immunofluorescence testing frequently reveals the intercellular deposition of Ig within the epidermis (a pemphigus-like pattern).[41] Blood and tissue eosinophilia are constant.

Methods of treatment are as described for feline indolent ulcer.

Feline Eosinophilic Granuloma

Eosinophilic granuloma (*linear granuloma*) is a common cutaneous, mucocutaneous, and oral mucosal lesion of cats. Clinically, most eosinophilic granulomas occur on the caudal thighs, on the face, and in the oral cavity (especially the tongue and palate). On the caudal thigh, the lesions are usually well circumscribed, raised, firm, yellowish to pink plaques with a distinctive linear configuration (see Fig 17:27 *B*). They are often discovered accidentally because they are usually nonpruritic. Lesions on the face and in the oral cavity have a papular to nodular configuration (see Fig. 17:27 *C*). Eosinophilic granuloma is the most common cause of lower lip swellings and nodules (pouting cats) and asymptomatic swollen chins (fat-chinned cats, *feline chin edema*) in the cat (see Fig. 17:27 *D*). When the surface of eosinophilic granulomas is eroded or ulcerated, a characteristic speckling with pinpoint white foci (corresponding to foci of collagen degeneration) may be seen. Peripheral lymphadenopathy may be present. Cats with eosinophilic granuloma may also have indolent ulcers, eosinophilic plaques, or both. Lesions that are histologically similar to eosinophilic granulomas occasionally occur in the conjunctiva.[45] There are no age or breed predilections, but females may be predisposed.

The differential diagnosis includes infectious bacterial or fungal granulomas and neoplasia. Biopsy reveals nodular to diffuse granulomatous dermatitis with multifocal areas of collagen degeneration (Fig. 17:30). Eosinophils and multinucleated histiocytic giant cells are common (Fig. 17:31), and flame figures may be seen. Mucinosis of the epidermis and hair follicle outer

Figure 17:27. *A,* Feline eosinophilic plaque. Raised, erythematous abdominal plaque. *B,* Typical eosinophilic granuloma on a white cat's rear leg with hair clipped away. The firm cordlike masses are slightly pink and not ulcerated, painful, or pruritic. *C,* Eosinophilic granuloma bilaterally located at the angles of the jaw behind the last molars. A metal mouth gag and plastic endotracheal tube can be seen. The ulcerated lesions have a fibronecrotic surface. Radiation therapy caused prompt remission. *D,* Feline eosinophilic granuloma. Pinkish nodule on the lower lip. *E,* Canine eosinophilic granuloma. Greenish brown mass on the ventrolateral aspect of the tongue near the commissure of the lips. (Courtesy J.O. Noxon.) *F,* Canine eosinophilic granuloma. Erythematous papules and nodules on the abdomen. *G,* Canine eosinophilic granuloma. Ulcerated nodule on prepuce. *H,* Canine eosinophilic granuloma. Ulcerated nodule on a foot.

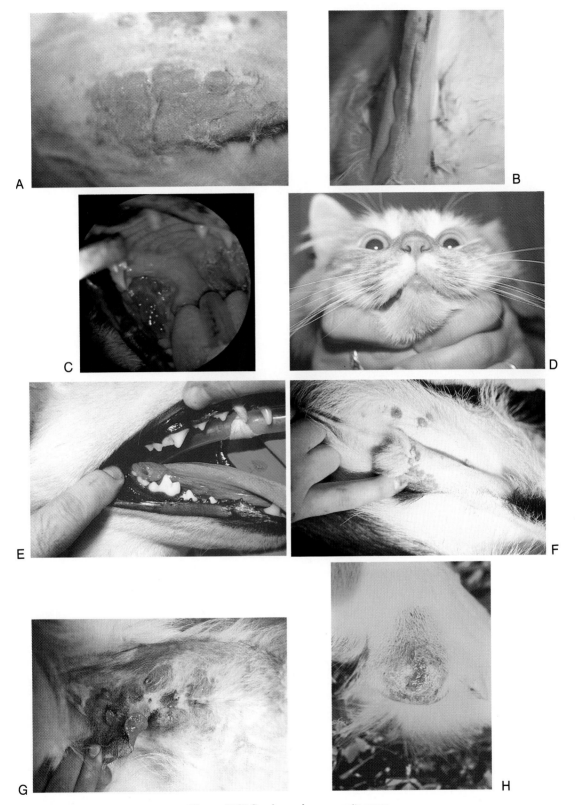

Figure 17:27 *See legend on opposite page*

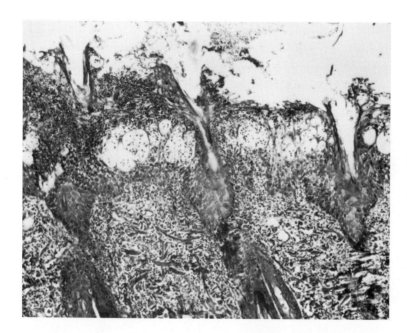

Figure 17:28. Feline eosinophilic plaque. Diffuse spongiosis and microvesicle or microvesicopustule formation in the epidermis.

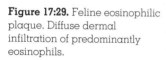

Figure 17:29. Feline eosinophilic plaque. Diffuse dermal infiltration of predominantly eosinophils.

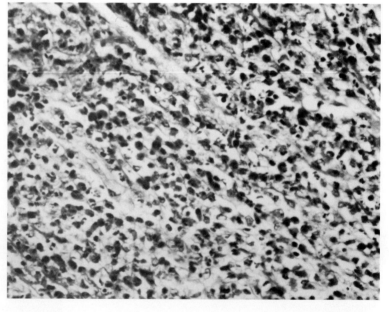

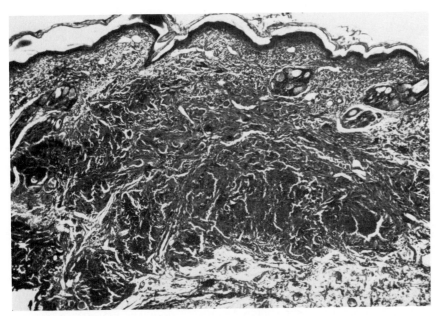

Figure 17:30. Feline eosinophilic granuloma. Granulomatous dermatitis associated with collagen degeneration. (From Scott, D. W.: Feline dermatology 1900–1978: A monograph, J. Am. Anim. Hosp. Assoc. 16:331, 1980.)

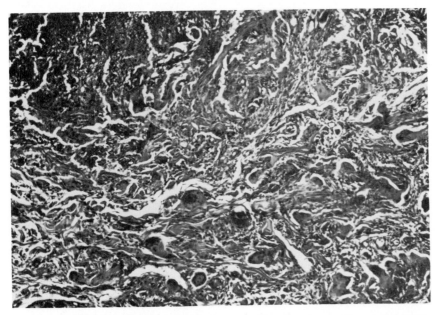

Figure 17:31. Feline eosinophilic granuloma. Granulomatous dermatitis associated with collagen degeneration and foreign-body giant cells. (High-power view of Fig. 17:30.)

root sheath, focal eosinophilic folliculitis or furunculosis, and focal eosinophilic panniculitis may be present. Older lesions are characterized by palisading granuloma formation around the foci of degenerate collagen. Eosinophils are less prominent in chronic lesions. Blood eosinophilia may be seen, especially with oral lesions. Carefully performed cultures are negative.

Methods of treatment are as described for feline indolent ulcer. Interestingly, many eosinophilic granulomas occurring in cats younger than 1 year of age spontaneously regress over a period of 3 to 5 months. Omega-3/omega-6 fatty acid–containing products (Derm Caps Liquid) are effective in some cases, and reduce glucocorticoid requirements in others (see Chap 3).

■ CANINE EOSINOPHILIC GRANULOMA

Eosinophilic granulomas are rare, idiopathic, nodular to plaquelike lesions associated with collagen degeneration in the oral cavity and skin of dogs[1, 3, 46–48]

Cause and Pathogenesis

The cause of cutaneous granulomas associated with collagen degeneration is poorly understood. In humans, occasional cases have been reported following insect bites, tuberculin tests, and other forms of trauma. Proposed pathomechanisms include vasculitis, microangiopathy, disorder of fibrinolysis, disorder of phagocytic function, disorder of catabolic enzyme release, and cell-mediated immune response. In dogs, no antecedent trauma or disease has been recognized, and cultures for bacteria, fungi, and viruses are negative. Macerated tissue from lesions produces no lesions in dogs that have been injected. The tissue eosinophilia, occasional blood eosinophilia, and glucocorticoid responsiveness of lesions have prompted speculation regarding a hypersensitivity state. In addition, the tendency of the oral form of the disease to occur in Siberian huskies has suggested a genetic basis for the disease. Some authors have reported the seasonal recurrence of cutaneous eosinophilic granulomas in dogs, suggesting that the condition may be a hypersensitivity reaction to pollens, molds, and insects.

Clinical Features

Although any age, breed, or sex of dog may be affected, eosinophilic granulomas occur most commonly in dogs less than 3 years of age (80 per cent of cases), Siberian huskies (76 per cent), and males (72 per cent). Eosinophilic granulomas occur most commonly in the oral cavity as ulcerated palatine plaques and vegetative lingual masses. The lingual masses often have a greenish brown hue (Fig. 17:27 *E*). Less commonly, they occur as multiple cutaneous papules, nodules, and plaques over the ventral abdomen, prepuce, and flanks (Fig. 17:27 *F, G, H*). The cutaneous lesions are usually nonpruritic and painless, and the dogs are otherwise healthy. Rarely, solitary lesions occur in the external ear canal.[49] There has been one report of a tracheal lesion.[50]

Diagnosis

The differential diagnosis includes granulomatous and neoplastic disorders. Diagnosis is based on biopsy. Characteristic histopathologic findings include variably sized foci of collagen degeneration, eosinophilic and histiocytic cellular infiltration, and palisading granulomas (Figs. 17:32 and 17:33). Flame figures may be seen. Properly performed cultures are negative, and blood eosinophilia is occasionally seen.

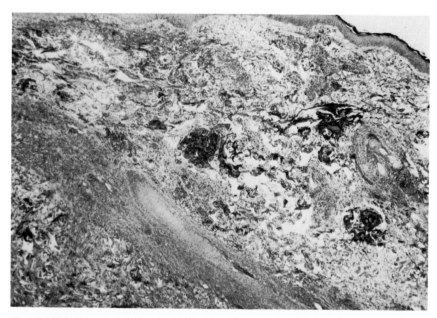

Figure 17:32. Canine eosinophilic granuloma. Granulomatous dermatitis associated with collagen degeneration.

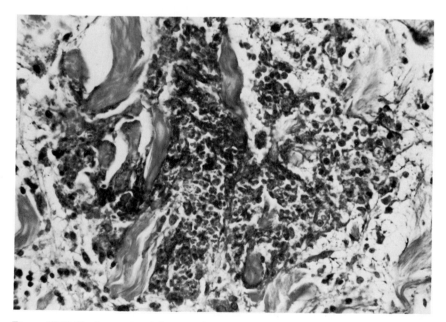

Figure 17:33. Canine eosinophilic granuloma. Focal collagen degeneration and accumulation of eosinophils.

Clinical Management

Canine eosinophilic granulomas are usually very glucocorticoid responsive. Seventy-eight per cent of the cases were treated with prednisolone or prednisone orally (0.5 to 2.2 mg/kg/day); their lesions regressed in 10 to 20 days, and no further therapy was needed. Some lesions undergo spontaneous remission, and some lesions are seasonally or chronically recurrent.

■ PANNICULITIS

Panniculitis is a multifactorial inflammatory condition of the subcutaneous fat, characterized by deep-seated cutaneous nodules that often become cystic and ulcerated and develop draining tracts. The disorder is uncommon in dogs and cats.[51]

Cause and Pathogenesis

The lipocyte (fat cell, adipocyte) is particularly vulnerable to trauma, ischemia, and neighboring inflammatory disease. In addition, damage to lipocytes results in the liberation of lipid, which undergoes hydrolysis into glycerol and fatty acids. Fatty acids are potent inflammatory agents, and they incite further inflammatory and granulomatous tissue reactions.

Multiple etiologic factors are involved in the genesis of panniculitis in human beings (Table 17:1). Many of these factors have yet to be recognized in dogs and cats, but this fact may only reflect lack of awareness. Infectious and nutritional causes of canine and feline panniculitis are discussed elsewhere (see Chaps. 4, 5, and 16) and are therefore not addressed here. This section concentrates on sterile forms of panniculitis.

Nodular panniculitis refers to sterile subcutaneous inflammatory nodules and is *not* a specific disease. It is a purely descriptive term, clinically representing the end result of several known and unknown etiologic factors.[51] *Weber-Christian panniculitis* has been a frequently misused term and does *not* exist as a specific disease. In dogs and cats, the majority of cases of sterile nodular panniculitis are solitary lesions of idiopathic origin. A few cases of lupus erythematosus panniculitis and erythema nodosum have been recognized in dogs (see Chap. 8).[1, 51]

Clinical Features

Panniculitis is manifested clinically as deep-seated cutaneous nodules. The lesions may occur singly or in crops; they are either localized to specific areas or generalized, and they vary from

Table 17:1. Differential Diagnosis of Human Panniculitis

Infectious
Bacterial,* mycobacterial,* actinomycetic,* fungal,* chlamydial, viral
Immunologic
Lupus erythematosus,* rheumatoid arthritis, drug eruption, erythema nodosum*
Physicochemical (factitial)
Trauma,* pressure, cold, foreign body* (e.g., post-subcutaneous injection of bulky, oily, or insoluble liquids)
Pancreatic disease
Inflammation,* neoplasia
Postglucocorticoid therapy
Vasculitis
Leukocytoclastic, periarteritis nodosa, thrombophlebitis, embolism*
Nutritional
Vitamin E deficiency*
Enteropathies
*Idiopathic**

*Recognized in dogs and cats.

a few millimeters to several centimeters in diameter. Nodules may be firm and well circumscribed, or soft and ill defined (Fig. 17:34 *A*). They are initially subcutaneous but may fix the overlying skin as they progress. The lesions may become cystic, ulcerate, and develop draining tracts that discharge an oily, yellowish brown to bloody substance (Fig. 17:34 *B* and *C*). The lesions may or may not be painful and often heal with depressed scars.

DOG

The majority (80 per cent) of dogs have a solitary lesion, most commonly over the ventrolateral chest, neck, and abdomen.[51] No age, breed, or sex predilections are apparent in dogs with solitary lesions.

Dogs with multiple lesions often have constitutional signs, including poor appetite, depression, lethargy, and pyrexia.[51–53] These signs are sometimes intermittent, heralding a new crop of skin lesions. A rare dog has arthralgias, abdominal pain, vomiting, or hepatosplenomegaly.[52, 53] In dogs with multiple skin lesions, the trunk is most commonly involved. There is no age or sex predilection, but dachshunds appear to be predisposed.

CAT

The majority (95 per cent) of cats have a solitary lesion, most commonly over the ventral abdomen and ventrolateral thorax (Fig. 17:34 *D*).[51] Cats with multiple lesions often have constitutional signs as described for dogs.[51, 52] No age, breed, or sex predilections are evident.

Diagnosis

Sterile nodular panniculitis is most commonly misdiagnosed as deep pyoderma, cutaneous cysts, or cutaneous neoplasms. Aspirates from intact lesions usually reveal numerous neutrophils, foamy macrophages, and no microorganisms (Fig. 17:35). Sudan stains may reveal extracellular and intracellular lipid droplets. Animals with multiple lesions and systemic illness often have a mild to moderate leukocytosis and neutrophilia, mild nonregenerative anemia, and elevated α_2, β_1, and β_2 fractions on serum protein electrophoresis.[52] Direct immunofluorescence testing may reveal the deposition of Ig and complement at the basement membrane zone.[52]

The diagnosis of panniculitis can be made only by biopsy, and excision biopsy is the *only* biopsy technique that is satisfactory for subcutaneous nodules.[1, 2] Punch biopsies fail to deliver tissue sufficient to be of diagnostic value in about 75 per cent of the cases. Panniculitis may be lobular, septal, or diffuse, or it may have a combination of these characteristics.[51] In addition, panniculitis may be granulomatous, pyogranulomatous, suppurative, eosinophilic, necrotizing, or fibrosing.[51] Thrombosis of subcuticular blood vessels, lymphoid nodules, and radial fat crystals may be seen.[51] The histopathologic pattern and cytomorphologic picture of the reactions has *little* diagnostic, therapeutic, or prognostic significance (Figs. 17:36 to 17:39). It is imperative to realize that most panniculitides, regardless of cause, look histologically identical. Thus, one cannot diagnose sterile nodular panniculitis from a biopsy specimen. Special stains and cultures are *always* indicated to rule out infectious agents, and polarized light examination is indicated to rule out foreign bodies.

If the panniculitis is predominantly lymphohistioplasmacytic, with or without concurrent neutrophilic vasculitis or interface dermatitis, or if other clinical signs suggest lupus erythematosus, other diagnostic tests may include antinuclear antibody and direct immunofluorescence testing of lesional skin (see Chap. 8). If a vasculitis is present, the diagnostic tests indicated may reflect the differential diagnosis of vasculitis (see Chap. 8). If the panniculitis is persistent and refractory or if the patient shows concurrent signs of gastrointestinal disease, pancreatic disease should be ruled out.

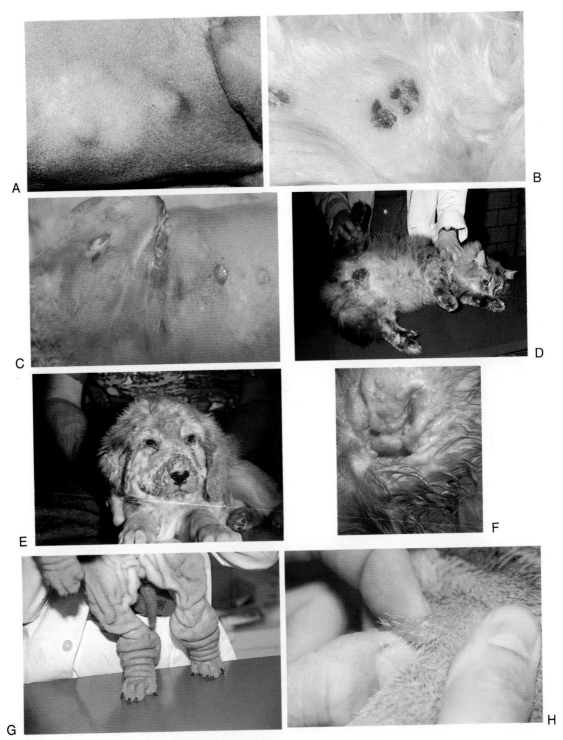

Figure 17:34 *See legend on opposite page*

Figure 17:35. Canine idiopathic sterile panniculitis. Cytologic examination reveals pyogranulomatous inflammation wherein neutrophils are nondegenerate, no microorganisms are seen, and macrophages contain numerous cytoplasmic vacuoles (lipophages).

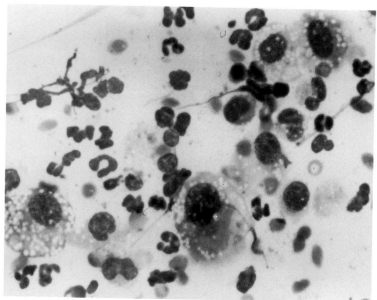

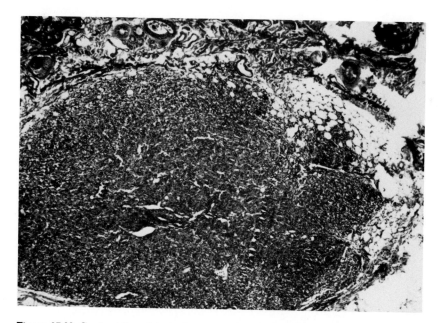

Figure 17:36. Canine idiopathic sterile panniculitis. Pyogranulomatous panniculitis.

Figure 17:34. *A,* Idiopathic sterile panniculitis in a dachshund. Two subcutaneous nodules on the trunk. *B,* Canine idiopathic sterile panniculitis. Subcutaneous nodule with multiple draining tracts. *C,* Feline panniculitis. Multiple fistulae on the ventral abdomen. *D,* Idiopathic sterile panniculitis in a cat. Ulcerated nodule in the groin. *E,* Juvenile cellulitis in a Golden retriever. Erythema, edema, exudation, crusting, and alopecia on the face and pinnae. *F,* Same dog as in *E.* Multiple pustules in the ear canal and on the pinna. *G,* Idiopathic mucinosis in a Chinese Shar Pei. Marked thickening and folding of the skin. *H,* Idiopathic mucinosis in a Chinese Shar Pei. Close-up of a mucinous vesicle.

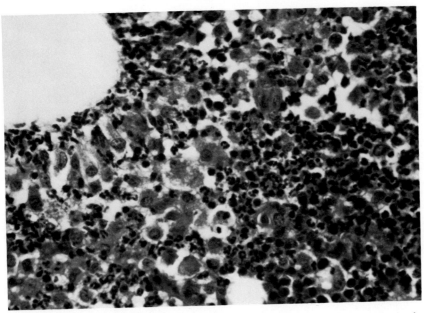

Figure 17:37. Canine idiopathic sterile panniculitis. Pyogranulomatous panniculitis with numerous foamy macrophages (lipophages).

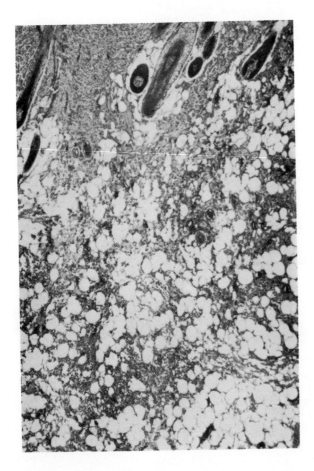

Figure 17:38. Feline idiopathic sterile panniculitis. Marked lobular panniculitis and fat necrosis. (From Scott, D. W.: Feline dermatology 1900–1978: A monograph. J. Am. Anim. Hosp. Assoc. 16:331, 1980.)

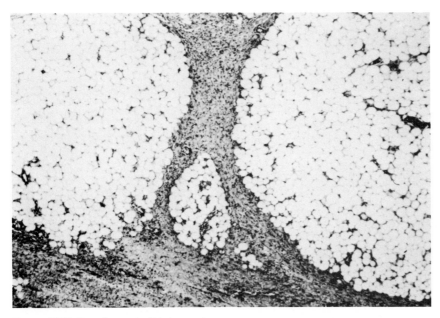

Figure 17:39. Septal panniculitis in a cat.

Erythema nodosum is characterized histologically by a *septal* panniculitis and is thought to represent a hypersensitivity reaction.[1, 2, 4] Thus, diagnostic considerations should include concurrent infections (e.g., bacterial endocarditis, coccidioidomycosis), neoplasia, and drug reactions.

Postinjection panniculitis is characterized by a discrete nodule that often has a necrotic center.[2, 53a, 53b] Surrounding the necrotic core is a layer of macrophages and often multinucleated histiocytic giant cells; there is an outer layer of intense lymphocytic and eosinophilic inflammation. In some cases, the presence of flocculent foreign debris is virtually diagnostic.

Traumatic panniculitis is characterized by a large central focus of lobular fat necrosis.[2] Lipocytes lack nuclei but retain their shape, creating ghosts or shells of fat cells. Ruptured lipocytes form large, cystic spaces. Interspersed and surrounding the devitalized lipocytes are scant inflammatory cells, predominantly foamy macrophages.

Clinical Management

Careful surgical excision of solitary lesions is usually curative.[51] Dogs and cats with multiple sterile panniculitis lesions usually respond well to systemic glucocorticoids.[51–53] Prednisolone or prednisone may be administered orally (2 mg/kg q24h in dogs, 4 mg/kg q24h in cats) until the lesions have regressed (in 3 to 8 weeks). Therapy should be stopped at that point, because many dogs, especially young dogs, enter long-term or permanent remission. In recurrent cases, alternate-day steroid therapy may be required for prolonged periods.

In a few canine and feline cases, good results have been obtained with oral vitamin E (dl-α-tocopherol acetate), 400 IU q12h.[1, 51] The vitamin E must be given at least 2 hours before or after a meal for maximum effectiveness. In humans, oral potassium iodide has been used successfully in cases of sterile nodular panniculitis;[4] one of the authors (DWS) has used this agent successfully in two dogs.

■ SUBCUTANEOUS FAT SCLEROSIS

Subcutaneous fat sclerosis has been described in a 1-year-old male domestic shorthair cat.[54] An inguinal abscess had been treated by surgical drainage and antibiotics 5 weeks prior to the

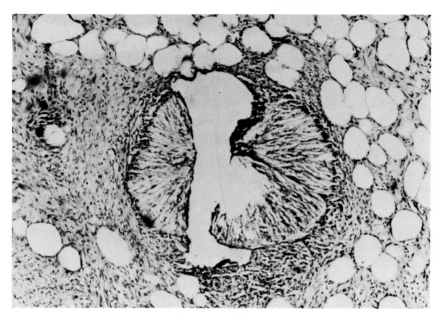

Figure 17:40. Sclerosing panniculitis in a cat. Fat crystal with radial configuration.

appearance of a rapidly growing abdominal subcutaneous mass. The mass was a firm, painless subcutaneous plaque that extended from the xiphoid process to the pelvic inlet and laterally to the lumbar processes. The borders were raised and distinct, and the normal overlying skin was cool, indurated, and adherent. The mass was large enough to restrict movement of the legs. Differential diagnosis included neoplasia, panniculitis, and nutritional steatitis. A hemogram and serum chemistry profile were normal. Bacterial and fungal cultures were negative. Oral treatment with prednisolone was not effective. Later, small subcutaneous satellite nodules could be palpated on the chest wall cranial to the mass.

On necropsy, the abdominal subcutaneous tissues were thickened, fibrous, and adhered to the dermis. Histopathologic findings revealed extensive subcutaneous fibrosis with minimal fat necrosis and inflammation. Within the subcutaneous fat, or within the fat-rich interstitial tissues of abdominal muscles, were bands of septal fibrosis, fat cells of increased size (fat micropseudocyst formation), and lipocytes containing needle-shaped fat clefts (fat crystals) (Fig. 17:40). Although a few scattered lymphocytes, histiocytes, and multinucleated histiocytic giant cells were found, and although there were isolated foci of neutrophils, the process was largely noninflammatory.

These findings are similar to two rare human disorders: sclerema neonatorum and subcutaneous fat necrosis of the newborn. The latter is indistinguishable from poststeroid panniculitis, but this cat had no history of corticosteroid administration.

■ CANINE JUVENILE CELLULITIS

Juvenile cellulitis (juvenile pyoderma, puppy strangles, juvenile sterile granulomatous dermatitis and lymphadenitis) is an uncommon granulomatous and pustular disorder of the face, pinnae, and submandibular lymph nodes of puppies.[2, 55–57]

Cause and Pathogenesis

The cause and pathogenesis are unknown. Heritability is supported by an increased occurrence in certain breeds and by familial histories of disease.[2, 55, 56] The occurrence of sterile granulomas and pustules that respond dramatically to glucocorticoids suggests an underlying immune dysfunction. Special stains and electron microscopic examination of tissues do not reveal microorganisms, and cultures are negative.[57] Attempts to transmit the disease with lesional tissues have been unsuccessful.[57]

Clinical Features

Puppies are affected between the ages of 3 weeks and 4 months, and one or several puppies in a litter may have the condition. Although numerous breeds have developed the disorder, Golden retrievers, dachshunds, and Gordon setters appear to be predisposed.[1, 2, 55–57] The initial abnormality noticed by most owners is an acutely swollen face, especially the eyelids, lips, and muzzle. Physical examination at this time reveals striking submandibular lymphadenopathy. Within 24 to 48 hours, papules and pustules develop rapidly, especially on the lips, muzzle, chin, bridge of the nose, and periocular area. Lesions typically fistulate, drain, and crust (see Fig. 17:34 *E*). A marked pustular otitis externa is often seen (see Fig. 17:34 *F*). Affected skin is usually painful but not pruritic. About 50 per cent of affected puppies are lethargic. Anorexia, pyrexia, and joint pain (sterile suppurative arthritis) are present in up to 25 per cent of the cases.

Occasional puppies have a concurrent sterile pyogranulomatous panniculitis with firm to fluctuant subcutaneous nodules that may be painful or fistulate. These nodules occur especially on the trunk or in the preputial or perianal areas.[1, 2, 52, 55–57]

Diagnosis

In very early cases, the differential diagnosis is angioedema (see chap. 8). However, angioedema is not accompanied by marked regional lymphadenopathy or systemic illness. After the dramatic inflammatory lesions have appeared, the differential diagnosis includes staphylococcal dermatitis, demodicosis, and drug eruption.

Cytologic examination of papulopustular lesions reveals pyogranulomatous inflammation with no microorganisms (Fig. 17:41). Carefully performed cultures are negative. Biopsies of early lesions reveal multiple discrete or confluent granulomas and pyogranulomas consisting of clusters of large epithelioid macrophages with variably sized cores of neutrophils (Fig.

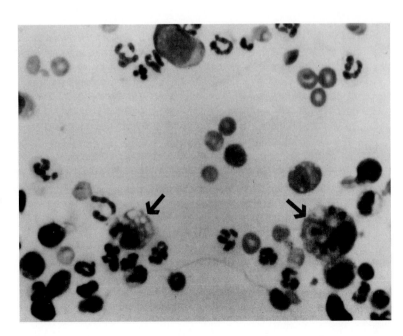

Figure 17:41. Juvenile cellulitis. Cytologic examination reveals pyogranulomatous inflammation wherein neutrophils appear nondegenerate and no microorganisms are seen. Note neutrophagocytosis by two macrophages *(arrows)*.

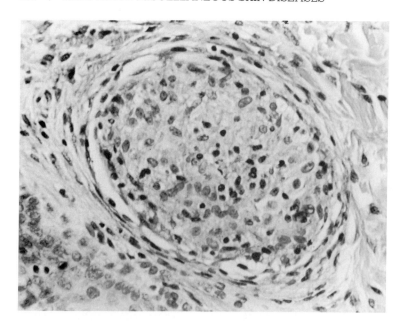

Figure 17:42. Juvenile cellulitis. Well-demarcated dermal granuloma from an early case.

17:42).[2, 57] Sebaceous glands and apocrine sweat glands may be obliterated. In later severe lesions, suppurative changes in the superficial dermis, in and around ruptured hair follicles, and in the subjacent panniculus are predominant (Fig. 17:43).

Total globulin levels, serum electrophoresis, immunoelectrophoresis, and bactericidal assays are normal.[1] Lymphocyte blastogenic responses to phytomitogens are suppressed in association with the presence of a serum suppressor factor.[1, 58]

Clinical Management

Early and aggressive therapy is indicated, because scarring can be severe. Large doses of glucocorticoids are the treatment of choice. Prednisone or prednisolone (2 mg/kg q24h orally)

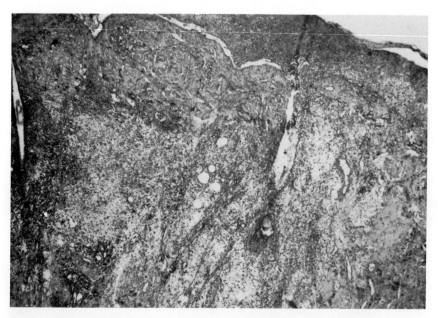

Figure 17:43. Juvenile cellulitis in a dog. Note diffuse cellulitis.

is administered daily until the disease is inactive (usually in 10 to 14 days). Dogs with an intercurrent truncal panniculitis may require a longer course of treatment to resolve all lesions. Some dogs respond much better to dexamethasone (0.2 mg/kg q24h orally). If there is cytologic or clinical evidence of secondary bacterial infection, bactericidal antibiotics (cephalexin, cefadroxil, amoxicillin clavulanate) should be given simultaneously. Topical therapy, especially wet soaks with aluminum acetate or magnesium sulfate (see Chap. 3) are useful, but puppies often find the restraint and pain undesirable, and the struggling and stress associated with the topical therapy become counterproductive. Relapses are virtually unheard of.

■ FELINE ULCERATIVE DERMATITIS WITH LINEAR SUBEPIDERMAL FIBROSIS

This is an uncommon feline dermatosis.[2, 59]

Cause and Pathogenesis

The cause and pathogenesis of this disorder are unknown. Trauma, injections, foreign bodies, and infectious agents do not appear to play a role.

Clinical Features

Any age, breed, or sex of cat may be affected. Typically, lesions are solitary and occur over the dorsal neck and shoulder area (Fig. 17:44). Crusted ulcers ½ to 1 cm in diameter enlarge slowly over a period of weeks to months. No pruritus and pain are present, and affected cats

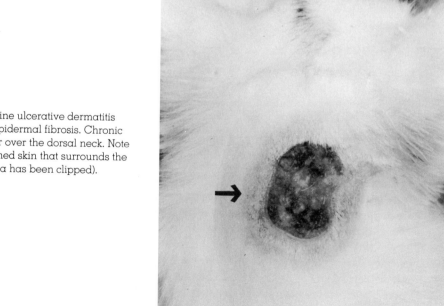

Figure 17:44. Feline ulcerative dermatitis with linear subepidermal fibrosis. Chronic nonhealing ulcer over the dorsal neck. Note the rim of thickened skin that surrounds the ulcer (*arrow; area has been clipped*).

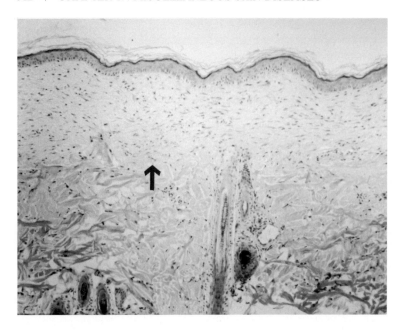

Figure 17:45. Feline ulcerative dermatitis with linear subepidermal fibrosis. Note the bandlike area of subepidermal fibrosis of the superficial dermis (arrow).

are otherwise healthy. These nonhealing ulcers typically have a thick, adherent, brown crust, and there is a rim of firm, thickened skin that surrounds the ulcer.

Diagnosis

The differential diagnosis includes trauma, injection reactions, burns, infections, panniculitis, and neoplasia (especially squamous cell carcinoma). Biopsy reveals ulcerative dermatitis with a rather mild, subjacent superficial perivascular to interstitial dermatitis. Eosinophils are not a prominent inflammatory cell type. The characteristic finding is a linear subepidermal band of superficial dermal fibrosis (Fig. 17:45) that extends peripherally from the ulcer to a distance of several pilosebaceous units.

Clinical Management

Either surgical excision or aggressive glucocorticoid therapy is usually curative. The recommended glucocorticoid protocol is 20 mg methylprednisolone acetate/cat subcutaneously, every 2 weeks until the cat is cured.

■ PERFORATING DERMATITIS

An unusual perforating dermatitis has been described in cats.[60] Multiple firm, conical, hyperkeratotic, yellowish brown lesions, 2 to 7 mm in diameter, are present over various areas of the body (Fig. 17:46). The lesions tend to cluster and form linear configurations. Pruritus and pain are not features. The lesions cannot easily be scraped or pulled off.

The differential diagnosis is that of a cutaneous horn (see Chap. 19). Biopsy reveals a superficial interstitial dermatitis, rich in eosinophils and mast cells, underlying a conical, exophytic projection from the skin surface (Fig. 17:47). The exophytic mass consists of necrotic cellular debris, strands of keratin, and numerous collagen fibers in varying degrees of degeneration. There is transepidermal elimination of collagen fibers, often vertically oriented, into the base of the surface mass (Fig. 17:48). Superficial and middle dermal collagen fibers show a segmental staining abnormality in Masson's trichrome-stained sections. With this stain, collagen fibers stain homogeneously blue. In perforating dermatitis, the collagen fibers show seg-

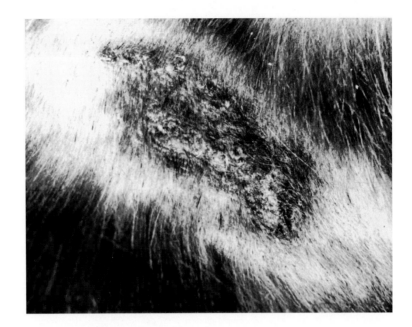

Figure 17:46. Perforating dermatitis over the hip of a cat. Note the linear arrangement of hyperkeratotic papules.

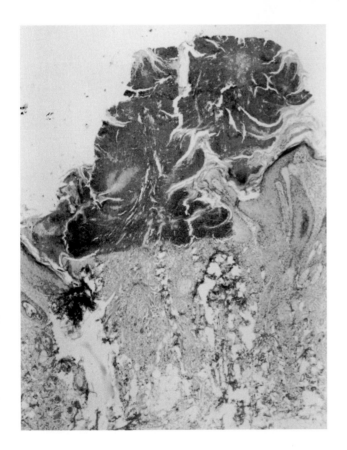

Figure 17:47. Perforating dermatitis in a cat. Exophytic conical mass containing degenerate collagen, inflammatory cells, and keratin.

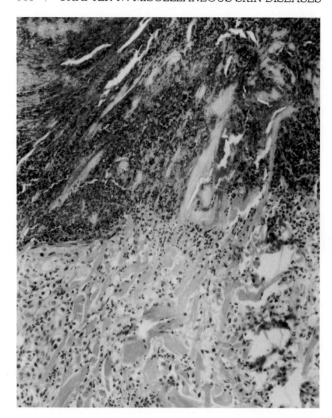

Figure 17:48. Perforating dermatitis in a cat. Vertical orientation of degenerate collagen fibers projecting into the exophytic surface mass.

mental red bands. This staining abnormality has been described in animals with cutaneous asthenia; it presumably indicates some kind of abnormality in collagen metabolism (synthesis, packing, degradation).

Clinical Management

Treatment with ascorbic acid (vitamin C), 100 mg q12h orally, resulted in resolution of the lesions within 30 days. However, when therapy was stopped, the lesions recurred within 8 months.

■ FELINE ACQUIRED SKIN FRAGILITY

This is a rare disorder with multiple etiologic factors. It is characterized by markedly thin and fragile skin.[2, 61, 62]

Cause and Pathogenesis

The pathogenesis of the cutaneous changes is unknown, and the cause appears to be multifactorial. Most reported cases have been associated with spontaneous or iatrogenic Cushing's syndrome (see Chap. 9), diabetes mellitus, or the excessive use of progestational compounds.[2] However, isolated cases have been reported in association with liver disease (lipidosis or cholangiocarcinoma) or nephrosis.[61, 62] Some cats have had normal serum biochemical profiles and adrenal function tests.[2]

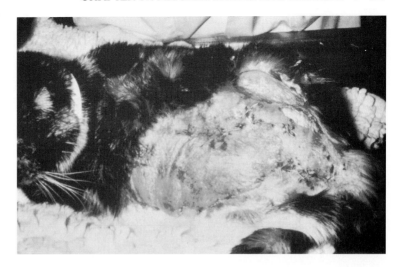

Figure 17:49. Feline acquired skin fragility. Extensive area of full-thickness skin loss over the trunk of a cushingoid cat. (Courtesy R. Rosychuk.)

Clinical Features

Most affected cats are middle-aged or older. The skin becomes markedly thin and is damaged readily by minor trauma. Extreme cutaneous friability leads to irregular tears and the shedding of large sheets of skin (Figs. 17:49 to 17:51). The skin may become so thin that it takes on a translucent quality. Partial alopecia may be seen.

Diagnosis

The differential diagnosis includes spontaneous and iatrogenic Cushing's syndrome and diabetes mellitus; appropriate laboratory tests should be performed. Similar signs are seen in some cats with cutaneous asthenia; in these cases, however, the abnormalities are present from birth.

Because of the extreme attenuation of the skin, biopsy is performed with difficulty. The tissue often folds and twists as wet tissue paper does and the dermis is severely atrophic. Dermal collagen fibers are very thin and disorganized (Figs. 17:52 and 17:53). Panniculus is

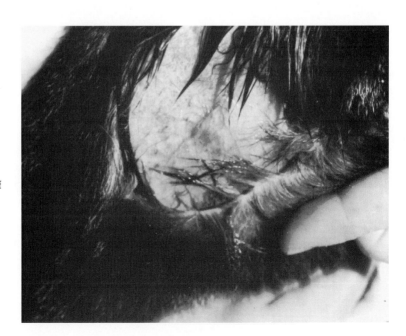

Figure 17:50. Feline acquired skin fragility. Large, full-thickness tear over the thorax of a cat with cholangiohepatitis.

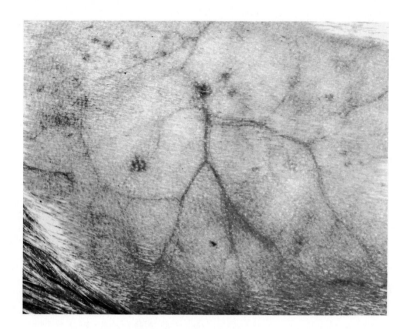

Figure 17:51. Feline acquired skin fragility. Remarkable thinning of truncal skin with resultant easy visualization of the underlying blood vessels in a cat with megestrol acetate–induced diabetes mellitus.

Figure 17:52. Feline acquired skin fragility. The dermis is very atrophic, and collagen fibers are attenuated, disorganized, and wispy in appearance.

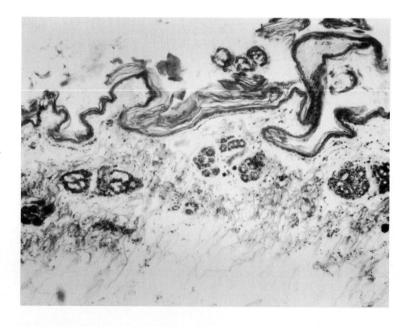

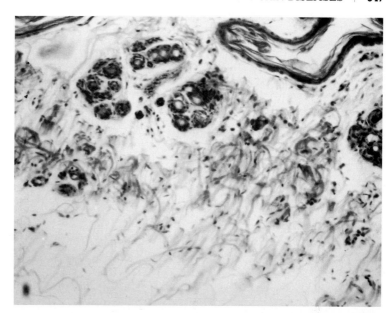

Figure 17:53. Feline acquired skin fragility. Note attenuated, disorganized, and wispy collagen fibers.

usually not present in biopsy specimens. The epidermis and hair follicles may be atrophied. Masson's trichrome-stained sections fail to show the segmental staining abnormality seen in cutaneous asthenia.

Clinical Management

Regardless of the underlying cause demonstrated, the prognosis is grave. The cats are very difficult to handle without skinning them. Surgical repair is usually unsuccessful and leads to more extensive damage.

■ IDIOPATHIC ULCERATIVE DERMATOSIS OF COLLIES AND SHETLAND SHEEPDOGS

This is a newly recognized, poorly understood syndrome that may represent a subgroup of canine familial dermatomyositis (see Chap. 11).[2] Transient vesicobullous eruptions lead to coalescing ulcerations with an undulating serpiginous border. The intertriginous areas of the inguinal and axillary regions are most commonly affected (Fig. 17:54). Lesions may involve the mucocutaneous junctions of the eyes, mouth, genitals, and anus. Concurrent myositis has been documented by electromyography in some affected dogs. This syndrome has been recognized only in adult collies and Shetland sheepdogs of either sex.

The differential diagnosis includes bullous pemphigoid, pemphigus vulgaris, systemic lupus erythematosus, and erythema multiforme. The results of antinuclear antibody tests and direct immunofluorescence tests are consistently negative.[2] Biopsy reveals hydropic interface dermatitis with prominent apoptosis of epidermal and superficial follicular basal cells (Fig. 17:55).[2] Apoptosis is less prominent in the suprabasilar areas of epithelium. Coalescent hydropic degeneration and apoptosis of basal cells lead to intrabasal vesicle and cleft formation, with resultant dermo-epidermal separation and ulceration.

Details of therapy are available (see Chap. 11).

■ IDIOPATHIC DIFFUSE LIPOMATOSIS

This condition is extremely rare in dogs and cats.[2, 63] Adult animals are presented for progressively enlarging skin folds, especially over the neck and trunk. The cutaneous abnormalities

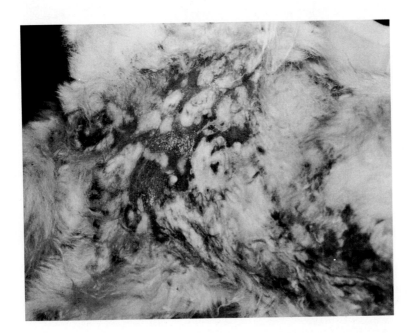

Figure 17:54. Idiopathic ulcerative dermatosis. Numerous well-demarcated, often serpiginous ulcers on the ventral abdomen of a collie.

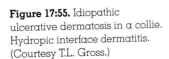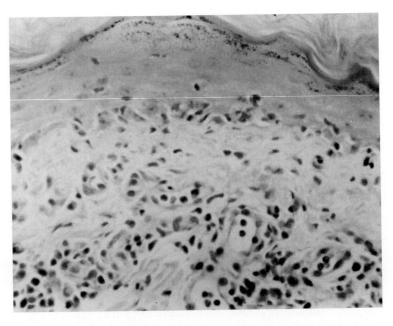

Figure 17:55. Idiopathic ulcerative dermatosis in a collie. Hydropic interface dermatitis. (Courtesy T.L. Gross.)

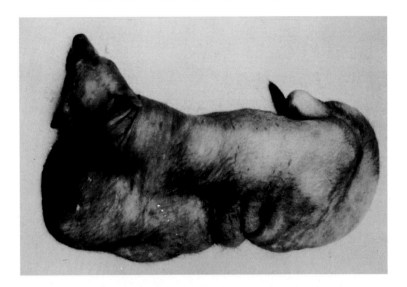

Figure 17:56. Idiopathic diffuse lipomatosis. Remarkable irregular proliferation of subcutaneous fat with resultant distortion of the body. (Courtesy L.A. Lima.)

are symmetric but may be more severe on one side of the body than on the other (Fig. 17:56). The skin folds are pendulous, thick, heavy, and blubbery. Skin overlying larger folds may be thin, hypotrichotic, and traumatized from contact with the environment.

Biopsy reveals a remarkable diffuse thickening of the panniculus (Fig. 17:57). Proliferating fat may resemble mature adipose tissue with mucinosis only of interlobular septae and with small numbers of primitive mesenchymal cells and lipoblasts present around blood vessels. In

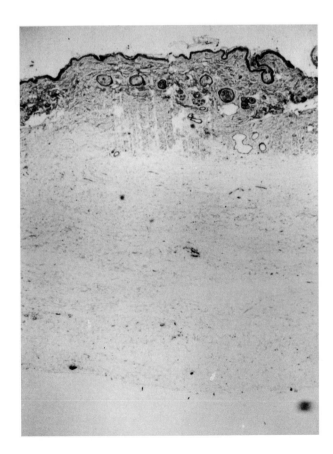

Figure 17:57. Idiopathic diffuse lipomatosis. The skin is markedly thickened because of the abnormal proliferation of lipocytes. Note the complete loss of the normal lobular-septal anatomy of the panniculus.

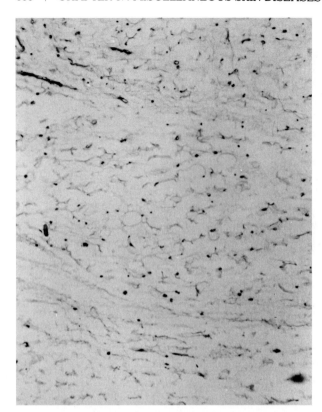

Figure 17:58. Idiopathic diffuse lipomatosis. Proliferation of often misshapen lipocytes.

other cases, the normal anatomy of the panniculus is lost in a proliferation of a mixture of normal-appearing and dysplastic lipocytes (Fig. 17:58).

There is no effective therapy.

■ IDIOPATHIC ACQUIRED CUTANEOUS LAXITY

An unusual dermal collagen disorder was reported in a 9-year-old male English setter[64] that had recently developed large folds of pendulous skin on both sides of the head and under the neck. The folds were composed of thin skin with a jelly-like subcutis, whereas other areas of the dog's body were covered with normal skin. On necropsy, the dermis in the affected areas was found to be only two thirds of the normal thickness, and the dermal collagen bundles were smaller than normal in diameter, fragmented, and widely separated by ground substance. The elastin was normal. The affected tissues contained areas of necrotic subcutaneous fat and vessels with endothelial swelling and a decreased lumen. No inflammation was observed. A vascular insufficiency was proposed as the cause.

■ IDIOPATHIC MUCINOSIS

Idiopathic mucinosis is rare in dogs, and occurs almost exclusively in the Chinese Shar Pei (see Chap. 11).[2, 65, 66] Abnormal deposition of mucin may be focal or diffuse and may vary from mild to severe.

Clinically, mucinosis may be manifested as generalized, thickened, puffy, nonpitting skin. Thickened folds are often most prominent over the face, neck, and limbs (Fig. 17:59; also see Fig. 17:34 *G*). Severe focal mucinosis is usually associated with some degree of generalized mucinosis. Multiloculated vesicles or bullae are seen (see Fig 17:34 *H*). When ruptured, these

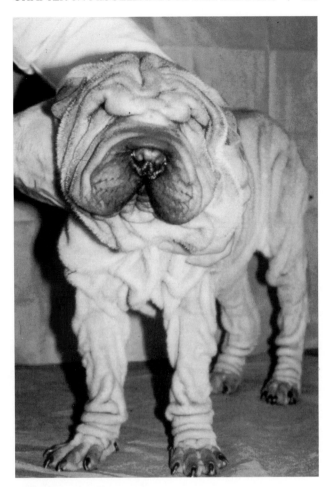

Figure 17:59. Idiopathic mucinosis of the Chinese Shar Pei. Note the remarkable thickening and folding of the skin. (Courtesy M. Paradis.)

lesions yield an acellular, clear, viscid, sticky, and stringy fluid. Affected dogs are not pruritic, do not have clinically inflamed skin, and are otherwise healthy.

An unusual focal mucinosis was reported in a 5-week-old Chow Chow cross puppy.[67] The puppy had pruritic, crusted, papular, and plaque-like lesions on the head and pinnae.

Idiopathic mucinosis occurs in young Chinese Shar Peis that do *not* have pruritus or clinically evident inflammation, and the diagnosis is straightforward in such cases. Biopsy reveals marked diffuse dermal mucinosis and mild perivascular accumulations of mast cells and eosinophils (Fig. 17:60 and 17:61). However, Chinese Shar Peis also develop localized and generalized mucinosis in conjunction with hypersensitivities (e.g., atopy, food hypersensitivity, flea bite hypersensitivity) and hypothyroidism. In these cases, typical signs of the primary disease are also apparent.

Some cases of idiopathic mucinosis in Chinese Shar Peis spontaneously resolve, or deflate, as the dogs age. Remarkable deflation also follows the administration of glucocorticoids.

■ WATERLINE DISEASE OF BLACK LABRADOR RETRIEVERS

Waterline disease is a poorly understood condition of black Labrador retrievers of either sex.[1] Affected dogs present with severe pruritus, secondary seborrhea, and alopecia of the legs and ventrum (Fig. 17:62), and occasionally, of the head. Scrapings and cultures are negative, as are responses to intradermal skin tests and hypoallergenic diets. The disorder is poorly responsive

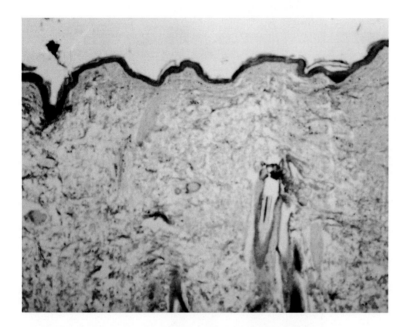

Figure 17:60. Idiopathic mucinosis of the Chinese Shar Pei. Diffuse dermal mucinosis with minimal inflammation.

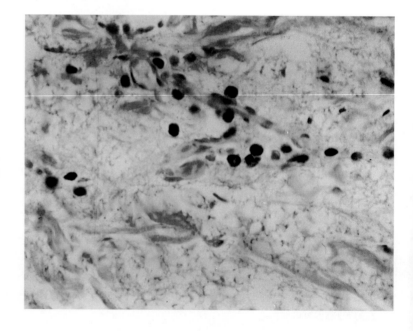

Figure 17:61. Idiopathic mucinosis of the Chinese Shar Pei. Close-up of mucinosis and perivascular mast cells.

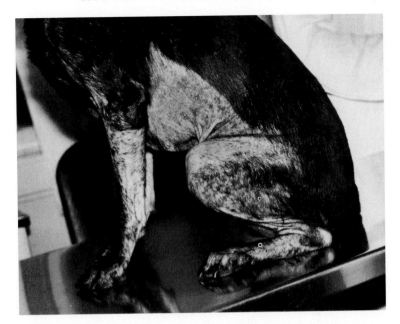

Figure 17:62. Waterline disease in a black Labrador retriever. Note remarkably well demarcated alopecia and dermatitis of the ventral aspect of the body.

to systemic glucocorticosteroids. The authors know of one case in which numerous *Malassezia* yeasts were found on scrapings. The condition responded to ketoconazole administration.

■ IDIOPATHIC PREAURICULAR ULCERATIVE DERMATITIS OF CATS

A pruritic, unilateral to bilateral, preauricular ulcerative dermatitis was reported in a 3-month-old kitten and two of its littermates.[68] The condition was unresponsive to glucocorticoids, antihistamines, fatty acids, antibiotics, and hypoallergenic diets. Isotretinoin (10 mg q24h orally) resulted in healing after 3 weeks. Further details were not given.

REFERENCES

General References
1. Muller, G.H., et al: Small Animal Dermatology, 4th ed. W.B. Saunders Co., Philadelphia, 1989.
2. Gross, T.L., et al.: Veterinary Dermatopathology. Mosby–Year Book, St. Louis, 1992.
3. Griffin, C.E., et al.: Current Veterinary Dermatology. Mosby–Year Book, St. Louis, 1993.
4. Fitzpatrick, T.B., et al.: Dermatology in General Medicine, 4th ed. McGraw-Hill, Inc., New York, 1993.

Canine Subcorneal Pustular Dermatosis
5. McKeever, P.J., Dahl, M.V.: A disease in dogs resembling human subcorneal pustular dermatosis. J. Am. Vet. Med. Assoc. 170:704, 1977.
6. Kalaher, K.M., Scott, D.W.: Subcorneal pustular dermatosis in dogs and in human beings: Comparative aspects. J. Am. Acad. Dermatol. 22:1023, 1990.
7. Clasper, M.: Successful use of gold in the treatment of a case of canine sub-corneal pustular dermatosis. N.Z. Vet. J. 39:65, 1991.
8. Grob, J.J., et al.: Role of tumor necrosis factor-α in Sneddon-Wilkinson subcorneal pustular dermatosis. J. Am. Acad. Dermatol. 25:944, 1991.

Feline Plasma Cell Pododermatitis
9. Scott, D.W.: Feline dermatology 1979–1982: Introspective retrospections. J. Am. Anim. Hosp. Assoc. 20:537, 1984.
10. Scott, D.W.: Feline dermatology 1983–1985: "The Secret Sits." J. Am. Anim. Hosp. Assoc. 23:255, 1987.
11. Taylor, J.E., Schmeitzel, L.P.: Plasma cell pododermatitis with chronic footpad hemorrhage in two cats. J. Am. Vet. Med. Assoc. 197:375, 1990.

Lichenoid Dermatoses
12. Buerger, R.M., Scott, D.W.: Lichenoid dermatitis in a cat: A case report. J. Am. Anim. Hosp. Assoc. 24:55, 1988.
13. Scott, D.W. Lichenoid reactions in the skin of dogs: Clinicopathologic correlations. J. Am. Anim. Hosp. Assoc. 20:305, 1984.

14. Scott, D.W.: Lichenoid dermatoses in dogs and cats. In: Kirk, R.W. (ed.): Current Veterinary Therapy X. W.B. Saunders Co., Philadelphia, 1989, p. 614.
15. Guaguère, E., Mialot, M.: Dermatite lichénoide idiopathique chez un Doberman. Prat. Méd. Chirurg. Anim. Comp. 26:355, 1991.

Canine Sterile Eosinophilic Pustulosis

16. Scott, D.W.: Sterile eosinophilic pustulosis in the dog. J. Am. Anim. Hosp. Assoc. 20:585, 1984.
17. Scott, D.W.: Sterile eosinophilic pustulosis in dog and man: Comparative aspects. J. Am. Acad. Dermatol. 16:1022, 1987.
18. Carlotti, D., et al.: La maladie d'Ofugi (pustulose éosinophilique stérile). Prat. Méd. Chirurg. Anim. Comp. 24:131, 1989.
19. Thomsen, M.K., et al.: Impairment of neutrophil functions in a dog with an eosinophilic dermatosis. Acta Vet. Scand. 32:519, 1991.
20. Craig, J.M.: A case of sterile eosinophilic pustulosis in a dog. Vet. Dermatol. Newsl. 15:11, 1993.
21. Scott, D.W., et al.: Sterile eosinophilic folliculitis in the cat: An unusual manifestation of feline allergic skin disease? Companion Anim. Pract. 19 (8&9): 6, 1989.

Feline Hypereosinophilic Syndrome

22. Scott, D.W., et al.: Hypereosinophilic syndrome in a cat. Feline Pract. 15:22, 1985.
23. Harvey, R.G.: Feline hypereosinophilia with cutaneous lesions. J. Small Anim. Pract. 31:453, 1990.
24. Neer, T.M.: Hypereosinophilic syndrome in cats. Comp. Cont. Educ. 13:549, 1991.

Idiopathic Sterile Granuloma and Pyogranuloma

25. Panich, R., et al.: Canine cutaneous sterile pyogranuloma/granuloma syndrome: A retrospective analysis of 29 cases (1976 to 1988). J. Am. Anim. Hosp. Assoc. 27:519, 1991.
26. Houston, D.M., et al.: A case of cutaneous sterile pyogranuloma/granuloma syndrome in a Golden retriever. Can. Vet. J. 34:121, 1993.
27. Scott, D.W., et al.: Idiopathic sterile granulomatous and pyogranulomatous dermatitis in cats. Vet. Dermatol. 1:129, 1990.
28. Scott, D.W., Noxon, J.O.: Sterile sarcoidal granulomatous skin disease in three dogs. Canine Pract. 15(3):11, 1990.

Granulomatous Sebaceous Adenitis

29. Scott, D.W.: Granulomatous sebaceous adenitis in dogs. J. Am. Anim. Hosp. Assoc. 22:631, 1986.
30. Rosser, E.J., Jr., et al.: Sebaceous adenitis with hyperkeratosis in the standard poodle: A discussion of 10 cases. J. Am. Anim. Hosp. Assoc. 23:341, 1987.
31. Scott, D.W.: Adénite sébacée pyogranulomateuse stérile chez un chat. Point Vét. 21:107, 1989.
32. Stewart, L.J, et al.: Isotretinoin in the treatment of sebaceous adenitis in two Vizslas. J. Am. Anim. Hosp. Assoc. 27:65, 1991.
33. Guaguère, E., et al.: Adénite sébacée granulomateuse. A propos de trois cas. Prat. Méd. Chirurg. Anim. Comp. 25:169, 1990.
34. Power, H.T., Ihrke, P.J.: Synthetic retinoids in veterinary dermatology. Vet. Clin. N. Am. (Small Anim. Pract.) 20:1525, 1990.
35. Carothers, M.A., et al.: Cyclosporine-responsive granulomatous sebaceous adenitis in a dog. J. Am. Vet. Med. Assoc. 198:1645, 1991.
36. Scott, D.W.: Sterile granulomatous sebaceous adenitis in dogs and cats. Vet. Ann. 33:236, 1993.
36a. Dunstan, R.W., Hargis, A.M.: The diagnosis of sebaceous adenitis in standard poodle dogs. In: Bonagura, J.D. (ed.). Kirk's Current Veterinary Therapy XII. W.B. Saunders Co., Philadelphia, 1995.

Localized Scleroderma

37. Scott, D.W.: Localized scleroderma (morphea) in two dogs. J. Am. Anim. Hosp. Assoc. 22:207, 1986.
38. Bourdeau, P., et al.: Observation d'un cas de sclérodermie localisée (morphée) chez un chien. Rev. Méd. Vét. 167:1121, 1990.

Feline Eosinophilic Granuloma Complex

39. Scott, D.W., et al.: Miliary dermatitis. A feline cutaneous reaction pattern. Proc. Ann. Kal Kan Sem. 2:11, 1986.
40. Von Tscharner, C., Bigler, B.: The eosinophilic granuloma complex. J. Small Anim. Pract. 30:228, 1989.
41. Moriello, K.A., et al.: Lack of autologous tissue transmission of eosinophilic plaques in cats. Am. J. Vet. Res. 51:995, 1990.
42. Mason, K.V., Evans, A.G.: Mosquito bite-caused eosinophilic dermatitis in cats. J. Am. Vet. Med. Assoc. 198:2086, 1991.
43. Power, H.T.: Eosinophilic granuloma in a family of specific pathogen-free cats. Proc. Annu. Memb. Meet. Am. Acad. Vet. Dermatol., Am. Coll. Vet. Dermatol. 6:45, 1990.
44. Paulsen, M.E., et al.: Feline eosinophilic keratitis: A review of 15 clinical cases. J. Am. Anim. Hosp. Assoc. 23:63, 1987.
45. Pentlarge, V.W.: Eosinophilic conjunctivitis in five cats. J. Am. Anim. Hosp. Assoc. 27:21, 1991.

Canine Eosinophilic Granuloma

46. Scott, D.W.: Cutaneous eosinophilic granulomas with collagen degeneration in the dog. J. Am. Anim. Hosp. Assoc. 19:529, 1983.
47. da Silva Curiel, J.M., et al.: Eosinophilic granuloma of the nasal skin in a dog. J. Am. Vet. Med. Assoc. 193:566, 1988.

48. Fontaine, J., et al.: Deux cas de granulomes éosinophiliques oraux chez un Husky Sibérien et un Malamute. Ann. Méd. Vét. 134:223, 1990.
49. Poulet, F.M., et al.: Focal proliferative eosinophilic dermatitis of the external ear canal in four dogs. Vet. Pathol. 28:171, 1991.
50. Brovida, D, Castagnaro, M.: Tracheal obstruction due to an eosinophilic granuloma in a dog: Surgical treatment and clinicopathological observations. J. Am. Anim. Hosp. Assoc. 28:8, 1992.

Panniculitis
51. Scott, D.W., Anderson, W.I.: Panniculitis in dogs and cats: A retrospective analysis of 78 cases. J. Am. Anim. Hosp. Assoc. 24:551, 1988.
52. Guaguère, E., et al.: Panniculite nodulaire stérile chez le chien. A propos de trois cas. Rev. Méd. Vét. 164:195, 1988.
53. Aoki, S., et al.: Nodular nonsuppurative panniculitis in a dog. J. Jpn. Vet. Med. Assoc. 41:659, 1988.
53a. Hendrick, M.J., Dunagan, C.A.: Focal necrotizing granulomatous panniculitis associated with subcutaneous injection of rabies vaccine in cats and dogs: 10 cases (1988–1989). J. Am. Vet. Med. Assoc. 198:304, 1991.
53b. Stanley, R.G., Jabara, A.G.: Chronic skin reaction to a combined feline rhinotracheitis virus (herpesvirus) and calicivirus vaccine. Aust. Vet. J. 65:128, 1988.

Subcutaneous Fat Sclerosis
54. Buerger, R.G., et al.: Subcutaneous fat sclerosis in a cat. Comp. Cont. Educ. 9:1198, 1987.

Canine Juvenile Cellulitis
55. White, S.D. et al.: Juvenile cellulitis in dogs: 15 cases (1979–1988). J. Am. Vet. Med. Assoc. 195:1609, 1989.
56. Mason, I.S., Jones, J: Juvenile cellulitis in Gordon Setters. Vet. Rec. 124:642, 1989.
57. Reimann, K.A., et al.: Clinicopathologic characteristics of canine juvenile cellulitis. Vet. Pathol. 26:499, 1989.
58. Barta, O., Oyekan, P.P.: Lymphocyte transformation test in veterinary clinical immunology. Comp. Immunol. Microbiol. Infect. Dis. 4:209, 1981.

Feline Ulcerative Dermatitis With Linear Subepidermal Fibrosis
59. Scott, D.W.: An unusual ulcerative dermatitis associated with linear subepidermal fibrosis in eight cats. Feline Pract. 18(3):8, 1990.

Perforating Dermatitis
60. Scott, D.W., Miller, W.H., Jr.: An unusual perforating dermatitis in a Siamese cat. Vet. Dermatol. 2:173, 1991.

Feline Acquired Skin Fragility
61. Diquelou, A., et al: Lipoïdose hépatique et syndrome de fragilité cutanée chez un chat. Prat. Méd. Chirurg. Anim. Comp. 26:151, 1991.
62. Regnier, A., Pieraggi, M.T.: Abnormal skin fragility in a cat with a cholangio-carcinoma. J. Small Anim. Pract. 30:419, 1989.

Idiopathic Diffuse Lipomatosis
63. Gilbert, P.A., et al.: Diffuse truncal lipomatosis in a dog. J. Am. Anim. Hosp. Assoc. 26:586, 1990.

Idiopathic Acquired Cutaneous Laxity
64. Pieraggi, M.T., et al.: An unusual dermal collagen disorder in a dog. J. Comp. Pathol. 96:289, 1986.

Idiopathic Mucinosis
65. Rosenkrantz, W.S., et al.: Idiopathic mucinosis in a dog. Companion Anim. Pract. 1:39, 1987.
66. Schäfer, H., Spieth, K.: Fallbericht: Idiopathische Muzinose bei einem Shar Pei. Kleintierpraxis 37:403, 1992.
67. Beale, K.M., et al.: Papular and plaque-like mucinosis in a puppy. Vet. Dermatol. 2:29, 1991.

Idiopathic Preauricular Ulcerative Dermatitis of Cats
68. Breen, P.T., Jeromin, A.M.: A case of feline idiopathic ulcerative dermatosis responding to isotretinoin. Dermatol. Dialogue, Spring/Summer 93, p. 6.

CHAPTER

18

Diseases of Eyelids, Claws, Anal Sacs, and Ear Canals

■

Chapter Outline

■ EYELID DISEASES

The eyelids are complex folds of skin susceptible to many structural and functional disorders. This discussion is limited to diseases that affect eyelids and not the eyeball, the conjunctiva, and the third eyelid, which are purely in the realm of the ophthalmologist.

Anatomy

Canine and feline eyelids consist of an upper eyelid, a lower eyelid, a row of cilia in the upper lid only, and a number of glands.[11a] Meibomian glands (tarsal glands)) are modified, large sebaceous gland units that produce a viscous, oily secretion. Zeis' glands are sebaceous glands associated with cilia. Moll's glands are modified apocrine sweat glands associated with cilia. In addition, accessory lacrimal glands in the eyelids discharge tears into the conjunctival sac and contribute to the precorneal film. The largest of these in the dog is the superficial gland of the membrana nicitans, also known (erroneously) as the Harder gland (or harderian gland).

The bacterial and fungal flora of the eyelids of normal dogs has been studied.[21, 31] The bacteria most commonly isolated include *Staphylococcus intermedius,* coagulase-negative staphylococci, and *Corynebacterium* spp. These are similar to the bacteria found on normal canine skin in many other locations (see Chap. 1). However, fungi were rarely isolated from eyelids, whereas they are commonly isolated from other areas of the skin.

Diseases

Because of the thin and delicate nature of the skin on the eyelid, its loosely attached subcutis, and the presence of a mucocutaneous junction at the eyelid margin, the eyelid and periocular area demonstrate exaggerated responses to numerous dermatologic conditions.[30] Because a normal eyelid margin is necessary for maintenance of tear film and protection of the cornea, abnormalities of the eyelid margin often produce signs of ocular discomfort and discharge. These signs can be the primary reason that the owner seeks veterinary care.

■ *Blepharitis.*   Inflammation of the eyelid is termed *blepharitis.*[11a, 11b] Often a mucous discharge is apparent. Many dermatoses may cause blepharitis or may be limited to the lids (Table 18:1).[3, 11] Some of these diseases are more likely to present with blepharitis only. In young dogs, localized *Demodex* infestation may appear on the lids (Fig. 18:1 *A*). Usually, only one eye and only part of the eyelid are involved. Alopecia with minimal inflammation may be seen. Periocular noninflammatory alopecia may also occur with topical ocular steroid reactions but is usually diffuse. Every year, the authors see a number of cases referred from ophthalmologists

Table 18:1. Diseases Limited to or That May First Present as Eyelid or Periocular Dermatoses

Demodicosis	Self-trauma resulting from ocular disease
Dermatophytosis	Lupus erythematosus
Malassezia dermatitis	Vitiligo
Bacterial folliculitis	Periocular leukotrichia (especially in Siamese cats)
Atopy (allergic inhalant dermatitis)	Solar dermatitis
Food hypersensitivity	Distemper
Zinc-responsive dermatosis	Topical steroid alopecia
Juvenile cellulitis	Drug eruption
Idiopathic periocular alopecia	

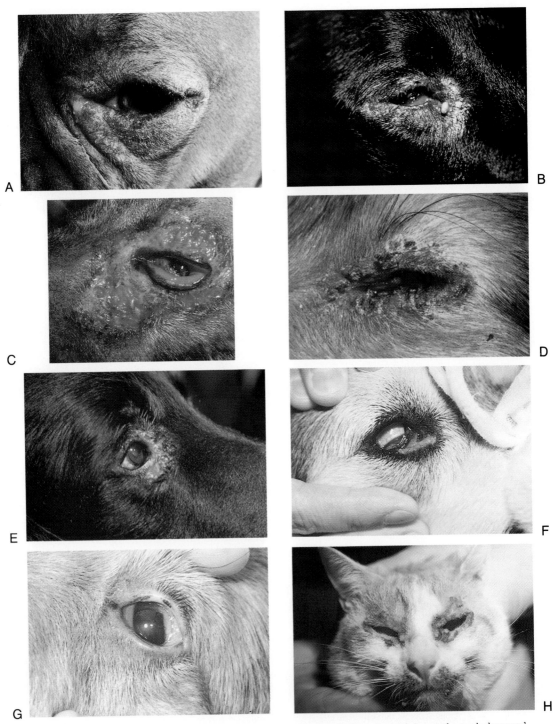

Figure 18:1. *A*, Marked focal alopecia due to demodectic blepharitis. *B*, Hypothyroid dog with staphylococcal blepharitis. *C*, Ulcerative blepharitis in a dog with mucocutaneous staphylococcal pyoderma. *D*, Dog with mycotic blepharitis due to *Trichophyton terrestre*. *E*, Ulcerative blepharitis in a dog with bullous pemphigoid. *F*, Ulcerative blepharitis in a dog with discoid lupus erythematosus. *G*, Depigmentation of eyelids in a dog with uveodermatologic syndrome. *H*, Severe blepharitis in a cat with hypereosinophilic syndrome.

because of chronic conjunctivitis and blepharitis due to atopy. Varying combinations of blepharitis with periocular alopecia, hyperpigmentation, and lichenification may result from chronic pruritus. Although other symptoms may be found on close examination, they often go unrecognized by the owner.

An idiopathic periocular crusting, occasionally associated with *Malassezia* or feline acne, may be seen in cats, particularly Persians. Idiopathic seborrhea and bacterial folliculitis in dogs and dermatophytes in dogs and cats (Fig. 18:1 *B* to *D*) may also cause scaling and crusting periocularly. Immune-mediated dermatoses have a mucocutaneous predilection and often involve the eyelids (Fig. 18:1 *E* to *G*). Other diseases are known for their periocular distribution, although they are not limited to that area (Fig. 18:1 *H*) (Table 18:2).[3]

An idiopathic chronic ulcerative blepharitis, localized to the medial canthal region, has been described in dachshunds, German shepherds, and Poodles.[1] Biopsy reveals a diffuse lymphoplasmacytic dermatitis. Response to topical or systemic glucocorticoids is excellent, but therapy must often be maintained for life.

Ulcers and nodules were seen on the eyelids of a dog with neosporosis.[11b]

■ *Entropion and Ectropion.* Entropion (inversion, or turning in) and ectropion (eversion, or turning out) of the lid margins are best corrected by surgery. Chronic conjunctivitis or other diseases of the eye that may result in distortion of the lids should also receive attention.

■ *Hordeolum (Stye).* This is an acute, painful pyogenic infection of a sebaceous gland of the eyelid. Two types are recognized. The external hordeolum (zeisian stye) involves the glands of Zeis and the cilia on the outer eyelid. The internal hordeolum (meibomian stye) involves the meibomian gland in the inner surface of the eyelid. The internal type is the most common hordeolum in dogs. Treatment consists of incising the abscess and applying an antibiotic ointment. Appropriate systemic antibiotics are useful when the hordeolum is caused by staphylococci.

■ *Chalazion.* A chronic inflammation of a meibomian gland, a chalazion appears externally on the skin surface of the lid as a painless nodule and internally on the palpebral conjunctiva as a yellow, smaller nodule. The irritation from the inner swelling causes conjunctivitis. Treatment consists of incision and curettage of accumulated sebaceous material. Large chalazia may be excised completely to prevent recurrence.

■ *Trichiasis.* This disorder is an abnormal position or direction of the cilia, resulting in epiphora, mucous ocular discharge, and sometimes corneal vascularization and even corneal ulceration. Treatment consists of meticulous electroepilation of the involved cilia.

■ *Distichiasis.* Animals with distichiasis display aberrant cilia on the lid. They may emerge from the openings of the meibomian glands or the inner lid margin. Electroepilation is the treatment of choice. Distichiasis has been reported in Poodles, boxers, Pekingese, German shepherds, Cocker spaniels, Shetland sheepdogs, and Bedlington and Yorkshire terriers, as well as in the Shih tzu, Pug, and St. Bernard.[33, 35, 37]

■ *Epiphora.* This disorder is common in Poodles (Fig. 18:2 *A*). The cause may be atresia, blockage of the nasal lacrimal system, or lid or membrana nictitans deformities.[6] Surgical correction of the lid problem or deepening of the lacrimal lake frequently permits improved function of the lower puncta. Correction of possible causes of chronic lacrimation from ocular irritation should also be implemented.

Table 18:2. Diseases That Affect the Eyelid or Periocular Area in Addition to Other Sites

Pemphigus foliaceus	Solar dermatitis
Pemphigus erythematosus	Vitiligo
Systemic lupus erythematosus	Hypereosinophilic syndrome
Discoid lupus erythematosus	Drug eruption
Uveodermatologic syndrome	Leishmaniasis
Canine familial dermatomyositis	Vasculitis
Canine necrolytic migratory erythema	Pemphigus vulgaris
Erythema multiforme	Bullous pemphigoid

■ *Tumors of the Eyelids.* These tumors are difficult to manage because of the problems with plastic repair after surgery or with protection of the globe, if radiation therapy is contemplated. In dogs, papillomas, sebaceous gland tumors, and melanocytic neoplasms are the most common (Fig. 18:2 *B*) (see Chap. 19). Basal cell tumors, mast cell tumors (Fig. 18:2 *C*), and epitheliotropic lymphoma (Fig. 18:2 *D*) are also found. In cats, squamous cell carcinoma is, by far, the most common.[47] A histiocytoma of the eyelid of a 10-month-old Afghan that regressed spontaneously has been reported.[20]

In older dogs, eyelid tumors are common (Table 18:3).[3] These can be adenomas and adenocarcinomas of Zeis' and Moll's glands as well as meibomian gland tumors. For treatment, surgical removal is indicated when the tumor is on the palpebral junction and touches the cornea. This can be accomplished by surgical excision, electrosurgery, or cryosurgery. Tumors that touch the conjunctiva and cause irritation (and sometimes ulceration) must be removed. It is important to remove the entire tumor; otherwise, it regrows. The surgery can be performed with a sedative (tranquilizer) plus local anesthesia. A small V-shaped incision exposes the entire tumor for removal and can be closed with one or two sutures. Animals with massive eyelid tumors that require removal of a large section of lid should be referred to an ophthalmologist, because correct plastic repair is necessary for proper lid function.

■ CLAW DISEASES

Claws may be affected by many of the diseases described in this text. However, dogs and cats presenting with claw disorders as the only dermatologic manifestation of disease are rarely encountered. Such dogs and cats accounted for approximately 1.3 per cent and 2.2 per cent, respectively, of all dogs and cats examined for dermatologic disease at one university teaching hospital.[61, 62]

Claws and their disorders have received little attention in veterinary medicine.[15, 61, 62] Reviews on canine and feline claw diseases have been published.[61, 62] The most commonly reported types of claw diseases are asymmetric and result from known or presumed trauma with or without secondary bacterial infection and onychodystrophy. The normal microanatomy

Figure 18:2. *A,* Epiphora. The chronic discharge of tears is common in Poodles and results in brown staining of the wet hair. (This phenomenon is seen anywhere that white hair is constantly wet.) *B,* Verrucous, hyperpigmented sebaceous gland hyperplasia on the lower eyelid. *C,* Mast cell tumor. Alopecic pink plaque on the upper eyelid of a cat. (Courtesy M. Paradis.) *D,* Epitheliotropic lymphoma. Depigmentation and erythematous papules on the eyelid of a dog. *E,* Bacterial paronychia with ulceration of the claw fold. Note the purulent exudate at the base of the nail. *F,* Onychomadesis in a dog with bacterial paronychia and hypothyroidism. *G,* Onychomycosis in a dog caused by *Trichophyton mentagrophytes.* Claws are grossly deformed, and there is secondary paronychia in the central toe. *H,* Clawbed *Malassezia* in an atopic dog. Brown discoloration on the claw in a dog with *Malassezia* paronychia.

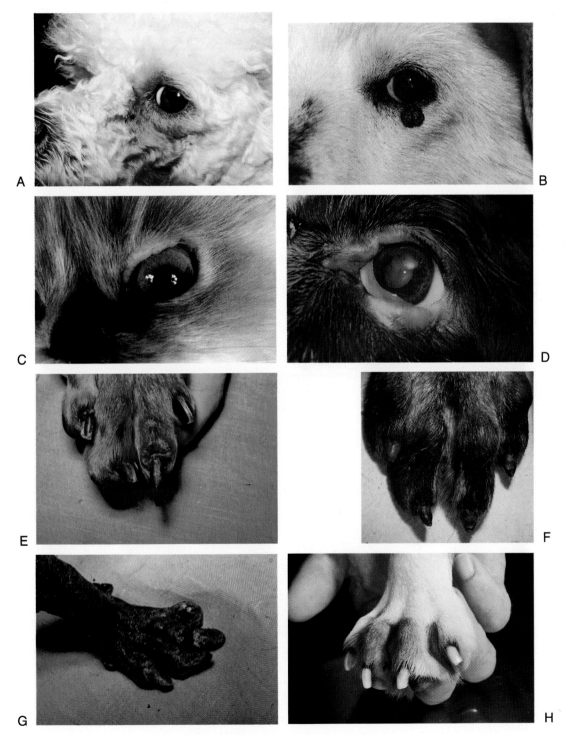

Figure 18:2 *See legend on opposite page*

Table 18:3. Neoplastic Conditions That May Affect the Eyelid or Periocular Area

Squamous cell carcinoma	Lymphoma
Actinic keratosis	Epitheliotropic lymphoma
Melanocytoma and melanoma	Papilloma
Sebaceous gland tumors	Mastocytoma
Fibrous histiocytoma	Histiocytoma
Dermoid	

of the canine claw has been studied,[49] but no in-depth microanatomic study of claw disorders has been published. Further work is warranted, because chronic claw diseases are debilitating for affected animals and frustrating for both veterinarians and owners.

Anatomy

The claw is a specialized structure that is a direct continuation of the dermis and epidermis (Fig. 18:3).[49, 62] The distal phalanx of each toe has a crescent-shaped dorsal process called the *ungual crest*. The dermis of adjacent skin is continuous with, and extends distally from, this bony process as the periosteum of the phalanx. It has a rich blood supply, which is the source

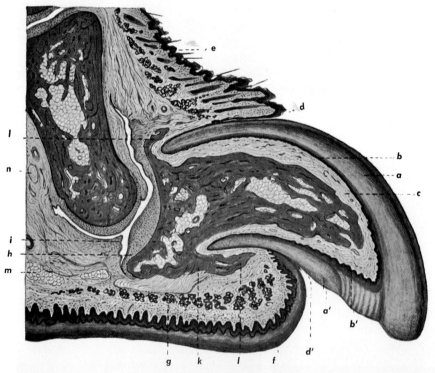

Figure 18:3. Midsagittal section through the claw of the dog: *a*, stratum corneum of the epidermis of the claw; *a'*, stratum corneum of the epidermis of the sole; *b,b'*, deep, noncornified epidermal layers of the dorsum and sole of the claw; *c*, corium (papillated in the area of the sole); *d*, claw fold; *d'*, limiting furrow separating the sole from the digital pad; *e*, skin with hair and glands; *f*, epidermis of the digital pad with stratum granulosum and lucidum; *g*, tubular glands in the digital pad; *h*, articular cartilage of the third phalanx; *i*, meniscus; *k*, Sharpey's fibers from a tendon insertion; *l*, ungual crest; *m*, fat cushion within the digital pad; *n*, lamellar corpuscle. (From Trautmann, A., Fiebiger, J.: Fundamentals of the Histology of Domestic Animals. Copyright 1952 by Cornell University. Reprinted by permission of Cornell University Press.)

of the profuse hemorrhage if the claw is trimmed too short. The structures constituting the claw are compressed laterally and may be divided into the coronary band, the ventral sole, and the lateral and medial walls. Most of the claw is formed from the coronary band and the dorsal ridge. In many areas, the dermis has fine papillae that project distally and interdigitate with soft epidermal lamellae.

The epidermis of adjacent skin is also continuous with that of the claw. The basal layer of the epidermis, supported by the dermis, is most active in the coronary band and dorsal ridge areas and causes growth in a circular fashion, producing a curved claw. This is why the claw may grow around into the volar surface of the footpad. The horny walls grow over the sole of the claw for the same reason. During the first 2 years of life, the claws of beagles grow an average of 1.9 mm/wk, but this rate declines with age. Rates of growth as slow as 0.8 mm/wk have been reported.[62]

The epidermis of the claw sole has distinct granular and clear layers, as well as the usual structures. However, the epidermis of the rest of the claw is largely composed of a thick horny layer that consists of flat cornified epidermal cells fused into a horny plate, with an absent stratum granulosum. On the ventral surface, the claw is separated from the footpad by a distinct furrow. This sole is relatively soft and is compressible. A fold of modified skin hides the dorsal junction of hairy skin and claw. This claw fold is free from hair on its inner surface and produces the thin stratum tectorium that is the outer layer of the proximal claw.

The claws of animals have important functions as prehensile, locomotor, and offensive and defensive organs. A dog's claws should be kept properly trimmed for good foot health and normal locomotion. Abnormal claws predispose the feet to trauma, strains, and pododermatitis. Because of the long growth cycle, the correction of abnormalities may necessitate 6 to 8 months of treatment.

A study on the microanatomy of the normal canine claw revealed that numerous intranuclear vacuoles are present in the keratinocytes of the stratum basale and stratum spinosum.[49] Additionally, focal areas of subepidermal clefting were frequently seen. These findings must be kept in mind when considering the diagnosis of interface dermatoses and dystrophies of the claw.

Certain terms are used specifically when describing claw abnormalities (Table 18:4).[62] Many of these abnormalities may be seen together in the same claw or in different claws of the same

Table 18:4. Terminology for Claw Disorders

Anonychia—absence of claws (usually congenital)
Brachyonychia—short claws
Leukonychia—whitening of claws
Macronychia—unusually large claws
Micronychia—unusually small claws, often shorter or narrower than normal
Onychalgia—claw pain
Onychauxis (hyperonychia)—simple hypertrophy of claws
Onychia (onychitis)—inflammation somewhere in the claw unit
Onychoclasis—breaking of claws
Onychocryptosis (onyxis)—ingrown claw
Onychodystrophy—abnormal claw formation
Onychogryphosis (onychogryposis)—hypertrophy and abnormal curvature of claws
Onychomadesis (onychoptosis)—sloughing of claws
Onychomalacia (hapalonychia)—softening of claws
Onychomycosis—fungal infection of claws
Onychorrhexis—longitudinal striations associated with brittleness and breaking of claws
Onychoschizia (onychoschisis)—splitting and/or lamination of claws, usually beginning distally
Onychopathy (onychosis)—disease or abnormality of claws
Pachyonychia—thickening of claws
Paronychia (perionychia)—inflammation or infection of claw folds
Platonychia—increased curvature of claws in long axis

From Scott, D.W., Miller, W.H., Jr.: Disorders of claws and clawbeds in dogs. Comp. Cont. Educ. 14:1448, 1992.

animal. Some conditions have little diagnostic specificity, although others may. For example, leukonychia with no other abnormalities is suggestive of vitiligo. Other changes that may affect claws include crusting or excessive keratinous, waxy deposits on the claws, staining of the claws (often to a brown or red color), and abnormally rapid growth rate. Inflammation of the claw fold and distal digit (paronychia) often lead to an abnormally rapid growth rate, which, in some cases, is associated with onychogryphosis. Varying degrees of lameness, pain on touch or palpation, pruritus, and regional lymphadenopathy may be present.

Diseases

A wide variety of diseases were recently shown to be associated with claw diseases in dogs (Table 18:5) and cats (Table 18:6).

TRAUMA

Trauma is the most common cause of claw disease seen in dogs and the second most common in cats.[61, 62] Usually, the trauma is physical, although chemical trauma due to substances such as fertilizers may occur. Trauma most commonly affects one or just a few claws (asymmetric claw disease). Occasionally, all four paws have multiple claws affected (symmetric claw disease), owing to trauma such as that induced by excessive running on hard (asphalt, concrete) surfaces and gravel. The resulting embedment of debris in the distal ends of the claws may cause secondary bacterial infections. Clipping too closely can also lead to injury from embedded debris or predispose the claws to secondary infections.

Table 18:5. Causes of Claw Disorders in 196 Dogs

Diagnosis	Number of Cases
Bacterial paronychia secondary to broken or torn claw	49
Bacterial paronychia, 1 paw, idiopathic	13
Bacterial paronychia, 4 paws, secondary to hypothyroidism	4
Bacterial paronychia, 4 paws, secondary to hyperadrenocorticism	2
Bacterial paronychia, front paws, secondary to atopy	1
Bacterial paronychia, 4 paws, recurrent, idiopathic	4
Broken or torn claw	44
Neoplasia	24
Demodicosis	3
Dermatophytosis (*Trichophyton mentagrophytes*)	3
Candidiasis secondary to diabetes mellitus	1
Blastomycosis	1
Geotrichosis	1
Cryptococcosis	1
Lupus erythematosus–like	7
Pemphigus foliaceus	2
Pemphigus vulgaris	2
Bullous pemphigoid	1
Epidermolysis bullosa	1
Onychodystrophy, idiopathic	18
Onychodystrophy or onychoschizia secondary to seborrhea	4
Onychodystrophy or onychorrhexis, idiopathic	9
Onychomadesis, 4 paws, with atrial fibrillation	1

From Scott, D.W., Miller, W.H., Jr.: Disorders of the claw and clawbed in dogs. Comp. Cont. Educ. 14:449, 1992.

Table 18:6. Causes of Claw Disorders in 65 Cats

Diagnosis	Number of Cases
Onychodystrophy (idiopathic)	23
Bacterial paronychia secondary to broken or torn claws	9
Broken or torn claws	8
Bacterial paronychia secondary to feline leukemia virus infection	7
Pemphigus foliaceus	3
Bacterial paronychia (recurrent, idiopathic)	2
Squamous cell carcinoma	2
Systemic lupus erythematosus	2
Bacterial paronychia secondary to acquired arteriovenous fistula	1
Bacterial paronychia secondary to diabetes mellitus	1
Bacterial paronychia secondary to iatrogenic Cushing's syndrome	1
Dermatophytosis from *Microsporum canis*	1
Cryptococcosis	1
Sporotrichosis	1
Eosinophilic plaque (atopy, presumptive)	1
Hemangiosarcoma	1
Metastatic bronchogenic carcinoma	1

From Scott, D.W., Miller, W.H. Jr.: Disorders of the claw and clawbeds in cats. Comp. Cont. Educ. 14:449, 1992.

INFECTIONS

Infectious causes of claw diseases are also common. Bacteria are most often incriminated, and bacterial infections should always be considered secondary (see Fig. 18:2 *E*). A search for an underlying cause should be made. If none is found, recurrences, especially when all four paws are involved, are likely and a guarded prognosis should be given. Trauma is the most common underlying cause. However, hypothyroidism, hyperadrenocorticism, diabetes mellitus, atopy, immune-mediated diseases, arteriovenous fistulae, other infectious agents, and dystrophy may be responsible (see Fig. 18:2 *F*). Purulent exudate within or under the claw is the preferred source of specimens for cytologic examination or culture and sensitivity testing.

Fungal infections, which are referred to as *onychomycosis*, may also occur (see Fig. 18:2 *G*). Dermatophytosis, particularly *Trichophyton* infection in the dog, blastomycosis, cryptococcosis, geotrichosis, and sporotrichosis have all been reported, although rarely. Lesions are not usually confined to the claws. Dermatophytes invade the claw keratin and, therefore, are usually associated with onychomalacia. Claws may be brittle and easily broken or powdered. *Malassezia* infection may affect only the claws.[23] Generally, these cases have mild paronychia with a brown, dry to slightly moist claw fold exudate that attaches to the claw. The claw becomes discolored brown-red (see Fig. 18:2 *H*). Often, these are atopic dogs, and the paw pruritus, due to *Malassezia* infection, may be the only symptom after successful control of the atopic disease.

Parasites may also result in claw diseases. Demodicosis may be accompanied by a paronychia that stimulates abnormal claw growth. *Ascaris* infection, hookworm dermatitis, and leishmaniasis have been reported causes of claw disease. Leishmaniasis is most commonly associated with onychogryphosis.

IMMUNE-MEDIATED DISEASES

Immune-mediated diseases often involve the claw fold, resulting in paronychia. In some cases, other claw changes, especially onychomadesis, may occur, and less commonly, only claw disease is seen. Lupus erythematosus, or a lupoid syndrome, appears to be the most common immune-mediated disease to cause abnormal claws (Fig. 18:4A).[55, 61, 62] When claw disease

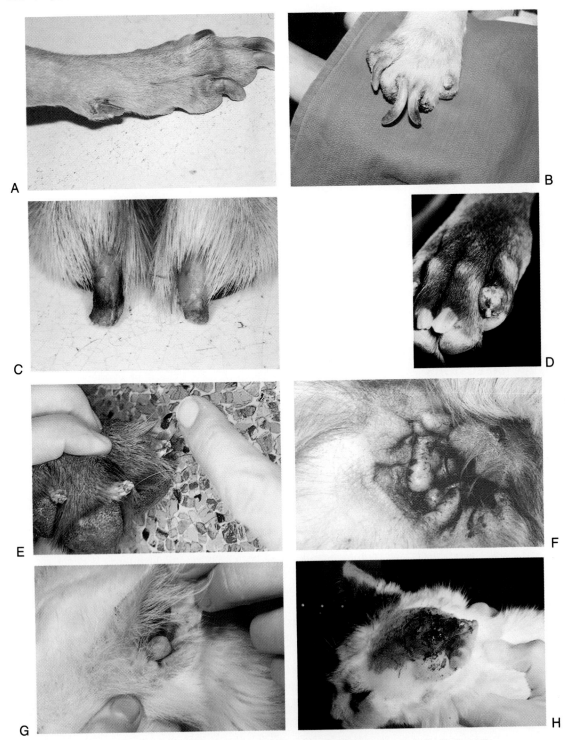

Figure 18:4. *A,* Onychogryposis in a dog with discoid lupus erythematosus. (Courtesy D. Carlotti.) *B,* Onychogryposis and onychomadesis in a dog with pemphigus foliaceus. *C,* A case of Raynaud-like disease in a dog. (Courtesy D. Carlotti.) *D,* Squamous cell carcinoma of the claw bed. *E,* A Rottweiler that developed concurrent claw dystrophy and vitiligo. Notice the depigmentation of the onycholytic claw. *F,* Idiopathic ceruminous otitis externa in a dog. *G,* Nasopharyngeal polyp. Blue polyp protruding from the ear of a cat with chronic otitis externa. *H,* Ceruminous gland carcinoma. Severe deformation and ulceration of the pinna of an aged cat.

alone is seen, lupus erythematosus and lupoid dermatosis, bullous pemphigoid, and pemphigus vulgaris are the most likely immune-mediated causes. With paronychia or footpad involvement, pemphigus foliaceus is most likely the underlying condition in both the dog and the cat (Fig. 18:4 *B*). Cold agglutinin disease and vasculitis have been reported to affect the claws. A form of vascular disease similar to Raynaud's disease in humans was recently described (Fig. 18:4 *C*).[10]

SYMMETRIC LUPOID ONYCHODYSTROPHY

A symmetric lupoid onychodystrophy has been described in dogs.[55, 60] German shepherd dogs appear to be predisposed. The dogs' ages ranged from 3 to 8 years. All dogs were presented for claw disease and were otherwise healthy. Typically, owners first noticed a single abnormal claw on two paws or more. However, within 2 to 9 weeks, every claw on all four paws was affected. The initial clinical sign was usually a separation at the claw bed and sloughing of one or more claws. After claws had been sloughed, regrowth was characterized by short, misshapen, dry, soft, brittle, often crumbling and discolored claws. Histopathologically, the disorder is characterized by hydropic and lichenoid interface dermatitis. Direct immunofluorescence testing did not reveal a lupus band. Response to omega-3 and omega-6 fatty acids (DVM Derm Caps) or systemic glucocorticoids was good.[60] In addition, the combination of tetracycline and niacinamide administered orally may be effective (see Chap. 3).[55] However, stopping treatment resulted in relapse.

NEOPLASIA

Neoplasia may also involve the claw or the distal digit (see Chap. 19). Usually, one claw is affected, although rarely multiple claws may be involved. Epithelial neoplasms are most common and include squamous cell carcinoma, subungual keratoacanthoma, inverted squamous papillomas, and eccrine carcinomas (Fig. 18:4 *D*). Eccrine carcinomas and squamous cell carcinomas in the claws of cats tend to be aggressive. Melanoma, mast cell tumors, osteosarcoma, lymphosarcoma, hemangiosarcoma, and metastatic carcinomas (especially from the lung) have all been reported.[10, 15, 61, 62]

ONYCHODYSTROPHY

Onychodystrophy is often diagnosed when multiple paws and claws are affected and other causes cannot be determined. These animals have secondary bacterial infections, so that improvement is seen with aggressive antimicrobial therapy. However, recurrence after discontinuation of appropriate therapy is routine. Certain breeds appear predisposed and include Siberian huskies, dachshunds, Rhodesian Ridgebacks, Rottweilers, and Cocker spaniels.[8, 10, 15, 49, 55] Cocker spaniels may have onychodystrophy as a manifestation of idiopathic seborrhea. The author (CEG) has also seen two cases in Welsh terriers. One owner, a breeder, reported that a littermate had a similar problem and other breeders, anecdotally, reported the same. Old dogs are prone to idiopathic onychodystrophy. Idiopathic onychomadesis is also described as a problem, particularly in the German shepherd, whippet, and English Springer spaniels.[15, 55, 62] This may also be a problem of the Rottweiler.[8] In one case, a Rottweiler had vitiligo and, concurrently, onycholysis (Fig. 18:4 *E*). These cases, besides having onychomadesis, are characterized by frequent secondary bacterial infections under the claw plate, onychoschizias, and onychorrhexis.

Miscellaneous causes of claw disease reported or seen by the authors include epidermolysis bullosa, dermatomyositis, drug eruption, ergotism, thallotoxicosis, linear epidermal nevi, nutritional deficiencies, disseminated intravascular coagulation, and necrolytic migratory erythema. Another situation that may occur is the development of permanent onychodystrophy after destruction of the basal cells of the germinative layers. Even though the infectious agent may be eliminated and the underlying or primary disease is cured or controlled, the claw continues to grow with a permanent deformity. If this area is prone to cracking, resultant infections may ensue.

Diagnosis

Because of the numerous causes of claw disease, it is obvious that a wide variety of diagnostic tests, or procedures, may be needed. These are often determined on the basis of history and physical examination findings. When only claw disease is present, a simpler approach may be warranted. In general, when only one or a few asymmetric claws are affected, the initial work-up may be limited to a complete history, physical examination, and cytologic evaluation of collected exudate or debris. Material from within the claw fold or under the claw should be obtained for evaluation. Cytologic examination is helpful in establishing the presence of bacterial or fungal infection (suppurative to pyogranulomatous to granulomatous inflammation, degenerate neutrophils, and phagocytosed microorganisms), pemphigus diseases (nondegenerate neutrophils or eosinophils and numerous acantholytic keratinocytes), and neoplasia.

If bacteria, yeast, or another cause is not identified, fungal cultures and skin scrapes are indicated. The presence of intracellular bacteria supports a diagnosis of bacterial disease, and trauma is the most likely inciting factor. If there is no evidence of neoplasia, initial trial antibiotic therapy is indicated. When multiple paws and claws are symmetrically affected, or when antibiotic therapy is ineffective, a work-up for underlying diseases should be begun. At this point, biopsy is often warranted.

Biopsy may be the only way of confirming a diagnosis of certain claw diseases, such as lupoid onychodystrophy, lupus erythematosus, vasculitis, pemphigus, pemphigoid, and neoplasia. Onychodystrophy, or idiopathic onychomadesis, should not be diagnosed without biopsy. In many instances, punch biopsy specimens and those taken elliptically with a scalpel fail to deliver the claw bed and, hence, the diagnosis. The claw bed is best visualized when the third phalanx is removed with the intact claw and the entire structure is sectioned longitudinally. The simple submission of an avulsed or sloughed claw for histopathologic examination is rarely of benefit.

Treatment

Prognosis is most accurately established and therapy is most accurately instigated when a specific diagnosis is determined. Bacterial infection, usually due to coagulase-positive staphylococci, is treated with the administration of systemic antibiotics (which may need to be continued for 4 to 6 months) and antibacterial agents and drawing soaks. In severe or refractory cases, it may be necessary to avulse the affected claws under general anesthesia. Onychomycosis, due to dermatophytosis, may be treated with long-term high-dose griseofulvin (50 to 75 mg/kg q12h) or ketoconazole (10 mg/kg q12h). Treatment should continue until all damaged claw has grown out and been trimmed off. This may take as long as 6 months, an expensive proposition in large dogs. Antifungal soaks may make the patient feel better and decrease contagion but are not effective therapy. Avulsing the claws may slightly speed resolution. Some cases continue to recur, and if so, surgical declawing may be preferred. This is also used as primary treatment in some cases, because of the cost of medical therapy and the likelihood of recurrences. Cases with permanent deformities may be prone to reinfection, and topical acrylic nail cements may be needed to protect the damaged area. The alternative is surgical declawing.

Perhaps the most frustrating cases are those with symmetric onychodystrophy with onychorrhexis, onychoschizia, and brittle claws in which the cause cannot be determined. Some breeds, such as the dachshund and Siberian husky, seem to be more prone to idiopathic onychodystrophy. In such cases, prophylactic trimming and filing of the claws and frequent application of acrylic nail cement can be helpful in preventing onychoschizia, pain, and secondary bacterial infection. Some cases may respond to long-term, repeated administration of gelatin; however, dystrophic changes recur when therapy is stopped. Gelatin is dosed empirically at 10 grains of capsules every 12 hours in dachshunds. Alternatively, one packet of Knox gelatin per 7 kg every 24 hours may be administered orally. These dogs should receive good-quality, high-protein diets. Biotin (5 mg/kg/d orally) has been reported to be deficient, at least in some dogs, and, therefore, may be helpful.[15]

■ ANAL SAC DISEASES

Three anal sac abnormalities are discussed here: impaction, chronic infection, and acute infection (abscessation).

Cause and Pathogenesis

Anal sacs are paired invaginations of the skin located between the internal and external sphincters of the anus. Each is connected to the surface by a single duct that opens at the mucocutaneous junction of the anus of the dog, but that opens on a pyramidal prominence 0.25 cm lateral to the anus of the cat. Most of each sac is lined with abundant large sebaceous glands, but the fundic portion of the canine sac has numerous apocrine glands. The total secretion of these glands is a brownish, oily fluid that has a characteristic disagreeable odor when expressed, or when infection or impaction occurs (Table 18:7). The odor or the fluid may have a function in social recognition among dogs. Normally, defecation causes compression of the sacs and expression of some of their contents. However, change in character of the secretion, oversecretion, or change in the muscle tone or fecal form may cause overfilling of the sacs, plugging of the ducts with resulting fermentation, inflammation, and infection. *Malassezia pachydermatis* is frequently isolated from normal and abnormal anal sacs.[27, 40]

Abnormalities of the anal sacs cause scooting, licking, biting, or rubbing the anus, and acute moist dermatitis from self-trauma may result in the surrounding region. Infected anal sacs are a focus of infection that has the potential for several untoward results. Some veterinarians are convinced that dogs licking the anal region in such cases transfer infection to the mouth with resultant tonsillitis, pharyngitis, and gagging, and only treatment of both areas (anal sacs and pharynx) has produced good results. In other cases, anal sac infection may be the source of antigen in dogs with widespread bacterial hypersensitivity.[2]

Anal sacs are probably vestigial structures that the ancestors of dogs and cats used as a spraying defense mechanism similar to that used by the skunk. Anal sac problems occur more

Table 18:7. Anal Sac Secretions

Color	Consistency	Odor	Disease Process
Straw	Thin liquid with small brownish flecks, or thick liquid pus	Pungent	None
Greenish yellow	Medium-thick liquid	Fetid	Infection
Red	Oily thick paste	Fetid	Infection
Clay	Dry paste	Mild	Impaction
Black	Dry or thick liquid	Mild	Chronic impaction

frequently in smaller breeds (under 15 kg), especially Poodles (Miniature and Toy), Chihuahuas, and seborrheic Cocker and English Springer spaniels. They are less common in German shepherds and giant breeds. There is no sex or age predisposition. The overall incidence was 2 per cent among the animals examined in a nonreferral hospital.[28] The anal sac is sometimes called the anal gland, which is an erroneous term that should not be used. There are, however, multiple perianal glands in the cutaneous border of the anus and modified sebaceous and apocrine cells in the lining and ducts of the anal sacs. The exact function of the anal sacs is unknown, and they are unnecessary for good health.

Clinical Features

The distended sacs can often be palpated just lateral to and below the midpoint of the anus (at 4 o'clock and 8 o'clock positions). Localized erythema, swelling, pain, and subsequent rupture and draining of an acutely infected sac may occur 1 to 2 cm lateral to the anus. The abscess is usually unilateral, and the course is short (7 to 10 days). Impaction and chronic infections may have a prolonged course (months) with many periods of quiescence and exacerbation.

Clinical Management

IMPACTIONS

Feline impactions usually occur without infection, and manual expression (by lateral external compression) usually relieves clinical signs for a relatively long time.[28, 63]

Canine impactions tend to recur. They should be gently but thoroughly expressed. This may have to be repeated several times at weekly intervals by gently placing a gloved finger in the posterior rectum and compressing the sac between the finger and the thumb (positioned lateral to the distended sac). A fetid brownish yellow or black discharge is expressed. If recurrence is frequent, the irrigation should be performed as for chronically infected anal sacs.

INFECTED ANAL SACS

Chronically infected anal sacs should be treated as any infection—by drainage. This need not be surgical. Frequent expression of the purulent or bloody exudate followed by instillation of an antibiotic solution may be curative. Inferior results are often obtained with this method because the tenderness of the region precludes thorough treatment. It is preferable to anesthetize the patient lightly and to lavage both sacs thoroughly with lactated Ringer's solution, using a blunt needle or cannula attached to a syringe. Ceruminolytic agents such as hexamethyltetracosane (Cerumenex) may also be useful as lavage fluids. After the sac is thoroughly flushed, it is important to instill an antibiotic cream, nitrofurazone solution, or a lotion containing antibiotic and corticosteroid in a ceruminolytic base (e.g., Liquachlor). This may be repeated in 5 to 7 days. If yeasts are involved, a solution containing nystatin (Panolog) may be used. If recurrence develops after initial response, surgical removal of the sacs is indicated.

An acutely infected anal sac (abscess) must be treated by liberal incision at the point of localization and by curettage and application of 5 to 7 per cent iodine solution (Lugol's solution). Healing occurs by granulation. If the anal sac abscess does not heal with the above treatments or if it recurs repeatedly, surgical excision of the anal sacs is indicated.

■ EXTERNAL EAR DISEASES

Otitis Externa

Otitis externa is inflammation of the ear canal, which may result from numerous causes. In most chronic cases, more than one cause is present. The most relevant classification scheme divides the causes of otitis externa into predisposing, primary, and perpetuating (Table 18:8). In every case, the clinician should identify as many factors as possible that may contribute to the otitis. Most chronic cases have at least one primary and several perpetuating causes, and failure to recognize and to correct one or more of these may lead to treatment failures.

PREDISPOSING FACTORS

Predisposing factors increase the risk of developing otitis externa.[5] They work in conjunction with primary causes or perpetuating factors to cause clinical disease. The most successful management of otitis externa necessitates that they be recognized and controlled whenever possible. Occasionally, dogs and cats present for chronic recurrent otitis that appears to have only excessive cerumen production as the underlying cause (Fig. 18:4 *F*). A variety of secondary bacterial or yeast infections occur. Work-ups reveal no underlying cause of these cases of idiopathic excessive cerumen production. In dogs with hairy ear canals prone to otitis externa, hair removal should be part of the management. However, in dogs without any ear disease or history of it, hair removal is not recommended by the authors. In fact, hair removal can precipitate or exacerbate otitis externa. Obstructive ear diseases often lead to otitis externa. Feline nasopharyngeal polyps and neoplasia in dogs are most often likely to cause this.

Feline nasopharyngeal polyps is a relatively uncommon inflammatory disease in cats.[32, 50] They may originate from the pharyngeal mucosa, the auditory (eustachian) tube, or the middle ear (Fig. 18:4 *G*). Although their etiology is unknown, inflammatory polyps may be congenital or secondary to viral or bacterial infections. A congenital cause has been proposed because polyps occur primarily in young cats and because they have been seen in sibling kittens. Feline calicivirus has been recovered from the tissues of several cats.

Nasopharyngeal polyps should be considered in the differential diagnosis of unilateral, medically resistant otitis externa or otitis media with or without respiratory signs. Otorrhea (dark brown ceruminous or purulent exudate) without signs of inflammation of the ear canal lining, head-shaking behavior, and a mass in the horizontal ear canal are the most common signs of external ear involvement. Middle ear involvement may cause head tilt, nystagmus, and disequilibrium.

Diagnosis is confirmed by examination of the ear and upper airway under anesthesia. Histopathologically, the lesion is a loose mass of connective tissue containing numerous blood vessels and mononuclear leukocytes, covered by an epithelium that may be stratified, nonkeratinized squamous, or simple to bilayered ciliated columnar. Treatment includes surgical removal of the polyp and, often, bulla osteotomy. Postsurgical complications include regrowth, persistent discharge, and transient Horner's syndrome.

Neoplasms of the ear include those capable of affecting the skin elsewhere, as well as primary neoplasms of ceruminous glands (see Chap. 19).[16, 56, 67] In the dog, the most common pinnal neoplasms are sebaceous gland tumors, histiocytomas, and mast cell tumors. In the cat, the most common pinnal neoplasms are squamous cell carcinoma, basal cell tumor, hemangiosarcoma, and melanocytic neoplasms.

The most common neoplasm of the ear canal is ceruminal gland in origin (Fig. 18:4 *H*).[41b, 41c] These neoplasms are more common in cats than in dogs. In the dog, the neoplasms are typically benign, whereas in the cat, they are malignant in about 50 per cent of cases. *Ceruminal gland neoplasms* typically occur in older animals and in one ear. Clinical signs include variable degrees of headshaking and ear-scratching behavior, otorrhea, an offensive necrotic odor, frequent secondary bacterial otitis externa, and even intermittent hemorrhage from the affected ear. Occasionally, ceruminal gland neoplasms present as bulging, ulcerative, draining masses below the ear in the parotid region. Otoscopic examination usually reveals a small (less than 1 cm in diameter), well-circumscribed, pinkish white, dome-shaped mass, with frequent ulceration, hemorrhage, and secondary infection. The only effective therapy is surgical excision, usually by lateral ear resection or total ablation of the ear canal. The best results are achieved

Table 18:8. Factors and Causes of Otitis Externa

Predisposing Factors	
Conformation	Stenotic canals
	Hair in canals
	Pendulous pinnae
	Hairy concave pinnae
Excessive moisture	Swimmer's ear
	High-humidity climate
Excessive cerumen production	Secondary to underlying diseases (especially hypersensitivities and keratinization defects)
	Primary (idiopathic)
Treatment effects	Trauma from cotton applicators
	Irritant topicals
	Superinfections by altering normal microflora
Obstructive ear disease	Neoplasms
	Polyps
	Granulomas (infectious, foreign body, sterile)
Systemic disease	Immune suppression or viral disease
	Debilitation
	Negative catabolic states

Primary Causes	
Parasites	*Otodectes cynotis*
	Demodex canis, D. cati, Sarcoptes scabiei, Notoedres cati
	Chiggers (especially *Eutrombicula*)
	Flies (especially *Stomoxys calcitrans*)
	Ticks (especially *Otobius megnini*)
	Fleas (especially *Echidnophaga gallinacea* and *Spilopsylla cuniculi*)
Microorganisms	Dermatophytes
	Sporothrix schenckii
Hypersensitivity diseases	Atopy
	Food hypersensitivity
	Contact hypersensitivity
	Drug reactions
Keratinization disorders	Primary idiopathic seborrhea
	Hypothyroidism
	Sex hormone imbalances
	Lipid-related conditions
Foreign bodies	Plants (especially foxtails)
	Hair
	Sand, dirt
	Hardened medications and secretions
Glandular disorders	Ceruminal gland hyperplasia
	Sebaceous gland hyperplasia or hypoplasia
	Altered secretion rate
	Altered type of secretions
Autoimmune diseases	Lupus erythematosus
	Pemphigus foliaceus
	Pemphigus erythematosus
	Cold agglutinin disease
Viral diseases	Distemper virus
Micellaneous conditions	Solar dermatitis
	Frostbite
	Vasculitis, vasculopathy
	Juvenile cellulitis
	Eosinophilic dermatitis or granuloma
	Sterile eosinophilic folliculitis
	Relapsing polychondritis

Table 18:8. Factors and Causes of Otitis Externa *Continued*

Perpetuating Factors

Bacteria	*S. intermedius*
	Proteus sp.
	Pseudomonas sp.
	Escherichia coli
	Klebsiella sp.
Yeast	*M. pachydermatis*
	Candida albicans
	Miscellaneous
Progressive pathologic changes	Hyperkeratosis
	Hyperplasia
	Epithelial folds
	Edema
	Apocrine gland hypertrophy or hyperplasia
	Hidradenitis
	Fibrosis
	Mineralization
Otitis media	Simple purulent
	Caseated or keratinous
	Cholesteatoma
	Proliferative
	Destructive osteomyelitis

*Modified from Griffin, C.E., et al.: Otitis externa and media. Current Veterinary Dermatology: The Art and Science of Therapy, Mosby–Year Book, 1993, p. 245.

with ear canal ablation and lateral bulla osteotomy.[41b, 41c] The recurrence rate is around 70 per cent with lateral ear resection.[41b, 41c]

PRIMARY CAUSES

Primary causes directly induce otitis externa. The most common causes seen by the authors are atopy, food hypersensitivity, keratinization disorders, and ear mites. It is critical to successful long-term management that a primary cause be found and controlled.

Parasites

A number of parasites have been associated with otitis externa (see Table 18:8). However, the ear mite *O. cynotis* is most common (see Chap. 6), being responsible for up to 50 per cent of the otitis externa cases diagnosed in cats and 5 to 10 per cent of the cases in dogs. Ear mites may initiate otitis externa but remain undetected. One reason is the difficulty that may occur in demonstrating the mites. As few as two or three mites can cause clinical otitis externa.[18] This may be explained by studies showing that ear mites can induce Arthus-type and immediate-type hypersensitivity reactions.[52, 69]

Another explanation is that the mites initiate the otitis externa and then leave the canal or are destroyed by the inflammation or the secondary infection. In recurrent cases of parasitic otitis externa, the possibility of other in-contact animals being asymptomatic carriers should be considered. Owing to variations in the time necessary for transmission from carrier to affected patient, the time of onset of hypersensitivity reactions, and the development of clinical signs noticeable by the owner, these diseases may present as rapidly or intermittently recurrent cases.[24]

Fly bites are a common cause of pinnal dermatitis during fly season (see Chap. 6). Pin-point ulcers that are rapidly covered by a black-red crust are typical (Fig. 18:5 *H*).

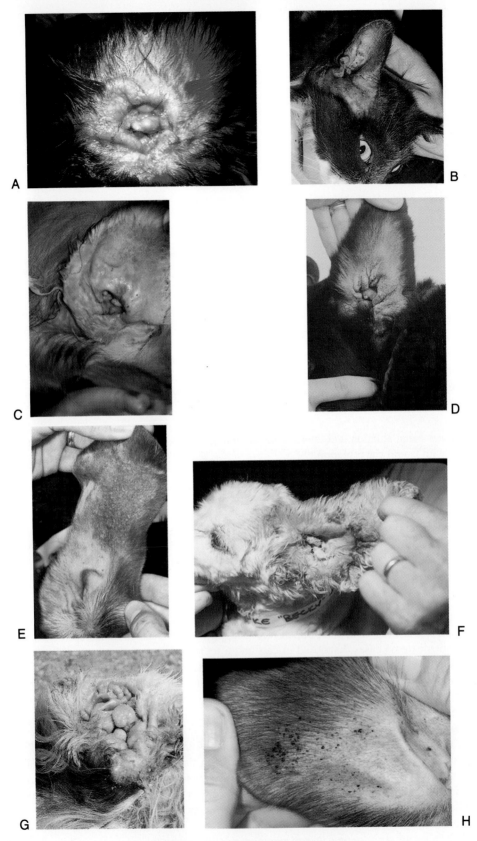

Figure 18:5 *See legend on opposite page*

Hypersensitivities

Atopy, food hypersensitivity, and contact hypersensitivity can all cause otitis externa (see Chap. 8). The otitis externa may be secondary to self-trauma, or the hypersensitivity reaction may involve the external ear canal. Atopy, as a result of its high incidence, is more frequently associated with otitis externa, which may be the only symptom in some cases.[24, 25, 59] Erythema of the pinna and vertical canal is a common feature of allergic otitis externa (Fig. 18:5 *A* and *B*).[24] Chronic inflammation may eventually lead to secondary bacterial or yeast infections.

Ear disease is present in up to 80 per cent of dogs and cats with food hypersensitivity, and food hypersensitivity is the second most common hypersensitivity reaction to affect the ear.

Contact hypersensitivity may result from medications (e.g., neomycin) used to treat otitis externa. In addition, vehicles such as propylene glycol can also be responsible for hypersensitive or irritant reactions in the ear.[24] Typically, these cases have an initial history of short-term response to therapy, and then when medication administration is continued, symptoms worsen. Another clinical clue is the development of erythema dorsally and ventrally to the external orifice, as the medications usually contact these areas as well. Therefore, changing medications on the basis of major medication ingredients may not alleviate a treatment reaction. Drug reactions may also involve the ear canal and the pinnae. This may be due to contact allergic or irritant effects. In other cases, systemic drug reactions, such as erythema multiforme, may affect the ear canal (Fig. 18:5 *C*).

Keratinization Disorders

The keratinization disorders generally present as chronic ceruminous otitis externa. Breeds prone to primary idiopathic seborrhea tend to have ceruminous otitis externa (see Chap. 13). Endocrinopathies, such as hypothyroidism and sex hormone imbalances (see Chap. 9), may result in chronic ceruminous otitis externa, most likely by altering keratinization and, possibly, glandular function (Fig. 18:5 *D*). Hypothyroidism is the most commonly encountered endocrinopathy involving the ear. Many times, the primary cause of the otitis externa is a disease that has some other historical or physical examination findings as a clue.

Foreign Bodies

Foreign bodies that enter the ear canal and become lodged usually result in otitis externa. Typically, it occurs unilaterally, although bilateral disease may occur. Most commonly, the dogs and cats have acute onset of headshaking and scratching at the ear or ears. There is no initial discharge; however, if immediate veterinary care is not sought, these cases may rapidly become secondarily infected and present with a purulent exudate.

Glandular Disorders

Glandular disorders are not well documented in the dog and cat. One study did show that Cocker spaniels with otitis had a greater surface area of glands in their ears than did Cocker spaniels without ear disease.[64] In addition, the author (CEG) has seen cases in dogs and cats that had chronic ceruminous otitis and also demonstrated histologic sebaceous gland hyperpla-

Figure 18:5. *A,* Allergic otitis externa in a dog with atopy. *B,* Contact hypersensitivity in a cat due to a topical product that contained neomycin. *C,* Erythema multiforme in a dog with severe ulceration of the ear canal. *Candida albicans* was found in cytologic studies and in otic cultures. *D,* Seborrheic otitis externa in a hypothyroid dog. *E,* Sterile eosinophilic pinnal folliculitis in a dog. *F, Pseudomonas* otitis externa in a Cocker spaniel with atopy and primary seborrhea. *G,* Proliferative otitis externa with numerous folds resulting. Similar changes are present in the vertical and horizontal canal. *H,* Classical fly bites *(Stomoxys calcitrans)* on the pinna of a dog.

sia. They had no other evidence of keratinization disorder or skin disease. Management necessitated that clients learn how to clean the ears on a routine basis.

Autoimmune Diseases

Autoimmune diseases may affect the ear canal but most commonly cause pinnal disease. Of the diseases listed in Table 18:8, the one most commonly seen is pemphigus foliaceus.

Viral Diseases

Viral diseases are known to cause otitis externa in humans but have rarely been incriminated in the dog. Canine distemper virus has been associated with otitis externa, but whether this is actually directly due to viral invasion of the ear or is secondary to debilitation, spread of respiratory infection, or immune suppression is unknown.

Miscellaneous Conditions

Canine sterile eosinophilic pinnal folliculitis is an uncommon idiopathic, nonseasonal, bilaterally symmetric pinnal dermatosis of dogs (Fig. 18:5 *E*).[57] Erythematous papules and crusts are present on the concave surface of the pinnae. Pruritus is variable. The ear canal is not involved.

Cytologic examination of papules reveals numerous eosinophils and no microorganisms. Biopsy reveals eosinophilic folliculitis and furunculosis. Cultures are negative. The condition is responsive to topical or oral glucocorticoids but usually recurs.

Canine proliferative eosinophilic otitis externa is an uncommon idiopathic inflammatory disorder of the ear canal of dogs.[51] Affected dogs have a history of chronic unilateral otitis externa. Otoscopic examination reveals solitary or multiple polypoid masses attached to the ear canal lining by a slender stalk. The masses obstruct the canal. Biopsy reveals a papillomatous, proliferative eosinophilic dermatitis or eosinophilic granuloma. Intraepidermal eosinophilic microabscesses are found. Some lesions contain multifocal areas of degenerate collagen and flame figures, with or without an accompanying palisading granuloma. Surgical excision may be curative or be followed by recurrence.

PERPETUATING FACTORS

Perpetuating factors prevent the resolution of otitis externa or otitis media. In chronic cases, one or more of these factors may be present and their recognition and management may be critical to a successful outcome. In early cases, treating the primary cause may be sufficient in controlling a case but, after the establishment of some perpetuating factors, additional treatment must be directed at them. Perpetuating factors may be the major cause of poor response to therapy, regardless of the predisposing factors and primary causes.

Bacteria and Yeast

Bacteria are rarely primary causes, therefore a diagnosis of bacterial otitis externa is usually not a complete diagnosis. *S. intermedius* and the gram-negative organisms *Pseudomonas* spp. (Fig. 18:5 *F*), *Proteus* spp., *E. coli*, and *Klebsiella* spp. are most commonly isolated as secondary pathogens (Table 18:9). The four gram-negative organisms are not routinely cultured from normal ears. After these organisms establish infection, they significantly contribute to the inflammation, damage and clinical signs.

M. pachydermatis is the most common yeast that contributes to otitis externa as a perpetuating factor. It is a budding yeast that has a peanut or bottle shape and may be found in as many as 36 per cent of normal canine ears.[9] It is a common complication with hypersensitivity

Table 18:9. Organisms Isolated From Normal Ear Canals and From Ears Affected With Otitis Externa

Organism	Clinically Normal Ear Canals			Ears With Otitis Externa			
	Grono, Frost (1969) %	Sampson et al. (1973) %	Marshall et al. (1974) %	Grono (Data to Be Published) %	Boyle, Grono (Data to Be Published) %	Sampson et al. (1973) %	Marshall et al. (1974) %
Coagulase-positive							
Staphylococcus	47.6	15	1.7	30.9	30.4	35.0	38.0
Malassezzia spp.	37.9	6	28.3	35.9	44.3	23.0	86.2
Pseudomonas spp.	2.4	4	0	34.6	16.5	5.0	16.4
Proteus spp.	1.6	0	0	20.8	9.9	5.0	8.6
Streptococcus spp.	0	2	0	7.4	4.3	5.0	8.6
Aspergillus	0	—	—	0.8	1.1	—	—

From Grono, L.R.: Otitis externa. In: Kirk, R.W. (ed.). Current Veterinary Therapy VII. W.B. Saunders Co., Philadelphia, 1980.

disorders and may result in a superinfection after antibiotic therapy. *M. pachydermatis* has been shown to be pathogenic when it or fluid is put in the ear canal.[41a] Two major phenotypes (large and small colony types) of *M. pachydermatis* have been described, but the significance of these is unknown.[28a] Oleic and linoleic acids were shown to be mycostatic, and the common fatty acids found in canine cerumen are margaric, stearic, oleic, and linoleic.[28a]

Although *M. pachydermatis* and *S. intermedius* are often isolated from normal ears, their occurrence is markedly higher in inflamed ears.[9] It has been proposed that *S. intermedius* produces a factor that stimulates the growth of *M. pachydermatis*.[9]

Otitis Media

Otitis media is inflammation of the tympanic bulla. It is usually associated with exudate, which is difficult to treat with topical therapy and often remains a source of infection and allows debris to reach the external ear canal via a ruptured tympanic membrane. In more advanced cases, the author (CEG) found keratin plugs developing within the tympanic cavity. The keratin may serve as a reservoir for bacteria and a source of inflammation. Eventually, mineralization, osteolysis, or osteomyelitis can occur, which may be observed radiographically.

It has been theorized that the tympanic membrane may stretch and extend into the tympanic cavity. Additionally, tympanic membranes readily heal, and therefore, otitis media may be present with an intact tympanic membrane. Tissue, including adnexal structures, which originated from the external ear canal, may be found in the middle ear cavity, even when the tympanic membrane appears intact.[39] The tympanic membrane often thickens in response to inflammation and may develop polyploid extensions of granulation tissue into the middle ear cavity, which, in some cases, form adhesions with the middle ear mucosa.

Aural cholesteatoma is a keratin-filled epidermoid cyst, located within the middle ear cavity. Aural cholesteatoma may occur in 11 per cent of the animals with chronic otitis media.[39] It has been postulated that cholesteatomas result when a pocket of tympanic membrane forms within the middle ear cavity. One predisposing factor may be spontaneous occlusion of the external ear canal from chronic proliferative changes leading to external ear canal stenosis.

Another response of the tympanic membrane is the development of a pocket that allows the impaction and sequestration of material from topical therapy. This may explain why some dogs appear to regrow their tympanic membrane rapidly after flushing of the false middle ear.[24] In contrast to dogs with ruptured tympanic membranes, these animals cannot have their middle ear flushed through the eustachian tube and are less susceptible to ototoxicity.

Progressive Pathologic Changes

The microanatomy of the canine and feline ear canal have been studied.[12, 14, 65] Chronic inflammation stimulates the skin lining the ear canal to undergo numerous changes, including epidermal hyperkeratosis and hyperplasia, dermal edema and fibrosis, apocrine (ceruminal) gland hyperplasia, and dilatation. Hidradenitis or inflammation of the apocrine glands may also occur. A study found that sebaceous glands do not atrophy as had been previously reported.[64] Morphometric analysis showed that breeds predisposed to otitis externa had an increased quantity of apocrine glands compared with the number of sebaceous glands and that dogs with otitis externa had an even greater area of apocrine glands. An occasional animal may have sebaceous gland hyperplasia.

These progressive changes cause a thickening of the skin, which eventually extends to both sides of the auricular cartilage. The swelling leads to stenosis of the canal lumen. More importantly, the skin is thrown into numerous folds, which inhibit effective cleaning and application of topical medications (Fig. 18:5 G). These folds act as sites for the accumulation of secretions and exudates and the perpetuation and protection of secondary microorganisms. The epidermis becomes thickened, and the hyperkeratotic stratum corneum increases the keratin debris that is exfoliated into the canal lumen. The increased secretions and epithelial debris favor the proliferation of bacteria and yeast.

CLINICAL FEATURES

Otitis externa is a common condition in dogs, perhaps accounting for 15 per cent of all the dogs presented for veterinary care.[4, 46] In cats, the incidence is much lower, perhaps 4 per cent.[4, 44, 45, 46, 58] The lower incidence in cats may be partially attributable to the upright position of the pinna and the relatively hairless ear canal.

The most common indication of otitis externa is aural pruritus or headshaking. As otitis externa progresses, a mild to marked exudate or malodor may develop. This is usually when the client presents the pet to the veterinarian. It is imperative that a thorough history, both general and dermatologic, be taken. If that is not done, many cases are unnecessarily misdiagnosed. History taking should include questions regarding predisposing factors. Additionally, the majority of cases of chronic ear disease have historical or physical evidence of the primary disease. The common indications that the underlying problem is a hypersensitivity disorder are seasonality and pruritus in other body locations. Keratinization disorders may have changes in coat quality, color, and density or scale formation. Pain when eating may be noticed in dogs with severe disease or in animals with otitis media that has progressed to involve the temporomandibular joint.[39]

PHYSICAL FINDINGS

Physical findings indicative of otitis externa include erythema, swelling, scaling, crusting, alopecia, broken hairs, head shyness, otic discharge (otorrhea), malodor, and pain on palpation of the auricular cartilage. Some animals attempt to scratch the ear with the ipsilateral hindpaw or shake the head during or after palpation of the ear canal. Lesions may involve the pinna and the skin caudal to the pinna on the head, on the lateral face, and around the vertical canal. Pyotraumatic dermatitis of the lateral face and aural hematomas are the lesions most commonly associated with aural pruritus, although clinical otitis externa may not be noticeable. Head tilt may be seen with either otitis externa or otitis media. However, concurrent facial nerve abnormalities (e.g., facial palsy and hemifacial spasm) or Horner's syndrome indicates otitis media, although facial palsy may also be seen with hypothyroidism and concurrent ceruminous otitis.

Palpation of the external ear canal and tympanic bulla may provide additional information. The thickness, firmness, and pliability of the vertical and horizontal canal should be determined. Thicker, firmer, and less pliable canals are associated with proliferative changes and support a more guarded prognosis. Mineralized canals are rock hard and can rarely be returned to normal or successfully managed with medical therapy.[24] Pain and palpable abnormalities of the tympanic bulla imply the presence of otitis media.

Erythema of the concave surface of the pinna with a normal convex surface is strongly suggestive of atopy or, less likely, food hypersensitivity. Early cases may have minimal erythema of the vertical canal with a normal horizontal canal. Cases that started with only ear canal disease and, after treatment, spread peripherally in rostral and ventral directions should make one suspect topical therapy reactions.

OTOSCOPIC EXAMINATION

The otoscopic examination is used to detect foreign bodies, to determine whether otitis media is present, and to assess what type of lesions, exudate, and progressive pathologic changes have occurred. If unilateral disease is present, the unaffected ear should be examined first. This decreases the possibility of the dog's experiencing pain and resisting examination of the second ear. Examining the unaffected ear first decreases the risk of spreading an infectious agent from the diseased ear to the unaffected ear. Having multiple otoscopic cones of varying sizes placed in cold sterilization containers allows one to use aseptic cones. One problem often encountered in practice is the extremely painful, ulcerated, swollen ear that one cannot adequately examine. Even with anesthesia, these cases may not be adequately examined, and it may be necessary to treat the animal and to reduce the swelling and inflammation, then have the patient return in 4 to 7 days so that an otoscopic examination can be properly performed.[24]

A record of lesions should be kept. Proliferative changes, the amount and type of discharge, and the presence of erythema or ulcers should be noted. Assessment of the tympanic membrane should be made and recorded.

The degree of canal stenosis should be determined, because changes in lumen size can be used to help monitor treatment. Is proliferation the result of diffuse thickening, or does the canal epithelium have a cobblestone appearance? The location of the stenosis should also be noted. Does it involve the horizontal canal, the vertical canal, or both?

The type of discharge can be used to help determine what primary or perpetuating factors may be involved. Dry coffee grounds–like debris is typical of ear mites. Moist brown discharge tends to be associated with staphylococcal and yeast infections. Purulent creamy to yellow exudates are often seen with gram-negative infections. Waxy, greasy, yellow to tan debris is typical of ceruminous otitis, sometimes with concurrent *Malassezia* infection. Ceruminous discharge is most often seen with keratinization, glandular conditions, and chronic hypersensitivity disorders.

DIAGNOSIS

A diagnosis of otitis externa is easily made from the history and the physical examination. Otitis media is much more difficult to diagnose, because many cases present with symptoms of only otitis externa. Evidence of inflammation of the tissue surrounding the middle ear or the inner ear usually indicates that otitis media has occurred. Even with otoscopic examination, many cases of otitis media may not be detected, and in cases with apparently intact diseased tympanic membranes, otitis media may be present. The tympanic membrane becomes opaque and white, gray, pinkish, or brown owing to disease and thickening. When this occurs and it loses its characteristic opalescent, fishscale appearance, it may resemble a keratinous plug.[24] In addition, middle ear changes, or the medial wall of the tympanic bulla, may be interpreted as a diseased, but intact tympanic membrane. An evaluation of tympanometry, otoscopy, and palpation findings revealed that, in inflamed ears, only tympanometry was accurate in determining the integrity of the tympanic membrane.[38] This study revealed that even after lavage of the ear canal, a satisfactory view of the tympanic membrane could be obtained in only 28 per cent of cases otoscopically examined while under anesthesia.

Radiography is indicated in suspected cases of otitis media and especially before surgical procedures involving the middle ear. However, radiography is helpful only when it demonstrates middle ear pathologic changes (e.g., fluid lines or changes in the osseous bulla); normal radiographs do not rule out the presence of otitis media.[54] Tympanometry appears valuable in the diagnosis of a ruptured tympanic membrane. Its value in clinically inflamed ears and ears with otitis media needs to be determined, although it appears preferable to previously described techniques.[38]

Palpation of the tympanic membrane with a blunt instrument has been shown to be inaccurate and causes a statistically significant incidence of damage to the tympanic membrane.[38] However, palpation and positioning of a soft feeding tube to help determine the presence or the location of the tympanic membrane is a valuable technique that may reveal false middle ear cavities.[24] The feeding tube is passed under visualization through a surgical otoscope head within the ear canal to the level where the tympanic membrane is expected to be located. In a normal ear, the tip of the tube remains visualized. In ears with false middle ear or ruptured tympanic membranes, the tube is passed beyond view and in a ventral direction below the normal plane of the horizontal canal.

Cytologic examination of discharge usually does not establish a definitive diagnosis, but it is valuable in determining what infectious agents, if any, are present. Cytologic study reveals any cocci (especially *Staphylococcus* and *Streptococcus*), rods (especially *Pseudomonas* and *Proteus*), other gram-positive or gram-negative organisms, budding yeasts (*Malassezia* and *Candida*), and mixed infections. The presence of white blood cells, as well as phagocytosis of bacteria, indicates that the body is responding to the infection and that treatment of the infection is warranted. The mere visualization of numerous bacteria in the absence of an inflammatory response and phagocytosis usually indicates only multiplication and colonization by the microorganism, *not* clinical infection. If there are toxic neutrophils, the ear canal must be flushed to remove the toxins.

Cytologic evaluation is the preferred method to ascertain the role of *Malassezia* in a particular case for two reasons. In one study, 18 per cent of the cases that had *Malassezia* detected by cytologic examination were sterile on culture by a commercial laboratory culturing specifically for *Malassezia* at 37°C (98.6°F).[24] Another blinded study compared the sensitivity of cytologic study versus culture for detecting bacteria or yeast in normal and otitic canine ears.[28b] The sensitivity of cytologic examination of cerumen for detection of gram-positive cocci, gram-negative rods, and yeasts was 84 per cent, 100 per cent, and 100 per cent, respectively. However, the sensitivity of the culture for detection of these organisms was 59 per cent, 69 per cent, and 50 per cent, respectively.

Histopathologic studies have been conducted on many dogs and cats with otitis externa.[13, 17, 67] Unfortunately, these have usually been animals with chronic disease in which the cause of the otitis externa was not specified. In general, there are variable degrees of epidermal, sebaceous gland, and ceruminal gland hyperplasia. The inflammation is usually interstitial, diffuse, or nodular in pattern, with lymphocytes, plasma cells, and mast cells usually predominating. Many cases show some degree of fibrosis and cystic dilatation of ceruminal glands. Suppurative epidermitis and hidradenitis may be seen.

CULTURE AND SENSITIVITY TESTING

The primary indication for culture and sensitivity testing is the presence of otitis media or severe otitis externa associated with rodlike bacteria when systemic therapy is going to be prescribed. Culture and sensitivity testing should not be done without cytologic evaluation, which demonstrates that bacteria and white blood cells (that are exhibiting degenerative changes and are phagocytosing the bacteria) are present in the discharge. Bacteria and yeasts usually multiply to large numbers in abnormal ear canals, and the mere ability to culture large numbers of one or more microorganisms does *not* demonstrate that these organisms are involved in the disease process. Samples should be taken from the horizontal canal whenever possible. If middle ear disease is present, it is often valuable to sample material from that site as well. There may not be a direct correlation between the results obtained for blood levels of systemically administered antibiotics and those for topical preparations used in the ear canal. When therapy is going to be limited to topical treatment, culture and sensitivity testing are rarely cost effective.

Depending on the primary diagnosis, many other tests may be needed to make a definitive diagnosis. Which tests are most cost effective and indicated depends on the history and complete physical examination findings.

TREATMENT

Therapy of otitis externa depends on identifying and controlling the predisposing and primary diseases whenever possible. In addition, cleaning the ear canals and the middle ear, applying topical therapies, and administering systemic medications may be necessary for the effective elimination or control of primary causes and perpetuating factors.

The administration of sedatives such as xylazine or ketamine and diazepam may be needed to allow adequate examination or treatment in some cases. Other animals require a general anesthetic. Many clients are reluctant to have their dogs anesthetized but are often more understanding if the need for getting the ears cleaned and completely examined is explained in detail.

Cleaning

Thorough cleaning of the ear canals is extremely important for the effective management of otitis externa. In chronic cases of otitis media or false middle ear, this includes cleaning that area. Cleaning is valuable for several reasons. Besides preventing effective therapy, the exudate may interfere with adequate examination, until it is cleaned out. Foreign bodies, especially small ones, are eliminated when ears are adequately cleaned. Pus and inflammatory debris can inactivate some medications (e.g., polymyxin). Thorough cleaning removes bacterial toxins, degenerating cellular debris, and free fatty acids, which decreases the stimulation for further inflammation. In proliferative conditions of the ear canals, thorough cleaning is one of the most valuable steps in management, just as it is in treating intertrigo (fold dermatitis).[24]

Ceruminolytic agents greatly facilitate and expedite the cleaning procedure. They include various types of surfactants, such as dioctyl sodium sulfosuccinate (docusate, DSS) or calcium sulfosuccinate, and detergents that act by emulsifying the waxes and lipids. Carbamide peroxide (Panoprep [Solvay]) is a slightly less potent ceruminolytic agent that acts as a humectant by releasing urea when activated. It releases oxygen, creating a foaming action that helps to break down or dislodge large clumps of debris. Carbamide peroxide is particularly helpful with more purulent exudates. The ceruminolytic Clear X ear cleansing solution (DVM Pharmaceuticals) combines DSS and carbamide peroxide, thus possessing the surfactant, humectant, and oxygen-producing effects of both ingredients. Propylene glycol, glycerin, and mineral oil have mild ceruminolytic effects and are best used for the relatively normal, slightly dirty ear.

Most ceruminolytics and detergents are contraindicated with a ruptured tympanum. Some disinfectant cleaners, such as chlorhexidine and iodophors, are also contraindicated with a ruptured tympanum.[19, 29] Frequently, the condition of the tympanic membrane cannot be determined until the ear canal has been cleaned. The probability of ototoxicity may be decreased by using ceruminolytics and flushing with water or sterile physiologic saline. Additional detergents, or disinfectants, are not used in the flushing water or saline unless an intact tympanum is noted. If the tympanum is ruptured, thorough rinsing of the ceruminolytics is mandatory. The use of ear loops, flushing the ear with water, or saline, or the use of a suction apparatus is the least ototoxic method of cleaning if a ruptured tympanum is suspected.

Cleaning Techniques

Several methods for removing the pus, debris, and emulsified waxes and lipids have been described. One of the easiest to set up, implement, and clean up is the use of a rubber ear bulb syringe. After the use of a ceruminolytic agent, repeated flushing with lukewarm water or saline removes most of the exudate. When the tympanic membrane is known to be intact, the use of a detergent or disinfectant solution may improve the results. A space should always be left between the rubber nipple and the canal orifice. This allows backflow and helps to prevent excessive pressure on the tympanic membrane. This procedure is not effective for cleaning false middle ears or the tympanic bulla. Ear curets or loops are helpful in removing debris lodged deep near the tympanum in cases of milder, waxy, crusty accumulation with small foreign bodies or leftover waxy debris. For larger foreign bodies or keratin plugs in the middle ear, an alligator forceps may be used. However, in most situations, an ear curet is preferred.

The ear curet is gently pulled along the epidermis to break loose any debris. This is less traumatic than using cotton swabs. Ear curets are placed down the ear canal through a surgical otoscope head. Under visualization, the loop is passed along the epithelium of the canal until the wax to be removed is reached. The loop is then rolled over the debris and gently pulled out of the canal. This method minimizes the risk of damaging an intact tympanum.

A feeding tube and a 12-ml syringe are effective for flushing the ear canal. Feeding tubes of various diameters, cut to different lengths, can be kept in cold sterilization. The tube, attached to a syringe filled with water or saline, is passed through a surgical otoscope head and cone and passed down the ear canal under visualization. After the tip is located at the desired point of the ear canal, the solution can be infused and then aspirated back out, along with the debris that was broken up. In severe cases, and whenever the tympanum is ruptured, flushing with a syringe and feeding tube is the most effective and safe flushing technique and is usually the method of choice.[24] This is a preferred method for drying the ear out as well, especially when there is no tympanum present.

Vestibular syndrome or deafness may occur after ear flushing, even when no ototoxic drugs are utilized. These side-effects are uncommon.

A suction apparatus is possibly the most effective method of cleaning ears, especially when thick, inspissated pus or keratin plugs are left in the middle ear. A Frazier suction tip works well. The tip can be positioned to exactly the desired location before initiating suction. When ceruminolytics must be avoided, the suction apparatus is effective in rapidly cleaning out the external ear canal and the middle ear cavity. The disadvantages are the lack of infusion of liquid, the limited access to the middle ear, and the time needed to clean the equipment.

Some clinicians use a dental water propulsion device (Water Pik). These devices rapidly clean the ear with multiple rapid pulses of water. There is no suction, and the time needed to set up and clean the equipment eliminates some of the advantages they seem to offer. It is not as effective in cleaning the middle ear as are the syringe and feeding tube. Care must be taken to avoid directing the pulsating stream directly onto a damaged tympanic membrane. The use of a curved water current defuser (Anthony Products) helps to avoid tympanic membrane damage.

After the flushing has been completed, the ear canal is dried, or in cases complicated by infection, a disinfectant may be applied to the canal. If the tympanum is ruptured, acetic acid at 2 to 5 per cent is preferred. A 5 per cent concentration of acetic acid may cause a slight burning sensation when it is applied to inflamed, eroded, or ulcerated epithelium and is best applied while the patient is still sedated.

After the ear is cleaned and relatively dry, topical medications or drying agents can be used. Most drying agents contain isopropyl alcohol and one or more of the following: boric acid, benzoic acid, salicylic acid, acetic acid, sulfur, and silicone dioxide. Veterinary products of this type include Clear X ear drying solution (DVM Pharmaceuticals), Oti-Clens (SmithKline Beecham), Epi-Otic (Allerderm), Oticare B (ARC Labs), Panodry (Solvay), Otic Clear (Butler Co.), and Domeboro Otic (Dome). These products can be used at home for prophylactic treatment of swimmer's ear and idiopathic excessive cerumen production and as a deodorizer. Alcohol and higher concentrations of the acids may be irritating or cause a burning sensation in ulcerated ears.

Modified drying products with less drying ingredients and more antimicrobial properties and mild ceruminolytic agents are available. Ingredients often combined with the drying agents achieve these effects and include propylene glycol, lanolin, glycerin, lactic acid, parachloro-metaxlenol, and chlorhexidine. Some of the veterinary products in this group include Epi-Otic (Allerderm), Oticlens A (ARC Labs), Oti-Fresh (Pan American), Nolvasan otic (Fort Dodge), and Chlorhexiderm flush (DVM Pharmaceuticals). These products are used most effectively in mildly dirty ears. Ears that have a mild objectionable odor to the client are helped by these products. They are not as helpful for clinical otitis externa, although they may be used for long-term management of milder cases of recurrent waxy otitis externa, after the inflammation is controlled. An advantage of these products is their lack of antibiotics or glucocorticoids, which may induce bacterial resistance or adrenal suppression, respectively.

In especially waxy or exudative ears, the client may need to clean the ears intermittently so that topical medications can be properly applied. In most chronic cases, the combination cleanser-dryers are not sufficient. In these cases, the client should be instructed in the use of the ear bulb syringe for home flushing and possibly the use of ceruminolytics.[24] These cases must be carefully selected. In general, the tympanum should be intact if ceruminolytics are going to be used. This is because the client may not be able to rinse adequately all residual drug, and repetitive application could be dangerous, especially if the agent is not being rinsed out. The client must be willing and able to try flushing, and the animal must be tolerant of the procedure. Many animals tolerate home flushing after the initial inflammation and pain are resolved. Therefore, this procedure is rarely recommended in acutely inflamed or ulcerated ears. Detergents are not routinely used for home flushing and necessitate thorough rinsing. The clients use cotton balls or swabs only in areas that they can *visualize, not down the ear canal.*

Topical Therapy

Numerous topical preparations for the external ear canal are available. Most of the ear products contain various combinations of glucocorticoids, antibiotics, antifungals, and parasiticides. Topical therapeutic agents are selected on the basis of the effects needed. As the case progresses, the patient should be monitored, and products changed accordingly. Each of these types of ingredients is discussed, but the clinician should be aware of the vehicle.

Vehicle

The base or type of vehicle should be considered when selecting a treatment of otitis externa. In general, dry, scaly, crusty lesions are benefitted by oil or ointment bases, which help to moisturize the skin. Moist, exudative conditions should be treated with solutions or lotions and not occlusive ointments or oils. Creams are frequently poor choices because the client may have difficulty in getting the medication to the horizontal canal. In addition, many clients find the application of fluid drops aesthetically more pleasing compared with the application of viscous materials or the need to insert an applicator down the ear canal.

Active Ingredients

Topical glucocorticoids are beneficial in most cases of otitis externa. Glucocorticoids have antipruritic and anti-inflammatory effects, decrease exudation and swelling, cause sebaceous gland atrophy, decrease glandular secretions, reduce scar tissue, and decrease proliferative changes, all of which help to promote drainage and ventilation. Because pain and pruritus are alleviated, the animal becomes easier to medicate. There are different types and potencies of topical glucocorticoids available, which the clinician should become familiar with. Moderately potent products, such as triamcinolone acetonide (Panolog [Solvay]) and dexamethasone (Tresaderm [MSD AgVet]) are absorbed systemically.[48] Treated dogs have elevated levels of liver enzymes and suppressed adrenal response to corticotropin (adrenocorticotropic hormone [ACTH]) stimulation. The systemic absorption of more potent topical glucocorticoids should make the clinician cautious of long-term treatment. The initial therapy or acute exacerbations may necessitate a potent topical glucocorticoid (fluocinolone, betamethasone, dexamethasone, or triamcinolone) but, after the inflammation or allergic reaction is controlled, prophylactic or long-term therapy should use the least potent topical glucocorticoid possible, such as products containing 0.5 or 1 per cent hydrocortisone such as Hydro B-1020, Epi-Otic HC (Allerderm), and Clear X ear drying solution (DVM Pharmaceuticals). In cases of otitis externa due to atopy or food hypersensitivity, the pinna is frequently affected and should be treated. Antibiotic agents are present in many topical ear products. Uncomplicated cases of allergic or ceruminous otitis externa may be managed by topical glucocorticoid application alone, and inappropriate use of topical antibiotics may cause a secondary superinfection or sensitization. All other concerns about the use of topical glucocorticoids should be considered (see Chap. 3).

Topical antibacterial agents are indicated when infection, whether primary or perpetuating, is present. The aminoglycosides—neomycin (Panolog, Tresaderm [MSD AgVet]), neomycin-polymyxin (Forte-topical [Upjohn]), and gentamicin (Gentocin otic solution, Otomax [Schering-Plough])—are potent topical antibiotics with good activity against pathogens usually found in otitis externa.[7, 26] Polymyxin B is inactivated by pus and should be used in only clean ears. Gram-negative, gentamicin-resistant infections may be successfully treated with injectable amikacin (50 mg/ml) applied at 3 to 5 drops in each ear every 12 hours. However, the aminoglycosides can be ototoxic with prolonged use or when used in animals with ruptured tympanums. Presoaking the ear with tromethamine–edetate disodium (TRIS EDTA) or mixing gentamicin at 3 mg/ml with TRIS EDTA increases the efficacy against gram-negative organisms. TRIS EDTA is made by mixing 6.05 gm of edetate disodium with 12 gm of tromethamine (Trizma) base and bring to 1 L by adding double-distilled water. The pH of this mixture is then adjusted to 8, usually by adding an acid such as hydrochloric acid. The pH-balanced solution should then be autoclaved so that sterilization is achieved. Topical enrofloxacin is made by adding 4 ml of the 2.27 per cent injectable enrofloxacin (Baytril [Miles]) to 8 to 12 ml of a liquid base (such as propylene glycol and water, Epiotic (Allerderm), or Clear X ear drying solution (DVM Pharmaceuticals) and may be useful in some cases of gram-negative infections. The risk of ototoxicity has not been evaluated.

Chloramphenicol (Liquichlor with Cerumene [EVSCO]) is frequently effective but may stimulate excessive granulation tissue in the middle ear.[24] Clients should also be careful not to contact chloramphenicol owing to the possibility of idiosyncratic bone marrow suppression. Using topical antibiotics that are not likely to be needed as systemic drugs may decrease the occurrence of resistant cases of otitis externa and otitis media. The more potent broad-spectrum antibiotics (gentamicin and chloramphenicol) should not be used as first-choice treatments so that resistant strains of bacteria are not created. Therefore, neomycin-polymyxin is preferred by the authors as a first-line topical antibiotic. Most topical antibiotics contain a glucocorticoid, and its potency may not always be desirable.

Topical antiseptics such as povidone-iodine, chlorhexidine, and acetic acid are helpful in the treatment of bacterial otitis externa. Acetic acid has been effective in the treatment of otitis externa in humans. It is believed that its activity is not completely due to the pH because other acidic products are not as effective in killing *Pseudomonas* and *Staphylococcus.* Acetic acid is most effective against *Pseudomonas,* with a 2 per cent solution being lethal within 1 minute of contact. *Staphylococcus* and *Streptococcus* can be killed within 5 minutes of contact with 5 per cent acetic acid solution. However, this concentration is occasionally irritating. Silver sulfadiazine at 1 per cent has been reported to be an effective antimicrobial in cases of otitis externa.[66] It is made by mixing 1 gm of silver sulfadiazine with 100 ml of sterile water and applying this solution at a dose of 0.5 ml per ear twice daily.

Antifungal agents are required in any case complicated or caused by the yeasts *Malassezia* and *Candida* or by dermatophytes. *Malassezia* and dermatophytes usually respond well to topical 1 per cent miconazole (Conofite lotion [Pitman-Moore]) or clotrimazole (Otomax [Schering-Plough]). In vitro testing has shown nystatin (Panalog) to be effective against *Malassezia.* Thiabendazole (Tresaderm [MSD AgVet]), although not effective in vitro, may work in some cases. Again, povidone-iodine or chlorhexidine is also effective. When bacteria and *Malassezia* are present together, the combination of gentocin, clotrimazole, and betamethasone (Otomax) is effective, as is povidone-iodine or chlorhexidine.

Parasiticidal agents are indicated in ear products for *Otodectes* and, less commonly, *Demodex, Otobius,* and trombiculid infestations. Most cases will respond to products containing pyrethrins; these include Cerumite (EVSCO), OtiCare M (ARC Labs), rotenone (Ear Miticide [Valco, Phoenix]), and thiabendazole (Tresaderm [MSD AgVet]). In addition to the use of an effective parasiticidal agent, two important points should be considered. First, many animals may be asymptomatic carriers of *Otodectes.* Because of this, all in-contact animals, both dogs and cats, must be treated. Second, *Otodectes* can be found on other body areas. Therefore, whole-body treatments with effective parasiticidals must be done. The life cycle of *Otodectes* necessitates that otic and body treatment be continued for at least 3 weeks, with a month being necessary in some cases. Some veterinarians recommend topical application of ivermectin (drops in the ears), especially in cats. Although this may be effective, one study showed that the recurrence rate was higher and the time to remission slower than with systemic therapy.[22] Amitraz (1 ml of amitraz in 29 ml of mineral oil) is also effective when applied as otic drops.

Systemic Therapy

Systemic therapy is indicated if otitis externa is severe or if otitis media is present, when owners cannot administer typical treatments, and, in some cases, when marked proliferative changes are present. Appropriate antibiotics or antifungals should be used until 1 week after a cure. Antibiotics that are known to penetrate bone or that have a good history of benefit in treating otitis media should be selected and given at doses that are at the high end of the recommended doses. Examples of antibiotics that are useful for otitis media include trimethoprim-sulfadiazine, 25 mg/kg every 12 hours; clindamycin (Antirobe), 7 to 10 mg/kg every 12 hours; cephalexin, 22 mg/kg every 12 hours; enrofloxacin (Baytril), 2.5 to 5 mg/kg every 12 hours. Pharmacokinetic studies suggest that a dose of 11 mg/kg of enrofloxacin every 12 hours may be necessary in some *Pseudomonas* infections.[68] Ketoconazole (Nizoral) at 10 mg/kg once daily, and up to twice daily, is given when otitis media is associated with *Malassezia.* Otoscopic examination is required before a patient can be considered cured.

Ivermectin, although not approved for this use in the United States, is an extremely effective systemic therapy for *Otodectes* infection. When given subcutaneously at 300 μg/kg and repeated three times at 10-day intervals, it eradicates the ear mites. This form of therapy treats the whole pet and eliminates a carrier state; therefore, it can be used to rule out *Otodectes* infection. In some recurrent cases, related to ear mites, the use of ivermectin in all the household pets was rewarding. *Collies and collie crosses should not be treated with ivermectin.* Shetland sheepdogs and Old English sheepdogs should be treated with great caution.

Systemic glucocorticoid therapy is indicated when there is markedly inflamed edematous otitis and when chronic pathologic changes cause marked stenosis of the canal lumen. Some cases of allergic otitis externa may be treated with systemic glucocorticoids, allowing the initial topical therapy to be a low-potency glucocorticoid product. Injectable dexamethasone is useful if only 2 to 3 days' action is required. For the uncommon case of stenosis primarily of the vertical canal, intralesional triamcinolone acetonide may be helpful.[24] Triamcinolone acetonide is particularly effective for inhibiting fibroblasts and reducing collagen production.

Isotretinoin (Accutane) and etretinate (Tegison) have been helpful in a limited number of cases of otitis externa. Isotretinoin was used in a few dogs and cats that had histologic evidence of sebaceous hyperplasia. Although it appeared to be helpful, its administration was stopped owing to side-effects or expense. Etretinate may be helpful in some animals with hyperproliferative forms of primary keratinization disorders. One study of etretinate in Cocker spaniels with primary keratinization disorders indicated that the ceruminous otitis externa in these dogs did not improve.[53] However, in these cases, other perpetuating factors were not adequately treated. When the ears are repetitively cleaned and concurrent infections are treated, etretinate may be more beneficial. Further work and studies with both these synthetic retinoids are indicated.

Surgery

Surgical procedures that may promote drainage or ventilation are described in most surgical textbooks. It should be emphasized that surgical procedures do not replace a thorough diagnostic work-up and that case selection should be done carefully. In cases with marked proliferative changes of the medial wall, surgical debridement is indicated.

Surgery is also indicated to alleviate stenosis of the canal, to remove tumors or polyps, and to manage medically resistant otitis media. It is imperative for the best results that the primary diagnosis is determined before surgery. Many animals have undergone surgical procedures only to continue to experience otitis externa. Although these cases may sometimes be easier to treat after the procedure, clients not properly educated about expectations may be unsatisfied with the results. Even cases that have been successfully ablated may have persistent pruritus and inflammation of the pinna.[24, 34]

Lateral ear canal resection eliminates the lateral wall of the vertical canal. It is successful in approximately 50 per cent of cases, and clients should be warned of the relatively high failure rate.[36] It is indicated when there is a stenotic vertical ear canal or when medical management is not effective and improvement of drainage and ease of topical application may help the medical management. It may decrease the humidity of the ear canal by up to 10 per cent. Contraindications are stenotic horizontal ear canals, otitis media, and severe proliferative disease or mineralization of the auricular cartilage.[37] The most important step is to make certain that the opening to the canal is as wide as possible and that there is skin-to-skin apposition to decrease scar tissue formation. The cartilage flap must be pulled ventrally, and skin-to-skin apposition should be obtained.

Vertical canal ablation may be indicated if the primary disease is limited to the vertical canal. This procedure removes a larger area of tissue and may reduce sensitivity that was associated with the medial wall of the vertical canal. A study reported improvement in 95 per cent of cases so treated.[43] Elimination of signs occurred in only 23 per cent, with the other cases requiring continued medical therapy. However, medical therapy was easier to carry out or was needed less frequently.[37, 43] It is not commonly recommended by the authors. When otitis media is present, other procedures are indicated. One should not amputate at the horizontal canal but at the last centimeter of the vertical canal. It is better to leave two drain boards, both dorsal and ventral.

Total ear canal ablation is often recommended in dogs with end-stage ear disease poorly or completely unresponsive to aggressive cleaning and medical therapy. In some animals with significant hearing loss that require frequent cleanings, this salvage procedure is less expensive and often preferable as a long-term solution. It is often combined with a bulla osteotomy and curettage of the tympanic bulla, which decreases the incidence of postoperative infections and fistula formation.[24, 37, 43] A major reason for not recommending total ablations has been the concern with hearing loss. Although this may be a problem in normal dogs, this is a minor concern in dogs with chronic diseases.[42]

Acquired Folding of the Pinna

Acquired folding of the pinnae (''flop-eared'' cats) has been reported in adult cats.[58a] All cats had a sudden, bilateral, lateral folding over of the distal 1/3 of the pinnae. The folded portion of the pinna was cool, thin, and palpably devoid of cartilage. All cats had received long-term (8 months to 2 years) daily applications of glucocorticoid-containing otic preparations. Serum cortisol responses to ACTH were depressed, suggesting the presence of iatrogenic secondary adrenocortical insufficiency and iatrogenic Cushing's syndrome. Stopping the glucocorticoid therapy did not result in any improvement of the pinnal folding.

REFERENCES

1. Abegneli, P.L.: Pathologie des paupières chez les carnivores domestiques. Rev. Méd. Vét. 165:217, 1989.
2. Anderson, R.K.: Anal sac disease and its related dermatoses. Comp. Cont. Educ. 6:829, 1984.
3. Angarano, D.W.: Dermatologic disorders of the eyelid and periocular region. In: Kirk, R.W. (ed.). Current Veterinary Therapy X. W.B. Saunders Co., Philadelphia, 1986, p. 678.
4. Ascher, F., et al.: Mise au point et étude expérimentale d'une formulation destinée au traitement des otites externes du chien et du chat. Parte 1: Epidémiologie et microbiologie. Prat. Méd. Chirurg. Anim. Cie. 1988.
5. August, J.R.: Diseases of the ear canal. In: Complete Manual of Ear Care. Veterinary Learning Systems, Princeton Junction, NJ, 1986.
6. Bistner, S.I.: Diseases of the nasolacrimal system. In: Kirk, R.W. (ed.). Current Veterinary Therapy V. W.B. Saunders Co., Philadelphia, 1974, p. 488.
7. Blue, J.L., Wooley, R.E.: Antibacterial sensitivity patterns of bacteria isolated from dogs with otitis externa. J. Am. Vet. Med. Assoc. 177:362, 1977.
8. Boord, M. Personal communication, 1993.
9. Bornand, V.: Bacteriologie et mycologie de l'otite externe du chien. Schweiz. Arch. Tierheilkd. 134:341, 1992.
10. Carlotti, D.: Nail diseases in the dog and cat: Differential diagnosis and treatment. Proceedings, William Dick Bicentenary, Edinburgh, July, 1993.
11. Charbonne, L., Clerc, B.: Les blepharites des carnivores domestiques. Point Vét. 20:33, 1988.
11a. de Geyer, G.: Dermatologie des paupières du chien et du chat. Première partie: étude générale. Prat. Méd. Chirurg. Anim. Cie. 28:605, 1993.
11b. de Geyer, G.: Dermatologie des paupières du chien et du chat. Deuxième partie: étude spéciale. Prat. Méd. Chirurg. Anim. Cie. 28:613, 1993.
12. Fernando, S.D.A.: A histological and histochemical study of the glands of the external auditory canal in the dog. Res. Vet. Sci. 7:116, 1966.
13. Fernando, S.D.A.: Certain histopathologic features of the external auditory meatus of the cat and dog with otitis externa. Am. J. Vet. Res. 28:278, 1967.
14. Fernando, S.D.A.: Microscopic anatomy and histochemistry of glands in the external auditory meatus of the cat (Felis domesticus). Am. J. Vet. Res. 26:1157, 1965.
15. Foil, C.S., Conroy, J. Dermatoses of claws, nails, and hoof. In: Von Tscharner, C., Halliwell, R.E.W. (eds.). Advances in Veterinary Dermatology I. Baillière Tindall, Philadelphia, 1990, p. 420.
16. Franc, M., et al.: Tumeurs du conduit auditif externe des carnivores. Rev. Méd. Vét. 132:733, 1981.
17. Fraser, G.: The histopathology of the external auditory meatus of the dog. J. Comp. Pathol. 71:253, 1961.
18. Frost, R.C.: Canine otoacariasis. J. Small Anim. Pract. 2:253, 1961.
19. Gallé, H.G., Venker-van Haagen, A.J.: Ototoxicity of the antiseptic combination chlorhexidine/cetrimide (Savlon): Effects on equilibrium and hearing. Vet. Quart. 8:56, 1986.
20. Gelatt, K.N.: Histiocytoma of the eyelid of a dog. Vet. Med. (S.A.C.) 70:305, 1975.
21. Gerdin, P.A., et al.: Survey and topographic distribution of bacterial and fungal microorganisms in eyes of clinically normal dogs. Canine Pract. 18(2):34, 1993.
22. Gram, D.: Treatment of ear mites (Otodectes cynotis) in cats: Comparison of subcutaneous and topical ivermectin. Proceedings, Am. Acad. Vet. Dermatol. Am. Coll. Vet. Dermatol., Scottsdale, AZ, 1991.
23. Griffin, C.E.: Claw diseases. Presentation, European School of Advanced Veterinary Studies, Luxembourg, 1994.
24. Griffin, C.E.: Otitis externa and media: In: Griffin, C.E., et al. (eds.). Current Veterinary Dermatology. Mosby–Year Book, St. Louis, 1993, p. 245.
25. Griffin, C.E.: Principles for treatment of the diseased ear canal. In: Complete Manual of Ear Care. Veterinary Learning Systems, Princeton Junction, NJ, 1986.
26. Grono, L.R.: Otitis externa. In: Kirk, R.W. (ed.). Current Veterinary Therapy VII. W.B. Saunders Co., Philadelphia, 1980.

27. Hajsig, M., Lukman, P.: *Pityrosporum pachydermatis (P. canis)* in the inflamed canine anal sacs. Vet. Archiv. 50:43, 1980.

28. Harvey, C.E.: Incidence and distribution of anal sac disease in the dog. J. Am. Anim. Hosp. Assoc. 10:573, 1974.

28a. Huang, H.P., Little, C.J.L.: Effects of fatty acids on the growth and composition of *Malassezia pachydermatis* and their relevance to canine otitis externa. Res. Vet. Sci. 55:119, 1993.

28b. Huang, H.P., et al.: The relationship between microbial numbers found on cytological examination and microbial growth density on culture of swabs from the external ear canal in dogs. Proc. Eur. Soc. Vet. Dermatol. 10:81, 1993.

29. Igarashi, Y., Oka, Y.: Vestibular ototoxicity following intratympanic applications of chlorhexidine gluconate in the cat. Arch. Otorhinolaryngol. 242:167, 1985.

30. Johnson, B.W., Campbell, K.L.: Dermatoses of the canine eyelid. Comp. Cont. Educ. 11:385, 1989.

31. Kakoma, I., et al.: Identification of staphylococci and micrococci from eyes of clinically normal dogs: Relative frequency of isolation, β-lactamase production, and selected antimicrobial sensitivity profiles. Canine Pract. 18(1):11, 1993.

32. Kapatkin, A.S., et al.: Results of surgery and long-term follow-up in 31 cats with nasopharyngeal polyps. J. Am. Anim. Hosp. Assoc. 26:387, 1990.

33. Ketring, K.L.: Diseases of the eyelids. In: Kirk, R.W. (ed.). Current Veterinary Therapy VII. W.B. Saunders Co., Philadelphia, 1980.

34. Krahwinkel, D.J., et al.: Effect of total ablation of the external acoustic meatus and bulla osteotomy on auditory function in dogs. J. Am. Vet. Med. Assoc. 202:949, 1993.

35. Lawson, D.D.: Canine distichiasis. J. Small Anim. Pract. 14:469, 1973.

36. Layton, C.E.: The role of lateral ear resection in managing chronic otitis externa. Semin. Vet. Med. Surg. (Small Anim.) 8(1):24, 1993.

37. Lenehan, T.A., Tarvin, G.: Personal communication, 1993.

38. Little, C.J.L., Lane, J.G.: An evaluation of tympanometry, otoscopy, and palpation for assessment of the canine tympanic membrane. Vet. Rec. 124:5, 1989.

39. Little, C.J.L., et al.: Inflammatory middle ear disease of the dog: The clinical and pathological features of cholesteatoma, a complication of otitis media. Vet. Rec. 128:319, 1991.

40. Lukman, P.: Nalazista glijvice *Pityrosporum canis* u organizuma zdravih i bolenith pasa. Vet. Archiv. 52:37, 1982.

41. Mansfield, P.D.: Ototoxicity in dogs and cats. Comp. Cont. Educ. 12:331, 1990.

41a. Mansfield, P.D., et al.: Infectivity of *Malassezia pachydermatis* in the external ear canal of dogs. J. Am. Anim. Hosp. Assoc. 26:97, 1990.

41b. Marino, D.J., et al.: Results of surgery and long-term follow-up in dogs with ceruminous gland adenocarcinoma. J. Am. Anim. Hosp. Assoc. 29:560, 1993.

41c. Marino, D.J., et al.: Results of surgery in cats with ceruminous gland adenocarcinoma. J. Am. Anim. Hosp. Assoc. 30:54, 1994.

42. Matthiesen, D.T., Scavelli, T.: Total ear canal ablation and lateral bulla osteotomy in 38 dogs. J. Am. Anim. Hosp. Assoc. 26:257, 1990.

43. McCarthy, R.J., Caywood, D.D.: Vertical ear canal resection for end-stage otitis externa in dogs. J. Am. Anim. Hosp. Assoc. 28:545, 1992.

44. McKeever, P.J, Richardson, H.W.: Otitis externa, part 2: Clinical appearance and diagnostic methods. Companion Anim. Pract. 2(8):25, 1988.

45. McKeever, P.J., Richardson, H.W.: Otitis externa, part 3: Ear cleaning and medical treatment. Companion Anim. Pract. 2(9):24, 1988.

46. McKeever, P.J., Torres, S.: Otitis externa, part 1: The ear and predisposing factors to otitis externa. Companion Anim. Pract. 2(7):7, 1988.

47. McLaughlin, S.A., et al.: Eyelid neoplasms in cats: A review of demographic data (1979 to 1989). J. Am. Anim. Hosp. Assoc. 29:63, 1993.

48. Moriello, K.A., et al.: Adrenocortical suppression associated with topical otic administration of glucocorticoids in dogs. J. Am. Vet. Med. Assoc. 193:329, 1988.

49. Mueller, R.S., et al.: Microanatomy of the canine claw. Vet. Dermatol. 4:5, 1993.

50. Pope, E.R.: Feline inflammatory polyps. Companion Anim. Pract. 19(1):33, 1989.

51. Poulet, F.M., et al.: Focal proliferative eosinophilic dermatitis of the external ear canal in four dogs. Vet. Pathol. 28:171, 1991.

52. Powell, M.B., et al.: Reaginic hypersensitivity in *Otodectes cynotis* infestation of cats and mode of feeding. Am. J. Vet. Res. 41:877, 1980.

53. Power, H.T., Ihrke, P.J.: Synthetic retinoids in veterinary dermatology. Vet. Clin. North Am. (Small Anim. Clin.) 20:1525, 1990.

54. Remedios, A.M., et al.: A comparison of radiographic versus surgical diagnosis of otitis media. J. Am. Anim. Hosp. Assoc. 27:183, 1991.

55. Rosychuk, R.A.W.: Diseases of the claw and claw fold. In: Bonagura, J.D. (ed.). Kirk's Current Veterinary Therapy XII. W.B. Saunders Co., Philadelphia, 1995.

56. Schulte, A.: Neoplasien im Ohr der Katze. Kleintier-Prax. 33:407, 1988.

57. Scott, D.W.: Canine sterile eosinophilic pinnal folliculitis. Companion Anim. Pract. 2(6):19, 1988.

58. Scott, D.W.: Feline dermatology 1900–1978: A monograph. J. Am. Anim. Hosp. Assoc. 16:331, 1980.

58a. Scott, D.W.: Feline dermatology 1986 to 1988: Looking to the 1990s through the eyes of many counsellors. J. Am. Anim. Hosp. Assoc. 26:515, 1990.

59. Scott, D.W.: Observations on canine atopy. J. Am. Anim. Hosp. Assoc. 17:91, 1981.

60. Scott, D.W., et al.: Symmetrical lupoid onychodystrophy in dogs: A retrospective analysis of 18 cases (1989–1993). J. Am. Anim. Hosp. Assoc. (accepted, 1994).

61. Scott, D.W., Miller, W.H.: Disorders of the claw and clawbed in cats. Comp. Cont. Educ. 14:449, 1992.
62. Scott, D.W., Miller, W.H.: Disorders of the claw and clawbed in dogs. Comp. Cont. Educ. 14:1448, 1992.
63. Seim, H.B.: Diseases of the anus and rectum. In: Kirk, R.W. (ed.). Current Veterinary Therapy IX. W.B. Saunders Co., Philadelphia, 1986.
64. Stout-Graham, M., et al.: Morphologic measurements of the external horizontal ear canal of dogs. Am. J. Vet. Res., 51:990, 1990.
65. Strickland, J.H., Calhoun, M.L.: The microscopic anatomy of the external ear of *Felis domesticus.* Am. J. Vet. Res. 21:845, 1960.
66. Thomas, M.L.: Development of a bacterial model for canine otitis externa. Proc. Annu. Memb. Meet. Am. Acad. Vet. Dermatol. Am. Coll. Vet. Dermatol. 6:28, 1990.
67. van der Gaag, I.: The pathology of the external ear canal in dogs and cats. Vet. Quart. 8:307, 1986.
68. Walker, R.D., et al.: Pharmacokinetic evaluation of enrofloxacin administered orally to healthy dogs. Am. J. Vet. Res. 53:2315, 1992.
69. Weisbroth, S.H., et al.: Immunopathology of naturally occurring otodectic otoacariasis in the domestic cat. J. Am. Vet. Med. Assoc., 165:1088, 1974.

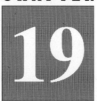
Neoplastic and Non-neoplastic Tumors

■

Chapter Outline

■ CUTANEOUS ONCOLOGY

Veterinary oncology has come into its own as a specialty. Detailed information on the etiopathogenesis and immunologic aspects of neoplasia is available in other publications,[4, 7, 8, 10, 12, 13] and is therefore not presented here. This chapter is an overview of canine and feline cutaneous neoplasia as well as non-neoplastic tumors.

The combined *incidence rates* (the number of new cases of a disease diagnosed in 1 year divided by the population at risk and expressed as cases per 100,000 of the population at risk) for benign and malignant neoplasms in dogs and cats were reported to be about 1077 and 188, respectively.[10, 12, 13, 31] Thus, dogs have about six times as many tumors as do cats. The incidence rates for canine and feline skin neoplasms are about 728 and 84, respectively.

The peak age period for neoplasm occurrence in dogs and cats is 6 to 14 years. The median ages for cutaneous neoplasm occurrence in dogs and cats are 10½ years and 12 years, respectively. The frequency of various skin neoplasms differs in dog and cat breeds (Table 19:1). Canine breeds that have the highest neoplasm incidence are the boxer, Scottish terrier, bull mastiff, Basset hound, Weimaraner, Kerry blue terrier, and Norwegian elkhound.[10, 12, 13, 17, 23, 31, 33] Siamese and Persians appear to be at risk for certain cutaneous neoplasms in cats.[4] The overall incidence of neoplasia is greater in female dogs than in male dogs (56 per cent versus

Table 19:1. Breed Predilections for Cutaneous Neoplasms and Non-neoplastic Lumps in the Dog and Cat

Papilloma	Cocker spaniel, Kerry blue terrier
Keratoacanthoma	Collie, German shepherd dog, Keeshond, Lhasa apso, Norwegian elkhound, Old English sheepdog, Yorkshire terrier
Squamous cell carcinoma	Scottish terrier, Pekingese, boxer, Poodle, Norwegian elkhound
Squamous cell carcinoma, glabrous, nonpigmented skin of trunk (actinic)	Dalmatian, bull terrier, American Staffordshire terrier, beagle
Squamous cell carcinoma, clawbed	Black Labrador retriever, Black Standard Poodle, Giant Schnauzer, dachshund, Bouvier des Flandres
Feline benign basal cell tumor	Persian, Himalayan
Basal cell carcinoma	Cocker spaniel, English Springer spaniel, Kerry blue terrier, Poodle, Shetland sheepdog, Siberian husky, Siamese cat
Trichoepithelioma	Cocker spaniel, English Springer spaniel, Basset hound, German shepherd dog, Golden retriever, Irish setter, Miniature Schnauzer, Standard Poodle, Persian cat
Tricholemmoma	Afghan hound
Pilomatrixoma	Kerry blue terrier, Old English sheepdog, Poodle
Trichoblastoma	Cocker spaniel, Poodle
Sebaceous gland tumors	Beagle, Cocker spaniel, dachshund, Irish setter, Lhasa apso, Malamute, Miniature Schnauzer, Poodle, Shih tzu, Siberian husky, Persian cat
Sweat gland tumors	Cocker spaniel, German shepherd dog, Golden retriever
Hepatoid gland tumors	Beagle, Cocker spaniel, English bulldog, German shepherd dog, Lhasa apso, Samoyed, Shih tzu, Siberian husky, Afghan hound, dachshund
Fibroma	Boston terrier, boxer, Doberman pinscher, fox terrier, Golden retriever
Fibropruritic nodule	German shepherd dog
Fibrosarcoma	Cocker spaniel, Doberman pinscher, Golden retriever
Myxoma or myxosarcoma	Doberman pinscher, German shepherd
Schwannoma	Fox terrier
Hemangioma	Airedale terrier, boxer, English Springer spaniel, German shepherd dog, Golden retriever
Hemangioma, glabrous, nonpigmented skin (actinic)	American Staffordshire terrier, Basset hound, beagle, Dalmation, English Springer spaniel, Greyhound, Saluki, whippet
Hemangiosarcoma	Bernese Mountain dog, boxer, German shepherd dog, Golden retriever
Hemangiosarcoma, glabrous, nonpigmented skin (actinic)	See actinic hemangioma
Hemangiopericytoma	Beagle, boxer, Cocker spaniel, collie, fox terrier, English Springer spaniel, German shepherd dog, Irish setter, Siberian husky
Lipoma	Cocker spaniel, dachshund, Doberman pinscher, Labrador retriever, Miniature Schnauzer, Weimaraner, Siamese cat
Liposarcoma	Brittany spaniel, dachshund, Shetland sheepdog
Mast cell tumor	American Staffordshire terrier, beagle, Boston terrier, boxer, bull terrier, dachshund, English bulldog, fox terrier, Golden retriever, Labrador retriever, Pug, Shar Pei, Weimaraner, Siamese cat
Lymphoma	Basset hound, boxer, Cocker spaniel, German shepherd dog, Golden retriever, Irish setter, Scottish terrier, St. Bernard
Plasmacytoma	Cocker spaniel
Histiocytoma	American Staffordshire terrier, Boston terrier, boxer, Cocker spaniel, dachshund, Doberman pinscher, English Springer spaniel, Great Dane, Labrador retriever, Miniature Schnauzer, Rottweiler, Scottish terrier, Shar Pei, Shetland sheepdog, West Highland white terrier
Malignant histiocytosis	Bernese Mountain dog
Systemic histiocytosis	Bernese Mountain dog
Cutaneous histiocytosis	Collie, Shetland sheepdog

Table 19:1. Breed Predilections for Cutaneous Neoplasms and Non-neoplastic Lumps in the Dog and Cat *Continued*

Benign fibrous histiocytoma	Collie, Golden retriever
Melanocytic tumors	Airedale terrier, Boston terrier, boxer, Chihuahua, Chow Chow, Cocker spaniel, Doberman pinscher, English Springer spaniel, Golden retriever, Irish setter, Irish terrier, Miniature Schnauzer, Scottish terrier
Follicular cyst	Boxer, Doberman pinscher, Miniature Schnauzer, Shih tzu
Dermoid cyst	Boxer, Kerry blue terrier, Rhodesian Ridgeback
Collagenous nevus	German shepherd dog
Vascular nevus, scrotal	Airedale terrier, Kerry blue terrier, Labrador retriever, Scottish terrier
Epidermal nevus	Miniature Schnauzer, Pug
Actinic keratosis	American Staffordshire terrier, Basset hound, beagle, bull terrier, Dalmation
Calcinosis circumscripta	Boston terrier, boxer, German shepherd dog
Focal mucinosis	Doberman pinscher, Shar Pei

44 per cent); in cats, however, male cats predominate (56 per cent versus 44 per cent) in most surveys.[10, 12, 34]

There are no completely satisfactory criteria for distinguishing benign neoplasms from certain proliferative inflammatory lesions and hyperplastic processes and for distinguishing benign from malignant neoplasms.[10, 12, 13] In general, malignant neoplasms are usually characterized by sudden onset, rapid growth, infiltration, recurrence, and metastasis. The most important criterion of malignancy is metastasis. In dogs, the number of malignant neoplasms is only about half the number of benign neoplasms.[10, 12, 13, 31] However, in cats, there are about three times as many malignant neoplasms as benign neoplasms.[10, 12, 13, 31, 34]

The skin is the most common site of occurrence of neoplasms in the dog (about 30 per cent of the total) and the second most common site in the cat (about 20 per cent of the total).* The most common skin neoplasm in dogs and cats varies somewhat from one report to another. In general, canine skin neoplasms may be broadly categorized as about 55 per cent mesenchymal, 40 per cent epithelial, and 5 per cent melanocytic in origin, and feline skin neoplasms as 50 per cent epithelial, 48 per cent mesenchymal, and 2 per cent melanocytic. In the dog, the most common skin neoplasms, in approximate descending order, are lipoma, sebaceous gland hyperplasia, mast cell tumor, histiocytoma, and papilloma (squamous papilloma and fibropapilloma). In the cat, the approximate order is basal cell tumor, squamous cell carcinoma, mast cell tumor, and fibrosarcoma.

The key to appropriate management and accurate prognosis of cutaneous neoplasms is specific diagnosis. This can be achieved only by biopsy and histologic evaluation. Exfoliative cytologic techniques (aspiration and impression smear) are easy and rapid and often provide valuable information about neoplastic cell type and differentiation. The techniques, methods, and interpretation used in cytologic studies have been beautifully described and illustrated (see Chap. 2).[41-44] However, exfoliative cytologic evaluation is inferior to and is no substitute for biopsy and histopathologic examination. Historical and clinical considerations often allow the experienced clinician to formulate an inclusive differential diagnosis on a cutaneous neoplasm, but variability renders such ''odds playing'' unreliable. In short, ''a lump is a lump'' until it is evaluated histologically.

The detailed histopathologic description of canine and feline cutaneous neoplasms is beyond the scope of this chapter. Only the histopathologic essence of individual neoplasms is presented here. For in-depth information and photomicrographic illustrations, the reader is referred to

---

*See references 10, 12–15, 18, 28, 31, and 34.

other texts on cutaneous neoplasia[4-6, 9, 10, 40] and the individual references cited for each neoplasm.

The use of markers—enzyme histochemical and immunohistochemical methods for identifying specific cell types—has increased and has been touted for the diagnosis of neoplastic conditions in dogs and cats.[45-58] Examples of these markers are presented in Chapter 2.

Clinical management of cutaneous neoplasms may include surgery, cryosurgery, electrosurgery, radiotherapy, chemotherapy, immunotherapy, hyperthermia, phototherapy, and combinations of these. Detailed information on the various treatment modalities is available in a number of excellent references.[2, 7, 8, 12, 13, 25a] Brief comments on treatment are included under clinical management for each tumor.

■ EPITHELIAL NEOPLASMS

Cutaneous Papilloma

CAUSE AND PATHOGENESIS

Since the mid 1980s, great advances have been made concerning the understanding and classification of papovaviruses in animals and humans.[64, 67, 68] Differentiation of papovavirus types by cleavage patterns produced by treating viral deoxyribonucleic acid (DNA) with restriction endonucleases and the in vitro hybridization of viral DNA have emphasized the heterogeneity of papovaviruses within animal genera. In dogs, at least three types of papovaviruses tend to have site specificity on the animal as well as histologic specificity.[32, 62, 65] A unique feline papillomavirus has been described.[63, 65]

The papillomaviruses are transmitted by direct and indirect (via fomites) contact. In general, infection occurs in damaged skin. The incubation period varies from 2 to 6 months.

CLINICAL FINDINGS

Dog

Cutaneous papillomas (warts and verrucae) are common in the dog,* and at least four syndromes are recognized clinically. *Canine viral papillomatosis* is common and affects young dogs with no apparent breed or sex predilection. Lesions are almost always multiple and affect the buccal mucosa, the tongue, the palate, the pharynx, the epiglottis, the lip, the skin, the eyelids, the conjunctiva, and the cornea (Fig. 19:1 *A*).[4, 11, 12, 69] The lesions begin as white, flat, smooth, shiny papules and plaques of a few millimeters in diameter and progress to whitish gray, pedunculated or cauliflower-like hyperkeratotic masses up to 3 cm in diameter.

Cutaneous papillomas occur in older dogs and are more common in male dogs, Cocker spaniels, and Kerry blue terriers.† Cutaneous papillomas may be single or multiple, occurring mainly on the head, the eyelids, and the feet (Fig. 19:1 *B* and *C*). They are usually pedunculated or cauliflower-like, firm to soft, well circumscribed, alopecic, and smooth to keratinous; they are usually less than 0.5 cm in diameter. These papillomas have not been definitely shown to be of viral origin.[6, 66, 67] *Cutaneous inverted papillomas* are seen in dogs 8 months to 3 years of age with no apparent breed or sex predilection.[62, 66a] Lesions occur commonly on the ventral abdomen and the groin; are small (1 to 2 cm in diameter), raised, and firm; and contain a central pore opening to the surface of the skin (Fig. 19:2). DNA hybridization studies with a canine viral papillomatosis virus probe revealed that cutaneous inverted papillomas are due to a different papillomavirus from that causing canine viral papillomas.

---

*See references 1, 4, 10–13, 18, 27, and 31.
†See references 1, 11, 12, 18, 27, 30, and 32.

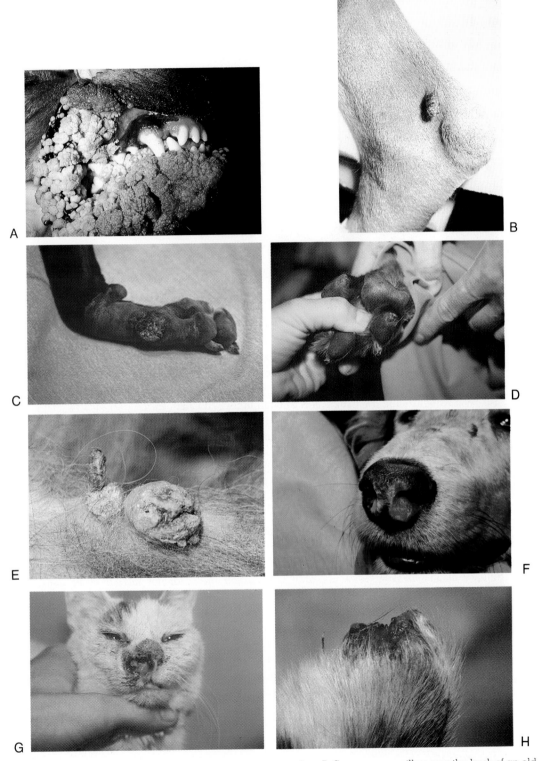

Figure 19:1. *A*, Severe oral viral papillomatosis in a young dog. *B*, Squamous papilloma on the hock of an old dog. *C*, Fibropapilloma on the paw of an old dog. *D*, Multiple squamous papillomas on the footpads of a young dog. *E*, Two keratoacanthomas on the dorsal neck of an Old English sheepdog. The lesion at the left has an overlying cutaneous horn. *F*, Squamous cell carcinoma on the nose of a collie. *G*, Squamous cell carcinoma on the nose of a cat. *H*, Squamous cell carcinoma on the tip of the pinna of a white cat.

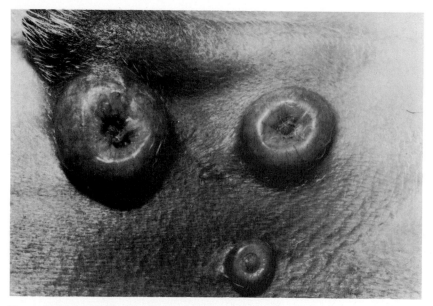

Figure 19:2. Inverted papillomas near the prepuce of a young dog.

Multiple papillomas have been recognized *on the footpads* of adult dogs.[94a] Lesions were firm, hyperkeratotic, and often hornlike in appearance. They occurred on multiple footpads of two paws or more (see Fig. 19:1 *D*). Larger lesions were associated with lameness. These papillomas have not been definitively shown to be caused by viruses. Multiple papillomas have also been recognized in the haired skin of adult dogs (see Chap. 7).

Occasionally, cutaneous horns may overlie papillomas.

Although cutaneous viral papillomas are usually benign, apparent transformation into squamous cell carcinoma has been recognized in a few canine cases.[11, 12] Some dogs treated with a live virus vaccine that was made from papillomavirus isolated from naturally occurring oral papillomas experienced squamous cell carcinomas at the sites of vaccine inoculation.[61, 69] Rare cases of viral papillomatosis have been completely unresponsive to treatment, perhaps owing to immunologic defects.[66]

Cat

Solitary cutaneous papillomas are rare in cats, and most are not known to be caused by papillomaviruses.[21, 26, 27, 34, 38, 63a] Lesions are seen in adult cats with no apparent breed, sex, or site predilection. The papillomas are solitary, pedunculated to cauliflower-like, well circumscribed, and hyperkeratotic; they are less than 0.5 cm in diameter. Papillomavirus-associated skin lesions were recently reported in aged male Persian cats,[63] as well as a cat seropositive for feline immunodeficiency virus.[65] Lesions were multiple on the head, the neck, the dorsal thorax, the abdomen, and the proximal limbs, and were characterized by black, greasy foci and raised, hyperkeratotic plaques 3 to 5 mm in diameter. In vitro studies revealed this papillomavirus to be a unique virus type.

Occasionally, cutaneous horns overlie papillomas.[34]

DIAGNOSIS

The differential diagnostic considerations in dogs incude keratoacanthoma and cutaneous horn, whereas in cats they include mast cell tumor and cutaneous horn. Histologically, papillomas may be divided into squamous and fibrous types.[4, 5, 9–12] Squamous papillomas (the most

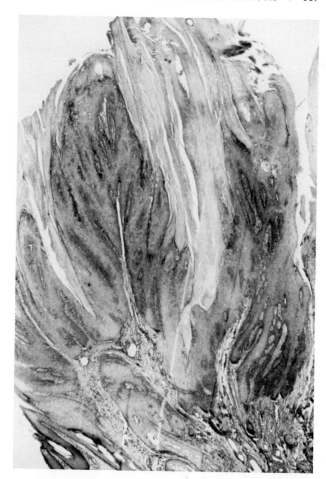

Figure 19:3. Canine viral squamous papilloma. Note papillomatosis and vacuolated keratinocytes.

common type) are characterized by papillated (exophytic papilloma) or plaquelike (verruca plana, or flat wart) epidermal hyperplasia and papillomatosis, with variable degrees of ballooning degeneration (koilocytosis) and giant, clumped, pleomorphic keratohyaline granules (Figs. 19:3 and 19:4).[4, 5, 9–11] Basophilic intranuclear inclusion bodies are variable findings. Inverted papillomas (endophytic papilloma) are cup-shaped lesions with a central core of keratin.[5, 62] The cup is lined by mature squamous epithelium with centripetal papillary projections, ballooning degeneration, abnormal keratohyaline granules, and variable intranuclear inclusion bodies. Idiopathic squamous papillomas are histologically identical to viral squamous papillomas, except they lack evidence of virus infection (ballooning degeneration, abnormal keratohyaline granules, and intranuclear inclusion bodies).[5] Fibropapilloma (fibrous polyp) is characterized by a fibroma-like proliferation of collagen with papillomatosis and papillated epidermal hyperplasia (Fig. 19:5). The feline viral papillomas were characterized by focal epidermal and follicular hyperplasia and hyperkeratosis, ballooning degeneration, abnormal keratohyaline granules, and intracytoplasmic inclusion bodies.[63, 65]

Papillomaviruses can be identified by immunohistochemical detection of papillomavirus structural antigens, electron microscopic detection of intranuclear and intracytoplasmic virus particles, and in situ hybridization detection of papillomavirus-specific DNA.[66a, 67, 68] Papillomas are positive for cytokeratin.[47, 57]

CLINICAL MANAGEMENT

Clinical management of cutaneous papillomas may include surgical excision, cryosurgery, electrosurgery, and observation without treatment.[10–13] Canine viral papillomatosis usually

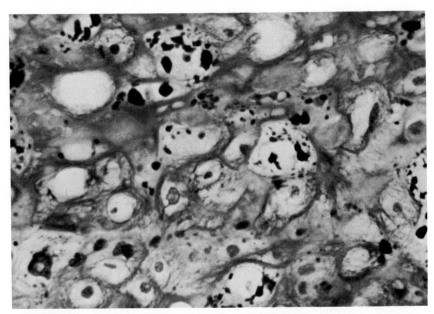

Figure 19:4. Canine viral squamous papilloma. Note ballooning degeneration and clumping of keratohyaline granules.

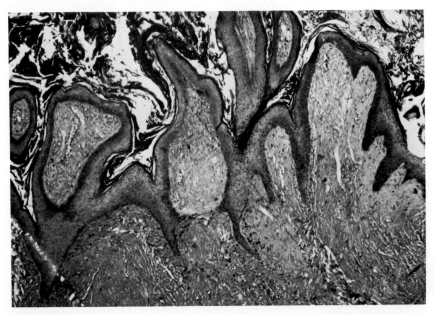

Figure 19:5. Canine fibropapilloma. Papillomatous proliferation of epidermis and fibroblasts.

undergoes spontaneous regression within about 3 months, and solid immunity follows experimental or natural infection. Autogenous or commercially produced wart vaccines and immunomodulating drugs (e.g., levamisole and thiabendazole) are without documented value. In certain cases with large masses of proliferating tissue, eating and maintaining oral hygiene may be facilitated by surgically removing some of the larger papillomas, which is usually performed by cryosurgery or electrosurgery. Reports have indicated that intralesional injections of bleomycin, 5-fluorouracil, or interferon, as well as the oral administration of levamisole or retinoids, are beneficial to humans with recalcitrant papillomas.[59, 60, 64] Retinoids have been reported to be effective in the treatment of canine inverted papillomas.[188a] Canine inverted papillomas have also been reported to regress spontaneously.[66a]

Keratoacanthoma

CAUSE AND PATHOGENESIS

Keratoacanthomas (intracutaneous cornifying epitheliomas, or infundibular keratinizing acanthomas) are uncommon benign neoplasms of the dog.[4, 10–13, 74] It has been suggested that these neoplasms are of hair follicle origin.[5] There are unsubstantiated references to the occurrence of keratoacanthomas in the cat. The cause of keratoacanthomas is unknown, although the generalized forms may have a hereditary basis in dogs and humans. Immunohistochemical studies failed to identify papillomavirus antigen.[62, 67]

CLINICAL FINDINGS

Usually, these neoplasms occur in dogs 5 years of age or younger. Male dogs are more commonly affected than female dogs. The incidence is higher in purebred dogs and particularly in the Norwegian elkhound and Keeshond, which are predisposed to the generalized form.[4, 10–13, 27, 74] However, the generalized form has also been recognized in the German shepherd dog and Old English sheepdog.[11, 12, 27] Collies, Lhasa apsos, and Yorkshire terriers are also reported to be at risk for the solitary form.[4, 11]

Although keratoacanthomas are usually solitary, they may be multiple in the Norwegian elkhound, Keeshond, German shepherd dog, and Old English sheepdog (see Fig. 19:1 *E*). Most tumors occur on the back, the neck, the thorax, and the limbs. There is considerable variation in the gross appearance of keratoacanthomas. Most of the tumors appear as firm to fluctuant, well-circumscribed dermal or subcutaneous masses varying from 0.5 to 4 cm in diameter, with a pore opening onto the skin surface that ranges from less than 1 mm to several millimeters in diameter. The opening usually contains a hard keratinized plug, varying from small and inconspicuous to large and hornlike. Superficial lesions with large keratinous plugs are easily mistaken for cutaneous horns. Some of the tumors are entirely dermal or subcutaneous, do not communicate with the surface of the skin, and are easily confused with cysts. Keratoacanthomas are not invasive or metastatic. However, in the generalized form (up to 50 lesions) a recurrent problem should be anticipated, because affected dogs tend to have new tumors at other sites throughout their lives.

DIAGNOSIS

The differential diagnostic considerations include papillomas, cutaneous horns, and cysts. Histopathologically, keratoacanthomas are characterized by a keratin-filled crypt in the dermis that opens to the skin surface (Fig. 19:6).[4, 5] The wall of the crypt is composed of a thick, complex, folded layer of well-differentiated stratified squamous epithelium, with columns of squamoid cells projecting peripherally from the basal surface of the wall and forming small epithelial nests (Fig. 19:7). The major histopathologic differential feature is the inverted

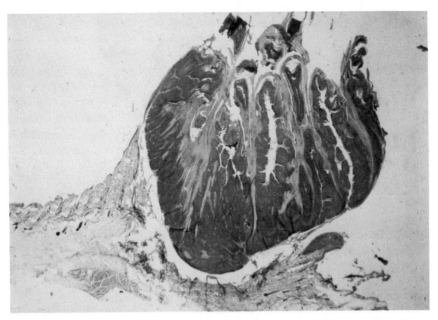

Figure 19:6. Canine keratoacanthoma. A central keratin-filled crypt opens to the skin surface.

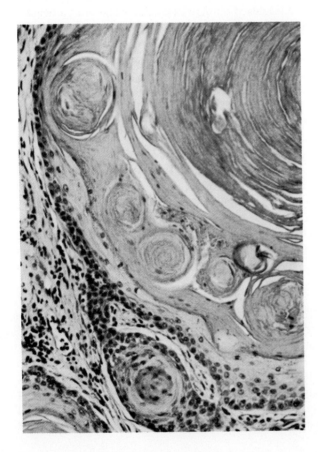

Figure 19:7. Canine keratoacanthoma. Note multiple horn cysts and projections of squamoid cells. (From Weiss, E., Frese, K.: VII. Tumors of the skin. Bull. World Health Organ. 50:79, 1974.)

papilloma.[5, 62] However, the keratoacanthoma does *not* have ballooning degeneration, abnormal keratohyaline granules, or intranuclear inclusion bodies. Keratoacanthomas are positive for cytokeratin.[45]

CLINICAL MANAGEMENT

Clinical management of keratoacanthomas may include surgical excision, cryotherapy, electrotherapy, and observation without treatment.[11-13] Chemotherapy with cyclophosphamide and prednisone and immunotherapy with autogenous vaccine or levamisole have been ineffective in dogs.[21] The oral administration of retinoids or intralesional injections of 5-fluorouracil or methotrexate have provided good results in the treatment of keratoacanthomas in humans.[3, 71] The oral administration of retinoids (isotretinoin or etretinate) has been successful for the treatment of multiple keratoacanthomas in some dogs.[70, 72, 188a] A good response is seen after 3 to 4 months of therapy, and treatment must be continued intermittently for life in most cases. Keratoacanthomas are also known to resolve spontaneously.[73]

Squamous Cell Carcinoma

Squamous cell carcinomas (epidermoid carcinomas) are common malignant neoplasms of the dog and cat, arising from keratinocytes.* The etiology of squamous cell carcinoma is not clear in all cases. Squamous cell carcinoma occurs most frequently in sun-damaged skin and may be preceded by actinic keratosis.† Thus, squamous cell carcinoma is seen more frequently in geographic areas characterized by long periods of intense sun exposure. Rarely, squamous cell carcinoma has been reported to arise from burn scars or chronic infectious processes.[12, 85, 90, 93] In humans, squamous cell carcinomas occasionally arise from burn and frostbite scars, radiation burns, and stasis dermatitis.[90] In a retrospective study,[68] papillomavirus structural antigens were demonstrated in five of nine canine cutaneous squamous cell carcinomas, suggesting that papillomaviruses have an etiologic role in this neoplasm. The results of similar studies were negative in the cat.[67, 68] Squamous cell carcinomas occurred at the site of injection of a live canine oral papillomavirus vaccine in some dogs.[4, 69]

CLINICAL FINDINGS

Dog

Squamous cell carcinoma occurs at an average age of 9 years, with no sex predilection, although puppies are rarely affected.[88] In general, Scottish terriers, Pekingese, boxers, Poodles, and Norwegian elkhounds are predisposed.[10-13, 99] Squamous cell carcinomas with clawbed origin are seen most commonly in black-coated dogs of large breeds, especially Labrador retriever, Standard Poodle, Giant Schnauzer, dachshund, and Bouvier des Flandres.‡ Short-coated breeds with white or piebald ventral coat and skin color (Dalmatian, American Staffordshire terrier, bull terrier, and beagle) have the highest incidence of solar-induced squamous cell carcinoma.[5, 11, 13, 91, 92] These dogs usually spend many hours a day lying in the sun. Nasal squamous cell carcinomas may rarely occur as a sequel to depigmentation associated with conditions such as discoid lupus erythematosus, pemphigus erythematosus, and vitiligo that result in increased susceptibility to actinic damage.

Lesions occur most commonly on the trunk, the limbs, the digits, the scrotum, the lips, and the nose (see Fig. 19:1 *F*) and may be proliferative or ulcerative. The proliferative types are

---

*See references 4, 5, 10–15, 18, 22, 25, 29, 31, and 34.
†See references 4, 5, 10–13, 82, 87, and 90–92.
‡See references 4, 10–13, 84a, 95, 96, and 98.

papillary masses of varying size, many of which have a cauliflower-like appearance. The surface tends to be ulcerated and bleeds easily. Cutaneous horns may develop on the surface of such lesions. The ulcerative types initially appear as shallow, crusted ulcers that become deep and crateriform. Squamous cell carcinomas are usually solitary, but they may be multiple on the trunk of sunbathing dogs or in the clawbeds of large, black-coated breeds. Dogs with clawbed (subungual) squamous cell carcinomas usually have a single affected digit, which is swollen and painful with a misshapen or absent claw and paronychial discharge, and they may experience multiple neoplasms in other digits during 2 to 4 years.

Cat

Squamous cell carcinoma occurs at an average age of 9 years, with no breed or sex predilection. White cats (short-haired or long-haired cats) have squamous cell carcinoma about 13 times as frequently as do other cats, owing to increased susceptibility to actinic damage.* The most common sites are the nose (see Fig. 19:1 *G*) (about 8 to 90 per cent of affected cats), the pinnae (Fig. 19:1 *H*) (about 50 per cent), and the eyelids (about 20 per cent).[4, 82a] Lesions may be proliferative or ulcerative (Fig. 19:8 *A*) and may occasionally have overlying cutaneous horns. Lesions are multiple in about 45 per cent of affected cats.[82a]

Generally, squamous cell carcinomas are locally invasive and slow to metastasize. In dogs and cats, squamous cell carcinomas arising from the digits appear to be more aggressive and may be misdiagnosed as paronychia or some form of pyoderma.

DIAGNOSIS

The differential diagnosis of solitary cutaneous squamous cell carcinomas includes numerous neoplastic and granulomatous disorders. Clawbed lesions are frequently misdiagnosed as infectious paronychia. Histologically, squamous cell carcinomas consist of irregular masses or cords of keratinocytes that proliferate downward and invade the dermis (Fig. 19:9 *A* and *B*).[4, 5, 9, 11, 12] Frequent findings include keratin formation, horn pearls, intercellular bridges, mitoses, and atypia (Fig. 19:10). Solar elastosis may occasionally be seen.[5, 89] The majority of squamous cell carcinomas in dogs and cats are of the well-differentiated, histopathologic subtype, but poorly differentiated, acantholytic (pseudoglandular), spindle cell, and clear cell varieties do occur.[5, 9, 11] Squamous cell carcinomas are positive for cytokeratin, and such examinations may be critical in establishing the true identity of spindle cell and clear cell varieties.[27, 45, 47, 54, 56]

CLINICAL MANAGEMENT

Squamous cell carcinomas are generally locally invasive but are slow to metastasize. Lesions of the clawbed appear to be more aggressive (about 70 per cent invade bony tissue of the third phalanx) and metastasize more frequently (up to 22 per cent to regional lymph node).[10–13, 84a, 95] In cats, the prognosis correlates with the degree of histopathologic differentiation but not with the anatomic site.[81] Fifty per cent of cats with poorly differentiated neoplasms were destroyed within 12 weeks, and the longest survival time was 20 weeks.

Clinical management of squamous cell carcinomas may include surgical excision, cryosurgery, electrosurgery, hyperthermia, and radiotherapy.[11–13, 82a] Cryosurgery was reported to provide a 1-year cure rate of 84 per cent in tumors of the nose, the pinna, and the eyelid in cats.[82a] Radiotherapy provided a 1-year cure rate of 62 per cent in nasal planum squamous cell carcinoma in cats.[83] Resection of the nasal planum yielded a good cosmetic effect in cats and a fair cosmetic effect in dogs with squamous cell carcinoma.[99a] Hyperthermia is often effective for the treatment of superficial cutaneous squamous cell carcinomas in cats and dogs. Photo-

---

*See references 10–13, 29, 34, 82a, 83, and 99a.

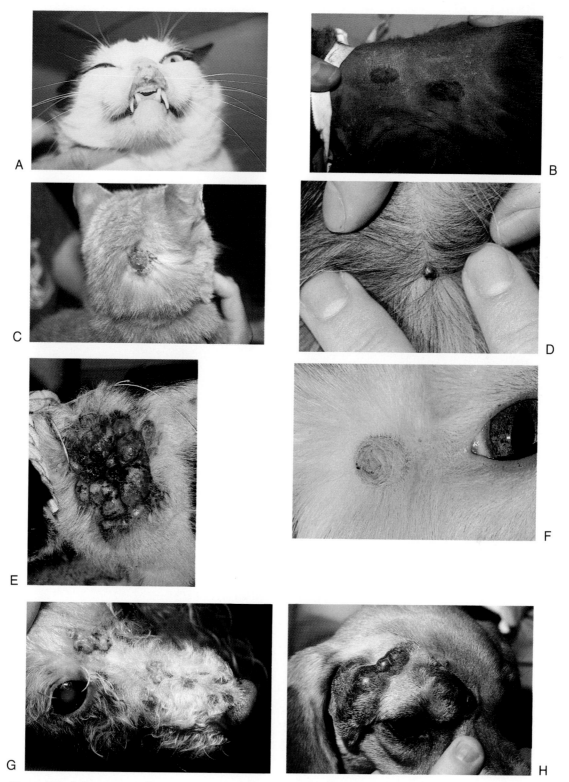

Figure 19:8. *A*, Squamous cell carcinoma on the upper lip of a cat. The carcinoma arose from a long-standing indolent ulcer. *B*, Bowen's disease in a cat. Multiple hyperpigmented, hyperkeratotic plaques over the shoulder (the area has been clipped). *C*, Basal cell tumor on the neck of a cat. *D*, Melanotic basal cell tumor on the rump of a cat. *E*, Multilobulated malignant trichoepithelioma over the lateral neck and shoulder of a dog. *F*, Dilated pore of Winer near the lateral canthus of a cat. Keratinous mass projecting from a surface pore. *G*, Multiple sebaceous gland hyperplasias on the face of a dog. *H*, Melanotic sebaceous epithelioma over the eye of a dog.

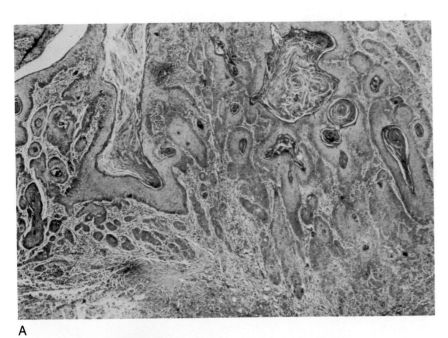

A

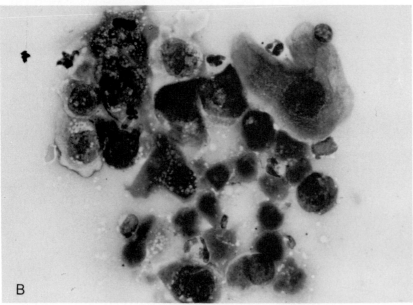

B

Figure 19:9 *A,* Canine squamous cell carcinoma. Irregular proliferation of keratinocytes with dermal invasion. *B,* Canine squamous cell carcinoma. Cytologic examination of aspirate shows a cluster of atypical keratinocytes. (Courtesy T. French.)

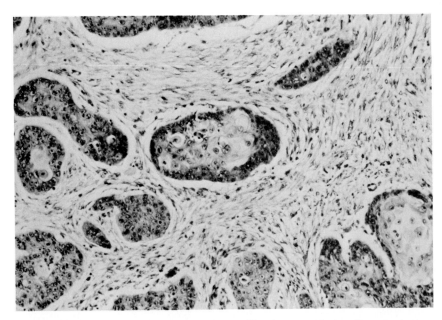

Figure 19:10. Canine squamous cell carcinoma. Note horn pearls, keratinocyte atypia, and desmoplasia.

dynamic therapy was successful in 63 per cent of feline nasal and aural squamous cell carcinomas.[96a] Chemotherapy with bleomycin, vincristine, hydroxyurea, cisplatin, benzaldehyde, thioproline, and oral retinoids has been generally ineffective.[11–13, 82, 84, 91, 92] In cats, the development of new squamous cell carcinomas is common because of continuing ultraviolet light exposure.[82a]

Multicentric Squamous Cell Carcinoma In Situ

CAUSE AND PATHOGENESIS

Multicentric squamous cell carcinoma in situ (Bowen's disease) is rare (in cats) to very rare (in dogs).[5, 80a, 86, 94] Exposure to ultraviolet light and arsenic are not causal factors.[94] Papillomavirus antigen has been demonstrated in the feline skin lesions by immunohistochemical methods.[94a] Thus, these carcinoma in situ lesions may be a malignant transformation of the viral papillomas described in cats.

CLINICAL FINDINGS

The condition is seen in older cats (10 years of age or older) and dogs. Lesions are multifocal, and in cats they occur most commonly over the head, neck, shoulder, and forelimbs.[80a, 94] Most lesions have occurred in thickly haired and darkly pigmented skin. They are initially characterized by well-circumscribed, melanotic, hyperkeratotic macules and plaques, 0.5 to 3 cm in diameter (see Fig. 19:8 *B*). Some lesions become almost verrucous. Later, the lesions become thick, crusted, ulcerated plaques, which tend to bleed easily. In dogs, the oral mucosa and the genitalia may be involved, and nodules may be seen in addition to the lesions described above for cats.[5, 86]

DIAGNOSIS

Histopathologically, well-circumscribed areas of irregular epidermal and superficial follicular hyperplasia and dysplasia are seen (Fig. 19:11).[5, 80a, 94] Keratinocyte size and appearance are

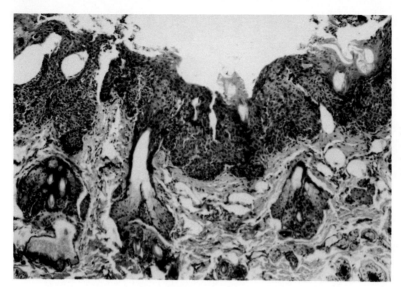

Figure 19:11. Bowen's disease in a cat. Marked dysplasia of the epidermis and follicular outer root sheaths.

highly variable, and mitotic figures are common in all cell layers. Orthokeratotic to parakeratotic hyperkeratosis is common, and a lichenoid inflammatory infiltrate may be seen. Immunohistochemical studies have demonstrated papillomavirus antigen within these lesions in cats.[94a]

CLINICAL MANAGEMENT

The mean course of disease, before animals are euthanized because of cosmetic concerns and owner frustration, is more than 2 years. No metastases have been recorded, although a footpad lesion invaded contiguous bone in one dog.[86] Lesions may wax and wane in size or, in some instances, individual lesions may disappear. However, multiple lesions are always present.

In dogs, the topical application of 5-fluorouracil caused regression of some lesions.[86] In cats, ^{90}Sr plesiotherapy (β-irradiation) was effective in healing thin lesions (less than 2 to 4 mm in thickness).[94] However, new lesions continued to develop, and thicker plaques did not respond. The oral administration of isotretinoin was ineffective in one cat.[94] In many instances, in otherwise healthy, asymptomatic animals, observation without therapy may be the most practical approach.

Basal Cell Tumors

The term *basal cell tumor* has been used in the veterinary literature to classify a large group of common neoplasms of dogs and cats presumed to be derived from basal epithelial cells of both epidermal and adnexal origin. Numerous histopathologic subclassifications have been applied to these neoplasms: medusa head, garland or ribbon, trabecular, solid, cystic, adenoid, basosquamous, and granular cell. In general, these various histopathologic types are often found within the same neoplasm and offer no useful clinical, prognostic, or therapeutic information.[27] Most veterinary basal cell tumors are benign and are *not* contiguous with the basal cell layer of the epidermis (medusa head, garland or ribbon, trabecular, adenoid, and granular cell types); these lesions generally show differentiation toward follicular structures and have been reclassified (see below).[5] The subclassifications solid basal cell tumor and basosquamous basal cell tumor are reported to be biologically aggressive in some instances; most of these lesions are probably true basal cell carcinomas.[5] The term basal cell tumor, borrowed from human dermatopathology, is now considered synonymous with basal cell carcinoma of low-grade malignancy. Some authors prefer the terms basal cell epithelioma and basaloma, both of which indicate the relatively good prognosis of the neoplasm.[5]

In conclusion, the term basal cell tumor appears to have limited usage in veterinary medicine and is retained for an uncommon, true basal cell neoplasm of cats that has no obvious adnexal features.[5]

BENIGN FELINE BASAL CELL TUMOR

■ *Cause and Pathogenesis.* These tumors are uncommon benign neoplasms of the cat that are thought to arise from the basal cells of the epidermis. The entire basal cell tumor category accounted for 11 to 30 per cent of all feline skin tumors in multiple surveys.* It is impossible to determine what proportion of these represents benign feline basal cell tumor.[5] The cause of basal cell tumors in cats is unknown. In humans, there is a strong correlation between exposure to ultraviolet light and the development of basal cell tumors.[3]

■ *Clinical Findings.* Basal cell tumors occur in adult cats with no sex predilection. Himalayan and Persian cats may be predisposed.[4] Usually, basal cell tumors are solitary, but they may occasionally be multiple.[77] The most common sites of occurrence are the head, the neck (Fig. 19:8C), the limbs, and the dorsal trunk.[4, 5] Basal cell tumors are usually firm, rounded, elevated, and well circumscribed; they are situated at the dermal-epidermal junction and are usually 1 to 2 cm in diameter. They are often melanotic (Fig. 19:8 D) and are frequently ulcerated and alopecic.

■ *Diagnosis.* Histopathologically, basal cell tumors are characterized by a well-circumscribed, symmetric proliferation of basaloid cells that has a fairly broad zone of connection to the overlying epidermis (Fig. 19:12 A and B).[4, 5] The tumor often has a lima bean–shaped silhouette, with the central indentation at the tumor surface. The basaloid cells are arranged in tightly packed lobules and trabeculae.

---

*See references 14, 18–21, 26, 29, 34, 38, and 76.

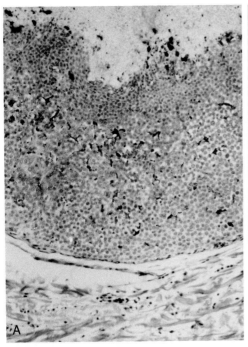

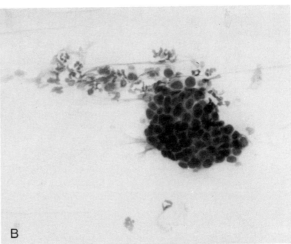

Figure 19:12 *A,* Feline basal cell tumor. Proliferation of basaloid cells and melanocytes. *B,* Feline basal cell tumor. Cytologic examination of aspirate shows typical clusters of monomorphic basaloid cells.

■ *Clinical Management.* Clinical management of basal cell tumors may include surgical excision, cryotherapy, electrosurgery, and observation without treatment.[11–13]

BASAL CELL CARCINOMA

■ *Cause and Pathogenesis.* Basal cell carcinomas are common (in cats) to uncommon (in dogs) low-grade malignancies arising from small, pluripotential epithelial cells within the basal cell layers of the epidermis and adnexae.[5, 9] Numerical incidence data are difficult to provide, because these neoplasms have been traditionally included in the broad category of basal cell tumor (see above). The cause of basal cell carcinomas in dogs and cats is unknown. In humans, there is a strong correlation between ultraviolet light exposure and the development of basal cell carcinomas.[3, 9]

■ *Clinical Findings.* Basal cell carcinomas occur in dogs and cats at an average age of 7 to 10 years and with no sex predilection.* Siamese cats, Cocker spaniels, Kerry blue terriers, Shetland sheepdogs, Siberian huskies, English Springer spaniels, and Poodles appear to be predisposed.† The tumors occur most commonly on the head, the neck, and the thorax. In cats, lesions occasionally occur on the nasal planum or the eyelids. Basal cell carcinomas are usually solitary, well circumscribed, firm to cystic, rounded, 0.5 to 10 cm in diameter, and commonly alopecic and ulcerated. Basal cell carcinomas are frequently melanotic.

■ *Diagnosis.* Three major histopathologic variants of basal cell carcinoma occur in dogs and cats: solid, keratinizing (basosquamous), and clear cell.[4, 5] *Solid basal cell carcinoma* is the most common subtype in cats and is characterized by circumscribed, irregular dermal masses comprising multiple basaloid cell aggregates embedded in a moderate stroma (desmoplasia). Mitotic activity is low to high, and atypical mitotic figures are common. Variable secondary features include cyst formation, melanization, adnexal differentiation, mucinosis, artifactual cleft formation between stroma and neoplastic cells, and cartilaginous metaplasia.[5, 9, 75]

Keratinizing basal cell carcinoma (basosquamous carcinoma) is the most common type in dogs and is characterized by an irregular dermal mass of basaloid cells having a plaquelike configuration, multifocal epidermal contiguity, and multiple areas of abrupt squamous differentiation and keratinization.[5]

Clear cell basal cell carcinoma is rare and is more commonly encountered in cats.[5] The overall architecture is identical to that of solid basal cell carcinoma, but the epithelial cells are large and polygonal and have water-clear or finely granular cytoplasm. Basal cell carcinomas are positive for cytokeratin.[45, 47, 56, 57] Papillomavirus antigen was not detected in feline basal cell carcinomas.[67]

■ *Clinical Management.* Clinical management of basal cell carcinomas may include surgical excision, electrosurgery, cryosurgery, and observation without therapy.[11–13] The incidence of recurrence and metastasis is very low.[75a] In humans, intralesional injections of interferon have been used to treat basal cell carcinoma.[79]

Hair Follicle Tumors

Previous surveys of hair follicle neoplasms in dogs and cats indicated that these neoplasms account for about 5 per cent and 1 per cent, respectively, of all skin neoplasms seen in these species.‡ The most common subtypes were trichoepithelioma and pilomatrixoma.[103] With the

---

*See references 4, 5, 11–13, 18, 29, 34, and 76.
†See references 4, 11–13, 18, 19, 76, and 80.
‡See references 18, 19, 21, 26, 27, 32, 103, and 104.

reclassification of so-called basal cell tumors (see above), it appears that the majority of previous reports of these neoplasms were examples of trichoblastoma.[5] Thus, neoplasms of hair follicle origin are much more common than previous veterinary literature suggested. Hair follicle tumors are positive for cytokeratin.[45]

TRICHOEPITHELIOMA

■ *Cause and Pathogenesis.* Trichoepitheliomas are uncommon benign neoplasms of dogs and cats that are thought to arise from keratinocytes that differentiate toward all three segments of the hair follicle.[4, 5, 32, 103] The cause of trichoepitheliomas in dogs and cats is unknown. In humans, a syndrome of multiple trichoepitheliomas is hereditary.[3, 9]

Usually, trichoepitheliomas occur in dogs and cats older than 5 years of age. No sex predilection appears to exist in either species. In cats, there is a predilection for Persians, and the neoplasms occur most commonly on the head, the limbs, and the tail.[4, 104] In dogs, there may be a predilection for the dorsal lumbar (see Fig. 19:8 *E*) and lateral thoracic and limb areas, and Golden retrievers, Basset hounds, German shepherd dogs, Cocker spaniels, Irish setters, English Springer spaniels, Miniature Schnauzers, and Standard Poodles may be predisposed.[4, 103]

Although these neoplasms are usually solitary, they may occasionally be multiple. They are solid or cystic, rounded, elevated, well circumscribed, and dermal-epidermal in position, ranging from 0.5 to 15 cm in diameter. Frequently, they become ulcerated and alopecic. Trichoepitheliomas are rarely invasive or metastatic.[11]

■ *Diagnosis.* Histopathologically, trichoepitheliomas vary considerably, depending on the degree of differentiation and whether the tumor is primarily related to the follicular sheath or the hair matrix (Fig. 19:13).[4, 32, 103] Frequent characteristics include horn cysts, lack of intercellular bridges (desmosomes), differentiation toward hair follicle–like structures, formation of abortive or rudimentary hairs, desmoplasia, inflammation, melanization, and shadow (ghost) cells.[103] Dystrophic mineralization or malignant transformation may be seen in up to 18 per

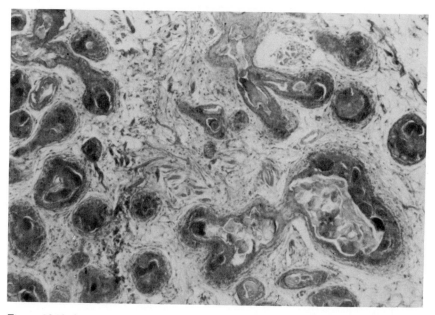

Figure 19:13. Canine trichoepithelioma. Disorganized proliferation of hair follicle–like structures and hairs.

cent of the cases.[103] A variant showing marked mucinous degeneration is most common in Golden retrievers.[103]

■ *Clinical Management.* Clinical management of trichoepitheliomas may include surgical excision, cryotherapy, electrosurgery, and observation without treatment.[11–13] Recurrence and metastasis are rare, in spite of histopathologic evidence of malignancy.[4, 103]

TRICHOLEMMOMA

■ *Cause and Pathogenesis.* Tricholemmomas are rare benign neoplasms of dogs and cats that arise from keratinocytes of the outer root sheath of hair follicles.[4, 5, 100, 103, 104] The cause of tricholemmomas is unknown. In humans, a syndrome of multiple tricholemmomas is hereditary.[3, 9]

■ *Clinical Findings.* In dogs, tricholemmomas occur at 5 to 13 years of age. There appears to be no sex predilection, but Afghan hounds may be predisposed. These neoplasms occur most commonly on the head and neck and are usually firm, ovoid, and 1 to 7 cm in diameter.

■ *Diagnosis.* Histopathologically, tricholemmomas are characterized by a nodular proliferation of keratinocytes, many of which are clear and have a positive reaction with periodic acid–Schiff (PAS) stain owing to their glycogen content (Fig. 19:14). The tumor lobules are surrounded by a distinct, often thickened basement membrane zone.

■ *Clinical Management.* Clinical management of tricholemmomas may include surgical excision, cryotherapy, electrosurgery, and observation without treatment.[11, 13, 103, 104]

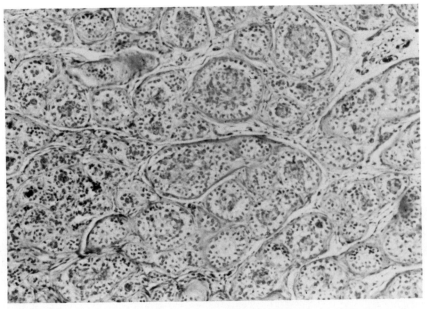

Figure 19:14. Canine tricholemmoma. Proliferation of predominantly clear, outer root sheath–like keratinocytes. Individual nodules are often surrounded by a distinct, thick basement membrane zone.

TRICHOFOLLICULOMA

■ *Cause and Pathogenesis.* Trichofolliculomas are rare benign neoplasms of dogs that are highly structured hamartomas of the pilosebaceous unit.[5, 9, 103] The cause of trichofolliculomas is unknown.

■ *Clinical Findings.* Trichofolliculomas occur in adult dogs with no apparent age, breed, sex, or site predilections. The lesions are solitary, dome-shaped, firm papules or nodules, often containing a central depression or pore that may exude sebaceous material or contain a tuft of hairs.

■ *Diagnosis.* Histopathologically, trichofolliculomas are characterized by a central large dilated or cystic follicle with smaller follicles or follicle-like structures that radiate outward from the central follicle into the surrounding connective tissue in an arborizing pattern (Fig. 19:15).

■ *Clinical Management.* Clinical management may include surgical excision and observation without treatment.[11, 103]

DILATED PORE OF WINER

■ *Cause and Pathogenesis.* Dilated pore of Winer is an uncommon benign follicular tumor of cats.[5, 102] The cause of this lesion is unknown, although most evidence favors a developmental

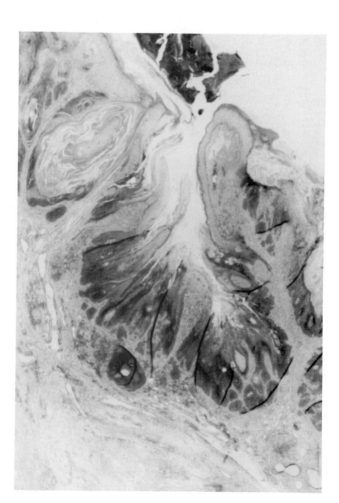

Figure 19:15. Canine trichofolliculoma. Central large hair follicle with numerous smaller abortive hair follicles radiating into the surrounding dermis.

origin arising from the combined forces of obstruction and intrafollicular pressure leading to hair follicle hyperplasia.

■ *Clinical Findings.* Dilated pore is seen in older cats with no apparent breed or sex predilection. The lesions are solitary and occur most frequently on the neck and the head (see Fig. 19:8*F*).[102] They are characterized by a well-demarcated, smooth, dermal-epidermal cyst-like structure with a central, keratin-filled wide-mouthed pore.

■ *Diagnosis.* Histopathologically, this disorder is characterized by a markedly dilated, keratinized, pilar infundibulum lined by an epithelium that is atrophic near the ostium but increasingly hyperplastic toward the base of the lesion (Fig. 19:16). The epithelium at the base shows psoriasiform hyperplasia with rete ridges and irregular, thin projections into the surrounding dermis (Fig. 19:17).

■ *Clinical Management.* Clinical management includes surgical excision and observation without treatment.

WARTY DYSKERATOMA

■ *Cause and Pathogenesis.* Warty dyskeratoma is a rare, benign, epithelial proliferation of dogs.[11, 101] Although warty dyskeratoma is believed by many investigators to arise from pilosebaceous structures, its occurrence in the oral cavity of humans has challenged traditional interpretations.[9]

■ *Clinical Findings.* Warty dyskeratoma occurs in dogs, but too few cases have been recognized to infer age, breed, sex, or site predilections. The lesions are solitary, wartlike papules or nodules with a hyperkeratotic umbilicated center.

■ *Diagnosis.* Histopathologically, warty dyskeratoma is characterized by a cup-shaped invagination connected with the surface by a keratin-filled channel (Fig. 19:18). The large invagina-

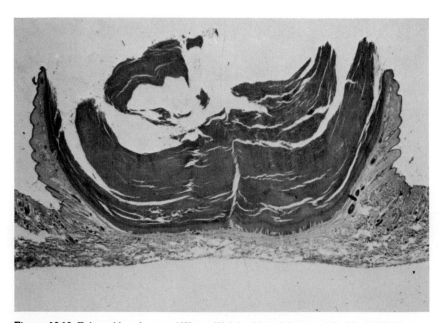

Figure 19:16. Feline dilated pore of Winer. Widely dilated, keratin-filled hair follicle.

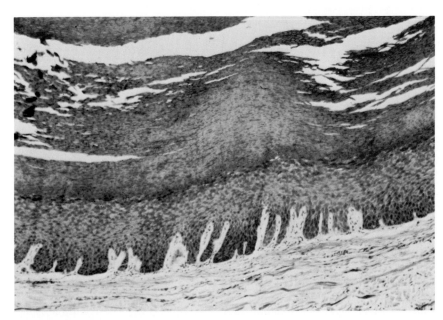

Figure 19:17. Close-up of Figure 19:16. The base of the lesion shows characteristic psoriasiform epithelial hyperplasia.

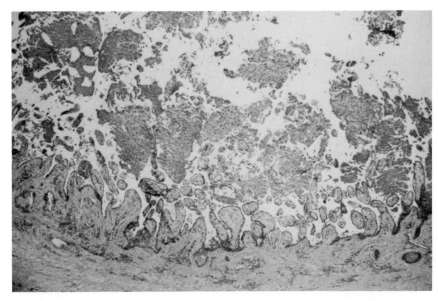

Figure 19:18. Canine warty dyskeratoma. The base of a keratin-filled mass shows multiple villi.

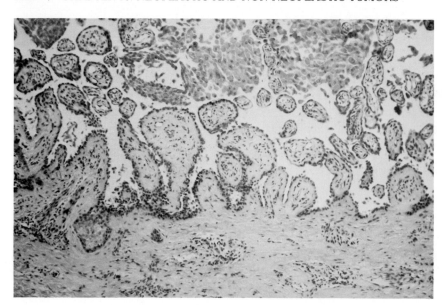

Figure 19:19. Close-up of Figure 19:18. Basal villi with a single layer of attached keratinocytes.

tion contains numerous acantholytic, dyskeratotic cells (Fig. 19:19). The lower portion of the invagination is occupied by numerous villi (elongated dermal papillae lined with a single layer of basal cells) (Fig. 19:20). Typical corps rounds (dyskeratotic acanthocytes with a pyknotic nucleus surrounded by a clear halo) can usually be found.

■ *Clinical Management.* Clinical management of warty dyskeratoma may include surgical excision and observation without treatment.

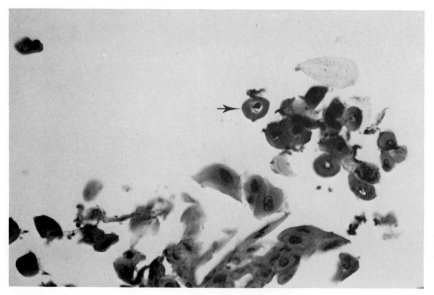

Figure 19:20. Close-up of Figure 19:18. Acantholytic cells and typical corps ronds (arrow).

PILOMATRIXOMA

■ *Cause and Pathogenesis.* Pilomatrixomas (pilomatricomas, or calcifying epitheliomas [of Malherbe]) are uncommon (in dogs) to rare (in cats) neoplasms and are thought to arise from the hair matrix.[4, 5, 9, 103, 104] The cause of pilomatrixomas is unknown.

■ *Clinical Findings.* Pilomatrixomas usually occur in dogs and cats older than 5 years of age.[4, 19, 103, 104, 106] There is no apparent sex predilection. Kerry blue terriers, Poodles, and Old English sheepdogs appear to be predisposed. Usually, pilomatrixomas are solitary. There may be site predilection to shoulders, lateral thorax, and back. Pilomatrixomas are solid to cystic, rounded, elevated, well circumscribed, and dermal to subcutaneous in position, and they range from 1 to 10 cm in diameter. They frequently become ulcerated and alopecic. Pilomatrixomas are rarely invasive or metastatic (matrical carcinoma).[4, 5, 10, 103, 105]

■ *Diagnosis.* Histopathologically, pilomatrixomas are characterized by a well-circumscribed, cystic, multilobulated, deep dermal to subcutaneous proliferation of basophilic cells (which resemble hair matrix cells) and shadow, or ghost, cells (fully keratinized, faintly eosinophilic cells with a central, unstained nucleus) (Fig. 19:21).[32, 103] Shadow cells are not pathognomonic, having been found in other hair follicle neoplasms, various keratinizing cysts, inflamed hair follicles, and chronic hyperkeratotic dermatoses.[11, 103] There is abrupt keratinization (no stratum granulosum), and the keratin is homogeneous, relatively amorphous, and nonfibrillar (tricho-lemmal keratin). A constant feature of pilomatrixomas is the occurrence of multiple dermal papilla-like structures within the basaloid cellular component (Fig. 19:22).[103] Other frequent but not constant features of pilomatrixomas are calcification within the areas of shadow cells, desmoplasia, and inflammation.[103]

■ *Clinical Management.* Clinical management of pilomatrixomas may include surgical excision, cryotherapy, and observation without treatment.[11–13, 103, 104]

TRICHOBLASTOMA

■ *Cause and Pathogenesis.* Trichoblastomas are common, usually benign neoplasms in dogs and cats, which are presumably derived from trichoblastic (primitive hair germ) epithelium.[5, 6, 9]

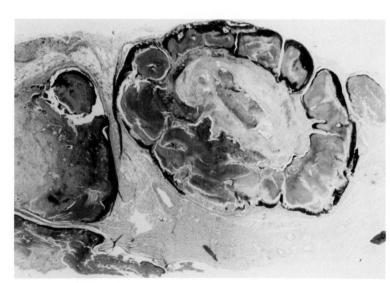

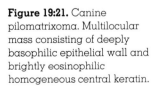

Figure 19:21. Canine pilomatrixoma. Multilocular mass consisting of deeply basophilic epithelial wall and brightly eosinophilic homogeneous central keratin.

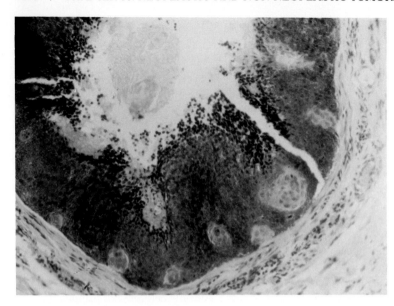

Figure 19:22. Close-up of Figure 19:21. Multiple dermal papilla-like structures within the basaloid wall of a neoplasm.

The incidence of these tumors in dogs is probably close to that previously reported under the term basal cell tumor (see above).[5] The incidence in cats is harder to estimate because cats have several types of neoplasms that are composed of small basaloid epithelial cells (to include benign feline basal cell tumor, apocrine ductular sweat gland neoplasms, and primitive hair follicle neoplasms).[5] The cause of trichoblastomas is unknown.

■ *Clinical Findings.* Trichoblastomas occur in dogs and cats older than 5 years of age.[5] No sex predilection is evident, but Poodles and Cocker spaniels may be overrepresented. Lesions are usually solitary, dome shaped, firm, 1 to 2 cm in diameter, and often alopecic, ulcerated, and melanotic. In dogs, lesions occur most commonly on the head and the neck, especially the base of the ear. In cats, lesions occur most commonly on the cranial half of the trunk. Metastasis is extremely rare.[100a]

■ *Diagnosis.* Trichoblastomas occur in three basic histopathologic subtypes: ribbon (garland, or medusa head), trabecular, and granular cell.[5] The ribbon type is most common in dogs, and characterized by basaloid cells arranged in branching, winding, and radiating columns with no epidermal contiguity (Fig. 19:23).[5] The trabecular type is most common in cats and is characterized by lobules and broad trabeculae of basaloid cells with prominent peripheral palisading and no epidermal contiguity.[5] The granular cell type is rare and is architecturally identical to the ribbon type of trichoblastoma, but many of the epithelial aggregates are composed entirely of larger cells with granular or vacuolated cytoplasm.[5, 78]

■ *Clinical Management.* Clinical management of trichoblastomas may include surgical excision, cryotherapy, and observation without treatment.[11–13]

Sebaceous Gland Tumors

CAUSE AND PATHOGENESIS

Sebaceous gland tumors are common (in dogs) to uncommon (in cats) epithelial growths arising from sebocytes.[4, 5, 19, 107–111] Their cause is unknown.

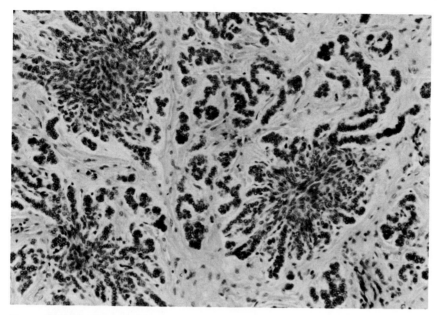

Figure 19:23. Canine trichoblastoma. Ribbon or medusoid type.

CLINICAL FINDINGS

Dog

Sebaceous gland tumors are common in dogs, accounting for 6 to 21 per cent of all canine skin tumors in multiple surveys.[107, 108] Affected dogs average 9 to 10 years of age, and there is no sex predilection. *Nodular sebaceous hyperplasias* account for about 53 per cent of the lesions and occur most commonly in beagles, Cocker spaniels, Poodles, dachshunds, and Miniature Schnauzers.[4, 108] The lesions are usually solitary (about 70 per cent of cases), well circumscribed, raised, smooth and greasy to hyperkeratotic, wartlike or cauliflower-like in appearance, pinkish to orangish, 3 mm to 7 cm in diameter, and frequently melanotic or ulcerated (see Fig. 19:8 *G*).[108] They occur most commonly on the limbs, the trunk, and the eyelids.

Sebaceous epitheliomas (basal cell carcinoma with sebaceous differentiation) account for about 37 per cent of sebaceous gland tumors and occur most commonly in Shih tzus, Lhasa apsos, Malamutes, Siberian huskies, and Irish setters.[108] The lesions are usually solitary (about 67 per cent of cases), well circumscribed, raised, smooth, and greasy to hyperkeratotic, wartlike or cauliflower-like in appearance, pinkish to orangish, 5 mm to 5 cm in diameter, and frequently ulcerated or melanotic.[108] They occur most commonly on the eyelids and the head (see Fig. 19:8 *H*).

Sebaceous adenomas account for about 8 per cent of sebaceous gland tumors and occur most commonly on the eyelids and the limbs (Fig. 19:24 *A*).[108] The appearance of the lesions is as described for sebaceous hyperplasia and sebaceous epithelioma (see above).

Sebaceous carcinoma accounts for only about 2 per cent of the tumors.[108] Lesions are solitary, nodular, 2.5 to 7.5 cm in diameter, and frequently ulcerated (Fig. 19:24 *B*). The head and the limbs are most commonly affected.[4] Cocker spaniels may be predisposed.[4]

Cat

Sebaceous gland tumors are uncommon in cats, accounting for about 3 per cent of all feline skin tumors.[4, 19, 109] Affected cats are usually 10 years of age or older; there is no apparent sex

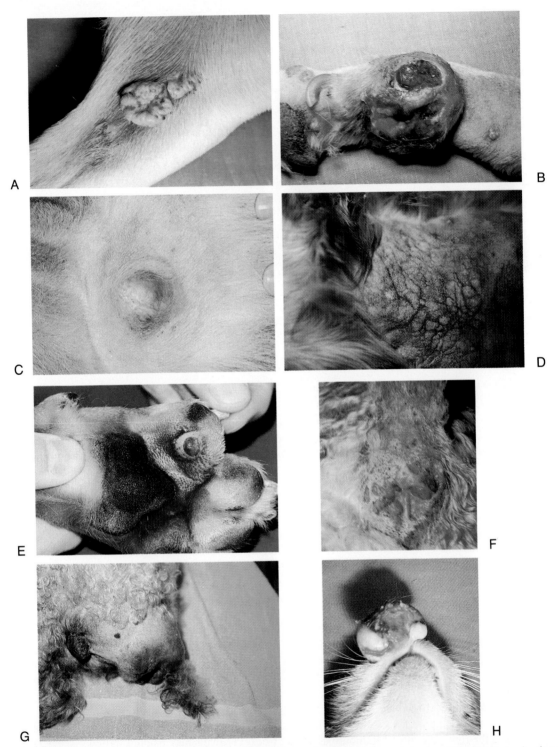

Figure 19:24. A, Sebaceous adenoma on the medial limb of a dog. B, Sebaceous carcinoma on the limb of a dog. C, Apocrine adenoma over the thorax of a dog. D, Apocrine carcinoma over the lateral neck and shoulder of a dog. E, Eccrine adenoma on the footpad of a dog. F, Hepatoid gland adenoma in the perianal region of a dog. G, Hepatoid gland carcinoma in a dog. H, Fibroma on the nose of a cat.

predilection. Persians may be predisposed.[4] Lesions are usually solitary and occur most commonly on the head, the neck, and the trunk. They are well circumscribed, raised, smooth and greasy to hyperkeratotic, wartlike to cauliflower-like in appearance, pinkish to orangish, and 0.5 to 1 cm in diameter. Nodular sebaceous hyperplasia accounts for about 67 per cent of all feline sebaceous gland tumors.[19, 109]

DIAGNOSIS

Histopathologically, sebaceous gland tumors are classified as nodular sebaceous hyperplasia (greatly enlarged sebaceous glands composed of numerous lobules grouped symmetrically around centrally located sebaceous ducts) (Fig. 19:25 *A* and *B*); sebaceous adenoma (lobules of sebaceous cells of irregular shape and size, which are asymmetrically arranged and well demarcated from the surrounding tissue and contain mostly mature sebocytes and fewer undifferentiated germinative cells); sebaceous epithelioma (tumor similar to basal cell tumor but containing mostly undifferentiated germinative cells and fewer mature sebocytes) (Fig. 19:26); and sebaceous carcinoma (tumor with pleomorphism and atypia) (Fig. 19:27).[5, 32, 108, 109] In a study, about 81 per cent of sebaceous epitheliomas and 54 per cent of sebaceous adenomas in dogs had areas of sebaceous hyperplasia peripheral to and often phasing into epitheliomatous or adenomatous areas, suggesting that sebaceous hyperplasia may be a precursor to the other lesions.[108] Sebaceous gland tumors are positive for cytokeratin.[45]

CLINICAL MANAGEMENT

Clinical management of sebaceous gland tumors may include surgical excision, cryotherapy, electrosurgery, and observation without treatment.[11, 13] Sebaceous gland neoplasms rarely recur after surgery, and sebaceous carcinomas rarely metastasize.[108, 109] Oral retinoids have been an effective treatment of sebaceous hyperplasia in humans[3] and a small number of dogs.[70, 72] Neither in dogs nor in cats were any clinical variables found to be useful predictors of the histopathologic type of sebaceous gland abnormality.[108, 109]

Sweat Gland Tumors

CAUSE AND PATHOGENESIS

Apocrine sweat gland tumors are uncommon growths in the dog and cat arising from the glandular or ductular components of apocrine sweat glands.[4, 5, 19, 27, 32, 114] Eccrine sweat gland tumors are rare in dogs and cats.[5, 19, 27, 32] The cause of sweat gland tumors is unknown.

CLINICAL FINDINGS

Dog

Apocrine sweat gland tumors may be benign or malignant in the dog.[4, 114] However, no clinical features are consistently helpful in distinguishing histologically benign from histologically malignant tumors.[114] These neoplasms generally occur in dogs that are 10 years of age or older, with no apparent sex predilection. Golden retrievers, Cocker spaniels, and German shepherd dogs may be predisposed.[4, 11, 114] Apocrine sweat gland neoplasms are usually solitary (about 93 per cent of cases), well circumscribed, firm, raised, 0.5 to 10 cm in diameter, and frequently ulcerated. Some tumors may be cystic and have a bluish or purplish tint when viewed through the overlying skin (see Fig. 19:24 *C*). Lesions occur most commonly on the neck, the head, the dorsal trunk, and the limbs.[4, 5, 27, 32, 114] Some apocrine sweat gland carcinomas are poorly circumscribed, infiltrative, plaquelike or ulcerative growths (see Fig. 19:24 *D*), especially in the

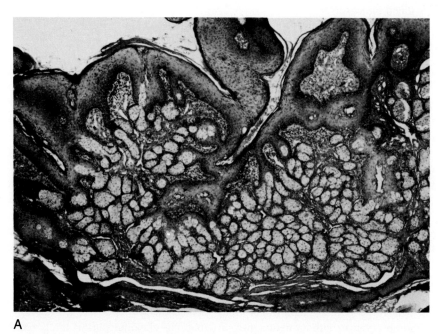

A

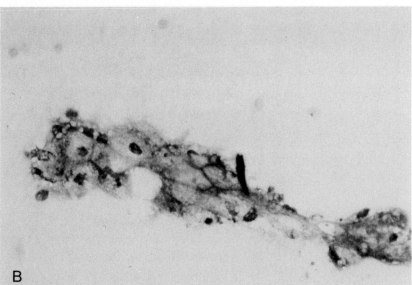

B

Figure 19:25. *A,* Nodular sebaceous hyperplasia in a dog. *B,* Nodular sebaceous hyperplasia in a dog. Cytologic examination of aspirate shows the typical clustering of highly lipidized sebocytes.

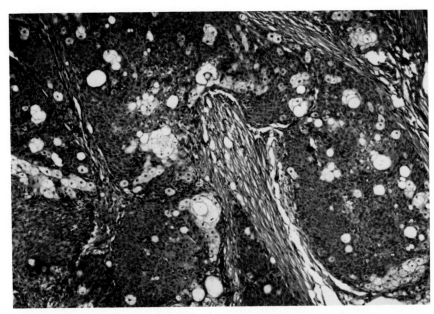

Figure 19:26. Canine sebaceous epithelioma. Proliferation of basaloid cells with frequent sebaceous differentiation.

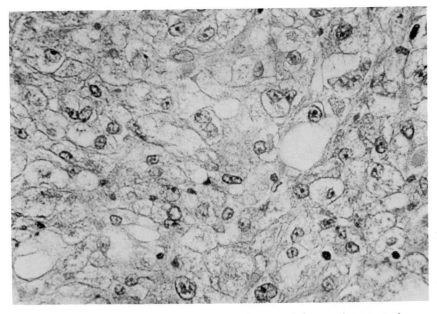

Figure 19:27. Canine sebaceous carcinoma. Proliferation of pleomorphic, atypical sebocytes.

ventral abdomen, proximal limb, or neck area, which may be misdiagnosed as pyotraumatic dermatitis or staphylococcal dermatitis.

Eccrine sweat gland tumors may be benign or malignant and are extremely rare.[5, 11, 27] The lesions are solitary, firm, well to poorly circumscribed, frequently ulcerated, and 1 to 3 cm in diameter; they occur on the footpads (see Fig. 19:24 *E*). Eccrine sweat gland carcinomas may present as a poorly defined swelling of the footpad and the digit.

Cat

Apocrine sweat gland tumors may be benign or malignant in cats.[4, 114] However, no clinical features are consistently helpful in distinguishing histologically benign from histologically malignant neoplasms.[114] These neoplasms generally occur in cats that are 10 years of age or older, with no apparent breed or sex predilection. Apocrine sweat gland carcinomas may be more frequent in the Siamese.[4] Apocrine sweat gland tumors are usually solitary (about 100 per cent of cases), well circumscribed, firm, raised, 0.3 to 3 cm in diameter, and frequently ulcerated. Some lesions may be cystic and have a bluish or purplish tint when viewed through the overlying skin. Lesions occur most commonly on the head (especially the cheek), the pinna, the neck, the axilla, the limb, and the tail.[4, 5, 19, 27, 29, 114] Dry gangrene and sloughing of the claws and distal phalanges on all paws was reported in a cat with metastatic apocrine sweat gland carcinoma.[115]

Eccrine sweat gland tumors are almost always malignant in cats and are extremely rare.[5, 19] Eccrine sweat gland carcinomas usually present as poorly defined swellings of the footpad and the digit and may affect multiple digits in cats. Ulceration is common.

DIAGNOSIS

The literature on histopathologic classification of sweat gland neoplasms is confusing and includes numerous subtypes: cystadenoma, glandular adenoma, ductular adenoma, syringoadenoma, spiradenoma, cylindroma, hidradenoma papilliferum, and carcinoma (solitary, papillary, tubular, glandular, ductular, mixed, clear cell, signet-ring) (Figs. 19:28 to 19:31).[4, 5, 10–12, 112–114]

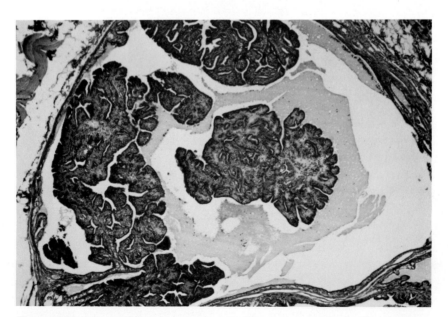

Figure 19:28. Feline papillary cystadenoma. Papillary processes, lined with a single row of cuboidal to columnar apocrine sweat gland cells, projecting into a cyst cavity containing amorphous secretory material.

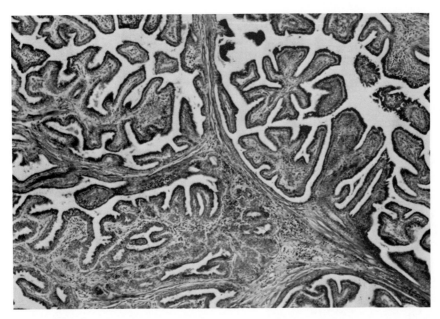

Figure 19:29. Canine papillary syringadenoma.

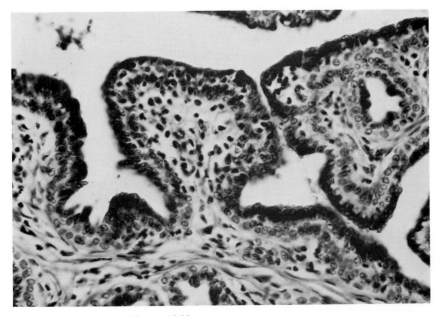

Figure 19:30. Close-up of Figure 19:29.

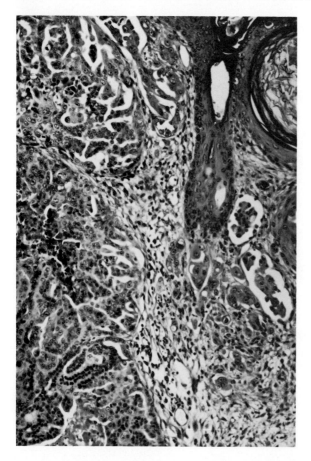

Figure 19:31. Canine apocrine carcinoma. Proliferation of atypical apocrine sweat gland cells in cords and glandular structures, with lymphatic invasion (right).

The clinical significance of these various histologic types is unknown. In one retrospective study, most apocrine sweat gland neoplasms in dogs (91 per cent) and cats (80 per cent) were histologically malignant.[114] Most carcinomas were the solid type, and there was no apparent relationship between the histopathologic subtype and clinical variables. In dogs, about 22 per cent of carcinomas showed lymphatic invasion (Fig. 19:32), and cartilaginous or osseous metaplasia was rarely seen. Apocrine sweat gland neoplasms are positive for cytokeratin.[45, 49]

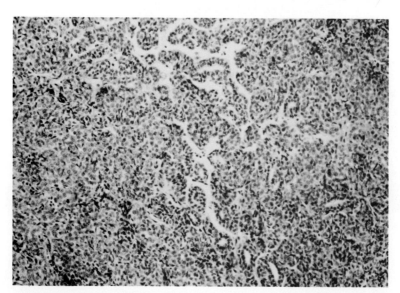

Figure 19:32. Canine eccrine adenoma.

Carcinomas, but not adenomas, were positive for carcinoembryonic antigen (in secretory cells) and vimentin (in myoepithelial cells).[49]

CLINICAL MANAGEMENT

Clinical management of sweat gland tumors may include surgical excision, cryosurgery, electrosurgery, and observation without treatment.[11–13] Although apocrine sweat gland carcinomas are occasionally reported to be highly invasive and rapidly metastatic,[12, 27, 32, 34] no instances of metastasis were documented in one retrospective study,[114] even though about 22 per cent of cases had histologically evident lymphatic invasion. Eccrine sweat gland carcinomas are aggressive and exhibit rapid metastasis to regional lymph nodes and subcutaneous tissues of the affected limb.[5]

Perianal Gland Tumors

CAUSE AND PATHOGENESIS

Perianal gland tumors, which are common in the dog, arise most frequently from hepatoid glands (perianal or circumanal glands and modified sebaceous glands) and less commonly from anal sac glands (apocrine glands of the anal sacs).* The cause of perianal gland tumors is unknown. However, the hepatoid glands and their tumors are known to be modulated by sex hormones.

CLINICAL FINDINGS

Hepatoid gland tumors occur in dogs at an average age of 11 years. Adenomas are about nine times more frequent in male than in female dogs. Carcinomas occur with equal frequency in male and female dogs. Cocker spaniels, English bulldogs, Samoyeds, Afghans, dachshunds, German shepherd dogs, beagles, Siberian huskies, Shih tzus, and Lhasa apsos are predisposed to the development of hepatoid gland tumors. Apocrine neoplasms of anal sac origin are most common in old female dogs and are often associated with pseudohyperparathyroidism.[4, 11–13, 116] Hepatoid gland neoplasms may be solitary or multiple. Most occur adjacent to the anus, but they may occur on the tail, perineum, prepuce, thigh, and dorsal lumbosacral area. The smaller (less than 1 cm in diameter) neoplasms are spherical or ovoid and tend to become multinodular and ulcerated as they become larger (up to 10 cm in diameter). Perianal neoplasms are usually firm, dermal-epidermal in location, and well circumscribed to poorly circumscribed.

Nodular hepatoid gland hyperplasia may occur as multiple discrete nodules of varying size that are impossible to distinguish from hepatoid gland adenomas (see Fig. 19:24 *F*) or as a diffuse bulging ring around the anus (Fig. 19:33). Most hepatoid gland tumors are benign.

Hepatoid gland carcinomas (see Fig. 19:24 *G*) tend to grow more rapidly, attain a larger size, and ulcerate more extensively than do adenomas. Dogs with lesions larger than 5 cm in diameter have an 11-fold higher risk of dying of tumor-related causes.[117] Metastasis, especially to the sacral and sublumbar lymph nodes,[4] occurs in up to 30 per cent of cases.

Apocrine tumors of anal sac origin are usually adenocarcinomas, present as a perineal mass (ventrolateral to the anus), and often produce pseudohyperparathyroidism. The tumors usually metastasize, especially to the sacral and sublumbar lymph nodes.[4, 116]

DIAGNOSIS

Histologically, perianal gland tumors are classified into two basic types: (1) perianal or hepatoid gland tumors (hyperplasia [Fig. 19:34], adenoma, and carcinoma) and (2) apocrine tumors of anal sac origin.† Perianal gland neoplasms are positive for cytokeratin.[45, 117a]

---

*See references 4, 5, 12, 16, 27, 32, 116, and 117.
†See references 4, 5, 11, 13, 32, 116, and 117.

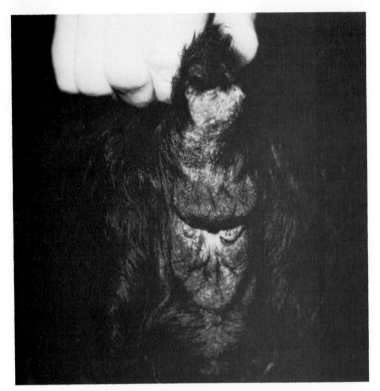

Figure 19:33. Diffuse hepatoid gland hyperplasia around the anus of a dog.

CLINICAL MANAGEMENT

Clinical management of perianal gland tumors may include surgical excision, cryosurgery, electrosurgery, radiotherapy, castration, and the administration of estrogens.[11–13] Castration is usually the treatment of choice for perianal (hepatoid) gland hyperplasias and adenomas, with 95 per cent of dogs responding well. Concurrent surgical excision is usually needed only with ulcerated or recurrent neoplasms in male dogs but is usually mandatory for perianal gland neoplasms in female dogs. Castration is not effective for carcinomas. Estrogen therapy is not usually recommended, because any tumor regressions induced are transient. Recurrence of

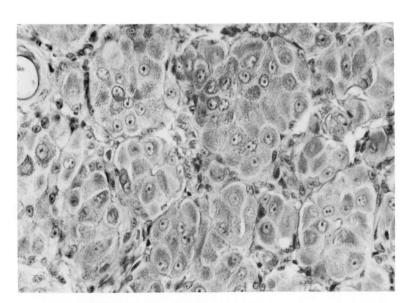

Figure 19:34. Canine hepatoid gland hyperplasia.

perianal hyperplasia or adenoma after surgical resection and castration, or occurrence of these lesions in female dogs, suggests that these animals should be evaluated for hyperadrenocorticism (elevated androgen levels, see Chap. 9).[11] Apocrine neoplasms of anal sac origin have a poor prognosis, as local recurrence and metastasis are common.[116]

Salivary Gland Tumors

Salivary gland neoplasms are rare in dogs and cats.[118] There are no apparent breed or sex predilections, and neoplasms generally occur in animals 10 years of age or older. Typical presentations include an ulcerated mass near the lateral commissure of the mouth and a subcutaneous mass caudoventral to the angle of the mandible or below the ear. The majority (85 per cent) of the neoplasms are malignant. Recurrence after surgery and metastasis are common.

■ MESENCHYMAL NEOPLASMS

Tumors of Fibroblast Origin

FIBROMA

■ *Cause and Pathogenesis.* Fibromas are uncommon benign neoplasms of the dog and cat arising from dermal or subcutaneous fibroblasts.[5, 11–13, 32] The cause of fibromas is unknown.

■ *Clinical Findings.* These neoplasms usually occur in older dogs and cats. There is no breed or sex predilection in cats. In dogs, however, fibromas are reported to occur most commonly in boxers, Boston terriers, Doberman pinschers, Golden retrievers, and fox terriers.[1, 4, 11–13, 18, 21a] Female animals are predisposed. Usually, these lesions are solitary (see Fig. 19:24 *H*) and may be more common on the limbs, flanks, and groin. They are usually well circumscribed, firm (fibroma durum) to soft (fibroma molle), dome shaped to pedunculated, dermal-epidermal to subcutaneous in location, and 1 to 5 cm in diameter. In dogs, fibromas may be melanotic, have a pinfeathered appearance, or both. In France, an unusual fibroma has been reported on the bridge of the nose in dogs.[51a] Although histologically benign, the neoplasm is locally aggressive, grows to a large size, and may invade the orbital cavity. Fibromas are noninvasive and nonmetastatic.

■ *Diagnosis.* Histologically, fibromas are characterized by whorls and interlacing bundles of fibroblasts and collagen fibers (Fig. 19:35 *A* and *B*).[5, 32] The neoplastic cells are usually fusiform, and mitoses are rare. Fibromas containing focal areas of mucinous or myxomatous degeneration are often called *fibromyxomas*. Fibromas are positive for vimentin.[45]

■ *Clinical Management.* Clinical management of fibromas may include surgical excision, cryosurgery, electrosurgery, and observation without treatment.[11–13]

DERMATOFIBROMA

■ *Cause and Pathogenesis.* Dermatofibromas are rare fibrocytic tumors in dogs and cats.[5] The cause is unknown, and there is controversy about whether the lesion is neoplastic or reactive.

■ *Clinical Findings.* Dermatofibromas appear as solitary, well-circumscribed, firm nodules that are usually less than 2 cm in diameter. The overlying epidermis is alopecic and thickened.

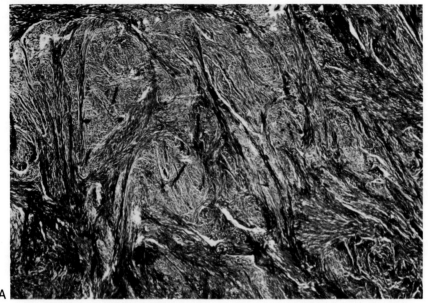

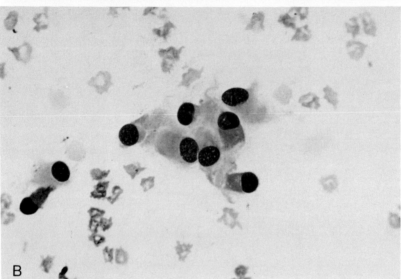

Figure 19:35 *A*, Canine fibroma. Interlacing proliferation of well-differentiated fibroblasts and collagen fibers. *B*, Canine fibroma. Cytologic examination of aspirate reveals small numbers of monomorphic fibroblasts.

Lesions occur most often on the head, and affected animals are usually younger than 5 years old.

■ ***Diagnosis.*** Histopathologically, dermatofibromas are characterized by spindle and stellate fibrocytic cells arranged in haphazard bundles and small whorls, interspersed with a moderate stroma composed of collagen fibers and bundles of varying thickness.[5]

■ ***Clinical Management.*** Clinical management of dermatofibromas may include surgical excision, cryosurgery, and observation without treatment.

FIBROVASCULAR PAPILLOMA

A fibrovascular papilloma (skin tag, keratin tag, skin polyp, acrochordon, fibroepithelial polyp, or soft fibroma) is an uncommon benign tumor of fibrovascular origin in dogs.[4, 5, 11] The cause of these growths is unknown, but they may be a proliferative response to trauma or focal furunculosis.

■ *Clinical Findings.* No sex predilection is established, but large and giant breeds appear to be predisposed, especially the Doberman pinscher and Labrador retriever.[4] The lesions may be solitary or multiple, filiform to pedunculated, smooth or hyperkeratotic, soft, and 2 to 5 mm in diameter by 1 to 2 cm in length (Fig. 19:36). Fibrovascular papillomas occur most commonly on bony prominences, the trunk, and the sternum.

■ *Diagnosis.* Histopathologically, fibrovascular papillomas are characterized by a fibrovascular core exhibiting papillomatosis and irregular hyperplasia of the overlying epidermis (Fig. 19:37).[5, 11]

■ *Clinical Management.* Clinical management of fibrovascular papillomas may include surgical excision, cryosurgery, electrosurgery, and observation without treatment.[11]

FIBROPRURITIC NODULE

■ *Cause and Pathogenesis.* The etiopathogenesis of fibropruritic nodules is unknown. However, they have been described only in conjunction with the chronic self-trauma of canine flea bite hypersensitivity.[5]

■ *Clinical Findings.* Fibropruritic nodules are most commonly seen in dogs older than 8 years of age and may be more common in German shepherd dogs and their crosses.[5] Multiple firm, sessile or pedunculated, alopecic nodules develop, which vary in size from 1 to 2 cm in diameter (Fig. 19:38 A). Lesions may be erythematous or hyperpigmented, smooth or hyperkeratotic, and are occasionally ulcerated. Fibropruritic nodules are located predominantly over the dorsal lumbosacral area of dogs with chronic flea bite hypersensitivity.

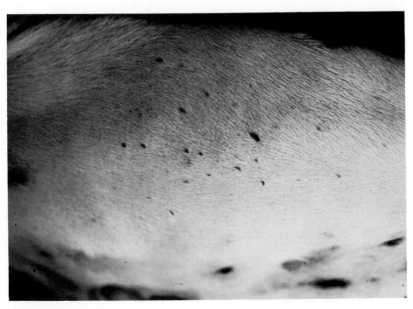

Figure 19:36. Multiple fibrovascular papillomas on the sternum of a dog.

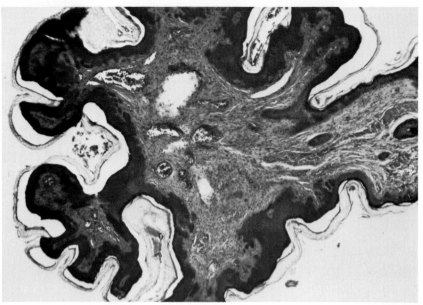

Figure 19:37. Canine fibrovascular papilloma. Papillomatous proliferation of epidermis and fibrovascular core.

■ *Diagnosis.* The clinical presentation is characteristic. Histopathologically, fibropruritic nodules are characterized by nodular dermal fibrosis, inflammation, and often, marked papillated epidermal hyperplasia (Fig. 19:39).

■ *Clinical Management.* The treatment of choice is surgical excision and controlling the associated flea bite hypersensitivity.

FIBROSARCOMA

■ *Cause and Pathogenesis.* Fibrosarcomas (fibroblastic spindle cell sarcomas) are common (in cats) to uncommon (in dogs) neoplasms arising from dermal or subcutaneous fibroblasts. The cause of fibrosarcomas in older animals is unknown. Some feline fibrosarcomas are virus induced.[11–13, 121] Such fibrosarcomas, and cell-free extracts derived from them, contain C-type virus particles. Cell-free extracts produce multicentric fibrosarcomas when injected into kittens and puppies. Cats older than 5 years appear to be more resistant to the oncogenic effects of this feline sarcoma virus (FeSV) and usually have no neoplasms or benign neoplasms that spontaneously regress. The FeSV is a mutant of the feline leukemia virus (FeLV), and cats with FeSV-induced fibrosarcomas are FeLV positive. FeSV is *not* associated with the solitary fibrosarcomas in old cats. It is believed that injection site reactions (especially with FeLV and rabies vaccines) may eventuate in fibrosarcomas in some cats, especially if vaccines are repeatedly given at the same site (cervical, interscapular).[4, 5, 120a, 121b]

■ *Clinical Findings*

■ *Dog.* Fibrosarcomas are uncommon in the dog.[5, 11–13] They occur in older and female dogs, and Cocker spaniels, Doberman pinschers, and Golden retrievers may be predisposed.[4, 11–13, 18, 21a] Fibrosarcomas are usually solitary, irregular and nodular in shape, firm to fleshy (see Fig. 19:38 *B*), poorly circumscribed, variably sized (1 to 15 cm in diameter), and subcutaneous in location. They are often ulcerated and alopecic. Lesions occur most commonly on the limbs

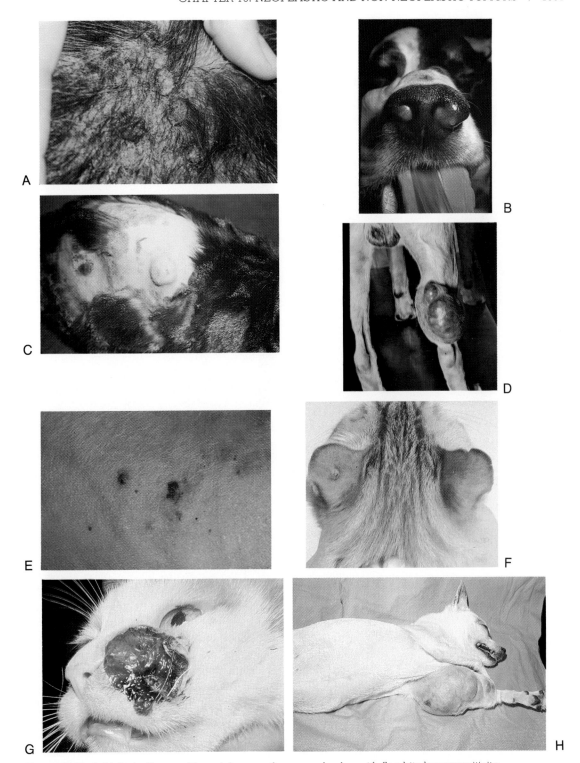

Figure 19:38. *A*, Multiple fibropruritic nodules over the rump of a dog with flea bite hypersensitivity. *B*, Fibrosarcoma. Fleshy masses involving both nostrils. (Courtesy J. Harvey.) *C*, Multiple fibrosarcomas over the trunk of a young, feline leukemia virus (FeLV)-positive cat. *D*, Schwannoma on the hock of a dog. *E*, Multiple solar-induced hemangiomas in a Saluki. (Courtesy A. Hargis.) *F*, Bluish hemangioma on the left pinna of a cat. *G*, Hemangiosarcoma on the face of a cat. *H*, Hemangiopericytoma on the proximal front limb of a dog.

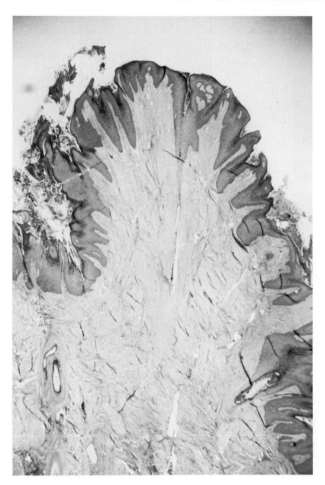

Figure 19:39. Canine fibropruritic nodule.

and the trunk. Immune-mediated thrombocytopenia has been reported in association with canine fibrosarcoma.

■ *Cat.* Fibrosarcomas are common in the cat.* FeSV-associated fibrosarcomas are seen in cats younger than 5 years of age and are usually multicentric (see Fig. 19:38 *C*).[4, 5, 11–13, 121] Fibrosarcomas that are *not* associated with FeSV are seen in older cats (average age 12 years) and are typically solitary. Lesions occur most commonly on the trunk, the distal limbs, and the pinnae. Postvaccination fibrosarcomas obviously occur on the sites of previous injections.[120a] The neoplasms are generally irregular and nodular in shape, firm to fleshy, poorly circumscribed, variably sized (1 to 15 cm in diameter), and subcutaneous (trunk and distal limbs) or dermal (pinnae and digits) in location. They are frequently alopecic and ulcerated. Most fibrosarcomas demonstrate rapid, infiltrative growth, with metastasis occurring in less than 20 per cent of the cases.[4, 122a]

■ *Diagnosis.* Histopathologically, fibrosarcomas are characterized by interwoven bundles of immature fibroblasts and moderate numbers of collagen fibers.[4, 5, 32] The neoplastic cells are usually fusiform, mitotic figures are common, and cellular atypia is pronounced (Fig. 19:40). Fibrosarcomas with focal areas of mucinous or myxomatous degeneration are often called *fibromyxosarcomas*. Fibrosarcomas are positive for vimentin.[45, 47, 54]

*See references 4, 5, 11–13, 21a, 26, 29, and 34.

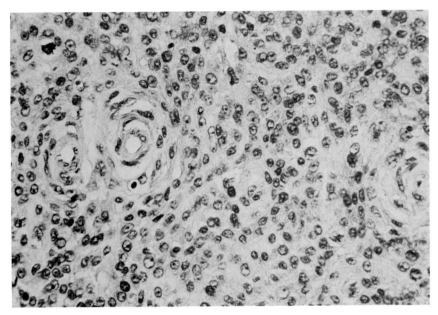

Figure 19:40. Canine fibrosarcoma. Proliferation of pleomorphic, atypical fibroblasts.

Fibrosarcomas arising in subcutaneous vaccination sites are accompanied by a lymphoid and granulomatous inflammatory response at the periphery, with epithelioid macrophages and multinucleate histiocytic giant cells, which have an amorphous gray-brown to bluish material within their cytoplasm.[4, 120a] Electron probe x-ray microanalysis revealed that the material was composed of aluminum and oxygen, and aluminum hydroxide and aluminum phosphate are used as adjuvants in some feline vaccines.[120a, 121b]

■ *Clinical Management.* The clinical management of choice for fibrosarcomas is wide surgical excision.[11–13, 22a] Radiotherapy, chemotherapy (with doxorubicin, cyclophosphamide, methotrexate, and vincristine), immunotherapy (with mixed bacterial vaccine and levamisole), and cryosurgery have been of limited benefit.[11–13, 122] Acemannan (Acemannan Immunostimulant) is a carbohydrate moiety that causes macrophages to secrete increased quantities of TNF-α, IL-1, and IFN.[25a, 121a] It has a conditional product license from the United States Department of Agriculture at this time. The product has been advocated (repeated intraperitoneal and intratumoral injections) for the treatment of fibrosarcoma in cats and dogs.[121a] However, efficacy and potency studies are still in progress. Most fibrosarcomas demonstrate rapid, infiltrative growth, frequent recurrence after surgery, and metastasis in less than 20 per cent of the cases.[4, 11–13, 21a, 122a]

In a study of 44 cats with fibrosarcomas, it was found that the mitotic index and tumor site correlated with prognosis, whereas histologic appearance, tumor size, and duration of tumor growth did not.[119] Cats with fibrosarcomas of the head, the back, or the limbs and with a mitotic index of 6 or greater had the poorest prognosis. In a study of 84 dogs with fibrosarcomas, the site of tumor occurrence, tumor size, and delay between detection of the tumor and surgical excision had little influence on the prognosis for recurrence or metastasis.[120] Mitotic index of the neoplasms had a significant predictive value for recurrence, postsurgical survival time, and metastasis.

Although epidemiologic evidence indicates that fibrosarcomas can arise at the site of previous vaccination, the incidence of this is rare, and the benefits afforded by the vaccines far outweigh the risks incurred with their administration.[121b]

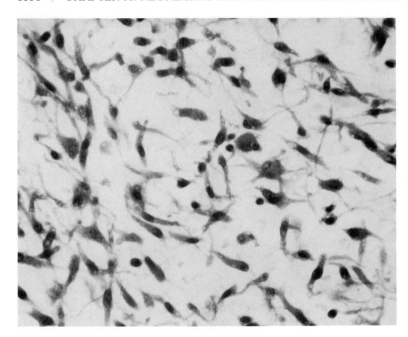

Figure 19:41. Feline myxosarcoma. Atypical fibroblasts (fusiform-to-stellate) with abundant ground substance (mucin).

MYXOMA AND MYXOSARCOMA

■ *Cause and Pathogenesis.*   Myxomas and myxosarcomas are rare neoplasms of the dog and cat arising from dermal or subcutaneous fibroblasts, the cause of which is unknown.[4, 5, 11–13, 21a, 32] Myxoma has been reported to develop at the site of a subcutaneous pacemaker in a dog.[123]

■ *Clinical Findings.*   These neoplasms usually occur in older dogs and cats, with no sex predilections. Doberman pinschers and German shepherd dogs may be predisposed.[4] These neoplasms may occur more frequently on the limbs, the back, or the groin.[4] They are usually solitary infiltrative growths that are soft, slimy, and poorly circumscribed and have no definite shape. Myxomas are benign. Myxosarcomas are malignant but apparently do not commonly metastasize.[86] Both neoplasms frequently recur after surgery, owing to their infiltrative growth patterns.

■ *Diagnosis.*   Histopathologically, myxomas and myxosarcomas are characterized by stellate to fusiform cells distributed in a vacuolated, basophilic, mucinous stroma that may be partitioned by collagenous connective tissue septae (Fig. 19:41).[5, 32] Myxomas and myxosarcomas are positive for vimentin.[52]

■ *Clinical Management.*   In clinical management, the therapy of choice for myxomas and myxosarcomas is radical surgical excision.[11–13, 22a]

NODULAR FASCIITIS

■ *Cause and Pathogenesis.*   Nodular fasciitis (pseudosarcomatous fasciitis) is a rare, benign, non-neoplastic growth of the dog and cat.[21a, 32, 51a] Nodular fasciitis is thought to represent a proliferative inflammatory process arising from the subcutaneous fascia and exhibiting a clinically aggressive behavior that suggests a locally invasive neoplasm.

■ *Clinical Findings.*   There are no age, breed, or sex predilections for dogs and cats. Nodular fasciitis can occur anywhere on the body but may favor the head, the face, and the eyelids. The masses are usually solitary, firm, poorly circumscribed, 0.2 to 5 cm in diameter, and subcutaneous in location. In humans, nodular fasciitis is self-limited, and thus, even if it is incompletely excised, it regresses. Cutaneous nodular fasciitis in dogs and cats is also benign, but spontaneous regression has not been reported.

■ *Diagnosis.* Histopathologically, nodular fasciitis is characterized by a poorly circumscribed, infiltrative proliferation of pleomorphic fibroblasts growing haphazardly in a highly vascularized stroma with varying amount of mucoid ground substance.[32] Mitoses and giant cells are common, and a chronic inflammatory infiltrate is often present.

■ *Clinical Management.* The clinical management of nodular fasciitis in dogs and cats has consisted of surgical excision.

Tumors of Neural Origin

SCHWANNOMA

■ *Cause and Pathogenesis.* Schwannomas (neurofibroma, neurilemoma, neurinoma, or perineural fibroblastoma) are rare neoplasms of the dog and cat arising from dermal or subcutaneous Schwann cells (nerve sheath).[4, 5, 11–13, 21a, 127] The cause of schwannomas is unknown.

There is much confusion about terminology concerning these neoplasms in the veterinary literature. In humans, there are at least two distinct clinical, histopathologic, and ultrastructural types of schwannomas,[9] neurofibroma and neurilemoma. There is histopathologic and ultrastructural evidence that the same two types occur in dogs and cats.[4] Unfortunately, most reports do not make this distinction and simply refer to them as *schwannomas* or *nerve sheath tumors;* consequently, meaningful clinicopathologic data on the two types do not exist.

■ *Clinical Findings.* Schwannomas usually occur in older dogs and cats, with no sex predilection. In cats, no breed predilection exists, but in dogs, the fox terrier may be predisposed. Schwannomas are usually solitary. They occur most commonly on the limbs, the head and the neck in cats but occur more commonly on the limbs, the head, and the tail in dogs (see Fig. 19:38 *D*).[4, 5, 11–13, 127] Schwannomas are firm (especially in dogs), well circumscribed to poorly circumscribed, often lobulated, variable in size, and dermal (especially in cats) to subcutaneous (especially in dogs) in location. They are often alopecic. Rarely, schwannomas may be plexiform (multinodular). There may be obvious nerve involvement with or without neurologic deficit. Some lesions are painful or pruritic and may be complicated by acral lick dermatitis.[127] Most schwannomas are malignant and recur frequently after surgery.

■ *Diagnosis.* Histopathologically, schwannomas are characterized by two patterns: (1) *neurofibroma*—faintly eosinophilic, thin, wavy fibers lying in loosely textured strands that extend in various directions, with spindle-shaped cells that may exhibit nuclear palisading (Fig. 19:42); and (2) *neurilemoma*—areas of spindle-shaped cells exhibiting nuclear palisading and twisting bands or rows (Antoni type A tissue), alternating with an edematous stroma containing relatively few haphazardly arranged cells (Antoni type B tissue) (Fig. 19:43).[4, 5, 11, 32] Benign and malignant histopathologic types are seen. Schwannomas are positive for vimentin and S-100 protein.[21a, 47, 54]

■ *Clinical Management.* The therapy of choice is surgical excision.[11–13, 22a, 127] Amputation may occasionally be necessary. Radiotherapy, chemotherapy, immunotherapy, and cryosurgery appear to be of minimal benefit. Schwannomas recur frequently after surgery but rarely metastasize.

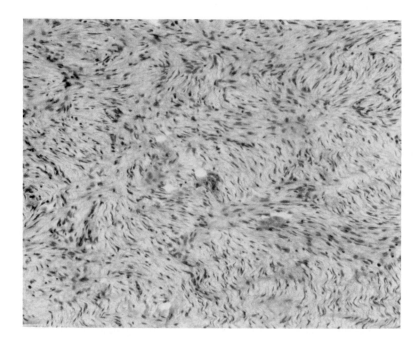

Figure 19:42. Canine schwannoma. Palisading spindle-shaped cells with fine, wavy fibers.

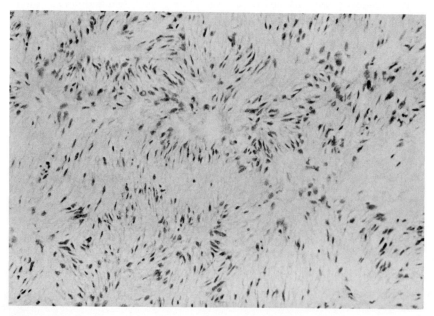

Figure 19:43. Canine schwannoma. Antoni A and B Type tissue.

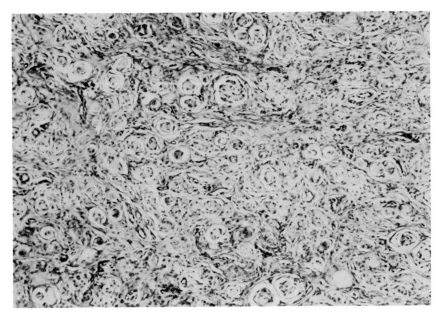

Figure 19:44. Canine neurothekeoma. Nests of neuroid tissue.

NEUROTHEKEOMA

■ *Cause and Pathogenesis.* Neurothekeomas are benign cutaneous neoplasms of Schwann cell origin.[5, 11] The cause of these neoplasms is unknown.

■ *Clinical Findings.* Neurothekeomas occur in dogs,[5, 11] but not enough cases have been seen to generate age, breed, or sex data. The lesions are solitary, firm, nodular, and subcutaneous to dermal in location. They occur on the legs and digits.

■ *Diagnosis.* Histopathologically, neurothekeomas are characterized by nests and cords of cells in a variably mucinous matrix (Fig. 19:44). Close relationship to small nerves may be seen.[5]

■ *Clinical Management.* Clinical management includes surgical excision.

GRANULAR CELL TUMOR

■ *Cause and Pathogenesis.* Granular cell tumors (granular cell myoblastoma, or granular cell schwannoma) are rare neoplasms of the dog and cat.[4, 11, 124, 124a, 127a, 128] Although the cell of origin is not established with certainty, current evidence suggests a neural source. In humans, granular cell tumors contain neuron-specific enolase and myelin basic protein.[9, 48] The cause of granular cell tumors is unknown.

■ *Clinical Findings.* Granular cell tumors have been reported in dogs from 2 to 13 years old, with no breed or sex predilection. Most of the neoplasms occurred as solitary, firm, round, well-circumscribed masses within the tongue. Other dogs had a solitary subcutaneous neoplasm near the shoulder or on the lip or ear, and one dog had multiple dermal-epidermal and subcutaneous malignant neoplasms with visceral metastasis (Fig. 19:45).[11, 124, 124a, 127a, 128] Most canine granular cell tumors have been benign. In cats, granular cell tumors have been seen on the tongue, vulva, and digits.[127a]

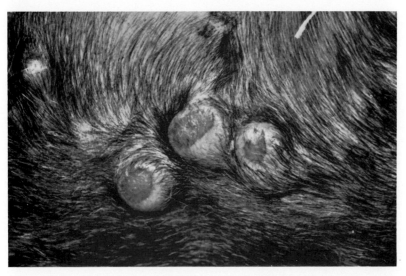

Figure 19:45. Malignant granular cell tumors on the thorax of a dog.

■ *Diagnosis.*   Histopathologically, granular cell tumors are characterized by a circumscribed mass of ovoid to polyhedral cells with central or eccentric nuclei and pale cytoplasm containing numerous small, faintly eosinophilic granules.[4, 11, 124, 124a, 127a, 128] The tumor cells may be arranged diffusely or in nests and rows (Fig. 19:46). The cytoplasmic granules are PAS positive. The pseudocarcinomatous hyperplasia that so frequently overlies granular cell tumors in humans is rarely seen in dogs. Canine granular cell tumors are positive for neuron-specific enolase and variably positive for vimentin and S-100 protein.[124, 124a, 127a]

■ *Clinical Management.*   The therapy of choice for granular cell tumors is surgical excision.[11–13]

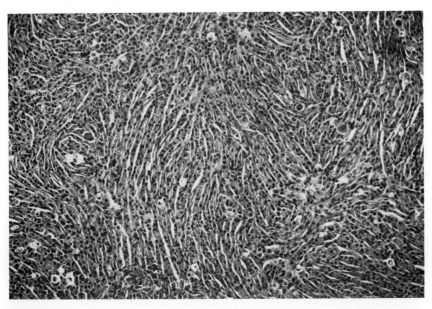

Figure 19:46. Canine malignant granular cell tumor. Cords and clusters of anaplastic cells with fine, eosinophilic cytoplasmic granules.

MENINGIOMA

■ *Cause and Pathogenesis.*   Primary cutaneous (extraneuraxial) meningioma is exceedingly rare in the dog.[126] Although the cause of these lesions is unknown, it is hypothesized that they originate from arachnoid cap cell rests displaced during embryogenesis into the skin.

■ *Clinical Findings.*   An 11-year-old Poodle had a firm, well-circumscribed, 3-cm-diameter, subcutaneous mass in the right hindleg that had been enlarging for several months.[126]

■ *Diagnosis.*   Histopathologically, meningiomas show a uniform and lobulated arrangement of solid masses of ovoid to elongated cells with eosinophilic cytoplasm.[126] Most cells form concentric whorls around central small capillary spaces that are often obliterated. Electron microscopy reveals characteristic delicate intracytoplasmic filaments.

■ *Clinical Management.*   Surgical excision is curative.

TAIL DOCK NEUROMA

■ *Cause and Pathogenesis.*   Tail dock neuroma occurs rarely in dogs as a sequela to cosmetic caudectomy.[4, 5, 125] Neuromas are a manifestation of traumatic or surgical nerve transection followed by disorganized proliferation of the proximal nerve stump because of poor apposition or the absence of the distal nerve segment.

■ *Clinical Findings.*   Historically, affected dogs have inflicted self-trauma to the tail since puppyhood, beginning soon after tail docking. Physical examination reveals a painful, alopecic, hyperpigmented, lichenified, excoriated dermatosis at the tip of the tail. The underlying connective tissue is thickened and firm. Cocker spaniels may be predisposed.

■ *Diagnosis.*   Histopathologic examination reveals axonal sprouting with secondary remyelination in a bed of fibrous connective tissue (Fig. 19:47).[5, 125]

■ *Clinical Management.*   Surgical excision is curative.

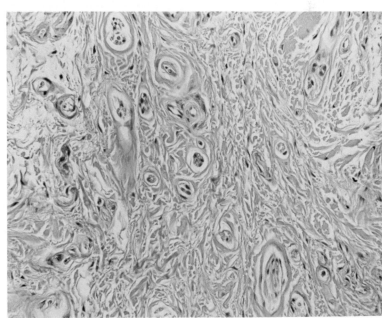

Figure 19:47. Canine tail dock neuroma. Axonal sprouting in a bed of fibrous connective tissue. (Courtesy T. Gross.)

Tumors of Vascular Origin

HEMANGIOMA

■ *Cause and Pathogenesis.* Hemangiomas (angiomas) are uncommon (in dogs) to rare (in cats) benign neoplasms arising from the endothelial cells of blood vessels.* The cause of most hemangiomas is unknown. C-type virus particles have been found in cells from a subcutaneous hemangioma in a cat.[34] Studies strongly suggested that chronic solar damage may be the cause of hemangiomas in the ventral glabrous skin of lightly pigmented, sparsely haired dogs.[5, 135, 135a]

■ *Clinical Findings*

■ *Dog.* Hemangiomas are more common than hemangiosarcomas and occur in dogs at an average age of 10 years with no sex predilection.[4, 5, 10–13, 135a] Dogs with lightly pigmented and sparsely haired ventral abdomen and thorax have an increased incidence of hemangiomas (see Fig. 19:38 *E*). Breeds at risk include boxer, Golden retriever, German shepherd dog, English Springer spaniel, Airedale terrier, whippet, Dalmatian, beagle, American Staffordshire (pit bull) terrier, Basset hound, Saluki, and English Pointer.[5, 18, 135a] Multiple, presumably solar-induced hemangiomas have been reported in related whippets.[135a] Hemangiomas are usually well circumscribed, firm to fluctuant, rounded, bluish to reddish black, 0.5 to 4 cm in diameter, and dermal to subcutaneous in location.

■ *Cat.* Hemangiomas are less common than hemangiosarcomas, usually occur in animals older than 10 years of age, and most often affect male animals.[5, 136b] Lesions are usually solitary and occur most commonly on the ears (see Fig. 19:38 *F*), the face, the neck, and the limbs. Hemangiomas are usually well circumscribed, firm to fluctuant, rounded, bluish to reddish black, 0.5 to 4 cm in diameter, and dermal to subcutaneous in location.

■ *Diagnosis.* Histologically, hemangiomas are characterized by the proliferation of blood-filled vascular spaces lined by single layers of well-differentiated endothelial cells.[4, 5, 32] Hemangiomas are often subclassified as cavernous or capillary, depending on the size of the vascular spaces and the amount of intervening fibrous tissues (Figs. 19:48 and 19:49).[4, 5, 32, 144] Solar-induced lesions are often less well circumscribed, and solar dermatitis and elastosis may be present.[5, 135a, 136b] Electron microscopy may be beneficial in determining the vascular origin of a neoplasm, as Weibel-Palade bodies are a specific cytoplasmic marker for endothelial cells.[129a] In addition, immunohistochemistry may be useful, because vimentin, factor VIII–related antigen, *Ulex europaeus* (UEA-1) lectin, and Type IV collagen and laminin are found in vascular proliferations.[45, 47, 51a, 58, 136b] Anemia, purpura, thrombocytopenia, hypofibrinogenemia, and findings associated with disseminated intravascular coagulation have been reported in conjunction with hemangiomas.[135]

■ *Clinical Management.* Clinical management of hemangiomas may include surgical excision, cryosurgery, electrosurgery, and observation without treatment.[11–13]

HEMANGIOSARCOMA

■ *Cause and Pathogenesis.* Hemangiosarcomas (angiosarcomas, or malignant hemangioendotheliomas) are uncommon malignant neoplasms of dogs and cats arising from the endothelial cells of blood vessels.[4, 5, 10–13] The cause of most hemangiosarcomas is unknown. In humans, they have been associated[3] with exposure to thorium dioxide, arsenicals, and vinyl chloride.[3]

---

*See references 4, 5, 10–13, 19, 21a, and 32.

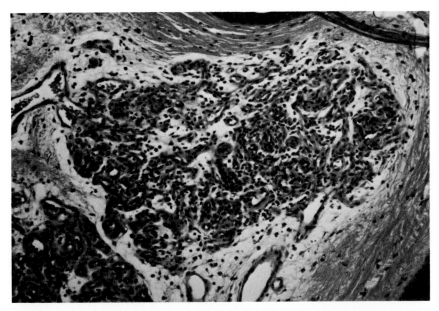

Figure 19:48. Canine capillary hemangioma. Superficial dermal proliferation of normal-appearing endothelial cells and blood vessels.

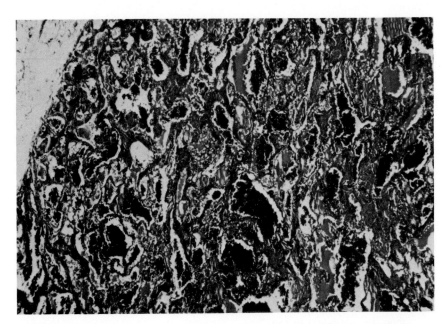

Figure 19:49. Canine cavernous hemangioma. Deep dermal proliferation of widely dilated, blood-filled vessels.

Studies strongly suggested that chronic solar damage may be the cause of hemangiosarcomas in the ventral glabrous skin of lightly pigmented, sparsely coated dogs[5, 135a] and on the pinnae of white-eared cats.[136b]

■ Clinical Findings

■ *Dog.* Hemangiosarcomas occur in dogs at an average of 10 years of age and with no apparent sex predilection. Typical hemangiosarcomas occur most commonly in German shepherd dogs, Golden retrievers, Bernese Mountain dogs, and boxers.[4, 11–13, 21a, 135b, 140a] Lesions are most commonly found on the trunk and the extremities. Whippets, Dalmatians, beagles, Greyhounds, American Staffordshire terriers, Basset hounds, Salukis, English Pointers, and other short-haired and light-skinned breeds are at increased risk for solar-induced hemangiosarcomas.[5, 135, 135a]

Solar-induced hemangiosarcomas are most common on the ventral thorax and the abdomen. Typical hemangiosarcomas are usually solitary, whereas solar-induced lesions may be multiple. Dermal hemangiosarcomas (more common in solar-associated lesions) are poorly circumscribed, red to dark blue plaques or nodules that are usually less than 2 cm in diameter. Subcutaneous hemangiosarcomas are poorly circumscribed, dark red or blue-black, spongy masses that can measure up to 10 cm in diameter. Alopecia, thickened skin, hemorrhage, and ulceration are common features of dermal or subcutaneous hemangiosarcomas.

■ *Cat.* Hemangiosarcomas usually occur in male cats older than 10 years of age.* There is no breed predilection. Lesions are usually solitary and occur most commonly on the head (see Fig. 19:38 *G*) and the pinna (especially in white-haired cats), on the limbs, and in the inguinal and axillary regions. Dermal hemangiosarcomas are poorly circumscribed, red to dark blue plaques or nodules that are usually less than 2 cm in diameter. Subcutaneous hemangiosarcomas are poorly circumscribed, dark red or blue-black, spongy masses that can measure up to 10 cm in diameter. Alopecia, thickened skin, hemorrhage, and ulceration are common features of dermal or subcutaneous hemangiosarcomas. A peripheral arteriovenous fistula was reported in a cat with a hemangiosarcoma of a limb.[136]

■ *Diagnosis.* Histopathologically, hemangiosarcomas are characterized by an invasive proliferation of atypical endothelial cells with areas of vascular space formation (Fig. 19:50).[4, 5, 32, 135a, 136b] Solar-induced lesions may have associated solar dermatitis and solar elastosis.[5, 135] Hemangiosarcomas are positive for vimentin, S-100 protein, factor VIII–related antigen, UEA-1 lectin, Type IV collagen, and laminin.† Anemia, purpura, thrombocytopenia, hypofibrinogenemia, and findings associated with disseminated intravascular coagulation have been reported in conjunction with hemangiosarcomas.[135, 138a]

■ *Clinical Management.* The therapy of choice for hemangiosarcomas is radical surgical excision.[11–13, 22a, 130] However, after *any* form of therapy, the prognosis for animals with hemangiosarcoma is poor, with local recurrence and metastasis being common. They are highly invasive and malignant in dogs, with an average survival time of 4 months after diagnosis.[129] In cats, hemangiosarcomas frequently recur after surgical excision but do not commonly metastasize.[19, 136b, 140] Palliative responses have been obtained in dogs with the concomitant administration of doxorubicin and vincristine.[134]

---

*See references 4, 5, 11–13, 21a, 29, and 136b.
†See references 45, 47, 48, 51a, 52, 58, and 136b.

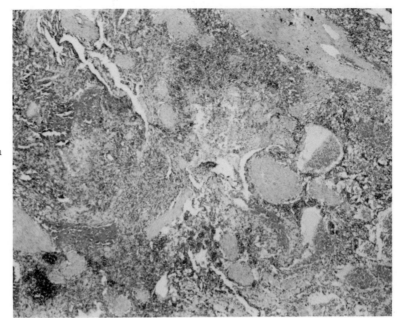

Figure 19:50. Canine hemangiosarcoma. Proliferation of atypical vascular structures associated with necrosis and hemorrhage.

HEMANGIOPERICYTOMA

■ *Cause and Pathogenesis.* Hemangiopericytomas (peritheliomas) are common neoplasms of the dog arising from vascular pericytes.* Rare cases of hemangiopericytoma in cats have been reported.[19] The cause of hemangiopericytomas is unknown. Trisomy 2 (three copies of chromosome 2) has been reported in three cases of canine hemangiopericytoma.[136a]

■ *Clinical Findings.* Hemangiopericytomas occur in dogs at a mean age of 7 to 10 years. Boxers, German shepherd dogs, Cocker spaniels, Springer spaniels, Irish setters, Siberian huskies, fox terriers, collies, and beagles are predisposed.[4, 11–13, 21a] There is no apparent sex predilection. Hemangiopericytomas are usually solitary and occur most commonly on the limbs (especially the stifle and elbow). They are usually firm, multinodular, well circumscribed, 2 to 25 cm in diameter, and dermal to subcutaneous in location (see Fig. 19:38 *H*). Alopecia, hyperpigmentation, and ulceration are common.

■ *Diagnosis.* Several patterns are associated with the hemangiopericytoma, and one pattern may predominate or several patterns may be identified within the same mass. This variable histopathologic appearance is considered unique to the hemangiopericytoma.[4] The classic pattern is the perivascular whorls (fingerprint pattern) of spindle-shaped to ovoid cells (Fig. 19:51 *A* and *B*).[4, 5, 11–13, 21a, 147] Other patterns include storiform, myxoid, and epithelioid. Hemangiopericytomas are positive for vimentin[45, 52] but negative for factor VIII–related antigen.[147]

■ *Clinical Management.* The therapy of choice for hemangiopericytomas is surgical excision or amputation.[10–13, 22a, 133, 138] Recurrent tumors have fewer whorls and look more like fibrosarcomas.[5, 133, 138] About 30 per cent or more of these neoplasms recur 4 months to 4 years after surgical excision, and about 60 per cent were reported to recur after surgery and orthovoltage radiation therapy.[130, 133, 138] In one study, tumors present for longer than 2 months before surgery

---

*See references 4, 5, 11–13, 21a, 133, 137, 138, and 147.

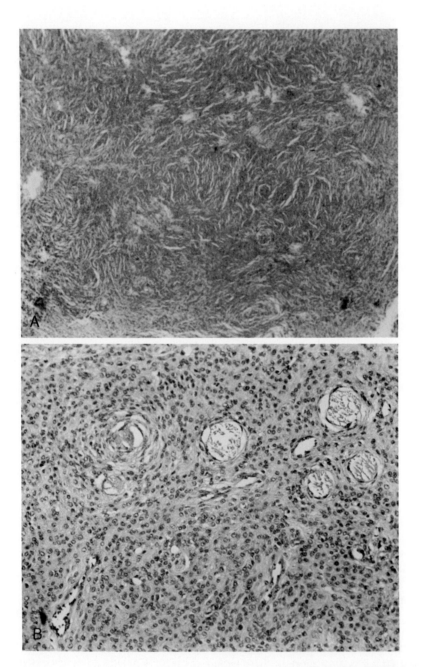

Figure 19:51 *A*, Canine hemangiopericytoma. Perivascular whorls of cells create a fingerprint-like appearance. *B*, Canine hemangiopericytoma. Perivascular proliferation of plump pericytes.

and tumors with increasing degrees of necrosis histologically had higher rates of recurrence.[138] Metastasis is rare.[21a, 133, 138]

ANGIOKERATOMA

Angiokeratomas are rare, benign superficial cutaneous telangiectases with an associated epithelial proliferation.[5, 11, 132] The cause of angiokeratoma is unknown.

■ *Clinical Findings.* Angiokeratomas occur on the conjunctiva and skin of dogs. The lesions are usually discrete, soft papules, 2 to 4 mm in diameter, that may be heavily melanized. Their color varies from red to black.

■ *Diagnosis.* Histopathologically, angiokeratomas are characterized by dilated and engorged superficial dermal blood vessels with a hyperplastic overlying epidermis (Fig. 19:52).[5, 11, 132]

■ *Clinical Management.* Clinical management of angiokeratomas includes surgical excision and observation without treatment.

LYMPHANGIOMA

■ *Cause and Pathogenesis.* Lymphangiomas (angiomas) are rare benign neoplasms of the dog and cat. They arise from the endothelial cells of lymphatic vessels.[4, 5, 11–13, 21a] Their cause is unknown, and some authors consider them hamartomas. Surgical trauma may occasionally be the cause.[146] The terminology used for benign lymphatic vessel lesions is confusing, with congenital lesions referred to as congenital lymphangioma, congenital lymphangiectasis, and lymphatic hamartoma. Acquired lesions are called acquired lymphangioma or lymphangiectasis.

■ *Clinical Findings.* Lymphangiomas have been reported in dogs and cats from younger than 1 to 8 years of age, with no apparent breed or sex predilection.[5, 11–13, 131, 137a, 141, 146] Lesions appear as fluctuant swellings up to 18 cm in diameter, which often appear poorly circumscribed

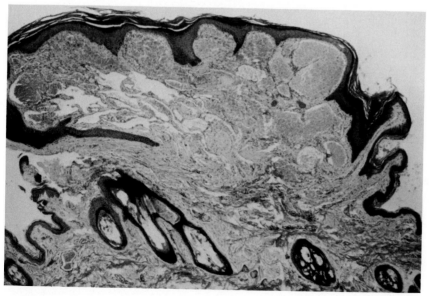

Figure 19:52. Canine angiokeratoma. Dilated, blood-filled superficial dermal vessels surrounded by hyperplastic epidermal collarettes.

(Fig. 19:53 *A*). Lymphangiomas may be accompanied by pitting edema and turgid vesicles (Fig. 19:53 *B*) and often drainage of a serous to milky fluid. Axillary and inguinal areas and limbs are most commonly affected.

■ *Diagnosis.* Histologically, lymphangiomas are characterized by a proliferation of variably sized, cavernous, angular vascular spaces. They are lined by a single layer of flattened endothelial cells and occur within the dermis, the subcutis, or both (Fig. 19:54).[4, 5, 11]

■ *Clinical Management.* The therapy of choice for lymphangiomas is surgical excision, but recurrence is common.[5] Radiation therapy was successful in a dog with recurring lymphangioma.[143] In another dog with an unresectable lymphangioma, the condition was controlled with intermittent administration of furosemide.[146]

LYMPHANGIOSARCOMA

■ *Cause and Pathogenesis.* Lymphangiosarcoma (angiosarcoma) is a rare malignant neoplasm arising from the endothelial cells of lymphatic vessels.[4, 5, 11–13, 19, 21a] The cause of lymphangiosarcoma is unknown, although in humans, the neoplasm often arises in areas of chronic lymphedema.[3, 9]

■ *Clinical Findings*

■ *Dog.* Lymphangiosarcoma has occurred in dogs younger than 1 to 11 years of age, with no apparent breed or sex predilection.[5, 139] Lesions are usually solitary, poorly circumscribed, fluctuant swellings up to 20 cm in diameter. Pitting edema, serous drainage, purpura, and ulceration may be present. The limbs and the ventral abdomen are most often affected.

■ *Cat.* Lymphangiosarcoma has occurred in adult and aged cats, with no apparent breed or sex predilection.[5, 11, 19, 142, 145] Lesions are typically a diffuse area of plaquelike thickening of the ventral abdomen (see Fig. 19:53 *C*) or draining tract to cystlike areas on a limb. Affected skin may be erythematous to purplish, is soft and spongy, and oozes a serosanguineous fluid (see Fig. 19:53 *D*).

■ *Diagnosis.* Histologically, lymphangiosarcoma is characterized by the proliferation of bizarre, atypical endothelial cells that tend to form variable-sized vascular spaces and surround collagen fibrils (Figs. 19:55 and 19:56). The neoplastic vessels are characterized by tortuous shapes, a lack of pericytes, and little or no blood. A pleomorphic inflammatory infiltrate is usually present.

■ *Clinical Management.* The treatment of choice is radical surgical excision or amputation.[11–13, 22a] Recurrence and metastasis are common in dogs.[5, 139] Local recurrence is common in cats, but metastasis is apparently uncommon.[5, 19]

Tumors of Adipose Origin

LIPOMA

■ *Cause and Pathogenesis.* Lipomas are common (in dogs) to uncommon (in cats) benign neoplasms arising from subcutaneous lipocytes (adipocytes).[4, 5, 10–13, 21a] The cause of lipomas is unknown.

■ *Clinical Findings.* Usually, these neoplasms occur in dogs and cats older than 8 years. There is no sex predilection in cats, but Siamese may be predisposed.[4] However, in dogs,

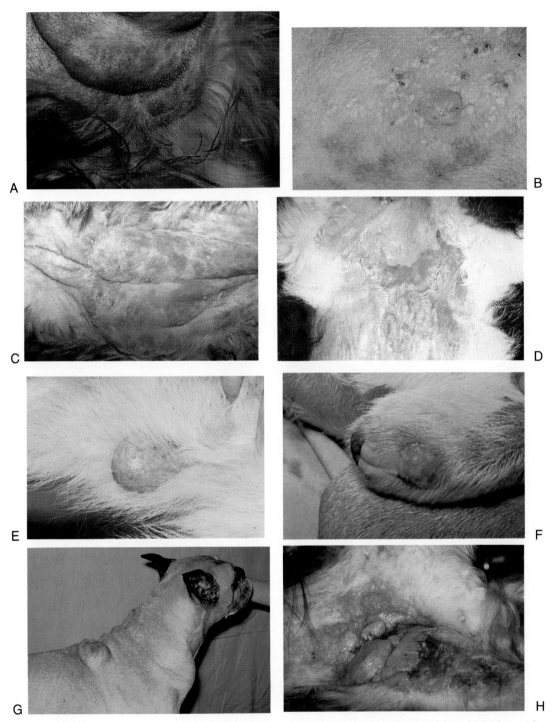

Figure 19:53. *A*, Canine lymphangioma. Purpuric mass in the groin. *B*, Canine lymphangioma. Multiple vesicles and bullae filled with clear-to-milky fluid on the medial thigh. *C*, Feline lymphangiosarcoma. Multiple purpuric, oozing plaques on the abdomen. *D*, Feline lymphangiosarcoma. Oozing, purpuric plaque. *E*, Canine lipoma. Soft, polypoid mass in the flank. *F*, Canine mast cell tumor. Two ulcerated plaques on the prepuce. *G*, Canine mast cell tumor. Multiple subcutaneous nodules over the withers. *H*, Canine mast cell tumor. Erythematous, edematous, and nodular lesions in the groin.

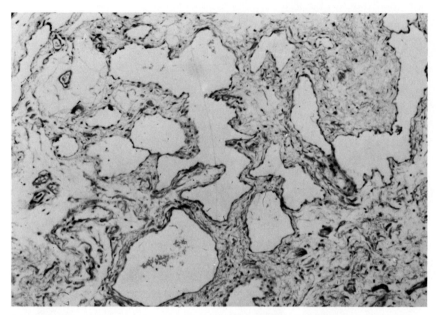

Figure 19:54. Canine lymphangioma. Proliferation of lymphatic vessels.

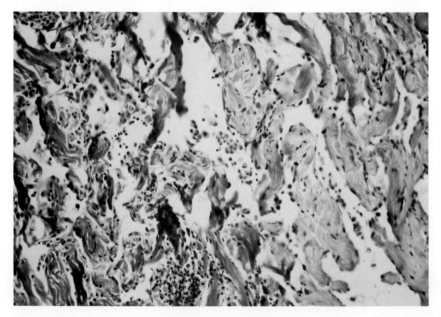

Figure 19:55. Feline lymphangiosarcoma. Atypical endothelial cells forming vessels and infiltrating between collagen bundles.

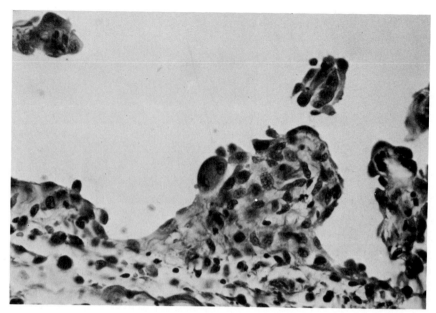

Figure 19:56. Close-up of Figure 19:55. Pleomorphic and atypical endothelial cells lining vessels and budding off into the vascular lumen.

lipomas are reported to occur more frequently in Cocker spaniels, dachshunds, Weimaraners, Doberman pinschers, Miniature Schnauzers, Labrador retrievers, and small terriers and in obese female dogs. Lipomas may be single or multiple and occur most often over the thorax, the brisket, the abdomen, and the proximal limbs (see Fig. 19:53 E). They are usually dome shaped or pedunculated, well circumscribed, soft to flabby, variable in size (1 to 30 cm in diameter), often multilobulated, and subcutaneous in location. Some lipomas are firm, owing to the presence of fibrous tissue, and are found to be fibrolipomas histologically.[5, 11, 21a] Some lipomas are painful and are found to be angiolipomas histologically.[11, 21a]

Infiltrative lipomas are uncommon in dogs and cats.[4, 5, 11, 148a, 149, 150] These tumors occur in middle-aged animals and have a predilection for female animals. Doberman pinschers and Labrador retrievers may be predisposed. Obesity does not appear to be a prerequisite. These tumors occur most frequently on the extremities, the thorax, and the neck. The neoplasms are large, poorly circumscribed, soft, deep subcutaneous masses that infiltrate adjacent muscle, fascia, tendon, joint capsule, and bone; they may cause dysfunction because of mechanical interference or pressure pain.[149a]

■ *Diagnosis.* Histologically, lipomas are characterized by a well-circumscribed proliferation of normal-appearing lipocytes (Figs 19:57 and 19:58).[4, 5, 32] Some neoplasms have a marked fibrous tissue component and are called *fibrolipomas. Infiltrative lipomas* are characterized by a poorly circumscribed proliferation of normal-appearing lipocytes that infiltrates surrounding tissues, especially muscle and collagen. *Angiolipomas* are characterized by mature adipose tissue with a complex, branching blood vascular component (Fig. 19:59). Lipomas are positive for vimentin.[45, 47, 54]

■ *Clinical Management.* The treatment of choice for all types of lipomas is surgical excision.[11–13] In obese animals, a restricted diet for a few weeks before surgery often reduces the size of the neoplasms and improves the definition from surrounding tissues. Small, asymptomatic lipomas are often merely observed, unless they grow large. Lipomas that are large can usually be easily peeled out, because they are well circumscribed and have a poor blood supply. The intratumoral injection of 10 per cent calcium chloride solution caused complete remission

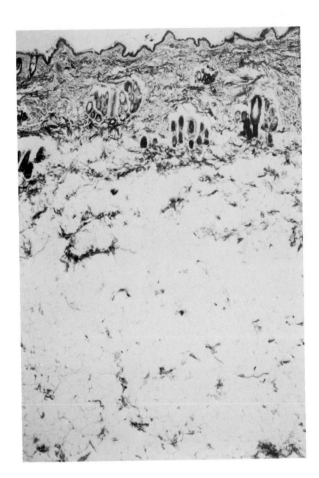

Figure 19:57. Feline lipoma. Proliferation of normal-appearing fat.

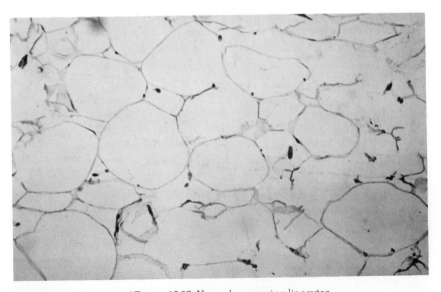

Figure 19:58. Close-up of Figure 19:57. Normal-appearing lipocytes.

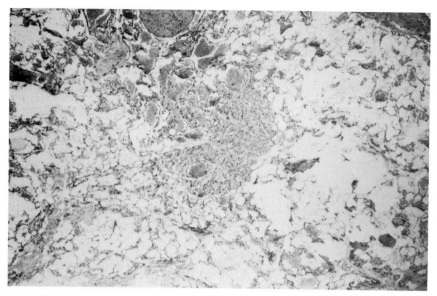

Figure 19:59. Canine angiolipoma. Proliferation of lipocytes with a central branching vascular component.

in 4 of 18 canine lipomas treated, with a 50 per cent reduction in size of the other 14 treated tumors.[148] Although infiltrative lipomas are not malignant, they necessitate radical surgical excision to prevent local recurrence, which still may occur in 36 per cent of the cases.[148a]

LIPOSARCOMA

■ *Cause and Pathogenesis.* Liposarcomas are rare malignant neoplasms of the dog and cat; they arise from subcutaneous lipoblasts.[4, 5, 11–13, 21a] The cause of liposarcomas is unknown, although they can be induced in cats by injection of FeLV.[11, 12, 152]

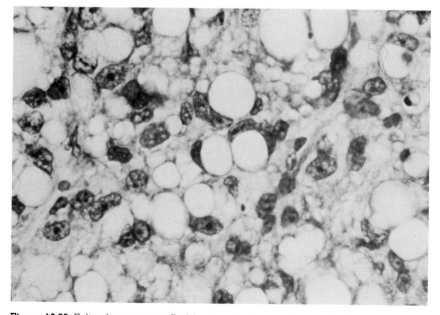

Figure 19:60. Feline liposarcoma. Proliferation of pleomorphic, atypical lipocytes.

■ *Clinical Findings.* Liposarcomas occur in dogs and cats at an average of about 10 years of age. In cats, there are no breed or sex predilections. In dogs, liposarcomas may be more common in dachshunds, Shetland sheepdogs, and Brittany spaniels and in male animals. Although they may be multiple, liposarcomas are usually solitary. In dogs, they occur most frequently on the ventral abdomen, the thorax, and the proximal limbs. Liposarcomas are usually poorly circumscribed, firm to fleshy, variable in size (1 to 10 cm in diameter), and subcutaneous in location. Liposarcomas are malignant and infiltrative but rarely metastasize.

■ *Diagnosis.* Histologically, liposarcomas are characterized by a cellular, infiltrative proliferation of atypical lipocytes with abundant, eosinophilic, finely vacuolated cytoplasm (Fig. 19:60).[4, 5, 32] Liposarcomas may be histologically well differentiated, pleomorphic, or myxoid.[5, 21a, 151] Liposarcomas are positive for vimentin and S-100 protein.[45, 47, 52, 54]

■ *Clinical Management.* The therapy of choice for liposarcomas is wide surgical excision.[22a]

Miscellaneous Mesenchymal Tumors

LEIOMYOMA AND LEIOMYOSARCOMA

■ *Cause and Pathogenesis.* Leiomyomas and leiomyosarcomas are extremely rare neoplasms of dogs and cats; they arise from smooth muscle cells of arrector pili muscles or cutaneous blood vessels.* The cause of these neoplasms is unknown.

■ *Clinical Findings.* These neoplasms are usually solitary, firm, well circumscribed, dermal-epidermal in location, and less than 2 cm in diameter. There are no reported age, breed, or sex predilections. They may occur more frequently on the groin, the vulva, the head, and the back (Fig. 19:61).

■ *Diagnosis.* Histopathologically, leiomyomas and leiomyosarcomas are characterized by interlacing bundles of smooth muscle fibers that tend to intersect at right angles (Fig. 19:62).[4, 5, 32] Cell nuclei are usually cigar shaped with rounded blunt ends. Masson trichrome stain is often helpful in distinguishing among tumors of muscle, collagen, and neural origin. Smooth muscle tumors are positive for vimentin, desmin, and S-100 protein.[47, 52, 54]

■ *Clinical Management.* The therapy of choice is surgical excision.[11–13]

RHABDOMYOMA AND RHABDOMYOSARCOMA

■ *Cause and Pathogenesis.* Rhabdomyomas and rhabdomyosarcomas are extremely rare neoplasms of dogs and cats that arise from skeletal muscle.[12, 152a, 152b] The cause of these neoplasms is unknown.

■ *Clinical Findings.* *Rhabdomyomas* were reported most commonly on the pinna in white-eared adult cats.[152b] The lesions were raised, firm, well-circumscribed, red-purple nodules, 1 to 2 cm in diameter, on the convex surface of the pinna. *Rhabdomyosarcomas* were described on the pinna and in the inguinal region of adult cats.[152a]

■ *Diagnosis.* Histopathologically, these neoplasms consist of whorls and bundles of elongated spindle-shaped cells.[152a, 152b] Phosphotungstic acid hematoxylin enhances the appearance

---

*See references 4, 5, 11–13, 19, 21a, and 32.

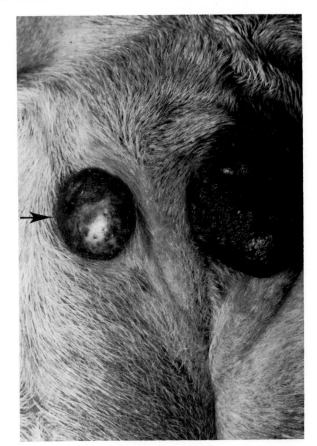

Figure 19:61. Canine leiomyoma. Pigmented nodule *(arrow)* lateral to the vulva.

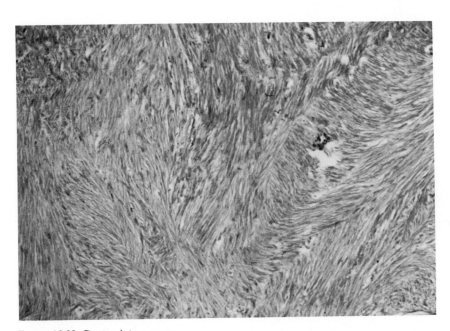

Figure 19:62. Canine leiomyoma.

of cross-striations in tumor cells and bundles. Skeletal muscle tumors are positive for desmin and vimentin.[152a]

■ *Clinical Management.* The therapy of choice is surgical excision.

OSTEOMA AND OSTEOSARCOMA

■ *Cause and Pathogenesis.* Extraskeletal osteomas and osteosarcomas are rare in dogs and cats.[4, 11, 152c] The cause of these neoplasms is unknown.

■ *Clinical Findings.* *Osteoma cutis* is reported in adult dogs and cats.[4, 11, 153] The lesions were solitary, discrete, firm nodules primarily involving proximal extremities (Fig. 19:63). Histopathologically, numerous trabeculae consisting of both woven and lamellar bone, normal osteocytes within lacunae, and multinucleate osteoclasts are seen (Fig. 19:64). Because osteoma-like changes may be seen in certain nevi and neoplasms or as heterotypic ossification in response to repeated tissue injury (chronic inflammation and calcinosis cutis), true osteomas must satisfy the following criteria: (1) growth unattached to periosteum or periarticular structures, (2) spontaneous occurrence (not secondary to trauma or inflammation), and (3) origin that is not developmental.

Extraskeletal osteosarcomas have been reported in the subcutaneous tissues (especially perianal, axillary, and proximal limb) of aged dogs and cats.[4, 11, 152c, 154] Metastatic lesions were present in most animals. Histopathologically, a proliferation of malignant osteoblasts and variable amounts of osteoid are seen (Fig. 19:65). Osteosarcomas are positive for vimentin.[45]

■ *Clinical Management.* The treatment of choice is surgical excision.[11]

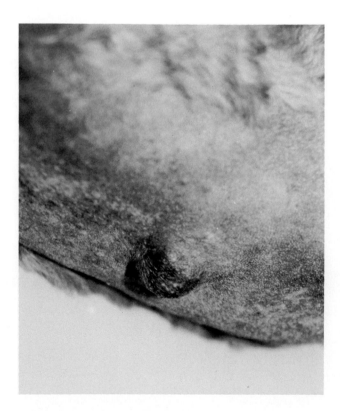

Figure 19:63. Canine osteoma. Solitary nodule on the ventral thorax (the area has been clipped).

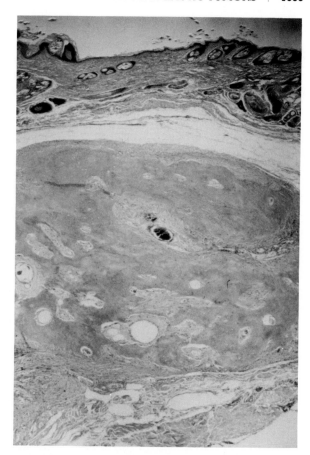

Figure 19:64. Feline osteoma. Bone formation in the subcutis.

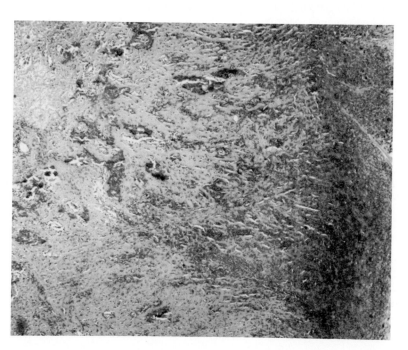

Figure 19:65. Canine osteosarcoma. Invasive proliferation of atypical osteoblasts and osteoid formation.

CHONDROMA AND CHONDROSARCOMA

■ *Cause and Pathogenesis.* Chondromas and chondrosarcomas are extremely rare skin neoplasms of the dog.[4, 154a] The cause of these neoplasms is unknown.

■ *Clinical Findings.* Primary cutaneous *chondroma* was diagnosed in a 10-year-old Labrador retriever.[4] The lesion was solitary, firm, 1 cm in diameter, and located on the head. Histologically, mature chondrocytes formed a nodule within the dermis and subcutis.

Primary cutaneous *chondrosarcomas* were diagnosed in a few dogs.[4, 154a] Lesions were solitary, firm, and multilobulated and occurred in the subcutaneous tissue of the neck, flank, groin, limb, and thorax. Histologically, malignant cells with chondroid differentiation formed nodules within the dermis and subcutis.

■ *Clinical Management.* The treatment of choice is surgical excision.

UNDIFFERENTIATED SARCOMA

■ *Cause and Pathogenesis.* Classification of some mesenchymal neoplasms may be difficult or impossible on histopathologic criteria.[5a, 11–13, 22a] Such anaplastic sarcomas are usually called *undifferentiated,* or *spindle cell, sarcomas.* Employing electron microscopy or immunohistochemical (marker) techniques greatly reduces the incidence of such diagnoses, but these are not always available to practitioners, nor are they always economically feasible.

■ *Clinical Findings.* Undifferentiated sarcomas usually occur in older dogs and cats and have the clinical features of fibrosarcomas, neurofibrosarcomas, and hemangiopericytomas. In cats, undifferentiated sarcoma has been reported to involve the footpads of one or more feet.[34] Affected cats are usually lame, and affected pads are soft, mushy, and painful and may be ulcerated.

In dogs, an undifferentiated sarcoma has been reported to affect the digit.[155] Affected dogs were 11 to 15 years old and had solitary, soft to firm, variably ulcerated masses involving a digit. Lesions were described as growing out of an ulcerated digital pad or occurring around a clawbed. The tumors caused lameness. Histologically, the tumors appeared to arise in the area of dense collagenous trabeculae located proximal to the fat pad and eccrine sweat glands. The tumor cells had some features of histiocytes: nuclear and cytoplasmic pleomorphism, frequent mitoses, and multinucleate tumor giant cells. Although most of these tumors had neoplastic cells in vessels, no recurrences or metastases were recorded. Tumor cells were positive for vimentin, but negative for desmin, S-100 protein, and histiocyte markers. Electron microscopic examination revealed 200- to 400-nm intracytoplasmic secretory granules. The authors concluded that this undifferentiated mesenchymal sarcoma resembled reports of so-called atypical histiocytoma.

■ *Clinical Management.* Radical surgical excision is the treatment of choice for undifferentiated sarcomas.[22a]

Mast Cell Tumor

CAUSE AND PATHOGENESIS

Mast cell tumors (mastocytomas, mast cell sarcomas, or mastocytoses) are common neoplasms of the dog and cat that arise from mast cells.* The cause of mast cell tumors is unknown. In

---

*See references 4, 5, 10–13, 27, 29, 159, and 169.

dogs, mast cell tumors have been experimentally transmitted using tissues and cell-free extracts, which suggests a viral cause. However, ultrastructural examination of mast cell tumors has only occasionally revealed viral particles. It has been theorized that boxers and Boston terriers possess oncogenes that are transmitted to offspring and combine with a genetically determined deficiency of immune surveillance to result in an increased incidence of mast cell tumors in these breeds. Rarely, canine mast cell tumor has been thought to arise within scars and chronic dermatoses.[11, 165] In cats, transmission studies with various mast cell tumor extracts failed to produce neoplasms in normal individuals. Multiple histiocytic mast cell tumors have been described in 6- to 8-week-old Siamese kittens in which multiple kittens of two litters (sired by the same tom) were affected, suggesting a genetic influence.[161]

CLINICAL FINDINGS

Dog

Mast cell tumors occur in dogs at an average age of 8 years but are rarely reported in puppies, too.[4, 5, 11–13, 24, 161a] There is no apparent sex predilection, but boxers, Boston terriers, English bulldogs, bull terriers, fox terriers, Staffordshire terriers, Labrador retrievers, dachshunds, beagles, Pugs, Golden retrievers, and Weimaraners are at increased risk. The clinical appearance of mast cell tumors is variable. Lesions may be firm to soft (see Fig. 19:53 *F*), papular to nodular to pedunculated, dermal to subcutaneous in location (see Fig. 19:53 *G*), well to poorly circumscribed, and skin colored to erythematous (see Fig. 19:53 *H*) to hyperpigmented (Fig. 19:66). They vary from a few millimeters to several centimeters in diameter. Some lesions may appear as urticarial swellings or diffuse areas of edema and inflammation resembling cellulitis (Fig. 19:67). Some neoplasms have a pinfeather appearance (Fig. 19:68) or are ulcerated. Palpation of some lesions may result in release of vasoactive substances and resultant local edema and inflammation. Flushing (sudden, symmetric, diffuse reddening of large areas of skin) has been rarely reported in dogs with mast cell tumors. Mast cell tumors are usually

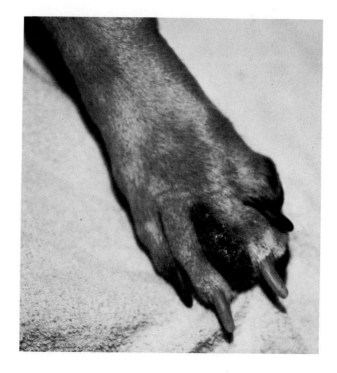

Figure 19:66. Canine mast cell tumor. Melanotic interdigital nodule.

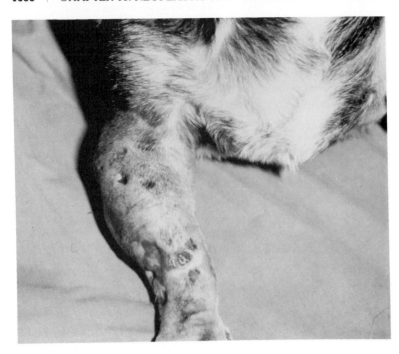

Figure 19:67. Canine mast cell tumor. Swollen, cellulitic-appearing forelimb. (Courtesy D. Angarano.)

solitary but may be multicentric either synchronously or sequentially. They occur most commonly on the caudal one half of the body (perineum, hindlimbs, and genitalia). Diffuse mast cell tumor produced gross distention and deformity of the hindlimbs in a Shar Pei.[179a] Noncutaneous symptoms that can be associated with mast cell tumors include gastric and duodenal ulcers, defective blood coagulation, and immune-mediated thrombocytopenia.[11–13, 162]

A case of cutaneous mastocytosis resembling *urticaria pigmentosa* was reported in a puppy.[161b] At 3 weeks of age, the dog had multiple cutaneous papules and nodules, pruritus, and lethargy. The lesions were generally alopecic, raised, pink to red, slightly firm, 1 to 5 cm in diameter, and especially numerous on the head, neck, legs, and perineum. By the time the dog was 27 weeks old, the condition resolved spontaneously.

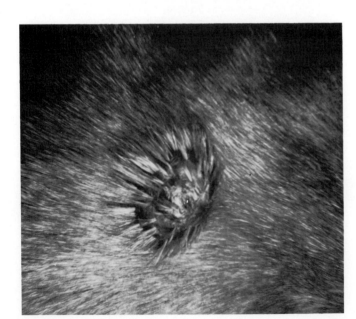

Figure 19:68. Canine mast cell tumor. Pin-feathered nodule over stifle region.

Urticaria pigmentosa-like disease was also reported in two adult dogs.[163a] Both had been affected since 6 months to 1 year of age. Papules and nodules would come and go over many areas of the body. Biopsies revealed the accumulation of well-differentiated mast cells in the superficial dermis and very few eosinophils. Occasionally, erythematous rashes that would progress to wheals or bullae would appear and disappear within hours. Traumatizing the lesions could produce sudden increase in size (edema), and stroking normal skin could result in a wheal-and-flare response. Both dogs were otherwise healthy and were followed for several years. The lesions were responsive to glucocorticoids, and to a combination of H_1- and H_2-blocking antihistamines.

Cat

Mast cell tumors occur in cats at an average age of 10 years.[4, 29, 159, 169] Male and Siamese cats are apparently predisposed.[4] Lesions occur most commonly on the head and the neck. The clinical appearance of mast cell tumors is variable: (1) multiple raised, soft, round, poorly demarcated, edematous, pinkish, variable-sized (0.5 to 5 cm in diameter) masses that are fixed to the overlying skin; (2) multiple raised, firm, round, well-circumscribed, white to yellow, small (2 to 10 mm in diameter) papules and nodules that are fixed to the overlying skin (Fig. 19:69 A); (3) single or multiple raised, firm, erythematous, well-circumscribed, variable-sized (1 to 7 cm in diameter) plaques (Fig. 19:69 B) that are frequently ulcerated and pruritic; and (4) solitary, firm to soft, well-circumscribed, variable-sized (0.3 to 3 cm in diameter), often alopecic dermal masses (Fig. 19:69 C).[34, 159, 169] A case of diffuse cutaneous mastocytosis in a 1-year-old cat was reported.[158] Generalized pruritus, papules, and erosions were present.

Urticaria pigmentosa is a proliferative mast cell disorder of humans.[3, 9] A syndrome with some clinicopathologic similarities to the human disorder has been seen in cats.[11] All cats have been young (younger than 1 year of age) Himalayans with asymptomatic macular erythema and hyperpigmentation around the mouth, chin, neck, and eyes. The condition regressed spontaneously after several months. Skin biopsies revealed hyperplastic superficial perivascular dermatitis with numerous mast cells and epidermal hypermelanosis.

A histiocytic subtype of mast cell tumor occurs primarily in Siamese cats from 6 weeks to 4 years of age.[5, 29, 161, 169] Multiple firm, pinkish papules occur primarily on the head and pinnae and eventually spontaneously regress.

Noncutaneous symptoms that may be associated with feline mast cell tumors include gastric and duodenal ulcers (thought to be histamine induced) and defective blood coagulation (thought to be heparin induced).

DIAGNOSIS

This is one tumor in which stained impression smears or aspirates are useful in establishing a tentative immediate diagnosis (Fig. 19:70).[41, 43] This procedure should not replace a complete histologic examination. Smears of cutaneous mast cell tumors in cats may reveal endocytosis of erythrocytes by the neoplastic mast cells.

Histologically, mast cell tumors are characterized by a diffuse to multinodular proliferation of mast cells (Figs. 19:71 and 19:72).[4, 5, 32] Frequent findings in canine mast cell tumors include tissue eosinophilia, focal areas of collagen degeneration, and a wide variety of vascular lesions (hyalinization, fibrinoid degeneration, and eosinophilic vasculitis) (Fig. 19:73). In cats, special caution is warranted to avoid confusing mast cell tumors with other round cell tumors and eosinophilic plaques. However, the striking tissue eosinophilia and collagen degeneration seen commonly in canine mast cell tumors is rare in cats.[4, 29, 159, 169] The histiocytic mast cell tumor in cats (especially Siamese) often has a granulomatous appearance, and the diagnosis can be confirmed only by electron microscopic demonstration of mast cell granules in some

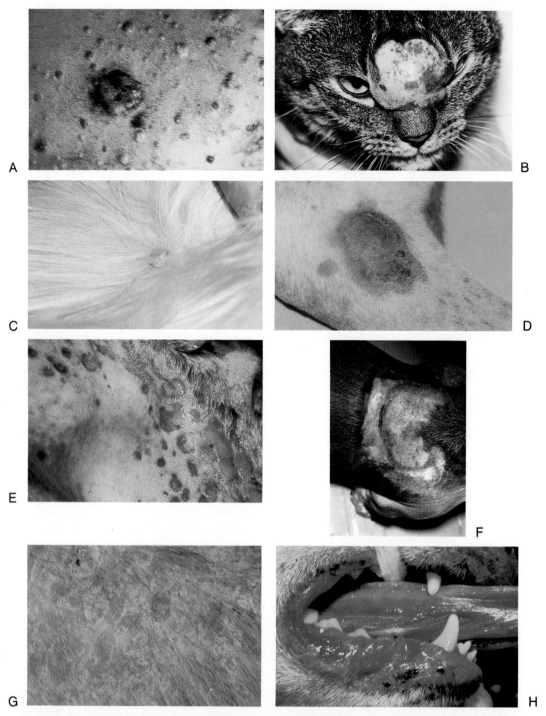

Figure 19:69. *A*, Feline mast cell tumor. Multiple papular-to-nodular lesions over the thorax (the area has been clipped). *B*, Feline mast cell tumor. Large, ulcerated nodule between the eyes. *C*, Feline mast cell tumor. Small, yellowish papule resembling a sebaceous gland tumor. *D*, Canine nonepitheliotropic lymphoma. Large erythematous plaque and multiple erythematous papules on a medial hind limb. *E*, Feline nonepitheliotropic lymphoma. Multiple erythematous plaques on the abdomen. *F*, Canine nonepitheliotropic lymphoma. Raised, erythematous lesion in the shape of an arc or C over the withers (the area has been shaved). *G*, Canine epitheliotropic lymphoma. Erythroderma, alopecia, and scales. *H*, Canine epitheliotropic lymphoma. Erythema, infiltration, and ulceration of the lips.

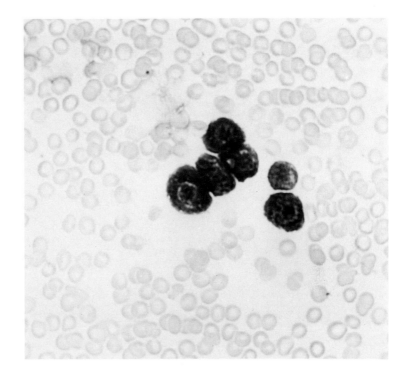

Figure 19:70. Canine mast cell tumor. Aspiration of a skin nodule reveals a clump of mast cells.

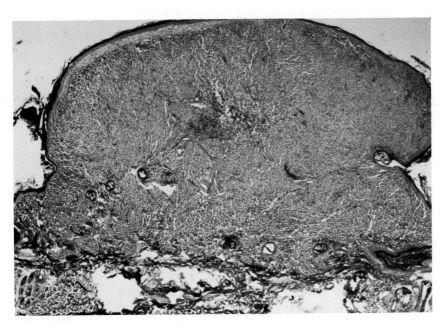

Figure 19:71. Feline mast cell tumor. Well-circumscribed, dome-shaped proliferation of mast cells.

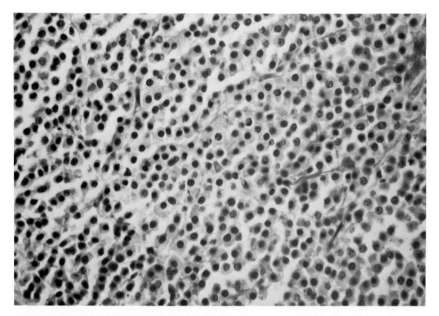

Figure 19:72. Close-up of Figure 19:71. Proliferation of monomorphous mast cells.

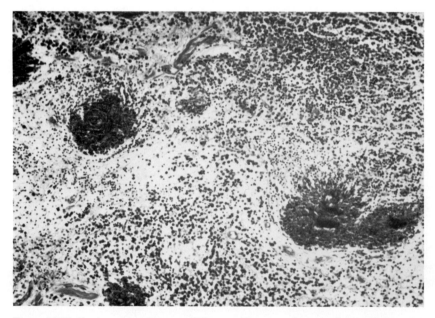

Figure 19:73. Canine mast cell tumor. Diffuse proliferation of mast cells, marked edema, and multifocal areas of collagenolysis.

Table 19:2. Histologic Classification of Mast Cell Tumors

Grade	Microscopic Description
High (anaplastic,[157] Grade I,[157] Grade III[164])	Highly cellular, indistinct cytoplasmic boundaries; irregular size and shape of nuclei, often frequent mitotic figures; low number of cytoplasmic granules
Intermediate (intermediate differentiation,[163] Grade II,[157] Grade II[164])	Closely packed cells with indistinct cytoplasmic boundaries; nucleus to cytoplasm ratio lower than that of high grade; mitotic figures infrequent; more granules than in high-grade tumors
Low (well differentiated,[163] Grade III,[157] Grade I[164])	Clearly defined cytoplasmic boundary with regular, spherical, or ovoid nucleus; mitotic figures rare; cytoplasmic granules large, deep staining, and plentiful

cases.[4, 5, 169] Mast cell tumors are positive for vimentin, α_1-antitrypsin, chymotrypsin-like protease, and dipeptidyl peptidase II.[51, 52, 55]

CLINICAL MANAGEMENT

Clinical management of mast cell tumors may include surgical excision, cryosurgery, electrosurgery, chemotherapy, radiotherapy, immunotherapy, and some combination of these.[11–13, 163b, 167, 168] In dogs, mast cell tumors should *always* be treated as potentially malignant neoplasms, because metastasis occurs in about 30 per cent of cases. Tumors arising from the perineum, the prepuce, the scrotum, and the digits appear to be more commonly aggressive and malignant. A histologic grading system (Table 19:2) and a clinical staging system (Table 19:3) have been developed for canine mast cell tumors. The recommended therapeutic approach for each canine mast cell tumor case is based on an amalgamation of these systems (Table 19:4). The clinical staging system is predicated on the results of studies of lymph node and bone marrow aspirates, as well as buffy coat examinations. However, mast cells may be found in lymph node and bone marrow aspirates from normal dogs,[156] as well as buffy coat smears from dogs with allergic and ectoparasitic skin disease.[160]

Early surgical excision is indicated in animals with a solitary neoplasm. Wide surgical margins, at least 3 cm between the palpable tumor and the incision, are recommended when possible. Approximately 50 per cent of canine mast cell tumors recur, even after a wide surgical excision.[11–13, 157] In dogs with mast cell tumors, the survival time is related to the degree of histologic differentiation.[157, 163, 164, 166] For animals with high-grade mast cell tumors, the mean survival time is 18 weeks after diagnosis; with intermediate-grade tumors, 28 weeks; and with

Table 19:3. Clinical Staging System for Mast Cell Tumors

Stage I	One tumor confined to the dermis without regional lymph node involvement
	a. Without systemic signs
	b. With systemic signs
Stage II	One tumor confined to dermis, with regional lymph node involvement
	a. Without systemic signs
	b. With systemic signs
Stage III	Multiple dermal tumors; large infiltrating tumors with or without regional node involvement
	a. Without systemic signs
	b. With systemic signs
Stage IV	Any tumor with distant metastasis or recurrence with metastasis

From Tams, T.R., Macy, D.W.: Canine mast cell tumors. Comp. Cont. Educ. 3:873, 1981.

Table 19:4. Suggested Treatment of Mast Cell Tumors Based on Clinical Stages

Stage	Treatment
I	Surgical excision only. (Surgery is defined as the excision of the tumor with a minimum margin of 3 cm between palpable tumor and the incision line; such excision should include regional lymph node when possible.)
II	Surgical excision plus radiation. (Radiation therapy is defined as the administration of 4000 rad divided into 10 fractions to be administered every other day for treatments.)
III	Intralesional steroids plus cimetidine. (Intralesional steroid is defined as the intralesional injection of 1 mg of triamcinolone for every centimeter diameter of tumor. This dose is to be administered every 2 weeks.)
IV	Systemic steroids* plus cimetidine.†

*A dose of 0.5 mg/kg of body weight of prednisolone to be administered every 24 to 48 hours.
†Cimetidine should be given daily at a dose of 4 mg/kg q6h.
From Tams, T.R., Macy, D.W.: Canine mast cell tumors. Comp. Cont. Educ. 3:876, 1981.

low-grade tumors, 51 weeks. However, some veterinary pathologists believe that tumor grade is often an unreliable prognostic indicator and are reluctant to grade these neoplasms.[4] DNA ploidy status of canine mast cells tumors was not found to be of prognostic significance.[155a]

In cats, the vast majority of cutaneous mast cell tumors are benign.[5, 29, 159, 169] A histologic grading system similar to that used in dogs was evaluated in feline mast cell tumors and found *not* to correlate with biological behavior.[159] The histiocytic mast cell tumor of cats, which is often characterized clinically by multiple cutaneous nodules in Siamese cats younger than 4 years, appears to undergo spontaneous remission frequently.[5, 29, 161, 169]

Chemotherapy has been advocated for disseminated mast cell tumors.[7, 8, 11–13] Administration of oral prednisolone or prednisone (0.5 mg/kg q24h) or intralesional triamcinolone (1 mg for every 1 cm of diameter of tumor) has been recommended (see Table 19:4). This treatment causes temporary regression of the tumors that may last several months. Combination chemotherapy (glucocorticoids plus cyclophosphamide, vincristine, or vinblastine, for example) has been recommended by some investigators, but no evidence suggests that this is superior to the use of glucocorticoids alone in dogs and cats. Cimetidine (4 mg/kg orally q6h) has been recommended in dogs with evidence of systemic or lymph node involvement or with evidence of gastrointestinal hemorrhage. Cimetidine acts by competitively inhibiting the action of histamine on the H_2 receptors of gastric parietal cells, thus reducing gastric acid output and concentration.

In dogs, there is a frequent tendency for local hemorrhage during surgery and delayed wound healing at the site of tumor removal.[4, 11–13] Cryosurgery or hyperthermia may precipitate a shocklike reaction in dogs that have not been pretreated with antihistamines.[4, 11, 13]

■ LYMPHOHISTIOCYTIC NEOPLASMS

Tumors of Lymphocytic Origin

LYMPHOMA

Cutaneous lymphoma (malignant lymphoma, lymphosarcoma, lymphoreticular neoplasm, lymphomatosis, or reticulum cell sarcoma) is an uncommon malignant neoplasm of the dog and cat.* In cats, the cause of most types of lymphoma is FeLV, although cats with cutaneous lymphoma are usually FeLV negative. In dogs, the cause of lymphoma is unknown, although (1) lymphoma can be transmitted to puppies by the injection of whole-cell preparations of

*See references 4, 5, 10–13, 174, 174a, 180, 183, and 188.

malignant lymphocytes, (2) C-type viruses were found in neoplastic cells from dogs with lymphoma, and (3) lymphoma has been induced in neonatal puppies by injections of FeLV.

Histologically and clinically, lymphoma can be divided into nonepitheliotropic and epitheliotropic forms. Nonepitheliotropic forms are typically of B lymphocyte origin, whereas epitheliotropic forms are of T lymphocyte origin.

Nonepitheliotropic Lymphoma

Nonepitheliotropic lymphoma occurs in older dogs and cats with no sex predilection.* In dogs, boxers, St. Bernards, Basset hounds, Irish setters, Cocker spaniels, German shepherd dogs, Golden retrievers, and Scottish terriers appear to be predisposed.

Nonepitheliotropic lymphoma is usually generalized or multifocal and has a variety of cutaneous manifestations. Nodules are present in virtually all cases; they are firm, dermal or subcutaneous, often alopecic and red to purple (see Fig. 19:69 D and E).[34, 172] Exfoliative erythroderma is present in about 20 per cent of cases, but pruritus and oral mucosal involvement are rare.[172] Occasionally, lesions are present in bizarre, arciform, or serpiginous shapes (see Fig. 19:69 F).[171] Rarely, dogs and cats may have solitary skin lesions. Affected animals usually have signs of systemic involvement. Rarely, nonepitheliotropic lymphoma is associated with monoclonal or biclonal gammopathies, serum hyperviscosity, or hypercalcemia.[7, 8, 11–13]

Histologically, nonepitheliotropic lymphomas are characterized by diffuse dermal and subcutaneous infiltration by malignant lymphocytes. These malignant lymphocytes are lymphocytic (well differentiated or poorly differentiated), lymphoblastic, or histiocytic in cytologic form (Figs. 19:74 to 19:76).[4, 5, 11–13]

Clinical management of nonepitheliotropic lymphoma is usually unsuccessful.[11–13, 171, 183] Traditional regimens of combined chemotherapy or chemoimmunotherapy may occasionally induce short-term (average, 8 months) remission. Rarely, surgical excision of a solitary cutaneous lymphoma lesion results in long-term remission or, perhaps, cure. The average survival from the onset of skin lesions to death (usually due to euthanasia) is about 4 months.[172]

Epitheliotropic Lymphoma

Epitheliotropic lymphoma is an uncommon cutaneous malignancy of dogs and cats.† Epitheliotropic lymphomas are usually of T lymphocyte origin.[170, 176, 185a, 186] In most instances, the cause of epitheliotropic lymphomas is unknown. There is controversy about whether human mycosis fungoides, the prototypic epitheliotropic (T cell) lymphoma, begins as a reactive process or as a neoplastic process.[3, 5, 179] In human adult T cell leukemia-lymphoma, the causative factor is believed to be the human T cell lymphotrophic virus type I.[3] Epitheliotropic lymphoma of dogs and cats is of unknown etiology, and all affected cats have been FeLV negative. Recently, tumor DNA was extracted from a cat with epitheliotropic T cell lymphoma, amplified for FeLV provirus by polymerase chain reaction, and shown to be positive.[185a] This study suggested that FeLV may be involved in the etiology of epitheliotropic T cell lymphoma in cats, even when cats test negative with commonly used methods of detecting FeLV antigen.

Cutaneous T cell lymphoma is characterized by a proliferation of T lymphocytes with phenotypic and functional properties of helper T cells.[3, 9, 179] Cutaneous T cell lymphoma encompasses a spectrum of disease, including mycosis fungoides and Sézary syndrome.

Mycosis Fungoides

In humans, mycosis fungoides is defined clinically and immunologically as a neoplasm of helper T cells.[3, 9] In dogs and cats, a T cell origin has been documented, but the functional properties of the cells have not been defined.[170, 176, 177a, 185a, 186]

---

*See references 4, 5, 10–13, 174, 174a, 180, 183, and 188.
†See references 4, 5, 170, 177a, 180, 182, 187, and 189.

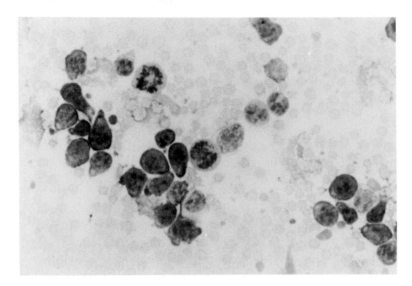

Figure 19:74. Canine epitheliotropic lymphoma. Aspirate from a skin nodule reveals pleomorphic, atypical lymphocytes.

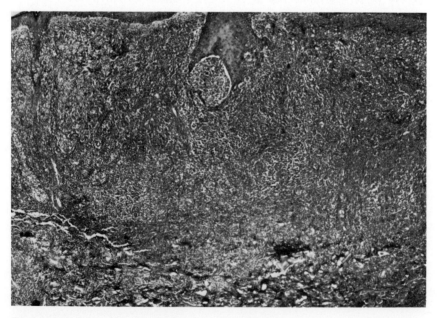

Figure 19:75. Feline nonepitheliotropic lymphoma. Diffuse dermal and subcutaneous infiltration of neoplastic lymphocytes.

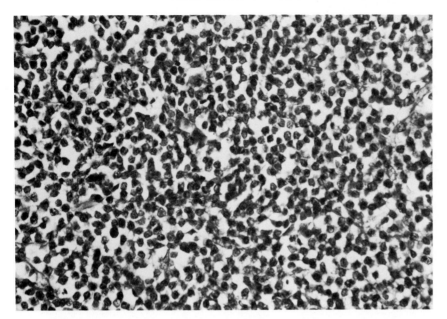

Figure 19:76. Close-up of Figure 19:75. Neoplastic lymphocytes.

In dogs and cats, mycosis fungoides usually affects older animals (average of 9 to 11 years), with no apparent breed or sex predilections. Four clinical presentations are described: (1) generalized pruritic erythema and scaling (exfoliative erythroderma) (see Fig. 19:69 *G*), usually misdiagnosed as allergy, scabies, or seborrhea; (2) mucocutaneous ulceration (see Fig. 19:69 *H*) and depigmentation (Fig. 19:77 *A*), usually misdiagnosed as immune-mediated disease (pemphigus vulgaris, bullous pemphigoid, or lupus erythematosus); (3) solitary or multiple cutaneous plaques or nodules (Fig. 19:77 *B* and *C*); and (4) infiltrative and ulcerative oral mucosal disease, usually misdiagnosed as a non-neoplastic, chronic stomatitis (Fig. 19:77 *D*).* Affected animals often have peripheral lymphadenopathy and signs of systemic illness. In cats, lesions may be initially well-circumscribed, annular areas of alopecia, erythema, and scaling (usually misdiagnosed as dermatophytosis or demodicosis) (Fig. 19:77 *E*).[170]

Histopathologically, mycosis fungoides is characterized by epitheliotropism, Pautrier microabscesses (focal accumulations of pleomorphic, atypical lymphocytes within the epithelium) (Figs. 19:78 and 19:79), and the presence of mycosis cells (large, 20- to 30-μm lymphocytes with hyperchromatic, indented or folded nuclei) and Sézary, or Lutzner, cells (smaller, 8- to 20-μm lymphocytes that have markedly hyperconvoluted nuclei with numerous finger-like projections, producing a classic cerebriform appearance).[4, 5, 170, 183b, 184, 185a] Often, a lichenoid band of pleomorphic lymphoid cells, with or without plasma cells, neutrophils, and eosinophils, is present in the superficial dermis and surrounding appendages. Epidermal mucinosis (acid mucopolysaccharides) and mild fibrosis of the immediate subepidermal superficial dermis may be seen. Electron microscopy reveals many tumor cells characterized by a high ratio of nucleus to cytoplasm, deep invaginations of the nuclear membrane (convoluted or cerebriform nucleus), a relatively wide rim of peripheral chromatin, a paucity of organelles, and peripheral cytoplasmic villi or projections (Fig. 19:80).[5, 170, 184] Direct immunofluorescence testing may show the intercellular deposition of immunoglobulin in the epithelium, falsely suggesting a diagnosis of pemphigus.[182, 184]

The prognosis for animals with canine and feline mycosis fungoides is grave.[170, 172, 187, 189] In dogs, the average survival time from the onset of skin lesions until death (usually due to

---

*See references 170, 172, 173, 178, 182, 184, 187, and 189.

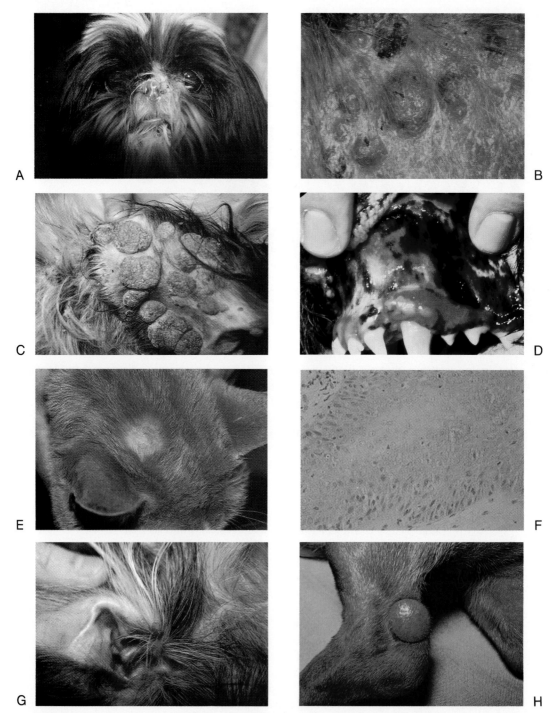

Figure 19:77. *A*, Canine epitheliotropic lymphoma. Depigmentation, infiltration, and mild erythema of the nose and lips. *B*, Canine epitheliotropic lymphoma. Numerous nodules, some of which are ulcerated and crusted, on a background of exfoliative erythroderma. *C*, Canine epitheliotropic lymphoma. Numerous cauliflower-like nodules on the pinna with background skin that appears normal. *D*, Canine epitheliotropic lymphoma. Infiltration and ulceration of the oral mucosa. *E*, Feline epitheliotropic lymphoma. Annular area of alopecia, scaling, and mild erythema on the head. *F*, Feline alopecia mucinosa. Note marked accumulation of blue mucin within the hair follicle outer root sheath. *G*, Canine plasmacytoma. Erythematous papule at the base of the ear. *H*, Canine histocytoma. Characteristic button tumor on the hock.

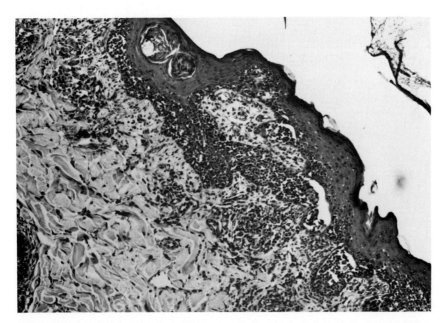

Figure 19:78. Canine epitheliotropic lymphoma. Infiltration of the lower portion of the epidermis with neoplastic lymphocytes.

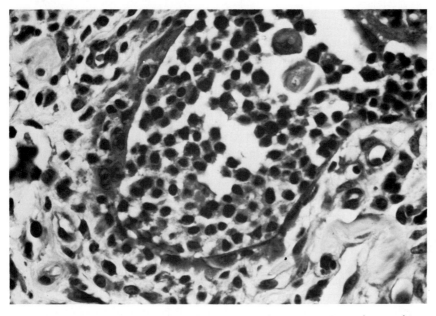

Figure 19:79. Close-up of Figure 19:78. Pautrier microabscess containing pleomorphic and atypical lymphocytes.

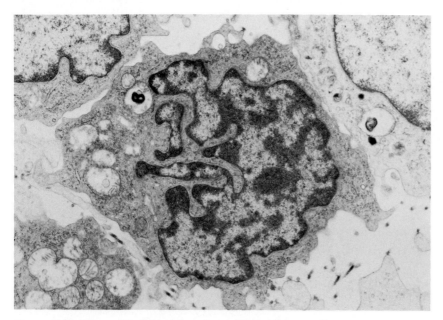

Figure 19:80. Feline epitheliotropic lymphoma. Typical Sézary cell.

euthanasia) is 5 to 10 months.[172, 173, 187, 189] Exceptionally, dogs and cats with mycosis fungoides may live for longer than 2 years after a diagnosis is made. Death is due to septicemia, metastatic lymphosarcoma, or euthanasia.

Therapy for mycosis fungoides in dogs and cats has usually been of little or no benefit.* Chemotherapy with various combinations of prednisolone, chlorambucil, vincristine, cyclophosphamide, doxorubicin, and methotrexate have occasionally produced some degree of clinical improvement for 1 to 5 months. Rarely, solitary nodules can be surgically excised, with long-term remissions or cures ensuing.[183, 187, 189]

The most commonly effective treatment of canine mycosis fungoides is the topical application of mechlorethamine (nitrogen mustard).[180, 183] Mechlorethamine hydrochloride, 10 mg, is dissolved in 50 ml of water and applied to the clipped surface (total body) two or three times weekly, until lesions have regressed. The solution is then applied as needed for maintenance (every 2 to 4 weeks). No signs of toxicity or drug hypersensitivity have been reported in dogs. Occasionally, dogs have experienced demodicosis. Because mechlorethamine is a potent sensitizing agent in humans, gloves should be worn when applying the drug, and the dog should not be handled for the first few hours after application. In addition, exposure to the powder form or vapors from the drug can produce burning of the eyes and throat. Although topical mechlorethamine appears to be useful for managing the "dermatitic" and plaque stages of mycosis fungoides, no evidence suggests that it alters in any way the ultimately fatal course of eventual systemic involvement. In addition, mechlorethamine is a topical carcinogen and cocarcinogen and may be associated with the subsequent development of cutaneous epithelial malignancies (squamous cell carcinoma and basal cell carcinoma), colon cancer, and Hodgkin's disease in humans.[179]

In humans, topical carmustine (BCNU) has been reported to be effective in mycosis fungoides, with fewer toxicities and hypersensitivity reactions than seen with topical mechlorethamine, and no development of secondary skin neoplasms.[179] Other therapies reported to be of benefit in humans with mycosis fungoides include the administration of oral retinoids or interferon, oral methoxsalen (8-methoxypsoralen) and subsequent exposure to ultraviolet A light (PUVA), cyclosporine, photophoresis, and electron beam therapy.[179] Retinoids (isotreti-

---

*See references 170, 172, 173, 177, 183, 183c, 187, 188a, and 189.

noin at 1 to 8 mg/kg/day; etretinate at 1 to 8 mg/kg/day) have occasionally been useful in dogs and cats with mycosis fungoides.[70, 71, 182, 188a] In one study, only about 50 per cent of the dogs with epitheliotropic and nonepitheliotropic cutaneous lymphoma that were treated with oral retinoids had a clinical improvement of more than 50 per cent.[188a] Survival time in these dogs varied from 5 to 17 months (mean, 11 months). Cyclosporine and omega-3 and omega-6 fatty acid–containing products have not been effective.[11, 182] About 50 per cent of the dogs with mycosis fungoides treated with peg L-asparaginase (weekly or biweekly injections of 30 U/kg intramuscularly or intraperitoneally) experienced a reduction in erythema and scaling.[181] However, there was no effect on plaques and tumors, and no indication that the treatment prolonged survival time.

Alopecia Mucinosa

In humans, alopecia mucinosa (follicular mucinosis) is characterized by well-demarcated areas of alopecia, fine scaling, and prominent hair follicle orifices, with or without slightly raised and mildly erythematous papules or plaques.[3, 9] There are three clinical patterns. The first, and most common, is seen in young adults; it is restricted to the head and neck, and it resolves in about 2 years. The second form is seen in a slightly older age group, lesions are more generalized, and resolution takes longer. The third form is seen in aged people, and plaques of mycosis fungoides eventually develop within the areas of alopecia. The pathogenic mechanism of alopecia mucinosa is unknown.

Alopecia mucinosa was recognized in two adult cats with asymptomatic, well-demarcated alopecia and fine scaling on the head, ears, and neck (Fig. 19:81).[36] Biopsy specimens initially revealed mucinosis of the epidermis and the hair follicle's outer root sheath (see Fig. 19:77 *F*). Several months later, both cats had plaques in the areas of alopecia. Biopsy results at this time were typical of mycosis fungoides. Both cats were lost to follow-up.

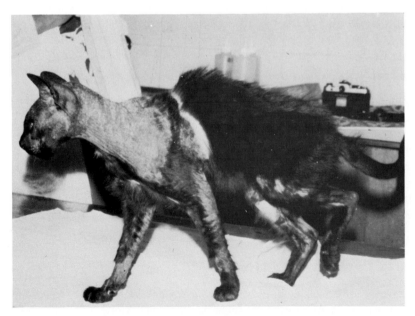

Figure 19:81. Feline alopecia mucinosa. Alopecia and scaling of head, neck, and front legs. (Courtesy V. Studdert.)

Sézary Syndrome

The Sézary syndrome is an epitheliotropic T cell lymphoma characterized by erythroderma (generalized erythema), pruritus, peripheral lymphadenopathy, and the presence of Sézary, or Lutzner, cells (see Mycosis Fungoides in this chapter) in the cutaneous infiltrate and in the peripheral blood.[3, 9, 179] Histopathologically, the skin biopsy specimens are usually indistinguishable from those in mycosis fungoides. Most authors believe that the Sézary syndrome and mycosis fungoides are variants of the same T cell lymphoma.

Sézary syndrome is extremely rare in dogs[175, 185] and cats.[183a] The animals had generalized pruritus, exfoliative erythroderma, multiple skin plaques and nodules, and lymphocytic leukemia. Skin biopsies revealed epitheliotropic lymphoma. Sézary-like cells were found in the peripheral blood and the skin. In humans, the Sézary syndrome has been treated with many modalities, a current favorite being chlorambucil and prednisone, administered orally.[3, 179] Dogs and cats usually do not respond to chemotherapy.

Pagetoid Reticulosis

In humans, pagetoid reticulosis (Woringer-Kolopp disease) is a controversial epitheliotropic lymphoma.[3, 9] There is controversy about (1) the cell of origin (T lymphocyte versus histiocyte), (2) the relative benignity or malignancy of the disease, and (3) the relationship of pagetoid reticulosis to mycosis fungoides. Pagetoid reticulosis in humans is usually characterized by (1) a solitary, often erythematous and scaly plaque or tumor on the distal extremities, (2) extreme epitheliotropism (no subepidermal component) featuring relatively monomorphous cells (polymorphous in mycosis fungoides) with peripheral halos, and (3) a relatively benign course wherein surgical excision or radiation therapy is curative.

A pagetoid reticulosis–like disease was described in dogs.[5, 187] However, many features of the canine disease were unlike those of the human disease: (1) clinical signs were generalized and indistinguishable from those of mycosis fungoides, (2) internal metastasis was recorded, and (3) subepidermal involvement with neoplastic cells was seen late in the disease. Early histopathologic findings included extreme epitheliotropism and monomorphous and haloed neoplastic round cells. So-called canine pagetoid reticulosis may be simply a variant of mycosis fungoides with more precise epitheliotropism and cellular monomorphism. Cases of focal Woringer-Kolopp–type disease have been reported in dogs, but no details were given.[5]

LYMPHOMATOID GRANULOMATOSIS

Lymphomatoid granulomatosis is a rare lymphohistiocytic proliferative disorder in dogs.[5] Most dogs have only visceral lesions. Occasional cutaneous involvement has been characterized by chronic, recurrent, punctate to crateriform ulcers that heal with scarring. Lesions involve the face, the eyelids, the mucocutaneous junctions, and the trunk. Biopsy reveals abrupt foci of full-thickness epidermal necrosis and ulceration overlying wedge-shaped zones of dermal necrosis.[5] A polymorphous lymphohistiocytic infiltrate invades blood vessel walls in the deep dermis and panniculus (Fig. 19:82), resulting in ischemic necrosis. Atypical large lymphocytes with pale cytoplasm and mitotic figures increase in number during the course of the disease. Successful therapy has not been reported.

PSEUDOLYMPHOMA

Pseudolymphomas have been defined as disorders in which a histologic picture suggesting malignant lymphoma stands in sharp contrast to benign biological behavior.[3, 190, 191] Cutaneous pseudolymphomas have been subclassified into simulators of B cell and T cell lymphomas. In humans, pseudolymphomas have been associated with reactions to sunlight, drugs, arthropods,

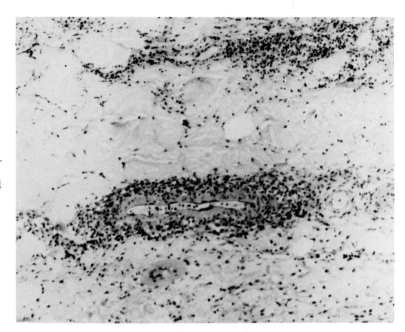

Figure 19:82. Canine lymphomatoid granulomatosis. Pleomorphic lymphohistiocytic cells infiltrating a deep dermal vessel. (Courtesy E. Walder.)

viruses, and contact allergens, as well as with idiopathy. Other authors prefer to reserve the term pseudolymphoma for benign, non-neoplastic but hyperplastic lymphoproliferative processes that mimic malignant lymphoma but that do not show adequate criteria for diagnosis of a specific disease and have a strong tendency for spontaneous regression. Thus, according to this definition, (1) pseudolymphomas are of unknown etiology and do not include specific disease entities of known cause and (2) pseudolymphomatous disorders of known cause are referred to as *pseudo-pseudolymphomas*!

Pseudolymphomas usually present as plaques or nodules, usually solitary, often erythematous, and occasionally ulcerated. Age, breed, sex, and site predilections are not clear in small animals. Animals with pseudolymphoma, regardless of the number of skin lesions or regional lymph node involvement, are typically otherwise healthy. Pseudolymphomas have been recognized in dogs and cats in association with arthropod (especially tick) bites, vaccinations, and drugs.[11, 190] A case of pseudolymphoma resembling pseudo-Hodgkin's disease was reported in a dog.[191] The dog had multiple, widespread, discrete, firm nodules and plaques that were alopecic and red-purple. Biopsy revealed a nodular to diffuse dermal and subcutaneous proliferation of pleomorphic and atypical lymphohistiocytic cells with numerous Reed-Sternberg cells (large cells with a multilobulated nucleus whose morphology is such that nuclear lobes appear to be ''kissing,'' or ''mirror images''). The disorder spontaneously resolved.

Histopathologically, the distinction between malignant lymphoma and pseudolymphoma of the skin is one of the most difficult problems in dermatopathology (Fig. 19:83).[9, 190] Major points of differentiation are presented in Table 19:5.

Treatment of pseudolymphoma is best directed at the underlying cause. Surgical excision of solitary lesions is usually curative.

CUTANEOUS PLASMACYTOMA

■ *Cause and Pathogenesis.* Cutaneous plasmacytomas (cutaneous extramedullary plasmacytomas) are uncommon in the dog and rare in the cat.[4, 5, 205–209] These neoplasms are of plasma cell origin and are rarely associated with multiple myeloma. The cause of cutaneous plasmacytomas is unknown. It is likely that these neoplasms were previously reported as reticulum cell sarcoma, atypical histiocytoma, or neuroendocrine tumor.

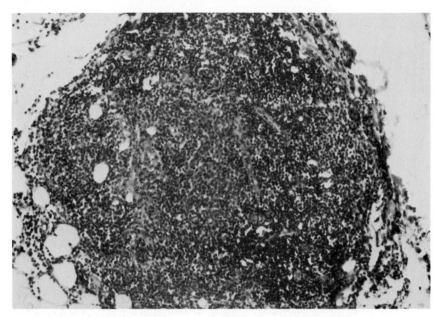

Figure 19:83. Canine pseudolymphoma. Nodular subcutaneous proliferation of normal lymphocytes and plasma cells.

■ *Clinical Findings.*   Cutaneous plasmacytomas occur in dogs at an average age of 10 years, there is no sex predilection, and Cocker spaniels may be predisposed.[4, 5, 205–207, 209] They are usually solitary and occur most commonly on the digits, the lips, and the ears (especially in the external ear canal) (see Fig. 19:77 *G*). Most plasmacytomas are well circumscribed, raised, smooth, firm to soft, pink to red, dermal in location, and 1 to 2 cm in diameter (range, 0.2 to 10 cm). Tumors in the ear canal are often polypoid, and those on digits are often ulcerated and hemorrhagic.

Plasmacytomas are extremely rare in cats, being reported on the lip and gingiva of aged animals.[208]

■ *Diagnosis.*   Histologically, plasmacytomas are characterized by sheets, packets, and cords of cells infiltrating the dermis and subcutis (Figs. 19:84 to 19:86).[5, 205a, 206–209] The neoplastic cells may be well differentiated or extremely pleomorphic and atypical. Amyloid is present in about 10 per cent of lesions.[4, 5, 210] Electron microscopy or immunohistochemical techniques may be required to confirm the plasma cell origin of the neoplastic cells. Immunohistochemical

Table 19:5. Histologic Criteria for the Differentiation of Malignant Lymphoma from Pseudolymphoma

Malignant Lymphoma	Pseudolymphoma
Cellular infiltrate greater in deep dermis (''bottom heavy'')	Cellular infiltrate greater in superficial dermis (''top heavy'')
Monomorphous cellular infiltrate	Polymorphous (mixed cell) cellular infiltrate
Medium-sized or large lymphocytes usually predominate	Small lymphocytes usually predominate
Germinal centers rare	Germinal centers common
Polychrome (tingible body) macrophages rare	Polychrome (tingible body) macrophages common
Necrosis en masse may be present	No necrosis en masse
Epithelial and vascular structures often involved	Epithelial and vascular structures spared
Cytologic atypia common	Cytologic atypia rare
Monoclonal immunocytologic pattern	Polyclonal immunocytologic pattern

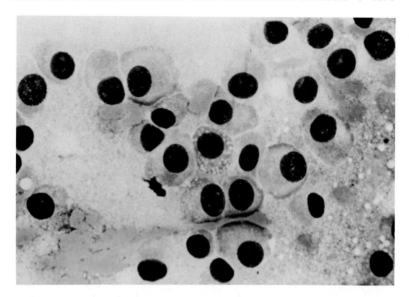

Figure 19:84. Canine plasmacytoma. Cytologic examination of aspirate shows pleomorphic plasma cells. (Courtesy T. French.)

studies have shown that most plasmacytomas are positive for immunoglobulin G heavy chains and λ light chains.[205, 205a, 207, 208, 210] Plasmacytomas are positive for vimentin,[205] and most stain with thioflavine T.[205a] Attempts to correlate DNA aneuploidy and oncoprotein content with histopathologic appearance and biologic behavior of canine plasmacytomas was fraught with false-positive and false-negative results.[206a]

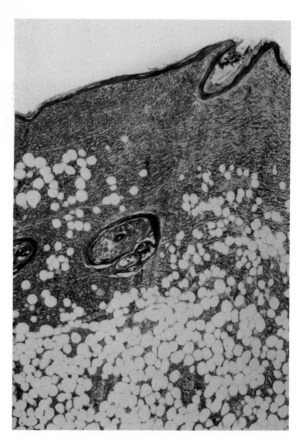

Figure 19:85. Canine plasmacytoma. Diffuse infiltration of dermis.

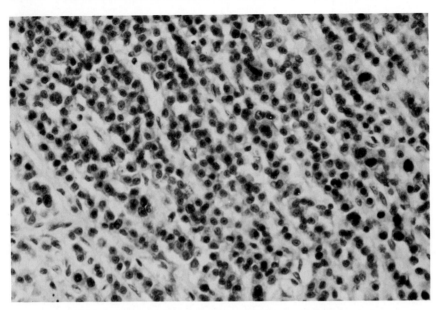

Figure 19:86. Close-up of Figure 19:85. Cordlike proliferation of pleomorphic, atypical plasma cells.

■ *Clinical Management.* The treatment of choice is surgical excision. Local recurrence and metastasis are rare.[4, 205, 206, 209] Some authors believe that plasmacytomas containing amyloid are more likely to recur after surgery.[4] A histologic grading system was of no benefit, as neoplasms exhibited benign biological behavior in spite of malignant histologic appearance.[5, 205, 209] Rarely, plasmacytomas may occur simultaneously with, or precede (by weeks to months), the development of multiple myeloma.[5, 11, 209]

Tumors of Histiocytic Origin

HISTIOCYTOMA

■ *Cause and Pathogenesis.* Histiocytomas are common benign neoplasms of the dog.[4, 5, 11–13, 27] They are rare in the cat.[19, 26] Their cause is unknown, although they are more likely a unique proliferation or reactive hyperplasia rather than a true neoplasm. Histiocytomas are derived from cells of monocyte-macrophage lineage, as supported by results of electron microscopy and enzyme histochemistry. An immunohistochemical study showed that histiocytomas are most likely of Langerhans' cell origin.[5, 191a]

■ *Clinical Findings.* Characteristically, histiocytomas affect young dogs, with about 50 per cent of cases occurring in dogs younger than 2 years.[4, 5, 11–13, 191b] However, old dogs may also be affected. Boxers, dachshunds, Cocker spaniels, Great Danes, Scottish terriers, Boston terriers, American Staffordshire terriers, Rottweilers, Shar Peis, West Highland white terriers,

Figure 19:87. *A,* Canine histiocytoma. Ulcerated nodule on a pinna. *B,* Canine systemic histiocytosis. Multiple erythematous papules, nodules, and plaques over the trunk (the area has been clipped). *C,* Same dog as in *B.* Infiltration, erythema, and depigmentation of the nose. *D,* Canine cutaneous histiocytosis. Multiple violaceous nodules over the lateral thorax (the area has been clipped). *E,* Canine malignant fibrous histiocytoma. Nodules on the bridge of the nose. *F,* Canine melanocytoma. Melanotic nodule on the lower eyelid. *G,* Canine melanoma. Melanotic nodule on the lip. *H,* Feline melanoma. Ulcerated, melanotic nodule on the ventral neck (the area has been clipped).

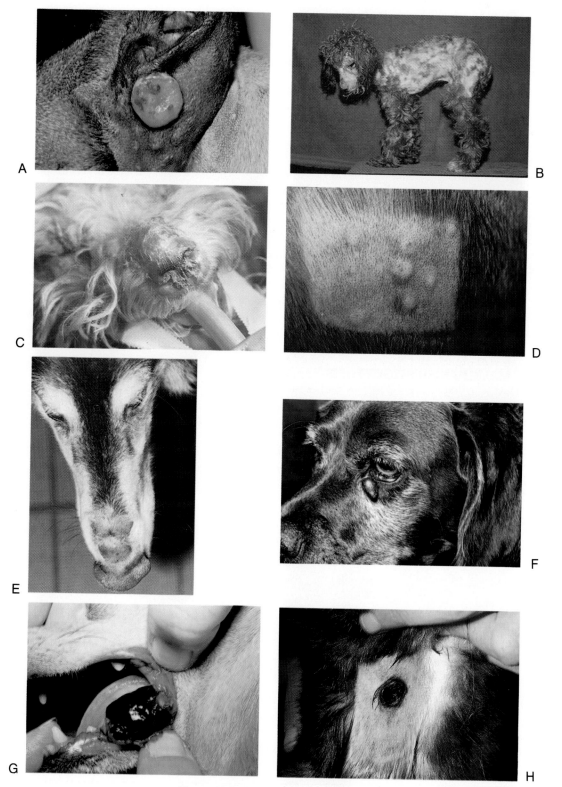

Figure 19:87 See legend on opposite page

Doberman pinschers, Labrador retrievers, Miniature Schnauzers, English Springer spaniels, and Shetland sheepdogs are predisposed. There is no sex predilection. Histiocytomas are usually solitary and occur most commonly on the head, the pinnae, and the limbs (Fig. 19:87 *A*; also see Fig. 19:77 *H*). They are usually small (less than 3 cm in diameter), firm, dome or button shaped, well circumscribed, dermal in location, and frequently ulcerated. Histiocytomas are fast growing but benign. The rare reports of alleged generalized histiocytomas in older dogs were not confirmed ultrastructurally or cytochemically and probably represent histiocytic lymphosarcoma, cutaneous histiocytosis, or pseudolymphoma.

■ *Diagnosis.* Histopathologically, histiocytomas are characterized by uniform sheets and cords of pleomorphic histiocytic cells infiltrating the dermis and subcutis and displacing the collagen fibers and adnexae (Figs. 19:88 to 19:90).[4, 5, 32] A characteristic feature of this neoplasm is a high mitotic index. Lymphocytic infiltration and areas of necrosis develop in regressing neoplasms. Canine Langerhans' cells are most specifically identified by monoclonal antibodies to CD1.[191a]

■ *Clinical Management.* Clinical management of histiocytomas may include surgical excision, cryosurgery, electrosurgery, and observation without treatment.[11–13] The majority of these neoplasms undergo spontaneous regression within 3 months. Lesions that are causing problems (pruritus, ulceration, and secondary infection), but are in areas where surgical excision is difficult, respond dramatically to the topical administration of a glucocorticoid in dimethyl sulfoxide.

MALIGNANT HISTIOCYTOSIS

■ *Cause and Pathogenesis.* Malignant histiocytosis is a rare, malignant neoplasm of histiocytic origin in dogs.[4, 11, 197a, 198, 199] The cause of the neoplasm is unknown.

■ *Clinical Findings.* Malignant histiocytosis has been recognized in several breeds of dogs with no sex predilection; typically, older animals are affected. This neoplasm has also been

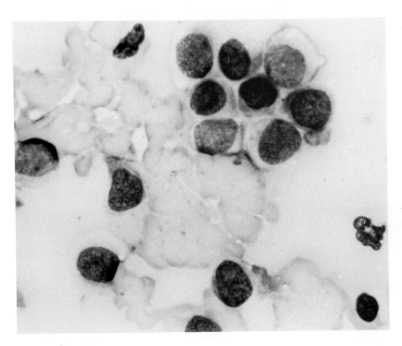

Figure 19:88. Canine histiocytoma. Aspirate of skin nodules shows numerous pleomorphic histiocytes. (Courtesy J. Blue.)

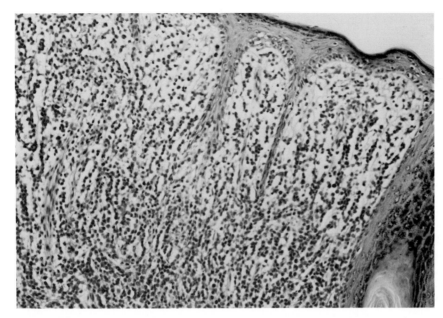

Figure 19:89. Canine histiocytoma. Diffuse infiltration of histiocytes with edema of superficial dermis and hyperplasia of overlying epidermis.

reported in closely related Bernese Mountain dogs, predominantly male dogs.[198] Cutaneous lesions are rarely seen and are characterized by multiple, firm, dermal to subcutaneous nodules anywhere on the body. Lesions may or may not be alopecic or ulcerated. Typical clinical signs of malignant histiocytosis include lethargy, weight loss, lymphadenopathy, hepatosplenomegaly, and pancytopenia. The course is rapidly progressive and invariably fatal.

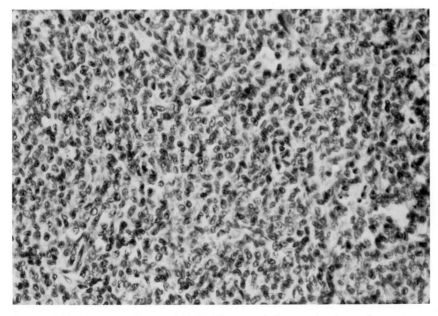

Figure 19:90. Close-up of Figure 19:89. Proliferation of pleomorphic, hyperchromatic histiocytes.

■ *Diagnosis.* Histopathologically, malignant histiocytosis is characterized by nodular to diffuse, deep dermal and subcutaneous infiltration, with cytologically atypical histiocytes exhibiting cytophagocytosis and high mitotic index (Fig. 19:91).[4, 197a, 198, 199] Tumor cells are positive for lysozyme, α_1-antitrypsin, and cathepsin B.[195a, 197a, 198]

■ *Clinical Management.* At present, there is no effective treatment.

SYSTEMIC HISTIOCYTOSIS

■ *Cause and Pathogenesis.* Systemic histiocytosis is a histiocytic proliferative disorder of dogs.[4, 53, 195–197] The cause of the condition is unknown.

■ *Clinical Findings.* Systemic histiocytosis was described in closely related Bernese Mountain dogs of 2 to 8 years of age, with male dogs predominating.[195, 196] An autosomal recessive mode of inheritance has been proposed.[195] The disorder has rarely been recognized in other breeds of dogs.[197] Clinical signs include anorexia, weight loss, respiratory stertor, and multiple cutaneous papules, plaques, nodules, and ulcers over the entire body, especially the muzzle, the nasal planum, the eyelids, and the scrotum (see Fig. 19:87 *B* and *C*). The course may be prolonged and fluctuating, with alternating episodes of exacerbation and remission, or rapidly progressive and fatal. Ultimately, most dogs were euthanized and showed histiocytic infiltration of multiple organ systems, especially lung, liver, spleen, bone marrow, and lymph nodes.

■ *Diagnosis.* Histopathologically, systemic histiocytosis is characterized by superficial and deep perivascular, nodular, or diffuse dermal and subcutaneous infiltrations of cytologically normal histiocytes (Fig. 19:92).[4, 5, 195, 197] Histiocytic cells also invade vascular walls, producing thrombosis and ischemic necrosis. Electron microscopic examination reveals typical histiocytes with convoluted nuclei, filopodia, and abundant lysosomes. Enzyme histochemical studies revealed that the cells were positive for typical histiocytic markers: acid phosphatase, nonspecific esterase, and lysozyme.[53, 195, 195a]

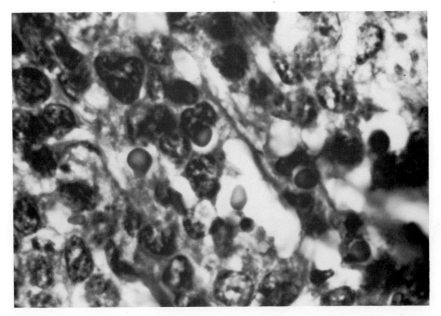

Figure 19:91. Canine malignant histiocytosis. Atypical histiocytes exhibiting erythrophagocytosis.

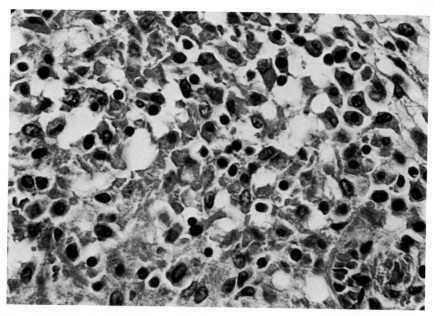

Figure 19:92. Canine systemic histiocytosis. Proliferation of normal-appearing histiocytes and occasional lymphocytes.

■ *Clinical Management.* Treatment with large doses of glucocorticoids and cytotoxic drugs has been generally ineffective. A preliminary report indicated that treatment with bovine thymosin fraction 5 may be beneficial.[195]

CUTANEOUS HISTIOCYTOSIS

■ *Cause and Pathogenesis.* Cutaneous histiocytosis is a benign histiocytic proliferative disorder of dogs.[4, 5, 191c, 192–194] The cause of the disorder is unknown.

■ *Clinical Findings.* Cutaneous histiocytosis occurs in dogs, with no apparent age or sex predilections. Collies and Shetland sheepdogs may be predisposed.[5] Lesions occur as multiple, erythematous, dermal or subcutaneous plaques or nodules, 1 to 5 cm in diameter, anywhere on the body (see Fig. 19:87 *D*). The lesions may occur in localized clusters or in a more generalized distribution. Some dogs have lesions limited to the nasal planum and nasal mucosa, producing a "clown nose" appearance.[5] Lesions often wax and wane and appear in new sites. Systemic involvement and lymphadenopathy are not reported.

■ *Diagnosis.* Histopathologically, cutaneous histiocytosis is characterized by nodular to diffuse dermal or subcutaneous infiltrations of cytologically normal histiocytes, lymphocytes, and neutrophils.[4, 5, 192] Electron microscopy reveals typical histiocytes, and enzyme histochemical studies show that the cells are positive for nonspecific esterase.

■ *Clinical Management.* Treatment with large doses of glucocorticoids and cytotoxic drugs usually produces remission. However, recurrences are common.[5, 194] One dog had a temporary response to the intraperitoneal injection of polyethylene glycol (PEG) modified L-asparaginase.[191c]

BENIGN FIBROUS HISTIOCYTOMA

■ *Cause and Pathogenesis.*   Benign fibrous histiocytomas are rare tumors of dogs and cats.[5,] [11, 21a, 200, 201] The cause of benign fibrous histiocytomas is unknown. These tumors may be reactive proliferations rather than true neoplasms.[5, 200]

■ *Clinical Findings.*   Fibrous histiocytomas occur most commonly in dogs 2 to 4 years of age, with no sex predilection. Collies and Golden retrievers appear to be predisposed.[5, 11] Cutaneous benign fibrous histiocytomas occur as solitary or multiple nodules and occur most commonly on the face, the legs, and the scrotum (Fig. 19:93). They are usually firm, well circumscribed, 0.5 to 7 cm in diameter, and dermal in location (Fig. 19:94). The overlying skin may be normal or alopecic. Histologically identical lesions occur in the cornea, with or without concurrent skin lesions (Fig. 19:95).[201] These neoplasms are benign.

■ *Diagnosis.*   Histologically, fibrous histiocytomas are characterized by poorly circumscribed cellular infiltrate permeated by a swirling stroma. The majority of cells are histiocytes and fibroblasts (Fig. 19:96).[5, 11, 201] Collagen formation is minimal. Lymphoid cells and plasma cells are commonly present, especially at the periphery of the masses.

■ *Clinical Management.*   Clinical management of fibrous histiocytomas may include surgical excision and the administration of glucocorticoids.[5, 11, 201] Sublesional injections of 10 to 40 mg of methylprednisolone may be effective for single lesions. Multiple lesions are best treated with prednisolone or prednisone, 2 to 4 mg/kg orally once daily until they have completely regressed (1 to 2 weeks). Recurrent lesions may necessitate long-term alternate-day steroid therapy. Some cases are initially unresponsive to, or become refractory to, systemic glucocorticoids. Azathioprine, 2 mg/kg orally every 48 hours, is usually effective in these cases.[11, 200]

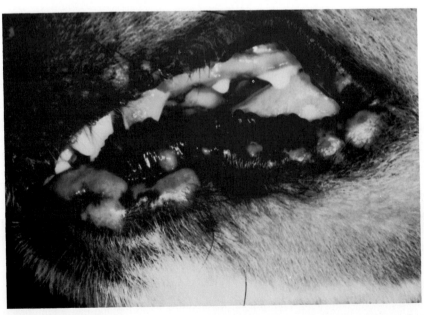

Figure 19:93. Canine benign fibrous histiocytoma. Multiple papules and nodules on the lower lip of a collie.

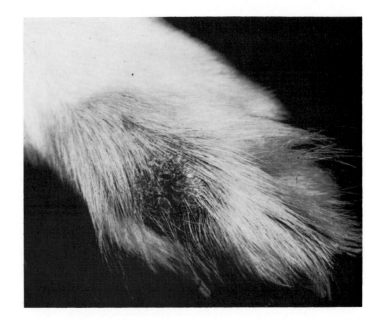

Figure 19:94. Canine benign fibrous histiocytoma. Nodule on the paw of a collie.

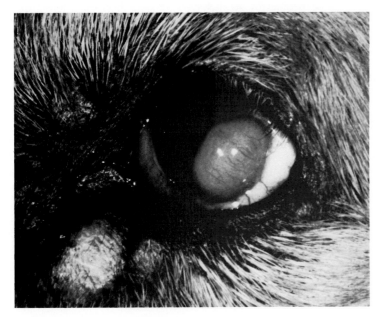

Figure 19:95. Canine benign fibrous histiocytoma. Nodule on the sclera of a collie.

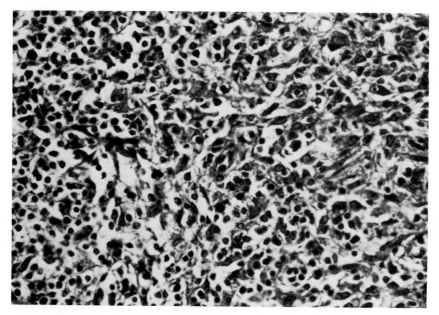

Figure 19:96. Canine benign fibrous histiocytoma. Proliferation of histiocytic and fibroblastic cells with intermingling lymphocytes.

MALIGNANT FIBROUS HISTIOCYTOMA

■ *Cause and Pathogenesis.* Malignant fibrous histiocytomas (extraskeletal giant cell tumors, giant cell tumors of soft parts, or dermatofibrosarcomas) are uncommon (in cats) to rare (in dogs) malignant neoplasms.* These neoplasms are believed to arise from undifferentiated mesenchymal cells. The cause of malignant fibrous histiocytomas is unknown.

■ *Clinical Findings.* Malignant fibrous histiocytomas occur in older cats and dogs, with no apparent breed or sex predilection. They are usually solitary, firm, poorly circumscribed, variable in size and shape, and dermal and subcutaneous in location (Fig. 19:97; also see Fig. 19:87 *E*). There is a predilection for the leg (especially the paw) and the shoulder.[4, 5, 27, 29, 202–204] These neoplasms are locally invasive (to muscle and bone) but apparently slow to metastasize.

■ *Diagnosis.* Histologically, malignant fibrous histiocytomas are characterized by an infiltrative mass composed of varying mixtures of pleomorphic histiocytes, fibroblasts, and multinucleate tumor giant cells (Fig. 19:98).[4, 5, 202–204] Mitotic figures and a storiform (''cartwheel'') arrangement of fibroblasts and histiocytes are common features. Recognized histologic subtypes include giant cell type, storiform-pleomorphic type, and dermatofibrosarcoma type.[5] Malignant fibrous histiocytomas are positive for vimentin, lysozyme, and α_1-antichymotrypsin.[45, 204a]

■ *Clinical Management.* The therapy of choice for malignant fibrous histiocytomas is radical surgical excision or amputation. Recurrence after surgical excision is common. Metastasis appears to be rare.[4, 202]

---

*See references 4, 5, 11, 13, 21a, 27, 29, and 202–204a.

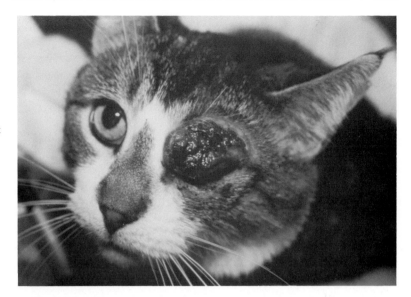

Figure 19:97. Feline malignant fibrous histiocytoma. Large, ulcerated mass originating in the periorbital region.

■ MELANOCYTIC NEOPLASMS

The nomenclature for melanocytic tumors is complex and confusing, with terms such as melanoma, malignant melanoma, melanosarcoma, melanocytoma, benign melanoma, melanocytic nevus, acquired nevus, and congenital nevus having uncertain meaning in certain contexts. The so-called nevus cell, which makes up the pigmented nevi of humans, is now known to be a melanocyte with slight histopathologic and biochemical alterations. On this basis, it has been suggested that all noncongenital, benign proliferations of melanocytes be designated *melanocytoma.*[5] The term *melanoma* is used in this text as synonymous with a malignant proliferation of melanocytes. In dogs, most cutaneous melanocytic neoplasms (about 70 per cent) are benign, whereas benign and malignant neoplasms occur with about equal frequency in cats.[19, 26, 34, 213, 215, 215a, 217]

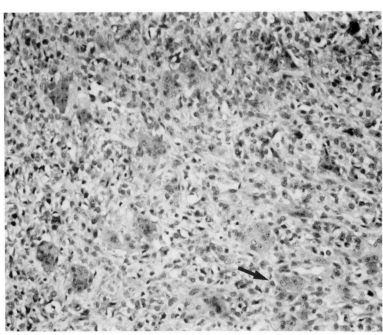

Figure 19:98. Feline malignant fibrous histiocytoma. Proliferation of atypical fibrohistiocytic cells and numerous atypical multinucleated histiocytic giant cells *(arrow).*

Melanocytic neoplasms are relatively common (in dogs) to uncommon (in cats) benign or malignant neoplasms arising from melanocytes and melanoblasts.[4, 5, 11–13] The cause of these neoplasms usually is unknown. In cats, melanomas have been produced with injections of FeSV.[11, 12] In humans, there is a correlation between exposure to ultraviolet light and the development of melanoma.[3] Canine melanomas can be transplanted to neonatal dogs (after treatment with antilymphocyte serum) and to nude mice.[217a]

Melanocytoma

CLINICAL FINDINGS

Dog

Melanocytomas occur in dogs at an average age of 9 years, with no sex predilection. Breeds reported to be at risk include Scottish terriers, Airedales, Boston terriers, Cocker spaniels, Springer spaniels, boxers, Golden retrievers, Irish setters, Irish terriers, Miniature Schnauzers, Doberman pinschers, Chihuahuas, and Chow Chows.[4, 5, 11–13, 212] Lesions are usually solitary and occur most frequently on the head (especially the eyelid and the muzzle) (see Fig. 19:87 *F*), the trunk, and the paws (especially interdigitally).[4, 5, 213, 245] They are usually well circumscribed, firm to fleshy, brown to black, 0.5 to 5 cm in diameter, and alopecic; they vary from dome shaped to pedunculated to papillomatous in appearance.

Cat

Melanocytomas occur in cats at an average age of 10 years, with no sex or breed predilections.[4, 5, 11–13, 215a, 217] Lesions are usually solitary and occur most commonly on the head (especially the pinna and the nose) and the neck.[4, 5, 11–13, 217] They are usually well circumscribed, firm to fleshy, brown to black, 0.5 to 4 cm in diameter, and alopecic and vary from dome shaped to pedunculated to papillomatous in appearance.

DIAGNOSIS

Histopathologically, melanocytomas are characterized by melanocytes in sheets, packets (nests and theques), and cords (Figs. 19:99 and 19:100).[4, 5, 32, 217, 245] The melanocytes may be predominantly epithelioid, spindle cell, or a combination of these two forms. Histologic subtypes include junctional, compound, and dermal.[5, 11] Rarely, the melanocytic proliferation is distinctly perifollicular (pilar neurocristic melanocytoma).[211] Melanocytomas are positive for vimentin.[5, 21a, 45, 55]

CLINICAL MANAGEMENT

The therapy of choice is radical surgical excision.[11–13] Up to 10 per cent of the dogs with histologically benign melanocytomas die of their disease (usually euthanasia performed for recurrence, metastasis, or both).[212, 213, 215] Regrettably, no clinical features reliably distinguish benign from malignant melanocytic proliferations.[245]

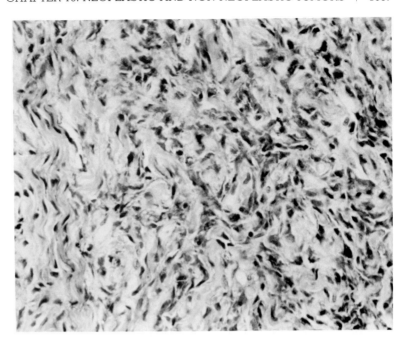

Figure 19:99. Feline melanocytoma. Proliferation of spindle-shaped melanocytes.

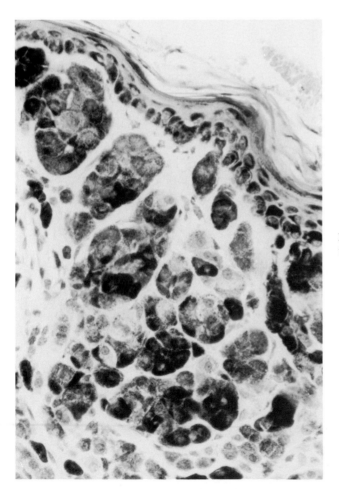

Figure 19:100. Feline melanocytoma. Multiple theques of epithelioid melanocytes.

Melanoma

CLINICAL FINDINGS

Dog

Melanomas occur in dogs at an average age of 9 years, with no sex predilection. Breeds reported to be at risk include those listed previously for melanocytoma.[4, 5, 11–13, 212] Lesions are usually solitary and occur most commonly on the head (Fig. 19:87 *G*), the limbs, the digits (including the clawbed), the scrotum, the lip, and the trunk.[4, 5, 11–13, 212, 245] They are variably circumscribed (well to poor), shaped (dome, plaque, and polypoid), and colored (gray, brown, and black) and range from 0.5 to 10 cm in diameter. Ulceration is common.

Cat

Melanomas occur in cats at an average age of 10 years, with no sex or breed predilections.[4, 5, 11–13, 19, 215a, 217] Lesions are usually solitary and occur most commonly on the head (especially the pinna, the eyelid, and the lip) and the neck (see Fig. 19:87 *H*).[4, 5, 11–13, 217] They are variably circumscribed and shaped (dome, plaque, and polypoid), and most are brown to black and vary from 0.5 to 4 cm in diameter. Ulceration is frequent.

DIAGNOSIS

Histopathologically, melanomas are characterized by atypical melanocytes in sheets, packets (nests and theques), and cords (Figs. 19:101 and 19:102).[4, 5, 32, 217, 245] The melanocytes may be predominantly epithelioid, spindle cell, or a combination of these two forms. Rarely, the melanocytic proliferation may be distinctly perifollicular (pilar neurocristic melanoma).[211] Clear cell (balloon cell) melanomas have been described.[5, 214] Melanomas are positive for vimentin and variably positive for S-100 protein and neuron-specific enolase.[5, 45, 54, 55]

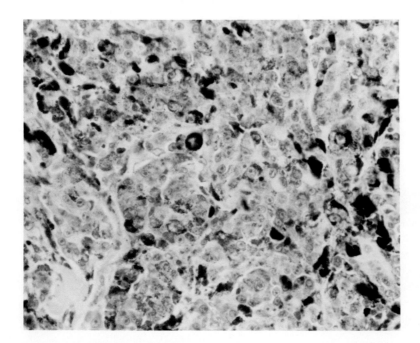

Figure 19:101. Feline melanoma. Proliferation of atypical epithelioid melanocytes.

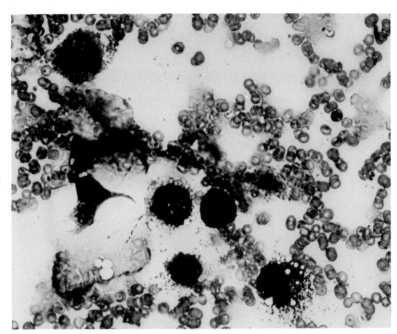

Figure 19:102. Canine melanoma. Cytologic examination of aspirate reveals several melanocytes.

CLINICAL MANAGEMENT

The therapy of choice is radical surgical excision.[11-13] Recurrence after surgery and metastasis are common.[4, 11-13, 213, 215] In one large study of surgically treated cutaneous melanomas in dogs, animals had a median survival time of 12 months and a death rate of 54 per cent within 2 years if their neoplasm was small, and a median survival time of 4 months and a death rate of 100 per cent within 2 years if their neoplasm was large.[213] The mean survival time of dogs with surgically treated oral melanomas was 3 months.[216] Regrettably, no clinical findings reliably distinguish melanomas from melanocytomas.[4, 217, 245] Histologic findings of high mitotic activity and marked cellular atypia may correlate with more aggressive biological behavior in canine melanomas,[5, 212, 213] whereas marked cellular atypia and high mitotic index suggest aggressive biological behavior in feline melanomas.[4, 217] One study in cats indicated that epithelioid cell–type neoplasms were more likely to be malignant,[4] whereas a second study failed to confirm this finding but suggested that lymphoplasmacytic inflammation indicated malignancy.[217]

■ MISCELLANEOUS CUTANEOUS NEOPLASMS

Transmissible Venereal Tumor

CAUSE AND PATHOGENESIS

The transmissible venereal tumor (infectious sarcoma, contagious venereal tumor, venereal granuloma, canine condyloma, transmissible lymphosarcoma, transmissible reticulum cell tumor, histiocytoma, or sticker tumor) is an uncommon benign to malignant neoplasm of the dog.[4, 11-13, 222, 225] The cell of origin is unknown. It is considered a naturally occurring allograft, with transmission occurring by transplantation of viable neoplastic cells to a susceptible host. The tumor cells contain 59 chromosomes, as compared with the normal canine complement of 78. A viral origin has been investigated but not verified. The neoplasm is usually transmitted by coitus but may be inoculated into multiple sites by licking, biting, and scratching. Transmission may be accomplished by subcutaneous, intravenous, and intraperitoneal injections and by skin or mucosal scarification (incubation period, about 3 weeks). Transmissible venereal tumor is more prevalent in tropical and subtropical areas.

Transmissible venereal tumor can grow for extended periods in an immunocompetent allogeneic host. During progressive growth of the tumor, cell-mediated immune responses to tumor cells are impaired, and serum antibodies are present that, when incubated with tumor cells, can block complement-mediated lysis of tumor cells by serum antibodies from dogs with regressing transmissible venereal tumors. Circulating immune complexes have been detected in dogs with transmissible venereal tumor, but the pathogenetic significance of this finding is unknown. Dogs experimentally rechallenged with transmissible venereal tumor cells mount a rapid T lymphocyte response, resulting in rapid tumor regression.[224]

Some investigators report that transmissible venereal tumors are usually benign in male dogs but that metastasis to regional lymph nodes is common in intact female dogs, suggesting that these tumors may be hormone dependent.[224a] Ovariectomy was reported to produce a rapid reduction in size of transmissible venereal tumors in bitches.[224b]

CLINICAL FINDINGS

Occurring in sexually active dogs (especially those young and unconfined), transmissible venereal tumor shows no apparent breed or sex predilection. Animals with poor health or immunosuppression for various reasons may be more likely to have metastatic lesions.[225] Neoplasms occur commonly on the external genitalia (penis and vagina) (Fig. 19:103 *A*) and the skin (especially the face and the limbs) (Fig. 19:104) and may be single or multiple, nodular, pedunculated, multilobular or cauliflower-like, firm or friable, 1 to 20 cm in diameter, and dermal-epidermal to subcutaneous in location, and they may frequently be ulcerated.

In experimental or laboratory dogs, these tumors frequently regress spontaneously. In one experimental dog colony, the neoplasm was transmitted through 40 generations, consisting of 564 dogs.[222] Neoplasms developed in 68 per cent of the dogs and spontaneously regressed permanently in 87 per cent of these dogs within 180 days. However, there is no such evidence of general benignity in the naturally occurring disease.[11, 223, 225] The overall frequency of spontaneous regression in naturally occurring cases of transmissible venereal tumor is unknown, and many instances of metastasis and extragenital occurrence have been reported.

DIAGNOSIS

Histopathologically, transmissible venereal tumor is characterized by compact masses or sheets of uniform round to polyhedral neoplastic cells, often growing in rows in a delicate stroma (Figs. 19:105 and 19:106).[4, 11, 32] Mitoses are plentiful. Tumors undergoing spontaneous regression display necrosis, increasing numbers of infiltrating leukocytes (especially lymphocytes), and increasing numbers of collagen bundles. Transmissible venereal tumors are positive for vimentin and negative for cytokeratin.[55, 223]

CLINICAL MANAGEMENT

Because of (1) the inconclusive evidence regarding spontaneous regression in naturally occurring neoplasms and (2) the numerous reports of metastasis, clinical management of transmissible venereal tumors is *always* indicated. Both radiotherapy and surgical excision have been successful, although recurrence after surgery is common.[11–13, 223, 225] Chemotherapy has also produced good results. Ninety-three per cent of dogs treated had complete regression of their neoplasms with no recurrence, after combination chemotherapy (vincristine, 0.0125 to 0.025 mg/kg intravenously weekly; cyclophosphamide, 1 mg/kg orally daily, or 50 mg/m^2 of body surface area (BSA) orally every other day; and methotrexate, 0.3 to 0.5 mg/kg intravenously weekly, or 2.5 mg/m^2 of BSA orally every other day).[11, 225] The average time to the point at

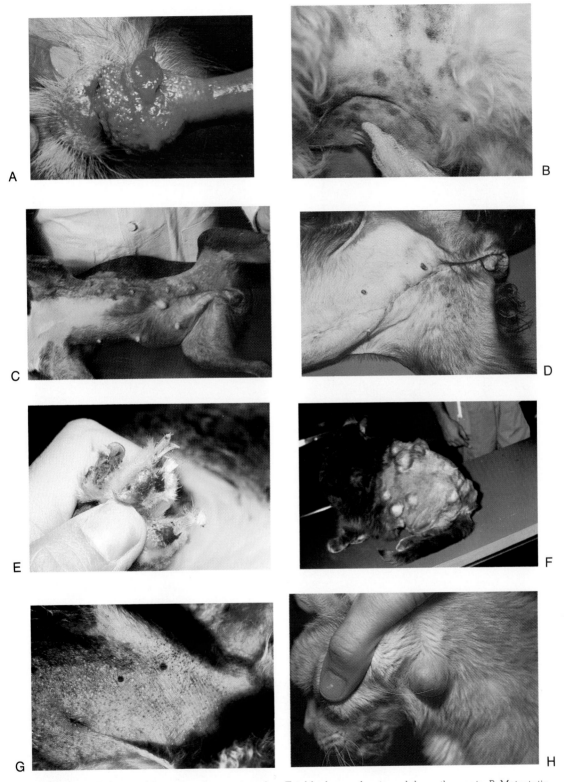

Figure 19:103. *A,* Transmissible venereal tumor in a dog. Friable, hemorrhagic nodule on the penis. *B,* Metastatic pharyngeal carcinoma in a dog. Purpuric plaques on the neck. *C,* Metastatic mammary adenocarcinoma in a dog. *D,* Metastatic colonic adenocarcinoma in a dog. Erythematous papules and plaques in the groin. *E,* Metastatic bronchiogenic carcinoma in a cat. Ulcerative paronychial lesions. *F,* Multiple follicular cysts in a cat. *G,* Multiple follicular cysts (milia) in the groin of a dog. *H,* Apocrine cyst on the neck of a cat.

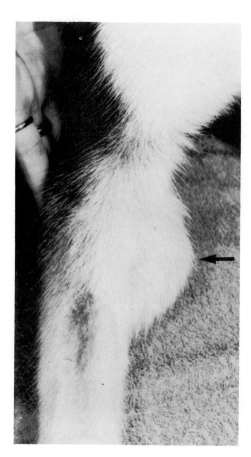

Figure 19:104. Transmissible venereal tumor in a dog. Subcutaneous nodule near the elbow.

Figure 19:105. Transmissible venereal tumor. Aspirate of skin nodule shows monomorphous population of large round cells with vacuolated cytoplasm. (Courtesy T. French.)

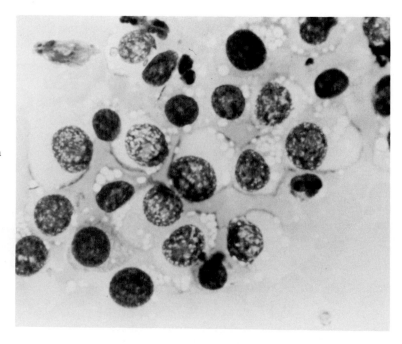

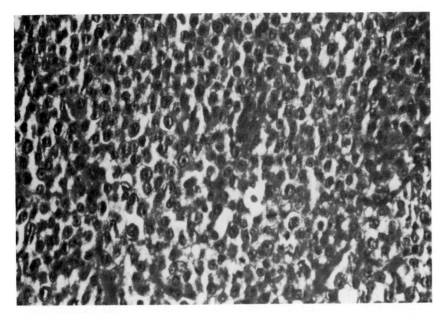

Figure 19:106. Transmissible venereal tumor. Sheets of neoplastic mononuclear cells with vesicular nuclei.

which no disease was evident was 4 to 6 weeks. Two of the dogs that were cured had regional lymph node metastasis. Eighty-two to 100 per cent of dogs treated with single-agent chemotherapy (vincristine, 0.025 mg/kg intravenously once weekly) underwent a complete remission within an average of 4 weeks.[11, 221, 221a, 225] Doxorubicin administered at a dosage of 0.5 mg/m² of BSA intravenously once weekly for an average of 6 weeks is also reported to be effective.[11, 225] Single-drug chemotherapy with cyclophosphamide or methotrexate was not effective.[221] Immunoadsorption of immune complexes with protein A, autogenous vaccine, levamisole, and intralesional bacille Calmette-Guérin vaccine is of unproven benefit.[11, 224c, 225]

Primary Cutaneous Neuroendocrine Tumor

CAUSE AND PATHOGENESIS

Primary cutaneous neuroendocrine tumors are rare neoplasms of dogs.[11, 218–220] The cause of these tumors is unknown. The cell of origin may be the Merkel cell, which, like this neoplasm, shows dual epithelial and neural differentiation.[9, 48] These neoplasms have probably been previously called "atypical histiocytomas."

CLINICAL FINDINGS

In dogs, primary cutaneous neuroendocrine tumors have been reported to be malignant and metastatic,[218] or benign with rare recurrence after surgery.[219, 220] Most dogs are older than 8 years of age, and most have solitary lesions, especially on the lips, the ears, or the digits.[219] The tumors are usually rapid growing, are 0.5 to 2.5 cm in diameter, and may be ulcerated. Neuroendocrine tumors may also occur in the oral cavity of dogs.[220]

DIAGNOSIS

Histopathologically, primary cutaneous neuroendocrine tumors are characterized by sheets, solid nests, or anastomosing trabeculae of uniformly round tumor cells with abundant amphophilic cytoplasm, hyperchromatic and vesicular nuclei, and frequent mitoses (Fig. 19:107).[5, 218–220] Giant and multinucleate tumor cells may be seen. Electron microscopic examination reveals characteristic cytoplasmic dense-core membrane-bound granules and a perinuclear whorl of intermediate filaments (Fig. 19:108). The characteristic cytoplasmic neurosecretory granules are lost in formalin-fixed tissues. Immunohistochemical studies have shown that the primary cutaneous neuroendocrine tumors of humans contain cytokeratin, neurofilament, neuron-specific enolase, and common epithelial antigen,[9, 48] but such studies have not been reported for canine neoplasms.

CLINICAL MANAGEMENT

Clinical management of these tumors is best accomplished with early radical surgical excision. The vast majority of dogs appear to be cured after surgery.

Epithelioid Sarcoma

CAUSE AND PATHOGENESIS

Epithelioid sarcoma is an extremely rare malignant neoplasm of dogs and cats that is probably epithelial in origin.[9, 21a, 35, 48, 225a] The cause of this tumor is unknown.

CLINICAL FINDINGS

Epithelioid sarcoma has been recognized in adult cats and dogs.[21a, 35, 225a] Lesions are solitary and occur on the limbs (Fig. 19:109). They begin as firm, poorly circumscribed, dermal or subcutaneous nodules that may ulcerate as they enlarge. Metastasis may occur.

DIAGNOSIS

Histopathologically, epithelioid sarcomas are characterized by a nodular arrangement of plump spindle cells and large, round to polygonal epithelioid cells (Fig. 19:110).[9, 35, 225a] Mitoses are

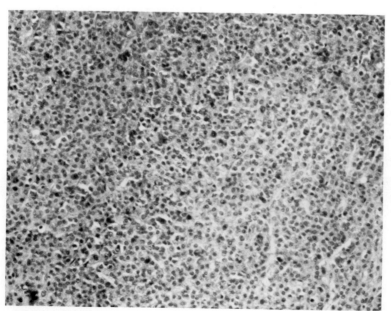

Figure 19:107. Canine neuroendocrine tumor. Infiltrate consisting of round tumor cells and frequent mitoses.

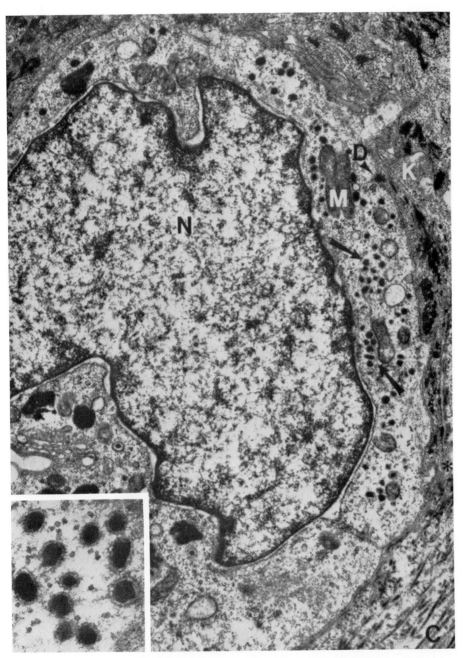

Figure 19:108. Merkel's cell. N, nucleus of a Merkel's cell; asterisk indicates basal lamina; M, mitochondria; arrows indicate specific granules of the Merkel's cell; D with pointer, desmosome between the Merkel cell and a keratinocyte (K); C, collagen with cross-striation (× 20,000). Inset: specific membrane-bound granules at higher magnification (× 75,000). (From Lever, W.F., Schaumburg-Lever, G.: Histopathology of the Skin, 7th ed. J.B. Lippincott Co., Philadelphia, 1990, p. 863.)

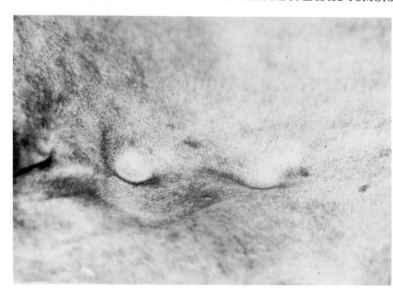

Figure 19:109. Feline epithelioid sarcoma. Two nodules in the axillary region.

frequent, and necrosis is characteristically present, especially in the center of large nodules (Fig. 19:111). In one dog, tumor cells were positive for vimentin and, focally, for desmin.[225a]

CLINICAL MANAGEMENT

The therapy of choice is early, radical surgical excision.

■ SECONDARY SKIN NEOPLASMS

Secondary skin neoplasms result from the metastasis of primary neoplasms in other organs to the skin. Secondary skin neoplasms are rare in dogs and cats. Circumscribed, solid, subcuta-

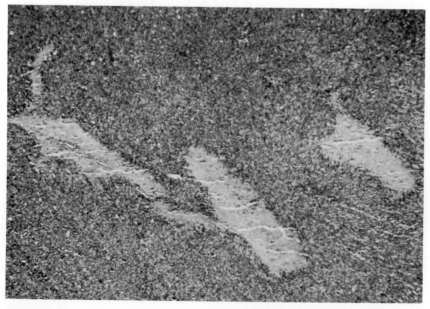

Figure 19:110. Feline epithelioid sarcoma. Multifocal area of necrosis within a neoplasm.

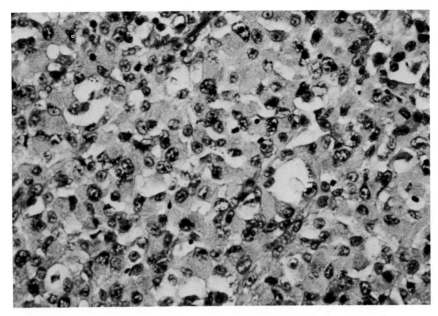

Figure 19:111. Close-up of Figure 19:110. Proliferation of pleomorphic, atypical epithelioid cells.

neous nodules were recognized on the heads of cats with metastatic mammary adenocarcinoma and gastric carcinoma.[11] Multiple purpuric papules, plaques, and nodules of the neck have been seen in dogs with metastatic pharyngeal carcinomas (see Fig. 19:103 *B*).[11] Nodular to ulcerative to edematous (pseudocellulitis, inflammatory carcinoma) lesions have been recognized in the inguinal skin of dogs and cats with metastatic mammary adenocarcinoma (see Fig. 19:103 *C*)[11, 235, 236] and colonic adenocarcinoma (Fig. 19:112; also see Fig. 19:103 *D*).[11, 232] Nodules in the umbilical skin have been recognized in dogs and cats with metastatic pancreatic ductal adeno-

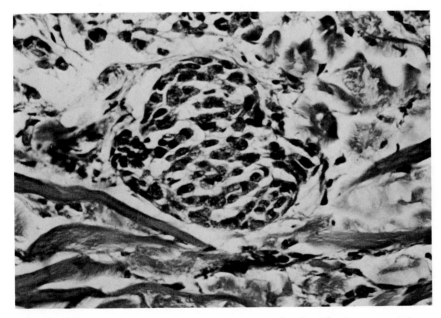

Figure 19:112. Metastatic colonic adenocarcinoma in a dog. Lymphatic metastasis in skin.

carcinoma, jejunal adenocarcinoma, and teratoma.[230] Ulcerative, destructive lesions on the digits (on multiple digits and multiple paws) have been seen in aged cats with asymptomatic bronchiogenic or squamous cell carcinomas of the lung (Fig. 19:113; also see Fig. 19:103 *E*).[97, 230a, 234]

Leukemia cutis is a dissemination of aggressive systemic leukemia to the skin. Cutaneous lesions seen with leukemia may be specific (leukemic infiltrates presenting as macules, papules, plaques, nodules, purpura, and ulcers) or nonspecific (infectious dermatoses, urticaria, erythema multiforme, exfoliative dermatitis, and pruritus). In dogs, leukemia cutis (patchy alopecia, erythema, and papules of the trunk) was reported with chronic lymphocytic leukemia.[229] Nonspecific skin lesions of leukemia (recurrent bacterial pyoderma) were reported in 9 per cent of a series of dogs with chronic lymphocytic leukemia.[233] Histopathologically, leukemia cutis is characterized by a perivascular, interstitial, lichenoid, or diffuse monomorphous infiltration of leukemia cells.[9, 11] The leukemia cells often infiltrate between collagen bundles.

Surgical transplantation of a neoplasm (tumor seeding) is rarely reported in dogs and cats.[226, 231] Lesions appear in the healed surgical incision through which the primary neoplasm was removed. Most cases involved urinary tract carcinomas.

A unique dermatosis has been seen in association with thymoma or thoracic lymphoma in cats.[94a, 227, 228] No breed or sex predilections are reported, and affected cats are adult to aged. Cutaneous lesions begin on the head, the pinnae, and the neck and rapidly generalize, resulting in an exfoliative erythroderma with oozing erosions and ulcers, which may be serpiginous. Histopathologically, the skin lesions are characterized by a hydropic to lichenoid interface reaction with pronounced single-cell to segmental necrosis of epidermal keratinocytes, resembling erythema multiforme (see Chap. 8).

A pancreatic paraneoplastic alopecia has recently been described in cats (see Chap. 10).

■ NON-NEOPLASTIC TUMORS

Cutaneous Cysts

A *cyst* is a non-neoplastic, simple saclike structure with an epithelial lining. Classification of cysts depends on identification of the lining epithelium or the pre-existing structure from which the cyst arose.

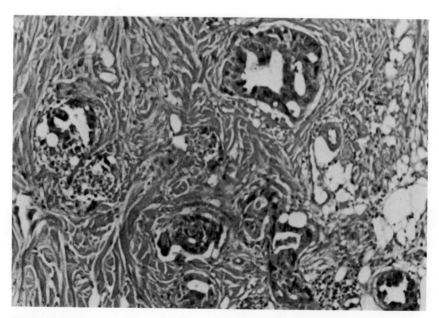

Figure 19:113. Metastatic bronchiogenic carcinoma in a cat. Metastatic lesions in dermis.

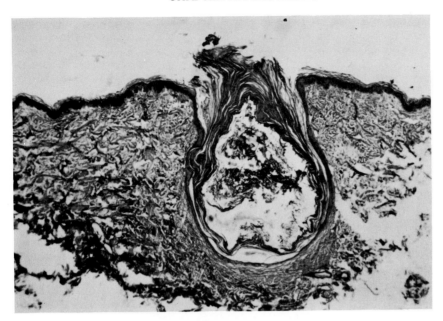

Figure 19:114. Canine follicular cyst (milium).

FOLLICULAR CYSTS

The majority of cutaneous cysts in the dog and cat are follicular in origin and can be further categorized by the level of the follicle from which they develop.[4, 5] Infundibular and isthmus-catagen (tricholemmal) cysts are common in dogs and uncommon in cats. Matrical cysts are uncommon in dogs and rare in cats. Hybrid cysts, which combine two or three types of follicular epithelium, are uncommon in dogs and cats.

Follicular cysts usually appear as solitary, well-circumscribed, round, smooth, firm to fluctuant lesions that are dermal to subcutaneous in location and 0.5 to 5 cm in diameter.[4, 5, 11] Occasional lesions may have a bluish hue. Lesions may open and discharge a yellowish, brownish, or grayish material that is caseous, cheesy, or doughy in consistency. There are no apparent age or sex predilections for solitary follicular cysts, and they occur most commonly on the head, the neck, the trunk (see Fig. 19:103 *F*), and the proximal limbs. Boxers, Doberman pinschers, Shih tzus, and Miniature Schnauzers may be predipsosed.[4] Rarely, follicular cysts appear as recurrent soft tissue swellings in the medial canthus of the eye.[238]

Multiple follicular cysts of presumed congenital origin occur on the dorsal midline of the head in young dogs and on pressure points (especially the elbow) of dogs, presumably resulting from chronic trauma, dermal fibrosis, and obstruction of follicular ostia.[5] Small (2 to 5 mm in diameter) follicular cysts (milia) may be seen as postinflammatory changes, especially in dogs.[11] They are usually white and grossly resemble pustules or calcinosis cutis (Fig. 19:114; also see Fig. 19:103 *G*). Multiple milia can also be seen in dogs that have received therapeutic levels of glucocorticoids for long periods.

All types of cysts may be complicated by rupture and resultant foreign body granuloma reaction and secondary bacterial infection. Such cysts often appear inflamed and infected grossly and may be painful, pruritic, or both.

The therapy of choice for most cutaneous cysts is surgical excision or observation without treatment. Cysts should *never* be squeezed hard or manually evacuated, as such procedures greatly increase the chance of expressing cyst contents into the dermis or subcutis and inciting foreign body reaction and infection.

Infundibular Cyst

Infundibular cysts have been previously called "epidermoid" or "epidermal inclusion" cysts by pathologists and "sebaceous cysts" or "wens" by clinicians.[5, 11, 239] They are characterized by a cyst wall that undergoes epidermal differentiation; a cyst cavity containing lamellar, often concentrically arranged keratin (Fig. 19:115); and often a connection to a rudimentary hair follicle if serial sections are employed.[5]

Isthmus-Catagen Cyst

Isthmus-catagen (trichilemmal) cysts are characterized by a cyst wall that undergoes trichilemmal differentiation (no granular layer) and a cyst cavity containing a more homogeneous, amorphous keratin (Fig. 19:116).[5, 242]

Matrical Cyst

Matrical cysts are characterized by a cyst wall of deeply basophilic, basaloid cells, which abruptly keratinize to form eosinophilic, amorphous keratin replete with ghost, or shadow, cells.[5]

Hybrid Cyst

Hybrid (mixed, or panfollicular) cysts are characterized by two or three types of follicular differentiation in the same lesion (Fig. 19:117).[5, 243]

DERMOID CYST

Dermoid cysts are rarely observed in dogs and cats.[4, 5, 11, 241, 244] They are developmental anomalies and are often congenital and hereditary. Dermoid cysts are most commonly reported in boxers, Kerry blue terriers, and Rhodesian Ridgebacks. In Rhodesian Ridgebacks and their

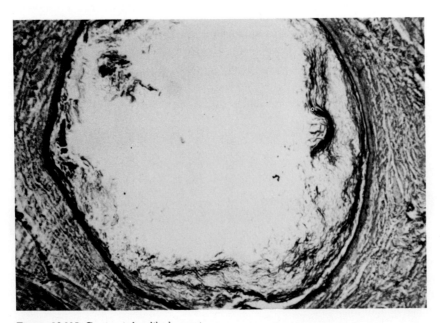

Figure 19:115. Canine infundibular cyst.

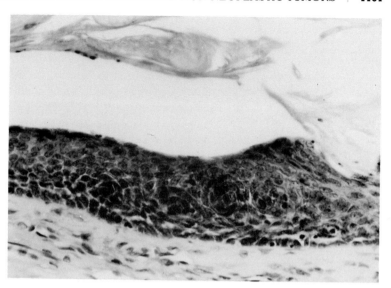

Figure 19:116. Canine isthmus-catagen (trichilemmal) cyst. Note trichilemmal differentiation of the cyst wall.

crosses, the condition (dermoid sinus, or pilonidal sinus) is thought to be inherited as a simple recessive trait (see Chap. 11).[5, 11, 244]

Lesions may be solitary or multiple and occur along the dorsal midline. Histopathologically, the lesions are characterized by a cyst wall that undergoes epidermal differentiation and contains well-developed small hair follicles, sebaceous glands, and occasionally apocrine sweat glands.[5, 11]

APOCRINE SWEAT GLAND CYST

Apocrine cysts are common in dogs and rare in cats.[4, 5, 11] There are no apparent breed or sex predilections, and affected animals are usually 6 years of age or older. They may be the result of sweat gland duct obstruction. Lesions are usually solitary, well-circumscribed, smooth, tense to fluctuant swellings, which are 0.5 to 3 cm in diameter. The overlying skin may be atrophic

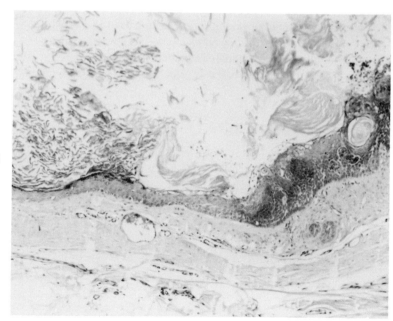

Figure 19:117. Canine hybrid cyst. Note combined epidermal (left) and trichilemmal (right) differentiation of the cyst wall.

and alopecic, and the lesions often appear bluish (see Fig. 19:103 *H*). Cyst contents are usually clear, watery, and acellular. Lesions occur most commonly on the head, the neck, and the limbs.[4]

Apocrine cystomatosis is a term used to describe a rare condition in dogs.[5, 11] Multiple clusters of cystically dilated apocrine sweat glands produce grouped vesicles and bullae, especially on the head and the neck (Fig. 19:118 *A*). The overlying skin is usually atrophic and alopecic, and the cysts may have a bluish to purplish tint.

Histopathologically, apocrine sweat gland cysts are made up of variable-sized dilated apocrine sweat glands (Figs. 19:119 and 19:120), which may occur as large solitary cysts, clusters of smaller cysts, or large cysts surrounded by smaller satellite cysts.[4, 5, 11]

The treatment of choice for apocrine cysts is surgical excision or observation without treatment. Solitary lesions may be aspirated but often recur within several weeks. There is at present no practical approach to the dog with apocrine cystomatosis.

SEBACEOUS GLAND CYST

Cysts that involve sebaceous structures are extremely rare in dogs and cats.[5] Sebaceous duct cysts appear as solitary, firm, dermal nodules that are less than 1 cm in diameter. There are no known age, breed, sex, or site predilections.

BRANCHIAL CYST

Branchial cysts are developmental defects arising from the second branchial cleft. They are extremely rare in dogs and cats.[4, 237, 240] There are no apparent age, breed, or sex predilections. Affected animals have a poorly circumscribed, firm to fluctuant swelling in the ventral cervical region. Histopathologically, branchial cysts are characterized by a thin-walled cyst lined by pseudostratified, nonciliated, columnar epithelial cells.[4] The treatment of choice is surgical excision or observation without therapy.

Nevi

A nevus (hamartoma) is a circumscribed developmental defect of the skin, characterized by hyperplasia of one or more skin components.[4, 5, 11, 252] They may or may not be congenital and are uncommonly reported in dogs and cats. The mechanism of nevus formation is not understood. A failure in the normal orderly embryonic inductive process has been theorized. In addition, the distribution of certain epidermal and vascular nevi has prompted speculation that a relationship to dermatomes or peripheral nerves exists. Finally, some nevi have a hereditary occurrence.

COLLAGENOUS NEVI

Collagenous nevi have been recognized in many breeds of dogs as solitary or multiple cutaneous lesions, especially on the head, neck, and proximal extremities (see Fig. 19:118 *B*).[5, 11, 248, 252] In German shepherd dogs, a syndrome of multiple, approximately symmetrically distributed collagenous nevi (so-called nodular dermatofibrosis) on the limbs (see Fig. 19:118 *C* and

Figure 19:118. *A*, Multiple apocrine sweat gland cysts in a dog. *B*, Solitary collagenous nevus in a Brittany spaniel. Firm, well-circumscribed, partially pin-feathered nodule over the thorax. *C*, Multiple collagenous nevi in a German shepherd dog. *D*, Multiple collagenous nevi on the paw of a German shepherd dog. *E*, Two small, melanotic organoid nevi in the preauricular area of a young cat. *F*, Congenital vascular nevus in the groin of a young dog. *G*, Congenital sebaceous nevus in the flank of a dog (the area has been clipped). *H*, Multiple hyperkeratotic, melanotic epidermal nevi in the flank of a young dog.

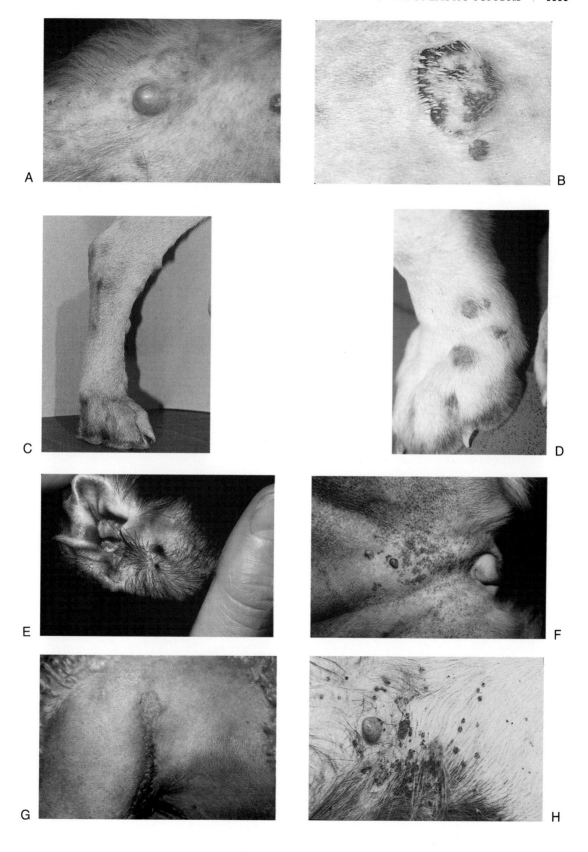

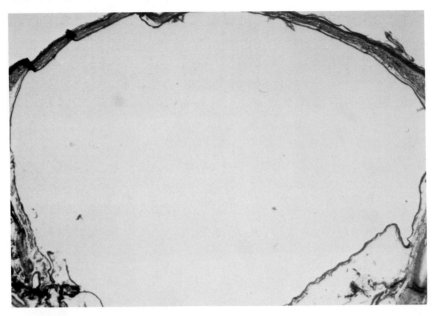

Figure 19:119. Canine apocrine sweat gland cyst.

D), head, neck, and ventral trunk has been described.[5, 11, 246, 247, 252] In these German shepherd dogs, the syndrome is autosomal dominant in inheritance and is characterized by the sudden onset of skin lesions at 3 to 5 years of age. These dogs almost always die of bilateral renal cystadenocarcinomas 3 to 5 years later. Female dogs frequently have multiple uterine leiomyomas. Most collagenous nevi are firm, well circumscribed, and 0.5 to 5 cm in diameter. Some lesions are alopecic, are hyperpigmented, and have pitted surfaces (''cobblestone'' or ''orange peel'' appearance). Lesions on the feet may ulcerate and cause pain and lameness.

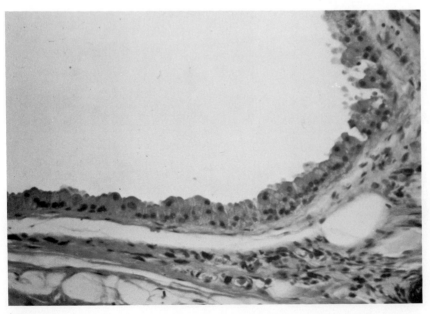

Figure 19:120. Close-up of Figure 19:119. Columnar glandular epithelium with apical budding.

Recently, a syndrome of regional collagenous nevi has been reported.[249a] Adult dogs develop nodular lesions on a limb or the face, that increase in number and spread to involve a large area of the limb, neck, and sternum.

Histopathologically, collagenous nevi are characterized by nodular areas of collagenous hyperplasia, which often displace adnexae and subcutaneous fat (Figs. 19:121 and 19:122). In clinical management, surgical excision or observation without therapy is usually employed.

ORGANOID NEVI

Organoid nevi are uncommonly reported in dogs and cats.[34, 250] Lesions are solitary, occasionally multiple, firm to mushy, 0.3 to 3 cm in diameter, and dome shaped to pedunculated. They occur primarily on the face, the head (see Fig. 19:118 *E*), and the proximal extremities. Linear organoid nevus occurred in a 1-week-old dog as linear, yellowish, crusty lesions on the head, neck, shoulders, and dorsolateral thorax.[250]

Focal adnexal dysplasia and adnexal nevi have been described in dogs.[4, 5, 253] These two conditions may, indeed, be identical. Lesions are solitary, firm, well circumscribed, and dome shaped to polypoid, and range from 1 to more than 4 cm in diameter. Larger lesions are frequently alopecic and ulcerated. The distal limbs (especially pressure points and interdigital areas) are most commonly involved. Affected dogs are generally middle aged or older, there is no sex predilection, and Doberman pinschers and Labrador retrievers may be predisposed.[4] The histopathologic findings of so-called focal adnexal dysplasia are similar to so-called folliculosebaceous hamartoma in humans, and the lesion is best classified as a nevus at present. Similarly, adnexal nevi consist of hyperplastic adnexae and fall under the category of organoid nevi.

Histopathologically, organoid nevi are characterized by hyperplasia of two or more skin components (Fig. 19:123). Focal adnexal dysplasia is characterized by circumscribed, dermal to subcutaneous nodules composed of loosely distributed, haphazardly arranged folliculosebaceous units and abundant collagen.[5, 253] Concurrent suppurative or pyogranulomatous inflammation is common. Adnexal nevi are composed of hyperplastic adnexae with frequent concurrent inflammation.[4] Therapeutic options include surgical excision and observation without treatment.

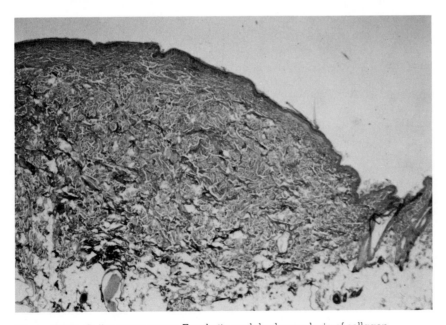

Figure 19:121. Collagenous nevus. Exophytic, nodular hyperplasia of collagen.

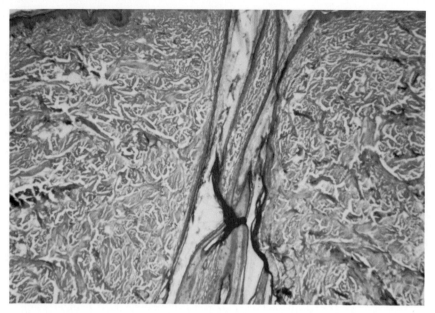

Figure 19:122. Close-up of Figure 19:121. Collagenous hyperplasia surrounding a hair follicle.

VASCULAR NEVI

Vascular nevi occur on the scrotum (varicose tumors of the scrotum, or scrotal vascular hamartoma) and occasionally elsewhere in dogs (see Fig. 19:118 *F*).[4, 5, 32, 254] They are most common in dogs older than middle age and in breeds with pigmented skin, such as Scottish terriers, Airedales, Kerry blue terriers, and Labrador retrievers. The lesions are characterized

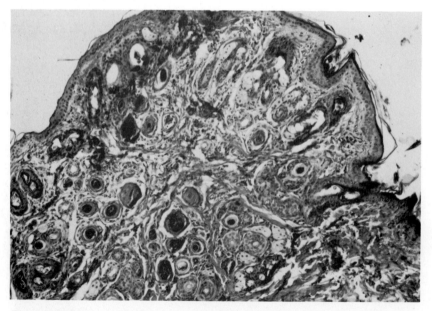

Figure 19:123. Organoid nevus. Dome-shaped mass consisting of an excess of hair follicles and sebaceous glands. (From Scott DW: Feline dermatology 1900–1978: A monograph. J.A.A.H.A. 16:331, 1980.)

by single or multiple, slowly enlarging and hyperpigmenting plaques on the scrotum. Periodic hemorrhage from the lesions may be seen. Vascular nevi are occasionally seen at other cutaneous sites.[22, 251] Histopathologically, the scrotal lesions are characterized by cavernous dilatation (telangiectasia) of blood vessels and epidermal melanosis. Therapeutic options include surgical excision and observation without treatment.

SEBACEOUS GLAND NEVI

Sebaceous gland nevi are rarely diagnosed in dogs.[4, 5, 252] They are usually solitary, alopecic, scaly plaques, less than 2 cm in diameter, with an irregular or papillated surface. A sebaceous gland nevus was recognized in a 1-year-old male Poodle.[252] The lesion had been present on the cranial right thigh since birth and had been slowly enlarging. It was linear, multinodular, alopecic, smooth, shiny, greasy, and orange-yellow (see Fig. 19:118*G*). Histopathologically, sebaceous gland nevi are characterized by sebaceous gland hyperplasia and overlying papillated epidermal hyperplasia (Fig. 19:124). Therapeutic options include surgical excision and observation without treatment.

APOCRINE SWEAT GLAND NEVI

Apocrine sweat gland nevi are rarely diagnosed in young dogs and cats.[4, 246a] Lesions have been solitary and located on the head and neck. Lesions may be bluish in color and fluctuant. Histologically, a linear to nodular proliferation of hyperplastic, dilated apocrine sweat glands is present in the deep dermis and subcutis. Therapeutic options include surgical excision and observation without treatment.

EPIDERMAL NEVI

Epidermal nevi are uncommonly diagnosed in dogs.[4, 5, 11, 252] These lesions usually occur in young adults, especially Pugs and Miniature Schnauzers, supporting a hereditary pathogenesis. Lesions previously reported as lentigines in Pugs (see Chap. 12) were probably epidermal nevi.

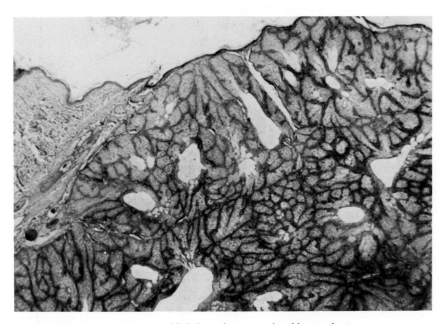

Figure 19:124. Sebaceous nevus. Nodular sebaceous gland hyperplasia.

Lesions are usually multiple, occasionally solitary, ovoid or circular plaques, hyperpigmented, scaly to papillomatous, and less than 2 cm in diameter. They occur most commonly on the ventral abdomen (see Fig. 19:118 *H*), the ventral thorax, and the medial limbs.

Epidermal nevi occurred in a 2-month-old male Miniature Schnauzer; the lesions developed as wavy, linear bands of closely set, hyperpigmented, hyperkeratotic papules and plaques over the trunk.[252] Inflammatory linear verrucous epidermal nevi were reported in three related Cocker spaniels.[254a] All dogs were female and had lesions before 6 months of age. Linear, pigmented verrucous lesions were noted most commonly on the lateral trunk, the footpads, and the ears. All lesions were moderately pruritic.

Histologic examination of epidermal nevi shows orthokeratotic hyperkeratosis, papillated epidermal hyperplasia, epidermal melanosis, and papillomatosis (Fig. 19:125). In some instances, granular degeneration of the epidermis is present.

Therapeutic options include surgical excision and observation without treatment. In three dogs with inflammatory linear verrucous epidermal nevus, improvement was achieved with the oral administration of isotretinoin or etretinate.[254a]

HAIR FOLLICLE NEVI

Hair follicle nevi are uncommonly diagnosed in dogs.[4, 5, 250] Lesions are solitary or multiple, hyperkeratotic, ovoid or linear plaques, especially on proximal extremities. Hairs arising from the lesions may be thick and brushlike. Histologically, hair follicles and hair shafts that are larger than normal are present in clusters. Therapeutic options include surgical excision and observation without treatment.

COMEDO NEVI

Comedo nevi are rarely diagnosed in dogs.[250] Lesions are solitary, well-circumscribed, annular areas of alopecia, hyperkeratosis, and clustered comedones. Schnauzer comedo syndrome is probably a more widespread form of comedo nevus (see Chap. 11). Histologically, there are clusters of dilated, hyperkeratotic hair follicles.

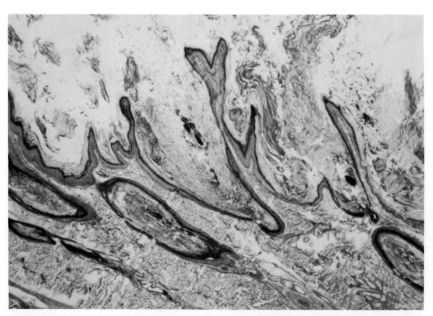

Figure 19:125. Epidermal nevus. Orthokeratotic hyperkeratosis, papillated epidermal hyperplasia, and papillomatosis.

Therapeutic options include surgical excision and observation without treatment. The oral administration of isotretinoin is effective treatment for the Schnauzer comedo syndrome (see Chap. 11).

PACINIAN CORPUSCLE NEVI

Pacinian corpuscle nevi are rarely reported in dogs and cats.[4] Numerous pacinian corpuscles are seen in the dermis and subcutis.

MELANOCYTIC NEVI

Although the term ''melanocytic nevus'' has been frequently employed in veterinary medicine,[5, 11, 32, 245, 249] it is preferable to call these lesions melanocytomas.

Keratoses

Keratoses are firm, elevated, circumscribed areas of reactive keratinocyte proliferation and excessive keratin production.[3, 5, 9, 11] Keratoses are uncommonly reported in dogs and cats.

ACTINIC KERATOSIS

Actinic (solar) keratoses occur in dogs and cats.[5, 11] They are caused by excessive exposure to ultraviolet light and occur more commonly in sunny areas of the world. Actinic keratoses may be single or multiple, appear in lightly haired and lightly pigmented skin, and vary in appearance from ill-defined areas of erythema, hyperkeratosis, and crusting to indurated, crusted, hyperkeratotic plaques varying from 0.3 to 5 cm in diameter (Fig. 19:126 *A*). Dalmatians, American Staffordshire terriers, beagles, Basset hounds, and bull terriers have an increased incidence of actinic keratoses. Histopathologically, they are characterized by atypia and dysplasia of the epidermis and superficial hair follicle epithelium, hyperkeratosis (especially parakeratotic), and occasionally solar elastosis of the underlying dermis (Fig. 19:127). Actinic keratoses are premalignant lesions capable of becoming invasive squamous cell carcinomas.

LICHENOID KERATOSIS

Lichenoid keratoses are rarely recognized in dogs.[5, 11, 255] Generally, solitary asymptomatic lesions are seen most commonly on the pinnae and groin of adult dogs. Lesions are well-circumscribed, erythematous, and scaly to markedly hyperkeratotic plaques or papillomas varying from 0.5 to 2 cm in diameter. Occasionally, multiple lesions are present on the lateral surface of the pinna (see Fig. 19:126 *B*).[255] Histologically, an irregular to papillated epidermal hyperplasia with overlying hyperkeratosis and an underlying subepidermal lichenoid band of inflammation are seen (Fig. 19:128). Therapeutic options include surgical excision or observation without treatment.

SEBORRHEIC KERATOSIS

Seborrheic keratoses are rarely recognized in dogs.[11, 256] The cause of seborrheic keratoses is unknown, and they have nothing to do with seborrhea. They may be single or multiple and have no apparent age, breed, sex, or site predilections. The lesions are elevated plaques and nodules with a hyperkeratotic, often greasy surface (see Fig. 19:126 *C*). They are frequently hyperpigmented. Histologically, seborrheic keratoses are characterized by hyperkeratosis, hyperplasia (basaloid and squamoid), and papillomatosis (Fig. 19:129). Therapeutic options include surgical excision and observation without treatment.

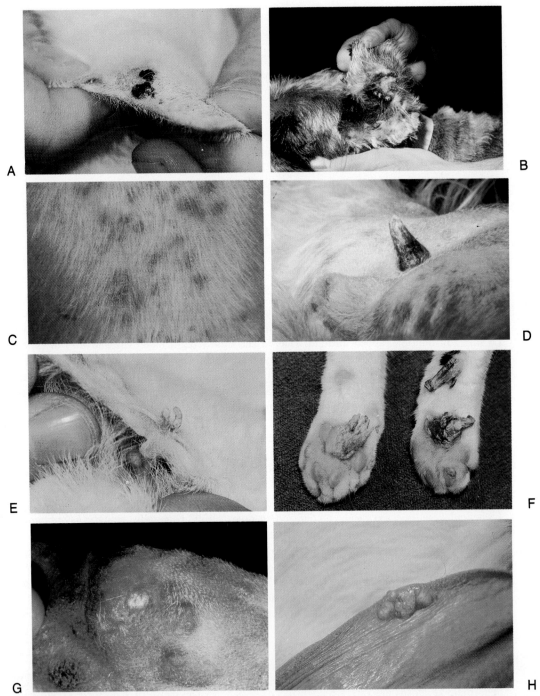

Figure 19:126. *A*, Feline actinic keratosis. Two crusted plaques on a background of solar dermatitis. *B*, Multiple melanotic lichenoid keratoses on the pinna of a miniature Schnauzer. *C*, Multiple brownish, greasy seborrheic keratoses over the back of a dog. *D*, Cutaneous horn cranial to the vulva. *E*, Two cutaneous horns on the pinna of a cat. *F*, Multiple cutaneous horns on the footpads of an FeLV-infected cat. *G*, Calcinosis circumscripta on the elbow of a dog. *H*, Calcinosis circumscripta on the tongue of a dog.

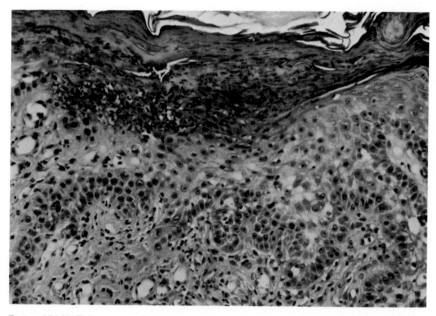

Figure 19:127. Feline actinic keratosis.

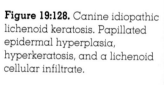

Figure 19:128. Canine idiopathic lichenoid keratosis. Papillated epidermal hyperplasia, hyperkeratosis, and a lichenoid cellular infiltrate.

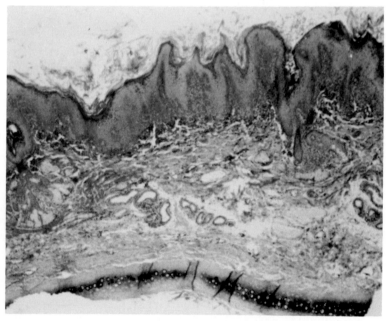

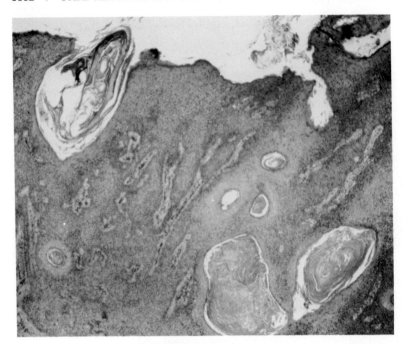

Figure 19:129. Canine seborrheic keratosis. Marked basaloid and squamoid hyperplasia with numerous horn cysts.

CUTANEOUS HORN

Cutaneous horns are uncommon in dogs and cats. The cause of cutaneous horns may be unknown, or they may originate from papillomas, basal cell tumors, squamous cell carcinomas, keratinous cysts, keratoacanthomas, or actinic keratoses. Cutaneous horns may be single or multiple and have no apparent age, sex, or site predilections. They are firm, hornlike projections of up to 5 cm in length (see Fig. 19:126 *D* and *E*). Multiple cutaneous horns have been seen on the footpads of cats with FeLV infection.[5, 35] Generally, multiple horns are seen on multiple footpads (see Fig. 19:126 *F*). Occasionally, lesions are seen on the face. Histopathologically, cutaneous horns are characterized by extensive, compact, laminated hyperkeratosis (Figs. 19:130 and 19:131). The base of a cutaneous horn must always be inspected for the possible underlying cause. FeLV-associated cutaneous horns in cats have been characterized by dyskeratosis and multinucleate epidermal giant cells (Fig. 19:132). Therapeutic options include surgical excision and observation without treatment.

Calcinosis Cutis

Calcinosis cutis is an uncommon disorder of the dog.[5, 11] Calcification of the skin may occur in a wide variety of unrelated disorders (Table 19:6). The complex biological process whereby inorganic ions are deposited as a solid phase in soft tissues is not understood. It is probable that abnormal skin calcifications are usually associated with collagen and elastin.

Metastatic calcinosis cutis is rarely seen in dogs and cats, and all cases have occurred in association with chronic renal disease.[5, 260, 264] Cutaneous lesions have been localized to the footpads. Affected pads are enlarged, painful, and firm; they are often ulcerated and discharge a chalky white, pasty to gritty material. Skin biopsy findings are identical to those reported for calcinosis circumscripta (see below). No therapy is beneficial. Although footpad lesions usually indicate metastatic calcinosis and renal disease, calcinosis circumscripta has been reported to affect one footpad of an otherwise healthy young German shepherd dog.[265] Surgical excision was curative.

Widespread calcinosis cutis has frequently been reported in dogs in association with naturally occurring or iatrogenic hyperglucocorticoidism (see Chap. 9). Cutaneous lesions consist

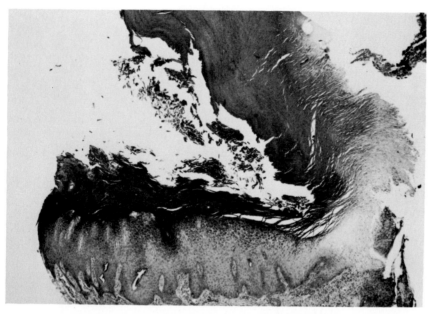

Figure 19:130. Feline cutaneous horn. Hornlike projection of dense keratin arising from hyperplastic, hypergranular, hyperkeratotic footpad epithelium.

Table 19:6. Causes of Calcinosis Cutis in Dogs

Dystrophic calcification (deposition of calcium salts in injured, degenerating, or dead tissue)
    Localized areas (calcinosis circumscripta)
        Inflammatory lesions (tuberculosis, foreign body granuloma, demodicosis, staphylococcal pododermatitis)
        Degenerative lesions (follicular cysts)
        Neoplastic lesions (pilomatrixoma, others)
    Widespread areas (calcinosis universalis)
        Hyperglucocorticoidism (naturally occurring or iatrogenic)
        Diabetes mellitus
        Percutaneous penetration of calcium

Idiopathic calcification (deposition of calcium salts with no appreciable tissue damage or demonstrable metabolic defect)
    Localized areas (idiopathic calcinosis circumscripta of large breed dogs)
    Widespread areas (idiopathic calcinosis universalis of young dogs)

Metastatic calcification (deposition of calcium salts associated with abnormal metabolism of calcium and phosphorus with demonstrable serum level changes)
    Chronic renal disease

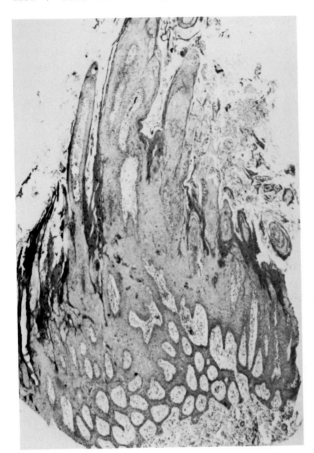

Figure 19:131. Feline cutaneous horn. Hornlike projection from the footpad of an FeLV-infected cat.

Figure 19:132. Close-up of Figure 19:131. Multinucleated keratinocytes (arrow).

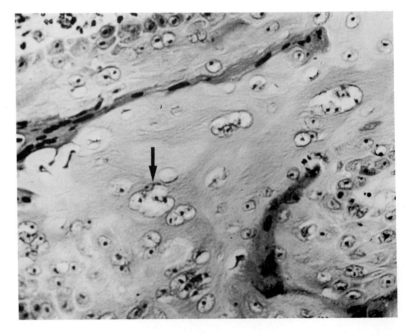

of papules, plaques, and nodules that are firm, often gritty, frequently ulcerated and secondarily infected, and yellowish white to pinkish yellow. These lesions may occur anywhere but are especially common along the dorsum and in the axillae and groin. Histologically, calcium salts are deposited along collagen and elastin fibers in the dermis and basement membrane zones and are frequently surrounded by a foreign body granuloma reaction. This form of calcinosis cutis in dogs is thought to be dystrophic in nature, because blood calcium and phosphorus levels are invariably normal. Correcting the hyperglucocorticoidism causes this type of calcinosis cutis to regress within 2 to 12 months. A syndrome of idiopathic calcinosis cutis grossly and histologically identical to glucocorticoid-associated calcinosis cutis has rarely been seen in healthy dogs younger than 1 year old.[5, 11] Lesions spontaneously regress within 1 year. Calcinosis cutis in dogs was reported to result from percutaneous penetration of calcium (contact with commercial hygroscopic landscaping products [see Chap. 15]). Spontaneous recovery followed avoidance of further contact with the substances.

CALCINOSIS CIRCUMSCRIPTA

■ *Cause and Pathogenesis.* Calcinosis circumscripta (kalkgicht, calcium gout, apocrine cystic calcinosis, or multiloculated subcutaneous granuloma) is uncommon in dogs and rare in cats.[5, 11, 258, 260, 264] In most cases, the cause is unknown. Because lesions most frequently occur over pressure points or sites of previous trauma, such as that incurred during ear cropping, the calcium deposition may be dystrophic.[5] The tendency for dystrophic mineralization may be enhanced by the active calcium metabolism of large, rapidly growing dogs.[5] Rarely, calcinosis circumscripta is reported to occur at the site of previous subcutaneous injections,[259, 261] from degeneration of pre-existing apocrine sweat gland cysts,[5] at the sites of previous bite wounds,[5] or at the site of polydioxanone sutures.[262] Although most affected animals are otherwise healthy, symmetric calcinosis circumscripta has been reported in dogs in association with hypertrophic osteodystrophy and idiopathic polyarthritis.[264]

■ *Clinical Findings.* Calcinosis circumscripta is seen most commonly in younger dogs (younger than 2 years of age) of either sex.[264] About 90 per cent of all reported cases have been in large breeds of dogs, and more than 50 per cent of cases have been in German shepherd dogs. Lesions are usually dome shaped, fluctuant or firm, and 0.5 to 7 cm in diameter. Initially, the overlying skin may be freely movable and covered with hair. As the lesions progress, however, ulceration frequently occurs, as does the discharge of a chalky white, pasty to gritty material. Lesions are usually single but occasionally multiple or bilaterally symmetric. They are most frequently seen over or near pressure points and bony prominences, especially the lateral metatarsal and phalangeal areas of the pelvic limb and the elbow (see Fig. 19:126 *G*).[264] They may also occur over the dorsal aspects of the fourth to sixth cervical vertebrae[263] or in the tongue (see Fig. 19:126 *H*).[264] Boxers and Boston terriers appear to be predisposed to lesions at the base of the pinna and on the cheek, respectively. Calcinosis circumscripta is extremely rare in cats.[258, 259]

■ *Diagnosis.* Histologically, calcinosis circumscripta is characterized by multifocal areas of granular amorphous material in the deep dermis and subcutis surrounded by a zone of granulomatous inflammation and separated by fibrous trabeculae (Figs. 19:133 and 19:134).[5, 264] Cartilaginous and osseous metaplasia, as well as transepidermal elimination of minerals, may be seen in some lesions. The amorphous masses are usually strongly PAS positive and Alcian blue positive.

■ *Clinical Management.* The treatment of choice is surgical excision. Recurrences or the development of new lesions after surgery is not reported.[264] Dogs with symmetric lesions (on

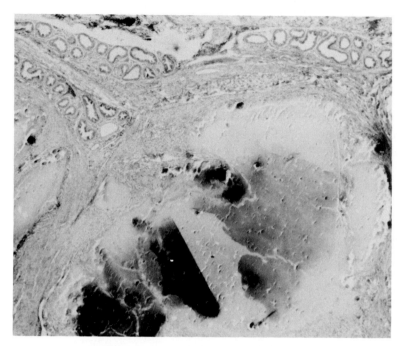

Figure 19:133. Canine calcinosis circumscripta. Nodular accumulations of mineral below the level of apocrine sweat glands.

Figure 19:134. Canine calcinosis circumscripta. Palisading granuloma surrounding a mineral deposit.

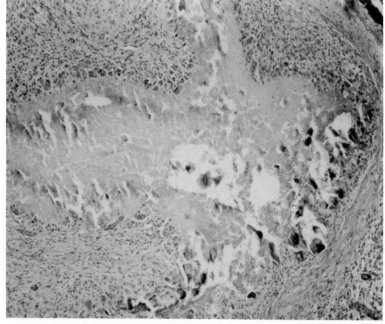

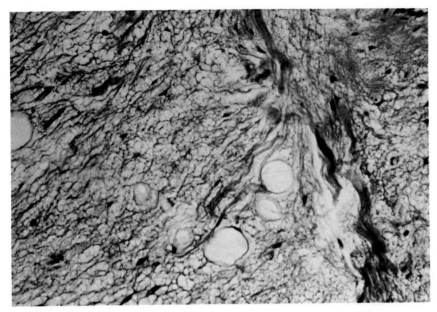

Figure 19:135. Canine focal cutaneous mucinosis. Diffuse dermal mucinosis.

scapulae and hips) in association with hypertrophic osteodystrophy or idiopathic polyarthritis had spontaneous remission of their calcinosis circumscripta as the associated disease became inactive.[264]

Cutaneous Mucinosis

Cutaneous mucinoses are a heterogeneous group of skin disorders characterized by the excessive accumulation or deposition of mucin (acid mucopolysaccharide) in the dermis or epithelial structures.[5, 11, 257] The mucinosis may be primary or secondary, or focal to diffuse. In dogs, cutaneous mucinosis may be seen with hypothyroidism, acromegaly, lupus erythematosus, dermatomyositis, and mycosis fungoides and as a normal finding in the Shar Pei. In cats, cutaneous mucinosis may be seen with alopecia mucinosa and mycosis fungoides.

Focal cutaneous mucinosis has rarely been reported in dogs.[257] Three dogs (two Doberman pinschers; all three females, 3 to 6 years old) had solitary, asymptomatic, firm and rubbery to soft nodules (1 to 3 cm in diameter) on the head or the leg. The primary histopathologic finding was an accumulation of excessive mucin (Alcian blue positive or colloidal iron positive) within the dermis or subcutis, which disrupted and separated collagen fibers (Fig. 19:135). In addition, a mild to extensive proliferation of fibroblasts and a mild lymphohistiocytic infiltrate were seen. Surgical excision was curative.

REFERENCES

General Textbook Sources
1. Bostock, D.E., Owen, L.N.: Neoplasia in the Cat, Dog, and Horse. Year Book Medical Publishers, Chicago, 1975.
2. Ettinger, S.J.: Textbook of Veterinary Internal Medicine: Diseases of the Dog and Cat, 3rd ed., Vol. 1. W.B. Saunders Co., Philadelphia, 1989.
3. Fitzpatrick, T.B., et al.: Dermatology in General Medicine IV. McGraw-Hill Book Co., New York, 1993.
4. Goldschmidt, M.H., Shofer, F.: Skin Tumors of the Dog and Cat. Pergamon Press, New York, 1992.
5. Gross, T.L., et al.: Veterinary Dermatopathology. A Macroscopic and Microscopic Evaluation of Canine and Feline Skin Disease. Mosby–Year Book, St. Louis, 1992.
5a. Hajdu, S.I.: Pathology of Soft Tissue Tumors. Lea & Febiger, Philadelphia, 1979.
6. Hashimoto, K., et al.: Tumors of Skin Appendages. Butterworth, London, 1987.

7. Kirk, R.W. (ed.): Current Veterinary Therapy X. W.B. Saunders Co., Philadelphia, 1989.
8. Kirk. R.W., Bonagura, J.D. (eds.): Current Veterinary Therapy XI. W.B. Saunders Co., Philadelphia, 1992.
9. Lever, W.F., Schaumburg-Lever, G.: Histopathology of the Skin VII. J.B. Lippincott Co., Philadelphia, 1990.
10. Moulton, J.E.: Tumors in Domestic Animals III. University of California Press, Berkeley, 1990.
11. Muller, G.H., et al.: Small Animal Dermatology, 4th ed. W.B. Saunders Co., Philadelphia, 1989.
12. Theilen, G.H., Madewell, B.R.: Veterinary Cancer Medicine II. Lea & Febiger, Philadelphia, 1987.
13. Withrow, S.J., MacEwen, E.G.: Clinical Veterinary Oncology. J.B. Lippincott Co., Philadelphia, 1989.

Survey Articles and Chapters

14. Bastianello, S.S.: A survey of neoplasia in domestic species over a 40-year period from 1935 to 1974 in the Republic of South Africa. V. Tumours occurring in the cat. Onderstepoort J. Vet. Res. 50:105, 1983.
15. Bastianello, S.S.: A survey of neoplasia in domestic species over a 40-year period from 1935–1974 in the Republic of South Africa. VI. Tumours occurring in dogs. Onderstepoort J. Vet. Res. 50:199, 1983.
16. Berrocal, A., et al.: Canine perineal tumours. J. Vet. Med. A 36:739, 1989.
17. Bostock, D.E.: Neoplasms of the skin and subcutaneous tissues in dogs and cats. Br. Vet. J. 142:1, 1986.
18. Brodey, R.S.: Canine and feline neoplasia. Adv. Vet. Sci. 14:309, 1970.
19. Carpenter, J.L., et al.: Tumors and tumor-like lesions. In: Holzworth, J. (ed.). Diseases of the Cat: Medicine and Surgery, Vol. 1. W.B. Saunders Co., Philadelphia, 1987, p. 413.
20. Cotchin, E.: Skin tumours of cats. Res. Vet. Sci. 2:353, 1961.
21. Crow, S.E., et al.: Skin tumors in dogs and cats. Dermatol. Rep. 3(1):1, 1984.
21a. Degorce, F., Parodi, A.L.: Tumeurs conjunctives des carnivores domestiques. Rec. Méd. Vét. 166:1043, 1990.
22. Finnie, J.W., Bostock, D.E.: Skin neoplasia in dogs. Aust. Vet. J. 55:602, 1979.
22a. Graham, J.C., O'Keefe, D.A.: Diagnosis and treatment of soft tissue sarcomas. Compend. Cont. Educ. 15:1627, 1993.
23. Head, K.W.: Some data concerning the distribution of skin tumors in domestic animals. In: Rook, A., Walton, G.S. (eds.). Comparative Physiology and Pathology of the Skin. F.A. Davis Co., Philadelphia, 1965, p. 613.
24. Keller, E.T., Madewell, B.R.: Locations and types of neoplasms in immature dogs: 69 cases (1964–1989). J. Am. Vet. Med. Assoc. 200:1530, 1992.
25. Ladds, P., et al.: Neoplasms of the skin of dogs in tropical Queensland. Aust. Vet. J. 60:87, 1983.
25a. MacEwen, E.G., Helfand, S.C.: Recent advances in the biologic therapy of cancer. Compend. Cont. Educ. 15:909, 1993.
26. Macy, D.W., Reynolds, H.A.: The incidence, characteristics, and clinical management of skin tumors of cats. J. Am. Anim. Hosp. Assoc. 17:1026, 1981.
27. Magnol, J.P.: Tumeurs cutanées du chien et du chat. Rec. Méd. Vét. 166:1061, 1990.
28. Mialot, M., Lagadic, M.: Epidémiologie descriptive des tumeurs du chien et du chat. Rec. Méd. Vét. 166:937, 1990.
29. Miller, M.A., et al.: Cutaneous neoplasia in 340 cats. Vet. Pathol. 28:389, 1991.
30. Nielsen, S.W., Cole, C.R.: Cutaneous epithelial neoplasms of the dog—A report of 153 cases. Am. J. Vet. Res. 21:931, 1960.
31. Priester, W.A.: Skin tumors in domestic animals. Data from twelve United States and Canadian colleges of veterinary medicine. J. Natl. Cancer Inst. 50:457, 1973.
32. Pulley, L.T., Stannard, A.A.: Tumors of the skin and soft tissues. In: Moulton, J.E. (ed.). Tumors in Domestic Animals III. University of California Press, Berkeley, 1990, p. 23.
33. Rothwell, T.L.W., et al.: Skin neoplasms of dogs in Sydney. Aust. Vet. J. 64:161, 1987.
34. Scott, D.W.: Feline dermatology 1900–1978: A monograph. J. Am. Anim. Hosp. Assoc. 16:331, 1980.
35. Scott, D.W.: Feline dermatology 1979–1982: Introspective retrospections. J. Am. Anim. Hosp. Assoc. 20:537, 1984.
36. Scott, D.W.: Feline dermatology 1983–1985: "The secret sits." J. Am. Anim. Hosp. Assoc. 23:255, 1987.
37. Scott, D.W.: Feline dermatology 1986–1988: Looking to the 1990s through the eyes of many counsellors. J. Am. Anim. Hosp. Assoc. 26:517, 1990.
38. Susaneck, S.J.: Feline skin tumors. Comp. Cont. Educ. 5:251, 1983.
39. Van Den Ingh, T.S.G.A.M.: Huidtumoren bij de Hond. Tijschr. Diergeneeskd. 98:538, 1973.
40. Yager, J.A., Scott, D.W.: The skin and appendages. In: Jubb, K.V.F., et al. (eds.). Pathology of Domestic Animals IV, Vol. 1. Academic Press, New York, 1993, p. 531.

Cytology

41. Barton, C.L.: Cytologic analysis of cutaneous neoplasia: An algorithmic approach. Comp. Cont. Educ. 9:20, 1987.
42. Carter, R.F., Valli, V.E.O.: Advances in the cytologic diagnosis of canine lymphoma. Semin. Vet. Med. Surg. (Small Anim.) 3:167, 1988.
43. Hall, R.L., MacWilliams, P.S.: The cytologic examination of cutaneous and subcutaneous masses. Semin. Vet. Med. Surg. (Small Anim.) 3:94, 1988.
44. Stirtzinger, T.: The cytologic diagnosis of mesenchymal tumors. Semin. Vet. Med. Surg. (Small Anim.) 3:157, 1988.

Immunohistochemistry

45. Andreasen, C.B., et al.: Intermediate filament staining in the cytologic and histologic diagnosis of canine skin and soft tissue tumors. Vet. Pathol. 25:343, 1988.
46. Brown, P.J.: Immunohistochemical localization of myoglobin in connective tissue in tumors in dogs. Vet. Pathol. 24:573, 1987.

47. Desnoyers, M.M., et al.: Immunohistochemical detection of intermediate filament proteins in formalin fixed normal and neoplastic tissues. Can. J. Vet. Res. 54:360, 1990.
48. Elias, J.W.: Immunohistopathology: A Practical Approach to Diagnosis. American Society of Clinical Pathologists, Chicago, 1990.
48a. Doherty, M.J., et al.: Immunoenzyme techniques in dermatopathology. J. Am. Acad. Dermatol. 20:827, 1989.
49. Ferrer, L., et al.: Immunocytochemical demonstration of intermediate filament proteins, S-100 protein and CEA in apocrine sweat glands and apocrine gland derived lesions of the dog. J. Vet. Med. A 37:569, 1990.
50. Fondevila, D., et al.: Immunohistochemical localization of S-100 protein and lysozyme in canine lymph nodes and lymphomas. J. Vet. Med. A 36:71, 1989.
51. Fondevila, D., et al.: Immunoreactivity of canine and feline mast cell tumours. Schweiz. Arch. Tierheilkd. 132:426, 1990.
51a. Magnol, J.P., et al.: Une nouvelle approche, diagnostique et pronostique des tumeurs des tissus mous du chien et du chat. Point Vét. 22:831, 1991.
52. Moore, A.S., et al.: Immunohistochemical evaluation of intermediate filament expression in canine and feline neoplasms. Am. J. Vet. Res. 50:88, 1989.
53. Moore, P.F.: Utilization of cytoplasmic lysozyme reactivity as a histiocytic marker in canine histiocytic disorders. Vet. Pathol. 23:757, 1986.
54. Rabanal, R.H., et al.: Immunocytochemical diagnosis of skin tumours of the dog with special reference to undifferentiated types. Res. Vet. Sci. 47:129, 1989.
55. Sandusky, G.E., et al.: Diagnostic immunohistochemistry of canine round cell tumors. Vet. Pathol. 24:495, 1987.
56. Sandusky, G.E., et al.: Immunocytochemical study of tissues from clinically normal dogs and of neoplasms using keratin monoclonal antibodies. Am. J. Vet. Res. 52:613, 1991.
57. Thoonen, H., et al.: Expression of cytokeratins in epithelial tumours of the dog investigated with monoclonal antibodies. Schweiz. Arch. Tierheilkd. 132:409, 1990.
58. Von Beust, B.R., et al.: Factor VIII–related antigen in canine endothelial neoplasms: An immunohistochemical study. Vet. Pathol. 25:251, 1988.

Papilloma
59. Amer, M., et al.: Verrucae treated by levamisole. Int. J. Dermatol. 30:738, 1991.
60. Amer, M., et al.: Therapeutic evaluation of intralesional injection of bleomycin sulfate in 143 resistant warts. J. Am. Acad. Dermatol. 18:1313, 1988.
61. Bregman, C.L., et al.: Cutaneous neoplasms in dogs associated with canine oral papillomavirus vaccine. Vet. Pathol. 24:477, 1987.
62. Campbell, K.L., et al.: Cutaneous inverted papillomas in dogs. Vet. Pathol. 25:67, 1988.
63. Carney, H.C., et al.: Papillomavirus infection of aged Persian cats. J. Vet. Diagn. Invest. 2:294, 1990.
63a. Carpenter, J.L., et al.: Cutaneous xanthogranuloma and viral papilloma on the eyelid of a cat. Vet. Dermatol. 3:187, 1992.
64. Cobb, M.W.: Human papillomavirus infection. J. Am. Acad. Dermatol. 22:547, 1990.
65. Egberink, H.F., et al.: Papillomavirus associated skin lesions in a cat seropositive for feline immunodeficiency virus. Vet. Microbiol. 31:117, 1992.
66. Mill, A.B., et al.: Concurrent hypothyroidism, IgM deficiency, impaired T-cell mitogen response, and multifocal cutaneous squamous papillomas in a dog. Canine Pract. 17(2):15, 1992.
66a. Shimada, A., et al.: Cutaneous papillomatosis associated with papillomavirus infection in a dog. J. Comp. Pathol. 108:103, 1993.
67. Sironi, G., et al.: Immunohistochemical detection of papillomavirus structural antigens in animal hyperplastic and neoplastic epithelial lesions. J. Vet. Med. A 37:760, 1990.
68. Sundberg, J.P., et al.: Immunoperoxidase localization of papillomaviruses in hyperplastic and neoplastic epithelial lesions of animals. Am. J. Vet. Res. 45:1441, 1984.
69. Sundberg, J.P., et al.: Cloning and characterization of a canine oral papillomavirus. Am. J. Vet. Res. 47:1142, 1986.

Keratoacanthoma
70. Kwochka, K.W.: Retinoids in dermatology. In: Kirk, R.W. (ed.). Current Veterinary Therapy X. W.B. Saunders Co., Philadelphia, 1989, p. 553.
71. Melton, J.L., et al.: Treatment of keratoacanthomas with intralesional methotrexate. J. Am. Acad. Dermatol. 25:1017, 1991.
72. Power, H.T., Ihrke, P.J.: Synthetic retinoids in veterinary dermatology. Vet. Clin. North Am. (Small Anim. Pract.) 20:1525, 1990.
73. Smith, D.A., Knottenbett, M.K.: Spontaneous regression of intracutaneous cornifying epitheliomata in a dog. J. Small Anim. Pract. 29:201, 1988.
74. Stannard, A.A., Pulley, L.T.: Intracutaneous cornifying epithelioma (keratoacanthoma) in the dog: A retrospective study of 25 cases. J. Am. Vet. Med. Assoc. 167:385, 1975.

Basal Cell Tumor
75. Anderson, W.I., Scott, D.W.: Cartilaginous metaplasia associated with a basal cell tumor in a dog. J. Comp. Pathol. 100:107, 1989.
75a. Day, D.G., et al.: Basal cell carcinoma in two cats. J. Am. Anim. Hosp. Assoc. 30:265, 1994.
76. Diters, R.W., Walsh, K.M.: Feline basal cell tumors: A review of 124 cases. Vet. Pathol. 21:51, 1984.
77. Fehrer, S.L., Lin, S.H.: Multicentric basal cell tumors in a cat. J. Am. Vet. Med. Assoc. 189:1469, 1986.

78. Seiler, R.J.: Granular basal cell tumors in the skin of three dogs: A distinct histopathologic entity. Vet. Pathol. 18:23, 1981.
79. Stenquist, B., et al.: Treatment of aggressive basal cell carcinoma with intralesional interferon. J. Am. Acad. Dermatol. 27:65, 1992.
80. Strafuss, A.C.: Basal cell tumors in dogs. J. Am. Vet. Med. Assoc. 169:322, 1976.

Squamous Cell Carcinoma

80a. Baer, K.E., Helton, K.: Multicentric squamous cell carcinoma in situ resembling Bowen's disease in cats. Vet. Pathol. 30:535, 1993.
81. Bostock, D.E.: Prognosis in cats bearing squamous cell carcinoma. J. Small Anim. Pract. 13:119, 1972.
82. Bourdeau, P.: Epithélioma spinocellulaire du chat. Point Vét. 19:55, 1987.
82a. Clarke, R.E.: Cryosurgical treatment of feline cutaneous squamous cell carcinoma. Aust. Vet. Practit. 21, 148, 1991.
83. Cox, N.R., et al.: Tumors of the nose and paranasal sinuses in cats: 32 cases with comparison to a national database (1977 through 1987). J. Am. Anim. Hosp. Assoc. 27:339, 1991.
84. Evans, A.G., et al.: A trial of 13-*cis*-retinoic acid for treatment of squamous cell carcinoma and preneoplastic lesions of the head in cats. Am. J. Vet. Res. 46:2553, 1985.
84a. Frese, K., et al.: Plattenepithelkarzinome der Zechen beim Hund. Dtsch. Tierarztl. Wochenschr. 90:359, 1983.
85. Gourley, I.M., et al.: Burn scar malignancy in a dog. J. Am. Vet. Med. Assoc. 180:1095, 1982.
86. Gross, T.L., Brimacomb, B.H.: Multifocal intraepidermal carcinoma in a dog histologically resembling Bowen's disease. Am. J. Dermatopathol. 8:509, 1986.
87. Hargis, A.M., Thomassen, R.W.: Solar keratosis (solar dermatosis, senile keratosis) and solar keratosis with squamous cell carcinoma. Am. J. Pathol. 94:193, 1979.
88. Haziroglu, M., Saylam, M.: Squamous cell carcinoma in a puppy. J. Comp. Pathol. 101:221, 1989.
89. Knowles, D.P., Hargis, A.M.: Solar elastosis associated with neoplasia in two Dalmatians. Vet. Pathol. 23:512, 1986.
90. Kwa, R.E., et al.: Biology of cutaneous squamous cell carcinoma. J. Am. Acad. Dermatol. 26:1, 1992.
91. Levine, N., et al.: Controlled localized heating and isotretinoin effects in canine squamous cell carcinoma. J. Am. Acad. Dermatol. 23:68, 1990.
92. Marks, S.L., et al.: Clinical evaluation of etretinate for the treatment of canine solar-induced squamous cell carcinoma and preneoplastic lesions. J. Am. Acad. Dermatol. 27:11, 1992.
93. Miller, W.H., Jr., Shanley, K.J.: Bilateral pinnal squamous cell carcinoma in a dog with chronic otitis externa. Vet. Dermatol. 2:37, 1991.
94. Miller, W.H., Jr., et al.: Multicentric squamous cell carcinoma in situ resembling Bowen's disease in five cats. Vet. Dermatol. 3:177, 1992.
94a. Miller, W.H., Jr., Scott, D.W.: Unpublished observations.
95. O'Brien, M.G., et al.: Treatment by digital amputation of subungual squamous cell carcinoma in dogs: 21 cases (1987–1988). J. Am. Vet. Med. Assoc. 201:759, 1992.
96. Paradis, M., et al.: Squamous cell carcinoma of the nail bed in three related Giant Schnauzers. Vet. Rec. 125:322, 1989.
96a. Peaston, A.E., et al.: Photodynamic therapy for nasal and aural squamous cell carcinoma in cats. J Am. Vet. Med. Assoc. 202:1261, 1993.
97. Scott, D.W., Miller, W.H., Jr.: Disorders of the claw and clawbed in cats. Comp. Cont. Educ. 14:449, 1992.
98. Scott, D.W., Miller, W.H., Jr.: Disorders of the claw and clawbed in dogs. Comp. Cont. Educ. 14:1448, 1992.
99. Strafuss, A.C., et al.: Squamous cell carcinoma in dogs. J. Am. Vet. Med. Assoc. 168:425, 1976.
99a. Withrow, S.J., Straw, R.C.: Resection of the nasal planum in nine cats and five dogs. J. Am. Anim. Hosp. Assoc. 26:219, 1990.

Hair Follicle Tumors

100. Diters, R.W., Goldschmidt, M.H.: Hair follicle tumors resembling tricholemmomas in six dogs. Vet. Pathol. 20:123, 1983.
100a. Fukui, K., et al.: [Two cases of canine malignant basal tumor]. J. Jpn. Vet. Med. Assoc. 45:856, 1992.
101. Hill, J.R.: Warty dyskeratoma in two dogs. Proc. Am. Acad. Vet. Dermatol. Am. Coll. Vet. Dermatol. 3, 1987.
102. Luther, P.B., et al.: The dilated pore of Winer—An overlooked cutaneous lesion of cats. J. Comp. Pathol. 101:375, 1989.
103. Scott, D.W., Anderson, W.I.: Canine hair follicle neoplasms: A retrospective analysis of 80 cases (1986–1987). Vet. Dermatol. 2:143, 1991.
104. Scott, D.W., Anderson, W.I.: Hair follicle neoplasms in three cats. Feline Pract. 19(3):14, 1991.
105. VanHamm, L., et al.: Metastatic pilomatrixoma presenting as paraplegia in a dog. J. Small Anim. Pract. 32:27, 1990.
106. Von Sandersleben, J.: Gutarige Epitheliale Neubildungen in der Haut des Hundes. Zentralbl. Vetinarmed. 8:702, 1964.

Sebaceous Gland Tumors

107. Finazzi, M., et al.: Reperti istologici su tumori delle ghiandole sebacee del cane. Clin. Vet. 110:123, 1987.
108. Scott, D.W., Anderson, W.I.: Canine sebaceous gland tumors: A retrospective analysis of 172 cases. Canine Pract. 15(1):19, 1990.
109. Scott, D.W., Anderson, W.I.: Feline sebaceous gland tumors: A retrospective analysis of nine cases. Feline Pract. 19(2):16, 1991.

110. Strafuss, A.C.: Sebaceous carcinoma in dogs. J. Am. Vet. Med. Assoc. 169:325, 1976.
111. Strafuss, A.C.: Sebaceous gland adenomas in dogs. J. Am. Vet. Med. Assoc. 169:640, 1976.

Sweat Gland Tumors
112. Christie, G.S., Jabara, A.G.: Canine sweat gland growths. Res. Vet. Sci. 5:237, 1964.
113. Jabara, A.G., Finnie, J.W.: Four cases of clear-cell hidradenocarcinomas in the dog. J. Comp. Pathol. 88:525, 1978.
114. Kalaher, K.M., et al.: Neoplasms of the apocrine sweat glands in 44 dogs and 10 cats. Vet. Rec. 127:400, 1990.
115. Meschter, C.L.: Disseminated sweat gland adenocarcinoma with acronecrosis in a cat. Cornell Vet. 81:195, 1991.

Perianal Gland Tumors
116. Ross, J.T., et al.: Adenocarcinoma of the apocrine glands of the anal sac in dogs: A review of 32 cases. J. Am. Anim. Hosp. Assoc. 27:349, 1991.
117. Vail, D.M., et al.: Perianal adenocarcinoma in the canine male: A retrospective study of 41 cases. J. Am. Anim. Hosp Assoc. 26:329, 1990.
117a. Vos, J.H., et al.: The expression of keratins, vimentin, neurofilament proteins, smooth muscle actin, neuron-specific enolase, and synaptophysin in tumors of the specific glands in the canine anal region. Vet. Pathol. 30:352, 1993.

Salivary Gland Tumors
118. Carberry, C.A., et al.: Salivary gland tumors in dogs and cats: A literature and case review. J. Am. Anim. Hosp. Assoc. 24:561, 1988.

Fibrosarcoma
119. Bostock, D.E., Dye, M.T.: Prognosis after surgical excision of fibrosarcomas in cats. J. Am. Vet. Med. Assoc. 175:727, 1979.
120. Bostock, D.E., Dye, M.T.: Prognosis after surgical excision of canine fibrous connective tissue sarcomas. Vet. Pathol. 17:581, 1980.
120a. Esplin, D.G., et al.: Post-vaccination sarcomas in cats. J. Am. Vet. Med. Assoc. 202:1245, 1993.
121. Harasen, G.L.G.: Multicentric fibrosarcoma in a cat and a review of the literature. Can. Vet. J. 24:207, 1984.
121a. Kent, E.M.: Use of an immunostimulant as an aid in treatment and management of fibrosarcoma in three cats. Feline Pract. 21:13, 1993.
121b. Kass, P.H., et al.: Epidemiologic evidence for a causal relation between vaccination and fibrosarcoma tumorigenesis in cats. J. Am. Vet. Med. Assoc. 203:396, 1993.
122. McChesney, S.L., et al.: Radiotherapy of soft tissue sarcomas in dogs. J. Am. Vet. Med. Assoc. 194:60, 1989.
122a. Stiglmair-Herb, M.T., Ortmann, U.: Die Fibrosarkome der Katze unter besonderer Berücksichtigung ihrer Dignitat. Kleintier-Prax. 32:75, 1978.

Myxoma
123. Rowland, P.H., et al.: Myxoma at the site of a subcutaneous pacemaker in a dog. J. Am. Anim. Hosp. Assoc. 27:649, 1991.

Neural Tumors
124. Geyer, C., et al.: Contribution to the histogenesis of granular cell tumours. Schweiz. Arch. Tierheilkd. 132:430, 1990.
124a. Geyer, C., et al.: Immunohistochemical and ultrastructural investigation of granular cell tumours in dog, cat, and horse. J. Vet. Med. B 39:485, 1992.
125. Gross, T.L., Carr, S.H.: Amputation neuroma of docked tails in dogs. Vet. Pathol. 27:61, 1990.
126. Herrera, G.A., Mendoza, A.: Primary canine cutaneous meningioma. Vet. Pathol. 18:127, 1981.
127. Moissonnier, P.: Les tumeurs des nerfs périphériques chez les carnivores. Point Vét. 22:149, 1990.
127a. Patniak, A.K.: Histologic and immunohistochemical studies of granular cell tumors in seven dogs, three cats, one horse, and one bird. Vet. Pathol. 30:176, 1993.
128. Turk, M.A.M., et al.: Canine granular cell tumor (myoblastoma): A report of four cases and review of the literature. J. Small Anim. Pract. 24:637, 1983.

Vascular Tumors
129. Brown, N.O., et al.: Canine hemangiosarcoma: Retrospective analysis of 104 cases. J. Am. Vet. Med. Assoc. 186:56, 1985.
129a. Carstens, P.H.B.: The Weibel-Palade body in the diagnosis of endothelial tumors. Ultrastruct. Pathol. 2:315, 1981.
130. Evans, S.M.: Canine hemangiosarcoma: A retrospective analysis of response to surgery and orthovoltage radiation. Vet. Radiol. 28:13, 1987.
131. Fossum, T.W., et al.: Generalized lymphangiectasis in a dog with subcutaneous chyle and lymphangioma. J. Am. Vet. Med. Assoc. 197:231, 1990.
132. George, C., Summers, B.A.: Angiokeratoma: A benign vascular tumor of the dog. J. Small Anim. Pract. 31:390, 1990.
133. Graves, G.M., et al.: Canine hemangiopericytoma: 23 cases (1967–1984). J. Am. Vet. Med. Assoc. 192:99, 1988.
134. Hammer, A.S., Couto, C.G.: Diagnosing and treating canine hemangiosarcoma. Vet. Med. 87:188, 1992.
135. Hargis, A.M., Feldman, B.F.: Evaluation of hemostatic defects secondary to vascular tumors in dogs: 11 cases (1983–1988). J. Am. Vet. Med. Assoc. 198:891, 1991.

135a. Hargis, A.M., et al.: A retrospective clinicopathologic study of 212 dogs with cutaneous hemangiomas and hemangiosarcomas. Vet. Pathol. 29:316, 1992.

135b. Kessler, M., Hammer, A.S.: Canines Hämangiosarkom: Diagnose und Therapie. Kleintier-Prax. 36:637, 1991.

136. Lewis, D.L., Harari, J.: Peripheral arteriovenous fistula associated with a subcutaneous hemangiosarcoma/hemangioma in a cat. Feline Pract. 20(1):27, 1992.

136a. Mayr, B., et al.: Trisomy 2 in three cases of canine haemangiopericytoma. Br. Vet. J. 148:113, 1992.

136b. Miller, M.A., et al.: Cutaneous vascular neoplasia in 15 cats: Clinical, morphologic, and immunohistochemical studies. Vet. Pathol. 29:329, 1992.

137. Mills, J.H.L, Nielsen, S.W.: Canine hemangiopericytoma: A survey of 200 tumors. J. Small Anim. Pract. 8:599, 1967.

137a. Post, K., et al.: Cutaneous lymphangioma in a young dog. Can. Vet. J. 32:747, 1991.

138. Postorino, N.C., et al.: Prognostic variables for canine hemangiopericytoma: 50 cases (1979–1984). J. Am. Anim. Hosp. Assoc. 24:501, 1988.

138a. Rishniw, M., Lewis, D.C.: Localized consumptive coagulopathy associated with cutaneous hemangiosarcoma in a dog. J. Am. Anim. Hosp. Assoc. 30:261, 1994.

139. Rudd, R.G., et al.: Lymphangiosarcoma in dogs. J. Am. Anim. Hosp. Assoc. 25:695, 1989.

140. Scavelli, T.D., et al.: Hemangiosarcoma in the cat: Retrospective evaluation of 31 surgical cases. J. Am. Vet. Med. Assoc. 187:817, 1987.

140a. Srebernik, N., Appleby, E.C.: Breed prevalence and sites of haemangioma and haemangiosarcoma in dogs. Vet. Rec. 129:408, 1991.

141. Stambaugh, J.E., et al.: Lymphangioma in 4 dogs. J. Am. Vet. Med. Assoc. 173:759, 1978.

142. Swayne, D.E., et al.: Lymphangiosarcoma and haemangiosarcoma in a cat. J. Comp. Pathol. 100:91, 1989.

143. Turrel, J.M., et al.: Response to radiation therapy of recurring lymphangioma in a dog. J. Am. Vet. Med. Assoc. 193:1432, 1988.

144. Vander Gaag, I., et al.: Canine capillary and combined capillary-cavernous haemangioma. J. Comp. Pathol. 101:69, 1989.

145. Walsh, K.M., Abbot, D.P.: Lymphangiosarcoma in two cats. J. Comp. Pathol. 94:611, 1984.

146. White, S.D., et al.: Acquired cutaneous lymphangiectasis in a dog. J. Am. Vet. Med. Assoc. 193:1093, 1988.

147. Xu, F.N.: Ultrastructure of canine hemangiopericytoma. Vet. Pathol. 23:643, 1986.

Adipose Tissue Tumors

148. Albers, G.W., Theilen, G.H.: Calcium chloride for treatment of subcutaneous lipomas in dogs. J. Am. Vet. Med. Assoc. 186:492, 1985.

148a. Bergman, P.J., et al.: Infiltrative lipoma in dogs: 16 cases (1981–1992). J. Am. Vet. Med. Assoc. 205:322, 1994.

149. Esplin, D.G.: Infiltrating lipoma in a cat. Feline Pract. 14(3):24, 1984.

149a. Frazier, K.S., et al.: Infiltrative lipoma in a canine stifle joint. J. Am. Anim. Hosp. Assoc. 29:81, 1993.

150. Kramek, B.A., et al.: Infiltrative lipoma in three dogs. J. Am. Vet. Med. Assoc. 186:81, 1985.

151. Messick, J.B., Radin, M.J.: Cytologic, histologic and ultrastructural characteristics of a canine myxoid liposarcoma. Vet. Pathol. 25:520, 1988.

152. Stephens, L.C., et al.: Virus-associated liposarcoma and malignant lymphoma in a kitten. J. Am. Vet. Med. Assoc. 183:123, 1983.

Rhabdomyoma and Rhabdomyosarcoma

152a. Martin de las Mulas, J., et al.: Desmin and vimentin immunocharacterization of feline muscle tumors. Vet. Pathol. 29:260, 1992.

152b. Roth, L.: Rhabdomyoma of the ear pinna in four cats. J. Comp. Pathol. 103:237, 1990.

Osteoma and Osteosarcoma

152c. Easton, C.B.: Extraskeletal osteosarcoma in a cat. J. Am. Anim. Hosp. Assoc. 30:59, 1994.

153. Jabara, A.G., Paton, J.S.: Extraskeletal osteoma in a cat. Aust. Vet. J. 61:405, 1984.

154. Kipnis, R.M., Conroy, J.D.: Canine extraskeletal osteosarcoma. Canine Pract. 17(1):34, 1992.

Chondroma and Chondrosarcoma

154a. Popovitch, C.A., et al.: Chondrosarcoma: a retrospective study of 97 dogs (1987–1990). J. Am. Anim. Hosp. Assoc. 30:81, 1994.

Undifferentiated Sarcomas

155. Carpenter, J.L., et al.: Distinctive unclassified mesenchymal tumor of the digit of dogs. Vet. Pathol. 28:396, 1991.

Mast Cell Tumor

155a. Ayl, R.D., et al.: Correlation of DNA ploidy to tumor histologic grade, clinical variables, and survival in dogs with mast cell tumors. Vet. Pathol. 29:386, 1992.

156. Bookbinder, P.F., et al.: Determination of the number of mast cells in lymph node, bone marrow, and buffy coat cytologic specimens from dogs. J. Am. Vet. Med. Assoc. 200:1648, 1992.

157. Bostock, D.E.: The prognosis following surgical removal of mastocytomas in dogs. J. Small Anim Pract. 14:27, 1973.

158. Brown, C.A., Chalmers, S.A.: Diffuse cutaneous mastocytosis in a cat. Vet. Pathol. 27:366, 1990.

159. Buerger, R.G., Scott, D.W.: Cutaneous mast cell neoplasia in the cat: 14 cases (1975–1985). J. Am. Vet. Med. Assoc. 190:1440, 1987.

160. Cayatte, S.M., et al.: Identification of mast cells in buffy coat preparations from dogs with inflammatory skin diseases. J. Am. Vet. Med. Assoc. (Accepted 1994).
161. Chastain, C.B., et al.: Benign cutaneous mastocytomas in two litters of Siamese kittens. J. Am. Vet. Med. Assoc. 193:959, 1988.
161a. Cole, W.: Mast cell tumor in a puppy. Can. Vet. J. 31:457, 1990.
161b. Davis, B.J., et al.: Cutaneous mastocytosis in a dog. Vet. Pathol. 29:363, 1992.
162. Fox, L.E., et al.: Plasma histamine and gastrin concentrations in 17 dogs with mast cell tumors. J. Vet. Intern. Med. 4:242, 1990.
163. Hottendorf, G.H., Nielsen, S.W.: Pathologic survey of 300 extirpated canine mastocytomas. Zentralbl. Veterinarmed [A]14:272, 1967.
163a. Jeromin, A.M., et al.: Urticaria pigmentosa–like disease in the dog. J. Am. Anim. Hosp. Assoc. 29:508, 1993.
163b. Legoretta, R.A., et al.: Use of hyperthermia and radiotherapy in treatment of a large mast cell sarcoma in a dog. J. Am. Vet. Med. Assoc. 193:1545, 1988.
164. Patnaik, A.K., et al.: Canine cutaneous mast cell tumor: Morphologic grading and survival time in 83 dogs. Vet. Pathol. 21:469, 1984.
165. Peterson, S.L.: Scar-associated canine mast cell tumor. Canine Pract. 12(2):23, 1985.
166. Thiel, W.: Mastzellentumoren bei Hunden-Auswertung pathologisch-histologischer Untersuchungsbefunde der Jahre 1980 bis 1986 mit Hinweis auf die TNM-Klassi fizierung von Tumoren bei Haustieren. Kleintier-Prax. 35:401, 1990.
167. Tinsley, P.E., Taylor, D.O.: Immunotherapy for multicentric malignant mastocytoma in a dog. Mod. Vet. Pract. 68:225, 1987.
168. Turrel, J.M., et al.: Prognostic factors for radiation treatment of mast cell tumors in 85 dogs. J. Am. Vet. Med. Assoc. 193:936, 1988.
169. Wilcock, B.P., et al.: The morphology and behavior of feline cutaneous mastocytomas. Vet. Pathol. 23:320, 1986.

Lymphoma
170. Baker, J.L., Scott, D.W.: Mycosis fungoides in two cats. J. Am. Anim. Hosp. Assoc. 25:97, 1989.
171. Beale, K.M., et al.: An unusual presentation of cutaneous lymphoma in two dogs. J. Am. Anim. Hosp. Assoc. 26:429, 1990.
172. Beale, K.M., Bolon, B.: Canine cutaneous lymphosarcoma: Epitheliotropic and non-epitheliotropic, a retrospective study. In: Ihrke, P.J., et al. (eds.). Advances in Veterinary Dermatology II. Pergamon Press, New York, 1993, p. 273.
173. Brain, P.H., Howlett, C.R.: Two cases of epidermotropic lymphoma in dogs. Aust. Vet. J. 68:247, 1991.
174. Buchet, B., et al.: Le lymphome malin du chien à la consultation de cancérologie de l'école nationale vétérinaire du Toulouse: Étude anatomoclinique. Prat. Méd. Chirurg. Anim. Cie. 24:233, 1989.
174a. Caciolo, P.L., et al.: Cutaneous lymphosarcoma in the cat: A report of nine cases. J. Am. Anim. Hosp. Assoc. 20:505, 1984.
175. Charpentier, F.R., et al.: Lymphome cutané épidermotrope chez un chien. Place nosologique. Essai de traitement. Prat. Méd. Chirurg. Anim. Cie. 23:321, 1988.
176. DeBoer, D.J., et al.: Mycosis fungoides in a dog: Demonstration of T-cell specificity and response to radiotherapy. J. Am. Anim. Hosp. Assoc. 26:566, 1990.
177. de Couliboeuf, F.: Cas clinique évoquant le mycosis fungoïde: Tentative de traitement par l'adriamycine et la prednisolone. Point Vét. 22:789, 1991.
177a. Ferrer, L., et al.: Detection of T lymphocytes in canine tissue embedded in paraffin wax by means of antibody to CD3 antigen. J. Comp. Pathol. 106:311, 1992.
178. Hewicker, M., et al.: Epidermotropes Lymphosarkom (Mycosis fungoides) bei einem Hund. Tierarztl. Prax. 18:633, 1990.
179. Holloway, K.B., et al.: Therapeutic alternatives in cutaneous T-cell lymphoma. J. Am. Acad. Dermatol. 27:367, 1992.
179a. Madewell, B.R., et al.: Cutaneous mastocytosis and mucinosis with gross deformity in a Shar pei dog. Vet. Dermatol. 3:171, 1992.
180. Miller, W.H., Jr.: Canine cutaneous lymphomas. In: Kirk, R.W. (ed.). Current Veterinary Therapy VII. W.B. Saunders Co., Philadelphia, 1980, p. 493.
181. Moriello, K.A., et al.: Peg L-asparaginase in the treatment of canine epitheliotropic lymphoma and histiocytic proliferative dermatitis. In: Ihrke, P.J., et al. (eds.). Advances in Veterinary Dermatology II. Pergamon Press, New York, 1993, p. 293.
182. Plant, J.D.: Would you have diagnosed cutaneous epitheliotropic lymphoma in these two cats? Vet. Med. 86:801, 1991.
183. Rosenthal, R.C., MacEwen, E.G.: Treatment of lymphoma in dogs. J. Am. Vet. Med. Assoc. 196:774, 1990.
183a. Schick, R.O., et al.: Cutaneous lymphosarcoma and leukemia in a cat. J. Am. Vet. Med. Assoc. 203:1155, 1993.
183b. Scott, D.W.: Lichenoid reactions in the skin of dogs: Clinicopathologic correlations. J. Am. Anim. Hosp. Assoc. 20:305, 1984.
183c. Shitaka, H., et al.: [Malignant lymphoma with skin lesions in a dog]. J. Jpn. Vet. Med. Assoc. 45:683, 1992.
184. Stoeckli, R., et al.: Canine epidermotropic lymphoma associated with the intercellular deposition of immunoglobulin on direct immunofluorescence testing. Companion Anim. Pract. 1(2):36, 1988.
185. Thrall, M.A., et al.: Cutaneous lymphosarcoma and leukemia in a dog, resembling Sézary syndrome in man. Vet. Pathol. 21:182, 1984.
185a. Tobey, J.C., et al.: Cutaneous T-cell lymphoma in a cat. J. Am. Vet. Med. Assoc. 204:606, 1994.
186. Tusjimoto, H., et al.: T-cell lymphoma in a dog with cutaneous lesions. Jpn. J. Vet. Sci. 45:543, 1983.

187. Walton, D.K.: Canine epidermotropic lymphoma (mycosis fungoides and pagetoid reticulosis). In: Kirk, R.W. (ed). Current Veterinary Therapy IX. W.B. Saunders Co., Philadelphia, 1986, p. 609.
188. Wellman, M.L., et al.: Lymphoma involving large granular lymphocytes in cats: 11 cases (1982–1991). J. Am. Vet. Med. Assoc. 201:1265, 1992.
188a. White, S.D., et al.: Use of isotretinoin and etretinate for the treatment of benign cutaneous neoplasia and cutaneous lymphoma in dogs. J. Am. Vet. Med. Assoc. 202:387, 1993.
189. Wilcock, B.P, Yager, J.A.: The behavior of epidermotropic lymphoma in 25 dogs. Can. Vet. J. 30:754, 1989.

Pseudolymphoma

190. Cerio, R., MacDonald, D.M.: Benign cutaneous lymphoid infiltrates. J. Cutan. Pathol. 12:442, 1985.
191. Miller, W.H., Jr., et al.: A spontaneously regressing pseudolymphoma in a dog resembling pseudo-Hodgkin's disease. Vet. Dermatol. 1:171, 1990.

Histiocytoma

191a. Moore, P.F., Schrenzel, M.D.: Canine cutaneous histiocytoma represents a Langerhans cell proliferative disorder based on immunophenotypic analysis. Proc. Am. Coll. Vet. Pathol. 42:119, 1991.
191b. Howard, E.B., Nielsen, S.W.: Cutaneous histiocytomas of dogs. Natl. Cancer Inst. Monogr. 32:321, 1969.

Cutaneous Histiocytosis

191c. Collins, B.K., et al.: Idiopathic granulomatous disease with occular adnexal and cutaneous involvement in a dog. J. Am. Vet. Med. Assoc. 201:313, 1992.
192. Mays, M.B.C., Bergeron, J.A.: Cutaneous histiocytosis in dogs. J. Am. Vet. Med. Assoc. 188:377, 1986.
193. Scott, D.W.: Canine cutaneous histiocytoses. In: Kirk, R.W. (ed.). Current Veterinary Therapy X. W.B. Saunders Co., Philadelphia, 1989, p. 625.
194. Thornton, R.N., Tisdall, C.J.: Multiple cutaneous histiocytosis in two dogs. N. Z. Vet. J. 36:192, 1988.

Systemic Histiocytosis

195. Moore, P.F.: Systemic histiocytosis of Bernese Mountain dogs. Vet. Pathol. 21:554, 1984.
195a. Moore, P.F.: Utilization of cytoplasmic lysozyme immunoreactivity as a histiocytic marker in canine histiocytic disorders. Vet. Pathol. 23:757, 1986.
196. Scherlie, P.H., Jr., et al.: Ocular manifestation of systemic histiocytosis in a dog. J. Am. Vet. Med. Assoc. 201:1229, 1992.
197. Scott, D.W., et al.: Systemic histiocytosis in two dogs. Canine Pract. 14(1):7, 1987.
197a. Hayden, D.W., et al.: Disseminated malignant histiocytosis in a Golden retriever: Clinicopathologic, ultrastructural, and immunohistochemical findings. Vet. Pathol. 30:256, 1993.

Malignant Histiocytosis

198. Moore, P.F., Rosin, A.: Malignant histiocytosis of Bernese Mountain dogs. Vet. Pathol. 23:1, 1986.
199. Scott, D.W., et al.: Lymphoreticular neoplasia in a dog resembling malignant histiocytosis (histiocytic medullary reticulosis) in man. Cornell Vet. 69:176, 1979.

Benign Fibrous Histiocytoma

200. Paulsen, M.E., et al.: Nodular granulomatous episclerokeratitis in dogs: 19 cases (1973–1985). J. Am. Vet. Med. Assoc. 190:1581, 1987.
201. Smith, J.S., et al.: Infiltrative corneal lesions resembling fibrous histiocytoma: Clinical and pathologic findings in six dogs and one cat. J. Am. Vet. Med. Assoc. 169:722, 1976.

Malignant Fibrous Histiocytoma

202. Gibson, K.L., et al.: Malignant fibrous histiocytoma in a cat. J. Am. Vet. Med. Assoc. 194:1443, 1989.
203. Legrand, J.J., et al.: Histiocytome fibreux malin chez un chat. Etude d'un cas clinique et comparison avec les données de la littérature. Prat. Méd. Chirurg. Anim. Cie. 22:401, 1987.
204. Thomas, J.B.: Malignant fibrous histiocytoma in a dog. Aust. Vet. J. 65:252, 1988.
204a. Thoolen, R.J.M.M., et al.: Malignant fibrous histiocytomas in dogs and cats: An immunohistochemical study. Res. Vet. Sci. 53:198, 1992.

Plasmacytoma

205. Baer, K.E., et al.: Cutaneous plasmacytomas in dogs: A morphologic and immunohistochemical study. Vet. Pathol. 26:216, 1989.
205a. Brunnert, S.R., Altman, N.H.: Identification of immunoglobulin light chains in canine extramedullary plasmacytomas by thioflavine T and immunohistochemistry. J. Vet. Diagn. Invest. 3:245, 1991.
206. Clark, G.N., et al.: Extramedullary plasmacytomas in dogs: Results of surgical excision in 131 cases. J. Am. Anim. Hosp. Assoc. 28:105, 1992.
206a. Frazier, K.S.: Analysis of DNA aneuploidy and C-myc oncoprotein content of canine plasma cell tumors using flow cytometry. Vet. Pathol. 30:505, 1993.
207. Kyriazidou, A., et al.: An immunohistochemical study of canine extramedullary plasma cell tumours. J. Comp. Pathol. 100:259, 1989.
208. Kyriazidou, A., et al.: Immunohistochemical staining with neoplastic and inflammatory plasma cell lesions in feline tissues. J. Comp. Pathol. 100:337, 1989.
209. Rakich, P.M., et al.: Mucocutaneous plasmacytomas in dogs: 75 cases (1980–1987). J. Am. Vet. Med. Assoc. 194:803, 1989.
210. Rowland, P.H., et al.: Cutaneous plasmacytomas with amyloid in six dogs. Vet. Pathol. 28:125, 1991.

Melanocytic Tumors

211. Anderson, W.I., et al.: Pilar neurocristic melanoma in four dogs. Vet. Rec. 123:517, 1988.
212. Bolon, B., et al.: Characteristics of canine melanomas and comparison of histology and DNA ploidy to their biologic behavior. Vet. Pathol. 27:96, 1990.
213. Bostock, D.E.: Prognosis after surgical excision of canine melanomas. Vet. Pathol. 16:32, 1979.
214. Diters, R.W., Walsh, K.M.: Cutaneous clear cell melanomas: A report of three cases. Vet. Pathol. 21:355, 1983.
215. Frese, K.: Verlaufsuntersuchungen beim Melanomen der Haut und der Mundschleimhaut des Hundes. Vet. Pathol. 15:461, 1978.
215a. Goldschmidt, M.H., et al.: Feline dermal melanoma: A retrospective study. In: Ihrke, P.J., et al. (eds.). Advances in Veterinary Dermatology II. Pergamon Press, New York, 1993, p. 285.
216. Harvey, H.J., et al.: Prognostic criteria for dogs with oral melanoma. J. Am. Vet. Med. Assoc. 178:580, 1981.
217. Miller, W.H., Jr., et al.: Feline cutaneous melanocytic neoplasms: A retrospective analysis of 43 cases (1979–1991). Vet. Dermatol. 4:19, 1993.

Neuroendocrine Tumor

218. Glick, A.D., et al.: Neuroendocrine carcinoma of the skin in a dog. Vet. Pathol. 20:761, 1983.
219. Nickoloff, B.J., et al.: Canine neuroendocrine carcinoma. A tumor resembling histiocytoma. Am. J. Dermatopathol. 7:579, 1985.
220. Whiteley, L.O., Leiningen, J.R.: Neuroendocrine (Merkel) cell tumors of the canine oral cavity. Vet. Pathol. 24:570, 1987.

Transmissible Venereal Tumor

221. Amber, E.I., et al.: Single-drug chemotherapy of canine transmissible venereal tumor with cyclophosphamide, methotrexate, or vincristine. J. Vet. Intern. Med. 4:144, 1990.
221a. Das, A.K., et al.: A clinical report on the efficacy of vincristine on canine transmissible venereal sarcoma. Indian Vet. J. 68:575, 1991.
222. Kavisin, A.G., Mann, F.C.: The transmissible venereal tumor of dogs. Observations on 40 generations of experimental transfers. Ann. N. Y. Acad. Sci. 54:1197, 1952.
223. Laging, C., Kroning, T.: Beobachtungen zum Ubertragbaren Venerischen Tumor (Sticker) beim Hund. Tierarztl. Prax. 17:85, 1989.
224. Mizuno, S., et al.: Role of lymphocytes in dogs experimentally re-challenged with canine transmissible sarcoma. Jpn. J. Vet. Sci. 51:86, 1989.
224a. Nandi, S.N., et al.: Incidence and histopathological observations on venereal lymphosarcoma in dogs in Calcutta area. Indian Vet. Med. J. 8:124, 1984.
224b. Nandi, S.N., et al.: Effect of ovariectomy on regression of transmissible venereal tumour in bitches. Indian J. Vet. Pathol. 12:97, 1988.
224c. Panchbhai, V.S., et al.: Use of autogenous vaccine in transmissible canine venereal tumour. Indian Vet. J. 67:983, 1990.
225. Vermooten, M.I.: Canine transmissible venereal tumour (TVT): A review. J. S. Afr. Vet. Assoc. 58:147, 1987.

Epithelioid Sarcoma

225a. Estrada, M.M., et al.: Epithelioid sarcoma in a dog. J. Comp. Pathol. 107:107, 1992.

Secondary Skin Neoplasms

226. Anderson, W.I., et al.: Presumptive subcutaneous surgical transplantation of a urinary bladder transitional cell carcinoma in a dog. Cornell Vet. 79:263, 1989.
227. Bonnard, P., Dralez, F.: A propos d'un cas de thymome chez un chat. Point Vét. 23:1089, 1993.
228. Carpenter, J.L., Holzworth, J.: Thymoma in 11 cats. J. Am. Vet. Med. Assoc. 181:248, 1982.
229. Couto, C.G., Sousa, C.: Chronic lymphocytic leukemia with cutaneous involvement in a dog. J. Am. Vet. Med. Assoc. 22:374, 1986.
230. Crowe, D.T., Todoroff, R.J.: Umbilical masses and discolorations as signs of intraabdominal disease. J. Am. Anim. Hosp. Assoc. 18:295, 1982.
230a. Estrada, M., Lagadic, M.: Métastases digitales d'un carcinome pulmonaire asymptomatique chez le chat. Etude d'une série de 11 cas. Prat. Méd. Chirurg. Anim. Cie. 27:791, 1992.
231. Gilson, S.D., Stone, E.A.: Surgically induced tumor seeding in eight dogs and two cats. J. Am. Vet. Med. Assoc. 196:1811, 1990.
232. Hampson, E.C.G.M., et al.: Cutaneous metastasis of a colonic carcinoma in a dog. J. Small Animal Pract. 31:155, 1990.
233. Leifer, C.E., Matus, R.E.: Chronic lymphocytic leukemia in the dog: 22 cases (1974–1984). J. Am. Vet. Med. Assoc. 189:214, 1986.
234. Scott-Moncrief, J.E., et al.: Pulmonary squamous cell carcinoma with multiple digital metastases in a cat. J. Small Anim. Pract. 30:696, 1989.
235. Susaneck, S.J., et al.: Inflammatory mammary carcinoma in the dog. J. Am. Anim. Hosp. Assoc. 19:971, 1983.
236. White, S.D., et al.: Cutaneous metastases of a mammary adenocarcinoma resembling eosinophilic plaques in a cat. Feline Pract. 15(1):27, 1985.

Cysts

237. Clark, D.M., et al.: Branchial cyst in a dog. J. Am. Vet. Med. Assoc. 194:67, 1989.
238. Davidson, H.J., Blanchard, G.L.: Periorbital epidermal cyst in the medial canthus of three dogs. J. Am. Vet. Med. Assoc. 198:271, 1991.

239. Fezer, G., Weiss, E.: Die zystischen Bildungen in der Haut der Haustiere. Arch. Exp. Vetinarmed. 23:60, 1969.
240. Joffe, D.J.: Branchial cyst in a cat. Can. Vet. J. 31:525, 1990.
241. Mann, G.E., Stratton, J.: Dermoid sinus in the Rhodesian Ridgeback. J. Small Anim. Pract. 7:631, 1966.
242. Scott, D.W., Anderson, W.I.: Cutaneous trichilemmal cysts in three dogs. Cornell Vet. 81:245, 1991.
243. Scott, D.W., Anderson, W.I.: Cutaneous hybrid cyst in four dogs. Cornell Vet. 81:19, 1991.
244. Selcer, E.A., et al.: Dermoid sinus in a Shih tzu and a boxer. J. Am. Anim. Hosp. Assoc. 20:634, 1984.

Nevi

245. Aronsohn, M.G., Carpenter, J.L.: Distal extremity melanocytic nevi and malignant melanomas in dogs. J. Am. Anim. Hosp. Assoc. 26:605, 1990.
246. Atlee, B.A., et al.: Nodular dermatofibrosis in German shepherd dogs as a marker for renal cystadenocarcinoma. J. Am. Anim. Hosp. Assoc. 27:481, 1991.
246a. de Geyer, G.: Dermatologie des paupières du chien et du chat. Première partie: Étude générale. Prat. Méd. Chirurg. Anim. Cie. 28:605, 1993.
247. Gilbert, P.A., et al.: Nodular dermatofibrosis and renal cystadenoma in a German shepherd dog. J. Am. Anim. Hosp. Assoc. 26:253, 1990.
248. Jones, B.R., et al.: Cutaneous collagen nodules in a dog. J. Small Anim. Pract. 26:445, 1985.
249. Kraft, I., Frese, K.: Histological studies on canine pigmented moles. J. Comp. Pathol. 86:143, 1976.
249a. Mays, M.B.C., et al.: Regional collagenous nevi in three dogs: Nevus, nodular dermatofibrosis, or something new? In: Ihrke, P.J., et al. (eds.). Advances in Veterinary Dermatology II. Pergamon Press, New York, 1993, p. 315.
250. Paradis, M., Scott, D.W.: Naevi récemment reconnus chez le chien: Naevus comédonien, naevus organoïde linéaire et naevus du follicule pileux. Point. Vét. 21:489, 1989.
251. Roudebush, P., MacDonald, J.M.: Mucocutaneous angiomatous hamartoma in a dog. J. Am. Anim. Hosp. Assoc. 20:168, 1984.
252. Scott, D.W., et al.: Nevi in the dog. J. Am. Anim. Hosp. Assoc. 20:505, 1984.
253. Walder, E.J., Gross, T.L.: Focal adnexal dysplasia (folliculo-sebaceous hamartoma). In: Ihrke, P.J., et al. (eds.). Advances in Veterinary Dermatology II. Pergamon Press, New York, 1993, p. 311.
254. Weipers, W.L., Jarrett, W.F.H.: Haemangioma of the scrotum of dogs. Vet. Rec. 66:106, 1954.
254a. White, S.D., et al.: Inflammatory linear verrucous epidermal nevus in four dogs. Vet. Dermatol. 3:107, 1993.

Keratoses

255. Anderson, W.I., et al.: Idiopathic benign lichenoid keratosis in the pinna of the ear in four dogs. Cornell Vet. 79:179, 1989.
256. Goldschmidt, M.H., Kunkle, G.: Inverted follicular keratosis in a dog. Vet. Pathol. 16:374, 1979.

Mucinosis

257. Dillberger, J.E., Altman, N.H.: Focal mucinosis in dogs: Seven cases and a review of cutaneous mucinoses of man and animals. Vet. Pathol. 23:132, 1986.

Calcinosis Circumscripta

258. Anderson, W.I., Scott, D.W.: Calcinosis circumscripta in a domestic short-haired cat. Cornell Vet. 77:348, 1987.
259. Berrocal, A., et al.: Calcinosis circumscripta in two cats. Feline Pract. 20(3):9, 1992.
260. Bohmer, E., et al.: Calcinosis cutis der Ballen bei einer Katze. Tierarztl. Prax. 19:88, 1991.
261. Ginel, P., et al.: Calcinosis circumscripta associated with medroxyprogesterone in two Poodle bitches. J. Am. Anim. Hosp. Assoc. 28:391, 1992.
262. Kirby, B.M., et al.: Calcinosis circumscripta associated with polydioxanone sutures in two young dogs. Vet. Surg. 18:216, 1989.
263. Lewis, D.G., Kelly, D.F.: Calcinosis circumscripta in dogs as a cause of spinal ataxia. J. Small Anim. Pract. 31:36, 1990.
264. Scott, D.W., Buerger, R.G.: Idiopathic calcinosis circumscripta in the dog: A retrospective analysis of 130 cases. J. Am. Anim. Hosp. Assoc. 24:651, 1988.
265. Stampley, A., Bellah, J.R.: Calcinosis circumscripta of the metacarpal pad in a young dog. J. Am. Vet. Med. Assoc. 196:113, 1990.

Dermatoses of Pet Rodents, Rabbits, and Ferrets

■

Chapter Outline

Owner complaints relative to skin problems in pet rodents, rabbits, and ferrets are commonly encountered in small animal practice.* Although much has been written about the dermatoses of the commonly kept exotic mammals, the material is often anecdotal or difficult to interpret. In particular, therapeutics in exotic animals is controversial because few of the drugs commonly used are approved for use in these species. In addition, because most treatments have evolved through a hit-and-miss approach,[3] there are great discrepancies in the literature concerning what drugs to use and at what dose to administer them.

Special caution is indicated with the use of antibiotics, as death due to direct toxic effects or alteration of the normal bacterial flora is common.[2–5, 12, 17] Especially in the guinea pig, antibiotics that specifically affect gram-positive organisms are contraindicated, and broad-spectrum antibiotics should be used.[106]

One drug that is commonly used in these species and that appears to be safe and effective in all ages is ivermectin.† The standard dose is 300 μg/kg given subcutaneously and repeated every 2 weeks until the disorder being treated is cured.

Special precautions must also be observed when using topical medications. First, these animals routinely remove topical agents through their grooming behaviors. Second, these small creatures are prone to hypothermia after shampooing and dipping. Thus, aqueous solutions should be kept at body temperature, and the animals must be kept warm and dry and away from drafts after treatment.

The structure and function of small exotic mammal skin are similar to those described in Chapter 1.‡ Hair growth in rodents (not guinea pigs) and rabbits occurs in periodic orderly waves originating on the ventrum between the front legs and spreading dorsally and caudally.§ In some rabbits, thickened patches of skin can be associated with the variation in hair growth cycles.[260] This is more common in young rabbits and becomes less obvious with increasing age. The mean thickness in these patches is 2 mm as compared with 1 mm in normal skin. Histologic examination of the patches reveals increased size of hair follicles and increased vascularity. Notable histologic differences include (1) the absence of apocrine sweat glands in rodents[2, 30] and (2) the structure of the tail epithelium of the mouse and rat, which features orthokeratosis with a stratum granulosum at the follicular osia and parakeratosis without a stratum granulosum in the interfollicular areas.[172, 192]

Hamsters have large glands on either flank, which are visible as dark brown patches that are more prominent in male animals.[2–5, 28, 33, 131] These flank or hip glands are sebaceous and are used for marking territory. In sexually aroused males, the haircoat over the glands becomes matted from secretions and readily visible, and the animals scratch the areas as if they were pruritic. These findings may be interpreted as signs of skin disease by some owners. Gerbils have a yellowish tan, midventral scent gland, which is also sebaceous, more prominent in male animals, and occasionally mistaken as a cutaneous abnormality.[2–5, 17, 33, 77b] Normal ferrets typically have visible accumulations of brownish cerumen around the external auditory meatus. In addition, normal ferrets can have several comedones on the tail.

Most rodents are burrowing animals that spend most of their time in the wild seeking food and escaping predators. When they are placed in sterile environments with ad libitum feeding and no danger of predators, they are left with little to do except to chew on themselves or on others. In addition, male rodents tend to be territorial and aggressive. Self-inflicted trauma or that inflicted on cagemates can be triggered or amplified by crowding.

---

*See references 3–5, 16, 18, 28, 31, 33, and 36.
†See references 3–5, 28, 33, 45, 60, 96, 113, and 228.
‡See references 30, 45, 77b, 87, 125, 140, 172, 231a, 233, 311, and 332.
§See references 2, 76a, 125, 131, 140, 144, 165, 179, 260, 297, and 315.

Some other normal behaviors may be misinterpreted as pruritus. A rabbit rubbing its mental, or chin, gland (which is sebaceous) on a cage or furniture is only marking its territory.[33] Likewise, a guinea pig scooting or dragging its perineal area on the ground is usually scent-marking, although in some male animals the glandular secretions can become impacted and cause irritation.[33] Male hamsters may clean and fuss with their flank glands.[33]

Staphylococci, especially *Staphylococcus aureus,* are frequently isolated from the skin, the ears, the nostrils, and the haircoat of rodents and rabbits.* Not surprisingly, *S. aureus* is a common opportunist and cause of skin infections in these species.

Finally, these small creatures, especially mice, rats, guinea pigs, and rabbits, are frequently used for studying models of human diseases (e.g., hereditary hypotrichoses and ichthyoses in mice and rats), for examining the pathogenesis of various dermatoses also seen in humans (e.g., contact hypersensitivity in guinea pigs and candidiasis in guinea pigs), for evaluating therapeutic agents used in various human dermatoses (e.g., treatment of *Malassezia* dermatitis in guinea pigs and the use of retinoids in rhino mice), for studying percutaneous absorption and various aspects of dermatopharmacology (e.g., the mouse tail assay for studying epidermal drug effects), and for screening the potential irritancy or sensitization of topical agents (e.g., the guinea pig Draize test for contact allergens and the rabbit skin test for topical irritants).[23a, 192, 229]

■ CHINCHILLA

In the wild, chinchillas keep their haircoats clean and healthy by bathing in fine volcanic dust.[39] A similar dust is commercially available (chinchilla dust, or Fuller's earth) and should be provided at least two or three times per week.[3, 36a] The dust is poured 5 to 10 cm deep in a metal pan and left in the animal's cage for about 30 minutes. Chinchillas deprived of their dust baths are prone to abnormalities of the haircoat and skin.

Fungal Infections

Dermatophytosis is uncommon in chinchillas.[3, 4, 37, 38] *Trichophyton mentagrophytes* is the most frequent cause, but *Microsporum gypseum* and *M. canis* are occasionally isolated. Lesions are most common around the eyes, the nares, and the mouth but may occur anywhere. Circumscribed areas of alopecia, broken hairs, and variable degrees of scaling, erythema, and crusting are seen. Secondary staphylococcal infection can occur and usually presents as cellulitis or abscess.[38]

Recommended therapy includes griseofulvin by mouth (50 mg/kg q24h) for 30 days and 15 to 30 ml of captan powder added to a clean dust bath once daily.[38, 39] This latter recommendation is suspect, as captan has been shown to be ineffective against *M. canis* (see Chap. 5).

Fur Chewing

Chinchillas may chew, pull out, and eat their fur during times of stress (gestation, travel, and shows), in the absence of dust baths and for unknown reasons.[3, 36a, 38, 39] When the fur chewing is idiopathic, it rarely ceases. It is believed that the idiopathic condition is a heritable trait, that no therapy is effective, and that the condition is best controlled by culling and selective breeding.[38, 39] Providing fresh alfalfa hay, giving proper chinchilla pellets, and reducing stress may help.

Fur-Slip

Fur-slip is a normal physiologic process whereby chinchillas appear to ''squirt'' or ''shoot'' some of their fur out.[38] This is a mechanism of self-defense, in which the chinchilla hopes to

---

*See references 2, 3, 5, 9, 12, 17, 18, 27, 28, 31, 33, 36, 74, 99, 116, 125, 131, 163, 252, 284, and 304.

leave a predator with a mouthful of fur as it escapes. Fur-slip is likely to occur when chinchillas are frightened or handled roughly. Chinchilla fur grows in tufts with up to 90 fibers per follicle and up to 1000 follicles/cm.[2, 38] Fur-slip affects spots 2 to 5 cm in diameter. Fur regrowth occurs within 3 months for some follicles and usually takes 5 months for an entire spot. However, regrowth is rarely a perfect fit and always looks patched.

Nutritional Disorders

Fatty acid deficiency results in generalized scaling, poor haircoat, reduced hair growth, and perhaps cutaneous ulcers in the chinchilla.[2, 36a]

Zinc deficiency may produce alopecia.[36a]

■ FERRET

Bacterial Infections

Bacterial skin infections are uncommon in the ferret and are usually caused by *S. aureus* or *Streptococcus* spp.* Infections are usually secondary to bite wounds (especially on the neck of female ferrets during breeding season, perpetrated by aggressive male animals as a prelude to coitus) or the pruritus associated with ectoparasites. There may be superficial and follicular lesions or deep abscesses and fistulae. Staphylococcal or streptococcal cellulitis of the neck may be associated with dental disease and mandibular osteomyelitis.[45] Diagnosis is based on cytologic examination. Treatment consists of a regimen of various combinations of topical antimicrobials (3 per cent hydrogen peroxide or 0.5 to 1 per cent chlorhexidine), surgical drainage, and the administration of systemic antibiotics (Table 20:1).

Actinomycosis ("lumpy jaw") is rarely reported in ferrets.[45, 69] Affected animals have nodules or abscesses in the neck, and fistulae and discharge of thick green-yellow pus may be seen.

Fungal Infections

Dermatophytosis appears to be rare in ferrets.† *M. canis* and *T. mentagrophytes* are the most common causes, and young animals are most frequently affected. Lesions consist of annular

---

*See references 4, 5, 12, 41, 43, 45, and 66.
†See references 3, 5, 12, 41, 43, 45, 60, 64, and 66.

Table 20:1. Common Therapeutic Agents in Small Mammals

Agent	Protocol
Antibiotics	
Ampicillin	5–10 mg/kg IM or PO q12h for 5–7 d (ferret, mouse, rat)
Cephaloridine	10–25 mg/kg IM or SC q24h for 5–7 d
Chloramphenicol succinate	30 mg/kg IM or SC q24h for 5–7 d
Chloramphenicol palmitate	50 mg/kg PO q12h for 5–7 d
Enrofloxacin	2.5 mg/kg PO q12h for 5–7 d
Gentamicin	5 mg/kg IM or SC q24h for 5 d
Sulfadiazine-trimethoprim	30 mg/kg SC q24h for 5–7 d
Sulfamethoxazole-trimethoprim	15 mg/kg PO q12h for 5–7 d
Tetracycline hydrochloride	20 mg/kg SC/PO q12h for 5–7 d
Antifungals	
Griseofulvin	25–50 mg/kg PO q24h for 4–6 wk
Antiparasitics	
Amitraz 250 ppm	Total body dip q2wk
Ivermectin	0.3 mg/kg SC q2wk
Lime sulfur 2%	Total body dip q7d

IM, intramuscularly; PO, orally; SC, subcutaneously.

areas of alopecia, broken hairs, scale, and varying degrees of erythema and crusting. Pruritus is usually absent. Diagnosis is confirmed by microscopic examination of affected hairs and fungal culture. Therapy consists of topical application of antifungal agents and environmental clean-up as described for cats. Griseofulvin is usually not needed. Dermatophytosis in ferrets is a potential zoonosis.

Blastomycosis was diagnosed in a ferret with chronic cutaneous plaques and ulcers.[55]

Histoplasmosis was diagnosed in a ferret with multiple subcutaneous nodules.[41]

Ectoparasites

Otodectic mange (ear mites) is common in ferrets.* Affected ferrets may manifest no clinical signs or variable degrees of excessive cerumen production. Pruritus, inflammation, and secondary bacterial infection are uncommon. Diagnosis is confirmed by finding *Otodectes cynotis* in ear swabs. Treatment is accomplished with topical acaricides or injectable ivermectin as described for cats. Ivermectin should be used with caution in pregnant jills.[43, 45] When ivermectin was administered at 2 to 4 weeks of gestation, an increased incidence of congenital defects, such as cleft palates, was seen. However, when ivermectin was administered after 4 weeks of gestation, no problems were noted.

Fleas (especially *Ctenocephalides felis felis*) are commonly found on ferrets.* Animals may be asymptomatic or have cutaneous reaction patterns similar to flea bite hypersensitivity in cats. Ferrets manifesting presumed flea bite hypersensitivity have a pruritic papulocrustous dermatitis over the rump, ventral abdomen, and caudomedial thighs, or a self-induced, symmetric alopecia over the rump, flanks, ventral abdomen, or medial thighs (fur-mowing) in which the skin appears normal. Treatment strategies must include the ferret; in-contact ferrets, cats, and dogs; and the environment, as described for cats.

Sarcoptic mange is uncommon in ferrets and has two clinical presentations: (1) intense pruritus and dermatitis over the face, the pinnae (Fig. 20:1 *A*), and the ventrum and (2) pruritic pododermatitis.† In the pododermatitis form, the feet are swollen, erythematous, and crusted, and the claws may be dystrophic. Affected ferrets may actually slough claws or digits. Diagnosis is confirmed by finding *Sarcoptes scabiei* mites in skin scrapings. However, mites can be extremely difficult to find, so response to miticidal therapy is often used as a diagnostic procedure. Treatment includes 2 per cent lime sulfur dips (weekly until 2 weeks after clinical cure) or ivermectin injections.

Ferrets housed outdoors may occasionally have cysts, abscesses, or fistulae in the neck associated with infestation by *Hypoderma* sp. or *Cuterebra* sp. larvae.[4, 41, 45] Treatment includes careful surgical removal of the larva and routine wound care.

Ticks may occasionally be found on ferrets, especially around the head and the ears.[43, 45] Treatment is as described for cats.

Ferrets can be experimentally infected with *Dracunculus insignis* and have been used as an animal model for studying dracunculiasis.[41a, 44a] Lesions consist of tender swellings, which abscess and develop fistulae. Lesions occur most commonly on the legs.

Viral Infections

The ferret is susceptible to canine distemper virus.[3, 5, 41, 43, 45, 63b] Typical cutaneous findings include an erythematous rash under the chin and in the inguinal region; brownish crusts on the chin, the nose, and the periocular area; and swollen, hyperkeratotic nose and footpads.

---

*See references 3–5, 33, 41, 43, 45, 58, 60, 63b, and 64.

†See references 3–5, 33, 41, 43, 45, 60, 63b, and 64.

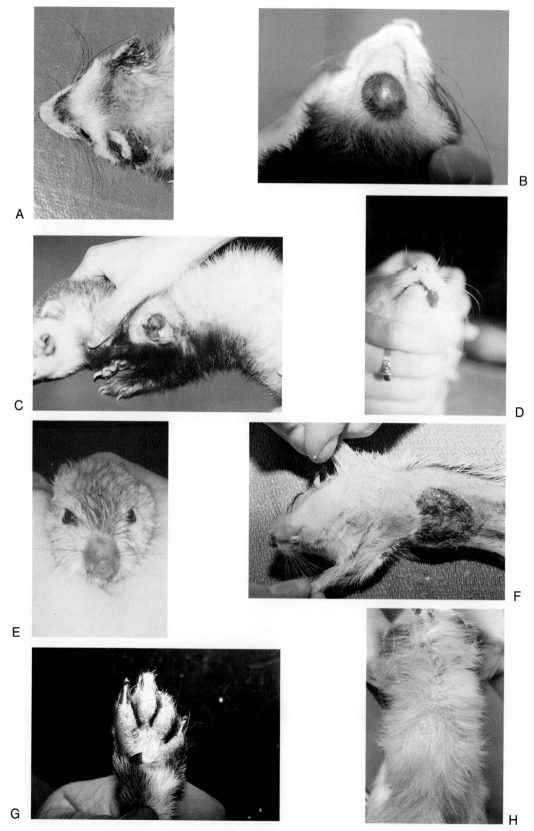

Figure 20:1 *See legend on opposite page*

Endocrine Disorders

ALOPECIA ASSOCIATED WITH ADRENOCORTICAL NEOPLASIA

Adrenocortical neoplasia is the most common cause of progressive bilaterally symmetric alopecia in the ferret.* The condition was previously diagnosed as hyperadrenocorticism or Cushing's syndrome. However, other classic clinical signs (polyuria, polydipsia, and polyphagia) and hematologic, biochemical, or urologic abnormalities associated with hyperadrenocorticism are rarely present. In addition, basal plasma cortisol levels are usually within the normal range,† and published adrenal function tests[47, 49, 51, 63, 63a] have not been useful in separating normal from diseased ferrets.[51] These considerations in concert with the common occurrence of vulvar enlargement in affected female ferrets suggest that the endocrine abnormality is in the adrenocortical production of sex hormones.[51, 67] Indeed, about 40 per cent of affected ferrets have elevated serum estradiol concentrations.[55a, 63a]

Clinical signs are usually seen between 2 and 5 years of age and most frequently in female ferrets. In most cases, clinical signs are first noted in the spring. The initial abnormality is a bilaterally symmetric, noninflammatory alopecia that usually begins on the tail and tail base (Fig. 20:3) and progresses to the ventral abdomen, caudomedial thighs, and lumbosacral region. In some animals, the alopecia may come and go. In such cases, clinical signs appear in the spring and spontaneously regress in the autumn. However, clinical signs recur with increasing severity each spring and eventually persist.[55a, 63a] Vulvar enlargement is common in female animals (Fig. 20:2). In more chronic cases, the back of the neck, top of the head (Fig. 20:4) and trunk become alopecic, and the body skin becomes thin and hypotonic (Fig. 20:5). Some animals are reported to be pruritic. Numerous comedones are occasionally found on the tail, and phlebectasias are commonly seen. Mammary gland hyperplasia has been reported, and stump pyometras are not uncommon.[55a, 57] The enlarged adrenal gland can be palpated in about 30 per cent of cases.

Diagnosis is confirmed by ultrasonographic examination or exploratory laparotomy.[42, 51, 54, 54a, 63a, 67] The vast majority of animals have an adenoma of the left adrenal. Rarely, both adrenals may be neoplastic, or an animal has a neoplasm in the remaining adrenal gland several months after the surgical removal of the initially neoplastic adrenal.[42, 51, 63a] Vaginal cytologic examination reveals changes indicative of estrus.[55a] Anemia and thrombocytopenia are rare.[63a] In one case,[55a] adrenal adenoma cells were immunohistochemically positive for estradiol.

In most animals, the treatment of choice is unilateral adrenalectomy. Clinical improvement is evident within 6 to 8 weeks, and complete recovery is usually seen within 5 months. Medical treatment has been used when surgery could not be performed, or when, after surgical removal of a neoplastic adrenal, the remaining adrenal gland also became neoplastic and clinical signs recurred.[42, 51] Mitotane (o,p'-DDD) has been used successfully at 50 mg orally, once daily for 7 days, then every 3 days until clinical cure. Administration of the drug is then stopped. If clinical signs recur, o,p'-DDD is given at a weekly maintenance dose of 50 mg. To facilitate administration, the o,p'-DDD is mixed with corn starch and 50-mg doses are put in gelatin capsules. Ketoconazole has been ineffective when given orally at 15 mg/kg every 12 hours.

---

*See references 4, 42, 51, 52, 54, 55a, 57, 61, 63a, 63b, and 67.
†See references 42, 45, 47, 49, 51, 61, 63, and 67.

Figure 20:1. *A,* Alopecia, crusts, and excoriations on the pinnae of a ferret with sarcoptic mange. *B,* Mast cell tumor on the lower jaw of a ferret. *C,* Sebaceous epithelioma on the shoulder of a ferret. *D,* Squamous cell carcinoma on the lip of a ferret. (Courtesy W. Gould.) *E,* Alopecia, crusting, and ulceration on the nose of a gerbil with "sore nose." *F,* Squamous cell carcinoma of the ventral scent gland in a gerbil. (Courtesy W. Gould.) *G,* Staphylococcal pododermatitis in a guinea pig. (Courtesy J. King.) *H,* Alopecia and thick crusts over the dorsum in a guinea pig with trixacariasis. (Courtesy E. Guaguère.)

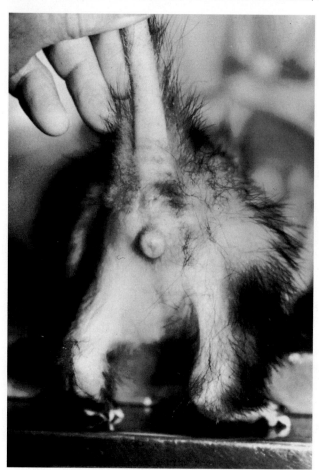

Figure 20:2. Symmetric alopecia and vulvar enlargement associated with an adrenal adenoma in a ferret (Courtesy W. Gould.)

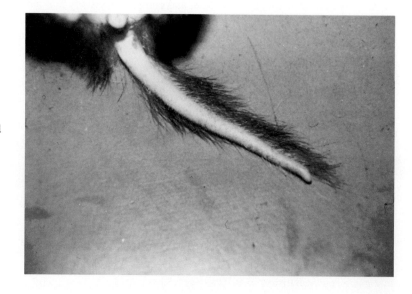

Figure 20:3. Alopecia of the tail in a ferret with an adrenal adenoma.

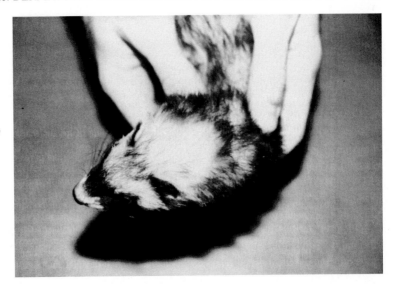

Figure 20:4. Alopecia over the top of the head of a ferret with an adrenal adenoma.

HYPERESTROGENISM

Hyperestrogenism is well recognized in the female ferret.* However, this disorder is currently rare because large-volume ferret breeders are neutering and descenting the animals at 6 weeks of age. An ovarian remnant may be suspected in a neutered female with signs of estrus.[63b] Jills allowed to remain in estrus during the breeding season are susceptible to the toxic effects of estrogen on bone marrow. Affected jills develop pancytopenia and varying degrees of alopecia. Clinical signs accompanying the pancytopenia include pale mucous membranes, petechial or ecchymotic hemorrhages, anorexia, depression, and weight loss. The alopecia is bilaterally symmetric, beginning on the tail, the perineum, the abdomen, the medial thighs, and the rump and progressing cranially (Fig. 20:6). Vulvar enlargement is a constant finding. Untreated animals die of infectious or hemorrhagic complications. Treatment is often unrewarding. Ovariohysterectomy; intravenous blood transfusions; administration of dexamethasone, anabolic steroids, and systemic antibiotics; and supportive care have rarely been reported to result in recovery, but transfusions may need to be repeated several times for 3 to 5 months.[41, 45, 65]

---

*See references 5, 40, 41, 45, 51, 53, 60, 63b, 65, 67, and 68.

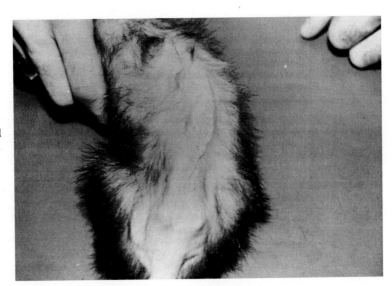

Figure 20:5. Truncal alopecia and hypotonic skin (note exaggerated wrinkling) in a ferret with an adrenal adenoma.

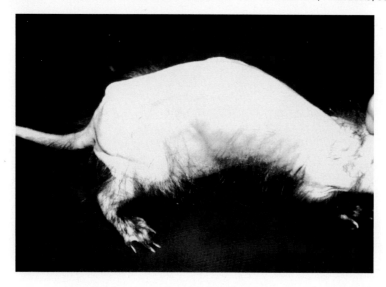

Figure 20:6. Alopecia of the trunk and tail in a jill with hyperestrogenism.

ALOPECIA ASSOCIATED WITH TESTICULAR NEOPLASIA

Testicular neoplasia is rare, as most large-volume breeders neuter male ferrets at 6 weeks of age. A sparse haircoat and a bald tail were reported in association with an interstitial cell carcinoma of the testicle in one ferret.[52] Total body alopecia and pruritus were reported in association with a testicular Sertoli's cell neoplasm in another ferret.[51]

BREEDING SEASON ALOPECIA

Breeding season alopecia is commonly seen, especially in the female and less frequently in the male ferret, during the period of sexual activity from March through August.[5, 45, 60, 64, 66, 67] Bilaterally symmetric alopecia affects the tail, the perineum, the ventral abdomen, the rump, and occasionally the periocular region and the paws. Affected ferrets are otherwise healthy, and spontaneous hair regrowth occurs in the fall.

SHEDDING

Seasonal shedding is seen in spring and early summer.[5, 45, 60, 67] Variable degrees of hypotrichosis or alopecia may be seen over the trunk and resolve spontaneously within a month or two.

TELOGEN DEFLUXION

Telogen defluxion is occasionally seen 2 to 3 months after a stressful circumstance (high fever, severe illness, surgery, and anesthesia).[67] Bilaterally symmetric hypotrichosis or alopecia is most prominent on the trunk (Figs. 20:7 and 20:8).

HYPOTHYROIDISM

Although anecdotal reports suggest that hypothyroidism is a common cause of endocrine-like alopecia in ferrets,[4] the authors and others[51] have never made such a diagnosis, and know of no documented cases. Some data have been published on basal serum thyroxine and triiodothyronine levels and thyroid function tests in normal ferrets.[45, 46, 49]

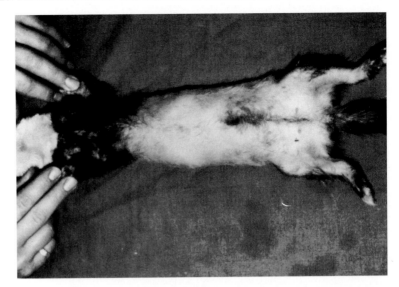

Figure 20:7. Telogen defluxion in a ferret. Alopecia of the ventral trunk and abdomen. (Courtesy M. Paradis.)

Miscellaneous Conditions

The skin of ferrets contains numerous sebaceous glands that produce copious amounts of secretions, which, in addition to giving the ferret its characteristic odor, also give the coat a greasy feeling.[5, 41, 43, 45, 60] The amount of secretion is greater in male ferrets. If these secretions are allowed to accumulate, they can stain the haircoat and the skin yellow and give them a dirty appearance. Castration and frequent bathing (once or twice weekly) can control this condition.

Some authors believe that the most common cause of alopecia and dull, dry haircoat in ferrets is poor dietary practices.[3] Food passage averages 3 to 4 hours in ferrets, thus diets high in protein and fat but low in fiber are important.

Biotin deficiency (from excessive feeding of raw eggs) can result in bilaterally symmetric alopecia in ferrets.[5, 41, 43, 45]

Severe intestinal parasitism (especially *Toxascaris leonina*) can produce variable degrees of hair loss and scaling in ferrets.[43]

Contact dermatitis can occur with frequent use of shampoos or insecticide sprays.[43]

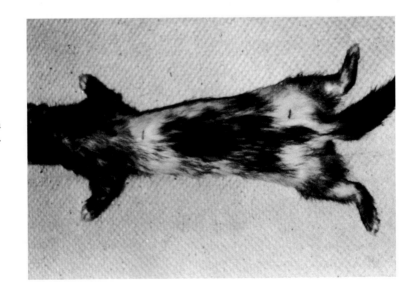

Figure 20:8. Telogen defluxion (same ferret as in Figure 20:7). Patchy alopecia of the dorsal trunk. (Courtesy M. Paradis.)

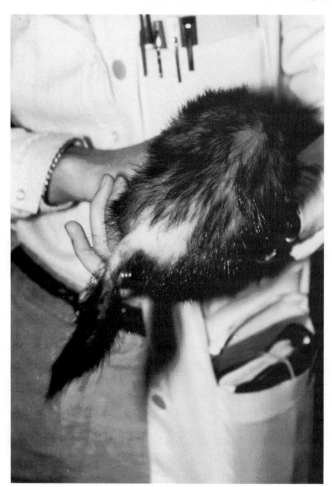

Figure 20:9. Self-induced alopecia over the rump of a ferret with a pruritic dermatosis resembling atopy.

Focal areas of alopecia have been seen at the site of previous injections.[43]

The authors have seen an occasional ferret with presumptive atopy. Affected animals manifested symmetric, nonlesional pruritus over the trunk, the rump (Fig. 20:9), and the paws. Fleas were not present, hypoallergenic diets were ineffective, and response to glucocorticoids or chlorpheniramine was good.

The *blue ferret syndrome* is an unusual idiopathic condition affecting ferrets of either sex, neutered or intact.[3] The abdominal skin shows bilaterally symmetric bluish discoloration. Affected ferrets are asymptomatic. The condition regresses spontaneously during a few weeks. In the authors' experience, this condition is most commonly seen in ferrets that have been clipped for surgery or access to veins during the resting phase of the hair cycle. The clipped area remains hairless for a long time, then suddenly begins to turn blue. It appears that hair follicles are making melanin, which will be incorporated into growing hairs. Soon after the ferret's skin turns blue, hair regrowth begins (within 1 to 2 weeks).

Neoplasia

Skin neoplasms appear to be fairly common in the ferret.* One of the most frequent of these is the mast cell tumor.[5, 44, 45, 52, 61a, 62, 63b] Lesions may be solitary or multiple and may come and go over time. Mast cell tumors present as papules or nodules (see Fig. 20:1 *B*), which vary from

*See references 3, 5, 20, 41, 44, 45, 52, 61a, and 62.

skin colored to yellow, brown, or red. They may be firm, soft, or cystic. Some lesions are pruritic. Lesions may occur anywhere but are most commonly reported on the neck and dorsal trunk. There is controversy in the literature concerning the biological behavior of mast cell tumors in the ferret, with some researchers suggesting that they are usually benign,[41, 61a] whereas other investigators claim that they are usually malignant and frequently metastatic.[52]

Basal cell tumors and sebaceous gland neoplasms (especially on the head, neck, limbs, tail and the shoulder [see Fig. 20:1 *C*]) are also common in ferrets.[44, 61a] Apocrine sweat gland carcinomas (especially on the tail and the groin), chondromas (especially on the tail), chondrosarcomas (especially on the tail), and squamous cell carcinomas (especially on the digit and the lip [see Fig. 20:1 *D*]) have also been reported on numerous occasions.* Other cutaneous neoplasms reported in ferrets include fibroma, fibrosarcoma, malignant fibrous histiocytoma, histiocytoma, hemangioma, hemangiosarcoma, neurofibroma, neurofibrosarcoma, myxosarcoma, lymphoma, and rhabdomyosarcoma.[5, 20, 44, 45, 61a]

The treatment of choice for cutaneous neoplasms is surgical excision.

■ GERBIL

Bacterial Infections

Bacterial skin infections, usually associated with *S. aureus,* are common in gerbils.[5, 17, 76b] These infections are virtually always secondary to other perhaps less obvious conditions, especially trauma (cage-related injuries and bite wounds), ectoparasite infestations, and accumulated harderian gland secretions.[5, 17] Infections resulting from cage-related injury are typically seen on the nose and the muzzle (from rubbing on the cage and equipment or burrowing in abrasive litter), whereas those caused by bite wounds typically occur around the head, the tail, the rump, and the perineal area. Those secondary to accumulated harderian gland secretion typically begin on the nose and the periocular area.[5, 17] Staphylococcal infections may be superficial (alopecia, erythema, oozing, crust, and scale) or deep (abscess, fistula, and ulcer), and are usually nonpruritic.

Treatment of bacterial dermatitis includes some combination of eliminating predisposing causes, daily topical cleaning with a 3 per cent hydrogen peroxide or 0.5 to 1 per cent chlorhexidine, and administration of systemic antibiotics (see Table 20:1).

Ectoparasites

Demodicosis has rarely been reported in gerbils.[5, 76] Lesions occurred on the face, the thorax, the abdomen, and the limbs and were characterized by alopecia, oozing, crusts, scales, and secondary bacterial infection. *Demodex merioni* was isolated in skin scrapings. Details concerning pathogenesis and treatment are presently unpublished.

Barbering

Although gerbils tolerate crowding better than do most rodents, they chew or "barber" the hair of cagemates.[5, 17] The affected areas appear clipped or shaved, and rarely are any actual skin lesions present. The dorsum of the tail and the top of the head are most frequently involved.

Bald Nose and Sore Nose

Bald nose describes a clinical condition common to the gerbil, which is characterized by alopecia on the muzzle and the dorsum of the nose.[3, 5, 17, 76a] There are usually no skin lesions.

---

*See references 3, 5, 20, 44, 45, 48, 50, 56, and 59.

The alopecia has been attributed to mechanical trauma associated with rubbing against cages and cage equipment and burrowing in abrasive bedding. Placing animals in a smooth-sided enclosure or aquarium with soft bedding such as shredded paper may be curative.

Bald nose may also be an early stage of the nasal dermatitis (*sore nose* [see Fig. 20:1 *E*]) associated with accumulated harderian gland secretion.* These secretions are rich in porphyrins and accumulate about the nasal and facial areas and apparently lead to the development of an irritant contact dermatitis and secondary staphylococcal infection. The animal's failure to groom the areas adequately leads to irritation, which can then lead to self-inflicted trauma and secondary infection. The stress of overcrowding and high humidity may contribute to the development or the severity of the condition. This condition is common in research colonies and commercial breeding colonies.

The earliest clinical sign is the accumulation of a reddish brown discharge and crust around the nose, the lips, and less frequently, the eyes. This porphyrin-rich secretion exhibits an orange fluorescence when viewed under ultraviolet light (Wood's light). There is frequently protrusion of the nictitans. This is followed by alopecia and, if not treated, dermatitis, pruritus, and secondary staphylococcal infections. Lesions can then spread to the paws, the legs, and the ventrum.

Therapy consists of topical or systemic antibiotic therapy for secondary staphylococcal infection, if present, and housing with access to sand. Surgical removal of the harderian gland is effective but less practical.[5, 70, 77]

Miscellaneous Conditions

An occasional litter of gerbils is born with abnormalities of hair growth and pigmentation.[5, 76a] Typically, the back is completely bald, the surrounding haircoat is thinned or patchily alopecic, and the haircoat shows profound leukotrichia. The majority of affected animals fail to thrive and die at the time of weaning. Surviving gerbils develop a normal haircoat as they mature. The etiopathogenesis of this condition is unknown.

The ventral scent gland in gerbils can become inflamed from being rubbed against wood chips or other abrasive bedding.[4] In addition, impaction of these glands can lead to self-mutilation.[4]

When relative humidity is greater than 50 per cent, the normally sleek and smooth gerbil haircoat often appears greasy and stands out.[3] Pine shavings can also cause this appearance.[3]

If a gerbil's tail skin is lost, the exposed tail becomes necrotic and sloughs off.[17a] Alternatively, the bare tail can be surgically removed where the skin stops.

Neoplasia

The skin is the second most common site of neoplasms in gerbils.[5, 69a, 73, 75, 77a] Skin neoplasms are typically seen in aged animals (2 to 4 years of age). The most commonly reported skin neoplasms in the gerbil are melanocytomas and melanomas (especially of the paw and the pinna),[5, 69a, 71, 72, 77a] sebaceous gland adenomas (especially of the ventral scent gland),[5, 69a, 77a] and squamous cell carcinoma (especially of the ventral scent gland [see Fig. 20:1 *F*] and the pinna).[5, 77a] Other reported skin neoplasms in gerbils include papilloma, fibrosarcoma, and neurofibroma.[5, 75]

Diagnosis of skin neoplasms is based on exfoliative cytologic study or biopsy, and the treatment of choice is surgical excision.

---

*See references 3, 5, 17, 33, 70, 74, and 77.

■ GUINEA PIG

Bacterial Infections

Bacterial skin infections are common in guinea pigs.* These infections are virtually always secondary to other factors, especially trauma (cage-related injuries and bite wounds) and ectoparasites. Those secondary to bite wounds are typically found around the head, the tail, the rump, and the genital area and are associated with *S. aureus*. Abscesses are occasionally associated with *Corynebacterium kutscheri, Streptococcus zooepidemicus* (especially abscesses on the neck), *Streptobacillus moniliformis,* or *Yersinia pseudotuberculosis.*[2, 5, 17, 78, 81] A staphylococcal cellulitis characterized by thickening and hyperkeratosis of the lips was associated with feeding of tough, fibrous hay.[116] Treatment of these infections includes elimination of predisposing factors, surgical drainage, daily topical applications of 3 per cent hydrogen peroxide or 0.5 per cent chlorhexidine, and systemic antibiotic administration (see Table 20:1).

An exfoliative dermatitis resembling staphylococcal scalded skin syndrome was reported in a guinea pig colony, chiefly among female animals in the late stages of gestation.[98] Bacterial contamination and the abrasive effects of rusty cage floors were suggested as initiating factors. Alopecia was first noted on the ventral abdomen. After a few days, the skin became acutely erythematous and painful. Affected skin subsequently fissured and large thick flakes were desquamated. The condition spontaneously resolved after a course of 10 to 14 days. *S. aureus* was isolated from the skin, the pharynx, the trachea, and nasal washings of affected animals. Skin biopsies revealed intragranular acantholysis and cleavage within the epidermis with minimal inflammation. An exfoliative toxin produced by the staphylococci was reported to cause the skin lesions.

The most common skin disease associated with *S. aureus* infection (occasionally *Corynebacterium pyogenes*) in the guinea pig is *pododermatitis* (bumble foot).† Predisposing factors include trauma to the footpad, poor sanitation, obesity, aging, and vitamin C deficiency. Affected animals react vigorously when the feet are palpated. The footpad is markedly enlarged, edematous, and erythematous (see Fig. 20:1 *G*). Crusts, ulcers, and hemorrhages may be present on the volar surfaces. In chronic or severe cases, the disease process extends to phalangeal and metatarsal or metacarpal bones and joints. Most guinea pigs with pododermatitis have a poor prognosis, as treatment is difficult and systemic amyloidosis is a frequent consequence of chronic infection. Pododermatitis can be prevented by frequently cleaning cages and changing bedding, using cages with smooth surfaces, instituting individual weight control, and providing routine foot care. Early lesions may respond to management changes and daily topical therapy (povidone-iodine or chlorhexidine scrubs, soaks, and ointments under a bandage). Extensive infections also necessitate systemic antibiotics (see Table 20:1).

Fungal Infections

Dermatophytosis is common in guinea pigs and is almost always caused by *T. mentagrophytes.*‡ This dermatophyte can be isolated from the skin and haircoat in up to 15 per cent of clinically normal guinea pigs.[1, 23, 92, 94, 99] Rarely, other dermatophytes, such as *M. canis, M. gypseum, M. audouinii,* and *T. verrucosum* can cause disease in guinea pigs.[84, 108, 114, 121, 124] Lesions typically begin as scaling, broken hairs, and alopecia on the nose, which spread to the periocular, forehead, and pinnal areas. In severe cases, the dorsal lumbosacral area is also affected, but the limbs (Fig. 20:10) and the ventrum are usually spared. Pruritus is usually minimal or absent. Some animals have more inflammatory lesions characterized by erythema, follicular papules, pustules, crusts, and pruritus. Diagnosis is confirmed by microscopic exami-

---

*See references 2–6, 12, 16–18, 31, 33, 36, 86, 98, 103, 106, 114, and 125.
†See references 2–6, 12, 16–18, 26, 28, 31, 33, 36, 99, 106, 108a, 114, and 118.
‡See references 2–5, 12, 16–18, 28, 31, 33, 36, 86, 99, 104, 106, and 107.

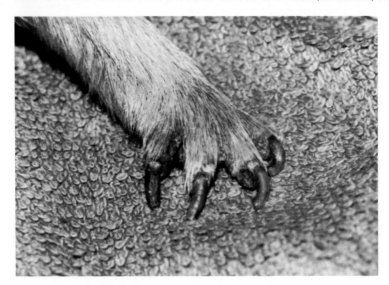

Figure 20:10. Alopecia, crust, and scale on the paw of a guinea pig with *T. mentagrophytes* infection.

nation of affected hairs and fungal culture. Treatment is usually accomplished with the topical application of antifungal agents (2 per cent lime sulfur, 1 per cent chlorhexidine, or 0.2 per cent enilconazole dips weekly until the animal is cured).* Griseofulvin is not usually needed but can be given at 25 mg/kg every 24 hours orally until the animal is cured.† The administration of griseofulvin should be avoided in pregnant animals.[5, 107] Dermatophytosis in guinea pigs is an important zoonosis.[21, 92, 94, 99, 107, 115]

Cryptococcosis was reported in a single guinea pig.[123] The animal had a plaque on the dorsum of the nose, which became crusted and ulcerated and spread into the nostrils. Skin biopsy was diagnostic, and the animal was euthanized.

Guinea pigs have been used as an experimental model for studying the pathogenesis of cutaneous *candidiasis*.[117] Skin lesions are readily produced by the application of *Candida albicans* under occlusion and consist of erythema, pustules, oozing, and crusts.

Guinea pigs have also been used as an experimental model for studying the pathogenesis and treatment of cutaneous *malasseziasis*.[122] Skin lesions are readily produced by the application of inocula of *Malassezia (Pityrosporum) ovale* and consist of erythema, edema, crusts, and scales.

Viral Infections

Hairless guinea pigs have been used as an experimental model for studying the pathogenesis of recurrent herpes simplex infection.[82] Intracutaneous inoculation of herpes simplex virus produces pustules and crusts, which spontaneously resolve and can be reactivated by local trauma.

Poxvirus–like virions were demonstrated during the electron microscopic examination of specimens from two guinea pigs with a chronic, crusting cheilitis.[87a]

Ectoparasites

Trixacarus (Caviacoptes) caviae is a burrowing sarcoptiform mite and, arguably, the most common cause of ectoparasitic skin disease of guinea pigs.‡ Trixacariasis is always the first

---

*See references 3–5, 28, 31, 33, 84, 86, 99, and 108.
†See references 4, 5, 28, 31, 33, 93, 99, 105, 106, 108, and 114.
‡See references 3–5, 10, 16, 17, 28, 31, 33, 85, 86, 88, 96, 99, 102, 106, 127, and 128.

differential diagnostic suspect in intense pruritus in guinea pigs. The mite is similar to *S. scabiei* in appearance but is smaller in size (average, 175 μm in length) and the female mite has a dorsal rather than terminal anus. *T. caviae* is similar in size and appearance to *Notoedres* spp. but differs by lacking prominent, sharp, dorsal cuticular spines. The areas most commonly affected include the dorsal neck and the thorax (see Fig. 20:1 *H*), but in severe cases, the entire body may be involved (Fig. 20:11 *A*).

Early clinical signs include pruritus, erythema, and traumatic alopecia. Chronic lesions include lichenification, hyperpigmentation, crusts, thick, whitish to yellowish scales (Fig. 20:11 *B*), and brittle, easily epilated hair. The extreme irritation and self-mutilation cause lethargy, anorexia, progressive emaciation, and death associated with bacterial infection or immune-mediated renal disease. Hyperesthesia, behavior such as furiously running in circles and blindly walking into objects, and seizures can be seen and may be triggered by examining the affected animal. Resorption of fetuses and abortion may be seen in breeding animals. Diagnosis may be confirmed by skin scrapings, but it is not unusual for these to be negative. Treatment consists of 2 per cent lime sulfur dips (once weekly until cure is achieved) or ivermectin injections.* *T. caviae* can temporarily infest humans, producing a pruritic papular dermatitis in areas contacted by the guinea pig (arms, thighs, and abdomen).†

Chirodiscoides caviae is the guinea pig fur mite.‡ Infestation is uncommon, and clinical disease is probably rare. Heavy infestations can cause pruritus, alopecia, erythema, scaling, and crusting, especially on the dorsolateral lumbosacral area (Fig. 20:11 *C*) and the perineum. Diagnosis is confirmed by the microscopic identification of the mites, which are often found attached to hair shafts. Treatment is as described for lice.

Other mites rarely reported to affect guinea pigs and produce clinical syndromes characterized by pruritus and dermatitis, which is most prominent on the face, the pinnae, and the dorsum, include *S. scabiei, Notoedres muris,* and *Myocoptes musculinus*.§ Diagnosis and treatment are as described for *T. caviae* infestation.

Lice are commonly encountered in guinea pigs.¶ The guinea pig may be parasitized by two different biting lice, with *Gliricola porcelli* (the slender guinea pig louse) being much more frequently encountered than *Gyropus ovalis* (the oval guinea pig louse). Most infestations occur without clinical signs, but heavy infestations may produce a roughened, disheveled haircoat, scaling, crusting, alopecia, and pruritus, especially around the ears and over the dorsum (Fig. 20:11 *D*). Heavy infestations are more commonly encountered in young animals and those with decreased resistance and under poor management. Diagnosis is confirmed by gross or microscopic visualization of lice or nits. Treatment can be accomplished with pyrethrin- or pyrethroid-containing flea powders or sprays approved for cats, 2 per cent lime sulfur dips, or ivermectin injections.[3–5, 28, 33] Cage sanitation is important.

Pelodera dermatitis is rarely reported in guinea pigs.[80, 119] Affected animals have ventral dermatitis consisting of erythema, papules, oozing, crusts, and alopecia. Skin scrapings and skin biopsy reveal the presence of the nematode *Pelodera strongyloides*. Removing contaminated bedding and maintaining a clean, dry cage environment are curative.

Cheyletiellosis is rarely reported in guinea pigs.[13, 99] Affected animals have scaling and variable degrees of hypotrichosis and pruritus on the dorsum. Skin scrapings reveal the mite *Cheyletiella parasitivorax*. Treatment is as described for rabbits.

Demodicosis is rare in guinea pigs.[7, 80, 95, 125] Lesions occur most commonly on the trunk (Fig. 20:12) and consist of alopecia, erythema, papules, and crusts. Pruritus is variable. Diagnosis is confirmed by finding numerous *Demodex caviae* mites in skin scrapings. Amitraz dips (250 ppm, every week until 4 weeks after skin scrapings are negative) are reported to be an effective treatment.[95]

---

*See references 3–5, 17, 28, 33, 85, 96, 102, and 106.
†See references 5, 28, 33, 85, 102, 127, and 128.
‡See references 2–5, 10, 15–18, 28, 31, 33, 83, 86, 99, 125, and 126.
§See references 2, 10, 15, 17, 31, 36, 91, 99, 125, and 128.
¶See references 2–5, 10, 15–18, 28, 30a, 31, 33, 99, 106, and 125.

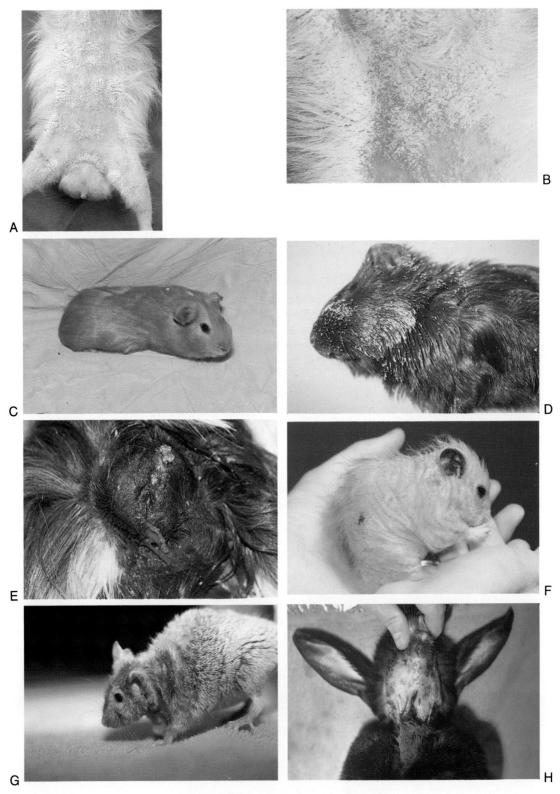

Figure 20:11 See legend on opposite page

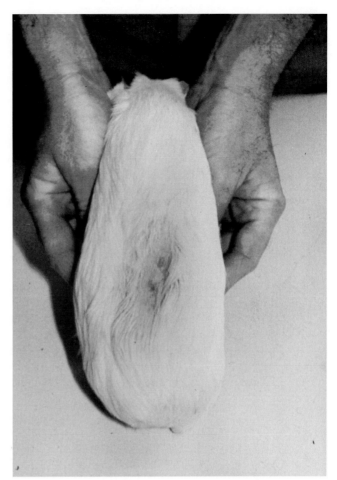

Figure 20:12. Alopecia and erythema over the back of a guinea pig with demodicosis. (Courtesy D. Carlotti.)

Fleas *(C. felis felis)* and ticks may be rarely encountered on guinea pigs.[5, 33, 97, 99] Treatment is as described for cats.

Nutritional Disorders

Nutritional deficiencies, other than vitamin C deficiency, are unlikely to be encountered in pet guinea pigs. Experimental production of nutritional deficiencies with resultant cutaneous abnormalities have been reported and are briefly mentioned here. Protein deficiency produces generalized alopecia.[2, 110] Fatty acid deficiency results in generalized alopecia, scaling, and dermatitis.[2, 34, 111] Pyridoxine deficiency produces alopecia, scaling, and dermatitis, which is most prominent on the limbs, the face, and the pinnae.[2, 112] Vitamin C deficiency is associated with

---

Figure 20:11. *A,* Alopecia, erythema, and thick, yellowish crusts on the ventrum of a guinea pig with trixacariasis. (Courtesy E. Guaguère.) *B,* Close-up of the thick, yellowish crusts on the skin of a guinea pig with trixacariasis. *C,* *Chirodiscoides caviae* infestation in a guinea pig. Note the uneven, clipped appearance of the haircoat over the caudal half of the body. *D,* Pediculosis in a guinea pig. Numerous nits can be seen over the face and neck. (Courtesy J. King.) *E,* Trichofolliculoma in a guinea pig. Hyperpigmented, ulcerated tumor over the dorsal lumbar area. (Courtesy W. Gould.) *F,* Epitheliotropic lymphoma in a hamster. Generalized alopecia, erythema, scaling, and exaggerated folds of skin. *G,* Severe self-inflicted alopecia and ulceration over the ear, neck, and shoulder in a mouse with *M. musculi* infestation. (Courtesy W. Gould.) *H,* Alopecia, erythema, crusts, and ulcers on the ventral neck of a rabbit with *Pseudomonas aeruginosa* infection.

cutaneous petechiae, ecchymoses, hematomas, generalized scaling, and a rough, unkempt haircoat.* Vitamin C deficiency is common and is most commonly seen in animals being fed a commercial rabbit chow or an outdated commercial guinea pig chow as the sole diet or in anorectic animals.

Miscellaneous Conditions

Telogen defluxion is frequently seen in the last trimester of pregnancy or during lactation.[5, 17, 31, 99, 106, 125] The alopecia is most prominent on the lumbosacral area and the flanks.

Marked shedding during stress is common in guinea pigs.[3] When guinea pigs are sick, it is often easy to epilate an entire area of haircoat when tenting the skin.

Guinea pigs establish male-dominated social hierarchies, and animals of low social ranking or young animals may lose considerable amounts of hair, especially on the head, the rump, the perineum, and the prepuce owing to barbering or receiving bite wounds.[5, 17, 31, 33, 106, 125] Ear chewing can be a problem, resulting in ear margin notches or actual cropping close to the head. Guinea pigs may also self-barber, producing hair loss in only those areas that they can reach with their mouth (the fur on the head, the neck, and the anterior shoulders is intact). Hair loss due to barbering appears irregular in length and clipped. The underlying skin is usually normal in appearance. In some cases, the addition of long-stemmed hay resolves the barbering, suggesting that the cause was boredom or a need for fiber.[5, 17, 31, 33, 125]

Necrosis of digits and paws is occasionally seen when owners put objects such as cloths and socks in cages with guinea pigs. Segments of these materials become wrapped around distal extremities and serve as constricting bands or tourniquets. Tissues distal to the constriction become swollen and painful, then necrotic, and then they slough (Fig. 20:13).

Thinning of the haircoat is common near the time of weaning in neonates and spontaneously resolves.[5, 125]

Hereditary hairlessness has been reported in guinea pigs (Fig. 20:14).[100, 109] Bilaterally symmetric alopecia has been seen in guinea pigs with cystic ovaries (Fig. 20:15).[4, 108a] Affected females usually present with progressive enlargement of the abdomen, and ovarian cysts are palpable as discrete, large, rounded masses in the dorsal middle abdomen. Ovariohysterectomy is curative.

Sebaceous glands are especially abundant around the anus, in the folds of the perianal and

*See references 2, 3, 17, 86, 99, 106, 108a, and 125.

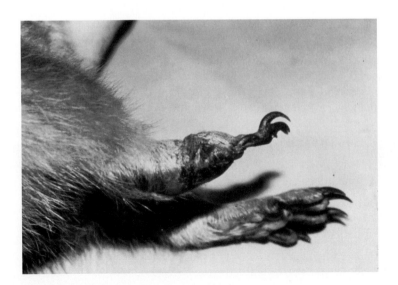

Figure 20:13. Necrosis and slough of the hindfoot of a guinea pig caused by a constricting band. (Courtes· G. Kollias.)

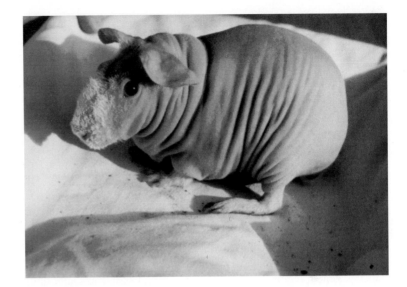

Figure 20:14. Congenital alopecia in a guinea pig. (Courtesy J. Gourreau.)

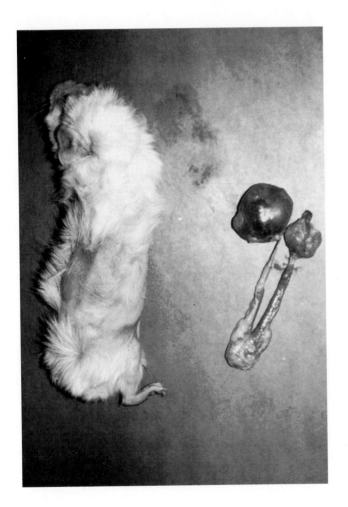

Figure 20:15. Truncal alopecia in a guinea pig associated with bilateral cystic ovaries. The cystic ovaries and uterus are on the right.

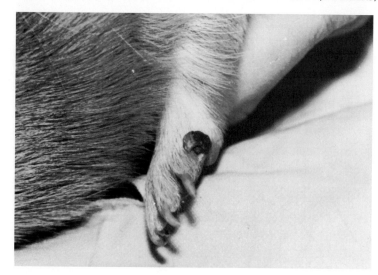

Figure 20:16. Cutaneous horn on the lateral digit of the left hindfoot of a guinea pig.

genital regions, and in the dorsal sacral skin, especially in sexually mature male animals.[5, 99, 125] Excessive accumulations of sebaceous debris, and occasionally bedding material and feces, may become entrapped in these folds or mat down the dorsal sacral haircoat. Intertrigo, secondary bacterial infections, and unpleasant odors may intervene in this situation. These areas should be cleaned as needed with 3 per cent hydrogen peroxide, 0.5 per cent chlorhexidine, or a mild astringent (aluminum subacetate) to prevent the aforementioned sequelae.

Heavy guinea pigs, especially those maintained in wire-bottom cages, frequently develop hyperkeratosis and cutaneous horns of the footpads (Fig. 20:16).[5, 99, 125] These horny growths are most commonly observed on the ventral aspect of the front paws. They can be removed with scissors and an emery file. Replacement of cage surfaces with smoother materials retards or prevents further hyperkeratoses.

Overgrown claws are a frequent problem in pet guinea pigs.[3, 106, 125] Frequent examination and trimming prevents traumatic and infectious complications.

Neoplasia

The skin is the second most common site of neoplasia in the guinea pig.* The most common cutaneous neoplasm is the trichofolliculoma.† This tumor is most commonly encountered as a benign, solitary lesion over the dorsal lumbar area (see Fig. 20:11 *E*). The overlying skin is usually alopecic and crusted. Frequently, a central pore is seen, through which keratinous material or dark, hemorrhagic exudate is discharged. Other cutaneous neoplasms reported in guinea pigs include sebaceous adenoma, fibroma, fibrosarcoma, lipoma, liposarcoma, schwannoma, and lymphoma.[2, 26, 90, 101, 125, 129]

■ HAMSTER

Bacterial Infections

Bacterial skin infections are uncommonly reported in hamsters. *S. aureus* and *Pasteurella pneumotropica* have been recovered from isolated cases of skin abscesses and bite wounds.[5, 17] Treatment of bacterial dermatitis includes elimination of predisposing causes, surgical drainage,

---

*See references 2, 3, 5, 17, 26, 90, 99, 101, 125, and 129.
†See references 3, 5, 17, 89, 90, 99, 120, 125, and 129.

daily topical cleaning with 3 per cent hydrogen peroxide or 0.5 per cent chlorhexidine, and occasionally systemic antibiotic administration (see Table 20:1).

Experimentally, the hamster is susceptible to infection with *Treponema pallidum* subsp. *endemicum*, the agent of endemic syphilis of humans.[141] Intradermal injection of the spirochete results in erythematous papules and ulcers, which eventually heal but are followed by perioral ulcers and an erythematous maculopapular rash on the paws and the trunk and death. This hamster syphilis has been proposed as a useful model for the study of the immune response, antibiotic therapy, and vaccination techniques in human venereal and congenital syphilis.

Fungal Infections

Dermatophytosis is rare in hamsters and is caused by *T. mentagrophytes*.* Diagnosis is confirmed by microscopic examination of affected hairs and fungal culture. Treatment is as described for the other rodents.

Ectoparasites

Demodicosis is the most common ectoparasitism of the hamster.† *Demodex criceti* and *D. aurati* are both normal residents of hamster skin.[146, 147] *D. aurati* is long and tapered (average, 180 μm long) and inhabits hair follicles, whereas *D. criceti* is short and stubby (average, 90 μm long) and inhabits the keratin and pits of the epidermal surface. Clinical demodicosis is seen in aged hamsters, is usually associated with *D. aurati,* and is usually associated with conditions that suppress immune responses (e.g., malnutrition, concurrent disease, cancer, and exposure to carcinogens).‡ Lesions are most commonly seen over the dorsal lumbosacral area but may be generalized. Moderate to severe alopecia is accompanied by variable degrees of scaling, erythema, and small hemorrhagic crusts. Pruritus is usually absent. Diagnosis is confirmed by skin scrapings. Treatment of demodicosis in hamsters has not been extensively evaluated or reported. The authors and others[4, 33] have had success with 250 ppm of amitraz applied as a whole-body dip once weekly until 4 weeks after skin scrapings are negative.

Notoedric mange is rarely reported in hamsters.[17, 33, 130, 131, 137] Lesions are characterized by thick yellowish crusts, erythema, and alopecia on the pinnae, the muzzle, the tail, the genitalia, and the paws. Pruritus is severe, and self-mutilation can be extreme. Diagnosis is confirmed by finding *Notoedres* sp. mites in skin scrapings. Treatment with 2 per cent lime sulfur dips (whole-body application weekly until two treatments after clinical cure) or ivermectin injections is effective.

S. scabiei, T. caviae, and *Ornithonyssus bacoti* are reported to be rare causes of pruritus and dermatitis in hamsters.[22, 91, 128] Clinical signs, diagnosis, and treatment are as described for notoedric mange.

Fleas *(C. felis felis)* are rarely encountered on hamsters.[5] Treatment is as described for cats.

Traumatic Alopecia and Dermatitis

Female hamsters are generally more aggressive than are males.[5, 142a] Aggressive behavior in male hamsters is testosterone dependent and is markedly reduced by castration.[5, 156a] The establishment of social dominance among male hamsters is positively correlated with the weight and size and degree of pigmentation of the flank glands.[134a, 149] Aggression-related bite wounds are most commonly seen around the head, the tail, and the perineal area. Aggression can produce severe wounding, such as the complete removal of the flank glands of the victim.[136]

---

*See references 2, 3, 5, 17, 28, 31, 33, and 158.
†See references 2, 5, 17, 33, 131, 135, 148, 152, and 157.
‡See references 5, 17, 33, 131, 135, and 152.

Nutritional Disorders

Nutritional deficiencies are unlikely to be seen in pet hamsters.* However, one author[17a] indicates that hair loss in hamsters is associated most often with continuous feeding of low protein (under 16 per cent) feed, such as are commonly found in pet stores. Experimental production of nutritional deficiencies with resultant cutaneous abnormalities have been reported and are briefly mentioned here. Pantothenic acid deficiency produces exfoliative dermatitis, depigmentation of the haircoat, and the accumulation of porphyrin-rich secretions around the nose, the mouth, and the eyes.[21, 155] Riboflavin deficiency produces alopecia, scaling, and dermatitis, which are most evident on the extremities.[21, 151] Pyridoxine deficiency results in generalized alopecia and depigmentation of the haircoat.[2, 154] Niacin deficiency produces a generalized alopecia.[2, 138] Fatty acid deficiency results in generalized alopecia, scaling, and the production of profuse amounts of cerumen.[2, 132] Copper deficiency results in alopecia and depigmentation.[2]

Miscellaneous Conditions

Foreign body granulomas associated with bedding consisting of wood shavings and sawdust were reported on the paws and the shoulders of hamsters.[143] The problem was eliminated by using shredded paper as bedding.

Swelling and pruritus of the face and the paws has been reported in several hamsters.[3] In all instances, owners had recently purchased a fresh bag of cedar or pine shavings produced by a leading pet company or bulk shavings from landscaping or nursery outlets. When affected animals were housed on plain newspaper, the lesions spontaneously regressed. Presumably, the shavings had been treated with some chemical that produced a contact dermatitis.

Hereditary hairlessness has been reported in hamsters.[145]

Hyperadrenocorticism is rarely reported in hamsters.[5, 131a] Clinical signs include bilaterally symmetric alopecia, hyperpigmentation, and thinning of the skin. The baseline plasma cortisol value in one affected hamster was elevated (approximately twofold increase) compared with that in one normal hamster. One hamster was treated with metyrapone (8 mg orally q24h for 1 month), and hair regrowth was complete after 12 weeks. A second hamster was treated with o,p'-DDD (5 mg orally q24h for 1 month), then metyrapone as described previously, and responded to neither drug. This hamster was euthanized, and a chromophobe adenoma of the hypophysis and bilateral adrenocortical hyperplasia were found at necropsy.

The flank scent glands of the hamster can become inflamed from being rubbed against wood chips or other abrasive cage equipment.[4] In addition, impaction of these glands can lead to self-mutilation.[4]

Ringtail is occasionally seen in the hamster (see Rat in this chapter).[2, 156, 181]

Neoplasia

Skin neoplasms are rare in hamsters.[2, 5, 17, 134, 142] The most frequently reported cutaneous neoplasms are melanomas and melanocytomas.[2, 5, 150] These tumors occur much more frequently in male hamsters and most commonly on the back, the head, the neck, and the flank gland.

Epitheliotropic lymphoma (mycosis fungoides) is the second most common cutaneous neoplasm of the hamster.[5, 139, 153] Affected animals have an exfoliative erythroderma (see Fig. 20:11 F), which is generally pruritic, and go on to manifest peripheral lymphadenopathy, lethargy, anorexia, emaciation, and death. Some animals also have cutaneous plaques and nodules (Fig. 20:17), which may become ulcerated and crusted. Light and electron microscopic examinations demonstrated an epitheliotropic lymphoma in which many cells show the typical features of Sézary cells.[139, 153] Immunohistochemical studies showed that the neoplastic cells are T lymphocytes.[139] Therapeutic trials have not been reported.

---

*See references 2–5, 12, 16–18, 26, 28, 31, and 33.

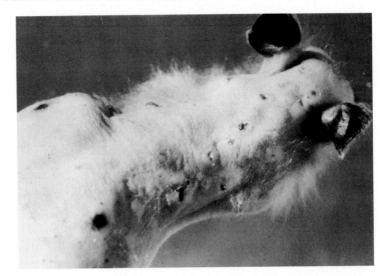

Figure 20:17. Epitheliotropic lymphoma in a hamster. Generalized alopecia and multiple crusted nodules and plaques.

Other cutaneous neoplasms reported in hamsters include basal cell carcinoma, squamous cell carcinoma, keratoacanthoma, papilloma, apocrine sweat gland adenoma, fibrosarcoma, and plasmacytoma.[2, 5, 133, 142]

■ MOUSE

Bacterial Infections

Bacterial skin infections are uncommon in pet mice, are usually caused by *S. aureus,* and are secondary to trauma (cage-related injuries and bite wounds) or self-inflicted (the pruritus associated with ectoparasites).* Infections resulting from cage-related injury are typically seen on the nose and the muzzle, whereas those associated with bite wounds typically occur around the head, the tail, the rump, and the perineal area. Staphylococcal infections may be superficial (alopecia, erythema, oozing, and crust) or deep (abscess, fistula, necrosis, and ulcer) and are usually nonpruritic. Other bacteria occasionally isolated from cutaneous abscesses and pyogranulomas in mice include *Streptococcus* sp., *P. pneumotropica, Actinobacillus* sp., *Actinomyces* sp., and *Klebsiella* sp.†

Treatment of bacterial dermatitis includes some combination of elimination of predisposing causes, surgical drainage, daily topical cleaning with 3 per cent hydrogen peroxide or 0.5 to 1 per cent chlorhexidine, and systemic antibiotic administration (see Table 20:1).

S. moniliformis is a rare cause of epizootics of edema and cyanosis of the extremities.[2, 17, 221]

C. kutscheri (murium) is a rare cause of epizootics of furunculosis and cutaneous pyogranulomas, which may progress to necrosis and sloughing of extremities.[2, 17, 224]

The mouse has been used as an experimental model for staphylococcal scalded skin syndrome.[180, 186]

Fungal Infections

Dermatophytosis is uncommon in mice and is usually caused by *T. mentagrophytes.*‡ This dermatophyte can be isolated from the haircoat of up to 60 per cent of clinically normal mice

---

*See references 2, 12, 17, 31, 36, 170, 174, 186, 203, 209, 214, 218, and 219.
†See references 2, 17, 203a, 206, 213, 215, 217, and 225.
‡See references 1–5, 8, 12, 16–18, 21, 23, 28, 31, 36, 164, 169, 183, 186, 199, and 210.

in pet shops and represents an important zoonosis. Lesions are most commonly seen on the face, the head, the tail, and the trunk and consist of annular areas of alopecia, broken hairs, scales, and variable degrees of erythema and crusting. Pruritus is usually minimal to absent. Diagnosis and treatment are as described for guinea pigs.

Viral Infections

Mouse pox (ectromelia) causes epizootics in research colonies but is rarely, if ever, seen in practice.* Skin lesions include a generalized papular dermatitis with eventual swelling, necrosis, ulceration, and even sloughing of digits, pinnae, and tail. Diagnosis is confirmed by skin biopsy, electron microscopic examination of crusts, and viral isolation of the orthopoxvirus.

Reovirus Type 3 infection of suckling mice causes severe illness and an oily haircoat.[2, 12, 17, 171] Animals that survive past weaning experience alopecia.

Sialodacryoadenitis virus infection causes eye rubbing and scratching, periorbital swelling, and red tears (chromodacryorrhea).[2, 12, 17a]

Ectoparasites

Myobia musculi is a mite commonly found on mice.† Some animals are asymptomatic carriers, whereas other animals show varying degrees of skin disease and pruritus. Severely inflammatory and pruritic forms of the infestation are associated with genetic susceptibility[176, 187, 227] and mite-related hypersensitivity reactions.[227] Immature mice or those that are immunocompromised may be more susceptible to severe forms of the disease. Clinical signs may be mild and include patchy alopecia, slight erythema, and minor scaling on the head and the muzzle. Other mice may show intense pruritus and self-mutilation of the face, the head, the pinnae, the neck, and the shoulders (see Fig. 20:11 *G*). Severely affected animals can become debilitated and die. Diagnosis is confirmed by skin scrapings. The treatment of choice is subcutaneous injections of ivermectin.[3, 4, 33, 228]

Myocoptes musculinus is a mite commonly found on mice.‡ Some animals are asymptomatic carriers, whereas others manifest varying degrees of skin disease and pruritus. Lesions are most severe on the back and the ventrum. Unlike the case with *M. musculi* infestations, severe ulceration is not seen with *M. musculinus* infestations. Diagnosis is confirmed by skin scrapings; however, the mites are often difficult to find. The treatment of choice is subcutaneous injections of ivermectin every 2 weeks until the animal is cured.[3, 4, 33, 228]

Other mites that are rarely found on mice include *Radfordia affinis, Psorergates simplex, O. bacoti, S. scabiei, N. muris,* and *Trichoecius romboutsi.*§

Fleas (especially *C. felis felis*) may be recovered from pet mice maintained in households frequented by dogs and cats.[2–5, 12, 17, 186]

The sucking louse, *Polyplax serrata,* is occasionally found on pet mice.¶ Some animals may be asymptomatic carriers, others manifest varying degrees of dermatitis and pruritus. Young animals, debilitated animals, and animals in poor management situations are more likely to be affected. Lice and related dermatoses are most commonly found on the neck and back. Treatment can be accomplished with topical insecticides or ivermectin injections.

---

*See references 2, 3, 5, 6, 12, 17, 36, 159, 182, 186, and 201.
†See references 2–5, 10, 12, 15–17, 28, 31, 33, 36, 160, 173, 186, 188, 191, 195, 208, 222, and 226.
‡See references 2–5, 10, 12, 15–17, 28, 31, 33, and 36.
§See references 2–5, 10, 12, 15–18, 22, 28, 31, 33, 185, and 186.
¶See references 2–5, 10, 12, 15–18, 28, 31, 33, 36, and 186.

Nutritional Disorders

Nutritional deficiencies are unlikely to be encountered in pet mice. Experimental production of nutritional deficiencies with resultant cutaneous abnormalities have been reported and are briefly mentioned here. Zinc deficiency produces exfoliative dermatitis, alopecia, and depigmentation of the haircoat.[2, 11, 35, 177] Pantothenic acid deficiency results in exfoliative dermatitis and depigmentation of the haircoat.[2, 205] Riboflavin deficiency produces alopecia, scaling, and dermatitis, especially on the extremities.[2, 196] Pyridoxine deficiency results in exfoliative dermatitis, especially on the face, the ears, the limbs, and the tail.[2, 161] Biotin deficiency causes exfoliative dermatitis.[2] Fatty acid deficiency produces an exfoliative dermatitis.[2, 29, 34, 178]

Miscellaneous Conditions

Male mice are aggressive.* Barbering and bite wounds are frequently seen, especially on the muzzle, the whiskers, the face, the head, the rump, the tail, and the perineum. These behaviors can be exacerbated by crowding, stress, and boredom. Mice frequently rub the hair off the muzzle as they stick their face through slotted feeders or wire bars.

Mice develop numerous types of hereditary hairlessness and keratinization defects, which are probably never seen by the practitioner.† Some of these conditions have been used as laboratory models for the study of various aspects of cutaneous pathophysiology and pharmacology, such as ichthyosis,[168, 186] asebia,[167, 190] rhino,[175, 200] blotchy (similar to the Menkes kinky hair syndrome in humans),[216] and flaky skin (similar to psoriasis in humans).[218a]

Ringtail is rarely reported in mice (see Rat in this chapter).[17, 25, 181] Idiopathic dry gangrene of the pinna is sporadically seen in young mice.[17, 162] The incidence appears to increase when the mice are exposed to cold temperatures and when the ears are traumatized by excessive grooming in attempts to remove lice. The condition progresses rapidly from initial erythema of the distal one third of the pinna to necrosis and slough. Rarely, the distal one third of the tail is also involved.

Perianal pruritus is seen in association with pinworms *(Syphacia obvelata).‡ Infected mice often mutilate the base of the tail. Diagnosis is confirmed by microscopic examination of strips of cellophane (Scotch) tape that have been applied to the perineum. The eggs of S. obvelata are banana shaped and about 30 μm by 150 μm. Treatment with ivermectin injections is* curative.

Neoplasia

Although mice are sensitive to the induction of various skin neoplasms by the topical or systemic administration of chemical carcinogens or ultraviolet light exposure, spontaneous skin neoplasms are rare.§ The most commonly reported cutaneous neoplasms are papilloma, squamous cell carcinoma, and fibrosarcoma. Other reported cutaneous neoplasms include hair follicle tumors, sebaceous gland tumors, mast cell tumors, melanomas, lymphomas, and a solitary epitheliotropic lymphoma resembling pagetoid reticulosis in humans.[158a]

■ RABBIT

Bacterial Infections

Pasteurellosis (snuffles) is the most common bacterial disease of the rabbit.¶ Most rabbits carry *Pasteurella multocida* asymptomatically in the nasal cavity, and under conditions of stress, the

---

*See references 2–5, 17, 28, 33, 193, 194, 197, 198, and 220.
†See references 2, 7, 17, 166–168, 175, 184, 186, 190, 200, 204, 218a, and 218b.
‡See references 2, 4, 10, 12, 17, 32, 33, and 36.
§See references 2, 3, 5, 6, 12, 17, 26, 186, 189, 211, and 223.
¶See references 2–5, 16–18, 252, 254a, 267, and 284.

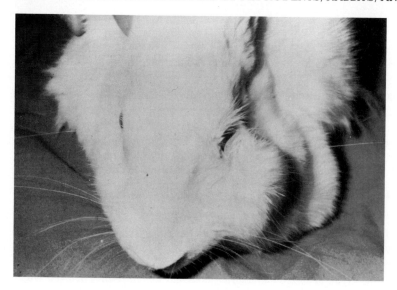

Figure 20:18. Large abscess on the left cheek of a rabbit with *P. multocida* infection. (Courtesy W. Gould.)

bacteria multiply and cause disease. Subcutaneous abscesses (Fig. 20:18) develop as a result of septicemia, external wound contamination, or direct extension from deeper sties. The abscesses are variable in size, are usually firm on palpation, and are filled with a thick, white to tan exudate. Diagnosis is confirmed by microscopic examination of direct smears of exudate and culture. In the rabbit, subcutaneous abscesses are due to pasteurellosis until proven otherwise. Other causes of abscesses include *S. aureus, Fusobacterium, Pseudomonas aeruginosa, Streptococcus* sp., and *C. pyogenes*.* Treatment consists of surgical drainage, topical antimicrobial application, and systemic antibiotic administration (see Table 20:1), or surgical excision.[254a]

Necrobacillosis (Schmorl's disease) is a sporadic bacterial infection of rabbits caused by *Fusobacterium necrophorum*.† It is characterized by inflammation, necrosis, ulceration, and abscessation, especially on the face, the head, and the neck. Diagnosis is confirmed by culture. Treatment is accomplished with surgical debridement, topical antimicrobials application, and systemic penicillin or tetracycline administration.

P. aeruginosa causes a *localized moist dermatitis (sore dewlap)* and, occasionally, subcutaneous abscess in areas of skin that are continuously wet.‡ The muzzle, the dewlap (see Fig. 20:11 *H*), the flank, and the haunches are most commonly involved. The affected skin is moist, erythematous, edematous, alopecic, and often ulcerated. The fur is often clumped, creating a spiked appearance. The most striking clinical feature is the blue-green color of the fur in animals with white fur, which is caused by a water-soluble pigment (pyocyanin) produced by the bacteria. Diagnosis is confirmed by microscopic examination of direct smears from oozing areas and culture. Treatment includes clipping, gentle cleaning, and application of astringents (aluminum acetate) and topical gentamicin sulfate ointment. Prevention is directed at removing the cause of continued wetness of the fur. Leaking water valves or water bottles should be replaced. Water bowls or pans should be replaced by water bottles with sipper tubes. Malocclusion of the teeth should be corrected to prevent drooling. Wet bedding should be changed more frequently.

Ulcerative pododermatitis (sore hocks) is a common disorder in rabbits.[2–5, 16–18, 252, 254a, 284] Genetic predilection is important, as large body size and thinner plantar fur pads are important predisposing factors. Unsanitary cage conditions, rough cage surfaces, and obesity also contrib-

---

*See references 2, 5, 12, 17, 18, 252, 254a, 281, and 284.
†See references 2, 3, 5, 16–18, 252, and 284.
‡See references 2–5, 16–18, 252, 263, 273, 284, and 288.

ute to pressure necrosis and secondary bacterial infection with *S. aureus.* Lesions commonly occur unilaterally or bilaterally on the plantar aspect of the metatarsal region or, less commonly, the volar surface of the metacarpal area. Focal inflammation, oozing, crusts, and alopecia progress to ulcers, hemorrhage, and abscesses. In severe infections, the disease may extend to the bony structures of the foot and result in septicemia. Treatment includes correction of predisposing conditions, surgical drainage, topical antimicrobial application, and systemic antibiotic administration (see Table 20:1). Severe cases usually do not respond.

Venereal spirochetosis (treponematosis, rabbit syphilis, or vent disease) is uncommon.* *Treponema cuniculi,* the causative spirochete, is transmitted by direct contact, especially mating. Cold environments appear to predispose to the disease. Because of the grooming, social, and sleeping habits of rabbits, lesions are frequently seen on the nose (Fig. 20:19 *A*), the lips, the chin, the face, the eyelids, the ears, and the paws as well as the genitalia. Lesions consist of vesicles, papules, erythema, edema, oozing, erosions, and brownish crusts. Focal ulcers and hemorrhage may be seen. Diagnosis is confirmed by skin biopsies, the Venereal Disease Research Laboratory (VDRL) slide test, and the rapid plasma reagin (RPR) card test. Treatment with penicillin G benzathine or penicillin G procaine is curative (42,000 IU/kg, subcutaneously, once a week for three treatments).

Fungal Infections

Dermatophytosis is common in rabbits.† *T. mentagrophytes* is the most common dermatophyte isolated, but *M. canis, M. gypseum, M. audouinii, T. verrucosum,* and *T. schoenleinii* have been reported.‡ *T. mentagrophytes* can be isolated from the haircoat and skin of up to 36 per cent of clinically normal rabbits, representing an important potential zoonosis.§ The disease is most common in the young and where husbandry and management are suboptimal. Lesions are characterized by patchy alopecia, broken hairs, erythema, and yellowish crusting and typically first appear on the bridge of the nose (Fig. 20:19 *B*), the eyelids, the pinnae, and the paws, and occasionally on many body sites. The condition is usually pruritic. Diagnosis and treatment are as described for the guinea pig.¶ Griseofulvin is teratogenic, and should not be used in breeding does.[33] A modified live *T. mentagrophytes* vaccine may prove useful in prophylaxis.[270]

Aspergillosis of the lungs and skin was reported in a whole litter of 4-week-old rabbits.[266] Multiple 1- to 2-mm papules were present all over the body. Histologically, the papules were cystic follicles distended with necrotic debris and dichotomously branching hyphae. *Aspergillus* sp. was isolated in culture. The animals were raised on moldy grass hay bedding material. A change in nesting materials prevented further occurrences.

Viral Infections

Myxomatosis is occasionally observed in domestic rabbits.|| The myxoma virus (a poxvirus) is transmitted from reservoir wild rabbit hosts by mosquitoes. There are several strains of virus with variable virulence. In domestic rabbits, severe disease and high mortality are frequently produced. Affected rabbits are febrile, lethargic, and depressed. In the acute form of the disease, there is edema and erythema of the anus, the genitalia, the lips, the nares, and the eyelids. Less virulent strains of the virus produce numerous skin tumors (Fig. 20:19 *C*). Myxomatosis appeared in the depilated skin of Angora rabbits.[246, 247] Lesions were a few millimeters to 3 cm in diameter, erythematous, and plaquelike and became hemorrhagic and necrotic. Morbidity was low and mortality infrequent. Diagnosis is based on distinctive clinical signs, biopsy, and

---

*See references 2–5, 16–18, 239–241, 252, and 284.
†See references 2, 3, 5, 12, 16–18, 28, 33, 230, 232, 245, 251, 252, 259, and 284.
‡See references 2, 3, 5, 16, 251, 272, 278, 279, 284, and 286.
§See references 1, 2, 16, 17, 21, 23, 245, and 284.
¶See references 2–5, 16, 17, 28, 33, 245, 248, 251, 252, 278, and 284.
||See references 2, 3, 5, 12, 16–18, 252, 265, and 284.

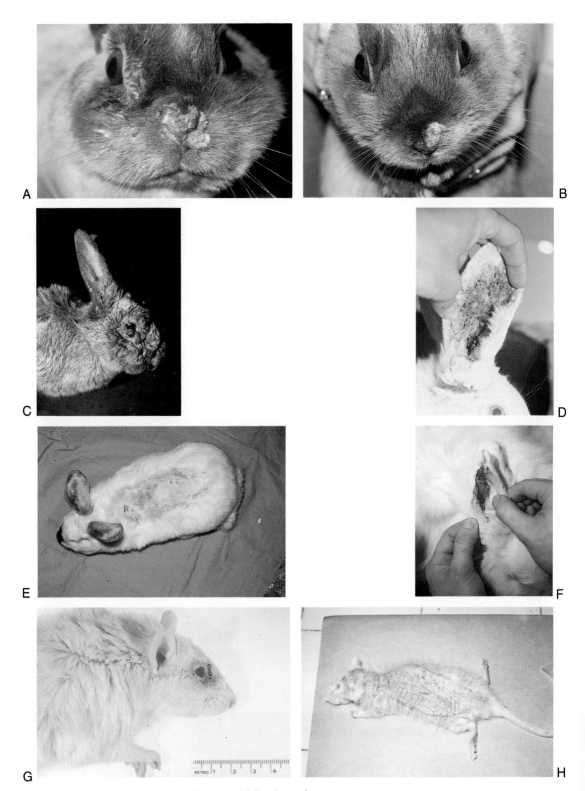

Figure 20:19 *See legend on opposite page*

virus isolation. There is no effective treatment, and control of insect vectors and screening of enclosures are paramount in endemic areas. Heterologous vaccine may be useful.

Rabbit pox is infrequently reported in domestic rabbits.* The causative poxvirus is closely related to vaccinia virus. Initial clinical signs of profuse nasal discharge, depression, and fever are followed in 4 to 5 days by a generalized, erythematous, macular to papular to nodular eruption. The rabbits have extensive edema of the face and perineum. Diagnosis is confirmed by biopsy and virus isolation.

Shope fibroma virus and Shope papilloma virus are oncogenic (see Neoplasia).

Ectoparasites

Psoroptes cuniculi, a nonburrowing mite, is the most common ectoparasite of the rabbit, and all rabbits should be considered infected until proven otherwise.† Rabbits are also susceptible to *P. ovis* (cattle and sheep).[289] *P. cuniculi* is transmitted by direct contact with infected rabbits, fomites, and contaminated environment. Starving mites survive up to 21 days off the host over the usual range of temperatures (5 to 30°C [41 to 86°F]) and relative humidities (20 to 75 per cent).[231] Crusts dislodged into the environment contain many mites. The mites pierce skin to feed, and hypersensitivity to mite-related antigens may be important in the pathogenesis of the dermatitis and pruritus.[250, 283]

P. cuniculi typically produces otitis externa (otoacariasis, ear canker, and ear mites) (Fig. 20:19 *D*). Affected rabbits shake their head and scratch at the head and ears. Alopecia, excoriations, and secondary bacterial infection may be present around the head and the neck. In early stages, a dry, whitish gray to tan crusty exudate forms inside the vertical ear canal. Later, a dry, crusty material with a layered appearance accumulates in the ear. A secondary bacterial infection may complicate the parasitic otitis externa, contributing to the foul odor and pain. Occasionally, mites may produce lesions on the face, the head, the neck, the limbs, the abdomen, and the back.[242a]

Diagnosis is confirmed by finding the mites in ear swabs or skin scrapings. In one report in which natural infections were studied and mite numbers were quantitated, affected animals harbored 40 to 100,000 mites per rabbit. The treatment of choice is the subcutaneous injection of ivermectin.‡ The cage and environment should be sanitized, and reducing the relative humidity to less than 20 per cent while increasing the temperature to 40°C (104°F) is of benefit in this regard.[231]

S. scabiei var. *cuniculi,* a burrowing mite, is a rare ectoparasite on rabbits in North America but is commonly found in some other parts of the world, such as Africa.§ Typical lesions include tan to yellow, often powdery crusts, alopecia, erythema, and excoriation on the muzzle, the lips, the bridge of the nose, the eyelids, the head, the margins of the pinna, the paws, and

---

*See references 2, 3, 5, 12, 16–18, 249, 252, and 284.
†See references 2–5, 12, 15–18, 28, 33, 231, 234, 242, 250, 252, 254a, 264, 276, and 284.
‡See references 3–5, 28, 33, 234, 242, 258a, 264, and 289.
§See references 2–5, 10, 12, 15–18, 28, 33, 252, 261, 262, 280, and 284.

Figure 20:19. *A,* Crusts on the nose of a rabbit with spirochetosis. (Courtesy G. Kollias.) *B,* Focal area of alopecia and crusting over the nose of a rabbit due to *T. mentagrophytes* infection. (Courtesy G. Kollias.) *C,* Multiple erythematous nodules and plaques around the eye, on the pinna, and on the muzzle of a rabbit with myxomatosis. (Courtesy G. Kollias.) *D,* Crusting and erythema of the lateral surface of the pinna of a rabbit with psoroptic mange. *E,* Crusts, scale, and focal ulcers over the dorsum of a rabbit with cheyletiellosis (area has been clipped). *F,* Frostbite in a rabbit. Note acrocyanosis and necrosis of the pinna. *G,* Orange-colored crust and discoloration of the hair around the eye of a rat with sialodacryoadenitis virus infection. (Courtesy J. King.) *H,* Extensive alopecia, erythema, crusting, and thickening of the skin of a rat with notoedric mange. (Courtesy E. Guaguère.)

the external genitalia. Pruritus is intense. Severe infestations can lead to anorexia, lethargy, emaciation, and death. These mites can transiently produce lesions in humans. Diagnosis is confirmed by finding *S. scabiei* mites in skin scrapings. However, mites are often difficult to demonstrate, and response to therapy is a frequently used diagnostic test. The treatment of choice is ivermectin.[5, 33, 261, 262, 280]

C. parasitovorax, a nonburrowing mite, is a common ectoparasite on rabbits.* Most rabbits harbor the mites without overt signs of skin disease. With heavy infestations or in hypersensitive hosts, a variably pruritic dermatosis is seen. Lesions consist of scaling, crusting, and variable degrees of erythema, alopecia, and greasiness over the withers, the back (Fig. 20:19 *E*), and the ventral abdomen. Occasionally, lesions are limited to the face.[237] These mites can produce skin lesions in humans. Diagnosis is confirmed by finding *C. parasitovorax* in skin scrapings or acetate tape preparations. The treatment of choice is ivermectin.

Listrophorus gibbus is a common fur mite of rabbits, which is rarely associated with clinical skin disease.† Most affected rabbits are asymptomatic. The mite is usually found attached to hair shafts, especially on the back, the groin, and the ventral abdomen. Occasional rabbits may manifest a variably pruritic, scaly, erythematous, alopecic dermatitis in the aforementioned sites. Some animals only manifest pruritus and traumatic alopecia with no skin lesions.[263a] Diagnosis is confirmed by finding *L. gibbus* in skin scrapings and acetate tape preparations. Treatment with pyrethrin- or pyrethroid-containing flea powders, 1 per cent selenium sulfide baths, or 2 per cent lime sulfur dips is curative.

Notoedres cati, a burrowing mite, is a rare ectoparasite on rabbits.‡ Clinical signs, diagnosis, and treatment are identical to those described for *S. scabiei.*

Fleas (especially *C. felis felis*) are occasionally found on rabbits, especially those in households with dogs and cats.‡ In the United States, rabbits may also be infested with *Cediopsylla simplex* (common Eastern rabbit flea), especially around the head and the neck, and *Odontopsyllus multispinosis* (giant Eastern rabbit flea), especially over the rump. Clinical signs, diagnosis, and therapy are as described for cats.

The rabbit sucking louse, *Haemodipsus ventricosus,* is uncommon in the United States.§ Pediculosis is usually associated with poor management. Lice are most commonly found on the dorsum and may produce intense pruritus. Severe infestations in debilitated animals may produce anemia, weakness, emaciation, and death. *H. ventricosus* is a vector of tularemia. Therapy is as described for cats.

Demodex cuniculi mites have been isolated from rabbits with generalized pruritus and scaling, but their pathogenic significance is in doubt.[253]

Members of the fly genus *Cuterebra* occasionally produce myiasis in domestic rabbits reared outdoors or in nonscreened enclosures.¶ Among those fly species reported in the United States are *Cuterebra cuniculi,* *C. buccata,* and *C. horripilum.* Larvae and, therefore, lesions appear in the summer and early fall. The incidence of infestation decreases with age, which correlates with the development of immediate and delayed-type hypersensitivity reactions to larval antigens.[5, 282, 284] *C. horripilum* prefers the ventral cervical region, whereas *C. buccata* larvae localize in the interscapular, axillary, inguinal, or rump area. Initial lesions include subcutaneous cystlike structures. As the larvae (warbles) enlarge, a ''breathing hole,'' or fistula, is produced. The surrounding haircoat is moist and matted, secondary bacterial infection is common, and the lesions are often painful. Treatment consists of surgical removal of the larvae (one should not crush or otherwise damage the larvae), routine wound care, and occasionally, administration of systemic antibiotics. Prevention and control are aimed at eliminating contact with the warble fly.

---

*See references 2–5, 10, 12, 13, 15–18, 28, 33, 235–237, 244, 252, 254a, and 284.
†See references 2–5, 10, 12, 15–18, 28, 33, 244, 252, 263a, 284, and 285.
‡See references 2–5, 10, 12, 15–18, 28, 33, 252, and 284.
§See references 2–5, 10, 15–18, 28, 33, 252, and 284.
¶See references 2–5, 10, 12–17, 252, 257, and 284.

Nutritional Disorders

Nutritional deficiencies are unlikely to be encountered in pet rabbits. Experimental production of nutritional deficiencies with resultant cutaneous abnormalities have been reported and are briefly presented here. Copper deficiency results in alopecia and a depigmented haircoat.[2, 275] Zinc deficiency produces alopecia, scaling, and a depigmented haircoat.[2, 274]

Miscellaneous Conditions

Several days before parturition, the female rabbit undergoes a generalized loosening of the fur.* The female rabbit pulls out mouthfuls of hair to line the nest. Hair loss is especially prominent on the abdomen and the chest. Some rabbits pull out fur as a behavioral vice.[2, 17] Other rabbits rub fur off against the cage surface or feeders.[17] Seasonal molts can result in haircoat irregularities and thinning.[17]

Hereditary alopecias (Fig. 20:20) are rarely described in rabbits[7] but are unlikely to be seen by practitioners.

Cutaneous asthenia was reported in two, 4-month-old New Zealand white rabbit siblings (male and female) (Fig. 20:21).[254] The animals had a history of repeated spontaneous skin tears and were covered with scars. The skin extensibility index (see Chap. 11) was 21 to 32 per cent in the affected rabbits as compared with a mean of 13 per cent in normal rabbits. Light microscopic examination was unremarkable, but electron microscopic examination revealed distorted and tangled collagen bundles with collagen fibrils being of different diameters and having a loose, frayed appearance.

Hutch burn is a contact dermatitis caused by urine scalding of the perineal region because of an unclean environment or an inability of the rabbit to void urine without soiling itself, such as after an orthopedic or neurologic injury.[3] Washing the area frequently with antimicrobial agents and applying a protectant cream, such as zinc oxide, are helpful.

Frostbite may be seen in rabbits that are suddenly exposed to cold climates without a period of acclimatization. Erythema, acrocyanosis, necrosis, and sloughing are typically seen on the pinna (see Fig. 20:19 *F*).

Both male and female rabbits possess two sebaceous scent glands on either side of the

---

*See references 2, 3, 5, 12, 17, 271, and 284.

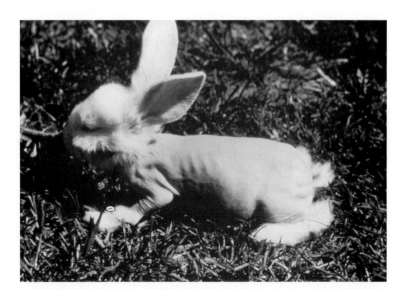

Figure 20:20. Congenital alopecia in a rabbit. (Courtesy J. Gourreau.)

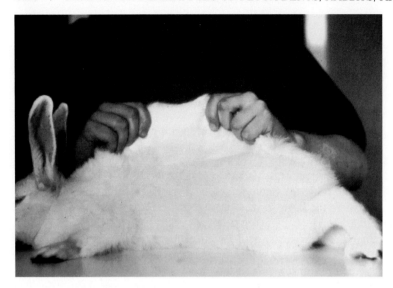

Figure 20:21. Hyperextensibility of the skin in a rabbit with cutaneous asthenia. (Courtesy R. Harvey.)

vulvar or testicular area that secrete a brown waxy debris.[3] This secretion can build up and can be easily removed by gentle traction or soap and water.

Facial eczema has been reported in young suckling rabbits.[18] The condition is sporadic and of unknown etiology. Areas of alopecia and slight erythema occur on the bridge of the nose and the periocular region. Affected animals are otherwise healthy. The condition responds rapidly to topical glucocorticoid therapy.

Neoplasia

Spontaneous nonviral cutaneous neoplasms are rare in rabbits.* Papilloma, basal cell carcinoma, squamous cell carcinoma, sebaceous carcinoma, osteosarcoma, and lymphoma have been reported.†

Shope papillomas are uncommon in domestic rabbits.‡ In the United States, the disease occurs in the Southwest and along the Mississippi River. Shope papilloma virus (a papovavirus) commonly infects wild rabbits, with insects serving as vectors. Lesions are characterized by multiple hornlike growths from a single site, especially about the eyelids and the pinnae. Removal of the papillomas usually results in healing, and recovered rabbits are resistant to reinfection. Spontaneous regression of lesions occurs within 12 months. Experimental infection of domestic rabbits resulted in malignant transformation to squamous cell carcinoma within 8 to 9 months in a high percentage of the inoculation sites. A program of screening animal enclosures and vector control should be instituted in endemic areas.

Shope fibromas are uncommon in domestic rabbits.§ Shope fibroma virus (a poxvirus) commonly infects wild rabbits in North and South America and is transmitted via insect vectors. Lesions consist of single or multiple flat, firm, subcutaneous nodules, especially on the genitals, the perineum, the ventral abdomen, the paw, the nose, the pinna, and the eyelid. Newborn rabbits are more susceptible than are older animals and have more extensive lesions. Experimentally infected adult rabbits often show spontaneous involution of their fibromas within 5 months through necrosis and sloughing. Mosquito eradication and enclosure screening is indicated to prevent infection in endemic areas.

*See references 2, 3, 5, 17, 20, 252, and 284.
†See references 2, 5, 17, 20, 252, 255, 256, 268, and 284.
‡See references 2, 3, 5, 12, 16–18, 252, and 284.
§See references 2, 3, 5, 16–18, 252, 258, 269, and 284.

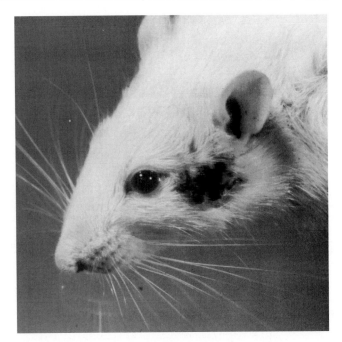

Figure 20:22. Staphylococcal dermatitis caudal to the eye in a rat. (Courtesy J. King).

■ RAT

Bacterial Infections

Bacterial skin infections are uncommon in pet rats, are usually caused by *S. aureus,* and are secondary to trauma (cage-related injuries and bite wounds) or self-inflicted (the pruritus associated with ectoparasites).* Rats are more resistant to experimental wound infection with *S. aureus* than are mice or hamsters.[9, 306] Infections resulting from cage-related injury are typically seen on the nose and the muzzle, whereas those associated with bite wounds typically occur around the head (Fig. 20:22), the tail, the rump, and the perineal area. Staphylococcal dermatitis may be superficial (alopecia, erythema, oozing, and crust) or deep (abscess, fistula, necrosis, and ulcer) and is usually nonpruritic. Other bacteria occasionally isolated from cutaneous abscesses and pyogranulomas in rats include *Streptococcus* sp., *P. pneumotropica, Klebsiella pneumoniae, P. aeruginosa,* and *Mycobacterium lepraemurium* (rat leprosy).†

Treatment of bacterial dermatitis includes some combination of elimination of predisposing causes, surgical drainage, daily topical cleaning with 3 per cent hydrogen peroxide or 0.5 to 1 per cent chlorhexidine, and systemic antibiotic administration (see Table 20:1).

S. moniliformis is a rare cause of epizootics of edema and cyanosis of the extremities.[2, 17, 318]

C. kutscheri (murium) is a rare cause of epizootics of furunculosis and cutaneous pyogranulomas, which may progress to necrosis and sloughing of extremities.[2, 17]

Fungal Infections

Dermatophytosis is rare in rats and is usually associated with *T. mentagrophytes.*‡ This dermatophyte can be isolated from the haircoat of clinically normal rats and is a potential zoonotic agent. Lesions are most commonly seen on the neck, the back, and the base of the tail and consist of annular areas of alopecia, broken hairs, scales, and variable degrees of erythema and

---

*See references 2–5, 12, 17, 18, 28, 31, 33, 36, 290, 291, 304, 309, 323, and 335.
†See references 2, 12, 17, 18, 314, 334, and 337.
‡See references 1–5, 8, 12, 16, 17, 21, 23, 28, 31, 33, 37, and 327.

crusting. Pruritus is usually minimal to absent. Diagnosis and treatment are as described for guinea pigs.

Viral Infections

Sialodacryoadenitis virus (a coronavirus) infection causes eye rubbing and scratching, periorbital swelling, and red tears (chromodacryorrhea) (see Fig. 20:19 G).[2, 4, 17, 298]

Poxvirus infection has been described in laboratory white rats.[320] Skin lesions consisted of erythematous papules, which became crusted and occurred mainly on the glabrous areas of the body (tail, paws, and muzzle). Sometimes, the affected portions of paws and tail underwent necrosis and sloughing. Diagnosis was confirmed by biopsy, electron microscopy, and viral isolation.

Ectoparasites

N. muris occasionally causes a severely pruritic dermatitis in rats.* Lesions are most commonly present on the pinnae, the nose, the paws, and the ventrum and consist of erythema, papules, yellowish hyperkeratotic crusts, and excoriations (see Fig. 20:19 *H*). Diagnosis is confirmed by skin scrapings. Treatment is accomplished with topical 2 per cent lime sulfur dips (once weekly until 2 weeks after cure) or subcutaneous injections of ivermectin.

Other mites that are rarely found on rats include *Radfordia ensifera*, *O. bacoti* (tropical rat mite), *S. scabiei*, *T. caviae*, *M. musculi*, and *Demodex* sp.†

Fleas (especially *C. felis felis*) may be recovered from pet rats maintained in households frequented by cats and dogs.[2–5, 12, 17]

The sucking louse, *Polyplax spinulosa*, is occasionally found on pet rats.‡ Some animals may be asymptomatic carriers, and other animals manifest varying degrees of dermatitis and pruritus. Young animals, debilitated animals, and animals in poor management situations are more likely to be affected. Lice and related dermatoses are most commonly found on the neck and back. Treatment can be accomplished with topical insecticides or ivermectin injections.

Nutritional Disorders

Nutritional deficiencies are unlikely to be encountered in pet rats. Experimental production of nutritional deficiencies with resultant cutaneous abnormalities has been reported, and these are briefly mentioned here. Zinc deficiency produces exfoliative dermatitis, alopecia, and depigmentation of the haircoat.[2, 11, 35] Pantothenic acid deficiency results in exfoliative dermatitis, depigmentation of the haircoat, and excessive harderian gland activity with increased porphyrin secretion resulting in red tears and blood-caked whiskers.[2, 292] Riboflavin deficiency produces alopecia, scaling, and dermatitis, especially on the extremities.[2] Pyridoxine deficiency results in exfoliative dermatitis, especially on the face, the ears, the limbs, and the tail.[2, 295, 305] Biotin deficiency causes exfoliative dermatitis and periocular alopecia.[2, 321] Niacin deficiency causes alopecia and excessive harderian gland activity, increased porphyrin secretion, and blood-caked whiskers.[2, 317] Essential fatty acid deficiency produces an exfoliative dermatitis and, occasionally, necrosis of the tail.[2, 29, 34] Protein deficiency causes alopecia, exfoliative dermatitis, and depigmentation of the haircoat.[2, 322]

Miscellaneous Conditions

Barbering and bite wounds are frequently seen when rats are housed together.§ These behaviors can be exacerbated by crowding, stress, and boredom. Areas most commonly affected include

---

*See references 2–5, 10, 12, 16, 17, 28, 33, 36, and 303.
†See references 2, 3, 5, 10, 28, 31, 33, 36, 91, 128, and 336.
‡See references 2, 3, 5, 10, 12, 16–18, 28, 31, 33, 36, and 328.
§See references 2–5, 12, 17, 36, 294, and 296.

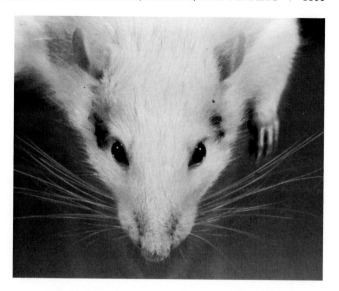

Figure 20:23. Bite wounds behind each eye in a rat. (Courtesy J. King.)

the muzzle, the whiskers, the face, the head (Fig. 20:23), the rump, the tail, and the perineum. Rats may also rub the hair off the muzzle as they stick their face through slotted feeders or wire bars.[290]

Rats have numerous types of hereditary hairlessness that are probably never seen by the practitioner (Fig. 20:24).*

Ringtail is a poorly understood condition seen in rats.† The incidence of the disorder increases as the relative humidity falls below 40 per cent and is especially common in young unweaned animals housed in cages with wire mesh bottoms, on hygroscopic bedding, and in rooms with excessive ventilation. In the northern hemisphere, most cases are seen from November to May, when heating systems often cause marked reductions in relative humidity. Some strains of rats seem more susceptible than others. The condition usually occurs after 2 months of reduced relative humidity. One or more annular constrictions develop in the tail, which becomes edematous, inflamed, and necrose distal to the constrictions (Fig. 20:25). Ringtail is prevented by maintaining a relative humidity of at least 50 per cent.

Perianal pruritus is seen in association with pinworms (Syphacia muris).‡ Infected rats occasionally mutilate the base of the tail. Diagnosis is confirmed by microscopic examination of strips of cellophane (Scotch) tape that have been applied to the perineum. The eggs of *S. muris* are banana shaped and about 30 μm by 150 μm. Ivermectin is effective treatment.

Auricular chondritis has been described in rats.[321a] The condition has occurred spontaneously and in association with the placement of metal ear tags or immunization with type II collagen. Typically, both ears are affected, although one ear may be affected days to weeks before the other. The pinnae are swollen, erythematous, and nodular, and they become thickened and deformed. Pain and pruritus are rare. Histologically, there is a multifocal granulomatous chondritis with progressive destruction of cartilage.

Systemic hair embolism has been reported subsequent to intravenous injections in rats.[317a] Cutaneous lesions consist of focal areas of necrosis and ulceration on the ventral aspect of the body. Histologic examination reveals granulomatous and necrotizing dermatitis and panniculitis, and intravascular hair shaft fragments.

The fur of the aged rat frequently turns yellow and becomes more coarse.[5] The cause is unknown.

*See references 6, 7, 299, 302, 311–313, 325, 326, 329, 330, and 334.
†See references 2–6, 12, 17, 18, 36, 300, 324, and 333.
‡See references 2, 4, 10, 12, 17, 32, 33, 36, and 293.

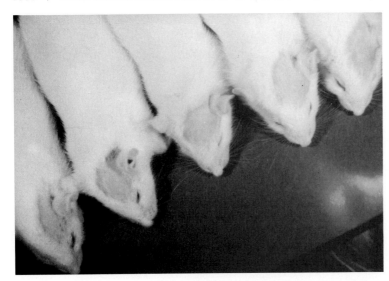

Figure 20:24. Congenital alopecia in a litter of rats. (Courtesy J. King.)

Figure 20:25. Ringtail in a rat. Necrosis of the distal portion of the tail. (Courtesy G. Kollias.)

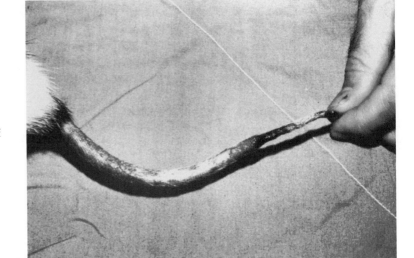

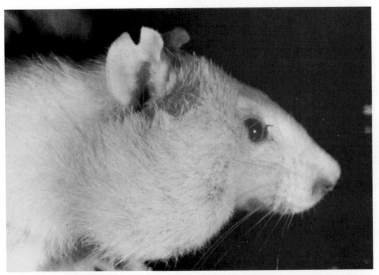

Figure 20:26. Large subcutaneous fibrosarcoma in the ventral neck of a rat. (Courtesy J. King.)

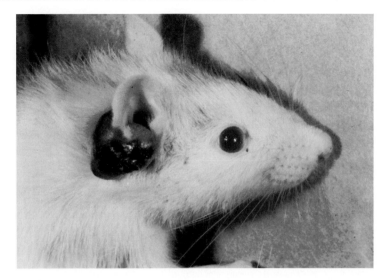

Figure 20:27. Large squamous cell carcinoma in the pinna of a rat. (Courtesy J. King.)

Neoplasia

Spontaneous cutaneous neoplasms are uncommon in rats.* Mesenchymal neoplasms are more common than are epithelial neoplasms. The most common are fibromas, fibrosarcomas (Fig. 20:26), and lipomas. The face, the shoulder, the flank, the tail, and the paws are typically affected. Other reported skin neoplasms in rats include papilloma, keratoacanthoma, sebaceous gland tumors, squamous cell carcinoma (Fig. 20:27), basal cell carcinoma, hair follicle tumors, hemangiosarcoma, melanoma, and malignant fibrous histiocytoma.

REFERENCES

1. Balsari, A., et al.: Dermatophytes in clinically healthy laboratory animals. Lab. Anim. 15:75, 1981.
2. Benirschke, K., et al.: Pathology of Laboratory Animals. Springer Verlag, New York, 1978.
3. Burgmann, P.: Dermatology of rabbits, rodents, and ferrets. In: Nesbitt, G.H., Ackerman, L.J. (eds.). Dermatology for the Small Animal Practitioner. Veterinary Learning Systems Co., Trenton, NJ, 1991, p. 205.
4. Burke, T.J.: Skin disorders of rodents, rabbits, and ferrets. In: Kirk, R.W., Bonagura, J.D. (eds.). Current Veterinary Therapy XI. W.B. Saunders Co., Philadelphia, 1992, p. 1170.
5. Collins, B.R.: Dermatologic disorders of common small nondomestic animals. In: Nesbitt, G.H. (ed.). Dermatology. Churchill Livingstone, New York, 1987, p. 235.
6. Cotchin, E., Row, F.J.C.: Pathology of Laboratory Rats and Mice. Blackwell Scientific Publications, Oxford, 1967.
7. David, L.T.: The external expression and comparative dermal histology of hereditary hairlessness in mammals. Z. Zellforsch. Mikrosk. Anat. 14:616, 1932.
8. Dolan, M.M., et al.: Ringworm epizootics in laboratory mice and rats: Experimental and accidental transmission of infection. J. Invest. Dermatol. 30:23, 1958.
9. Donnelly, T.M., Stark, D.M.: Susceptibility of laboratory rats, hamsters, and mice to wound infection with *Staphylococcus aureus*. Am. J. Vet. Res. 46:2634, 1985.
10. Flynn, R.J.: Parasites of Laboratory Animals. Iowa State University Press, Ames, IA, 1973.
11. Forbes, R.M.: Use of laboratory animals to define physiological functions and bioavailability of zinc. Fed. Proc. 43:2835, 1984.
12. Fox, J.G., et al.: Laboratory Animal Medicine. Academic Press, Orlando, FL, 1984.
13. Geary, M.: *Cheyletiella* mites in rabbits and guinea pigs. Vet. Dermatol. Newsl. 1:6, 1976.
14. Gibson, T.E.: Parasites of laboratory animals transmissible to man. Lab. Anim. 1:17, 1967.
15. Griffiths, H.J.: Some common parasites of small laboratory animals. Lab. Anim. 5:123, 1971.
16. Guittin, P.: Médecine des lapins et rongeurs de compagnie. Rec. Méd. Vét. 162:363, 1986.
17. Harkness, J.E., Wagner, J.E.: The Biology and Medicine of Rabbits and Rodents III. Lea & Febiger, Philadelphia, 1989.
17a. Harkness, J.E.: Small rodents. Vet. Clin. North Am. (Small Anim. Pract.) 24:89, 1994.
18. Hime, J.M., O'Donoghue, P.N.: Handbook of Diseases of Laboratory Animals. Heinemann Veterinary Books, London, 1979.
19. Jacobson, E.R., Kollias, G.V.: Exotic Animals. Churchill Livingstone, New York, 1988.
20. Kaiser, H.E.: Neoplasms—Comparative Pathology of Growth in Animals, Plants, and Man. Williams & Wilkins Co., Baltimore, 1981.

*See references 2, 3, 5, 6, 12, 17, 20, 26, 307, 308, 310, 316, 319, and 331.

21. Kaplan, W., et al.: Recent developments on animal ringworm and their public health implications. Ann. N. Y. Acad. Sci. 70:177, 1958.
22. Keefe, T.J., et al.: *Ornithonyssus bacoti* infestation in mouse and hamster colonies. Lab. Anim. Care 14:366, 1964.
23. Lopez-Martinez, R., et al.: Dermatophytes isolated from laboratory animals. Mycopathologia 88:111, 1984.
23a. Marzulli, F.N., Maibach, H.I.: Dermatotoxicology and Pharmacology. John Wiley & Sons, New York, 1977.
24. McKellar, Q.A., et al.: Clinical and pharmacological properties of ivermectin in rabbits and guinea pigs. Vet. Rec. 130:71, 1992.
25. Nelson, J.B.: The problems of disease and quality in laboratory animals. J. Med. Educ. 35:34, 1960.
26. Ribelin, W.E., McCoy, J.R.: Pathology of Laboratory Animals. Charles C Thomas, Springfield, IL, 1965.
27. Rountree, P.M., et al.: Nasal carriage of *Staphylococcus aureus* by various domestic and laboratory animals. J. Pathol. Bacteriol. 72:319, 1956.
28. Schuchman, S.M.: Individual care and treatment of rabbits, mice, rats, guinea pigs, hamsters, and gerbils. In: Kirk, R.W. (ed.). Current Veterinary Therapy X. W.B. Saunders Co., Philadelphia, 1989, p. 738.
29. Sinclair, H.M.: Essential fatty acids in perspective. Hum. Nutr. Clin. Nutr. 38C:245, 1984.
30. Sokolov, V.E.: Mammal Skin. University of California Press, Berkeley, 1982.
30a. Soulsby, E.J.L: Helminths, Arthropods, and Protozoa of Domesticated Animals VII. Lea & Febiger, Philadelphia, 1982.
31. Sparrow, S.: Diseases of pet rodents. J. Small Anim. Pract. 21:1, 1980.
32. Taffs, L.F.: Pinworm infections in laboratory rodents: A review. Lab. Anim. 10:1, 1976.
33. Timm, K.I.: Pruritus in rabbits, rodents, and ferrets. Vet. Clin. North Am. (Small Anim. Pract.) 18:1077, 1988.
34. Tinoco, J.: Dietary requirements and functions of α-linolenic acid in animals. Prog. Lipid Res. 21:1, 1982.
35. Underwood, E.J.: Trace Elements in Human and Animal Nutrition IV. Academic Press, New York, 1977.
36. Wagner, J.E., Farrar, P.L.: Husbandry and medicine of small rodents. Vet. Clin. North Am. (Small Anim. Pract.) 17:1061, 1987.

Chinchilla

36a. Hoefer, H.L.: Chinchillas. Vet. Clin. North Am. (Small Anim. Pract.) 24:103, 1994.
37. Morganti, L., et al.: *Microsporum gypseum* infection in chinchillas. Sabouraudia 8:39, 1970.
38. Rees, R.G.: Some conditions of the skin and fur of *Chinchilla lanigera.* J. Small Anim. Pract. 4:213, 1963.
39. Zeinert, K.: Husbandry of chinchillas. Vet. Med. (S.A.C.) 78:1292, 1983.

Ferret

40. Bernard, S.L., et al.: Estrogen-induced bone marrow depression in ferrets. Am. J. Vet. Res. 44:657, 1983.
41. Besch-Williford, C.L.: Biology and medicine of the ferret. Vet. Clin. North Am. (Small Anim. Pract.) 17:1155, 1987.
41a. Brandt, F.W., Eberhard, M.L.: Distribution, behavior, and course of patency of *Dracunculus insignis* in experimentally infected ferrets. J. Parasitol. 76:515, 1990.
42. Brown, S.A.: Management of adrenal and pancreatic neoplasia in the ferret. Proc. Eastern States Vet. Conf. 5:580, 1991.
43. Cooper, J.E.: Skin diseases of ferrets. Vet. Ann. 30:325, 1990.
44. Dillberger, J.E., et al.: Neoplasia in ferrets: 11 cases and a review. J. Comp. Pathol. 100:162, 1989.
44a. Eberhard, M.L., et al.: Chemoprophylactic drug trials for treatment of dracunculiasis using the *Dracunculus insignis*–ferret model. J. Helminthol. 64:79, 1990.
45. Fox, J.G.: Biology and Diseases of the Ferret. Lea & Febiger, Philadelphia, 1988.
46. Garibaldi, B.A., et al.: Serum thyroxine (T4) and tri-iodothyronine (T3) radioimmunoassay values in the normal ferret. Lab. Anim. Sci. 38:455, 1988.
47. Garibaldi, B.A., et al.: Serum cortisol radioimmunoassay values in the normal ferret and response to ACTH and dexamethasone suppression tests. Lab. Anim. Sci. 38:452, 1988.
48. Hamilton, T.A., et al.: Bleomycin chemotherapy for metastatic squamous cell carcinoma in a ferret. J. Am. Vet. Med. Assoc. 198:107, 1991.
49. Heard, D.J., et al.: Thyroid and adrenal function tests in adult male ferrets. Am. J. Vet. Res. 51:32, 1990.
50. Hendrick, M., Goldschmidt, M.H.: Chondrosarcoma of the tail of ferrets *(Mustela putorius furo).* Vet. Pathol. 24:272, 1987.
51. Hillyer, E.: Ferret endocrinology. In: Kirk, R.W., Bonagura, J.D. (eds.). Current Veterinary Therapy XI. W.B. Saunders Co., Philadelphia, 1992, p. 1185.
52. Jenkins, J.R.: Multiple concurrent neoplasia and metabolic diseases in the ferret: Selected cases. Proc. Eastern States Vet. Conf. 5:582, 1991.
53. Kociba, G.J., Caputo, C.A.: Aplastic anemia associated with estrus in pet ferrets. J. Am. Vet. Med. Assoc. 178:1293, 1981.
54. Kuper, D.S., Bauck, L.: Hyperadrenocorticism in a ferret: Diagnosis (using ultrasound) and treatment. J. Small Exotic Anim. Med. 1:66, 1991.
54a. Lawrence, H.J., et al.: Unilateral adrenalectomy as a treatment for adrenocortical tumors in ferrets: Five cases (1990–1992). J. Am. Vet. Med. Assoc. 203:267, 1993.
55. Lenhard, A.: Blastomycosis in a ferret. J. Am. Vet. Med. Assoc. 186:70, 1985.
55a. Lipman, N.S., et al.: Estradiol-17β–secreting adrenocortical tumor in a ferret. J. Am. Vet. Med. Assoc. 203:1552, 1993.
56. Miller, T.A., et al.: Recurrent adenocarcinoma in a ferret. J. Am. Vet. Med. Assoc. 187:829, 1985.
57. Mor, N., et al.: Concurrent mammary gland hyperplasia and adrenocortical carcinoma in a domestic ferret. J. Am. Vet. Med. Assoc. 201:1911, 1992.

58. Nie, I.A., Pick, C.R.: Infestation of a colony of ferrets with ear mites *(Otodectes cynotis)* and its control. J. Inst. Anim. Techn. 29:63, 1978.

59. Olsen, G.H.: Disseminated cutaneous squamous cell carcinoma in a ferret. J. Am. Vet. Med. Assoc. 186:702, 1985.

60. Paradis, M.: Guide du furet domestique. Méd. Vét. Québec 17:63, 1987.

61. Paradis, M., et al.: Hyperadrenocorticism in association with an adrenocortical adenoma in a pet ferret. Can. Vet. J. 30:60, 1989.

61a. Parker, G.A., Picut, C.A.: Histopathologic features and post-surgical sequelae of 57 cutaneous neoplasms in ferrets (mustelaputorius furo L.). Vet. Pathol. 30:499, 1993.

62. Poonacha, K.B., et al.: Cutaneous mastocytoma in a ferret. J. Am. Vet. Med. Assoc. 185:442, 1984.

63. Rosenthal, K.L., et al.: Evaluation of plasma cortisol and corticosterone responses to synthetic adrenocorticotropic hormone administration in ferrets. Am. J. Vet. Res. 54:29, 1993.

63a. Rosenthal, K.L., et al.: Hyperadrenocorticism associated with adrenocortical tumor or nodular hyperplasia of the adrenal gland in ferrets: 50 cases (1987–1991). J. Am. Vet. Med. Assoc. 203:271, 1993.

63b. Rosenthal, K.L.: Ferrets. Vet. Clin. North Am. (Small Anim. Pract.) 24:1, 1994.

64. Ryland, L.M., Gorham, J.R.: The ferret and its diseases. J. Am. Vet. Med. Assoc. 173:1154, 1978.

65. Ryland, L.M.: Remission of estrus-associated anemia following ovariohysterectomy and multiple blood transfusions in a ferret. J. Am. Vet. Med. Assoc. 181:820, 1982.

66. Ryland, L.M., et al.: A clinical guide to the pet ferret. Comp. Cont. Educ. 5:25, 1983.

67. Scott, D.W., et al.: Bilaterally symmetric alopecia associated with an adrenocortical adenoma in a pet ferret. Vet. Dermatol. 2:165, 1991.

68. Sherrill, A., Gorham, J.R.: Bone marrow hypoplasia associated with estrus in ferrets. Lab. Anim. Sci. 35:280, 1985.

69. Skulski, G., Symmers, W.S.C.: Actinomycosis and torulosis in the ferret. J. Comp. Pathol. 64:306, 1954.

Gerbil

69a. Benit, K.F., Kramer, A.W.: Spontaneous tumors in the Mongolian gerbil. Lab. Anim. Care 15:281, 1965.

70. Bresnahan, J.F., et al.: Nasal dermatitis and the Mongolian gerbil. Lab. Anim. Sci. 33:258, 1983.

71. Cramlet, S.H., et al.: Malignant melanoma in a black gerbil *(Meriones unguiculatus)*. Lab. Anim. Sci. 24:545, 1974.

72. Handler, A.H., et al.: Oncogenic studies on the Mongolian gerbil. Cancer Res. 26:844, 1966.

73. Meckley, P.E., Zwicker, G.M.: Naturally-occurring neoplasms in the Mongolian gerbil, *Meriones unguiculatus*. Lab. Anim. 13:203, 1979.

74. Peckham, J.C., et al.: Staphylococcal dermatitis in Mongolian gerbils *(Meriones unguiculatus)*. Lab. Anim. Sci. 24:43, 1974.

75. Ringler, D.H., et al.: Spontaneous neoplasms in aging *Gerbillinae*. Lab. Anim. Sci. 22:231, 1972.

76. Schwartzbrott, S.S., et al.: Demodicosis in the Mongolian gerbil *(Meriones unguiculatus):* A case report. Lab. Anim. Sci. 24:666, 1974.

76a. Schwentker, V.: Care and Maintenance of the Mongolian Gerbil. Tumblebrook Farm, Brant Lake, N.Y. 1967.

76b. Solomon, H.F., et al.: A survey of staphylococci isolated from the laboratory gerbil. Lab. Anim. Sci. 40:316, 1990.

77. Thiessen, D.D., et al.: Harderian gland involvement in facial lesions in the Mongolian gerbil. J. Am. Vet. Med. Assoc. 181:1375, 1982.

77a. Vincent, A.L., Ash, L.R.: Further observations on spontaneous neoplasms in the Mongolian gerbil *(Meriones unguiculatus)*. Lab. Anim. Sci. 28:297, 1978.

77b. Williams, W.M.: The Anatomy of the Mongolian Gerbil *(Meriones unguiculatus)*. Tumblebrook Farm, Brant Lake, N.Y. 1974.

Guinea Pig

78. Aldred, P., et al.: The isolation of *Streptobacillus moniliformis* from the cervical abscesses of guinea pigs. Lab. Anim. 8:275, 1974.

79. Bacigalupo, J., et al.: *Demodex caviae* n. sp. Rev. Med. Vet. Buenos Aires 36:149, 1954.

80. Bagnall, B.: Nematode dermatitis in guinea pigs. Vet. Dermatol. Newsl. 1:7, 1976.

81. Bishop, L.M.: Study of an outbreak of pseudotuberculosis in guinea pigs (cavies) due to *B. pseudotuberculosis rodentium*. Cornell Vet. 22:1, 1932.

82. Bobrowski, P.J., et al.: Latent herpes simplex virus reactivation in the guinea pig. An animal model for recurrent disease. Int. J. Dermatol. 30:29, 1991.

83. Bourdeau, P.: Quel est votre diagnostic? Point Vét. 19:275, 1987.

84. Bourdeau, P., Guaguère, E.: Vrai et faux parasitisme chez un cobaye atteint de dermatose. Point Vét. 19:155, 1987.

85. Bourdeau, P., Guaguère, E.: La gale du cobaye à *Trixacarus (Caviacoptes) caviae*. A propos d'un cas avec contaminations humaines. Rec. Méd. Vét. 161:397, 1985.

86. Clifford, D.R.: What the practicing veterinarian should know about guinea pigs. Vet. Med. (S.A.C.) 68:678, 1973.

87. Cooper, G., Schiller, A.L.: Anatomy of the Guinea Pig. Harvard University Press, Cambridge, MA, 1975.

87a. Culley, D.: Poxvirus as a cause of cheilitis in the guinea pig. Vet. Dermatol. News. 15:15, 1993.

88. Dorrenstein, G.M., et al.: *Trixacarus caviae (Acari: Sarcoptidae)* as a cause of mange in guinea pigs and papular urticaria in man. Vet. Parasitol. 5:389, 1979.

89. Ediger, R.D., et al.: Trichofolliculoma of the guinea pig. J. Natl. Cancer Inst. 46:517, 1971.

90. Ediger, R.O., Kovatch, R.M.: Spontaneous tumors in the Dankin-Hartley guinea pig. J. Natl. Cancer Inst. 56:293, 1976.
91. Enigk, K., et al.: Die *Sarcoptesräude* des Goldhamsters. Z. Parasitenkd. 15:25, 1961.
92. Fuentes, C.A., et al.: *Trichophyton mentagrophytes* from apparently healthy guinea pigs. Arch. Dermatol. Syphilol. 71:478, 1955.
93. Gentles, J.C.: Experimental ringworm in guinea pigs: Oral treatment with griseofulvin. Nature 182:476, 1958.
94. Gip, L., et al.: Occurrence of *Trichophyton mentagrophytes* var. *asteroides* on hairs of guinea pigs without ringworm lesions. Acta Dermatovenereol. 44:208, 1964.
95. Häfeli, W.: Demodikose beim Meerschweinchen. Kleintier-Prax. 34:337, 1989.
96. Harvey, R.G.: Use of ivermectin for guinea pig mange. Vet. Rec. 120:351, 1987.
97. Hunt, L.M.: Guinea pig—*Amblyomma americanum* animal systemic insecticide test. Proc. Entomol. Soc. Am. 7:253, 1983.
98. Ishihara, C.: An exfoliative skin disease in guinea pigs due to *Staphylococcus aureus*. Lab. Anim. Sci. 30:552, 1980.
99. Jornet-Boullery, M., Bourdeau, P.: Le cobaye. 2ᵉ partie: Pathologie. Point Vét. 18:141, 1986.
100. Kamun, J.: Incidence and morphology of the thymus in hairless guinea pigs. Acta Vet. Brno. 56:19, 1987.
101. Kitchen, D.N., et al.: A report of 14 spontaneous tumors of the guinea pig. Lab. Anim. Sci.. 25:92, 1975.
102. Kummel, B.A., et al.: *Trixacarus caviae* infestation of guinea pigs. J. Am. Vet. Med. Assoc. 177:903, 1980.
103. Lee, K.J., et al.: Prepucial dermatitis in male guinea pigs *(Cavia porcellus)*. Lab. Anim. Sci. 28:99, 1978.
104. Menges, R.W., et al.: An epizootic of ringworm among guinea pigs caused by *Trichophyton mentagrophytes*. J. Am. Vet. Med. Assoc. 128:495, 1956.
105. Menges, R.W., et al.: Therapeutic studies on ringworm infected guinea pigs. J. Invest. Dermatol. 28:233, 1957.
106. Peters, L.J.: The guinea pig: An overview part II. Comp. Cont. Educ. 3:403, 1981.
107. Pombier, E.C., et al.: An epizootic outbreak of ringworm in a guinea pig colony caused by *Trichophyton mentagrophytes*. Lab. Anim. 9:215, 1975.
108. Post, K., Saunders, T.R.: Topical treatment of experimental ringworm in guinea pigs with griseofulvin in dimethylsulfoxide. Can. Vet. J. 20:45, 1979.
108a. Quesenberry, K.E.: Guinea pigs. Vet. Clin. North Am. (Small Anim. Pract.) 24:67, 1994.
109. Reed, C., et al.: A new guinea pig mutant with abnormal hair production and immunodeficiency. Lab. Anim. Sci. 29:744, 1979.
110. Reid, M.E., Von Sallmann, L.: Nutritional studies with the guinea pig. VI. Tryptophan with ample dietary niacin. J. Nutr. 70:329, 1960.
111. Reid, M.E., Martin, M.G.: Nutritional studies with the guinea pig. V. Effects of deficiency of fat or unsaturated fatty acids. J. Nutr. 67:611, 1959.
112. Reid, M.E.: Nutritional studies with the guinea pig. XI. Pyroxidine. Proc. Soc. Exp. Biol. Med. 116:289, 1964.
113. Richardson, V.: Ivermectin in guinea pigs. Vet. Rec. 130:432, 1992.
114. Rigby, C.: Natural infections of guinea pigs. Lab. Anim. 10:119, 1976.
115. Smith, J.M., et al.: Animals as a reservoir of human ringworm in New Zealand. Aust. J. Dermatol. 10:169, 1969.
116. Smith, M.W.: Staphylococcal cheilitis in the guinea pig. J. Small Anim. Pract. 18:47, 1977.
117. Sohnle, P.D., et al.: Mechanisms involved in elimination of organisms from experimental cutaneous *Candida albicans* infections in guinea pigs. J. Immunol. 117:525, 1976.
118. Taylor, J.I., et al.: Chronic pododermatitis in guinea pigs, a case report. Lab. Anim. Sci. 21:944, 1971.
119. Todd, K.S., et al.: *Pelodera strongyloides* dermatitis in a guinea pig. (S.A.C.) 77:1400, 1982.
120. Tuch, E., et al.: Trichofolliculom beim Meerschweinchen. Kleintier-Prax. 24:237, 1979.
121. Van Cutsem, J., Janssen, P.A.J.: Experimental systemic dermatophytosis. J. Invest. Dermatol. 83:26, 1984.
122. Van Cutsem, J., et al.: The in vitro antifungal activity of ketoconazole, zinc pyrithione, and selenium sulfide against *Pityrosporum* and their efficacy as a shampoo in the treatment of experimental pityrosporosis in guinea pigs. J. Am. Acad. Dermatol. 22:993, 1990.
123. Van Herck, H., et al.: Dermal cryptococcosis in a guinea pig. Lab. Anim. 22:88, 1988.
124. Vogel, R.A., Timpe, A.: Spontaneous *Microsporum audouinii* infection in a guinea pig. J. Invest. Dermatol 28:311, 1957.
125. Wagner, J.E., et al.: The Biology of the Guinea Pig. Academic Press, New York, 1976.
126. Wagner, J.E., et al.: *Chirodiscoides caviae* infestation in guinea pigs. Lab. Anim. Sci. 22:750, 1972.
127. Zajac, A., et al.: Mange caused by *Trixacarus caviae* in guinea pigs. J. Am. Vet. Med. Assoc. 177:900, 1980.
128. Zenoble, R.D., et al.: Sarcoptic mite infestation in a colony of guinea pigs. J. Am. Vet. Med. Assoc. 177:898, 1980.
129. Zwart, P., et al.: Cutaneous tumors in the guinea pig. Lab. Anim. 15:375, 1981.

Hamster

130. Baies, A., et al.: *Notoedres* scabies of the golden hamster. Z. Versuchsteirkd. 1:251, 1968.
131. Battles, A.H.: The biology, care, and diseases of the Syrian hamster. Comp. Cont. Educ. 7:815, 1985.
131a. Bauck, L.B., et al.: Hyperadrenocorticism in three teddy bear hamsters. Can. Vet. J. 25:247, 1984.
132. Christensen, F., Dam, H.: A new symptom of fat deficiency in hamsters: Profuse secretion of cerumen. Acta Physiol. Scand. 27:204, 1953.
133. Cooper, J.E., et al.: Tumors in Russian hamsters *(Phodopus sungorus)*. Vet. Rec. 128:335, 1991.
134. Deerberg, F., et al.: Spontaneous mortality and incidence of spontaneous tumors in Han CHIN hamsters. Z. Versuchstierd. 29:129, 1987.
134a. Drickamer, I.C., et al.: Predictors of dominance in the male golden hamster. Anim. Behav. 21:557, 1973.
135. Estes, P.C., et al.: Demodectic mange in the golden hamster. Lab. Anim. Sci. 21:825, 1971.

136. Frisk, C.S., et al.: Unusual aggressive behavior in the male golden hamster. Lab. Anim. Sci. 27:682, 1977.
137. Fulton, J.D.: The treatment of *Notoedres* infections in golden hamsters *(Mesocricetus auratus)* with dimethyl diphenylene disulphide (Mitigal) and tetraethyl-thiuram monosulphide. Vet. Rec. 55:219, 1943.
138. Hamilton, J.W., Hogan, A.G.: Nutritional requirements of the Syrian hamster. J. Nutr. 27:213, 1944.
139. Harvey, R.G., et al.: Epidermotropic cutaneous T-cell lymphoma (mycosis fungoides) in Syrian hamsters *(Mesocricetus auratus).* A report of six cases and the demonstration of T-cell specificity. Vet. Dermatol. 3:13, 1992.
140. Hoffman, R.A., et al.: The Golden Hamster. Iowa State University Press, Ames, IA, 1968.
141. Kajdacsy-Balla, A., et al.: Syphilis in the Syrian hamster. A model of human venereal and congenital syphilis. Am. J. Pathol. 126:599, 1987.
142. Kesterson, J.W., Carlton, W.W.: Multiple malignant neoplasms in a golden hamster. A case report and literature survey. Lab. Anim. Care 2:220, 1970.
142a. Marques, D.M., Valenstern, E.S.: Individual differences in aggressiveness of female hamsters: Response to intact and castrated males and to females. Anim. Behav. 25:131, 1977.
143. Meshorer, A.: Leg lesions in hamsters caused by wood shavings. Lab. Anim. Sci. 26:828, 1976.
144. Musser, T.K., et al.: The hair cycle of the Syrian golden hamster *(Mesocricetus auratus).* Lab. Anim. Sci. 40:68, 1980.
145. Nixon, C.W.: Hereditary hairlessness in the Syrian golden hamster. J. Hered. 63:215, 1972.
146. Nutting, W.B.: *Demodex aurati* sp. nov. and *D. criceti,* ectoparasites of the golden hamster *(Mesocricetus auratus).* Parasitology 51:515, 1961.
147. Nutting, W.B., Rauch, H.: Distribution of *Demodex aurati* in the host *(Mesocricetus auratus)* skin complex. J. Parasitol. 49:323, 1963.
148. Owen, D., Young, C.: The occurrence of *Demodex aurati* and *Demodex criceti* in the Syrian hamster *(Mesocricetus auratus)* in the United Kingdom. Vet. Rec. 92:282, 1973.
149. Payne, A.P., et al.: Agonistic behaviour between pairs of hamsters of the same and opposite sex in a neutral observation area. Behaviour 36:259, 1970.
150. Rosenberg, J.C., et al.: The malignant melanoma of hamsters. I. Pathologic characteristics of a transplanstable melanotic and amelanotic tumor. Cancer Res. 21:627, 1961.
151. Routh, J.J., Houchin, O.B.: Some nutritional requirements of the hamster. Fed. Proc. 1:191, 1942.
152. Sarashina, T., et al.: Demodicosis in the golden hamster. Jpn. J. Vet. Sci. 48:619, 1986.
153. Saunders, G.K., Scott, D.W.: Cutaneous lymphoma resembling mycosis fungoides in the Syrian hamster *(Mesocricetus auratus).* Lab. Anim. Sci. 38:616, 1988.
154. Schwartzman, G., Strauss, L.: Vitamin B$_6$ deficiency in the Syrian hamster. J. Nutr. 38:131, 1949.
155. Schweigert, B.S., et al.: Effect of feeding polyoxyethylene monostearates on growth rate and gross pathology of weanling hamsters. Proc. Soc. Exp. Biol. Med. 73:427, 1950.
156. Stuhlmann, R.A., et al.: Ringtail in *Mystromys albicaudatus.* A case report. Lab. Anim. Sci. 21:585, 1971.
156a. Vandenbergh, J.G.: The effects of gonadal hormones on the aggressive behavior of adult golden hamsters *(Mesocricetus auratus).* Anim. Behav. 19:589, 1971.
157. Van Ham, M., et al.: Simultaneous parasitization of the golden hamster with two species of *Demodex: D. criceti* and *D. aurati.* Refuah Vet. 36:21, 1979.
158. Young, C.: *Trichophyton mentagrophytes* infection of the Djungarian hamster *(Phodopus sungorus).* Vet. Rec. 93:287, 1974.

Mouse

158a. Abbott, D.P., et al.: A condition resembling pagetoid reticulosis in a laboratory mouse. Lab. Anim. 25:153, 1991.
159. Allen, A.M., et al.: Pathology and diagnosis of mousepox. Lab. Anim. Sci. 31:599, 1981.
160. Bean-Knudsen, D.E., et al.: Evaluation of the control of *Myobia musculi* in laboratory mice with permethrin. Lab. Anim. Sci. 36:268, 1986.
161. Beck, E.M., et al.: The nutrition of the mouse. IX. Studies on pyridoxine and thiouracil. Yale J. Biol. Med. 23:190, 1950.
162. Bell, J.F., et al.: Dry gangrene of the ear in white mice. Lab. Anim. 4:245, 1970.
163. Blackmore, D.K., et al.: The apparent transmission of staphylococci of human origin to laboratory animals. J. Comp. Pathol. 80:645, 1970.
164. Blank, F.: Favus of mice. Can. J. Microbiol. 3:885, 1957.
165. Borum, K.: Hair pattern and hair succession in the mouse. Acta Pathol. Microbiol. Scand. 34:521, 1954.
166. Brooke, H.C.: Hairless mice. J. Hered. 17:173, 1926.
167. Brown, W.R., et al.: An hypothesis on the cause of chronic epidermal hyperproliferation in asebia mice. Clin. Exp. Dermatol. 13:74, 1988.
168. Carter, T.C., Phillips, R.S.: Ichthyosis, a new recessive mutant in the house mouse. J. Hered. 41:297, 1950.
169. Cetin, E.T., et al.: Epizootic of *Trichophyton mentagrophytes* (interdigitale) in white mice. Pathol. Microbiol. 28:839, 1965.
170. Clarke, M.C., et al.: The occurrence in mice of facial and mandibular abscesses associated with *Staphylococcus aureus.* Lab. Anim. 12:121, 1978.
171. Cook, I.: Reovirus Type 3 infection in laboratory mice. Aust. J. Exp. Biol. Med. Sci. 41:651, 1963.
172. Cook, NM.: The Anatomy of the Laboratory Mouse. Academic Press, New York, 1965.
173. Cook, R.: Murine mange: The control of *Mycoptes musculinis* and *Myobia musculi* infestations. Br. Vet. J. 109:113, 1953.
174. Cover, C.E., et al.: Ear tag induced *Staphylococcus* infection in mice. Lab. Anim. 23:229, 1989.
175. Davies, A.E., et al.: The rhino mutant mouse as an experimental tool. Trans N. Y. Acad. Sci. 33:680, 1971.

176. Dawson, D.V., et al.: Genetic control of susceptibility to mite-associated ulcerative dermatitis. Lab. Anim. Sci. 36:262, 1986.
177. Day, H.G., et al.: Some effects of dietary zinc deficiency in the mouse. J. Nutr. 33:27, 1947.
178. Decker, A.B., et al.: Chronic essential fatty acid deficiency in mice. J. Nutr. 41:507, 1950.
179. Dry, F.W.: The coat of the mouse (*Mus musculus*). J. Genet. 16:287, 1926.
180. Elias, P.M., et al.: Staphylococcal toxic epidermal necrolysis (TEN): The expanded mouse model. J. Invest. Dermatol. 63:467, 1974.
181. Ellison, G.T.H., et al.: Ringtail in the pouched mouse (*Saccostomus campestris*). Lab. Anim. 24:205, 1990.
182. Fenner, F.: Mousepox (infectious ectromelia of mice); A review. J. Immunol. 63:341, 1949.
183. Fischman, O., et al.: *Trichophyton mentagrophytes* infection in laboratory white mice. Mycopathologia 59:113, 1976.
184. Flanagan, S.P.: "Nude," a new hairless gene with pleiotropic effects in the mouse. Genet. Res. 8:295, 1966.
185. Flynn, R.J., et al.: Nidification of a mite (*Psorergates simplex*, Tyrrell, 1883; *Myobiidae*) in the skin of mice. J. Parasitol. 42:49, 1956.
186. Foster, H.L., et al.: The Mouse in Biomedical Research. Academic Press, New York, 1982.
187. Friedman, S., et al.: The parasitic ecology of the rodent mite *Myobia musculi*. II. Genetic factors. Lab. Anim. Sci. 25:440, 1975.
188. Friedman, S., et al.: The parasitic ecology of the rodent mite *Myobia musculi*. IV. Life cycle. Lab. Anim. Sci. 27:34, 1977.
189. Gardner, M.B., et al.: Spontaneous tumors of aging wild house mice. Incidence, pathology, and C-type virus expression. J. Natl. Cancer Inst. 50:719, 1973.
190. Gates, A.H., Karasek, M.: Hereditary absence of sebaceous glands in the mouse. Science 148:1471, 1965.
191. Green, C.J., et al.: Control of mange mites in a large mouse colony. Lab. Anim. 8:245, 1974.
192. Kietzmann, M., et al.: The mouse epidermis as a model in skin pharmacology: Influence of age and sex on epidermal metabolic reactions and their circadian rhythms. Lab. Anim. 24:321, 1990.
193. Koopman, J.P., et al.: Tail lesions in C3H/He mice. Lab. Anim. 18:106, 1984.
194. Les, E.P.: A disease related to cage population density: Tail lesions of C3H/H3J mice. Lab. Anim. Sci. 22:56, 1972.
195. Levine, J.F., et al.: House mouse mites infesting laboratory rodents. Lab. Anim. Sci. 34:393, 1984.
196. Lippincott, S.W., Morris, H.P.: Pathologic changes associated with riboflavin deficiency in the mouse. J. Natl. Cancer Inst. 2:601, 1942.
197. Litterst, C.L.: Mechanically self-induced muzzle alopecia in mice. Lab. Anim. Sci. 24:806, 1974.
198. Long, S.Y.: Hair nibbling and whisker trimming as indications of social hierarchy in mice. Anim. Behav. 28:10, 1972.
199. MacKenzie, D.W.R.: *Trichophyton mentagrophytes* in mice: Infection of humans and incidence among laboratory animals. Sabouraudia 1:178, 1961.
200. Mann, S.J.: Hair loss and cyst formation in hairless and rhino mutant mice. Anat. Rec. 170:485, 1971.
201. Manning, P.J., et al.: Clinical, pathologic, and serologic features of an epizootic of mousepox in Minnesota. Lab. Anim. Sci. 31:574, 1981.
202. Maronpot, R.R., Chavannes, J.M.: Dacryoadenitis, conjunctivitis, and facial dermatitis of the mouse. Lab. Anim. Sci. 27:277, 1977.
203. McBride, D.F., et al.: An outbreak of staphylococcal furunculosis in nude mice. Lab. Anim. Sci. 31:270, 1981.
204. Moriwaki, K.: Activity change of phosphatases in the skin of hairless mutant mice during development. Physiol. Zool. 35:193, 1962.
205. Morris, H.P., Lippincott, S.W.: The effect of pantothenic acid on growth and maintenance of life in mice of the C3H strain. J. Natl. Cancer Inst. 2:29, 1941.
206. Mullink, J.W.: A case of actinomycosis in a male NZW mouse. Z. Versuchstierkd. 10:225, 1968.
207. Murray, M.D.: The ecology of the louse *Polyplax serrata* (Burm.) on the mouse *Mus musculus* L. Aust. J. Zool. 9:1, 1961.
208. Needham, J.R.: The control of mange mites (*Myobia musculi* and *Mycoptes musculinis*) in a conventional mouse colony. J. Inst. Anim. Techn. 29:1, 1978.
209. Nutini, L.G., et al.: Effect of diet and strain difference on the virulence of *Staphylococcus aureus* for mice. Appl. Microbiol. 13:614, 1965.
210. Parrish, H.H., et al.: Ringworm epizootic in mice. Br. J. Exp. Pathol. 12:209, 1931.
211. Peters, R.L., et al.: Incidence of spontaneous neoplasms in breeding and retired breeder B ALB/cCR mice throughout the natural life span. Int. J. Cancer 10:273, 1972.
212. Rogers, J.A.: Histopathogenesis of mouse pox. II. Cutaneous infection. Br. J. Exp. Pathol. 43:462, 1962.
213. Schreemilch, H.S.: A naturally acquired infection of laboratory mice and *Klebsiella* capsule Type 6. Lab. Anim. 10:305, 1976.
214. Shults, F.S., et al.: Staphylococcal botryomycosis in a specific-pathogen-free mouse colony. Lab. Anim. Sci. 23:36, 1973.
215. Simpson, W., Simmons, D.J.C.: Two *Actinobacillus* species isolated from laboratory rodents. Lab. Anim. 14:15, 1980.
216. Starcher, B., et al.: Abnormal cellular copper metabolism in the blotchy mouse. J. Nutr. 108:1229, 1978.
217. Stewart, D.D., et al.: An epizootic of necrotic dermatitis in laboratory mice caused by Lancefield Group G streptococci. Lab. Anim. Sci. 25:296, 1975.
218. Stowe, H.D., et al.: A debilitating fatal murine dermatitis. Lab. Anim. Sci. 21:892, 1971.
218a. Sundberg, J.P., et al.: Inherited mouse mutations as models of human adnexal, cornification, and papulosquamous dermatoses. J. Invest. Dermatol. 95:62S, 1990.

218b. Sundberg, J.P., Schultz, L.D.: Inherited mouse mutations: Models for the study of alopecia. J. Invest. Dermatol. 96:95S, 1991.

219. Taylor, D.M., Neal, D.L.: An infected eczematous condition in mice: Methods of treatment. Lab. Anim. 14:325, 1980.

220. Thornberg, L.P., et al.: The pathogenesis of the alopecia due to hair chewing in mice. Lab. Anim. Sci. 23:843, 1973.

221. Van Rooyen, C.E.: The biology, pathogenesis, and classification of *Streptobacillus moniliformis.* J. Pathol. Bacteriol. 43:455, 1936.

222. Wagner, J.E.: Control of mouse ectoparasites with resin vaporizer strips containing Vapona. Lab. Anim. Care 19:804, 1969.

223. Ward, J.M., et al.: Neoplastic and non-neoplastic lesions in aging (C57BL/6NxC3H/HEN) F1 (B6C3F1) mice. J. Natl. Cancer Inst. 63:849, 1979.

224. Weisbroth, S.H., et al.: *Corynebacterium kutscheri* infection in the mouse. I. Report of an outbreak, bacteriology, and pathology of spontaneous infections. Lab. Anim. Sci. 18:451, 1968.

225. Weisbroth, S.H., et al.: *Pasteurella pneumotropica* abscess syndrome in a mouse colony. J. Am. Vet. Med. Assoc. 155:1206, 1969.

226. Weisbroth, S.H., et al.: The parasitic ecology of the rodent mite *Myobia musculi.* I. Grooming factors. Lab. Anim. Sci. 24:510, 1974.

227. Weisbroth, S.H., et al.: The parasitic ecology of the rodent mite *Myobia musculi.* III. Lesions in certain host strains. Lab. Anim. Sci. 26:725, 1976.

228. Wing, S.R., et al.: Effect of ivermectin on murine mites. J. Am. Vet. Med. Assoc. 187:1191, 1985.

229. Wrench, R.: Scale prophylaxis. A new antiparakeratotic assay. Arch. Dermatol. 117:213, 1981.

Rabbit

230. Alteras, I., Cojocaru, I.: Human infection by *Trichophyton mentagrophytes* from rabbits. Mykosen 12:543, 1969.

231. Arlian, L.G., et al.: Infectivity of *Psoroptes cuniculi* in rabbits. Am. J. Vet. Res. 42:1782, 1981.

231a. Arvy, L., More, J.: Atlas d'Histologie du Lapin. Librairie Maloine, Paris, 1975.

232. Banks, K.L., et al.: Naturally occurring dermatomycosis in the rabbit. J. Am. Vet. Med. Assoc. 151:926, 1967.

233. Barone, R., et al.: Atlas d'Anatomie du Lapin. Masson, Paris, 1973.

234. Bowman, D.D., et al.: Effect of ivermectin on the control of ear mites *(Psoroptes cuniculi)* in naturally infested rabbits. Am. J. Vet. Res. 53:105, 1992.

235. Bronswijk, J.E.M.H., de Kreek, E.J.: *Cheyletiella (Acari: Cheyletiellidae)* of dog, cat, and domesticated rabbit, a review. J. Med. Entomol. 13:315, 1976.

236. Clark, J.D., et al.: *Cheyletiella parasitivorax* (Megnin), a parasitic mite causing mange in the domestic rabbit. J. Parasitol. 62:125, 1976.

237. Cloyd, G.G., et al.: Facial alopecia in the rabbit associated with *Cheyletiella parasitivorax.* Lab. Anim. Sci. 26:801, 1976.

238. Culbertson, J.T.: Antibody production by the rabbit against an ectoparasite. Proc. Soc. Exp. Biol. Med. 32:1239, 1935.

239. Cunliffe-Beamer, T.L., Fox, R.R.: Venereal spirochetosis of rabbits: Description and diagnosis. Lab. Anim. Sci. 31:366, 1981.

240. Cunliffe-Beamer, T.L., Fox, R.R.: Venereal spirochetosis of rabbits: Epizootiology. Lab. Anim. Sci. 31:372, 1981.

241. Cunliffe-Beamer, T.L., Fox, R.R.: Venereal spirochetosis of rabbits: Eradication. Lab. Anim. Sci. 31:379, 1981.

242. Curtis, S.K., et al.: Use of ivermectin for treatment of ear mite infestation in rabbits. J. Am. Vet. Med. Assoc. 196:1139, 1990.

242a. Curtis, S.K.: Moist dermatitis on the hind quarters of a rabbit. Lab. Anim. Sci. 41:623, 1991.

243. Fisher, W.F.: Detection of serum antibodies to psoroptic mite antigens in rabbits infested with *Psoroptes cuniculi* or *P. ovis (Acari: Psoroptidae)* by enzyme-linked immunosorbent assay and immunodiffusion. J. Med. Entomol. 20:257, 1983.

244. Flatt, R.E., et al.: A survey of fur mites in domestic rabbits. Lab. Anim. Sci. 26:758, 1976.

245. Franklin, C.L., et al.: Treatment of *Trichophyton mentagrophytes* infection in rabbits. J. Am. Vet. Med. Assoc. 198:1625, 1991.

246. Ganière, J.P., et al.: Myxomatosis of the depilated Angora rabbit. A preliminary study. Vet. Dermatol. 2:11, 1991.

247. Ganière, J.P., et al.: Etude clinique et expérimentale de la myxomatose du lapin Angora. Point Vét. 22:187, 1990.

248. Gentles, J.C.: Experimental ringworm in guinea pigs: Oral treatment with griseofulvin. Nature 182:476, 1958.

249. Greene, H.S.N.: Rabbit pox. I. Clinical manifestations and cause of the disease. J. Exp. Med. 60:427, 1934.

250. Guillot, F.S., Wright, F.C.: Evaluation of possible factors affecting degree of ear canker and numbers of psoroptic mites in rabbits. Southwest. Entomol. 6:245, 1981.

251. Hagen, K.W.: Ringworm in domestic rabbits: Oral treatment with griseofulvin. Lab. Anim. Care 19:635, 1969.

252. Harkness, J.E.: Rabbit husbandry and medicine. Vet. Clin. North Am. (Small Anim. Pract.) 17:1019, 1987.

253. Harvey, R.G.: *Demodex cuniculi* in dwarf rabbits *(Orycytolagus cuniculus).* J. Small Anim. Pract. 31:204, 1990.

254. Harvey, R.G., et al.: A connective tissue defect in two rabbits similar to the Ehlers-Danlos syndrome. Vet. Rec. 126:130, 1990.

254a. Hillyer, E.V.: Pet rabbits. Vet. Clin. North Am. (Small Anim. Pract.) 24:25, 1994.

255. Hinton, M., Regan, M.: Cutaneous lymphosarcoma in a rabbit. Vet. Rec. 103:140, 1978.

256. Hoover, J.P., et al.: Osteogenic sarcoma with subcutaneous involvement in a rabbit. J. Am. Vet. Med. Assoc. 189:1156, 1986.

257. Jacobson, H.A., et al.: Bot fly miasis of the cotton tail rabbit, *Sylvilagus floridanus mallurus* in Virginia with some biology of the parasite, *Cuterebra buccata.* J. Wildlife Dis. 14:56, 1978.

258. Joiner, G.N., et al.: An epizootic of Shope fibromatosis in a commercial rabbitry. J. Am. Vet. Med. Assoc. 159:1583, 1971.

258a. Kurtis, S.K., Brooks, D.L.: Eradication of ear mites from naturally infested conventional research rabbits using ivermectin. Lab. Anim. Sci. 40:406, 1990.

259. Kuttin, E.S., et al.: *Trichophyton mentagrophytes* infection in rabbits successfully treated with a polyvinyl iodine solution. Lab. Anim. Sci. 26:960, 1976.

260. Marcella, K.L., et al.: Raised skin patches. Lab. Anim. 15:13, 1986.

261. Mbuya-Mimbanga, M., Gamperl, H.J.: Essai de traitement à l'ivermectine de la gale sarcoptique chez les lapins. Rev. Elév. Méd. Vét. Pays Trop. 41:55, 1988.

262. Nfi, A.N.: Ivomec, a treatment against rabbit mange. Rev. Elév. Méd. Vét. Pays Trop. 45:37, 1992.

263. O'Donoghue, P.N., Whatley, B.F.: *Pseudomonas aeruginosa* in rabbit fur. Lab. Anim. 5:251, 1971.

263a. Patel, A., Robinson, K.J.E.: Dermatosis associated with *Listrophorus gibbus* in the rabbit. J. Small Anim. Pract. 34:409, 1993.

264. Pathak, K.M.L., Kapoor, M.: Efficacy of ivermectin against *Psoroptes* in rabbits. Ind. J. Anim. Health 29:189, 1990.

265. Patton, N.M., et al.: Myxomatosis in domestic rabbits in Oregon. J. Am. Vet. Med. Assoc. 171:560, 1977.

266. Patton, N.M.: Cutaneous and pulmonary aspergillosis in rabbits. Lab. Anim. Sci. 25:347, 1975.

267. Petkus, A.R., et al.: Experimental chronic *Pasteurella multocida* infection of subcutaneous chambers in the rabbit. Lab. Anim. Sci. 29:749, 1979.

268. Port, C.D., Sidor, M.A.: A sebaceous gland carcinoma in a rabbit. Lab. Anim. Sci. 28:215, 1978.

269. Pulley, L.T., Shively, J.N.: Naturally occurring infectious fibroma in the domestic rabbit. Vet. Pathol. 10:509, 1973.

269a. Roy, T., et al.: Effect of ivermectin against sarcoptic mange in rabbits. Ind. J. Anim. Health 30:93, 1991.

270. Sarkisov, A.K., et al.: [Specific prevention of trichophytosis in fur-bearing animals]. Veterinariya (Moscow) 7:37, 1981.

271. Sawin, P.B., et al.: Maternal behavior in the rabbit: Hair loosening during gestation. Am. J. Physiol. 198:1099, 1960.

272. Saxena, S.P., et al.: *Microsporum canis* infection in a rabbit. Sabouraudia 8:235, 1970.

273. Schoenbaum, M.: *Pseudomonas aeruginosa* in rabbit fur. Lab. Anim. 15:5, 1981.

274. Shaw, N.A., et al.: Zinc deficiency in female rabbits. Lab. Anim. 8:1, 1974.

275. Smith, S.E., Ellis, G.H.: Copper deficiency in rabbits. Arch. Biochem. 15:81, 1947.

276. Sweatman, G.K.: On the life history and validity of the species in *Psoroptes,* a genus of mange mites. Can. J. Zool. 36:905, 1958.

277. Uhlír, J.: Humoral and cellular immune response of rabbits to *Psoroptes cuniculi,* the rabbit scab mite. Vet. Parasitol. 40:325, 1991.

278. Van Cutsem, J., et al.: Treatment with enilconazole* spray of dermatophytosis in rabbit farms. Mykosen 28:400, 1985.

279. Vogtsberger, L.M., et al.: Spontaneous dermatophytosis due to *Microsporum canis* in rabbits. Lab. Anim. Sci. 36:294, 1986.

280. Ward, G.S., et al.: What's your diagnosis? Crusty lesions. Lab. Anim. 19:19, 1985.

281. Ward, G.S., et al.: Inflammatory exostosis and abscessation associated with *Fusobacterium nucleatum* in a rabbit. Lab. Anim. Sci. 31:280, 1981.

282. Weisbroth, S.H., et al.: Immune and pathologic consequences of spontaneous cutaneous myiasis in domestic rabbits *(Oryctolagus cuniculus).* Lab. Anim. Sci. 23:241, 1973.

283. Weisbroth, S.H., et al.: Immunopathology of psoroptic otitis in laboratory rabbits. Proc. Fed. Am. Soc Exp. Biol. 31:614, 1972.

284. Weisbroth, S.H., et al.: The Biology of the Laboratory Rabbit. Academic Press, New York, 1974.

285. Weisbroth, S.H., et al.: *Listrophorus gibbus (Acarina: Listrophoridae).* An unusual parasitic mite from laboratory rabbits *(Oryctolagus cuniculus)* in the United States. J. Parasitol. 57:438, 1971.

286. Weisbroth, S.H., Scher, S.: *Microsporum gypseum* dermatophytosis in a rabbit. J. Am. Vet. Med. Assoc. 159:629, 1971.

287. Weisbroth, S.H., et al.: Immune and pathologic consequences of spontaneous *Cuterebra* myiasis in domestic rabbits *(Oryctolagus cuniculus).* Lab. Anim. Sci. 23:241, 1973.

288. Williams, C.S.F., et al.: Sore dewlap: *Pseudomonas aeruginosa* on rabbit fur and skin. Vet. Med. (S.A.C.) 70:954, 1975.

289. Wright, F.C., et al.: Comparative efficacy of injection routes and doses of ivermectin against *Psoroptes* in rabbits. Am. J. Vet. Res 46:752, 1985.

Rat

290. Andrews, E.J.: Muzzle trauma in the rat associated with the use of feeding cups. Lab. Anim. Sci. 27:278, 1977.

291. Ash, G.W.: An epidemic of chronic skin ulceration in rats. Lab. Anim. 5:115, 1971.

292. Barboriak, J.J., et al.: Pantothenic acid requirement of the growing and adult rat. J. Nutr. 61:13, 1957.

293. Battles, A.H., et al.: Efficacy of ivermectin against natural infection of *Syphacia muris* in rats. Lab. Anim. Sci. 37:791, 1987.

294. Beare-Rogers, J.L., et al.: Alopecia in rats housed in groups. Lab. Anim. 7:237, 1973.

295. Beaton, G.H., Chaney, M.C.: Vitamin B6 requirement of the male albino rat. J. Nutr. 87:125, 1965.

296. Bresnahan, J.F., et al.: Facial hair harboring in rats. Lab. Anim. Sci. 33:290, 1983.

297. Butcher, E.O.: The hair cycle in the albino rat. Anat. Rec. 61:15, 1934.
298. Carthew, P., Slingr, R.P.: Diagnosis of sialodacryoadenitis virus infection of rats in a virulent enzootic outbreak. Lab. Anim. 15:339, 1981.
299. Castle, W.E., et al.: Three new mutations of the rat. J. Hered. 46:9, 1955.
300. Dikshit, P.K., Sriramachari, S.: Caudal necrosis in suckling rats. Nature 181:63, 1958.
301. Dolan, M.M., Fendrick, A.J.: Incidence of *Trichophyton mentagrophytes* infections in laboratory rats. Proc. Anim. Care Panel 9:161, 1959.
302. Festing, M.F.W., et al.: An athymic nude mutation in the rat. Nature 274:365, 1978.
303. Flynn, R.J.: *Notoedres muris* infestation in rats. Proc. Anim. Care Panel 10:69, 1960.
304. Fox, J.G., et al.: Ulcerative dermatitis in the rat. Lab. Anim. Sci. 27:671, 1977.
305. Goldberger, J., Lillie, R.D.: A note on an experimental pellagralike condition in the albino rat. Public Health Rep. 41:1025, 1926.
306. Goldschmidt, F.: Reproducible topical staphylococcal infection in rats. Appl. Microbiol. 23:130, 1972.
307. Goodman, D.G., et al.: Neoplastic and non-neoplastic lesions in aging F344 rats. Toxicol. Appl. Pharmacol. 48:237, 1979.
308. Goodman, D.G., et al.: Neoplastic and non-neoplastic lesions in aging Osborne-Mendel rats. Toxicol. Appl. Pharmacol. 55:433, 1980.
309. Hard, G.C.: Staphylococcal infection of the tail of the laboratory rat. Lab. Anim. Care 16:421, 1966.
310. Henderson, J.D.: Cutaneous horn in a laboratory rat. Vet. Med. (S.A.C.) 70:141, 1975.
311. Herbel, R., Stromberg, M.W.: Anatomy of the Laboratory Rat. Williams & Wilkins Co., Baltimore, 1976.
312. Inazu, M., et al.: Characteristics of a new hairless mutation (bald) in rats. Lab. Anim. Sci. 34:577, 1984.
313. Inazu, M., et al.: Morphologic characteristics of the skin of bald mutant rats. Lab. Anim. Sci. 34:584, 1984.
314. Jackson, N.N., et al.: Naturally acquired infections of *Klebsiella pneumoniae* in Wistar rats. Lab. Anim. 14:357, 1980.
315. Johnson, E.: Quantitative studies of hair growth in the albino rat. Normal males and females. Endocrinology 16:337, 1958.
316. Kaspareit-Rittinghausen, J., et al.: Mortality and incidence of spontaneous neoplasms in BD II/Han rats. Z. Versuchstierkd. 30:209, 1987.
317. Krehl, W.A., et al.: Factors affecting the dietary niacin and tryptophane requirement of the growing rat. J. Nutr. 31:85, 1946.
317a. LaRegina, M.C., et al.: Skin infarction in rats. Lab. Anim. Sci. 43:99, 1993.
318. Lerner, E.M., Sokoloff, L.: The pathogenesis of bone and joint infection produced in rats by *Streptobacillus moniliformis*. Arch. Pathol. 67:20, 1959.
319. MacKenzie, W.F., Garner, F.M.: Comparison of neoplasms in six sources of rats. J. Natl. Cancer Inst. 50:1243, 1973.
320. Marennikova, S.S., et al.: Pox infection in white rats. Lab. Anim. 12:33, 1978.
321. Marchetti, M., Testoni, S.: Relationship between biotin and vitamin B12. J. Nutr. 84:249, 1964.
321a. Meingassner, J.G.: Sympathetic auricular chondritis in rats. A model of autoimmune disease. Lab. Anim. 25:68, 1991.
322. Meister, A.: Biochemistry of Amino Acids. Academic Press, New York, 1957.
323. Morrow, D.T., et al.: Poditis in the rat as a complication of experiments in exercise physiology. Lab. Anim. Sci. 27:679, 1977.
324. Njaa, L.R., et al.: Effect of relative humidity on rat breeding and ringtail. Nature 180:290, 1957.
325. Ohno, T., et al.: "Atrichosis," a new hairless gene with cyst formation in rats. Experientia 37:126, 1981.
326. Palm, J., et al.: "Fuzzy," a hypotrichotic mutant in linkage group I of the Norwegian rat. J. Hered. 67:284, 1976.
327. Povar, M.L.: Ringworm *(Trichophyton mentagrophytes)* infection in a colony of albino Norway rats. Lab. Anim. Care 15:264, 1965.
328. Pratt, H.D., Karp, H.: Notes on the rat lice *Polyplax spinulosa* (Burmeister) and *Hoplopleura oenomydis* (Ferris). J. Parasitol. 39:495, 1953.
329. Roberts, E., et al.: Hereditary hypotrichosis in the rat. J. Invest. Dermatol. 3:1, 1940.
330. Roberts, E.: Inheritance of hypotrichosis in rats. Anat. Rec. 29:141, 1924.
331. Schardein, J.L., et al.: Spontaneous tumors in Holtzman-Source rats of various ages. Pathol. Vet. 5:238, 1968.
332. Smith, E.M., Calhoun, M.L.: The Microscopic Anatomy of the White Rat: A Photographic Atlas. Iowa State Press, Ames, IA, 1968.
333. Totton, M.: Ringtail in newborn Norway rats—A study of the effect of environmental temperature and humidity on incidence. J. Hygiene 56:190, 1958.
334. Van der Schaff, A., et al.: *Pasteurella pneumotropica* as a causal microorganism of multiple subcutaneous abscesses in a colony of Wistar rats. Z. Versuchstierkd. 12:356, 1970.
335. Wagner, J.E., et al.: Self-trauma and *Staphylococcus aureus* in ulcerative dermatitis of rats. J. Am. Vet. Med. Assoc. 170:839, 1977.
336. Walberg, J.A., et al.: Demodicosis in laboratory rats *(Rattus norvegicus)*. Lab. Anim. Sci. 31:60, 1981.
337. Wyard, D.S., Jones, A.M.: *Pseudomonas aeruginosa* infection in rats following implantation of an indwelling jugular catheter. Lab. Anim. Care 17:261, 1967.

21

Chronology of Veterinary Dermatology (1900–1995)

■

An overview of the history of veterinary dermatology, Historical Highlights—Ancient and Modern, can be found in Chapter 90, pages 711 to 735, of the second edition of this book (1976). This material was updated for the third edition of this book (1983). Because the historical material is unchanged, it is not repeated in the fifth edition. Instead, the chronology is given here and updated to 1995.

1900 Joseph Bayer and Eugene Fröhner of Vienna, Austria, persuaded Hugo Schindelka to write a book on skin diseases of domestic animals.

1903 Publication of the first book on veterinary dermatology *Hautkrankheiten bei Haustieren* (Skin Diseases of Domestic Animals) by Hugo Schindelka at Vienna.

1908 Publication of the second and final edition of Schindelka's book *Hautkrankheiten bei Haustieren.*

1910 Publication of the first book on comparative dermatology *Die Vergleichende Pathologie der Haut* (The Comparative Pathology of the Skin) by Julius Heller at Berlin, Germany.

1926 Publication of *Animal Dermatology* by Leblois in France.

1930 Publication of the book *Course in Skin Diseases of Domestic Animals* by N.N. Bogdanov at Moscow.

1931 Publication of *Die Klinik der Wichtigsten Tierdermatosen* (The Clinic of the Most Important Animal Dermatoses) by Julius Heller at Berlin, Germany.

1931 Publication of *Veterinari Dermatologie* by Frantisek Kral (Frank Kral) at Brno, Czechoslovakia.

1948 Frank Kral emigrated to the United States and joined the faculty of the School of Veterinary Medicine, University of Pennsylvania in Philadelphia. He formed the Veterinary Dermatology Clinic, which was the first teaching unit of animal skin diseases in the United States.

1953 Publication of *Veterinary Dermatology* by Frank Kral and Benjamin J. Novak, first veterinary dermatologic book in English: a complete revision, expansion and translation of Kral's 1931 book (325 pages).

1958 Formation of the Dermatology Subcommittee of the Committee on General Medicine of the American Animal Hospital Association on April 23, 1958. R.W. Worley and G.H. Muller, Cochairmen: first organization of veterinary dermatology.

1958 E.M. Farber appoints G.H. Muller to the clinical faculty of Stanford University's Dermatology Department and establishes the first center of comparative dermatology in America.

1959 R.M. Schwartzman obtains the first Ph.D. degree in Veterinary Dermatology and shortly thereafter joins F. Kral's veterinary dermatology section at the University of Pennsylvania.

1959 Formation of the Dermatology Committee of the American Animal Hospital Association on February 5, 1959. G.H. Muller, Chairman. Committee functioned for 7 years.

1959 Publication of the *Compendium of Veterinary Dermatology* by Frank Kral. Hand-out for Kral's cross-country symposia in 1959 (69 pages).

1962 Publication of *A Comparative Study of Skin Diseases of Dog and Man* by Robert M. Schwartzman and Milton Orkin: the first book in English on comparative dermatology (365 pages).

1963 Transatlantic Conference on Canine and Feline Dermatology at Chicago and London on April 26, 1963. Knowles, Muller, and Schwartzman for the United States; Singleton, Joshua, and Wilkinson for England.

1964 Publication of section on Dermatologic Diseases (edited by G.H. Muller) in R.W. Kirk's *Current Veterinary Therapy*. Revised and updated in all subsequent editions.

1964 Publication of chapter on "Feline diseases of the skin" by J.D. Conroy in *Feline Medicine.*

1964 The American Academy of Veterinary Dermatology was organized at Philadelphia by Conroy, Kral (President), Muller, and Schwartzman.

1964 Symposium on Comparative Physiology and Pathology of the Skin at London, England, in April, 1964. A.J. Rook and G.S. Walton, Chairmen. Proceedings were published in 1965.

1964 Publication of *Veterinary and Comparative Dermatology* by F. Kral and R.M. Schwartzman: a revision and expansion of Kral and Novak's *Veterinary Dermatology* (444 pages).

1964 First Symposium on Comparative Dermatology sponsored by the American Academy of Dermatology at Chicago on December 8, 1964. Milton Orkin was chairman of this and the next three symposia.

1965 Second Symposium on Comparative Dermatology, December 7, 1965, at Chicago.

1965 Publication of *Comparative Physiology and Pathology of the Skin* by A.J. Rook and G.S. Walton.

1966 Third Symposium on Comparative Dermatology, December 5, 1966, at Miami, Florida.

1966 Symposium on Skin Diseases Common to Man and Animals at Palm Springs, California, on November 2, 1966. Orkin and Muller, Cochairmen.

1967 Fourth Symposium on Comparative Dermatology, December 4, 1967, at Chicago.

1967 Publication of *Atlas of Canine and Feline Dermatoses* by R.M. Schwartzman and Frank Kral.

1968 Publication of the atlas *Canine Skin Lesions* by G.H. Muller.

1968 J.D. Conroy receives a Ph.D. degree and thereby launches the first career devoted exclusively to veterinary dermatohistopathology in America.

1969 Publication of *Small Animal Dermatology* by G.H. Muller and R.W. Kirk (485 pages): the first complete textbook devoted exclusively to skin diseases of dogs and cats. Used as a textbook by many schools of veterinary medicine. Translated into Japanese and French and reprinted in Taiwan.

1970 Formation of an organizing committee of the American College of Veterinary Dermatologists consisting of Blakemore, Conroy, Muller (Chairman), Schwartzman, Kirk, and Kral.

1973 The formation of the *Task Force on Comparative Dermatology* as part of the *National Program for Dermatology* of the *American Academy of Dermatology.*

1974 Publication of the atlas *Feline Skin Lesions* by G.H. Muller.

1974 Publication of a stereoscopic atlas of *Clinical Dermatology of Small Animals* by G.G. Doering and H.E. Jensen (211 pages).

1974 Dermatology Specialty Group of the American College of Veterinary Internal Medicine (ACVIM) receives approval of the Advisory Board of Veterinary Specialties of the American Veterinary Medical Association (AVMA) on April 5, 1974.

1974 The first meeting of the Dermatology Specialty Group of the ACVIM was held on April 20, 1974, at San Francisco.

1974 The Dermatology Specialty Group was officially recognized by receiving probationary approval of the ACVIM and Council of Education of the AVMA on July 20, 1974, at Denver, Colorado.

1976 Formation of the British Veterinary Dermatology Study Group on February 20, 1976. Honorary Secretary Brian G. Bagnal; committee members Michael R. Geary, Raymond Hopes, David H. Lloyd, and Keith L. Thoday.

1976 Publication of the *Veterinary Dermatology Newsletter* (Vol. 1, No. 1) in May 1976 by the British Veterinary Dermatology Study Group.

1976 Publication of the second edition of *Small Animal Dermatology* by G.H. Muller and R.W. Kirk (809 pages). Translated into Italian.

1979 Publication of *The Skin and Internal Disease* (edited by G.H. Muller), the Veterinary Clinics of North America, 1979, W.B. Saunders Company (152 pages).

1980 Publication of *Feline Dermatology 1900–1978: A Monograph* by D.W. Scott (128 pages).

1980 Frank Kral deceased September 7, 1980.

1981 Formation of a French veterinary dermatologic organization: Groupe D'Étude en Dermatologie des Animaux de Compagnie (GEDAC). President Pierre Fourrier, Secretary Didier Carlotti.

1981 Publication of *Canine Dermatoses* by J.M. Keep (Australia).

1981 Publication of *Feline Dermatoses* by J.M. Keep (Australia).

1981 Publication of *Equine Dermatoses* by R.R. Pascoe (Australia).

1982 On March 9, 1982, the American Board of Veterinary Specialties of the AVMA granted probationary approval to the American College of Veterinary Dermatology as a certifying body in Veterinary Dermatology. This group replaces the Dermatology Specialty Group of the ACVIM. The organizing committee of the American College of Veterinary Dermatology consists of Doctors J.C. Blakemore, J.D. Conroy, R.E.W. Halliwell, G.H. Muller, and E. Small.

1982 The American College of Veterinary Dermatology was approved by the Council of Education of the AVMA on April 23, 1982, and approved by the House of Delegates of the AVMA on July 20, 1982. The charter members of the group are the diplomates of the ACVIM (Dermatology) listed under 1981. There were 24 diplomates at the end of 1982.

1982 Formation of a German veterinary dermatology organization called the "Freundeskreis Hautkrankheiten Interessierter Tierärtzte." The organizing members are H. Koch (President), B. Beardi, G. Feslev, H. Gehrig, G. Kasa, F. Kasa, G.H. Muller, and C. Terling. The first meeting was held on October 12, 1982, at Birkenfeld, West Germany. The name of this organization was later changed to Arbeitskreis Veterinär Dermatologie.

1983 Publication of the third edition of *Small Animal Dermatology* by G.H. Muller, R.W. Kirk, and D.W. Scott (889 pages). Translated into Portuguese and Japanese.

1983 Publication of *Canine and Feline Dermatology: A Systematic Approach* by G.H. Nesbitt (244 pages).

1983 Publication of *Atlas of Skin Diseases of the Horse* by L.F. Montes and J.T. Vaughan.

1984 Formation of the European Society of Veterinary Dermatology (ESVD) on September 18, 1984. President Hans Koch (Germany), Vice President Ton Willemse (Holland), Secretary David Lloyd (England), Treasurer Didier Carlotti (France), Membership Secretary Pierre Fourrier (France), Meeting Secretary Claudia Von Tscharner (Switzerland). Honorary Members Richard Halliwell, Peter Ihrke, Robert Kirk, George Muller, and Danny Scott (USA).

1984 Formation of an Australian veterinary dermatology organization began; started informally that year under the auspices of the Australian College of Veterinary Scientists. It granted full fellowship by examination in veterinary dermatology to Kenneth V. Mason on August 28, 1984. Two other veterinarians, George Wilkinson and Susan Shaw, are qualified in internal medicine and practicing veterinary dermatology within university organizations.

1984 Publication of *Equine Dermatoses* by R.R. Pascoe (Australia).

1984 Publication of *Skin Diseases of the Pig* by R.D.A. Cameron (Australia).

1985 Publication of the *Color Atlas of Small Animal Dermatology* by G.T. Wilkinson (272 pages), Australia.

1986 Publication of *Skin Diseases in the Dog and Cat* by D.I. Grant (187 pages), England.

1986 Formation of the Canadian Academy of Veterinary Dermatology. President Lowell Ackerman, Secretary B.P. Pukay.

1987 Publication of *Contemporary Issues in Small Animal Practice: Dermatology,* Vol. 8, New York (332 pages) (edited by G.H. Nesbitt).

1987 Formation, on October 23, of the Italian Veterinary Dermatology Group as part of the Italian Small Animal Veterinary Association (SCIVAC). President, Alessandra Fondati.

1987 Publication of *Atlas of Skin Diseases in Dogs and Cats* by F. Kristensen (Denmark).

1988 Publication of *Large Animal Dermatology* by D.W. Scott (487 pages).

1988 Publication of *Vanliga Hudsjukdomar Hos Hund Och Katt* by B. Öhlén (Sweden).

1988 Publication of *Pruritus* (edited by S.D. White), the Veterinary Clinics of North America, 1988, W.B. Saunders Company (143 pages).

1989 Publication of the fourth edition of *Small Animal Dermatology* by G.H. Muller, R.W. Kirk, and D.W. Scott (1007 pages). Translated into German.

1989 Publication of first issue of *Veterinary Dermatology,* an international journal devoted to dermatology.

1989 Publication of *Skin Infection in Domestic Animals* by A. Chatterjee (India).

1989 Publication of *Allergic Skin Diseases of Dogs and Cats* by L.M. Reedy and W.H. Miller, Jr.

1989 Publication of *Skin Diseases of Cattle* by D.I. Bryden (Australia).

1989 Publication of *Practical Canine Dermatology* by L.J. Ackerman.

1989 Publication of *Practical Feline Dermatology* by L.J. Ackerman.

1989 Publication of *Practical Equine Dermatology* by L.J. Ackerman.

1989 The First World Congress in Veterinary Dermatology was held in September at Dijon, France.

1990 Publication of *Small Animal Allergy. A Practical Guide* by E. Baker.

1990 Publication of *Color Atlas of Small Animal Dermatology* by B.A. Kummel.

1990 Publication of *Advances in Veterinary Dermatology,* Vol. I, by C. von Tscharner and R.E.W. Halliwell.

1990 Publication of *Common Skin Diseases in Dogs and Cats* by B. Öhlén (Sweden).

1990 Publication of *A Colour Atlas of Equine Dermatology* by R.R. Pascoe (Australia).

1990 Publication of *Canine and Feline Dermatology* by K.P. Baker and L.R. Thomsett (United Kingdom).

1990 Publication of *Advances in Clinical Dermatology* (edited by D.J. DeBoer), the Veterinary Clinics of North America, 1990, W.B. Saunders Company (310 pages).

1991 Publication of *Clinical Dermatology of Dogs and Cats* by T. Willemse (Netherlands).

1991 Publication of *Les Dermites Allergiques du Chien et du Chat* by P. Prélaud (France).

1991 Publication of second edition of *Skin Diseases in the Dog and Cat* by D.I. Grant (United Kingdom).

1991 Publication of *Dermatology for the Small Animal Practitioner* by G.H. Nesbitt and L.J. Ackerman.

1991 Publication of *Techniques Diagnostiques en Dermatologie des Carnivores* by E. Guaguére (France).

1992 Publication of *Skin Tumors of the Dog and Cat* by M.H. Goldschmidt and F.S. Shofer.

1992 Publication of *Veterinary Dermatopathology. A Macroscopic and Microscopic Evaluation of Canine and Feline Skin Diseases* by T.L. Gross, P.J. Ihrke, and E.J. Walder.

1992 The Second World Congress in Veterinary Dermatology was held in May at Montreal, Quebec.

1992 The European College of Veterinary Dermatology was granted approval as a certifying body in veterinary dermatology, and the following individuals were elected as Invited Specialists (''grandfathers''): D. Carlotti, R. Halliwell, H. Koch, D. Lloyd, K. Thoday, and T. Willemse.

1993 Publication of *Current Veterinary Dermatology. The Science and Art of Therapy* by C.E. Griffin, K.W. Kwochka, and J.M. MacDonald.

1993 Publication of *Manual of Small Animal Dermatology* by P.H. Locke, R.G. Harvey, and I.S. Mason (United Kingdom).

1993 Publication of second edition of *Color Atlas of Small Animal Dermatology* by G.T. Wilkinson (United Kingdom).

1993 Publication of *Advances in Veterinary Dermatology,* Vol. II, by P.J. Ihrke, I.S. Mason, and S.D. White.

1994 Publication of *Color Atlas and Text of Surgical Pathology of the Dog and Cat.* Dermatopathology and Skin Tumors by J.A. Yager and B.P. Wilcock.

1995 Publication of the fifth edition of *Muller and Kirk's Small Animal Dermatology* by D.W. Scott, W.H. Miller, and C.E. Griffin.

Index

■

Note: Page numbers in *italics* refer to illustrations; page numbers followed by t refer to tables.

ISBN 0-7216-4850-9